*The
Encyclopedic
Handbook
of
Private
Practice*

The
Encyclopedic
Handbook of

PRIVATE
PRACTICE

ERIC MARGENAU, PH.D.
Editor-in-Chief

ASSOCIATE EDITORS

Neil Ribner, Ph.D. ◇
Reuben Silver, Ph.D. ◇
George Stricker, Ph.D. ◇
Charles Patrick Ewing, J.D., Ph.D. ◇
Richard Robertiello, M.D. ◇

GARDNER PRESS, INC.

New York   London   Sydney

GARDNER PRESS, INC.
19 Union Square West
New York, New York 10003

All foreign orders except Canada and South America to:

Afterhurst Limited
Chancery House
319 City Road
London, N1, England

Library of Congress Cataloging-in-Publication Data

The Encyclopedia handbook of private practice.

    Includes index.
    1. Psychotherapy—Practice. 2. Mental health
services—Marketing. I. Margenau, Eric.
[DNLM: 1. Private Practice. W 89 E56]
RC465.5.E46 1989   616.89'0068   87-19624
ISBN 0-89876-151-4

PRINTED IN THE UNITED STATES OF AMERICA

Book Design by Raymond Solomon

*This book is lovingly dedicated,
in memorium,
to my parents, Dvo and Ernest Margenau*

CONTENTS

PART II. FINANCIAL AND ECONOMIC MANAGEMENT
REUBEN SILVER, PH.D., EDITOR

PART III. EMOTIONAL ISSUES
GEORGE STRICKER, PH.D., EDITOR

PART IV. LEGAL AND ETHICAL ISSUES
CHARLES PATRICK EWING, J.D., PH.D., EDITOR

PART V. PHILOSOPHICAL, THEORETICAL AND TECHNICAL ISSUES
RICHARD ROBERTIELLO, M.D., EDITOR

Contributors

David Adams, Ph.D.
Atlanta Medical and Neurological
Psychology/Psychiatry
Atlanta, Georgia

James C. Beck, M.D., Ph.D.
Cambridge Court Clinic
Harvard Medical School
Cambridge, Massachusetts

J. G. Benedict, Ph.D.
Private Practice, Denver, Colorado
Denver University School of
Professional Psychology

Thomas Edward Bratter, Ed.D.
The John Dewey Academy
Great Barrington, Mass.
Union Graduate School
Yellow Springs, Ohio

Lois Brien, Ph.D.
School of Psychology & Human Behavior
National University, San Diego, CA

David Brinks, Ph.D.
University of Toledo, Toledo, Ohio

Stanley L. Brodsky, Ph.D.
University of Alabama
Tuscaloosa, Alabama

Mathilda B. Cantor, Ph.D.
Private Practice, Phoenix, Arizona

Phyllis Caroff, D.S.W.
Hunter College School of Social Work
Private Practice, New York, NY

Carol P. Chanco, A.C.S.W.
Private Practice, New York, New York

Rosalie Chapman, Ph.D.
Private Practice, San Diego, California

David Clayson, Ph.D.
The New York Hospital-
Cornell Medical Center
New York, New York

Howard M. Cohen, Ph.D.
State University of New York
New Paltz, New York

Ronald Jay Cohen, Ph.D.
St. John's University
Independent Consultant
Spring Valley, New York

Grace Conlee
The Grace Conlee Company
San Diego, California

Sheila Coonerty, Ph.D.
Private Practice, Little Neck, NY
Long Island University
Brooklyn, New York

Dale Lee Coovert, Ph.D.
Bay Pines VA Medical Center
University of South Florida
Tampa, Florida

Diana Cort, M.S.W.
Private Practice, Forest Hills, NY
Senior Option Service
Allendale, New Jersey

Alan D. Davidson, Ph.D.
Private Practice, San Diego, California

James V. DeLeo, Ph.D.
California School of Professional
Psychology, University of San Diego
San Diego, California

Leonard J. Deutsch, M.D., P.C.
College of Physicians and Surgeons
Columbia University
Private Practice, New York, NY

Cecille Dillon, Ph.D.
Private Practice, Huntington Beach, CA

Patricia M. Dvonch, Ph.D.
Options Associates, Inc.
New York, New York

Jayne Eliach, R.N., M.S.
Employee Assistance Program
Consortium, New York, NY

Michael F. Enright, Ph.D.
Private Practice, Jackson, Wyoming
St. John's Hospital, Jackson, Wyoming

**Elisabeth G. Everett, M.S.W.,
B.C.D., L.I.C.S.W.**
Private Practice, Arlington, Mass.

**Charles Patrick Ewing,
J.D., Ph.D.**
University at Buffalo
State University of New York
Buffalo, New York

Sheri Fenster, Ph.D.
Private Practice, New York, NY and
Baldwin, New York
Adelphi University, Garden City, NY

A. Steven Frankel, Ph.D.
Family and Child Therapeutic Services,
Inc., Torrance, California

Herbert Freundenberger, Ph.D.
Private Practice, New York, NY

Marion Gedney, Ph.D.
Private Practice, New York, NY
Rutgers Graduate School of Applied
and Professional Psychology
New Brunswick, New Jersey

Minna Marder Genn, Ed.M.
Private Practice, New York, NY and
Tenafly, New Jersey

Richard N. Gevirtz, Ph.D.
California School of Professional
Psychology, San Diego, CA

J. Roy Gillis, M.A.
Metropolitan Toronto Forensic Service
Clarke Institute of Psychiatry
Toronto, Ontario, Canada

Jerold R. Gold, Ph.D.
Private Practice, Little Neck, New York
Yeshiva University, New York, NY

Carl Goldberg, Ph.D.
Albert Einstein College of Medicine
New York, NY
Private Practice, New York, NY

Robert H. Goldstein, Ph.D.
University of Rochester School of
Medicine and Dentistry
Rochester, New York

Leonard Haas, Ph.D.
University of Utah
Salt Lake City, Utah

Carmi Harari, Ed.D.
Humanistic Psychology Center of
New York, NY
Interactions, New City, New York

David E. Hartman, Ph.D.
Cook County Hospital, Chicago, Illinois
Private Practice, Chicago, Illinois

David Howard, Ph.D.
Counseling Center of Thousand Oaks
Thousand Oaks, California

Joan Howard, M.A.
Counseling Center of Thousand Oaks
Thousand Oaks, California

James W. Hull, Ph.D.
New York Hospital-Cornell
Medical Center
White Plains, New York

Leonard A. Jason, Ph.D.
DePaul University, Chicago, Illinois

John Kachorek, Ph.D.
Private Practice, Encinitas, California

Robert H. Keisner, Ph.D.
C.W. Post College of Long Island
University, Brookville, New York
New York State Board of Psychology
Private Practice, Syosset, New York

Richard R. Kilburg, Ph.D.
The Johns Hopkins University
Baltimore, Maryland

Theodore Kurtz, M.A.
Private Practice, New York, NY

Robert C. Lane, Ph.D.
Adelphi University, Garden City, NY
New York Center for Psychoanalytic
Training, Long Island, New York

James F. Lassiter, Ph.D.
Adelphi University, Garden City, NY
Mental Health Management Associates,
Inc., Amityville, New York

Anna C. Lee, Ph.D.
Private Practice
Lisbon and Cascals, Portugal

Mark H. Lewin, Ph.D.
Upstate Psychological Service Center, P.C.
Rochester, New York

Harold Linder, Ph.D.
Nova University
Fort Lauderdale, Florida

Karen L. Lombardi, Ph.D.
Adelphi University, Garden City, NY

Eric Margenau, Ph.D.
Private Practice, New York, NY
Center for Sports Psychology,
New York, New York
Hackettestown, New Jersey

William E. Mariano, J.D.
Mariano and Wolman, P.C.
New York, New York

Ninalee F. May, Ed.D.
Private Practice, New York, New York
Fair Haven, New Jersey

Carroll L. Meek, Ph.D.
Private Practice, Pullman, Washington

Robert Mendelsohn, Ph.D.
Adelphi University, Garden City, New York

David J. Miller, Ph.D.
VA Medical Center
University of Pittsburgh School of
Medicine, Pittsburgh, Pennsylvania

David Monroe Miller,* M.B.A.
College of Human Services
New York, New York
*(Deceased)

James K. Morrison, Ph.D.
Private Practice, Latham, New York

William C. Normand, M.D.
Albert Einstein College of Medicine
Bronx-Lebanon Hospital Center
New York, New York

E. Warren O'Meara, Ph.D.
Private Practice, San Diego, California

Suzanne Phillips, Psy.D.
Private Practice, Northport, New York
Adelphi University, Garden City, NY

Martin S. Pollens, M.S.W.
Private Practice
North Tarrytown, New York City, and
New Windsor, New York

Kenneth S. Pope, Ph.D.
Los Angeles, California

Estelle R. G. Rapoport, Ph.D.
Private Practice, Roslyn Heights, NY
Adelphi University, Garden City, NY

Neil Ribner, Ph.D.
California School of Professional
Psychology, San Diego, California

Donald Robbins, C.P.A., Ph.D.
Private Practice, Little Neck, New York

Edwin S. Robbins, M.D.
New York University Medical Center
Bellevue Hospital Center
New York, New York

Lillian Robbins, Ph.D.
Rutgers University, Newark, New Jersey

Richard Robertiello, M.D.
Private Practice, New York, New York

Richard Rogers, Ph.D.
Metropolitan Toronto Forensic Service
Clarke Institute of Psychiatry
Toronto, Ontario, Canada

Max Rosenbaum, Ph.D.
Private Practice, New York, New York

**Waleed Anthony Salameh,
Ph.D.**
San Diego Institute for Integrative
Psychotherapy, San Diego, California

Richard M. Samuels, Ph.D.
Private Practice
Human Insights, Oradell, New Jersey

Gerald Schoenewolf, Ph.D.
Private Practice, New York, New York

Joseph E. Schumacher, Ph.D.
The University of Alabama
Tuscaloosa, Alabama

Robin B. Shafran, Ph.D.
William Alanson White Institute
New York, New York

David L. Shapiro, Ph.D.
Private Practice, Washington, D.C.

**Esther Siegel, Ed.D., R.N.,
Ed.M.**
Private Practice, New York, New York

Reuben Silver, Ph.D.
Albany Medical College
Albany, New York

Frederick J. Smith, Ph.D.
Albany Medical Colelge
Albany, New York

Lucy B. Smith, C.S.W.
Private Practice, New York, New York

Malka Sternberg, Ed.D., M.S.W.
Hunter College School of Social Work
New York, New York

George Stricker, Ph.D.
Adelphi University, Garden City, New York

Jo Claire Sullivan, B.A.
San Diego, California

Michael Thackrey, Ph.D.
California School of Professional
Psychology, Fresno, California

Sheldon Travin, M.D.
Bronx-Lebanon Hospital Center
Albert Einstein College of Medicine
New York, New York

Donald Viglione, Ph.D.
California School of Professional
Psychology, San Diego, California

Steven Walfish, Ph.D.
Private Practice
University of South Florida
Tampa, Florida

Peggy Watkins-Ferrell, M.A.
DePaul University, Chicago, Illinois

Wilhelm Wedin, Ph.D.
Clinical Director, Gay Psychotherapy
New York, New York

Robert D. Weitz, Ph.D.
Private Practice, Boca Raton, Florida

Robert Wishnoff, Ph.D.
Human Resource Associates
Albany, New York

Lawrence T. Woodburn, Ph.D.
California Consulting Group
Solana Beach, California

Rogers H. Wright, Ph.D.
Private Practice
Long Beach and San Diego, California

PREFACE

As is true with most health practitioners in private practice, nowhere in the lengthy course of my formal education was there ever offered a section addressing the issues, problems, and practical considerations involved in providing treatment services in a private practice setting. Most likely this is due to an unstated convention that mental health treatment is concerned with service or medicine—certainly not business. As such, it should not be denigrated by being discussed from such a pragmatic perspective. However, there is much more to surviving, let alone succeeding, in private practice than clinical expertise. Clinical skills are essential but they are only a prerequisite to succeeding in the unique context of the private practice setting. It is the goal of this book to cover the broad range of factors outside of training that effect the success of the private practice endeavor.

The enormous size and comprehensive scope of this ambitious undertaking has, to a large extent, dictated the format. The book is a collection of contributions by a group of highly experienced and knowledgable authors from diverse backgrounds. Though my twenty years of experience as a psychologist and psychotherapist has been brought to bear in the conceptualizing, organizing, and overseeing of the project, it is left to the therapists, lawyers, accountants and other professionals to provide the "nitty-gritty" content that is necessary to function effectively, profitably, and happily in private practice.

This volume is directed to all those who participate in the private practice of psychotherapy and mental health services. Given the complexity and the increasingly wide spectrum of the area, it is no longer sufficient to address the disciplines of psychology, psychiatry, and social work exclusively. *The Encyclopedic Handbook of Private Practice* contains specific information that will facilitate the practices of psychoanalysts, hypnotherapists, sex therapists, marriage and family counselors, as well as others who have found that the private practice setting is conducive to their specializations. The competitive nature of the field requires that every practitioner—beginning or seasoned—be in touch with changing developments and varied alternatives. This has determined the breadth of the book.

Five major themes with respect to building, maintaining, expanding, and enjoying private practice are considered. The first two parts of the book deal with the fundamental specifics of practice management, and financial and economic issues. Parts three, four, and five present discussions of legal, ethical, philosophical, and emotional aspects. Taken as a whole, the book presents a detailed, applications-oriented source for those considering, beginning, or maintaining a private practice. I believe that the information imparted offers the necessary basis from which to identify options, take advantage of opportunities, define personal and professional needs, and thereby to function at the highest level possible.

Eric Margenau, Ph.D.

ACKNOWLEDGEMENTS

A book such as this could only be completed with the work of countless people. Its size and comprehensiveness required years of continual pursuit of information. For that I would like to acknowledge the work of two people. Suzi Tucker was the Editorial Assistant throughout this book's inception and formative stages and Nell Porter easily took over where she left off and shepharded the project through its completion. In addition, of course, countless hours were spent by my colleagues, the Associate Editors, each of whom was responsible for overseeing a section that easily could have been a book by itself. To them I am greatly appreciative. Likewise, an enormous amount of work was contributed by Gardner Spungin, whose years of experience in conceptualizing and executing valuable texts for the Mental Health community is without peer. Finally, I would like to express my gratitude to Sidney Solomon, whose tireless efforts in producing the actual book you are reading right now cannot adequately be measured. For a job well done, thank you, Sidney.

Part
One

Practice
Management

Neil Ribner, Ph.D.
Editor

S E C T I O N

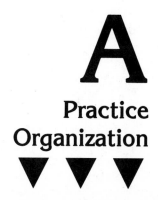

A

**Practice
Organization**

C H A P T E R

1

SOLE PROPRIETORSHIP

Rosalie Chapman, Ph.D.

S ole proprietorship is the practice of psychology independent of an employer or organization. A sole proprietor is a business owner and operator in addition to being a psychologist. It is important to realize that there is a blend of major career roles here. Unless business management is effective and efficient, the psychology practice will not flourish. Likewise, unless independent psychological services are top quality, all of the business expertise in the world will not support a practice in the long run.

There are different practice models for sole proprietorship. That is, the psychologist operating as a sole proprietor works in the following possible ways

- Solo practice with no staff or associates
- Practice involving support staff contractors or employees
- Practice involving practitioner employees/assistants
- Sharing of overhead with other practitioner associates

Whatever the model, the key issue is that the sole proprietor accepts the dual roles of healer/practitioner and business owner/manager. Each of these roles must be understood, fulfilled, and managed in the best interests of the practitioner, given his or her own professional and personal life-style goals.

This discussion focuses on sole proprietorship as a full-time job or a major source of income. For those for whom private practice is a part-time job or a supplementary income source, the material may be applicable on a selective basis only.

CRITERIA FOR SOLE PROPRIETORSHIP— IS IT FOR YOU?

Criteria

- I am willing and able to manage a business independently.
- I can plan budgetary requirements, taking into consideration business and personal expenses.
- I can plan and forecast the economic and political factors affecting my business as accurately as possible.

- I am willing and able to handle all decisions about patient diagnosis, and treatment, and management.
- I am licensed and qualified to provide top-quality and ethical psychological services, including seeking supervision when needed.
- I can define and handle my specialty areas of clinical expertise and provide quality services.
- I can ensure quality referral for all persons with treatment needs outside of my areas of expertise.
- I am willing to balance professional skills and entrepreneurial skills in my practice to the best of my ability.
- I am willing to work many hours alone.
- I am prepared to recognize when I need help and to get it.
- I am able to manage independent structuring of my time.
- I am prepared to fit solo practice into my life-style.

This checklist is provided to inspire your thoughtful consideration of major issues concerning the implementation of a private practice of psychology. Think over the issues clearly. The rest of the material in this chapter furnishes the information and resources necessary to enable you to pursue your concerns to their logical conclusion.

ESTABLISHING A SOLE PROPRIETORSHIP

There are several major areas that are essential to setting up a well-functioning practice. For me, the psychologist needs to know how effectively to adapt sound business principles to the practice of psychology.

Licensure

The first step is to acquire a state license to practice as a psychologist; this is obtained from state licensing authorities. A business license is also necessary, obtainable from city officials in the locale of your practice. These licenses must be kept current, and should be displayed in your office.

Business Record System

It is important to think about all of your business records that need to be kept in terms of setting up a comprehensive system for maximum efficiency. Use of a computer system is essential in order to preserve valuable time and energy. In this regard, computer software packages available that are called "practice managers" or "office managers."

You must decide how you want to handle your office management. You can do your own office management, own the hardware and software but hire an employee to do the work, or contract out the office management operations. In the long run, having your own system and using an employee is probably the most cost-effective and easiest way to ensure quality control.

When setting up your computerized system components, it is necessary to consider the following:

1. Billing system—including record keeping and processing of bills, insurance forms, and any reports that are required.
2. Collections—deciding how to handle these and whether an outside agency will be used.
3. Practice management statistics—including analysis of various parameters of data about your practice on a monthly basis, such as cash flow, outstanding accounts, and referral sources.
4. Business bookkeeping—including monthly budgetary analysis.
5. Personal accounting—separating business from personal funds and expenses for tax purposes as well as business planning.
6. Budget planning—including monthly financial planning such as setting aside quarterly income tax funds and retirement plan contributions.
7. Secretarial functions—including word processing and appointment keeping and any other secretarial operations that are routinely used.
8. Client data systems—the fact that client data can be stored on the computer much more conveniently than in cumbersome charts.
9. Psychological testing and report writing—choosing from the variety of different software packages available for these functions depending on what is routinely used in your practice.

It is important to keep in mind that practice management is time consuming. If it is not done comprehensively and competently, it can become a source of severe stress and financial difficulty.

Business Contracts

It is essential to set up specific business contracts in writing for arrangements made with anyone involved in your business, which should be signed by all parties concerned. Such contracts eliminate potential misunderstanding, clarifies the exact nature of what services or monies are being exchanged, and simplify matters for any legal proceedings that may become necessary. It is worthwhile to hire an attorney to review the forms used for such contracts. The usual forms needed include:

1. Employee job descriptions and financial arrangements
2. Services of contractors
3. Contracts with clients, which should include:
     a. adequate identifying information such as driver's license and relevant identification cards
     b. signature accepting responsibility for treatment and payment for treatment
     c. payment agreement specifying what fees will be paid, and when and how they will be paid, including consequences of payment delinquency

> d. treatment contract — some practitioners like to use a written statement of what treatment is being provided, including client commitment agreement

Insurance

Adequate insurance coverage is necessary in a sole proprietorship. Professional liability insurance can be purchased through your professional organization, as can disability insurance — which should be considered since, as a sole proprietor, you must provide your own benefits. Personal liability insurance is also needed. It would also be wise to purchase an additional umbrella policy in the unlikely case of major disaster. Group medical insurance plans may be available through your affiliated professional organization as well.

As a sole proprietor, you are completely responsible for all business arrangements you make and their consequences. It is well worth the time and effort required to set these up specifically and efficiently, having printed forms available for each transaction. If these steps are not taken, problems will eventually arise.

PRACTICE FORMAT

Deciding on the proper practice format shapes the operation of the entire practice. The practice format must fit in with one's professional needs as well as one's individual life-style. What may be comfortable for one practitioner may not suit another. Following are some common practice formats.

Renting an Office

Rental may be the best choice for a practitioner who is comfortable using someone else's space. It has the advantages of paying a flat fee per month and not having to be responsible for the details of property maintenance. The disadvantages are that you are somewhat at the mercy of the landlord regarding quality of property maintenance, and that rents are subject to increase.

Owning an Office

Many sole proprietors elect to purchase office space, often also acting as a landlord and renting part of the space to others. This is a good move to reduce overhead and obviously has the advantages of a property investment. In addition, it offers the opportunity to receive rents as supplementary income. Purchasing space would entail knowledge of real estate, and consideration of how long it is anticipated that the real estate would be used to house the office practice.

Latchkey Office

This arrangement involves renting an already existing office, including all amenities specified, on a flat-fee basis. In essence, another practitioner agrees to rent furnished office space together with use of equipment, facilities, and supplies, as agreed upon by the two parties. The office is used at prearranged hours.

An advantage of this arrangement is that office maintenance and support services are covered and you can concentrate your energy on clinical services. A disadvantage is that you must rely on the landlord to provide consistent, quality support services that meet your needs.

House/Home Office

Some sole practitioners elect to arrange office space inside or adjacent to their private residence for use as an office. It is important that the individual practitioner be completely comfortable with this idea before making this decision. Although this arrangement may be less expensive and have some tax benefits, it may restrict one's family life. Clients may have more knowledge about the doctor's personal life than is appropriate, and there is always the risk of the family being exposed to dangerous clients.

Business Manager Format

Some sole proprietors view their role much more clearly as a business manager than as a clinician. They elect to have a large practice, spending most of their time soliciting business and managing the practice while employees do all of the clinical work. Although the sole proprietor does very little of the actual clinical work in this model, it is every bit as important for him or her to possess a high level of current clinical expertise, because the sole responsibility still rests on the business owner to deliver and maintain quality control of competent and ethical services. In this model, the sole proprietor must be a good judge of people and possess the skills to have a comprehensive grasp of all aspects of the business.

Whatever the practice format that is chosen, it is essential to put all arrangements in writing, specifying the exact nature of the contract. Both parties should sign this contract.

OFFICE FACILITIES

Office facilities must be comfortable and conducive to relaxation and stress reduction for both the practitioner and the client. No matter how well you plan your office in advance, you have to live with it for awhile to determine what works best for you. You learn from experience what is helpful and what hinders efficient functioning. Clients are also a good source of feedback. Flexibility in planning is a good idea, to leave room for necessary modifications.

Office Layout

There are several facets of office layout to consider.

1. Comfort with entering and exiting. The traffic pattern should be taken

into consideration. For example, clients may be upset and desire privacy and anonymity in the waiting area. The traffic pattern should include sensitivity to confidentiality.

2. Waiting room layout. There are several considerations here, such as size, privacy, comfort, and what to provide for client use, such as magazines, coffee, play area, etc. Remember that the waiting room establishes the image of your practice and things such as orderliness, currency of magazines, tastefulness of decorations, cleanliness, style of decoration, degree of formality, and amenities project a nonverbal message to clients about the environment they are entering.

3. Office staff area. This area should enhance client care by being accessible to the client, yet respectful of the client's confidentiality. A noisy or messy staff area can detract from the client's comfort level or sense of confidence in the services offered. The client should find it easy to obtain any assistance needed from office staff.

4. The therapy area. This area should be comfortable, quiet, and pleasant. It is a good idea to offer several seats from which the client may choose, depending on whether he or she would like to sit on a couch, or a straight-backed chair, or curl up informally in a large chair. Clients also vary regarding the distance they like to sit from the practitioner. It is unwise for the practitioner to sit behind a desk, which creates a barrier to communication. Display of credentials should be tasteful. The office is a nonverbal expression of yourself and the services you offer.

5. Specialty facilities. Specialty facilities may be needed, such as a computer area, biofeedback or testing area, children's area, or staff lounge. Plan carefully for what you need.

Accessibility and Parking

Geographical access to the office is an important factor. Consider how easy it is to find the office, how complicated it may be to get there, and how long it may take. Parking is also very important. Time is at a premium in most of their lives. Handicapped access is also necessary.

Office Equipment and Supplies

Once the office format and mode of operations are determined, decisions about office equipment and supplies need to be made. Arrangements are also essential regarding what services will be purchased by contract. The following items should be considered.

1. Reception and secretarial services — in-house or contracted by an independent party
    a. Computer facilities and affiliated supplies
    b. Typewriters
    c. Billing systems and forms and postage
    d. Copier

    e. Office paperwork materials
        Printed forms
        Letterhead stationery
        Business cards
        Appointment cards
        Mailing materials and postage
        Paper
        File folders
        Pens and pencils
        Memo pads
        Appointment book
        Testing materials
        Billing paperwork materials
          Forms
          Credit card equipment
        Tape-recording facilities
        Miscellaneous client handout materials
        Other miscellaneous paper forms and supplies
   f. Client amenities
        Tissues
        Bathroom facilities
        Coffee or other refreshments
 2. Telephone setup and message/answering systems

With regard to the last item, it is important to decide who will answer your telephone and how your messages will be handled. The options are to have your telephone answered by a receptionist, an answering service, an answering machine, or a voice mailbox paging company.

Some people consider it important to have a receptionist answer every call. If a sensitive and well-trained psychologically minded person is available to do this job, it is probably preferable to do so, provided one can afford such services.

This writer has found the voice mailbox superior to an answering machine or answering service. The voice mailbox answers the telephone with a recorded message and pages you as each caller hangs up the telephone. Calls can be returned on a timely basis. Other practitioners prefer an answering service, which provides personal telephone response. Still others feel comfortable using an answering machine.

The key to using a telephone answering and message service system is to establish an accessible and dependable method for your clients and business associates. People need to feel that they are able to contact you when they need to speak to you.

Whatever telephone communication you establish, it is important to describe the system to your clients and associates. Once they are familiar with the system, and are assured that it works consistently, communication is likely to be effective. If you inform your clients about what to expect from your message communication system, they are likely to respect it and use it effectively.

Personnel and Staff Policies

Following is a checklist to consider in hiring office personnel. Many people err by hiring office personnel who are "nice" people, in the belief that therefore they will be competent. It is important to look beyond the essential "nice" personality, which is a requirement, but is only one facet of doing a competent job.

An employee must demonstrate competency in the specific office skills for which he or she is being hired. Skills required for the job should be outlined, and actual skill performance assessed by a job trial before hiring the employee. Specific skills to assess include:

1. Ability to greet and interact appropriately with clients.
2. Ability to interact sensitively on the telephone and careful response to instruction about handling phone calls.
3. Good public relations skills, including projection of a professional attitude.
4. All necessary secretarial skills, including typing, word processing, editing, and other computer skills.
5. Bookkeeping, billing, and collection skills as needed by the practice requirements.
6. Personality characteristics:
    a. Makes very few mistakes — is meticulous.
    b. Is psychologically minded.
    c. Maintains confidentiality — clients, business associates, and co-workers and in personal life.
    d. Has good personal grooming.
    e. Is punctual and reliable.
    f. Follows directions dependably.
    g. Is able to function independently within the limits specified.
    h. Is able to deal with erratic behavior on the part of clients in a businesslike manner without taking it personally.

OFFICE PROCEDURES

One critically important step for the sole proprietor is to establish thorough and effective office procedures. How efficiently this is done can spell the difference between success and failure. In contrast to the procedures of a clinic or other organization, the sole proprietor has much more control over what transactions take place and how well they are enforced.

The sole proprietor can monitor all treatment and billing arrangements that are being made with each client. Assuming that the proper contracts are made, the results can be personally followed. For example, if a client is not getting the treatment results he or she is seeking, the issue can be directly addressed. In other instances, if the client is defaulting on payments, the issue can be addressed directly between the practitioner and the client rather than making it a "system" issue.

Very often, the practitioner can be overly concerned with the delivery of clinical services in therapy, and can overlook the methods and transactions necessary to run the business of psychological services. Specific arrangements must be made for the following client services.

1. How is initial telephone contact made with a client?
2. How are appointments made?
3. What reception and guidance are available at first contact?
4. How are specific financial arrangements made?
5. How are specific treatment contracts made?
6. What system is set up for the orderly handling of routine paperwork?
7. How are psychological testing arrangements made?
8. What are telephone call policies?
9. What specific cancellation procedures are made?
10. What other client policies are needed, and how are they communicated to the client?

Client Records

1. What are the appointment book procedures?
2. What is the system for client charts?
3. How are provisions for release of information handled?
4. How is client correspondence handled?
5. What documentation is kept about client transactions that may be subject to legal proceedings?
6. What documentation is kept about client transactions that is normally required for insurance information?

Billing and Finances

1. What billing arrangements are made and how is this done?
2. What is the system for routine daily collections?
3. What monthly billing system is used and how is it implemented?
4. What are the specific insurance billing arrangements?
5. What measures are established for practice analysis dimensions and monthly financial summaries?
6. What budgeting system is implemented in the practice?

REFERRALS

The backbone of a private practice is the assurance of referrals on a steady basis. Most sole proprietors, unless they are unusually well known, need to devote significant attention to the process of establishing and maintaining referrals.

It is a mistake to assume that if you are good at the work you do, the referrals will come in. Albeit that competent work is essential, it is not sufficient to ensure adequate numbers of referrals in today's health-care market and the current economic pressures on individuals and businesses.

A conscientious business-oriented plan must be devised to develop and maintain referral sources. A major key is identification of the specific types of referrals that are sought. Once they are identified, a strategy can be developed that concentrates on three major areas:

1. Developing new referral sources.
2. Maintaining old referral sources.
3. Maximizing referrals from current and past clients.

New Referrals

New referrals involve identification of target clients and how to communicate with them. Once you identify target areas, it is important to concentrate on developing public visibility, liaisons, networking, and any formal organization connections between you and the population you want to reach. It is important to impart information to persons needing your services in a tasteful and ethical manner. This information can be communicated in the following ways.

1. Distributing brochures describing services and availability.
2. Calling facilities and organizations needing your services and offering consultation, speaking, or compatible services.
3. Networking with individuals who care about the same issues as you do. Establishing ongoing contacts is a key activity.
4. Becoming socially involved with persons and agencies with whom you feel comfortable and can establish informal confidence referral networks.
5. Becoming affiliated with agencies as a consultant, speaker, or supervisor with which you can generate confidence as a teacher and referral source.
6. Informing professional organiations to which you belong about your professional expertise, and becoming known among peers for your professional competence.

Maintaining Old Referral Sources

The maintenance of ongoing referral sources is very important. Often referral sources do not know whether their referral has made the effort to contact you, and they do not know whether the referral is valuable to their clients. The following communications with referral sources are suggested.

1. Written acknowledgment of referral, and initial evaluation and treatment impressions.
2. Written "thank you" for referral, and an offer to cooperate with treatment in any way possible, with suggestions, if recommended.
3. Establishment of appropriate regular contact mechanisms with ongoing referral parties concerning communication, exchange of necessary information, and provision of needed feedback for legal, professional, or other purposes.
4. Regular and ongoing involvement in professional organizations pertaining to areas of professional expertise.
5. Political involvement in practice-relevant issues insofar as you are knowledgeabe, skilled, and willing to deal with this inevitable facet of independent practice.

Former Client Referrals

These have often been said to be the most productive referral source. Clients who have received successful treatment value it highly. They describe their treatment results to others on a very personal level. Personal endorsement is very effective in producing highly motivated clients. Satisfied clients are happy to endorse your services and should be rewarded with a "thank you" when they do so.

ADVANTAGES AND DISADVANTAGES
OF SOLE PROPRIETORSHIP

Sole proprietorship has advantages as well as disadvantages. It is useful to take a look at the major trade-offs one must consider. Following is a partial list of priority concerns:

Control Over Services and Time Schedule
versus Time-Limited Working Hours

As a sole proprietor, you decide what services you offer and what hours you work. You have complete control over your schedule in contrast to employment or group practice, where you are assigned specific services, duties, and hours. For example, you can start or end the day early or late as needed. Schedule accommodations may be made for people needing late appointments after their own working hours. Vacations may be scheduled during seasons of the year when business is lighter.

Variable Income Potential versus Fixed Income

As a sole proprietor, income potential exceeds that of a salaried job, but there are more risks involved. Some months may be slow and others more productive. Often it seems that there is no discernible reason for income fluctuations. For example, there are often unexpected delays in receiving third-party payments. Collection problems can arise. Economic fluctuations and the changing health-care market can affect people's ability to afford psychological treatment.

This is a situation with which the sole proprietor needs to be able to live both financially and emotionally. It is a trade-off for a lower income with the security of a fixed salary and benefits.

Responsibility for Professional Competence

The sole proprietor is singularly responsible for all of his or her actions with clients. He or she is personally liable for the consequences of professional ethics, decisions, and actions. One must be comfortable with taking this level of responsibility and be prepared to deal with any mistakes or differences of opinion that may arise with clients. For example, if a client is dissatisfied with some aspect of treatment or policy, he or she deals directly with you.

An advantage is that the opportunity for control over policies and procedures is present. You can change and adjust any policies that do not fit the needs of your practice.

Responsibility for All Business Transactions

The sole proprietor is responsible for all of the business aspects of the practice, including planning, implementation, and follow-up of business strategies. One must be willing to attend to this facet of the business of psychological services; there is no built-in "department" to handle this. For example, if referrals drop off, if the computer makes errors, if there are cash-flow problems or any difficulties with business procedures, the practitioner must personally arrange for the handling of these problems.

Professional Isolation versus Involvement

The sole proprietor is vulnerable to professional isolation. When one's job is to visit with client after client for several hours per day, even if groups are seen, there is a tendency to need time alone at the end of the day to relax from the work of therapy. When the day is mostly filled with work and includes very little peer contact, coupled with the need to relax emotionally and physically at the end of the day, feelings of isolation can develop. One must be prepared to work independently and to compensate for isolation vulnerability by building in peer contacts and social contacts through professional meetings and other social activities. If attention is not paid to this factor, burnout is an added vulnerability.

No Benefits versus Salaried or Group Practice Benefits

The sole proprietor literally provides his or her own benefits. Private insurance coverage must be secured. There are no paid vacation or sick days. There are no bonuses. When you work, you get paid; when you do not work, you do not get paid.

The advantages of sole proprietorship in general revolve around independence and personal responsibility. These can be very attractive to a person who feels good about controlling the work situation and is willing to handle all of the situations and problems that arise.

The disadvantages of sole proprietorship relate to the need to work hard for many hours to handle all of the responsibilities that go beyond direct service to clients. The price of the freedom in practice is the assumption of the simultaneous job of business manager, a nonpaying position.

Sole proprietorship requires a competent, independent, and entrepreneurial clinician who is a self-starter and has a high energy level. For such a person, a sole proprietorship can be highly rewarding. The personal satisfaction and freedom can more than compensate for the work that goes into the achievement of business success.

In the future, the private practice of psychology will probably undergo dramatic change. Current trends in health care indicate increasing cutbacks on mental health insurance benefits and a growing number of the health maintenance organizations type of health service providers, many of which exclude or limit psychological services. It has become necessary for the sole proprietor to be aware of these trends and to consider their effects on business security. Diversification of services and professional roles is a current response of many sole proprietors to the changing future of private health care.

REFERENCES

Barker, R. (1982). *The business of psychotherapy.* New York: Columbia University Press.

Browning, C. (1982). *Private practice handbook* (wnd ed.) Los Alamitos, CA: Duncliff's International.

Levin, A. (1983). *The private practice of psychotherapy.* New york: Collier Macmillan.

Mone, L. (1983). *Private practice: A professional business.* La Jolla, CA: Elm Press.

Pressman, R. (1984). *Microcomputers and the private practitioner.* Homewood, IL: Dow Jones-Irwin.

Pressman, R. (1979). *Private Practice: A handbook for the independent mental health practitioner.* New York: Gardner Press.

Psychotherapy in Private Practice: The Journal for the Independent Practitioner. Binghamton, NY: Haworth Press, published quarterly.

Rubenstein, E., & Lorr, M. (Eds.) (1954). *Survey of clinical practice in psychology.* New York: International Universities Press.

Schimberg, E. (1979). *The handbook of private practice in psychology.* New York: Brunner/Mazel.

CHAPTER
2

GROUP PRACTICE

David Howard, Ph.D., and Joan Howard, M.A.

Our Story

We began our marriage, family and child counselor (MFCC) careers as husband and wife with solo practices. Two of us operated out of a single office with an attached waiting room. We scheduled client hours carefully, as space limitations allowed only one of us to see a client during a given hour.

After approximately a year, we explored the idea of joining an existing group practice in a community closer to our residence. Joining such a group with a number of offices offered us the opportunity to see our patients at the same time without having to take turns using only one office. Our longer-range plan inlcuded a gradual phasing out of our solo practices in our original location and the building of new practices in a more convenient location.

We began to check into already established centers, and also with therapists who might be interested in collaborating with us. The group practice we eventually joined consisted of several partners, all licensed MFCCs. The group had a renter program that offered a buy-in option, a feature that was not available with other practices in the area.

Becoming acquainted over time with potential new partners seemed appropriate for all involved. A "trial marriage" of sorts was established for one year. During this period, we paid rent to the group's corporation and received a limited number of referrals that were based on our own speciality areas..

Rent consisted of a flat fee per month for unlimited usage of one office. However, we had the option of using other offices and a group room if they were available, so we had more flexibility than with our previous arrangement of being restricted to one office.

It became apparent to us that we would need to become better known in the community in order to expand our clientele. We joined local civic organizations and became actively involved on committees. Getting out in the community with other business people was an opportunity to let them know about our services as we worked together on various projects. We also joined charitable organizations and established a local chapter of a statewide non-profit mutual support group that has since grown to national prominence. We also did volunteer work in the schools. All of these activities allowed us to make contacts and reap professional as well as personal benefits. Our involvement generated good will and helped build our reputation.

After a year, we decided to "buy in" to the center, becoming owners in the corporation. At that time, we believed that working together closely with other mental health professionals on joint projects would be mutually beneficial financially, professionally, and personally. To do that and feel as if we were reaping the rewards as owners of an entity seemed attractive. We believed in the potential of this entity, and it was already established as a corporation. Our private practices would grow better and faster if we were a part of the ownership. It seemd to us that we would benefit if we were more fully on the rotational system for new clients and had more to say about the direction of the organization.

A buy-in fee was set by the partners based on an amount roughly equal to what each of them had originally invested in the corporation in order to secure the lease, buy furniture, etc., plus an amount that they believed was the current value of goodwill of the corporation. Negotiations took place around the amount of the buy-in fee, agreement was reached, a deposit was made, and a monthly payment plan was established. This monthly fee payment was in addition to the fluctuating monthly overhead costs paid by all corporate shareholders.

Overhead was divided equally by the partners and included the lease payment plus telephone, copying machine, office personnel, and other miscellaneous expenses required for the ongoing operation of the corporation.

The overall financial impact of becoming owners in the group practice seemed negligible. We anticipated an increase in referrals to us as owners, and this did happen, although to a lesser extent than we had expected. What was not negligible was the increased amount of time required to participate in the kind of decision making that affected us in the corporation.

Weekly meetings and biannual, longe-range planning retreats seemed necessary and desirable. However, as a result of the partners diversity of goals, styles, opinions, and approaches to running a business, the operating porcess was often very time consuming.

After a time, two owners asked to be bought out by the others. We viewed the change positively, and the remaining owners felt that there was now more commonality. In an effort to build on that commmonality, a reorganization took place that involved the establishment of common goals. In addition, we experimented with pooling all income in an effort to free us creatively to be the best we could be as individuals. We thought that this would in turn result in growth for the center. We thought that if we worked collectively, we would all be much more responsible for making the business work, and even grow.

The office was relocated in order to give us more space. We had bigger dreams, developed brochures, and hired consultants to advise us on how to increase our business. We were investing time and money in marketing and programs.

We functioned approximately a year in the pooled income mode until we realized we were not operating as successfully as we had hoped. A state of decision-making paralysis resulted because, ironically, our energies were consumed by administrative duties. The result was that programs moved ahead slowly or never got off the ground, so that little or no income was derived from them.

The experiment in communal practice turned into a systemic crisis as the corporate income dropped to a painfully low level. We realized that changes needed to be made if we wanted the business to survive.

We had made several critical errors. First, we had established a business with all owners having equal decision-making power, and although each owner was in charge of a program, he or she did not have complete autonomy for directing it. In addition, none of the program directors were commissioned to establish performance standards and ways of measuring the results in terms of monetary value to the group. Accountability had not been built into our system.

We set about devising a new organizational plan. Pooling of income was stopped. We let go of our joint ownership of programs by transferring the ownership to individual partners. Each partner would be responsible to himself or herself for the functioning and development of his or her program, and would be liable for expenses while retaining net profits.

A new way to pay monthly expenses was devised. We assessed our need in terms of how much space we would use. Income was more directly tied into use of the space for some partners than for others. Therefore, we decided that we would charge ourselves "room rent," which would be based on the actual amount of client hours during prime time (3p.m.–9p.m., Monday through Thursday). As we did not want to remove the incentive for any of us to use our office, we had free of use of our offices during downtime (any time that was not considered prime time). Renters would pay a minimum amount per month. In addition, we charged renters for prime time and downtime usage; however, the charge for downtime was half the charge for prime time. Whatever monies were left from room rent and renter income, after paying the monthly expenses, would be applied to the monthly lease payment. The balance for the lease would be divided equally among the partners.

Like us, many psychotherapists wish to associate with others in order to utilize office space more economically or to purchase shared services or equipment. Some practitioners desire regular, on-site contact with others for professional growth or mutual support. Our experience has led us to believe that these kinds of objectives can be met most efficently through a formalized but loose association, utilizing rental agreements or partnership agreements that do not involve the comingling of income.

There are, however, partnerships in which the practice of pooled income works effectively. It is essential that the approach used to divide income and expenses is one that is equitable for all without becoming unnecessarily complex and, therefore, costly. The concept of accountability, which we discussed previously as not having been built into our pooled income experiment, is important. One therapist's work style may be to have a heavy schedule of individual sessions in the office. A partner's style may be to focus on employee assistance programs through corporations where the work schedule is drastically different. Another partner may emphasize public relations in order to increase awareness of services offered by the center. All may be contributing ot the success of the business; however, methods of measurement will vary. Partners must meet and maintain a certain production quota in order for income to be drawn from the group.

Common methods of meeting the quota are by utilizing money or points as the measurement of value. Points are assigned to activities based on relative merit to development and maintenance of the business entity.

It may be necessary to hire a management consultant or a lawyer to assist in developing a method of dividing income that is fair and will allow for individual potentials and styles. Expenditures in the initial stages of a business for the development of financial procedures will be money well spent when compared with the financial complexities and possible ruined relationships that can result from neglecting this important aspect.

MAINTAINING INDIVIDUAL IDENTITY

Identity is a major issue in all types of group practices. When deciding to create, join, or bring new members into a practice, careful attention must be paid to this matter. In our practice, we think that it is necessary to have a common background as well as a specialty. This affords us the ability to cover for each other internally, when needed, and also allows for the strength of diversity. At our center, all of us are marriage, family, and child counselors, yet we all have specialized training in such areas as adolescent counseling, stepfamily issues, hypnotherapy, and the like.

Our individual practices are separate and we come together only on very specific, time-limited joint projects. Having our private practice and progams functioning autonomously allows us to maintain our individual identities. This type of organizational structure holds practitioners together and, at the same time, allows them ample room for self-identification.

In advertising, we recommend that therapists list themselves both individually and as a group. Here again, this offers the advantage of both group and individual recognition. All forms of identification can be handled in this way. Names on stationery, on office doors, and directories can reflect the group identity, and that of each individual, and their specialty.

In our group setting, we have carefully chosen members for their professional specialty that will enhance their value to group identity. When considering associating with others or bringing in new associates, it is important to consider their individual specialties, as these contribute in a significant way to the group identity.

An optional approach to the commonality we have chosen is the multiple-discipline approach. For example, it can be advantageous for an MFCC to associate with a clinical psychologist who specializes in testing as well as a psychiatrist who consults, hospitalizes, prescribes medication, and can supervise the work on site.

Our approach has been to develop these complimentary associations in an informal manner. When a client requires psychiatric evaluation, we contact psychiatrists referred to us by medical professionals. Usually the psychiatrist is willing to work with us by screening the patient for possible hospitalization or for the purpose of prescribing and monitoring medications.

OFFICE PROCEDURES

A group structure that is complicated by private practice calls for well-organized office procedures. First, we strongly recommend that some one person control the office. In a small group, this person would be a combination secretary, bookkeeper, and office manager. Having the group's bookkeeping done by someone outside the ownership circle provides for more objectivity and smoother communication within the group.

Our office manager prepares monthly, quarterly, and annual reports for cash-flow information, as well as profit and loss statements. All financial records are kept by the office manager in a central location. We contract separately with the manager for individual services, such as bookkeeping, secretarial, and special reports. All of our individual practice files are kept in our separate offices and we maintain these ourselves.

The flow of work to be accomplished by the office manager often requires the setting of priorities. When an overload situation occurs, the manager informs us and we meet together to develop possible solutions. At times it has been necessary to send work out. For example, we have found that special, large mailings can be handled most efficiently by direct-mail firms. Or temporary office help can be hired to handle time-consuming typing projects.

In cases where the partnership feels it cannot afford the services of office personnel, the partners can take turns in the routine answering of the telephone during office hours. In very small group practices, this task is often handled exclusively by an answering service or answering machine.

Handling client referrals is easier than it may seem. Since we recommend that private practices be advertised separately, calls will usually come into the office requesting the services of a specific person. If a client responds to a group ad, a referral by specialty can be made. Cases of presenting problems that do not fit anyone in particular may be handled on a rotational basis, with partners working on a rotational basis to screen these incoming calls.

With the advent of modern technology, confidentiality problems may arise, particularly around the use of copying machines and computers. Often, papers are generated from these machines that are casually discarded in the waste basket or are used for scratch paper in the office or at home. It is necessary to destroy all client records before they leave the office.

SCHEDULES

We recommend that a master schedule be maintained for all the room space in the office and that it be kept in a central location. In our group, the partners sign up on Thursdays for space they need for the coming week. Renters may sign up on Fridays. This system works well for everyone, and also creates a permanent record of the time used by each of us.

Time is billed to each user on a per-hour basis as the group practice holds the contract for our office space. We refer to this as "room rent" (as described previously). Each person thus has the financial responsibility for his or her part of the group commitments and his or her own private practice.

Another model for scheduling that is commonly used successfully involves the partners' contracting for a fixed amount of space for which they are financially rsponsible. Used time can be contracted for among partners on an "as-needed" basis.

TAKING IN NEW PEOPLE

There are two methods of bringing new therapists into a group practice. They may be hired or they may be brought in as full partners.

For example, if the practice is experiencing a period of heavy client flow, it may be practical to hire someone on a straight salary or for an amount averaging less per client-hour than the charges to the client. The employed therapist may, on his or her own time see self-referrals, using space as available in the center and paying a set fee (hourly rental) for the use of the office.

The advantage to the center of this kind of an arrangement is that clients do not have to be turned away, and additional income is realized. The advantages to the incoming therapist are that an income is received without paying monthly rent or overhead expense, and it is a method of building a new practice.

A disadvantage for the center in hiring is that employees present special circumstances in several areas. With employees come the need for providing for the bookkeeping for withholding taxes, holidays, vacation, sick leave, retirement, and other fringe benefits. Also required is malpractice insurance and responsibility for supervision.

Does the group really need another partner and for what purpose? This becomes a crucial question to address when making a decision about adding to the group. Often people have wanted to buy into our group, and we address the proposal cautiously. The following factors are assessed when considering an additional partner:

1. Does the person relate well to the existing group?
2. Are the goals of the potential partner compatible with the goals of the other partners?
3. Does the person bring in a complimentary expertise that will be of value to the group practice?
4. Does the clientele the person will attract fit well with the current mix of clientele?
5. Will the new mix of partners maintain the ability to cover for each other in emergencies and during vacations?

On the basis of our experience, we recommend that, when a new therapist is brought into the group practice, he or she come in as a fully self-sustaining partner. That is, the therapist is not dependent on the center to provide referrals for clientele. Joining the group as a partner requires legal agreements to be made and a lawyer and/or management consultant is required to facilitate the process. In the state of California, any changes in the ownership of the corporation are required to be reported to the state.

Laws and licensing agency guidelines pertaining to group practice vary from state to state, and, in time, change. We recommend that the reader investigate all guidelines and laws that may apply, and consider all suggestions made in this chapter in light of applicable local and state laws and guidelines.

3

WORKING WITH PRIVATE MENTAL HEALTH CENTERS

Lawrence T. Woodburn, Ph.D.

INTRODUCTION

Private mental health centers provide a unique opportunity for psychologists to practice supervisory and administrative skills. The term "private mental health centers" covers a wide variety of agencies. For the purpose of this chapter, the term will be defined as follows: "A multi-disciplinary agency which is not a branch of a governmental entity, which offers mental health services to the general public." Thus, a "private mental health center" might be a proprietary corporation, a non-profit corporation, a partnership, or an individually-owned business. Likewise, a private mental health center might provide inpatient, outpatient, residential, or educative services, or any combination thereof. In spite of the diversity of private mental health centers, they tend to have certain commonalities:

1. Direct service is largely provided by B.A., M.A., or paraprofessional counselors.
2. An administrative hierarchy exists which is separate from the service providers.
3. Funding comes both from clients' fees and contracts marketed to government or private businesses.
4. The role of the psychologist is primarily training and supervision of staff counselors.

Most private mental health centers employ only one psychologist either full or part time. That one psychologist seldom provides any direct service, but rather is responsible for supervising and training the staff counselors. Consequently, when we talk about practice organization and basic procedures and skills for working with private mental health centers, we are referring primarily to supervision and training procedures.

PRACTICE ORGANIZATION

There are two basic strategies for a psychologist to break into working in private mental health centers: (1) seek employment at an existing agency; or

(2) create your own agency. Each of these strategies has certain advantages and disadvantages.

The primary advantage of applying to an existing agency, of course, is that the psychologist avoids the problems, long hours, and economic frustrations of developing the agency from scratch. The disadvantage is that the agency philosophy and agency needs might not be a good match for the skills of the psychologist. Emphasizing the skills in the following section of this chapter would be a good beginning for a psychologist to "sell" himself or herself to an agency. However, I would recommend that a job applicant learn as much about the individual agency as possible by conversing with staff counselors, so that he or she could custom design a skill package accordingly.

The primary advantage of creating one's own agency is, of course, greater control and autonomy. A private mental health center can be incorporated quite easily as either a non-profit or proprietary corporation. Government funding sources tend to favor non-profit status so that alternative is probably preferable.

To become a non-profit corporation, a mental health center must file articles of incorporation and by-laws of the corporation with the State, Department of Corporations, or Secretary of State, or equivalent organization. Format for submission can be obtained directly from the appropriate state office. An attorney with expertise in corporate law can file all the necessary documents, usually for a fee of $500 or less. Perhaps an even more expedient method for incorporating is to obtain the articles of incorporation and by-laws of another non-profit corporation and simply modify them with the new names, etc. Most of the legal jargon and format can be copied verbatim. For a non-profit corporation to also be exempt from federal taxes, an additional form must be submitted to the I.R.S. This is the Tax Exempt Status form, and it can be obtained from an I.R.S. office. The federal government may require 6 to 8 months to act on Tax Exempt status, so application should be made well in advance of obtaining funding.

Funding from private mental health centers comes from a variety of sources, and the psychologist who forms his or her own agency must be creative at pursuing new funding leads. Some funding comes directly from client fees. However, it is difficult for an agency to function without some additional funding. The following are some suggestions for funding needs:

1. County Mental Health contracts.
2. Commerce Business Weekly—contracts for federal government services.
3. Employee assistance program contracts to private industry.
4. Local Health Maintenance Organizaiton mental health subcontracts.

BASIC PROCEDURES

The following is a typical job description for a psychologist in a private mental health center:

Consulting Psychologist

Job description:

1. 24-hour on-call availability to staff.

2. Supervises all full-time staff and interns.
3. Provides teambuilding process group for all staff.
4. Develops, coordinates, and implements in-service training.
5. Assists in program development.
6. Provides psychological testing and assessment when necessary.
7. Attends all staff meetings.
8. Presides over weekly Utilization Review Committees for all clients.
9. Reviews all charts and ensures that all entries are appropriate. Countersigns those entries by all personnel not cleared to sign chart entries: volunteers, etc. He or she is to be responsible for all diagnoses and treatment plans by approving them when signing the diagnosis/mental status sheet.

From this job description, there flows certain skills which are essential for a psychologist to be effective in a private mental health center setting. The first of these is *supervision.* All staff counselors are required to be under individual supervision on a weekly basis. I consider any topic which is even remotely work-related to be fair game for supervision. Thus, supervision topics might include a discussion of a particularly difficult client, clarification of a diagnostic category, discussion of a conflict with another staff counselor, examinations of counter-transference issues, explorations of frustrations over management procedures, or explorations of a personal problem which interferes with work. Maintaining confidentiality of supervision sessions is extremely important. I stress that supervision is just as confidential as a therapy session, as long as the counselor is not a clear and present danger to staff, others, or the agency.

I have found that the best style of supervision is a balance between didactic and experiential supervision. Most counselors want to "gain knowledge" from their supervisor, so some didactic teaching is important. Likewise, most counselors wish to learn more about themselves, so some experiential work is important. Interestingly, counselors who resist one or the other of these methods usually become problematical. Those who resist didactic supervision tend to be narcissistic and overidentify with the clients. Consequently, providing a balance between experiential and didactic supervision also meets the needs of the agency in terms of identifying potential problems.

The model for supervision which I find provides this balance between didactic and experiential styles is the "equilateral triangle" method. In this approach, one conceptualizes the supervision hour as an equilateral triangle with the following dimensions:

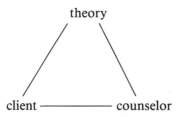

The session then is equally divided among discussing client dynamics, theoretical concerns, and counselor issues and dynamics. A good format for facilitating such discussion is shown in the case presentation format below. Counselors are given the case presentation format at the beginning of their employment and asked to prepare a case for supervision at least once per month.

Case Presentation

1. Presenting problem
2. Three (3) sentences on history
3. Diagnosis
4. Impressions of client
    — reality testing
    — defenses
    — strengths
5. Treatment goals
6. Specific interventions used
    — relationship to overall goals
    — theoretical orientation
    — indications and contraindications
    — how to follow-up
7. Ethical and legal issues
8. Immediacy issues
    — how client reacts to therapist
    — therapist's feelings about client
    — personal issues aroused

A few additional comments on supervision: the counselor is given responsibility for asking for what he or she wants from the supervision session. To be most effective, the supervisor needs to provide positive feedback rather than just criticism. When confrontation is necessary, it should be behavioral rather than personal. Additionally, the supervisor should give "homework" assignments to assist counselors in following up on new awareness.

The second skill which is essential for a psychologist to be effective in a private mental health center setting is the ability to provide *staff training*. Staff training generally occurs through two different processes: an intensive 3- to 5-day training for new employees, offered quarterly or semi-annually, and in-service training at regularly scheduled staff meetings.

Training for new employees is designed to ensure that all counselors attain a minimum level of skill and consistency. This is particularly important since counselors at most private mental health centers come from a variety of different backgrounds and orientations. As long as counselors adhere to certain minimum standards, the most diverse theoretical orientations can be accommodated.

The emphasis in the 3-day training is on practicality. Theoretical material used is translated directly into usable intervention techniques. The training package I use consists of modules and was designed originally for an inpatient setting. The outline is as follows:

3-Day Training For New Employees

   I. Philosophy of the Agency
  II. 3-Phase Eclectic Model of Counseling (Carkhuff and Egan)
     a) Responsive Phase
     b) Initiative Phase
     c) Action Phase
 III. Treatment Planning and Charting
     a) Objectively measurable
     b) S.O.A.P. format
 IV. Suicide Assessment
  V. Treating the Violent Client
     a) Theoretical concerns
     b) 6-Step model for the violent crisis
     c) Long-term treatment planning
 VI. Treatment Implications of Various Diagnosis Groups
VII. Treating the Borderline
     a) Theory
     b) Contraindicated interventions
     c) Effective interentions
VIII. Treating the Paranoid
     a) Theory
     b) Contraindicated interventions
     c) Effective interventions
 IX. Treating the Bipolar
     a) Theory
     b) Contraindicated interventions
     c) Effective interventions
  X. Treating the Antisocial
     a) Theory
     b) Contraindicated interventions
     c) Effective interventions

I have found the "Treatment Implications of Various Diagnostic Groups" to be particularly helpful, as it provides a quick reference for concrete treatment guidelines to which counselors can refer. This module is outlined in detail, in table titled, **Treatment Implications of Various Diagnosis Groups.**

In-service training at regularly scheduled staff meetings consists of a 1-1.5 hour workshop format offered every month at the conclusion of the administrative portion of the staff meeting. The psychologist is in charge of coordinating the training and may either present the training or arrange outside speakers with specialized areas of expertise. The psychologist generally solicits staff input every 6 months for desired in-service training topics. Any of the 10 modules from the 3-day training might be repeated as the need arises. Additional popular topics include:

Treatment Implications of Various Diagnosis Groups

DX Category	Preferred Defense	Treatment	
		Contra-indicated	Indicated
Schizophrenia	regression	regressive techniques	present focus/ structure/respond to a part of message
Histrionic	repression	over nurture/ cover	cognitive/R.E.T.
Paranoid	projection	confrontation/ touching	respond to a part of message
Bipolar	denial	catharsis	cognitive
Obsessive/ compulsive	intellectual- ization	cognitive	Gestalt
Borderline	splitting	confrontation touching catharsis genuineness	create benign environment/ make process comments/ask process questions
Anti-social	rationalization	too much empathy	paradox/ confrontation

1. Adult children of alcoholics
2. Group leadership styles
3. Structural family therapy
4. AIDS
5. Eating disorders
6. Medication side effects
7. Drug abuse and treatment
8. Suicide assessment

A third necessary skill for a psychologist in a private mental health center is the ability to provide *team–building*. The success of a private mental health center rests largely on the ability of the staff counselors to function as a team. To do so is not always easy, for a number of reasons. First, mental health jobs are usually high stress and low pay. This combination tends to exacerbate petty disagreements and rivalries amongst staff. Additionally, the administrative staff is generally removed from direct client contact (and also higher paid) and this creates an "us–them" attitude. Counselors themselves also tend to be somewhat competitive by nature and what begins as an honest disagreement over a treatment strategy can quickly become a personal rivalry. At times a particular staff member can be cast in the role of scapegoat.

In order to deal with these dynamics effectively, the psychologist must be knowledgeable in the areas of group dynamics and family therapy. (Indeed, an agency often resembles a dysfunctional family!) Team–building then becomes an ongoing process, and the psychologist must be active and creative in structuring exercises which foster group cohesion and clear communication.

I implement team–building through three different channels (although there is nothing "magic" about this format). First and most basically, I present a stress reduction seminar (1/2 day) on an annual basis. If properly structured, the seminar will provide not only techniques for dealing with stress, but also an opportunity to discuss job stress issues in small groups, as illustrated in the following outline.

Stress Reduction Seminar

    I. Origins of Stress – Normal and Exaggerated
   II. Stress Effects on the Body
  III. Scoring of Stress Questionnaires
  IV. Symptoms of Stress
   V. Stress in the Workplace
  VI. Stress Reduction Techniques
      A. Logistical techniques
         1. Multiple Stressor Theory
         2. Predictability Model
      B. Cognitive Techniques
         1. Rational Emotive Therapy
         2. Cognitive Reframing
      C. Relaxation Techniques
         1. Progressive Muscle Relaxation
         2. Biofeedback
         3. Imagery and Self-Hypnosis

The second phase of team–building is done in semi-annual "team–building marathons," which are half-day sessions held off the facility. The psychologist is responsible for providing structured exercises which promote group cohesion or conflict resolution. Some of the formats which I have found useful are:

1. Most effective/least effective behavior
2. Satir's incongruent communication exercises
3. Empathic response triads
4. Unfinished business visualizations

The third phase of teambuilding is done in the form of staff process groups. These are 1/2- to 1-1/2- hour groups at the end of the monthly staff meetings. These groups are unstructured, with the psychologist assuming the role of group facilitator by reflecting the group dynamics and clearing up communications.

Psychologists who work in private mental health centers also need to develop *administrative skills.* In a sense, the psychologist is the liaison person between the counseling staff and administrative hierarchy, much like middle management in industrial settings. One of the administrative duties is that the psychologist reviews all treatment plans and diagnoses for appropriateness. He or she also presides over utilization review committee meetings, at which cases are discussed and need for continued treatment evaluated. The psychologist is also on call 24 hours per day by "beeper" for counselors to consult. Proposal writing to obtain additional funding or new programs is also a valuable skill for a psychologist in a private mental health center setting.

PROBLEMS AND DISADVANTAGES

The private mental health center as a workplace presents several disadvantages for a psychologist which should be addressed. The psychologist tends to be the "person of last resort" for staff counselors' dissatisfactions and conflicts. To do the job properly, the psychologist provides a safe emotional release for all counselors, yet generally has no such vehicle for personal stress management. This is partly due to the fact that there is generally only one psychologist in a given mental health center and partly due to the fact that content of supervision sessions is bound by rules of confidentiality.

This sense of isolation is compounded by the fact that the psychologist often does not get acknowledgement from administration for superior performance and abilities but rather is simply expected to "keep the counselors satisfied." One must remember that a private mental health center is, after all, a business and that business values sometimes conflict with more humanistic values. Counselors are chronically overworked and underpaid; this is simply a political and economic fact which the psychologist is powerless to change. Consequently, the psychologist must be satisfied with providing more instrinsic reinforcement to counselors, such as a cohesive environment and supervision which results in career enhancement.

An additional disadvantage of working in a privae mental health center is the possible instability of funding and consequent lack of job security. This again creates a sense of powerlessness which one might not experience as a sole practitioner. However, this sense is sometimes alleviated if the psychologist also assists with writing proposals and program development.

The middle management position of the psychologist is inherently challenging. Counselors often have very valid suggestions and complaints which go unheard by administration. Similarly, administrators may have valid feedback for a counselor, only to find that the counselor has discounted the feedback as being "a set-up." The psychologist is often called upon to communicate such messages and to mediate conflicts which go unresolved. Again, the psychologist must be adept at communicating and reframing.

In spite of these disadvantages (and at times even *because* of them) private mental health centers can provide a rewarding work setting for psychologists. The type of person who would function well in this position would have to be autonomous, an excellent communicator, and well versed in group and family dynamics. In addition, he or she would need to develop a personal stress management system and a high tolerance for ambiguity.

REFERENCES

Blanck, G., & Blanck, R. (1974).*Ego psychology: Theory and practice.* New York: Columbia University Press.
Community Research Foundation. (1981). *Staff Procedure Manual.*
Egan, Gerald. (1975). *The skilled helper.* Bellmont, CA: Wadsworth Co.
Satir, Virginia. (1972). *Peoplemaking.* Palo Alto: Science and Behavior Books.

C H A P T E R

4

THE AFFILIATED HOSPITAL PRACTICE

E. Warren O'Meara, Ph.D.

T he private mental health practitioner today is faced with many perplexing choices in establishing his or her practice. This chapter will focus primarily on helping the practitioner understand and develop a hospital practice and will advise on affiliations with other professionals. The competition for patients and the ever-diminishing mental health dollar is creating intense competition for patients, which has made it necessary for the mental health practitioner to affiliate with other professionals and institutions as a means of survival. The most contested and highly volatile issue today is that of hospital practice for clinical psychologists and other nonmedical mental practitioners. As this subject is so important to all non-medical practitioners, we will begin by exploring this issue.

Clinical psychologists were the first nonmedical practitioners to explore and be granted hospital privileges. Therefore, relevant historical facts will be presented in order that all nonmedical practitioners may understand the difficulties and serious problems that arise when entering the traditional medical arena. It is the author's hope that the reader, regardless of professional background, will gain from the experiences that clinical psychologists as a profession have had to endure, and that the information in this overview will be helpful to all nonmedical private practitioners.

Traditionally, the nonmedical private practitioner was relegated to outpatient services almost exclusively, or to extremely controlled inpatient services. However, an increasing need for short-term hospitalizations for persons seen on an outpatient basis, and the need for private practitioners to be involved in their patients' hospitalization, are clincially relevant to the continuity of care. The hospital practice is taking on an entirely new meaning for the nonmedical health practitioner, both clinically and politically. For example, the new focal point for national and state organizations is the right of the clinical psychologist to practice in hospital settings independently—that is, without supervision from physicians. On the national level, the American Psychological Association's Division 42 (Psychologists in Independent Practice) has formed a committee on hospital practice. The division was formed, in part, because approximately 35 states have laws or regulations that prevent psychologists from obtaining full medical staff privileges.

In California, for example, the California State Psychological Association (CSPA) and the California Association of Psychology Providers have already tested the legitimacy of the physicians' "exclusive" right to hospitalize and to control nonmedical decisions. The court's view of a psychologist's right to independent practice in a hospital setting has been upheld to date. Currently, all appeals regarding this decision have been fueled by the Psychiatric and Hospital Association in the state of California. This situation is creating tremendous tension between the two professions.

California is an excellent example of what can be done for psychologists and other nonmedical mental health practitioners everywhere in order to gain the rights and privileges that are necessary to practice independently and to provide patients with the highest standard of care. In 1969, the CSPA Executive Board made a commitment to formally oppose the supervision of psychologists by psychiatrists. The board further asserted that psychologists need to have, and should have, full voting privileges in hospitals. In 1974, the CSPA's task force on the psychologist's role in hospitals was formally established. It reviewed all state regulations and JCAH guidelines. The study concluded that organized medicine had been using the existing law and regulations for protection of interdisciplinary competition and economics. Status and control, rather than quality of patient care, were essential issues. The board concluded that the psychologist's role would have to be formally encoded in law to ensure professional autonomy, including the ability to manage a patient's care and to bill independently of psychiatrists. In 1975, the bill was introduced in the state senate. The senate bill included psychologists to be on hospital staffs. However, in 1976, the JCAH Board of Commissioners was petitioned to change its position on psychology. At the same time, the California Association for the Advancement of Psychology formally requested that the Federal Trade Commission prohibit the JCAH from excluding psychologists from hospital staffs as a violation of federal antitrust law.

However, court and regulation battles continued and, in 1978, despite heavy opposition by California's medical and hospital associations, the state Health and Safety Code was amended, allowing psychologists to continue their work in hospital settings. In 1980, the Code was amended again, specifically authorizing the appointment of clinical psychologists to medical staffs and prohibiting discrimination against them in the delivery of services within the scope of their licensure.

Although these laws and regulations were being changed, very few hospitals were enacting them. In 1984, a strike force composed of Division One of the CSPA incorporated independently as the California Association of Psychology Providers (CAPP) and pursued the issues legally. CAPP filed suit in 1984 challenging the validity of psychologists' deletion from medical staffs. The motion for summary judgment to invalidate the discriminatory regulations was granted and, in October 1985, the Department of Health Services reinstated the original version of the provision allowing psychologists to practice independently in hospital settings. This action resulted in further problems between the professional associations, leading to, in January 1986, a court-issued order charging the Department of Health Services with the responsibility of enforcing the law of prohibiting discrimination against psychologists on the medical staff of hospitals. The order placed ultimate responsibility for the psychological care of hospitalized patients and the authority to admit and discharge patients within the legal scope of the practice of licensed psychologists in California. This new directive led to further complications between the state psychiatric and hospital associations' willingness to enact these new provisions. In March 1986, they launched a series of legal attacks designed to negate the regulations, all of which were denied and are currently under appeal.

The new law simply allows psychologists, within the scope of their licensure, to be responsible for the diagnostic formulation of each patient admitted to the hospital under their care. Furthermore, the psychologist is responsible for the development and implementation of each patient's treatment plan. This significant change in law/regulation now allows the California psychologist to enter an area that was once held exclusively for psychiatrists, the hospital. In addition, the law opened the door to hospital practice not only to clinical psychologists, but also to allied health provessionals — clinical social workers, marriage and family therapists, and nurse practitioners. However, each of these groups is regulated very differently and the reader is encouraged to check the bylaws of any hospital where he or she may wish to become affiliated. Many hospitals in California have yet to enact the new regulations requiring that psychologists may practice independently because both professions are trying to work out an amenable solution. Physicians argue, justifiably, that psychologists' training in hospitals is not standardized. However, psychologists could force hospital compliance through legal procedures. Psychologists and other nonmedical mental health practitioners in California are having their patience tested to the limit.

In response, many hospitals have begun to design programs for psychologists and other nomedical practitioners where they may learn hospital standards and procedures. For example, experienced clinical psychologists have developed peer inpatient proctoring programs that allow for adequate training in inpatient procedures for psychologists interested in practicing in hospitals. For other, allied mental health practitioners, however, very little has been done to formalize hospital procedures for their particular expertise. The reader is invited to explore existing procedures that have been successfully utilized for clinical psychologists and to extrapolate any relevant material. Additionally, in order to help physicians feel more comfortable, cotherapy models are being developed to help educate both professionals. However, this approach would be utilized only as a temporary compromise until the appellate courts decide the merits of the lower court's decision.

The major concern to both professions is patient care and responsibility. The prevailing view in most institutions is that clinical and legal responsibilities are shared, regardless of professional background. In the case of any suspected malpractice, one can be sure that both the nommedical and the medical person will be held potentially equally liable. Any knwoeldgeable personal injury attorney should be able to supply details.

From a therapeutic standpoint, very little has been written on the cotherapy model in the hospital setting. There is certainly a great need for continued research efforts in this area. Many hospitals are hesitant to grant psychologists and other nonmedical practitioners full privileges because of their lack of "hospital experience." The basis of this argument is that the nonmedical professional does not have formal training in multidisciplinary settings. The argument is a shallow one; for example, most nonmedical practitioners have had to coordinate treatment plans with physicians, teachers, or other social organizations in order to provide the best possible care for their patients in an outpatient setting. Training programs are being designed as a means to help orient the nonmedical practitioner to his or her new role in the hospital setting. For example, bylaws are being changed to accommodate psychologists in the inpatient health center, although slowly and cautiously.

The author has worked as a coleader on a cotherapy model treatment team and has been responsible for taking histories, conducting mental status examinations, and seeing patients two to three times per week in the hospital. Psychologists and psychiatrists often meet in informal cosupervision of cases on which they are collaborating. The experience of many psychologists working within this framework has been successful. Patients have also reported satisfaction with the cotherapy model. To allow psychologists to practice within this model, if only temporarily, will ease physicians' and administrators' apprehensions and permit both professions to interact more efficiently for the benefit of the patient.

As this model becomes more successful with the use of psychologists, it is certain that other nonmedical mental health practitioners will be able to utilize similar models designed specifically to their needs. However, in California, it is, without a doubt, the hottest professional issue facing psychologists, psychiatrists, and hospital administrators. On the sidelines are other nonmedical mental health practitioners who will certainly take advantage of all the work that psychologists have done in terms of leading the way to a more open door policy in psychiatric hospitals. It is a legal arena of turf battles and the legal lines are being drawn. It is now up to the courts to decide the outcome, which many observers feel will be positive for nonmedical practitioners.

Interested practitioners should contact their local state psychological association to ascertain the legal/regulatory issues. Admission to a medical staff is a fairly simple process, beginning with an application to that medical staff. Most hospitals require various limits of malpractice insurance and cardiopulmonary resuscitation training. In addition, one should be able to prove prior hospital practice through recommendations from administrators or other mental health practitioners who are knowledgeable of one's professional work in these settings. For practitioners who have had little hospital experience, most hospitals today are providing excellent education programs to help make the transition easier. Many of these programs include peer supervision, a cotherapy model, and a proctoring model. Most of these programs include a year of informal supervision. At the end of the training or proctoring period, the proctor and the proctoree are both reviewed by the peer review committee, which is made up of medical and nonmedical mental health practitioners. A decision is then made by that committee as to whether or not further proctoring is indicated or whether the practitioner can practice independently in the hospital setting.

The affiliated practice extends far beyond the hospital practice. For example, psychologists and attorneys have become closely associated. The two professions have teamed together in jury selection decisions where the attorney consults the psychologist in matters of juror personalities and how they may affect an outcome. Forensic psychology is an ever-broadening area due to psychologists' asserting their expertise in legal opinions. However, this has not been an easy task, because psychiatrists have also had a long-standing interest in this area of practice. In addition, allied mental health practitioners are usually limited and must exhibit their specific expertise; for example, it would be very difficult for a marriage, family, and child therapist to show his or her forensic conclusions via psychological testing, unless that professional could prove extensive testing background. Other allied health professionals are usually used in child custody cases and cases of emotional and physical abuse. Legally, the issue is somewhat similar to the hospital medical staff issue; however, state legislators appear to be more open to forensic reform. The area of personal injury evaluation and treatment is expanding rapidly and provides excellent referrals. Practitioners who are interested in the forensic field should contact their state or local forensic organization. Further training is often required, so be prepared to spend time meeting stringent requirements.

Practitioners are also affiliating with physicians directly. Both professionals often practice in the same office, and interoffice referrals are common. Another benefit to the mental health practitioner is less isolation, which can become a burnout issue. The mental health practitioner who also wishes to build his or her practice by affiliating with a physician needs to identify the specialty and to locate a physician. Fourth- or fifth-year medical residents in formal training programs may be excellent candidates as they soon will be starting their own practice.

With the advent of health maintenance organizations (HMOs) and preferred provider organizations (PPOs), nonmedical practitioners are finding new challenges in terms of assuring their ability to practice independently. Many of these organizations have been formed exclusively around the medical practitioner, to the point that some HMOs exclude everyone else. In response, nonmedical practitioners have successfully formed their own PPOs. The interested mental health practitioner needs to contact the local or state psychological organization to locate these organizations in his or her locality.

In conclusion, the independent practitioner is facing an ever-changing market climate. Expanding one's horizons often results in some frustrating legal maneuvering or professional "lockout." The need to be resourceful and creative is essential. The breadth of issues is cumbersome, however, attainable with our continued perseverance. The interdisciplinary team (affiliated) is the future. We can no longer depend on the traditional, often oppressive, past and present. The reader is encouraged to join relevant professional organizations that have their germane clinical and political interests at hand.

REFERENCES

Amundson, J., Carpenter, L., & Morin, S. (1986). Legislative committee 1986 annual report. *Newsletter, The California Psychologist, 21* (6).

Berg, M. (1986). Toward a diagnostic alliance between psychiatrist and psychologist. *American Psychologist, 41* (1).

Cummings, N. (1986). The dismantling of our health system: Strategies for the survival of psychological practice. *American Psychologist, 41* (4).

Kingsbury, S. (1987). Cognitive differences between clinical psychologists and psychiatrists. *American Psychologist, 31* (2).

Newman, C.J. (1987). Wearing us down. *California Association of Psychology Providers, 5* (1).

Undwigsen, K. (1987). Hospital practice in psychology: The California experience. *American Psychological Association Practitioner, 1* (1).

Walker, E.C. (1980). Continuing professional development. In Eugene Walker (Ed.), *Clinical Practice of psychology.* New York: Pergamon Press.

5

PART-TIME PRIVATE PRACTICE

Neil G. Ribner, Ph.D.

M ost of the issues facing the therapist in full-time private practice are also those that must be faced by the part-time practitioner. This chapter will highlight some of the unique aspects of being in part-time practice as well as well as describe the overlapping issues.

THE SEEDS OF A PART-TIME PRACTICE

Like many practitioners, I started my career as a salaried employee. While collecting postgraduate hours for licensure, and even immediately after getting licensed, working for a salary seemed the safest, most reasonable alternative. Advice from mentors that one "cannot just hang up a shingle and expect clients to stand in line" was taken seriously, particularly with loans to repay and family commitments having been made. In addition, the costs of starting a practice were prohibitive so soon after graduate school, and doubts about "who would refer to me" were strong as I was inexperienced and not well known.

Even for therapists with no financial burdens or family constraints, the prospect of making a secure, steady income after graduate school often is appealing. Thus, most take jobs in clinics, schools, or community agencies, and dutifully put in eight hours a day for 50 weeks a year. Then they get itchy—for more money, more flexibility, more varied experiences.

Working at a clinic or agency fills one's clinical hours, but the clients often seem unmotivated or noninsightful, and the type of clientele seems to fall within a narrow range of diagnoses. I recall that after working for several years in college counseling centers, I swore that the next client whose presenting complaint was an "identity crisis" would drive me to find a new profession! When an intake presented with marital issues or looked a bit schizophrenic, the staff would fight for rights to work with that person. Also, in these settings, one always has to account for what one is doing—if not to a supervisor, then to the county or state. "Clinical time" often becomes "filling out forms" time. In academia, of course, there is no direct clinical work. One can supervise interns, teach courses in assessment and therapy, and even do therapy research without ever seeing a patient.

Then there is the money issue. What seemed like a huge salary to someone just coming out of graduate school is now just enough to get by, and the prospect of doing some private work becomes more and more appealing. The fantasy is that in private practice you can do what you want to do (i.e., therapy) with the kinds of people you want to do it with (i.e., motivated clients in your specialty area) without anyone looking over your shoulder (i.e., no tally sheets to fill out), and get paid many times more than what you are already getting paid! The reality is that it is not that simple.

PART-TIME VS. FULL-TIME PRACTICE

After one works at a salaried job for a while, the opportunity to do private practice often presents itself. Patients who no longer are eligible for clinical services want to see you privately. People who have heard you give a lecture want to have their family start therapy. Students have friends they think would work well with you. So the idea of an independent practice is not as far-fetched as it once seemed. But the old doubts linger. Can I make it on my own? What if I find I don't like it — can I get my old job back? Am I ready to give up all the benefits of my current job?

Rather than dive in head first, a therapist can go more slowly. Some of the hesitancy is a reality shared by the fledgling full-time practitioner; that is, leaving the security of the known for the insecurity of private practice. Some of the fear is personal. However, making the shift into full-time practice involves many risks, such as time, money, and personal factors, that are not as great when moving into part-time practice. Also, the combination of a part-time job and part-time practice can provide the best of both worlds.

If one maintains a part-time job while doing part-time private practice, one has the following advantages.

1. *Income Security.* While practicing part-time, your job provides a steady income. Knowing you can count on a regular check each month takes some of the anxiety out of cash flow worries. Albeit much lower on an hourly basis than private practice income, salary keeps coming in even while one is sick or on vacation.

2. *Employee Benefits.* Having at least half-time salaried job gives you the fringe benefits of a full-time employee: health insurance, pension plan, paid vacation and sick leave, and so on. These can be particularly useful when one is starting out in private practice, as the costs would be an enormous percentage of one's gross income.

3. *Referrals.* Although the guidelines for avoiding conflict of interest must be clear, maintaining a salaried job keeps you visible to a number of people — students, other professionals, the general public — where the possiblity of referrals exists.

4. *Client selection.* Not depending on income from private practice to meet bills allows you to be more selective in the types of clients with whom you work. Private practice, per se, may allow you this freedom, but it is much more difficult to turn away patients when you count on their fees to pay the mortgage.

5. *Enhancing job skills.* Maintaining a practice can give you valuable experiences that may enable you to do your salaried job much better. For example, seeing one's own clients gives one's teaching and supervision a liveliness

that cannot be obtained anywhere else. It also keeps you in touch with trends in client complaints, insurance issues, assessment and diagnostic issues, and the like.

The following are benefits of a part-time practice whether or not you maintain a part-time salaried job.

1. *Free Time*. Being in practice on a part-time basis allows you to utilize the rest of your time as you choose. Some of this may go to a salaried job, and some might go toward other professional activities, such as writing, consulting, research, or presenting educational seminars. Aside from professional work, you can also have more time for leisure-time activities, hobbies, and child care. As my wife is employed full time, we share in the raising of our three children. My part-time practice allows me to schedule patients when my wife is at home, and usually to be at home when the children get out of school.

2. *Guarding against burnout.* The image of seeing eight to ten patients a day, five or six days a week, has burnout written all over it. No wonder most East Coast analysts take the entire month of August off. Maintaining a part-time practice, however, allows one to engage in a variety of both professional and leisure-time activities. I may spend two to three hours each day with patients, two to three hours in teaching or supervision, two to three hours in writing, consulting, or research, and two to three (daytime) hours with my children. The dread that I sometimes felt on the morning of a 10-patient day no longer exists.

3. *Not being an entrepreneur.* It may seem odd to call not being something a benefit, yet limiting one's practice does have the advantage of "not being" an entrepreneur. To be a successful full-time practitioner, one must learn to develop a business attitude. This is never taught in graduate school, and often runs counter to the humanitarian attitude with which most people enter the profession. For many therapists, developing the entrepreneurial attitude is very difficult. In part-time practice, however, one can usually maintain a small caseload without doing too much hustling. The business attitude would help, and, clearly, some business sense is necessary even in part-time practice; but it is not as much of an issue as it is in full-time practice.

Potential Negative Aspects of a Part-time Practice

"And behind every silver lining is a cloud." Although part-time practice offers many of the aforementioned benefits, there are some aspects to watch so that they do not become disadvantages.

1. *Becoming dependent on the income.* What starts out as "extra" income can become money needed to pay the bills. Once this happens, one loses some of the advantages of part-time practice. Although part of your income is still secure if you maintain your salaried job, the portion from private practice is not. Cancellations by clients can cause as much worry about how to pay this month's mortgage as it does for the full-time practitioner; and it can cause more anxiety, as the latter will make more money and thus have more reserve than the part-timer. Counting on the income may also make it difficult to turn

patients away, or to maintain a schedule of other activities.

2. *Time pressures.* Particularly if one has a salaried job that takes up time, one may not be as available to private clients as would be desirable. One could easily fall into a schedule of seeing clients after one's salaried job (evenings) and on weekends, despite initial plans to use these times for personal activities.

3. *Isolation.* It may be difficult to feel you are part of a group if you are at your private office part-time. Of course, most private practitioners, even those in practice full-time, complain of feeling isolated. But this may especially true if one is physically not in the office more than a few hours each week.

4. *Financial burden.* Although you are in practice only part-time, you still have most of the same costs as a full-time practitioner, including business license, furniture and equipment, rental of office space, telephone and answering service, secretarial tasks, advertising, professional memberships, and malpractice insurance. There are ways to cut down on these expenses; however, the percentage of income spent on overhead is usually much greater than if one were in practice full-time.

5. *Professional identity.* It is not unusual or someone to remark to me, "Oh, I didn't know you saw patients. I thought you just taught!" Full-time practitioners are known as therapists; part-timers may be known more as teachers or administrators or agency staff, not as being in private practice. Even when it is known that you have a part-time practice, referral sources may be more inlcined to refer to therapists whom they believe to be more available. As one physician told me, "I'd like to know you were more accessible when I called, not that you were teaching and would get back to me in several hours." As ridiculous as this sounds in terms of actual logistics, it is perception that counts.

6. *Not knowing when to say no.* Good work brings more work. If you do quality work with your patients, then the referrals keep coming, from both referral sources and former clients. Turning away a client may become a difficult task, particularly if you come to depend upon the income. What initially seems reasonable, say 10 to 15 hours of practice, can begin to creep up to 20 hours or more. Maintaining the advantages of a part-time practice means learning to say No.

DECISIONS TO BE MADE

Once one has decided to go into a part-time practice, several decisions need to be made. Many of these are identical to the decisions that must be made by the full-time therapist, such as office space and design, marketing, and record keeping. There are, however, some unique aspects within each decision that pertain specifically to the part-timer.

Hours in Practice

The first major decision that needs to be made is, how many hours per week will you devote to your private practice? The number of hours you are employed elsewhere is an obvious consideration, leaving you just so many hours per week that are available for private work. Another consideration is your salaried-work schedule; that is, how many "prime" hours (usually after 4 p.m.) are available for practice?

Money is, of course, an additional factor. Is it important or necessary for you to supplement your salary with a certain income from private practice? How many hours of private work each week will net this income?

How many hours can you conceivably manage—physically, emotionally, spiritually—without creating burnout for yourself? As described above, good work usually means more referrals, and if you do not learn to limit your practice, you may find yourself working the equivalent of two full-time jobs.

Yet another factor in deciding on the number of hours per week of private practice is the amount of time that is necesary and desirable for family and leisure-time activities. A friend of mine jogs and works out every morning, limiting her practice to afternoons and evenings. I do a good portion of child care while my wife works, keeping my practice limited to a set number of hours each week.

Setting Priorities

In addition to deciding how many hours you will devote to each activity, you must prioritize these in terms of both professional realities and personal needs and interests. With regards to the former, it is likely that patients would prefer to come in after work, in the evenings, or on Saturdays. Groups and families almost always have to be seen at these times. As for personal needs and interests, are there activities in which you can participate only at certain times of the day, such as concerts, classes, or sporting events? Do you schedule late-afternoon clients or spend the time coaching your child's soccer team? Do you work on Saturdays or keep that as a "family day?" Do you do groups two evenings per week or take cooking or aerobics classes?

Setting priorities, and sticking to them, can be a difficult process. Knowing that you cannot see a patient at a particular hour because of a teaching commitment may have a very different feel than not seeing the patient because you have agreed to pick up the children at school. Each part-time practitioner needs to set priorities in advance, so that personal activities and commitments become as sacred as professional ones.

Renting an Office

The part-time therapist must decide on the type of rental arrangement that best suits his or her needs. Many therapists will rent you either their office or a furnished office in their suite by the hour, small block of time, or day. This can be very cost efficient if you know exactly how many hours you need the office, and the specific times you need it. Some professionals are very flexible about this; a physician from whom I once rented space had a free office in his suite, and allowed me to use it whenever I needed it, with no prior scheduling. Others are very rigid about such arrangements; a friend is renting space that she can have only on Thursdays, and must pay for it a month in advance whether or not she uses it.

If flexibiltiy is desirable, or you plan to do up to a half-time practice, you may find it more cost effective to rent your own space, and then, perhaps, to sublet your office to other part-timers who need space for fewer hours. After I rented my own office, I sublet to one therapist on Wednesday evenings, and to another for blocks during the day when I knew I would be teaching. Given the income from the sublets, I wound up paying no more than I would have if I had subleased someone else's office, and I had the flexibility I wanted as well as the freedom to design and decorate the office as I saw fit. I also had a more solid view of myself as a private practitioner, as this was my office that others were renting.

Support Staff and Equipment

For the part-time practitioner, there is a proportionately smaller need for staff and equipment than for the full-time therapist. Is it more cost effective, then, to hire a secretary, or to contract out secretarial services as needed? How much typing, filing, and billing will you have? Can you do these yourself? It takes me approximately 10 minutes per client per month to do billing myself. I can also type efficiently, so I prefer to type letters and reports myself on a word processor; this takes approximately two hours per week, although it would take more time for a therapist who does a lot of testing and evaluations. One therapist, for example, hires a secretary for three to four hours every two weeks, as he prefers to have someone else do his typing and billing. An answering service costs as much whether it picks up all your calls or only after normal business hours; although not as personal or efficient as a secretary, it is considerably cheaper!

As for equipment, there are probably some things you cannot do without, and others that are optional. If you do evaluations, testing equipment is necessary. A standard library should be sufficient: WAIS-R and WISC-R kits, Rorschach blots, TAT cards, Bender-Gestalt, MMPI tests and answer sheets, Sentence Completion blanks. Other tests are optional, depending on one's interests and expertise: Halstead-Reitan battery, Stanford-Binet and other developmental tests, Kaufman Assessment Battery for Children, Wide-Range Achievement Test, and so on. A standard reference library should also suffice: *DSM-III* manual, *Physician's Desk Reference*, test manuals and books on interpretation (such as *Diagnostic Psychological Testing* by Rapaport , Gill, and Schaeffer). What other books one includes depends once again on interests: individual, group, or family therapy, neuropsychological assessment, child development. Biofeedback equipment may be important for the behavioral medicine practitioner; play equipment for the child clinician.

In terms of office equipment, is your practice large enough to warrant a typewriter? A computer? A copying machine? For most part-timers, a huge investment in these items is not necessary. Typing may be contracted out, and copying can be done at a copy center. I have an arrangement with another office in the building to use its copying machine whenever needed, at a nominal cost.

There are other items that are essential regardless of the number of hours in practice, such as business cards, letterhead and billing stationary, envelopes, file folders and cabinet, ledger cards, and note pads and pens. They can range in price from the standard, least expensive types to personalized, expensive ones.

Telephone and Answering Service

Depending on how much they will be utilized, the part-timer can choose among some creative options. You can have your office number on a call-forwarding system, so that it rings in your house even if you do not have an actual phone in the office. You can also share a telephone number and answering service with another therapist; a colleague and I did this when we both rented separate offices part-time in the same suite. The arrangement worked very well, except when we both wanted to use the phone at the same time.

Working Alone or in a Group

The advantages and disadvantages of sole and group practice are elucidated elsewhere in this book. Like the full-time therapist, the part-timer must decide what arrangement is best. A unique facet of being a part-timer, though, is that even if you are part of a group, or share a suite of offices with others, you may be present much less than the others. Although this factor may not pose a problem, it can leave you feeling "out" of the group. On the other hand, if you use your office for writing, research, supervision, and so on, you may actually be present as much as the others, and have the concomitant advantages of being in a group.

Professional Ethics

This issue is not so much a decision to be made as a caution for the part-time practitioner about maintaining professional ethics. Being in practice part-time does not, in any way, mean you can compromise your ethics. Just as much care and professionalism must go into your work as would if you were a full-time therapist. Seeing patients as a secondary job does not mean that one's standards of care can be given a low priority.

The part-timer may face another dilemma—that of conflict of interest. If you maintain a salaried job, you must be very clear about keeping it separate from your practice—not taking clinic patients into your practice, not seeing students in therapy, not giving your secretary at school or the clinic your private typing. Any activities that are questionable, such as which patients can be in your practice or whether manuscripts can be typed by your school secretary, should be discussed with colleagues and supervisors so that appropriate decisions can be made.

CONCLUSION

The decision to enter part-time practice has its advantages and disadvantages, and there are many factors to consider before making the commitment. This chapter, it is hoped, has clarified some of these factors, and given the reader a place to start and a design for doing so.

REFERENCES

American Psychiatric Association. *Diagnostic and statistical manual of mental disorders,* 3rd ed. (1980). Washington, D.C.: Author, 1980.

Browning, C. (1982) *Private practice handbook.* Los Almamitos, Calif.: Duncliff's International.

Lachar, D. (1980). *The MMPI: Clinical assessment and automated interpretation.* Los Angeles: Western Psychological Services.

Mone, L. (1983). *Private practice: A professional business.* La Jolla, Calif.: Elm Press.

Ogdon, D. (1981). *Psychodiagnostics and personality assessment.* Los Angeles: Western Psycholgical Services.

(1987),*Physicians's desk reference,* (41st ed.) Oradell, J.J.: E. Barnhart.

Pressman, R. (1979). *Private Practice: A handbook for the mental health practitioner.* New York: Gardner Press.

Rapaport, D., Gill, M.M., & Schafer, R. (1968). *Diagnostic psychological testing.* New York: International Universities Press.

AFFILIATION

Neil G. Ribner, Ph.D., Associate Professor, California School of Professional Psychology-San Diego, Private Practice, La Jolla, California

S E C T I O N

B

Basic
Procedures

CHAPTER

6

CRITICAL EQUATIONS IN LAUNCHING A CLINICAL PRACTICE

Waleed Anthony Salameh, Ph.D.

"Wisdom is the failure of all body systems except the brain."

It has been said that one swallow does not a summer make. Along the same trajectory, it can be said that one license does not a practice make. Being a licensed mental health practitioner is only one of the elements involved in launching a private clinical practice. The purpose of this chapter is to discuss two other factors that enter into the clinical practice equation: (1) the operational factor—the nuts-and-bolts professional structure necessary for managing a clinical practice; and (2) the attitudinal factor—the psychological issues and personal orientation related to being a private practitioner.

GETTING DOWN TO BUSINESS: OPERATIONAL AND MANAGERIAL ASPECTS OF LAUNCHING A CLINICAL PRACTICE

Office Location

Where should you locate your practice? A good choice would be a well-known part of town where other health or business professionals are located. Your office should be easily accessible from the major freeways in your geographic area and the building should be modern and well maintained. If you opt to buy an old house and renovate it or to buy a condominium office in a business building, its location should also be in a well-recognized part of town and you should expect to expend personal effort and financial resources to maintain the building of which you are the owner or part-owner. If you decide to rent an office you would want to ensure that your lease includes a clause stating that the building owners are responsible for maintaining the building in respectable shape. You may want to walk around the building before you sign your lease to make sure that it is up to your professional expectations and the image you want to project. It is best to sign at least a one-year lease with a fixed monthly rent, so that you can be protected from arbitrary rent increases.

Two other winning qualities you need to look for in a building are good parking facilities and handicapped access. There should be ample parking space available throughout the day—your patients will be discouraged if they have to go through a parking ordeal every time they come to your office. Handicapped access is also important, especially if you intend to do neuropsychological testing or psychotherapeutic work with head-injured or physically handiapped individuals. The proximity of other health professionals in the building or nearby, the ambient level of noise, and the overall safety of the building location are three additional factors to take into account.

Office Layout and Furniture

Once you have located the right office, how do you go about setting it up for patient consultations? First, the size of your office could range from 350 to 900 square feet. The office should be divided into three areas: (1) patient waiting room; (2) secretarial, filing, and equipment area; and (3) consulting room. Let us examine the setup for each of these areas.

Patient Waiting Room   This area should always be neat and uncluttered. Some of your professional cards should be available here for your patients' reference. You can have magazines such as *Time, Newsweek, People, Connoisseur, The Smithsonian, Architectural Digest, Psychology Today,* and the *Berkeley Wellness Newsletter,* available for patients to read. Subscribing to a good children's magazine and having children's books and toys available would also be a good idea if you work with children. Overall, your waiting room should project an informal, relaxed environment. The waiting room furniture should include one or two comfortable couches, an end table for your professional cards and magazines, and some comfortable chairs, and should be enhanced by some nicely framed prints. In order to avoid a dungeonlike atmosphere, the waiting room should be well-lighted.

Secretarial, Filing, and Equipment Area   This area should contain a desk with matching credenza, at least two file cabinets, a typewriter and telephone, a small refrigerator for food refueling on busy office days, and a copying machine. Owning a copying machine can save copying expenses while reducing time-consuming trips to the copy store. Other items located in this area include wall shelves on which to put supplies and references, a coffee maker, space for a computer or word processor in case you decide to buy one, a good adjustable chair for your secretary, and a large work table on which to lay materials.

Consulting Room   The consulting room is important because it is the most intimate reflection of your professional identity. An academic-looking room with too many diplomas and books displayed tends to intimidate patients. Rather, a sensible choice of your important credentials and one bookcase for professional books would be sufficient. The consulting room should be large enough to accommodate eight to ten individuals. You will need this space for family and group work. Your consulting room should have your desk at one end with matching credenza and lateral file against the wall, one or two swivel chairs with matching side chairs, a large sectional sofa and love seat, and an end table with a lamp. The accent should be on comfort.

Your office should include original artwork that denotes your personal taste. For instance, my consulting office is decorated with African and Asiatic wood statuettes and figurines, as I like the warm tone of wood sculpture. Your consulting room should also have one or two plants for a lively touch. Another important item is a quartz clock to maintain punctuality in your appointments. Finally, your consulting room should be sound proofed to safeguard the confidentiality of your interactions with patients. If you occupy a large office, you may designate some of your office space for use as a children's play therapy area, a testing area, or a group therapy area.

Office Equipment and Supplies

Your office equipment usually falls into two categories: test materials and office supplies. Test materials include adult test forms and answer sheets, test scoring materials, and psychological tests for children. Office supplies include a modern telephone system, professional stationery and cards, appointment book and patient appointment cards, personal data sheet for new patients to fill out, billing statements, ledger cards, pendaflex hanging folders, insurance forms, and a reference library containing the standard reference volumes necessary for clinical work (*the third revised edition of the Diagnostic and Statistical Manual-III, American Psychological Association-Ethical Principles of Psychologists,* and other standard references). Your office budget should be apportioned monthly in different percentages for each category of necessary materials, going in descending order from the most important items to the least important ones.

Basic Business Outlook

In order to start your office, you will need a business license from the city in which you are located — to be renewed every year for a small fee. A certified public accountant (CPA) can advise you as to the relevance of incorporation for your particular situation. Most important, your business outlook and procedures should be kept as simple as possible. If you become caught up in a clutter of complicated procedures, you will soon be discouraged and stop keeping track of your end of things.

A good business outlook includes maintaining daily income and expense sheets. The income sheet lists your daily income from all sources, and the expense sheet lists your daily office expenses. Your overhead has to be kept low so that your expenses do not eat up your income. On the other hand, you will also need to monitor your fee-collection procedures so that your income can reflect the hard work you do. Tracking down insurance payments, monitoring collection problems, and sending prompt billing statements to insurance companies constitute one of your secretary's primary tasks. Make certain that your secretary has a file copy of all billings and correspondence with patients or insurance companies. Moreover, it would be preferable for you to provide some direct supervision over the insurance claims and collections procedures to verify that insurance claims are properly completed. If your practice may be likened to a ship, then you would be the captain at the ship's helm, steering it in the right direction.

Office Infrastructure and Resource Team

One of the most important decisions you will ever make in private practice concerns your office infrastructure, that is, the people you hire to represent you and help carry out your office work. The first such individual is your secretary. Your secretary is your ambassador to the world: to patients, to referral sources, to insurance companies. Your secretary needs to be recruited carefully and paid fairly. Four of the most important assets of that person are technical know-how (typing, billing, computer operation), patience (can wait on the phone for insurance company answers), persistence (stays with a task until it is completed), and a pleasant interpersonal disposition (makes patients feel at ease, can help reduce instead of increase tension in relating to others). An angry, overly friendly, or short-tempered secretary can quickly project a negative image of your office. Depending on the size of your practice, your secretary can take care of your billing or you may need an extra person to do it. It is best that all billing originate from your office and be done by someone who knows your office procedures. Some clinicians hire outside billing services to do their billing, but, for the same fees, one could just as well hire an inhouse secretary. When you start your practice, you can hire a part-time secretary and increase his or her work hours as your work increases.

When you are not available to answer the telephone, such duties can be assigned to your secretary, an answering machine, or an answering service. Answering machines are becoming much more accepted as media of communication between individuals, and have the advantage of message accuracy and privacy. An answering service is more complex, and some are better than others. If you opt for an answering service, you may want to check the professional grapevine and find out which answering service is utilized by your local professional association or your colleagues.

The other important component of your office infrastructure is your resource team, which is a group of professionals who advise you on matters on which are you not an expert. You will need a lawyer to consult with on legal issues related to your practice, a CPA to consult with on financial matters, and an insurance specialist to provide you and your office staff with appropriate medical and life insurance and personal disability coverage. In many instances, your resource team can save you time and energy by providing quick and concise answers to questions that may otherwise take up too much professional time to research on one's own.

Setting Fees

Fee setting is a cardinal issue for the clinician in private practice. In setting your fees, you need to take the following factors into account.

1. Your fee has to be proportionate to the average fee for professional psychotherapeutic and psychodiagnostic services in your community.

2. Your professional *time* is your biggest asset. It should be used judiciously.

3. Your degree of success in private practice will probably be positively cor-

related to your degree of flexibility. Different patients have different needs.

4. It is necessary to develop a certain degree of differentiation in your professional fee structure as you determine your fees for group psychotherapy, individual psychotherapy, and family psychotherapy. Professional fees are also affected by the length of time spent with the patient for each procedure, and by whether the procedure was conducted at your office or at a different location (hospital, attorney's office for deposition, expert testimony, on-site professional consultations).

5. Your fee structure will have to be reviewed periodically to take into account the rate of inflation, the steady rise in the cost of materials and supplies, your rent increases, and the cost of insurance. In general, it would be advisable to review your fees once or twice a year. If fee increases are warranted, then they need to be reasonable and your patients should be informed about them in advance, at least one month before implementation of the new fee structure.

In the clinical community, the topic of fee setting usually causes considerable apprehension. In discussing this topic with colleagues, I have noticed emotional reactions that include guilt, anger, embarrassment, shame, secretiveness, and denial. Many psychotherapists behave as though discussing professional fees is taboo. It might be helpful to evaluate the cost of psychotherapeutic services with respect to other expenses. Let us assume that an average cost for a psychotherapeutic treatment intervention with an individual, including initial evaluation, some psychological testing, and a psychotherapeutic program, would be approximately $3,000, or roughly equal to the cost of a used car, ulcer or cataract surgery, or an appendectomy. On the other hand, a good dune buggy would cost no less than $4,000, and a small leisure boat would cost about $8,000.

Let us now look at what individuals in different professions charge for their services per hour. Table 1 compares average hourly fees for moderately successful individuals in different occupations:

Table 1. Comparison of Average Hourly Fees in Different Occupations

Profession	Hourly Rate ($)
Senior police officers and firefighters	15– 25
Hairdressers	20– 40
Plumbers	30– 50
Airline pilots	65– 85
Real estate appraisers	50– 125
Race car drivers	100– 200
Lawyers	100– 250
Interior designers	100– 300
Acting and voice coaches	100– 350
Entertainers and models	100–2,000

As the table shows, the use of the term "expensive" to describe a particular item or professional service depends on how one spells relief. We do not have to be apologetic about discussing our fees with patients. Our professional services provide significant relief from emotional pain and can radically change the direction and quality of our patients' lives. Moreover, for the patient, the experience of psychotherapy is an investment in himself or herself, which can result in personal and work-related success with relief from the paralysis engendered by repetitive maladaptive patterns. Patients need to be clearly informed about the cost and potential dividends of psychotherapy. They have the right to ask for relevant information, and we have the responsibility of setting reasonable fees that reflect the value of our level of training, expertise, and the expenditure of running a private practice.

Specialty Areas and Professional Training

An expert distinguishes himself in the professional battlefield by the special skills he has in wielding specific instruments. A clinician distinguishes himself or herself in the clinical field by the specialty areas or techniques that make his or her services unique. It is understood that most clinicians can do psychotherapy, for example. Therefore, you need to develop specialized skills beyond a general or generic orientation — perhaps in psychodiagnostics, neuropsychological testing, biofeedback, clinical hypnosis, or doing psychotherapy with a specific patient population. Your previous training and experience might help orient you in specific directions, but regardless of whether you have a predetermined area (or areas) of clinical engagement, it makes excellent business and professional sense to invest in furthering your training by developing focused areas of clinical interest. Such training could take the form of intensive weekend workshops, continuing education, correspondence courses, courses at local institutes or universities, attendance at annual professional conferences, or one to two weeks professionally approved summer seminars focusing on particular areas of clinical work.

Improving your professional skills is a lifelong process that will continue to have positive repercussions for your work, your patients, and your business. This process will help you feel refreshed and reduce your stress. Furthermore, you will also be identified in your community as someone who has a special handle on a particular aspect of clinical work. Of course, this does not mean that you will cease being a generalist; it just means that you are interested in being more than an average clinician.

ATTITUDE REDIRECTION:
THE JOURNEY TO EVERESTLAND

Private practice is a new reality that requires a change in personal attitudes. It presents the clinician with unique dilemmas on unfamiliar grounds. In a university or public-sector position, one is usually provided with a general structure of the duties to be carried out and some form of supervisory control. In contrast, the clinician in private practice has to begin building a new attitudinal architecture that will ensure continued motivation and personal success. There are no clear guidelines to be followed and no supervisors or department chairpersons to set the course of one's work. Most clinicians are usually ill-equipped to tackle this situation, and the author does not know of any university course to date that directly addresses the issue of attitude redirection in private practice. As developed by the author, the concept of "attitude redirection" (Salameh, in press) refers to a retooling of personal resources to successfully confront the challenges facing an individual at a particular personal milestone. With regard to the private practice milestone, attitude redirection is indicated in the following areas.

Going Beyond The Academic Stance

Most clinicians were intellelctually raised in academia. They have persevered through the rigors of a Ph.D. dissertation or other advanced graduate degree. It is quite difficult to leave the habits and styles associated with "the academia family" in order to move to "the private practice family." Many personal tensions and doubts can accompany this transition, which must be made gradually. There are palpable differences that distinguish an academic identity from a clinical identity, and many identity pangs in between. This is certainly not to say that an academician cannot have clinical interests or that a clinician cannot have academic interests. It simply means that each of these persons spends his or her time doing different things. Table 2 delineates some of the differences between the academic and clinical perspectives.

Table 2. Differences Between Academic and Clinical Perspectives

Facet	Academic Perspective	Clinical Perspective
Writing	Writing is inspired by theoretical concepts or controlled laboratory experiments.	Writing is inspired by clinical interventions with patients.
Support staff	Support staff is provided and paid for by institution.	Has to screen, hire, supervise, and pay own support staff.
Time	Time is usually a constant without exact limitations.	Has to control own time for optimal productivity.
Hierarchical structure	Is responsible to department chairperson or dean.	Is responsible to self.
Financial compensation	Financial renumeration is provided by institution.	Has to generate own financial renumeration.

Table 2. Differences Between Academic and Clinical Perspectives

Facet	Academic Perspective	Clinical Perspective
Legal Exposure	Narrow window of legal exposure due to relative safety of academic environment and liability protection provided by academic institutions.	Wide window of legal exposure due to increasingly litigious clinical environment and the necessity to provide one's own liability coverage.
Communication style	Expresses abstract ideas from which applications may be deduced.	Expresses concrete ideas with links to direct everyday patient behavior.
Personal appearance	This is an irrelevant variable.	This is an important variable in interactions with patients and the public.
Professional interactions	Interacts with colleagues usually for administrative and research purposes.	Must network with colleagues in own profession and in other professions for clinical and professional reasons.
Learning style	Learns about field mostly through research and readings.	Learns about field mostly through interactions with patients.
Scientific paradigm	Science is above utility; has a theoretical view of science	Applicability is the cornerstone of science; has an applied view of science.
Verbal skills	Not a primary variable; can communicate by numerical means or by publishing research results.	Crucial to success. Must be able to explain knowledge and convey important concepts in simple words.

Developing A New Personal Outlook

The clinician in private practice needs to fortify certain personal qualities that are quite useful in assuring success in the private practice setting. Table 3 identifies and defines such qualities.

Adopting A Humorous Perspective

Running a private practice does not have to be a solemn task. Solemnity is not synonymous with personal effectiveness or seriousness about one's

Table 3. Useful Qualities For The Private Practitioner

Quality	Definition
Flexibility	If one option does not materialize, try another. Keep your windows open. We always have more than one choice.
Innovation	Take reasonable risks with new developments. Look at practice issues from new angles.
Goal Directedness	Take a stand to set your life's course. Recognize the difference between primary and secondary goals. Have specific daily, weekly, monthly, and yearly goals.
Clear-Headedness	Make your thoughts visible. Allow other individuals inside your brain so they can see what you have in mind.
Diplomacy	Do not burn your bridges to others. It is appropriate and desirable to send "Thank you" notes when you receive new referrals. It is also advisable to let others save face with you in case of a mishap. Your courtesy will be appreciated.
Self-Respect	Respect your expertise. Use your potential wisely. Know both what you are capable of doing and what you cannot do.
Persistence	"It ain't over till it's over" (Yogi Berra). Keep at projects until they become fruitful. Do not give up too soon. Make the extra effort. Impatient boys and girls miss dessert.
Self-Reliance	Do not wait for others to make things happen in your life. Get your own typewriter and test materials, and your own office.
Simplicity	Go for simple, effective solutions. Individual effectiveness is directly related to the ability to simplify seemingly complex tasks.
Balance	Do not allow work to overwhelm you. Develop a sense of proportion. Avoid perfectionism. Perfectionism provokes self-criticism as well as undue criticism of others, which ultimately provokes exhaustion and emotional bankruptcy. Best is the enemy of good.
Punctuality	Time is the fuel of productivity. Stick to beginning and ending times. Do not delay or make others wait.

Table 3. Useful Qualities For The Private Practitioner

Quality	Definition
Availability	Be accessible to patients at all times (through answering service, etc.). Also, have some office hours that fit with patients' needs (some evenings, early mornings, etc.).
Commitment	Reduce factors that can interfere with your commitment to patient's welfare: burnout, not updating your expertise and skills, countertransference issues, tardiness, lateness with reports, not filing insurance claims properly, etc.
Ethics	Ethics is about integrity, mutuality, respect, reliability, and professionalism. Ethics makes good clinical and business sense.
Surefootedness	Do not wobble. If a decision is needed and appropriate, make it.

work. Humor can help the clinician do his or her work more seriously and more energetically. At the personal level, humor can be an antidote to stress and burnout. The daily requirements of attending to patients, ensuring that the office is running efficiently, and answering correspondence can all combine to create a feeling of being overburdened. Humor comes to the rescue by reminding us not to take ourselves too seriously. All unnecessary burdens can be taken to the 'Burden Recycling Center.'

At the interpersonal level, humor bridges the distance between two people. It is a powerful way of breaking defensive barriers and a refreshing means of conveying information. Using humor with patients helps us to help them without delivering sermons (see Fry & Salameh, 1987; Salameh, 1986, 1987). Humor also represents a self-help model for patients. It is best received by most patients when the therapist has developed a good level of trust and a constructive working alliance with the patient. Once an adequate rapport has been established, humor can be utilized with patients experiencing a variety of emotional problems. For example, humor is particularly effective with obsessives to highlight their absurd worries and to illustrate how they count the minutes instead of living them. Humor can also be used with depressives to help them explore a more cheerful outlook on life, and with character disorders to accentuate recurring manipulations. Moreover, for those patients who equate emotional honesty with pain, humor can convey the message that it is liberating and enjoyable to express honest emotion. For those patients who function in the "should" mode, humor can encourage an acceptance of their real, as opposed to ideal, needs.

On the other hand, special care needs to be taken in using humorous interventions with severely disturbed psychotics, with borderline patients, or with paranoid and manic-depressive patients, who may sometimes misinterpret or deform the therapist's humor. However, a serene and cheerful approach in working with these patients can still impart a feeling of hope and human warmth while allowing them the freedom to bring forth their own sense of humor. In addition, therapists may need to exercise cautious judgment in using humor with individuals who have been victims of a recent trauma or who are hypersensitive because of an impending disconcerting event, such as divorce, severe physical illness, or other major life transitions.

The following steps are suggested in using therapeutic humor with any patient: (1) Take a brief history of the patient's past and present experiences with humor. Are such experiences negatively tainted or are they constructive in scope? What are the patient's feelings surrounding these humor experiences? (2) Ask the patient for his or her favorite joke or about a recent enjoyable or humorous experience. (3) Move on to situational humor (humor about current events, the weather, news items). (4) Use self-directed humor by communicating to the patient some personal humorous experiences that may be of relevance to the patient's own issues. (5) Once a sense of mutual trust has been established, allowing for more relaxed interactions, one can proceed to unobtrusive patient-directed humor (humor related to the patient's own dilemmas, paradoxes, absurd patterns, or maladaptive behaviors). Of course, patients can also be encouraged throughout treatment to unburden themselves of unnecessary solemnity and to develop their own humorous perspectives. (6) It is important to emphasize that the type of humor discussed here is constructive humor, not sarcasm, putdowns, or other mutilations of humor that deprecate the individual's sense of self-worth.

Humor carries a soothing message of lightheartedness and alleviation. It teaches us that misery is optional in many instances. It prevents us from becoming "pestimists" (a new term coined by the author to identify a personality characteristic combining pessimism and pestilence).

There is a Sufi story about Mulla Nasrudin who was invited to deliver a sermon to a congregation of the faithful. Mulla Nasrudin asks the congregation, "Will those of you who know what my sermon will be about raise your hands?" Half of the congregated faithful raise their hands. Mulla then asks, "Will those of you who do not know what my sermon will be about raise your hands?" The other half of the congregated faithful raise their hands. As he steps down from the pulpit, Mulla Nasrudin comments, "Then let those of you who know tell those of you who do not know."

Educating Patients About Psychotherapy

Both prospective patients and the general public harbor certain erroneous misconceptions about therapists and psychotherapy. Their preconceived beliefs and apprehensions can either inhibit them from seeking psychotherapeutic help or hinder them from achieving desired benefits when in treatment. The clinician in private practice needs to acknowledge his or her role as an educator regarding the professional services that he or she offers. This educational responsibility might be called upon in the consulting room, in interactions with other professionals, in a social context, or in any other number of unexpected situations. We owe it to our patients to decode our profession to them and to respond to their questions with patience, empathy, and understanding.

Some of our patients' misconceptions or erroneous beliefs about psychotherapy can constitute formidable blocks to treatment if they are not addressed in the early phase of psychotherapy, preferably in the first two sessions.

A recent survey of the beliefs about psychotherapy held by individuals seeking therapeutic help (Halgin & Weaver, 1986) supports the beneficial effect of responding directly to commonly shared fears about psychotherapy early in treatment. Table 4 presents some common myths about psychotherapy (phrased as patient questions) as opposed to the objective realities that dispel these myths (phrased as therapist answers).

Table 4. Myths and Realities About Psychotherapy

Myth (Patient's Question)	Reality (Therapist's Answer)
I will become eternally dependent on my therapist. I will see my therapist for the rest of life.	The goal of psychotherapy is to end your dependency on other people, including your psychotherapist. The ultimate goal of your therapy is that you will no longer need your therapist.
I will be broke because of the cost. I will never be able to afford psychotherapy.	In many instances, your health insurance plan will cover a part of your treatment. You will only be responsible for the part of your treatment that is not covered by your insurance company. The part of your treatment you end up paying for is considered a medical expense, which can be deducted on your yearly tax returns to the extent that it exceeds 7.5 percent of your yearly adjusted gross income. Furthermore, your psychotherapeutic treatment is an investment in yourself, which, when effective, will result in personal success at many levels of your life
Everyone will know all the bad things about me if I pursue therapy.	Your psychotherapy is protected by the laws of confidentiality. The material you bring up in psychotherapy stays between you and your psychotherapist. The only exception to this is if you are a danger to yourself or others, or if you have committed an act of sexual or physical abuse. In these instances, your therapist must take certain precautions to protect you or others by reporting these incidents to the appropriate agencies. if you are a minor, there may be instances where your parents would have the right to know about some of the material you bring up in therapy because they are your legal guardians. However, your therapist will usually make an agreement with

Table 4. Myths And Realities About Psychotherapy

	your parents before you begin therapy about the confidentiality of your treatment with him or her.
People will think I am crazy if I see a psychotherapist.	Being in psychotherapy is not a crazy action. It is the most rational solution for dealing with a problematic situation. Seeking psychotherapeutic help shows that you recognize the need to tackle your conflicts and want to work toward improving your emotional life.
Psychotherapy is too costly.	When you think of costs, consider the cost of your conflicts in terms of your emotional pain and subjective suffering, your loss of productivity, the effect of your stress and anxiety on your physical health, and the way your emotional conflicts affect your work and family relationships.
My friends and family can help me. I don't need psychotherapy to have someone talk to me when my friends can do the same thing.	Your friends and family are important and can help you up to a point. However, they do not have the extensive clinical training and technical knowledge that a licensed psychotherapist possesses to help you. In other words, your friends and family are not experts in the field of emotional illness. A licensed psychotherapist provides an objective point of view based on scientific training and knowledge. You would not, for example, ask a good friend to perform eye surgery on you if your friend was not an eye surgeon.
I will get better eventually anyway.	According to existing research on psychotherapy outcome, psychotherapy accelerates and focuses change. Turning off the alarm will not put out the fire. It may not be in your best interest to wait years to get better, and even then your conflicts will resurface if they have not been addressed at their core. The sense of relief provided by psychotherapeutic intervention is emotionally liberating. Moreover, psychotherapy makes sense. It provides you with a new framework for tackling present problems and offers new tools for addressing potential problems that may come up after you complete your psychotherapeutic work.
I will have to lie on the couch and be psycho-	Psychoanalysis is only one of the many available forms of psychotherapy. Other

Table 4. Myths And Realities About Psychotherapy

analyzed while you take notes.	psychotherapeutic approaches include focused psychotherapy, behavior therapy, cognitive therapy, and family therapy.
I'll never be able to know which psycho-therapist is the best one for me. There are so many psychothera-pists out there.	Your best bet is to go with your guts. Ask yourself during your initial session if you feel comfortable with the therapist. If you do not feel moderately comfortable during the first session, chances are you will not be able to work with that individual. Also, feel free to ask all the questions you need to ask to make up your mind about therapy. You have the right to ask your therapist about the exact nature of his or her academic training, the universities he or she attended, any particular specialty areas, the psychotherapeutic ap-proach he or she follows, and what the exact fees for treatment would be. If your psycho-therapist avoids answering your questions or is irritated by your inquiries, then you should probably seek help elsewhere.
Therapy lasts forever. It is too inconvenient and too lengthy.	Some recently developed forms of psychother-apy are not lengthy by definition. For exam-ple, strategic family therapy, short-term psy-chotherapy, and cognitive therapy are all time-limited therapies and do not require a long-term time commitment
All psychotherapists look the same to me. I wouldn't know which one to consult.	Not all psychotherapists are created the same. First, there are differentiations among clinical psychologists, psychiatrists, marriage and family therapists, and licensed social workers. Each of these professions requires a different type of training. You can find out about their exact training backgrounds by contacting the respective professional organizations. First, you need to make certain that the therapist you are seeking is a licensed psychotherapist. Second, you need to seek a therapist who is a specialist in the particular condition for which you need help. For example, a child therapist would be indicated if your child is having problems. A family therapy expert would be appropriate if you were having family prob-lems. A therapist specializing in eating dis-orders would be appropriate if you were anorexic or bulimic. The third consideration is

Table 4. Myths And Realities About Psychotherapy

	the specific type of psychotherapy you need: individual therapy, couple therapy, family therapy, group therapy, or some combination of these modalities. Your therapist will be able to help you determine your needs in this respect.
Some important people in my life may disapprove of me if I start a psychotherapeutic program.	Others cannot live your life for you. If you are feeling the need to seek therapeutic help, then this usually means that you have reached your personal ceiling of frustration and disappointment in dealing with repetitive maladaptive patterns or conflicts. Important others in your life will eventually appreciate the positive changes generated from your therapeutic experience. Psychotherapy helps you develop your self-reliance within the context of better relationships with others.
What happens if I have strongly negative feelings toward my therapist right in the middle of therapy?	In many cases, your negative feelings about the therapist may indicate that you are zeroing in on a highly important therapeutic issue that is creating emotional ambivalence within you. Your feelings toward your therapist are a crucial part of therapy and can be a significant tool for self-understanding. It is crucial that you do not keep your negative feelings to yourself but bring them up directly with your therapist. Therapy is one place where there should be no secrets.

Developing A Working Alliance With Patients

The purpose of psychotherapy is to provide the patient with a corrective emotional experience. At a practical level, the patient will get a definite flavor of this corrective emotional experience in the way that he or she is treated by the therapist each time they meet. It is important that the clinician make an effort to build a solid working alliance with patients, with the readiness to examine and monitor the factors that may hamper such an alliance. Showing appreciation, respect, encouragement, and concern for the patient are part of the overall gestalt that manifests this positive alliance. Being punctual and ethical with patients represents yet another facet of this alliance. These basic, rudimentary building blocks constitute a cardinal part of psychotherapy because a large part of therapy is about relationships.

Due to dysfunctional behavioral scenarios dating back to childhood family experiences, many individuals come to treatment expecting an antagonistic or conflictual relationship with a judgmental therapist whom they fear will ignore their sensitivities. For instance, a highly anxious and suspicious patient rapidly developed a positive working alliance with the author, which she felt was greatly facilitated by the fact that the author gave her detailed and clear instructions about finding the author's office when she called to make her first appointment. Since one of the underlying themes in her life was that she felt slighted by others, the simple act of giving her detailed directions made her feel respected and attended to.

Along the same lines, the author usually prefaces his psychotherapeutic work by relating the following to patients during the first therapy session.

> It is important for you to know that I am your ally, totally on your side, and that we are cooperating, working together to tackle your problems. My orientation is not to judge you, but rather to help you clarify your available choices: where you are now, and where you can go from here if you so decide. I respect the courage you have shown today by seeking treatment for intimate issues that are usually hard to talk about. I will do my best to support you and help you feel comfortable throughout our working together. I encourage you to share with me whatever feelings you may have at any time about myself, your therapy, or other issues. The consulting room is like a sanctuary where you can express your innermost feelings or secrets without fear of rejection. If I make a humorous comment or a certain statement that isn't clear to you, you might want to ask me what I meant by my statement so that things can make sense as we go along.

Statements similar to these can prevent many misunderstandings and create a constructive emotional and cognitive framework within which therapeutic interventions not only will be welcomed, but will also receive favorable consideration. There is no reason for patients to feel that they are stepping into enemy territory when they seek therapeutic help.

The First Session

The initial evaluation session with the patient is of primary importance and requires special handling by the clinician as it sets the tone for the rest of the treatment. It will be quite difficult to alter the imprint that the first session leaves on the patient's mind and emotions in subsequent sessions. Furthermore, there may not be any subsequent sessions if the first session is mishandled. Therefore, the thrust of the first session is to establish a constructive therapeutic imprint that will serve as a dependable basis for future therapeutic developments. The following initial evaluation procedure has been found to be fruitful with most patients.

1. The session begins by putting the patient at ease, for example, "Did you have a hard time finding the office?

2. The patient is asked to identify his or her goals in seeking treatment. The therapist verifies that he or she clearly understands the patient's goals.

3. The therapist specifies his or her impressions of the patient and proposes additional therapeutic goals to be addressed during the course of therapy. The therapist also assesses at this time whether the patient is a good candidate for the particular therapeutic approach that the therapist utilizes, and voices the patient's constructive resources that can be marshalled to help in the process of change.

4. The patient has the opportunity at this point to respond to the therapist's impressions and additional goals. Patient and therapist then reach a mutual agreement on the therapeutic goals.

5. The therapist determines and communicates to the patient an estimated number of sessions needed to achieve the agreed-upon therapeutic goals. The number of sessions would vary according to each patient's individual needs.

6. The therapist explains his or her therapeutic perspective in simple terms, including how the patient can participate in specific ways to facilitate treatment within this therapeutic perspective. Office policies are also explained at this time (changes in appointment times, missed sessions, professional fees, vacation schedules, phone calls and emergencies, etc.), and any patient questions or concerns are duly answered.

7. The patient is asked whether he or she feels comfortable with the therapist and can make a commitment to treatment for the estimated number of sessions.

8. The session concludes with an attempt to decode the patient's emotional and cognitive impression of his or her interaction with the therapist: "What is your overall impression about this session?" "I wonder what you will feel when you leave this room?"

Self-Determination

The last item under the rubric of attitude redirection is the concept of self-determination. The launching of a private practice casts the clinician against the horizon of his or her possibilities. Private practice represents a context within which the clinician becomes acutely aware of both limitations and talents. The freedom offered by the private practice setting can be dizzying, and the risks can trigger more than a fleeting feeling of insecurity. Given such a terrain, self-determination requires that the clinician identify his or her ultimate concerns, and rely mostly on personal resources to achieve desired goals. Rescuer fantasies tend to fall short at this life juncture. The author's favorite metaphor for this theme is the statement, "It is now time to get your own cow." However, it is relieving and refreshing to know that every individual has numerous personal resources of which he or she is not consciously aware.

ATTITUDE REDIRECTION PERSONAL CHECKLIST

Once the structural foundations for launching a private practice have been clearly demarcated, it might be useful for the reader to anchor this structure at a personal level. Table 5 presents an Attitude Redirection Personal Checklist. The reader is invited to rate himself or herself on each of the attitude redirection dimensions presented on a scale from 1 to 5: 1—unsatisfactory, 2—improvement needed, 3—satisfactory, 4—good, 5—excellent. This self-rating process can be repeated six months later, one year later, and two years later. The table also includes a personal commentary section for the reader to specifically note what he or she needs to do more of or less of with respect to each of the attitude redirection dimensions.

CONCLUSION

This chapter has presented a blueprint for launching a private practice based on two foundations: operational structure and attitude redirection. In the author's perspective, these two elements are intimately intertwined in the quest for establishing a productive private practice — attitude redirection is insufficient without operational structure, and vice versa. The only remaining factor needed to make this equation potent is action.

There is a Cherokee story about a young warrior who wants to challenge the authority of the tribe's elder. He captures a bird and hides it between the palms of his hands. His strategy is to ask the elder if the bird is dead or alive. If the elder answers that the bird is alive, the warrior's plan is to suffocate it; if the answer is that the bird is dead, then the warrior will let it live. Thus, the elder is disproved in either case. The warrior goes to the elder with his

Table 5. Attitude Redirection Personal Checklist

Attitude Redirection Dimension	*Self Rating* 5=Excellent, 4=Good, 3=Satisfactory, 2=Improvement Needed, 1=Unsatisfactory					
	Initial Date____	6 Months Later. Date____	1 Year Later. Date ____	2 Years Later. Date____	Need to Do More of	Need to Do Less Of
Operational Factors						
Specialty areas and professional training						
Going beyond the adacemic stance						
Developing a new personal outlook						
Adopting a humorous perspective						
Educating patients about psychotherapy						
Developing a working alliance with patients						
The first session						
Self-determination						

hands cupped over the bird and asks: "Old man, is the bird dead or alive?" The old sage smiles compassionately as he replies: "The bird, my son, is in your hands."

REFERENCES

Fry, W.F., Jr., & Salameh, W.A. (Eds.) (1987). *Handbook of humor and psychotherapy: Advances in the clinical use of humor.* Sarasota, Fla.: Professional Resource Exchange, Inc.

Halgin, R.P., & Weaver, D.D. (1986). Salient beliefs about obtaining psychotherapy. *Psychotherapy in Private Practice, 4,* 23–31.

Salameh, W.A. (1986). The effective use of humor in psychotherapy. In *Innovations in clinical practice: A source book* (Vol. 5), pp. 157–175. P.A. Keller & L.G. Ritt (Eds.), Sarasota, Fla.: Professional Resource Exchange, Inc.

Salameh, W.A. (1987). Humor as a form of indirect hypnotic communication. In *Hypnotic and strategic interventions: Principles and practice,* pp. 133–188. M. Yapko (Ed.), New York: Irvington.

Salameh, W.A. (In press). The hidden dimension—developing your emotional intelligence.

CHAPTER
7

OFFICE DESIGN

Lois Brien, Ph.D.
National University, San Diego, CA

A n architect who specialized in designing office space for psychotherapists was contracted by a psychiatrist to plan and execute a house with
an office according to prescription. When it was finished, the architect took
his 24-year-old daughter to see the office and asked her, "What do you think
this man does?" She promptly replied, "He's a judge!" Truly, the professional
office is a reflection of both the occupant and the occupation.

Designers and architects know that offices reflect the user and that they
can convey certain personality characteristics, such as your sense of humor
and whether you are organized or creative or simply sloppy, as well as other
strengths and weaknesses. People tend to make their offices places where they
can be themselves. Sheldon Roth (1987), a psychiatrist, points out that given
the stressful nature of the process of conducting psychotherapy, the therapist
should make sure that the office setting maximizes his or her sense of comfort and security. He further states: "The office is a window on the person
of the therapist—a place where the client can know something about the
therapist instead of only the other way around."

Your office not only tells about you, but it acts upon you and your clients.
Its colors, appointments, and general ambience can shape what occurs there.
Given the possibility of so much interaction between office design and persons using the offices, not enough analysis of the influence of the office has
been attempted. As Ryan (1979) put it, "We treat space somewhat as we treat
sex; it is there but we do not talk about it."

A review of the literature turns up only a few relevant works. Amira and
Abramowitz (1979) studied 82 undergraduates viewing simulated therapy
segments under two conditions of contextual formality. Varying the tradi-
tionalism of the therapist's attire and office was not found to have an effect
on how the students viewed their experience (including how they viewed the
therapist's performance) in two interview analogues, although there was a
trend toward subjects' attitudes being more positive when the therapist was
casually dressed in the formal room, and viewing the therapist as more competent when the interview took place in the more formal room.

Bloom et al. (1977) and Trautt view the physical environment as one of
four factors contributing to psychotherapeutic effects, and so they studied the
interaction of gender pairing and office decor and their effects on therapist
credibility. There was demonstrated interaction between office decor and

therapist gender and the perception of therapist credibility. That is, subjects consistently perceived a female therapist in the traditional professional office as more credible and a male therapist in the "humanistic" (less formal) office as more credible. The authors conclude that:

> It may be possible to utilize environmental factors to enhance a therapist's credibility. For male therapists this might be accomplished in an environment that suggests warmth, sensitivity, and caring. Factors that help create such an environment are therapist sitting fairly close to the client, absence of a desk between therapist and client, and poignant sayings on the wall. For female therapists, competence may be potentiated by an office environment that suggests professional quality, training, and experience.

Wittington (1985) surveyed her past clients who had been treated in their homes as opposed to an office setting. She states that there appear to be no differences in length and patterns of service between office and house practice. Her bias in the direction of home service, however, may have influenced her conclusions.

There is an entire literature on color research that was only cursorily considered for this discussion, mainly from the fields of architecture (Kunishima & Yanase, 1985) and retailing (Bellizzi et al., 1983). Generally, colors seem to interact with affect in some ways. Colors attract shoppers differently, and activity levels and brightness of colors may be related. Aaronson (1971) found the color red to be the most activating, with blue being the most tranquilizing. Purple, which is a mixture of red and blue, fell somewhere in between. Activity seems also to be greatly affected by brightness, with higher levels of activity associated with brighter colors.

The psychoanalytic view of the iconography of the analyst's office is presented by Kurtz (1986), who construes it to be a purely creative act that gives "expression to the most primitive elements in [the analyst's] personality." He describes Freud's office as a "virtual museum," with walls covered with all types of framed artwork and surfaces literally covered with memorabilia. As Kurtz put it, "The room was a sensory plenum," and he partly explains that, by means of the museum, Freud gathered and displayed the lost past, a past that was otherwise inaccessible. But perhaps more importantly, he saw Freud's relationship to his room as the embodiment of the symbiotic relationship as its "patterned totality included the occupant himself." Further, he contrasted the *process* of psychotherapy with the *frame* of psychotherapy. The former was the therapeutic alliance, which is made with the healthiest part of the patient, and the latter (the frame or office space) is the alliance established with the most psychotic or symbiotic part of the patient's personality. The frame or space provides for the necessary regression.

Moses (1985) commented on Milton M. Berger's offices as she waited to interview him for an article, noting that waiting rooms always reflect some aspect of their owners, even those that attempt complete neutrality. She describes Dr. Berger's room as reflecting "the central quality of the man" and as exuding

> a quiet comfortable clutter. The walls are filled with lithographs, posters and photographs. . . .Cartoons line the side of one wall. The room

itself is filled with furniture, stacks of magazines and videotapes. There is a large vase with dried flowers and a few scattered jade plants. The room is filled almost to overflow, and seated there, I felt that I was about to become acquainted with a man who fills every moment of his day as well.

And then,

the office seems like a much larger version of the waiting room. It brims over with books, equipment, videotapes, papers and furniture. It is a large and inviting room. . . .The rooms had conveyed what I was to experience over and over again — a sense of urgency and an energy that could hardly be contained.

TYPE OF OFFICE SETTING

The first choice to be made is what sort of office setting one wants. Should the offices be in a modern multistory steel and glass commercial building or in an old, one-story house with small garden areas and trees, or should one seek some combination of the two? One almost needs to have been a patient to appreciate the importance of office setting and design. All possible settings have their advantages and disadvantages and all convey somewhat different messages to the client. What is often essential in psychotherapy is the provision of an environment within which the client may feel safe enough to regress. Blanck and Blanck (1986) talk about providing a "benign environment." Sometimes the individual office supports regression but the larger setting, the building, does not. In the case of the slick, commercial-looking building, a client reported that he became aware of wanting to look "normal" when he came out of the office into the hallway and elevator areas, not weepy and red-eyed. He found that he pulled himself together, interrupting the mood of the just-finished therapy hour. Such abrupt finishing may not further therapeutic aims. Gestalt therapists, in particular, have long been aware of this need for time at the end of a piece of work for its integration. Even the anticipation of leaving the therapy office and entering the surrounding environment may affect the in-office therapy. One of the author's clients would start to become anxious and depressed about halfway through each session as he became aware of the time getting shorter before he had to leave. Further, clients are often heard to complain of the emotional problems they have in carrying on practical affairs directly after a therapy session. An environment that can provide the most postsession quiet and alone time may function best to facilitate integration of the work done in that session.

Some therapists find that the appearance of affluence which the setting suggests may be important in terms of therapist credibility. This, in turn, may facilitate within the client the development of feelings of hope and trust in the therapist, as well as making him or her more willing to pay the fees — "With an office as well appointed as this, the therapist must be worth it."

In addition, one setting may be preferred over another depending upon the therapeutic discipline with which one is allied. Humanistic therapists often gravitate toward homey, informal environments, whereas analytical therapists may prefer more neutral surroundings. The former offices are more likely to have family pictures and personal collectibles, and the latter to have only degrees or licenses displayed, to be decorated in subdued colors, and to be sparsely furnished. It may not be only that one setting is more appealing to one kind of therapist, but different aspects of the therapist may be acted out in the different environments. For example, a therapist may be more in touch with his or her less rigid personality characteristics in an informal office setting. Conversely, the more formal or neutral setting might bring out a therapist's more conservative or austere side. What is probably most germane, however, is the idea of congruence. That is, the office setting should support whatever message the therapist is sending to the client. As Osmond (1975) stated, "The physical setting should show congruence with what the persons are trying to achieve there." One must pay attention to whether the physical space facilitates or inhibits the growth experience for the client.

It is often an advantage to occupy a building used only or primarily by therapists, as angry monologues or loud crying might be upsetting to nonprofessional tenants. Most inappropriate neighbors would be restaurants or shops. The author once had an office on a second floor, overlooking a garden cafe. During one session, a client repeatedly yelled "Leave me alone!" as she confronted her mother in fantasy. Soon there was a knock on the door—a police officer. A customer in the cafe had assumed that someone was in trouble up there.

Even the outside view from the windows must be considered as a variable in therapy. The setting should definitely convey that the therapist and client are alone, have complete privacy, and are not distracted by the outside environment (Jacobs, 1987). Imagine looking out on a busy street intersection, a children's playground, or an auto repair shop—all are distracting visually as well as auditorially. A colleague of mine told of having to stop talking for about one minute in the middle of several of her sessions each day to allow a fast train to go by—the train's passing shook the building and made a deafening noise.

DESIGN OF SEPARATE ROOMS

After the building has been chosen, there are usually three areas of the office to be designed for the practice of psychotherapy: the office for individual or couples work, the room for families or groups, and the waiting room. Sometimes there are additional spaces, such as a playroom or area for children, a kitchen for coffee and snacks, and a room or area for a receptionist or secretary. Each of these spaces has its special considerations.

The individual office should be large enough so that the client and therapist do not have to sit knee to knee. Therapist–client physical distance is an important variable and clients need to have the freedom to choose this distance and to alter it as their needs change. Ryan (1979) cites some literature pertinent to distance as it is related to personality and gender. In general, the more dependent and submissive patients prefer a greater distance from the therapist, whereas more self-assured patients prefer a middle distance.

The furniture should include a couch for lying on or for two people to sit together on, and chairs, probably of the swivel type. This allows for the observation of action between individuals and couples.

· The height of the chairs and couches, including the therapist's chair, is also an important variable. A message about status may be conveyed by, for instance, the client's seat being lower than the therapist's. Not to be overlooked is the fact that chairs are often too high to be sat in comfortably, especially by women. It seems that most furniture is designed to fit the average male height. In my present office, I have scaled all of the furniture down to 15 inches (for chairs) and 25 inches (for tables or desks) from the floor. This allows for all people, regardless of height, to sit with their feet comfortably on the floor. All of the furniture, however, is adjustable for height and can be easily raised if necessary.

Tables or desks should not be placed between the therapist and clients as this usually represents distancing and a barrier to empathy. O'Hara (1987) recalls a comment by Ronald Laing at a conference to the effect that Carl Rogers caused a revolution in psychology by coming out from behind his desk and sitting face to face with his clients, in identical chairs, in his living room!

Colors should be commensurate with the effects desired, and wall decor and art objects or collectibles should be considered in terms of what messages the therapist wants to convey to the client. As previously discussed, colors appear to influence mood. If you are trying for a very neutral environment, then pale colors that are cool, such as blue and green, might be used. But if you work in a cognitive way with depressives, for instance, you may want to consider more activating colors such as stronger hues or red.

What goes on the walls or shelves should be pleasing to look at but not too personal. Pictures of family should be avoided as they may invoke painful transference episodes so common to the borderline patient. Pictures of well-known therapist/mentors can be accommodated by most patients. One's major degrees and licenses should also be displayed. I will never forget a colleague's office that I rented temporarily. All four walls were literally covered with framed licenses, degrees, awards, professional memberships, short courses, honors from service clubs, board memberships, and certificates of attendance at various functions. What was instantly communicated to me was this person's tremendous self-absorption! As a client, I believe I would have felt quite unnoticed.

Of course, there is the ubiquitous box of tissues and a well-placed clock so that you do not need to glance furtively at your watch to see how the hour is progressing.

A word about plants—if your office is not used every day and does not have much direct sunlight, it is probably not a good idea to include live plants in your decor. Nothing looks quite as unesthetic as browning and dry or dropping foliage. Try the new silk plants instead; many of them (especially ficus and other green leafy varieties) are very realistic.

Lighting must also be attended to, with strong overhead lighting avoided as it disturbs the regressive possibilities for the client. Also to be avoided is glare from the windows or the hypnotic effect often produced by having to look directly into a Venetian blind or a miniblind; these are distractions.

Ventilation in this room is especially important as the therapist may get sleepy and inattentive in a poorly ventilated space. If there are no windows to open, a ceiling fan can be helpful. You can also keep the air conditioner on fan only.

The acoustics of this room, and all of the rooms, need attention, as clients must feel free to express themselves without the fear of being overheard. Privacy is essential to the establishment of a therapeutic alliance, and this, in turn, is a necessary condition for psychotherapy to proceed and be successful. Also, the issue of confidentiality is an important one in psychotherapy, and intruding noises and voices from the outside do nothing to support this practice. Extra soundproofing can be provided through the use of solid-core doors, extension of interior walls up to the roof of the building (beyond the ceiling), and a device that fits on the bottom of doors that drops down to cover the distance between the bottom of the door and carpet when the door is opened wider than 20 percent. Soundproofing is especially important between offices and the waiting room.

If you are using technical equipment such as video cameras and monitors, such equipment can be built into drawers with cameras wall mounted so that they are unobtrusive and do not impede the primary action between client and therapist.

The group room should have 10 to 12 individual movable chairs; couches are not particularly functional in this setting. Some large floor pillows might be desired to allow for flexibility in seating. All rooms should be fully carpeted for maximum comfort.

The waiting room should have individual chairs only and a table for magazines. The reading material should be appropriate to the therapeutic environment and in good condition and current. Some publishers will provide free subscriptions for office waiting rooms, such as *MS.* magazine and *Psychology Today.* Soft background music can be a mood-setting addition to this environment and can also function to mask any sounds from the offices. Recordings of waves and other nature sounds will function in the same capacity. This room should be quiet so that clients can begin to regress. In such a place, the outside world begins to fade away, preparing the client for the session to come.

Psychoanalytical therapists recognize the difficulty that clients may have upon emerging from the therapy room into the waiting room where they may encounter other patients. Feelings of jealousy, embarrassment, and resentment are common. If it can be provided, a separate exit from the therapy space would be helpful.

A sense often overlooked when planning office space is that of smell. Older spaces may have unpleasant smells ingrained as the result of activities of previous occupants, perhaps from animals or cooking. New spaces may have construction odors. You may spray your rooms with appropriate scents, burn incense, or repaint to overcome such odors. In any event, the odors associated with your office will communicate meanings to your clients.

A special office consideration is whether you will provide coffee, tea, and snacks for clients. Although this practice entails some additional expense and space, it is often experienced by clients as nurturance and could further therapeutic goals. (The author will never forget the mint tea and honey served her in the kitchen after each "rolfing" session!)

If a special space is provided for children's therapy or play, it needs to be set up somewhat differently from the other rooms described. There should be no carpeting, allowing for the making of "messes" with paints and other play materials, especially for children involved in play therapy. The floor can be covered with easily washable vinyl. The room should look as different as possible from the child's home so as to inhibit those behaviors the child expresses at home that are considered troublesome and to facilitate the use of different behaviors in the office.

A general consideration when designing office space is that of parking. Ample parking must be provided for both therapists and clients so that energy is not dissipated needlessly on driving around looking for a place to put one's car. Such provision will also help both therapist and client to hold to their allotted time schedules.

Other aspects of space design that interface with therapeutic functioning are those alluded to by some of the social psychologists. Goffman (1967) discusses how people can be "persuaded" to think or behave in certain ways depending on what may be present in the environment, such as diplomas, books, and bric-a-brac. Kozol (1961) considers the symbolic meanings that surroundings have for the individual in his discussion of the impact, symbolically, on the students of the old and shabby furnishings and acoutrements in Boston's segregated public schools in the 1960s. A supervisee commented on how depressing her work environment was and wondered about the messages being conveyed to her clients. It was a fairly typical mental health outpatient facility furnished with hand-me-down furniture—shabby, unmatched, not color coordinated, and painted off-white or light green. Such a setting informs the client that what is done here is not very important and that the therapist does not consider the client very important either, or more care would be taken to provide a comfortable, attractive environment that would facilitate the therapy process.

Designing the office space is a complex undertaking that both affects and is affected by the type and process of therapy. Choices involve the overall setting (i.e. the building itself), and the design of specific rooms according to their function. With regard to these rooms, one must decide upon the style, type, and placement of furniture; the use of color and wall and incidental decor; the use of plants and music; and questions of lighting, acoustics, and ventilation. All of these variables interact with the person of the therapist and the messages he or she wishes to convey to the client. The therapeutic spaces both act upon and are acted upon by the players involved. Kurtz (1956) says it most impressively:

> Patient and analyst may be said to be allied, in a loose sense, in their mutual creation of a shared space within the analytic situation—comparable to the shared space created by actors and audience in the theatre. . . . The ideal analyst would be a corner capable of molding and remolding itself to fit the shape of each new patient. In actuality, his flexibility is limited, so that some fits are impossible, many are adequate, and a few are nearly perfect.

Certainly, rich research opportunities exist for determining, especially, the relationships among these variables and treatment efficacy and outcomes.

REFERENCES

Aaronson, B.S. (1971). Color Perception and Affect. *American Journal of Clinical Hypnosis, 14 (1),* 38–43.

Amira, S., & Abromowitz, S.J. (1979). Therapeutic Attraction as a Function of Therapist Attire and Office Furnishings. *Journal of Consulting and Clinical Psychology, 47 (1),* 198–200.

Bellizzi, J.A., Crowley, A.E., & Hasty, R.W. (1983). The Effects of Color in Store Design. *Journal of Retailing, 59 (1),* 21–45.

Bloom, L.J., Weigel, P.W., & Trauit, G.M. (Oct. 1977). Therapeutic Factors in Psychotherapy: Effects of Office Decor and Subject-Therapist Sex Pairing on the Perception of Credibility. *Journal of Consulting and Clinical Psychology, 45 (5),* 867–873.

Goffman, E. (1982). *Asylums,* New York: Houghton-Mifflin.

Jacobs, D. (1987). Personal Communication.

Kozol, J. *Death at an Early Age.* New York: Anchorage Books.

Kunishima, M., & Yanase, T. Visual Effects of Wall Colours in Living Rooms. *Ergonomics, June, 28 (6),* 869–882.

Kurtz, S.A. (1986). The Analyst's Space. *Psychoanalytic Review, 73 (1),* 41–55.

Moses, L.N. (1985). Moving His Growing Edge Forward: An Interview with Milton M. Berger, M.D. *Group, 9 (1),* 46–53.

O'Hara, M. (1987). Personal Communication.

Osmond, H. Function as a Basis of Psychiatric Ward Design. *Mental Hospitals, 8,* 23–29.

Roth, S. (1987). *Psychotherapy: The Art of Wooing Nature.* New York: Jason Aronson.

Ryan, W.P. (1979). Therapist's Office As a Treatment Variable. *Psychological Reports, 45,* 671–675.

Whittington, R. (1985). Psychotherapy in the Client's Chosen Environment. *Psychotherapy in Private Practice, 3 (1).* 1–7.

8

OFFICE PERSONNEL AND SERVICE

James V. DeLeo, Ph.D.

There comes a time when most practitioners move beyond doing their own office work and decide to hire help. This decision is usually made with the expectation that the hiring of a person will relieve the practitioner of such routine clerical duties as typing, answering the phone, making appointments, bookkeeping, filing, and billing. In making this decision, the practitioner has moved into the domain of management with its accompanying responsibilities, including the efficient use of (1) people, (2) time, (3) materials, (4) equipment, and (5) money. In fulfilling these responsibilities, the practitioner must develop the management skills of planning, organizing, delegating, training, controlling, motivating, and evaluating. No matter how small or large the practice, these skills are generally considered essential to the management process.

This chapter concerns itself with the management of office personnel and services and so will focus on the application of these skills to this area.

PLANNING

Planning is generally defined as the process whereby we direct our thinking toward achieving an end. Plans are guideposts for action. When properly done, planning forces the practitioner to pause and take an objective look at his or her practice. Planning also forces critical and analytical thinking about resources. Finally, the plan as formulated becomes an orderly statement of goals and procedures, thereby affording an invaluable tool for training and communication. Because planning implies mental formulation, it precedes doing.

With regard to office personnel and service, the practitioner's first task is to plan for the process of recruitment, selection, and evaluation by preparing a position description. The position description is derived from the needs of the practitioner and the office. As such, it states the general and specific tasks to be accomplished along with the appropriate educational, experiential, and skill requirements of the job. The writing of the position description in this way forces the practitioner to examine the nature of the job and to set realistic performance expectations. Once written, the position description can be reviewed by colleagues for issues of integration and clarity. In reviewing the position description, it sometimes becomes obvious that the practitioner's expectations are unrealistic and beyond the scope of any one person. Obviously, it is better to discover this need during the planning stage when something can be done about it. For example, it is not uncommon for a practitioner to realize too late that what is wanted is a receptionist with a warm, ingratiating manner; a highly efficient secretary who can type clinical reports; and a full-charge bookkeeper. During the planning stage of writing the job description, it is possible to identify these needs and prioritize them in considering interested applicants.

The adopted position description can serve as the basis for a wage and salary survey. In a wage and salary survey, the practitioner attempts to ascertain a competitive median salary for the position. Local newspapers, employment agencies, other practitioners, and state employment agencies can be invaluable resources in arriving at a competitive salary range. The median salary generally reflects the going rate for an individual with all the expected competencies. The range allows for flexibility in bringing in people with less than the desired experience or with exceptional skills.

Once completed, the wage and salary survey provides the practitioner with a dollar amount that can be budgeted. This figure, along with the amount allotted for benefits, forms the basis for the annual personnel budget. This budget is reviewed periodically to allow for salary adjustments and/or merit increases. The personnel budget goes beyond the salary paid to employees and includes benefits. Federal and state law provide for mandated benefits as delineated in the Fair Labor and Standards Act. These benefits cover such issues as overtime payment, payment for training, and related provisions. State laws usually provide for issues related to lunch and rest breaks. In view of the complexity of these regulations, it behooves the practitioner to consult a colleague with regard to their application in a specific state.

With the position description adopted and the wage and salary figure determined, the practitioner can plan for the recruitment, selection, hiring, and evaluating parts of the process.

RECRUITMENT

Recruitment ensures that the position is made known to as many people as possible in the applicant pool. This is best accomplished through advertisements in local newspapers, association newsletters, announcements forwarded to local business colleges, and discussions with friends and colleagues. Recruitment and selection procedures are subject to state and federal law concerning equal employment, and every practitioner must become acquainted with the basics of these regulations as they govern employment.

Some practitioners elect to avoid the problems related to the recruitment process (i.e., the placement of advertisements, answering telephone inquiries) and work through an employment agency. Two factors come into play here: (1) the fee to the agency, and (2) the effectiveness of the agency. Before making this decision, and as part of the planning process, the practitioner would do well to contact a number of local agencies.

Many practitioners arrange to have résumés, along with cover letters and salary requirements, forwarded to either a post office box or the office.

Materials are then screened against the position requirements.

In planning for the selection, the practitioner can prepare a checklist of criteria by which to evaluate each candidate, together with a series of questions that are directly relevant to the position description. Some practitioners make the position description available to the applicant in advance of the interview to ensure a focus during the interview. It is generally agreed that references are valuable tools in helping to make the final employment decision. The practitioner should plan to check two of the references provided by the applicant to acquire information concerning the applicant's strengths and limitations with regard to performing the required tasks.

Before the selection interview, some practitioners have the applicant complete a standard employment application. Such applications, which are generally available at office supply stores, serve to amplify an applicant's résumé. The résumé, cover letter, and application form then become part of the applicant file.

At the risk of belaboring the obvious, an employment interview is not a clinical interview. The employment interview is designed to help the practitioner and applicant assess the degree of "fit" between the needs of the office as described in the position description and the skills, experiences, and needs of the applicant. Federal and state law have delineated what can and cannot be asked during an employment interview. Some of these guidelines are evident, but others are not. For example, questions with regard to a person's marital status, age, ethnic origin, or religion are considered irrelevant for most positions and so should not be asked. The *caveat* mentioned above bears repeating: consult a colleague with expertise in this area and review state laws and guidelines.

The offer of a position requires a mutual understanding between the practitioner and the applicant concerning the terms of employment. Some practitioners put the offer of employment in writing, thereby specifying such issues as date employment is to begin, starting salary, benefits, work hours, and duration of probationary period. Although it is assumed that all these issues are discussed during the employment interview, it is good practice to confirm them in writing.

It should be made clear to the applicant that the probationary period is mutual, which means that either the applicant or the practitioner can terminate the relationship without prejudice. This agreement makes it clear that the probationary period (usually three months) is a training time. It is incumbent upon the practitioner to train the applicant carefully in the office practices and procedures. During the first week of employment, it is advisable for the practitioner to meet twice daily with the applicant to go over what needs to be done and how to do it, and to provide feedback concerning work accomplished. At the end of the probationary period, it is important that the practitioner meet with the employee and provide an appraisal of his or her performance. For example, an employee may be rated on punctuality, adherence to office policies and policies, telephone courtesy, cooperation with colleagues, quality and quantity of work, and job knowledge.

An employee appraisal must be based upon an examination of the relationship between the employee's behavior and mutually agreed upon standards of accomplishment. The manner in which an appraisal is conducted is directly related to the practitioner's management style. Thus, the more directive a management style, the more direct is the appraisal. Support and understanding on the part of the practitioner will provide security and recognition for the employee, thereby increasing the likelihood that he or she will experience the situation as a learning conference. As the employee learns and grows into the position, the practitioner can delegate more work.

DELEGATION

Delegation can be defined as the willingness of the practitioner to accept and support the making of decisions and the taking of actions by his or her employees. There are five steps in proper delegation: assigning priorities to jobs, separating personal jobs from delegatable ones, determining who is capable of doing the job, delegating the assignment, and controlling the assignment so as to ensure its execution and completion.

In assigning priorities, the practitioner must consider the relative importance of the tasks and set appropriate deadlines. This is best done in consultation with the employee. This consultation sets the tone for participative management, which increases the employee's commitment to the practice.

"Delegate as much as possible" is the catch phrase. In separating personal jobs from delegatable ones, the practitioner must commit himself or herself to doing only those tasks that require the practitioner's personal attention.

The best way to control the assignment once it is properly delegated is to provide help when necessary, allowing for feedback and clarification. The practitioner must provide a means of accountability through written or oral reports. Upon completion of the assignment, the practitioner should provide for an evaluation, commenting on the work in terms of quality and quantity.

As mentioned at the outset, the practitioner who decides to hire office personnel has made a decision to become a manager. The management skills of planning, organizing, delegating, training, controlling, and evaluating are essential tools. Motivating employees and assisting them to achieve job satisfaction are the final skills discussed in this chapter.

Of the many approaches to improving employee motivation, two will be considered here: goal setting and job design.

GOAL SETTING

In goal setting, the practitioner assigns specific, challenging goals and encourages the employee to do his or her best. Simple as such a procedure sounds, it is rarely followed in small office situations. Research done by Latham and Locke (1979) and Garland (1982) confirm the dramatic results produced by this technique. In studying goal levels and task performance, Garland hired students to perform a creative task—listing as many objects as they could that could be described by a given adjective. Before setting goals, participants listed an average of about 7.5 objects. In one condition in which an easy goal was set, performance dropped to a little more than six objects. In another condition when a more difficult goal of 14 objects was set, performance increased to a little more than eight objects.

JOB DESIGN AND ENRICHMENT

Fredrick Herzberg (1959) developed the idea of job design and job enrichment as a way of motivating people to work effectively. Job design refers to the practice of expanding the content of a job by increasing the number and variety of tasks assigned to a person. Job enrichment refers to giving people not only more tasks, but more tasks at a higher level, allowing them to have greater control over their work.

As the employee progresses, the practitioner is challenged to use these techniques to increase the employee's job satisfaction and level of commitment to the practice and the people served.

So far, the discussion has centered on basic dimensions of a private practice. These dimensions must be reviewed against such factors as the size of the practice: individual, group, or small clinic.

Many individual practices are characterized by a simple functional design in which one or two people perform specialized functions or tasks such as billing and clerical-receptionist activities. In such settings, there is the advantage of routine activities that can be shared by all members of the practice in times of need. In addition, such a design provides for economies of scale and avoids unnecessary duplication. The major problem here is finding one or two people who can combine what are sometimes disparate skills: dealing with figures and dealing with people. Thus the job requirements may become conflictual, causing interpersonal tension and organizational conflict.

As a practice grows in terms of the number of practitioners, the design must change accordingly and a matrix design must be considered. In such a design, a dual system of authority is established. There are private practitioners with authority and responsibility for their particular client load, and there are also office or business managers with authority and responsibility for particular functions, such as billing, marketing, or bookkeeping. The result is that some people have two bosses — the practitioner and the office manager. A key advantage of such a design is the flexible use of human and organizational resources. An apparent disadvantage is the frustration and stress produced by having two bosses and the potential conflict of these two supervisors with each other. Considering, however, that practices must constantly attempt to stretch their financial and human resources, a matrix design is the most viable approach in meeting the needs of clients, practitioners, and staff.

REFERENCES

Garland, H. (1982). Goal levels and task performance: A compelling replication of some compelling results. *Journal of Applied Psychology, 67,* 245–248.

Herzberg, F., Mausner, B., & Snyderman, B. (1959). *The motivation to work.* New York: Wiley.

Latham, G.P., & Locke, E.A. (1979). Goal setting: A motivational technique that works. *Organizational dynamics, 8(2),* 68–80.

9

PLAY THERAPY ROOM: SPACE AND DESIGN

Cecile Dillon, Ph.D.

INTRODUCTION

The design of the physical environment of the play therapy room has an important relationship to the creation of a therapeutic environment. Psychotherapists who employ play techniques when working with children up to the ages of 10 or 12, either individually or in a group situation, usually have access to a play therapy room. However, in contrast to the relatively large volume of literature describing different play techniques, comparatively little has been written about the physical environment where child play therapy takes place.

In the early history of psychoanalysis, child psychotherapy was not performed in any special rooms and so a room especially equipped for play techniques may be the sign of the modern psychotherapy era. In addition, different factors combine to produce a psychotherapeutic environment. Thus, the physical environment of the play therapy room may be discussed in combination with other factors that produce the psychotherapeutic environment — such as the personality, training, experience, and theoretical orientation of the therapist. Further, the type of patients to be treated and their presenting problems have an effect on the setting in which psychotherapy takes place. Since the psychotherapeutic environment is a very complex phenomenon, invariably derived from a number of factors that directly and indirectly influence each other, it may be difficult to isolate and discuss only the physical environment without commenting on these other factors.

This chapter will deal with a number of concerns that the psychotherapist, office manager, or administrator might have and some basic facts one needs to know when confronted with the task of setting up a new play therapy room.

THE SETTING FOR PLAY THERAPY

If play is to be utilized effectively in psychotherapy, a setting that allows for reasonable expression and communication through play is necessary, although the real need may vary with the age and personality of the child requiring the treatment. The organization of the setting and the selection of its play materials can be as individual and resourceful as the personality of the psychotherapist. A general rule of thumb is that the setting for play therapy will reflect the priorities of the therapist who is using the setting as well as his or her patients.

Therapists who utilize play techniques in their work with prelatency and early-latency children either should have a separate room set up for play therapy or have play materials available in the regular consultation room. Further, when consultation with a child takes place in a school, day-care center, hospital, or any other facility where there is no particular space assigned for play therapy, the therapist can carry the playroom, as some affectionately refer to the play therapy room, in a bag or a suitcase.

Play Therapy Room Design and Furniture

When the therapist moves into a new office, it is necessary to design the office to fit the therapist's needs for the practice of psychotherapy. This may involve remodeling existing space or planning the arrangement of newly constructed space. After the spaces for a waiting room and consultation room have been established, the play therapy room often is created from what is left. The therapist who does individual psychotherapy can use a space as small as eight feet by eight feet for the play therapy room as long as the door opens outward. On the other hand, dimensions exceeding 144 square feet may be a warning that the space is not being used effectively. If possible, the room should have a window.

Since psychotherapy cannot be conducted in a space where confidentiality is not secured, control of sound from other rooms is an important aspect of the design. Also, background music often provided in offices can be distracting in a play therapy room and it should be disconnected.

Before deciding on covering for floor and walls, furniture, and so forth, the therapist should examine the color schemes that will be used throughout the office. Walls painted in bright, cheerful colors are the most economical and easiest to keep clean. If the therapist's practice requires that floor covering in the play therapy room be different from the rest of the office, several options are available. Industrial carpeting, which is glued to the floor, can stand up to tremendous amounts of wear and tear and can easily be cleaned. Vinyl and tile floors are other options. An ideal setting would include a sink with hot and cold running water; however, the plumbing cost for this can be eliminated by using bottled water.

Furniture in the play therapy room needs to be comfortable and simple. At least two chairs, one for the therapist and one for the child, and a child-size activity table seem to be all that is required. Shelves with play materials should be easily accessible so children can choose material that they want by themselves. A sandbox and wooden workbench may also be desirable. Also, a file cabinet with a lock and a small desk with a chair can be included if there is a need and space allows.

In a private practice, effective utilization of space may be very crucial, and so it is not unusual for the room set aside for play to be limited in size. Azarnoff and Flegall (1975) have made the following suggestions that may be helpful in creating more space in the play therapy room.

1. Remove all furniture except for one comfortable chair.
2. Utilize wall shelves to display play materials, leaving space below for chairs and play activities.
3. Install a wall table (16 inches by 20 inches) made of 1-inch-thick, easy-to-clean Formica with heavy-duty spring hinges. Snap it open when needed for board games, writing, painting, and so forth. When not in use it is folded down, flush to the wall for storage without using floor space.
4. Attach a painting easel with the bottom on a hinge to the wall so that a chair can be brought to it when in use.

If the room affords plenty of space, these space savers still may be used, but many of the following suggestions can also be implemented.

1. Establish centers of interest, such as building materials or sand boxes, to give the child a wider selection of play areas.
2. Provide an activity table for those children who need structural play or who want to produce something.
3. Design a sink and work counter at a child's elbow level for such activities as pasting, clay work, and painting.
4. Use floor covering that can be easily washed or vacuumed, but is warm enough to sit or lie down upon.
5. Design an observation room, to enable the supervising staff, consultant on the case, or even parents to observe the session without disturbing the child.
6. Establish a storage space where drawings or pictures of children's work can be saved. Some therapists compile a photo album of a child's work for their own reference.

Play Space In The Consulting Room

The therapist may prefer to set up the play area in the regular consulting room. The reason for choosing to do so can be as simple as a preference to work with children and parents together in the same room or the fact that the therapist is working with children too old for the play therapy room but not completely ready for talk therapy. Also, when office space is limited, a separate play therapy room may not be an option.

The consulting room should be large enough to accommodate a setting for necessary play materials and an area suitable for their use. Usually, the consulting room would be a rectangular room with a ratio of 4:3 between the long wall and short wall, although a square room or a somewhat longer room may also be functional. When the therapist has only one consulting room with a variety of furniture, including a desk, file cabinet, chair, and play materials, then a space 12 feet by 20 feet to 16 feet by 16 feet may be adequate. Great care will have to be taken to indicate the boundaries of various parts of the room by use of rugs, room dividers, furniture groupings, and so on. If rugs are being used, it is important that they lie flat to prevent any possible hazard for the therapist and the patients. Office equipment, such as computer, typewriter, dictation equipment, and calculators, should be protected, if not from the patient's view, then at least from the patient's reach. This may be accomplished by having a folding desk or a built-in closet. Play materials could be available as needed from a cabinet, shelves, or a cart on wheels. A storage space should be available when the cart with play items is not in use.

SELECTION OF PLAY MATERIALS

It is the therapist's responsibility to evaluate the play material before it is introduced into the play therapy room. Therefore, the therapist must become familiar with different types of play materials as well as knowledgeable regarding types of behavior and feelings each material tends to elicit from children. A review of the literature provides us with some general guidelines regarding the selection of play materials. Nelson (1966) suggests three types that should be considered: (1) materials that may be used in a number of ways, such as clay and paints; (2) materials that encourage communication, such as a toy telephone; and (3) materials that elicit the expression of aggression, such as toy guns. Whereas Ginott (1961) recommends that play material should (1) assist in the establishment of rapport with the child, (2) encourage catharsis, (3) enhance the opportunity for insight, (4) allow for reality testing; and (5) provide for sublimation, Gumaer (1984) simply stresses that play material should be safe, durable, and inexpensive.

Regardless of a therapist's theoretical orientation, different play materials should be chosen for their ability to convey children's communication. Play materials, in and by themselves, are not sufficient to produce a therapeutic effect. However, the child psychotherapist may find such materials especially helpful with youngsters who find it difficult accurately to express their thoughts and feelings in words, but who can do so in a play therapy setting, where they are encouraged to play with dolls, blocks, clay, paints, and the like. In a distant and somewhat indirect way, play materials can provide the child with a way to express feelings, concerns, and interests. For example, dolls, small animals, and puppets can evoke issues concerning the child's family. The child may express feelings and concerns to the point of imitating the words and tone of voice in which she or he has been addressed, information the child might not have been able to communicate without the use of play items.

The therapist's theoretical approach to play therapy will determine what emphasis will be placed on certain play materials. For example, if the therapist is aiming for regressive play, the physical setting needs to be conducive to such play. The presence of such items as finger paints, clay, and water will encourage the child to engage in regressive play. On the other hand, according to Klein (1975), toys suitable for the psychoanalytic play technique include mainly small-size items, such as wooden men and women, cars, trains, airplanes, animals, houses with fences, paper, scissors, knife, glue, string, and paints. The number of toys and their variety will enable the child to express a wide range of fantasies and experiences.

Other important considerations in the selection of materials for the play therapy room are the developmental level of the children in treatment and the potential of play materials to facilitate their growth. According to Carek (1972), a therapist needs to make available play materials that will enhance attainment of the therapist's particular goal in the therapy of children treated. For example, play materials like wet and dry sand lend themselves to more regressive types of play whereas materials like puppets, dolls with a house and furnishings, cars, and so forth enhance the child's need for self-expression. For the times when it is necessary to get into more ocmpetitive games between the child and the therapist, a variety of board games, checkers, or cards may be more appropriate.

Play therapists tend to prefer simple play media to more complex ones for a number of reasons. First, the more basic the play material is, the more the child will be able to project upon it. In this way, play material can encourage the creative use of imagination and fantasy, which in turn elicit the child's view of self, family, and his or her environment. A second reason for wanting simple play materials is a practical one. Most play therapy sessions, especially ones in a private practice, are limited in time and space. While it is possible in ongoing play therapy to work on a project that may extend over weeks, or even months, such play is not possible in other contexts, such as in an assessment session or when play materials need to be available for other patients. Further, simple play materials can be easily used by children of different emotional and chronological development with little or no instruction.

In addition, psychotherapists should use materials that are capable of providing long-lasting service in the play therapy room. For example, the dollhouse should be made of natural hard wood with removable and variable partitions and should be furnished with solid wooden furniture that, when tossed around, will not break. The doll family should be as unbreakable as possible, outfitted with removable clothes, and able to move and sit.

Under special circumstances, as when a sibling is born or a child will be going to the hospital or seems to be experiencing a life transition (such as a move to a new city, the parents' divorce or a parent's remarriage, a death in the family, or sexual molestation), materials that may help the child deal with the situation may be included in the play therapy room. For the sexually abused child, anatomically correct dolls might be supplied. A doll family with a new baby can be available for the displaced sibling. For the child undergoing surgery, the therapist can offer materials to play "doctor" and "hospital." Two different dollhouses with at least two sets of families seem to be appropriate for children dealing with issues related to divorce and the remarriage of one or both parents. The therapist, through use of materials guaranteed to elicit some focused responses, may confront the child with life situations that the child has to face while providing the child with the support necessary for release, mastery, and a sense of fulfillment.

The capacity for distribution and the management of cleanup are also important criteria in selecting play materials. When planning a play area, the amount of space available has to be taken into account, as well as the accessibility of water, soap, and other cleaning resources. Time also can become an important factor when selecting play materials. Some materials require more time for preparation and cleanup than is allowed for the activity itself. It appears that drawing is one of the most productive media as it is easily accessed, is easy to use, and is easy to clean up.

Since not all therapists have unlimited budgets for play materials or work in settings most advantageous for play therapy, it is often necessary to find a compromise between ideal materials and those that are feasible within realistic constraints. It should be stressed that it is the therapeutic experience rather than the play materials that assists children toward therapeutic growth and change. Therefore, any item that is interesting to the child and can enhance the therapeutic interaction between the therapist and the child can be a valuable addition to the play equipment.

AVAILABLE PLAY MATERIALS

When the therapist must be highly selective about what materials to use, it is necessary to be aware of the various possibilities in order to make the best possible choices. It is helpful for a therapist to receive catalogs from commercial distributors on a regular basis in order to keep up with new developments in play materials. Considering the great number of play materials currently available for furnishing the play therapy room, they can be broken down into seven major categories.

Pretend Play Materials

Play with dolls, a dollhouse including furnishings, animals, puppets, and so forth is a medium that allows the child to play and talk out conflicted issues related to the child's family, roles in the family, unfulfilled dependency needs, and so on. By staging "a pretend family," the child plays out personal feelings and attitudes toward family members. The wooden dollhouse in the play therapy room should be ready to be furnished and decorated. The furniture, also preferably made of wood, should be scaled to fit the house and should resemble everyday furniture in a kitchen, bathroom, bedroom, child's room, living room, and dining room. The doll family should include mother, father, brother, sister, baby, and grandparents to allow the child to deal with as many family figures as possible.

A large wooden box (29½ by 20½ inches, approximately) filled with dry or wet sand placed on a sturdy stand (31½ inches high) provides the child with another setting in which to play with dolls, animals, cars, trucks, airplanes, and the like. Sand can be snow, rain, water, or earth where items can disappear or be buried. Sand also can be thrown out or molded into hills, meadows, rivers, and lakes. It can be a setting for a war where toy soldiers get killed or a background for a friendly farmhouse. The child's imagination is the limit to the use of the sand box with additional play items.

Pretend work may include work with puppets. Hand or finger puppets should include all possible family members, as well as animal characters with large movable mouths for easy animation, such as dragons, lions, ducks, rabbits, dogs, frogs, and skunks. Here, again, due to the anonymity of the puppets, the child can relax and deal with the complex problems of family relationships.

Art Materials

The therapist should be familiar not only with the many types of art materials available, but also with the particular characteristics of each and with the appropriate tools and surfaces. A sufficient nontoxic variety of paints, colors, sizes and types of paper, clay, felt-tip pens, pencils, and the like should be provided for the child. It is important to realize that children lacking fine motor coordination may experience frustration in drawing or in painting with brushes. However, they can enjoy crayons and finger paints. "Finger crayons," which are very easy to hold and simple to manipulate, are nonsmear and come in many bright colors.

Other drawing materials often found in play therapy rooms include soft, hard, colored, and charcoal pencils, as well as a variety of pens, from scented, erasable ballpoint to felt-tip. Also, many different kinds of ink and watercolor markers are now available for drawing activities.

Painting materials are also diversified. Tempera may be found in blocks, liquid, and powder form. Finger paints can be created in different textures, using a variety of available bases, such as soap flakes or liquid detergent. There is also the commercially prepared variety in moist, foam, or powder form ready to use either with fingers or brush. Finally, there are more expensive paints such as oils and acrylics that are available in tubes or as liquids.

Surfaces on which children can draw or paint can be papers of various weights, textures, colors, and sizes; different kinds of cardboards; canvases; masonite; and wood.

In addition to drawing and painting materials, play therapy rooms often are equipped with modeling materials, the most common of which is clay. There are many kinds of clays, from those that are fired in a kiln to those designed to be baked in a kitchen oven or air-dried. Further, it is also necessary to know about clay with a water base, which hardens, as well as about oil-base clay, which does not become hard and is available in a variety of colors and degrees of pliability. Clay may be used successfully with children in a number of ways. The child can mold it into different objects of anger by hand or can use sculpting tools, a rolling pin, and shape cutters. Then these objects can be thrown away, cut, stabbed, or pounded on. Clay can also be used to create images of love, such as a heart or a breast.

A play therapy room supplied with art materials should also have an easel. An easel may either be portable, for use on a desk, a table top, or the floor, or be a full-size double adjustable one with panels that double as a chalkboard. A plastic tray, with washable surface and raised edges, helps keep mess to a minimum, as does a clean vinyl paint smock that protects clothing.

Building Materials

When psychotherapy starts to deal with integrative issues, the child begins to organize motor and mental fields into constructive patterns. It is not unusual for the child to turn to materials like blocks, puzzles, string, glue, or tape to tell the therapist how things are "put together," or what may get lost or left behind. A number of materials can be used for this purpose, from stiff paper to wire, yarn, and wood. Tools that may be necessary are scissors, different kinds of dull knives, a stapler, string, rubber bands, clips, and adhesive materials. Also, a great variety of blocks may be available from light, fiberboard building blocks to brightly colored magnetic ones that can be assembled in an infinite number of ways. Nesting items are also valuable for this purpose.

Games

According to Berlin (1986), the therapist may find it necessary to use games in the play therapy room to establish therapeutic contact with the child who grew up in an environment that stressed action rather than verbal communication. A number of structured games, such as "Life," "Social Security," "Ungame," and Gardner's "Talking, Feeling, Doing Game," have been developed to make the expression of thoughts and feelings easier. For the times when a child is working on competitive issues, such games as checkers, chess, "Aggravation," and tic-tac-toe seem to be more appropriate to allow the child to experience the rules and feelings of fair or unfair play.

Materials For Bibliotherapy

In general, using children's literature in psychotherapy involves selecting materials or activities that employ written (books, journals, magazines, etc.) or spoken (films, film strips, audiotapes, videotapes, etc.) words to enhance the therapeutic process. At an appropriate time, the therapist suggests the use of bibliotherapy materials to the child. When employing bibliotherapy, it is extremely important to be aware of both the child's personal characteristics, such as age, sex, problem issues, and reading interest and ability, and comprehension and literature characteristics, such as length, plot, and reading level. The words can be provided by the therapist or by the child. When the child provides the words, the story can be told to the therapist or written down. For children who cannot write effectively, or for the times when words will be recorded, a tape recorder or video recorder can be used. Also, the child can dictate his or her material to the therapist.

Most questions regarding how bibliotherapy material should be used and when it should be introduced still remain unanswered. However, a rule of thumb is that a child should have access to a world of children's literature in a play therapy room. Children often lack the necessary verbal skills to express their thoughts and feelings accurately. In addition, they may be so traumatized that they are unable to discuss their problems directly. In such cases, recorded materials about sex, drugs, crime, death, divorce, remarriage, and so forth may be less intrusive than the spoken words. Information in all these areas has gradually become a part of the mainstream of children's literature, and today's children are more knowledgeable about those matters than any previous generations. Pardeck and Pardeck (1984) offer a wide list of books available for bibliotherapy.

Music Materials

Music is a nonthreatening medium through which feelings can be experienced as well as expressed. Depending on the therapist's background, exposure to music, and experience, music can be used as a supplement to words. A rhythm band consisting of a tambourine, a pair of brass cymbals, triangles with strikers, jingle clog, and drum set, along with xylo-bells, keyboard, cassette, and record collection of traditional children's songs for listening or singing along, can be helpful in bringing the world of music into the play therapy room.

Audio And Video Recording Equipment

During the past decade, the lower cost and increased availability of recording equipment have resulted in its greater use in play therapy rooms. The basic audio and video media may include such equipment as cassette player and recorder, videotape recorder, several different types of microphones, polaroid camera, lamps and lights, and a monitor or television set. Although audio and video media are nothing more than advanced technology, and as such cannot replace the therapist, they can be a valuable therapeutic adjunct in the hands of any therapist.

Heilveil (1983) points out that there are several ways to incorporate audio and video equipment into child psychotherapy. First, the equipment can be used as a standard feedback technique, whereby a portion of or an entire therapeutic session is played back to the child. Gardner (1975), who uses audio and video recorders in connection with his mutual storytelling technique, recommends to his patients that they record the whole therapy hour and listen or view the tape between sessions. This practice, Gardner explains, reinforces therapeutic messages and deepens the intensity of the therapeutic experience. Further, Gardner views recording media advantageously as he finds it to be free from the distracting stimuli built into more traditional play materials, such as dolls and puppets, around which stories are told in child psychotherapy. Although Gardner uses videotape recordings with all of his patients, current research regarding the benefits of videotape feedback for children across diagnostic categories is not available.

A second strategy for incorporating audio and video equipment may be to use videotaped models to help the child to learn more adaptive behaviors. Understanding the child's level of cognitive and emotional development may be crucial in determining whether or not videotape usage could benefit the child by advancing the child's development. Third, a video camera and recorder may be used as advanced technological toys in the play therapy room, giving the child an opportunity to experience feelings of being in control when trying to direct and produce projects of his or her interest. Finally, video games, besides providing great exercise for improving the child's eye-hand coordination, can also be used successfully in place of the more traditional competitive board games. It goes without saying that the use of audio and video equipment communicates to the child that the therapist is actively involved in staying in touch with modern times and new developments.

Although it may be obvious, it is important to point out that all recording equipment needs to be completely visible to the child. Usually a child coming into the play therapy room will notice equipment and will question its purpose within the first few sessions. Any covert use of recording equipment may lead to distrust and destroy the accomplishments of psychotherapy. Furthermore, before recording equipment is used with the child, it will be necessary to obtain permission from the child's parent or guardian. Both the child and the parent should be told how tapes made during the therapy sessions will be used. Usually, verbal permission is sufficient in a private office setting as long as the child and the parent are assured that the recorded tape will not be shown to anyone else. When the recorded tapes are made for teaching, research, or demonstration purposes, it is necessary to obtain permission in written form. Finally, it is the therapist's ethical and legal concern for the child's welfare that will decide whether or not taped material should be shown to others even if written permission is on file.

LIMIT SETTING IN THE PLAY THERAPY ROOM

Most therapists agree that certain limits are necessary in the play therapy room and will deal with setting the limits by using methods with which they are most comfortable. Some therapists may curtail verbal activity, especially if it interferes with consultations going on in other rooms, while others may not. However, almost all therapists set limits on different nonverbal behaviors. Ginott and Lebol (1969) point out that for the therapist who has a special room for child psychotherapy, the limits may be as simple as (1) property in the room cannot be destroyed, and (2) anyone in the room cannot be harmed. However, when the therapist uses a regular consultation room with play materials in it, the setting in itself requires a number of limits in order to protect carpeting, furniture, the desk and items in drawers, books, telephone, and so forth.

If the selection of play materials is inappropriate for the child's developmental level, the child may become too excited and overstimulated. Therefore, it is the therapist's responsibility to help the child control himself or herself by limiting the available selection of toys and other play materials and by clearly stating the simple ground rules for behavior in the play therapy room. Cooper and Wanerman (1977) suggest that having two of each type of toy is especially helpful in this situation as the therapist can suggest with words and in action how one might use these materials differently. Allowing the child to "act out" aggressive feelings by breaking and destroying play materials rarely proves therapeutic. Such activity can be overly stimulating in itself and may produce feelings of guilt and fear of retaliation. Furthermore, besides giving the child a nonverbal message that the play therapy room is not "a safe place," it also can be too expensive.

The general goal would be to bring the child for each session into a play therapy room that always looks the same, although to achieve this in practice may be at times difficult. Therefore, certain requirements should be established so that the child and the therapist can easily locate items they want to use. Besides keeping the room in order, it is necessary to keep a constant check on the play materials. The play items are usually reserved for use only in the play therapy room. Most psychotherapists do not allow children to remove any items from the room except for the child's own drawings or paintings, while others prefer to evaluate each case on an individual basis. In addition, the child is not permitted to add any of his or her personal items. Broken items should be fixed or replaced as soon as possible. A child may notice an item, without initially playing with it, only to decide to integrate that item into play at some later time. The fact that items are not available for the child when the child is ready for them will tell the child that the stability of the room equipment is not appreciated and that the individual items are not important.

The psychotherapist has the responsibility to leave the play therapy room clean and orderly so that one child's play does not influence the child who follows. For example, if the child makes a mess and dumps play items everywhere, it is the therapist's job to make sure the room is cleaned. The therapist can either enlist the child's assistance in cleaning up the room, or have the child leave the session a few minutes early and clean up the mess alone. In addition, sand should always be left smooth and free of any play items. All pictures just drawn should be removed from the room and other items produced during the session should be taken apart at the end of each session after the child leaves, so that the room is always the same when the child walks in. Produced items may be saved from one psychotherapy session to the next if the child requests it, and if circumstances allow. When the play therapy room is available for unsupervised play between the scheduled appointments, it is the therapist's responsibility to inspect the room before each psychotherapy session.

Due to the nature of some play materials such as paints and clay, both the child and the therapist should be provided with smocks to protect their clothing. This practice allows the child the freedom to use the materials without worrying about soiling clothing, and also allows the therapist to remain emotionally accepting of the child regardless of the produced mess.

SUMMARY

This chapter is concerned with providing the reader with the wide range of existing possibilities for setting up a physical environment for play psychotherapy—the play therapy room. Material that is discussed applies and is valid regardless of the therapist's theoretical orientation. What emerges from this review is that there are a few simple answers to these complex issues, and that there is a great deal that can be done within the scope of present resources to create a setting that can facilitate therapeutic goals and objectives. When confronted with the task of setting up the play therapy room, every therapist will work around limitations that may include (1) the therapist's theoretical approach to the therapeutic use of play, (2) idiosyncratic tendencies and needs of each child, (3) available space, and (4) budget. However, one of the most important limitations is the therapist's knowledge about what certain play materials can and cannot do and how they relate to the developmental level of each child in terms of difficulty and symbolic meaning. This awareness about play materials has to be gained through substantial personal experience, preferably under the direct supervision of an expert in the area of play psychotherapy.

REFERENCES

Azarnoff, P., & Flegal, S. (1975). *Pediatric play program: Developing a therapeutic play program for children in medical setting.* Springfield, IL: Charles C. Thomas.

Berlin, I.N. (1986). The use of competitive games in play therapy. In C.E. Schaefer and S.E. Reid (Eds.), *Game play: The therapeutic use of childhood games.* New York: John Wiley & Sons.

Carek, D.J. (1972). *Principles of child psychotherapy.* Springfield, IL: Charles C. Thomas.

Cooper, S., & Wanerman, L. (1977). *Children in treatment: A primer for beginning psychotherapists.* New York: Brunner/Mazel.

Gardner, R.A. (1975). *Psychotherapeutic approaches to the resistant child.* New York: Jason Aronson.

Ginott, H.G. (1961). *Group psychotherapy with children.* New York: McGraw-Hill.

Ginott, H.G., & Lebo, D. (1969). Most and least used play therapy limits. In C. Schaefer (Ed.), *The therapeutic use of child's play.* New York: Jason Aronson.

Gumaer, J. (1944). *Counseling and therapy for children.* New York: Free Press.

Heilveil, I. (1983). *Video in mental health practice: An activities handbook.* New York: Springer Publishing Company.

Klein, M. (1975). *The psycho-analysis of children.* London, England: Hogarth Press.

Nelson, R. (1966). Elementary school counseling with unstructured play media. *Personnel and Guidance Journal, 1,* 24–27.

Pardeck, J.A., & Pardeck, J.J. (1984). *Young people with problems: A guide to bibliotherapy.* Westport, CT: Greenwood Press.

Pressman, R.M. (1979). *Private practice: A handbook for the independent mental health practitioner.* New York: Gardner Press.

Robbins, A. (1987). *The artist as therapist.* New York: Human Sciences Press.

APPENDIX A

Checklist for Play Therapy Room Evaluation

Look over the entire room and answer the following questions.

	Not Observed	*Unsatis-factory*	*Satis-factory*
1. Does each selection of play items welcome the child?	___	___	___
2. Does each area (creative, building, etc.) suggest its function by its content and arrangement?	___	___	___
3. Are the items that belong together displayed together?	___	___	___
4. Does the number of play items allow the room to be properly organized?	___	___	___
5. Are there enough play items to allow variety in play?	___	___	___
6. Do windows assure complete privacy?	___	___	___
7. Is the sink accessible to the area where creative play is done?	___	___	___

APPENDIX A

	Not Observed	*Unsatis-factory*	*Satis-factory*
8. Is the child able to reach play equipment easily?	_____	_____	_____
9. Is a safe foot-stepladder available in the room?	_____	_____	_____
10. Are cleaning supplies easily available?	_____	_____	_____
11. Is cleaning up from the unsupervised play handled well?	_____	_____	_____
12. Do more than one therapist use the room and play items?	_____	_____	_____
13. Is maintenance of the room and play items handled well?	_____	_____	_____
14. Are smocks available for the child and the therapist?	_____	_____	_____

APPENDIX B

Basic Rules Regarding The Play Materials

The following rules are adapted from Cooper and Wanerman (1977).

1. Create a comfortable therapeutic atmosphere so that play materials allow the child to express himself or herself.

2. All therapists in the office may use the same play materials. However, during any particular therapeutic session, the play materials belong to that particular therapist.

3. Each therapist should know the values and the limits of each item that he or she uses.

4. Each new play item should be prepared and assessed for its potential before it is introduced to the child. If the child knows that he or she is the first to use a new item, the child may overvalue it and reject the other ones.

5. Whenever possible, have duplicate pieces of play equipment in order to encourage interaction and communication between the therapist and the child.

6. Play materials will break and get dirty. When possible, the therapist may repair broken items in the child's presence so that the child may learn that some things are repairable.

7. Although it is not customary to let children remove play items from the play therapy room, under some circumstances (vacation, holidays, etc.) it may be of clinical value to allow the child to remove an item as long as the overall therapy room setup is not disturbed.

APPENDIX C

List Of Play Materials

The following suggestions are offered for equipping the basic play therapy room.

1. Two nursing bottles.
2. Dollhouse complete with furniture and doll family of grandparents, parents, children, and a baby.
3. A large rag doll.
4. Playhouse materials, including table, chairs, cot, doll bed, stove, dishes, pots and pans, spoons, and knives and forks.
5. Toy telephone.
6. Play money.
7. A puppet stage with family of puppets and community figures, such as police officer, fire fighter, doctor.
8. Wet and dry sandboxes.
9. Miniature replicas of people; houses; animals, both wild and domestic; trees; bridges; fences; cars and trucks, including an ambulance, police and fire equipment, a tow truck, and passenger cars.
10. Army green plastic war toys, including two to three dozen soldiers, four to five tanks, trucks, jeeps, and fired guns.
11. Plastic miniature cowboys and Indians.
12. Water, running or bottled.
13. An easel with nontoxic art materials, including paints, pencils, pens, crayons, and colored chalk.
14. Drawing paper, finger-painting paper, old newspapers, cutting paper, and several journals with pictures.
15. A clay board, nonhardening modeling clay and plastcene.
16. Paste, glue, stapler, and tape.
17. Dart gun with rubber darts.
18. Pounding bench.
19. Tinker toy, Legoes, Lincoln logs, blocks, or similar construction material.
20. Punching bag.
21. Yatzee, dominoes, checkers, chess, and cards.
22. A variety of competitive board games—Aggravation, Sorry, Battleship, Connect Four, and so on.
23. A variety of communication board games—Reunion, Social Security, Ungame, and so on.
24. Nerf balls.
25. Plastic or rubber knife, scissors, string, rubber bands, paper and card clips.
26. Cleaning equipment—small basin, broom, mop, rag, and paper towels.

APPENDIX D

Recommended Resources

The following establishments specialize in psychotherapy instruments and equipment, communication games, and books for parents, children, and mental health professionals. Information regarding their products is free upon request.

1. Childcraft Educational Corporation
   20 Kilmer Road
   Edison, NJ 08813

2. Constructive Playthings
   1227 East 119th Street
   Grandview, MO 64030
   816/761-5900 or 1-800/255-6124

3. Uniquity
   215 Fourth Street
   P.O. Box 6
   Galt, CA 95632
   209/745-2111

4. Creative Therapeutics
   P.O. Box R
   Cresskill, NJ 07626-0317

5. For Challenged Kids by Mattel, Inc.
   15930 East Valley Boulevard
   City of Industry, CA 91744

6. Jason, Inc.
   317 East Front Street
   Grand Ledge, MI 48837
   517/627-5135

S E C T I O N

C

Logistics

C H A P T E R
10

RECORD KEEPING

John Kachorek, Ph.D.

During my first days of internship in clinical psychology, I entered an office shared with my colleagues and was immediately confronted with an 8½- by 11-inch photocopy of a line drawing of a toddler sitting on a toilet; beside him was an overly large roll of toilet paper. The caption read: "The job isn't over 'til the paperwork is done."

The clinical psychologist for some unknown reason has long had the reputation of being averse to paperwork — and, unfortunately, this failing often causes personal discomfort. This chapter reviews the psychologist's paperwork responsibilities in the following areas: (1) practice records, (2) financial records, (3) clinical records, and (4) ethical responsibilities. The clinical literature reviewed in preparation for this chapter is relatively devoid of the clear mandates and specific guidelines that appear to be more available to our colleagues in other clinical areas or in psychological research. The chapter is the compilation of personal experience with the support of cited published material.

PRACTICE RECORDS

In general, practice records include the original and/or copies of materials necessary to operate a well-functioning business. Among practice records are the individual's appointment book, a log of phone contacts, practice correspondence, blank practice forms, contracts, rental agreements, service contracts, warranties, and copies of any material related to the public's awareness of the practice (i.e., copies of announcement, newspaper articles, etc.). Practice records might even include photographs of office space before and after setup for insurance documentation. In general, the practice records, if complete, would allow an outside observer to get a general overview of the type and the nature of the practice.

The appointment book is probably the central feature of the practice records, and most therapists utilize their appointment books or calendars as guidelines for scheduled and routine activities. The choice of an appointment book is a matter of personal taste; however, it should afford, at a glance, the opportunity to assess quickly what time is being utilized, how it is utilized, and what time remains available. Clinicians often use their appointment books also to record incoming and outgoing telephone calls and as daily activity planners. Appointment books are readily available commercially, although there are also books designed by clinicians that allow space for record-keeping functions, including whether the client arrived for the appointment, the nature of the appointment, and the charge.*

More therapists are discovering the advantage of maintaining an ongoing log of their telephone contacts. Although most therapists, unlike other professionals, currently do not charge for time spent in routine telephone consultation, many are beginning to recognize this as a billable service. The phone log, if a therapist chooses to utilize one, would include the date and time of the contact with the individual, a brief statement of the nature of the contact, and possibly whether this service would be billed and at what charge. When a phone log is used in this manner, it also becomes a part of a financial record. It has the potential to become a significant part of a client's clinical record, especially during litigation.

Practice correspondence can be as limited or as voluminous as is the individual's practice or personal style. Practice correspondece, which is differentiated from "clinical correspondence," includes letters of introduction to referral sources, copies of media coverage and/or announcements, copies of mailing lists of potential nonclient contacts, copies of lease agreements, service contracts, equipment purchases, and test and psychological services catalogs. Therapists frequently file their appointment books and phone logs from the previous year with their practice records in order to be able to refer easily to past events.

FINANCIAL RECORDS

The delivery of psychological and/or psychotherapeutic services is a business. While many psychologists have trained in public institutions where financial record keeping was not one of their tasks, failure to document and maintain financial records appropriately may sound the death knell for a clinician's practice, reputation, and livelihood. Insurance companies indicate that the destruction of a small business's records by fire, theft, and so forth is the most frequent cause of business failure.

Accurate financial records are a necessity if the business of "psychological services" is to be a success, in order to be fully accountable to one's clientele and to protect oneself in financial audits. Audits, by the Internal Revenue Service (IRS) or third-party payers and/or contracting organizations, are becoming increasingly frequent.

Financial records are generally broken down into the two major areas of expenditures and income.

Expenditures

The expenditures of a small practice might be easily documented in the check register of the business checkbook. Larger practices will require more complex record-keeping systems, possibly pegboard systems or computerized accounting systems. In all cases, the basic principle and issue remain the same: document the outflow of money necessary to maintain the practice. Although

---

*See *Publications for Practitioners,* Ohio Psychology Publishing Co., 131 North High Street, #300, Columbus, OH 43215-3003.

a canceled check is usually considered a legal document for IRS purposes and sufficient documentation for most individuals, checks that are not for services clearly of a business nature (i.e., a check written to a psychological test publisher) may not be sufficient proof to an auditor that the expense was truly for the business. As such, further documentation, including bills or statements that provide the information to document the business nature of the expense, generally must accompany the canceled check.

For even the smallest of practices, it is in the practitioner's best interest to maintain a separate business checking account, and, if needed, a separate business credit card. Neither should ever be used for personal purposes. A solo practitioner who is unincorporated might deposit his or her practice income into the business account and then, for personal (nonbusiness) expenses, write checks to the personal account at regular intervals. Any comingling of business and personal monies is regarded as poor business practice by auditors, and is likely to raise additional questions concerning the possibility of other poor business practices. The accuracy and the completeness of practice records will help the clinician to sleep easily when faced with an audit. It should be noted that, according to reports in the popular press, the IRS has targeted the small independent business person, who has high opportunity to hide income, as a primary audit target.

Income

Ideally, the therapist provides a service, the therapist is paid for the service, and both the client and the therapist are satisfied with the exchange. At that point, the payment—whether in the form of cash, check, or credit-card charge—must be recorded in some form of ledger to document the transaction. This documentation generally includes the date, type, and cost of service; for whom the service was rendered; the amount of payment received; and any other financial credits. This posting of financial documentation is necessary to allow clients to be reimbursed by their insurance carrier and to document their expenditures for their record keeping, and to provide the practitioner with a good understanding of income and accounts receivable. These records also provide the basis for the independent practitioner to make appropriate estimates of quarterly income-tax liability in order to avoid large end-of-the-year payments, and possibly underpayment of estimated tax. Depending on the size of the practice, there are many ways to record services and income. For the smaller practices, a simple ledger card system updated manually is sufficient to meet IRS, client, and practitioner requirements (see Appendix A). Larger practices, however, may require more complicated documentation systems, necessitating a personal computer with general ledger packages and automated invoicing and insurance billing. But, whatever the system, it will still involve the time-consuming entry of data, whether by hand or by keystroke. However, the pain of not having an accurate system far outweighs the hassle of maintaining such a system, especially if provided for by a paid bookkeeper.

CLINICAL RECORDS

The *Standards for Provider of Psychological Services* (APA, 1977) and the *Specialty Guidelines for the Delivery of Services* (APA, 1981) were developed by the American Psychological Association (APA) to provide potential users and other interested groups with essential information about services available from psychologists. The guidelines are intended to "educate the public, the profession, and other interested parties regarding specialty professional practices." Additionally, "they are meant to provide guidance to providers, users, and sanctioners, regarding the best judgment of the profession on these matters." The Specialty Guidelines have "been established by the APA as a means of self-regulation to protect the public interest." Also, "these guidelines represent the profession's best judgment of the conditions, credentials and experience that contribute to competent professional practice."

The Standards and Specialty Guidelines both indicate that it is the standdard of practice for a psychologist to maintain clinical records. Both the Standards and the Specialty Guidelines state: "Accurate, current, and pertinent documentation shall be made of essential psychological services provided." The interpretation of this directive is that, "Records kept of psychological services may include, but not be limited to, identifying data, dates of service, types of services, and significant actions taken." It goes on to indicate that the "provider of psychological services shall insure that the essential information concerning services rendered is appropriately recorded within a reasonable time of their completion." The Specialty Guidelines also adds that records kept of clinical psychological services may include information concerning outcome at termination. Both the Standards and the Specialty Guidelines go on to discuss the record retention and disposition policy recommended by the APA, which will be discussed in the following sections.

In spite of what appears to be the clear mandate of the APA concerning record keeping, there seem to be many psychologists who do not concur or follow these recommendations. Apparently they do not do so either out of ignorance, or out of a disregard for the APA's stance that these guidelines are intended to be used by sanctioners. The reasons given for the failure to keep accurate and pertinent documentation run the gamut from a sincere attempt to protect a client's confidentiality at all costs, including possible legal jeopardy, to the clinician's disregard for the client's welfare in the interest of expediency. Allan Gerson (1987) has said that in an informal study of 100 psychologists in California, he discovered a five-to-three ratio of those who take notes (make a clinical record) versus those who do not. He found that analytic therapists, traditionally trained, tend to take more notes than eclectic therapists; also, 60 percent of his sample said they kept permanent records, whereas 40 percent of his sample did not keep records after termination. He quotes one therapist as saying, "My notes are roughly progress notes, little content, generally illegible by others, and meaningless after a few months have elapsed. All this to preserve confidentiality."

Dr. Gerson also discusses his survey results in light of recent court actions, in which, for example, inadequate record keeping contributed to a successful court action against a psychologist by establishing a "lack of care." The court found, "Said record did not conform to the standards of the community. . . ." Apparently, the court, in interpreting the standards of the community, also saw fit to evaluate whether or not a therapist's record keeping meets minimum community standards. At a recent symposium concerning avoidance of malpractice, Kenneth Austin (1987), a psychologist and a former member of the ethics committee of the California State Psychology Association, stated that failure to keep records is in itself grounds for a malpractice charge. In addition to clear APA directives, there also is now "case law" establishing the need for appropriate clinical record keeping.

Given that record keeping is an important component of service delivery, several questions arise:

Why are records kept?
Who has access to these records?
What should be put into these records?
Who may view these records?
Who are these records for?
How long shall these records be kept?

These issues will be discussed later in this chapter. Here, the general issue of clinical record keeping will be briefly addressed.

As discussed above, the financial record documents date, type of service (individual therapy and so forth), charge, and payment; the clinical record, however, needs to provide more information. Several "systems" for record keeping have been discussed in the literature, including the SOAP (subjective, objective, assessment, plan) record keeping system, strict behavioral systems, and many individualized variations, usually learned in training placements. It is the belief of this author that record keeping must be more than perfunctory in order to meet basic minimum requirements established by a professional organization or reviewing body. The clinical records provide an essential, and at times crucial, baseline of information concerning the patient. Accurate and complete clinical records might provide essential documentation of a patient's functioning, which later might be utilized as the baseline for exploring the development of physical and emotional problems. Psychotherapeutic services successfully offered and then terminated without appropriate records implies that the client might never again need psychological services. As such, the absence of records robs future therapists of the opportunity to understand the patient from the accurate perspective of the past. Admittedly, some schools of thought hold that the "present" and the "here and now" are most important. While not disagreeing, it should be noted that an accurate and complete record provides for the therapist, and possibly for the client, a portrayal of what the "here and now" was at that time in the past. Additionally, a complete record in the hands of a future therapist might help the client to recognize the significant gains that have been made and maintained over time. It may also, in the hands of an astute clinician, provide significant clues for successful therapy on behalf of the client in the present. Finally, an accurate and complete record may also provide crucial information necessary in litigation or some other form of hindsight investigation, including psychological autopsy, establishment of claims of health, and as a potential record for the patient's own utilization at a later time.

In the clinical record, most often kept in a simple manila folder, either handwritten or typewritten notes should be kept, along with other clinically related material. It is the belief of this author that financial documentation regarding the client may also be kept in the clinical record since it is a component of the clinical behavior of the individual. Additionally, the material that should go into the clinical record or chart should include the "face sheet," any "informed consent" documentation, all the psychological testing protocols, previously obtained psychotherapy and medical records, correspondence concerning the client, other correspondence that the client bring to sessions as part of the referral or therapeutic process, and significant events in the client's life that might be reported in the media, etc. The face sheet (see Appendix A) would generally include the name, address, and relevant demographic information concerning the patient. It may include specific statements, preferably in the patient's own handwriting, of his or her problem on admission. It may also include other specifically relevant information, such as the source of referral, special problems, physical health, and the names of the physician and family members.

A feature that is becoming more and more important in the clinical record is that of documenting the patient's "informed consent" (see Appendix A). Informed consent is the concept that suggests that the client is provided all the information that might potentially affect the decision to participate in psychological services offered. While most psychologists recognize that the client needs to have certain information regarding services, this information is often limited to statements concerning fees and office procedures. It is now becoming more accepted that other information about services provided should be clarified early in the therapeutic process. Informed consent suggests that therapists discuss with clients not only the issues of fees and procedures, but also vacations, insurance billing, medication, hospitalization, "after-hours" services, confidentiality and limits thereto, client and therapist expectations, and means for resolving misperceptions. Although this and other information might be legitimately discussed with any client early in therapy, one must also question the legitimacy of utilizing the client's time on behalf of these client–therapist issues. One approach finding favor with more therapists, especially in our litigious culture, is to present these factors in writing to the client before the second session, requesting that the client read, and sign a statement that he or she has read, the information provided. If this is done, the informed consent document should also be a part of the client's clinical record.

There is no universally accepted format for maintaining records, and several formats have been proposed in the literature. The following format is considered to be a model that would meet the requirements of most clinical schools of thought. The clinical record then includes not only the information from the client and other sources (see above), but also the thoughts and ideas of the clinician concerning the patient's needs and the plan for amelioration of these needs. This is the crucial part of the record, as it reflects the thinking of the clinician providing the services. The clinical record then should include the following components.

1. Initial evaluation
2. Progress notes
3. Discharge or termination notes

Initial Evaluation

In the initial evaluation, the clinician should make comments about the following areas.

1. Identifying information
2. Reasons for referral and presenting problem(s)
3. Relevant history and relevant issues
4. A formulation of the individual's clinical state
5. An initial treatment plan

The utilization of this model is effecive whether a clinician is following a dynamic or a more behavioral model.

Progress Notes

The most important feature of the clinical record is the clinician's documentation of the services provided. The clinician who fails to keep adequate clinical records is doing a disservice to self as well as to clients. In general, it is believed that the maintenance of adequate clinical records is more than worth the time that it entails, although most clinicians discover that they must set aside specific times for adequate record keeping. Failure to do so often leads to records that are incomplete, weak, or contaminated with distortions from other clients and other experiences. Traditionally, clinicians have hand-recorded their notes and these "progress notes" have been kept in chronological order in a patient's chart. Some clinicians record their notes during the session, but most do so later. Writing notes after each session allows the clinician to evaluate the progress of therapy and to recognize themes that might have been overlooked during the interactions with the client. Other therapists dictate progress notes, which are later transcribed onto "transcription strips" that may then be entered into the patient's record. If this transcription is completed after every session, there is less likelihood of contamination by other thoughts, memories, and experiences.

Progress notes enable the clinician to trace the clinical interactions with the patient. The initial progress notes would elaborate on and highlight issues that were developed in the initial evaluation, and would also afford the clinician the opportunity to "fine-tune" the treatment plan and add information that so often comes later in the therapeutic contact. Additionally, the progress notes are an appropriate place to discuss alterations in the initial treatment plan, the patient's response to the treatment plan, and significant other variables that affect the course and the outcome of treatment.

Termination Notes

The termination note is a summary statement. It includes the patient's identity, the nature of the problems, the types of treatment and the patient's response to it, and anticipated problems or prognosis. In the clinical record, the termination note is most often overlooked, especially if thereapy has progressed smoothly. However, termination notes play an important part in the clinical record and serve to document the reason for termination, especially when the clinical contact is terminated as a result of some external incident or some major interference in therapy. Frequently, a progress note becomes a de facto termination note by the nature of what is included.

To summarize, the clinical record is an important part of the treatment of an individual. It serves as the basis for providing continuity of care and increased understanding of the patient as well as an opportunity for the clinician to document the observations of the client for either personal or external review. Possibly of greatest importance is that it is a baseline of patient functioning.

ETHICAL ISSUES IN RECORD KEEPING

Confidentiality has long been the cornerstone of the therapist–patient professional relationship. Confidentiality of communication between patient and therapist, in addition to being ethically mandated, is often legally mandated, with certain exceptions, as well as by states issuing licenses for therapists to practice. Clients expect, for the most part, their communications with the therapist to be kept secret, and therapists build their special place in society in part on that privilege. Any record keeping that exists increases the possibility that the confidential relationship between therapist and client might be discovered and might jeopardize not only the relationship, but the welfare of both parties. States, and the public in general, expect that records be pertinent concerning a patient's care, and there is the parallel expectation that these records be kept confidential until appropriate release-of-information procedures are followed. Any release of information by the patient or the legal guardian of the patient should be carried out only after appropriate informed consent. Often, however, the release of the client's clinical record is ordered by a court when it judges that the "common good" is more important than the individual's right to maintain confidentiality. Additionally, laws have been established that reduce the person's right to "claim privilege" (i.e., insist that the communications between therapist and patient remain secret) if they enter into certain kinds of activities that jeopardize the welfare of another party. Among examples of interactions that limit a person's right to claim privilege are malpractice litigation, personal injury suits, other torts, or cases where the person's psychological contact was to aid in the commission of a crime (see California Evidence Code).

The fact that records are maintained makes it possible that these records may eventually be obtained, legitimately or illegitimately—and, in fact, attorneys will often characterize their need for records as an important part of the "discovery" process. Consequently, the content of records, their accuracy, and their relevance are of significant importance. Additionally, issues concerning ownership of the records, under what conditions an individual may have access to them, and how long records should be kept are also important and might affect a patient's welfare in many ways (see Keith-Spiegel, 1985).

It is important that the clinician become familiar with the licensing laws governing his or her own practice. These laws may or may not provide specific guidelines for record retention; however, should specific guidelines not be provided, the therapist is encouraged to work with an attorney who is knowledgeable in health law, and especially in mental-health law, to assess whether there might be "case law" or other precedent that might establish the basic requirements for record keeping in the individual's own state or local jurisdiction. In addition, records should meet the minimum requirements and guidelines established by one's national professional organization.

What one does with the records once they are created may be as important as or more important than what was originally put into the records. In general, it is thought by most observers that the actual physical record is the property of the therapist; however, most people also believe that the content of the record is the property of the patient. It is also important that therapists recognize that the content of the records may potentially be harmful to the client. Certainly the law in many states recognizes this potential harm, and ethical codes, as well as the law, provide procedures whereby therapists can release information to the patient, or the patient's guardian or representative, in such a way as to make it as nonthreatening and as usable as possible (see Health and Safety Code, 1982). Should this not be possible, therapists are encouraged to release the information only to other persons who have the ability, by training or experience, and also the trust of the patient, to interpret the data appropriately. Releasing information to individuals other than the patient or the patient's legal representative without the appropriate signed informed consent puts the therapist in significant legal jeopardy.

REFERENCES

American Psychological Association. (1981). *Specialty guidelines for the delivery of services.* Washington, DC: Author.

American Psychological Association. (1977). *Standards for providers of psychological services.* Washington, DC: Author.

Austin, K. (1987). *The California Psychologist, 22*(3), 13.

Conidaris, M., Ely, D., & Erickson, J. (1986). *California laws for psychotherapists.* New York: Harcourt, Brace, Jovanovich.

Gerson, A. (1987). The independent practitioner. *Bulletin of the Division of Psychologists in Independent Practice,* Division 42 of the American Psychological Association, *7*(1), 3.

Keith-Spiegel, P., & Koocher, G. (1985). *Ethics in psychology.* New York: Random House.

State of California, Board of Medical Quality Assurance. (1986). *Laws, rules and regulations relating to the practice of psychology.*

APPENDIX A

CONTRACT FOR PSYCHOLOGICAL SERVICES*

I, _____, agree to join with Dr. John Kachorek
each _____ from _____ to _____ at _____.
During these _____ 45–50 minute sessions, we will direct our mutual efforts
toward these goals.

1.

2.

3.

I agree to pay _____ per session for the use of his training, skills and experience
as a psychologist and psychotherapist. This fee is payable _____.
I understand that I am fully responsible for the fee and that Dr. Kachorek will cooperate with my insurance company in its reimbursal program. I also recognize that
psychological services provided by phone are billed at the same rate as our face to face
sessions.

If I am not satisfied with the progress we make toward these goals, I may renegotiate
this contract providing I give Dr. Kachorek seven (7) days notice of my desire. If I fail
to attend a scheduled session without 48 hours forewarning I remain financially responsible for that missed session; the exception to this standard is when I am unforeseeably
and/or unavoidably prevented from attending by accident or illness.

At the end of _____ sessions, Dr. Kachorek and I agree to renegotiate this contract. We include the possibility that the stated goals may have changed. I understand
that this agreement does not guarantee that we will attain the above goals, however,
it does constitute an offer on my part of pay Dr. Kachorek for access to his resources
as a psychologist and his willingness to apply those psychological resources in good
faith.

I further stipulate that this agreement will become a part of the psychological record
which is accessible to the parties at will, but to no other person without my written
consent. Dr. Kachorek will respect my right to maintain the confidentiality of any information communicated by me or obtained from me during our work together.

I give/do not give my persmission to Dr. Kachorek to audiotape sessions for his review.
However, he will not publish, communicate or otherwise disclose, without my written consent, any such information, which, if disclosed, would injure me in any way.

Client's Signature _____

Therapist's Signature _____

Date _____

*Patterned after a model contract developed by the Health Research Group, a Ralph Nader
group. See *American Psychologist,* January, 1979, p. 8.

JOHN KACHOREK PH.D.
CLINICAL AND CONSULTING PSYCHOLOGY
220 SECOND ST.
ENCINITAS, CA 92024

619–942–3194   PA 5055

Welcome to my practice. I am pleased to have the opportunity to serve you and hope that this handout will provide information helpful in making an informed decision concerning my services. Please ask questions at any time.

I am a psychologist and have been in general practice for over 15 years. I have training and experience in a number of areas including individual, family and group therapies for children, adolescents and adults. I have also had extensive training in personality assessment. If our work together leads to problems beyond my expertise, I will help you to obtain the necessary services from the appropriate specialist. My resume is available for review.

APPOINTMENTS:

My services are by appointment only. The length of the appintment time varies on the basis of services provided. Individual therapy is generally scheduled for 45 to 50 minutes, and this is known as the "clinical hour." Because the appointment is reserved for you, it is necessary to charge for appointments which are not cancelled 24 hours in advance, unless in fact they are occasioned by circumstances which we would both define as an emergency. Failure to provide a 24 hour notice of cancellation generally means that some other person is not able to use that appointment time. Appointments are scheduled during the usual office hours: 8:00 a.m. to 6:00 p.m., Monday through Friday.

MESSAGES:

As we work together, you will notice that I do not accept phone calls while I am with my clients. During those times and at other times during the day or evening, my calls are answered electronically. I check for messages frequently during the day, and I am able to return 90 to 95 percent of my calls the same day. If we anticipate that greater availability is necessary, special arrangements can be made for therapeutic services.

INITIAL CONTACT:

Our initial appointment is often called an "initial evaluation." This appointment is scheduled for you to discuss your concerns and problems from your point of view. There may be time during this appointment to obtain historical and other background data or this information may be gathered at subsequent sessions. In times of crises, the usual format of an "initial evaluation" is not followed in the hope that the time might be used to resolve or relieve the immediate crisis. As part of the "initial evaluation" new clients are requested to complete at least one questionnaire concerning their beliefs, experiences, thoughts and feelings which will then be scored using statistical norms. The results of this "psychological test" will allow me to "measure" your concerns and problems.

TREATMENT:

I expect and encourage you to obtain knowledge of the procedures, goals, and possible side-effects of psychotherapy. I expect to make our professional contact one where you receive the maximum benefit, and I will also keep you informed about alternatives to psychotherapy. Psychotherapy may be tremendously beneficial for some individuals while, at the same time, there are some risks. The risks may include the experience of intense and unwanted feelings, including: sadness, anger, fear, guilt or anxiety. It is important to remember that these feelings may be natural and normal and are an important part of the therapy process. Other risks of therapy might include: recalling unpleasant life events, facing unpleasant thoughts and beliefs, increased awareness of feelings, values, and experiences, alteration of an individual's ability or desire to deal effectively and harmoniously with others in relationships. In therapy, major life decisions are sometimes made, including: decisions involving separation within families, development of other types of relationships, changing employment settings and changing lifestyles. These decisions are a legitimate outcome of the therapy experience as a reult of an individual's calling into question many of their beliefs and values. As your therapist, I will be available to discuss any of your assumptions, problems, or possible negative side effects of our work together.

OTHER PSYCHOLOGICAL SERVICES:

While the majority of my time is spent in providing psychotherapeutic services, at times other psychological services are provided. These include psychological assessment and diagnosis, mediation, facilitation and problem solving in emotionally charged situations, including: divorce, child custody and other human relationships; consultation to individuals seeking to have questions answered about other members of their family, friends, and so on. If these services are provided, I will inform the client as to whether or not insurance carriers typically reimburse for these services. Psychological services provided by phone are available and are often a legitimate ancillary service.

Infrequently, a patient's distress remains or becomes so high that hospitalization or the use of medication must be considered. Psychologists are not physicians, and consequently do not prescribe medication; however, at times psychologists may treat patients in hospitals if they have "privileges" at the hospital. In cases where medication or hospitalization may be required, this will be discussed in advance with the client and, if necessary, with other responsible individuals. I work with several psychiatrists in the area, and we often collaborate on issues of medication, hospitalization and second opinion; in this way the client who has these needs is better served. It is generally the case that my clients utilize the services of a psychiatrist as a "consultant" while continuing psychological therapy with me.

PSYCHOLOGICAL ASSESSMENT:

In addition to the psychological test administered as a part of the "initial evaluation," it is often beneficial to conduct a "formal" psychological assessment and/or testing in the early stages of therapeutic services or in consultation for others. The decision to assess using psychological instruments will be discussed with the client in advance, and the discussion will include the nature of the tests to be utilized, the rationale for the testing and, if warranted, the results of the testing. Accurate and valid results are obtained from psychological assessment and testing only when the client is willing to cooperate, motivated to do "well" and naive to the "right answers." As such, professional ethics and California law mandate that the psychological tests themselves are not to be distributed to clients at any time. It may be necessary to schedule a three to four hour block of time in order to accomplish a single "testing" and it is important to recognize that the psychologist may spend an hour in test scoring, data interpretation, and report writing for every hour spent in face-to-face contact with and for the client. If requested, the results of the testing will be discussed. A written report can also be provided; however, written reports require additional time to prepare and are more expensive to the client.

TERMINATION:

Termination of psychotherapy may occur any time and may be initiated by either the client or the therapist. I request that if a decision is being made to terminate, that there be a minimum of a seven day notice in order that a final termination session(s) may be scheduled to explore the reasons for termination. Termination itself can be a constructive, useful process. If any referral is warranted, it will be made at that time.

CLIENT'S RIGHTS:

At any time, my clients may question and/or refuse therapeutic or diagnostic procedures or methods, or gain whatever information they wish to know about the process and course of therapy. Clients are also assured of confidentiality which is protected by both ethical practice and by California law. There are, however, important exceptions to confidentiality that are legally mandated. In general terms, these exceptions include: (1) the law requires that I notify relevant others if I judge that a client has an intention to harm another individual; (2) I am also obliged by the law to report any incidence of suspected child abuse, neglect, or molestation in order to protect the children involved; (3) in legal cases, I or my records may be subpoenaed by the court. Confidentiality will be respected in all cases, except as noted above, and in those additional cases where in my clinical judgment the maintenance of confidentiality is, in fact, destructive to the individual. In those situations, I will inform my clients of my judgment and they will have the final decision as to whether I maintain confidentiality. Included in this information packet is a form which allows me to discuss your evaluation and/or treatment with others. Please complete this "Release of Information" form with the name and address of those individuals. If you wish, you may also limit the time of release validity by an expiration date, or limit what I have your permission to discuss, by simply writing in the space entitled "Limits."

CLIENTS WHO ARE DEPENDENTS:

If you are requesting my services as the guardian or parent of a child, or the guardian of a dependent adult, the same general practice as outlined above will apply. However, as your child's psychologist, it is important that your child is able to completely trust me. As such, I keep confidential what your child says in the same way that I keep confidential what an adult says. As the parent or guardian, you have the right and responsibility to question and understand the nature of my activities and progress with your child, and I must use my clinical discretion as to what is an appropriate disclosure. In general, I will not release specific information that the child provides to me; however, I feel it appropriate to discuss with you, the parent or guardian, your child's progress and your participation in their treatment.

CHARGES:

The charges for my services are based on the usual, customary, and reasonable fee profiles for this area. My charges are $95.00 per 45 to 50 minute clinical hour. The fee also includes my time on your behalf, including: record keeping and preparation. I encourage you to discuss fees at any time, and my clients are expected to pay for services when provided unless arrangements have been made in advance. I request that your check for payment be made out in advance so that our entire time may be spent attending to your concerns. When my psychological report is sent to a third party, payment in full is necessary prior to release of my findings. Other charges are based on the fee discussed above, and you are requested to read and sign the attached "Schedule of Charges" to choose your preferred payment option.

INSURANCE:

If you have a health insurance plan, your visits may be reimbursed by your insurance company. Since you have a contract with your health insurance carrier, it has been my experience that they are more responsive to you, the insured, than to me, the provider. Therefore, I prefer that you file your own insurance claim, but I will be glad to assist you. Insurance forms that require information from me must first be completely filled out in all the applicable places by you. This office will then complete our section. Your insurance company probably requires diagnostic and treatment information before reimbursing you. I will release that information to them with your permission. If you wish, I will be happy to discuss with you the "diagnosis" that I am releasing to your insurance carrier. While a client's diagnosis is very sensitive information and in is generally treated as such by insurance carriers, I cannot guarantee how any particular insurance carrier or employer respects this information. If you prefer that I do not release information to your insurance carrier for reimbursement purposes, or if your insurance carrier fails to reimburse you in a manner which you expected, you will remain responsible for the fee for services.

Many individuals are members of preferred provider plans with whom I have contractual obligations. Please inform me in advance should you be eligible for these contracted services to prevent insurance billing mistakes which may jeopardize your utilization of these plans.

I again welcome you to our work together, and anticipate that it will be mutually beneficial.

John J. Kachorek, Ph.D.

I have read the above material and agree to abide by its terms.

		Copy:
Signature	Date	

Effective Date: 1/04/89

JOHN KACHOREK PH.D.
CLINICAL AND CONSULTING PSYCHOLOGY
220 SECOND ST.
ENCINITAS, CA 92024

619-942-3194   PA 5055

TO MY CLIENTS:

Periodically, you or an attorney on your behalf may request that I make a court appearance in order to testify as an expert regarding services that I have provided to you or to your children. While psychological services are most often "cooperative" experiences, court proceedings are most often adversarial experiences.

When called to testify, I must answer all the questions posed by either side and/or the judge as honestly and truthfully as possible, and at times I may therefore say things that are painful for others to accept. My court appearance may lead to psychological distress on behalf of the parties and/or in other ways injure the relationship that has previously existed between us. Please take this into consideration if you think that you might wish to have me make a court appearance.

My fee for court appearances is between $500 and $600 per half day. The fee is based on the amount of time that I anticipate will be needed to review my records in advance so that I might be able to answer the questions asked of me accurately, as well as the amount of time that is cancelled out of my normal schedule in order to make the appearance. It is not unusual that much time might be "wasted" waiting around in the hallways of the court before being actually called to the stand. Nevertheless, I have cancelled appointments in order to be available for the testimony. Additionally, there is always the possibility that I may be scheduled for a court appearance in the morning, consequently cancelling out my morning appointments, only to be sent home after a couple of hours and then recalled later that afternoon or on another date. Should this occur, my fee for the reapparance is $500. Additional preparation, unless the rescheduled date is far in the future, is generally not necessary.

Requesting or being subpoenaed to appear in court is expensive and may also be emotionally difficult. Please consider this and discuss this with your attorney and with me in advance. If you wish to have me appear, my expert witness fee, consistent with California law, is required in advance. Should reappearance be required, that fee is also expected in advance.

Sincerely,

John J. Kachorek, Ph.D.

JOHN J. KACHOREK, PH.D.
Clinical and Consulting Psychology
PA5055

*CLIENT QUESTIONNAIRE**

Name of Patient:_____Today's Date:_____
Address: _____

Telephone(s): _____ / _____ Social Security No. _____
                 (home)   (work)
Age:_____Birth Date:_____Marital Status:_____
Occupation: _____
Education: _____
Briefly describe your reason for seeking help: _____

Who suggested you contact this office? _____
When were you last examined by a physician? _____
Name of Physician: _____ Phone: _____
List any major health problems for which you currently receive treatment: _____

List any medications you are now taking: _____

Have you ever received psychiatric or psychological help or counseling of any kind before?
_____ If you have, please explain: _____

List the members of your family and all others in your home:

Name(s)	Age/Birth Date	Relationship	Occupation

Please circle any of the following problems which pertain to you:

Nervousness	Depression	Fears
Shyness	Sexual Problems	Suicidal Thoughts
Separation	Divorce	Finances
Drug Use	Alcohol Use	Friends
Anger	Self-Control	Unhappiness
Sleep	Stress	Work
Relaxation	Headaches	Tiredness
Legal Matters	Memory	Ambition
Energy	Insomnia	Making Decisions
Loneliness	Inferiority Feelings	Concentration
Education	Career Choices	Health Problems
Temper	Nightmares	Marriage
Children	Appetite	Stomach Trouble
Bowel Troubles	Being a Parent	My Thoughts

If you believe insurance may cover a portion of your visits here, please complete the following information:_____

Insurance Company	Policy Holder	Group & Policy Number(s)

Name of Responsible Party: _____

Address: _____ City: _____

Phone: _____Social Security No: _____ Driver's License No.: _____

Employer:_____

Address: _____

_____ Phone: _____

May we contact you at work? _____ May we leave messages for you at work? _____

Name of person(s) to be contacted in case of emergency:

_____ Phone: _____

_____ Phone: _____

_____ Date: _____
(Signature of Responsible Party

*Published with Permission from *Innovations in Clinical Practice: A Sourcebook,* Vol. I; Professional Resource Exchange, Inc., Sarasota, Florida.

NAME					ACCOUNT NO.				
ADDRESS					SHEET NO.				
DATE	I T E M S	Folio	✔	DEBITS	✔	CREDITS	DR. OR CR.	BALANCE	

Published with Permission from *Innovations in Clinical Practice: A Sourcebook,* Vol. I; Professional Resource Exchange, Inc., Sarasota, Florida.

S E C T I O N

D

**The Referral
System**

C H A P T E R
11

THE REFERRAL MYSTIQUE

Alan D. Davidson, Ph.D.

P robably since Sigmund Freud first opened his practice in Vienna, psycho-therapists have been struggling with the question of building, maintaining, and enhancing a referral base. The practitioner in the late 20th century faces almost the same challenges that Freud and his contemporaries dealt with in Victorian Europe. Certainly, the names, styles of organization, and revolutionary changes seen in the provision of mental health services in the past decade do not change what must be considered an indisputable bottom line: The basis of any truly successful private practice is the steady and consistent flow of new referrals into the practitioner's office.

Much is currently being written (Bernstein, 1986) about the future of health-care delivery in the United States—which only intensifies the problem for the private practitioner as more and more consumers go to the large institutional health-care providers for services. With the increasingly competitive nature of private practice, the practitioner would be well advised to recognize that, as in Freud's time, the flow of referrals is based on the scope and extent of the practitioner's name recognition, reputation and accessibility in the community. Although the value of marketing, advertising, and other promotional activities has been well publicized, an essential rule for the private practitioner continues to be that the success of the practice will be determined by the extent to which the practitioner can become established and known in the community as a provider of high-quality services.

As organized health-care delivery utilizing a large corporate model becomes more extensive, it will become increasingly vital for the private practitioner to establish a wide base of professional recognition and the appropriate inhouse systems to sustain the acquisition of new clients. It appears inescapable that the private practitioner will need to, at least in part, approach the practice as an entrepreneurial venture. The idea may be somewhat distasteful to some, but the private practice of psychotherapy is first and foremost a business and thus will be most successful when it is dealt with as a business.

In 1987, some 400 health maintenance organizations (HMOs) were in existence, serving approximately 20 million consumers. By 1990, it is predicted that over 700 HMOs will be providing service for almost 70 million people, or approximately 40 percent of the entire population of the United States (as reported in the *Register Report,* Feb. 1987). Thus, as the provider pool of psychotherapists expands, the well of potential clients from which these private practitioners will draw becomes smaller at an alarming rate. The real challenge to the private practitioner in the next 25 years will be to develop new and creative ways to establish and maintain a broad-based private practice referral network while remaining within realistic and ethical boundaries.

The question may simply boil down to, "How does a new or even established practitioner expand his or her reputation throughout the community?" The objective is to be known by a large number of people so that when the need for psychological services arises, the private practitioner enjoys what those in marketing refer to as "top-of-mind" recognition — that is, will be the first practitioner whose name comes to mind when someone requires professional assistance.

It is a well-known principle in sales and marketing that one must "ask for the order" at some juncture. Ethical constraints and professionalism make this process one that requires delicacy and diplomacy. The difference between ethical referral request and outright solicitation may appear a fine line to some. Certainly, the responsibility of the practitioner will be to give the referral source sufficient information on which to base appropriate and consistent referrals. The most basic definition of an ethical referral (Fields, 1982) requires that the referral be obviously necessary for the well-being of the client and that the service will be provided in such a way as to meet the standards of quality care in the community. The only reward to the referral source will be the knowledge that the client will receive high-quality treatment by a skilled practitioner.

Solicitation often carries a negative connotation and implies an active attempt on the part of the practitioner to solicit business, typically before a trusting and ongoing relationship is developed between the referral source and the practitioner. While financial considerations and method of remuneration are important issues, they should remain secondary in terms of the development of such a relationship.

Perhaps the greatest challenge faced by the new practitioner is simply getting started in a community, especially if the practitioner did not attend graduate school in the area and so is a stranger in a new marketplace. One's ability, exposure, and credibility-enhancing behavior are the cornerstones of establishing a solid referral base. At the outset, a new practitioner may want to consider a part-time teaching post or even a full-time or part-time position in a community mental health center, hospital, or clinic to begin the process of becoming familiar with the community. At some point, however, a clinician must begin to make known his or her availability as a private practitioner.

Sending a formal announcement to possible referral sources can be the most logical way to begin. Potential referrers need to know (1) that you are in private practice, (2) where the practice is located, (3) what subspecialities you are offering, and (4) that you are accepting new clients. In some areas, with only a dozen or so established practitioners, this is a relatively straightforward process. However, in large urban areas where practitioners can number in the hundreds or thousands, it is obviously more complex.

A good way to begin is by making up a mailing list of all those individuals who know the practitioner and have at least an initial respect for the practitioner's work. Obviously, such individuals need to be in a position eventually to refer clients, and may include such mental health gatekeepers as teachers, attorneys, physicians in general practice, and members of the clergy. In addition to the formal announcement, a brief, personalized note explaining the scope of your practice can be valuable. Colleagues, as well as potential referrers, may not be aware that you want new referrals. Even the practitioner who has been established for a number of years may fail to maintain ongoing relationships with referral sources and be surprised when the flow of referrals begins to dry up. These sources often need to be "massaged" (Goodstein, 1986)—that is, they need to have ongoing contact with the practitioner to realize that the practitioner continues to be interested in providing care for those who may require it.

Practitioners who expect to maintain flourishing private practices need to keep their names alive in the minds of both their colleagues and the public. Previous clients also should be included among those receiving professional announcements, reprints of articles, or seasonal communications such as Christmas cards. Frequently, it appears that the busiest practitioners are the ones who follow up on the concept of "top-of-mind" name recognition. For example, an extremely successful psychiatrist in the large southern California city in which this author practices always sends me a personalized holiday greeting at the end of the year. He includes a brief handwritten "thank you" for the referrals that I have sent him during the year and notes that he continues to be available for both medication consultations and psychoanalysis. This practitioner recognizes that these are two services that I, as a psychologist, do not provide, and thus his notation as to his availability in no way conflicts with my own need to develop and maintain my own private practice.

The merits of advertising for psychotherapists (Koocher, 1977) are currently being widely debated. Certainly, some people have benefited from advertising, whereas others report no particular gain. There is also the risk that advertising will have a boomerang effect by suggesting that the practitioner is unable to fill his or her appointment book by referrals alone. Advertising, if used at all, must be professional as well as modest. Scientific caution and avoidance of direct solicitation of clients are essential. One difficulty with advertising is that it eliminates the personal knowledge of you and your skills considered to be essential by some referral sources.

Although controversy exists as to the advisability and value of advertising for mental health practitioners, public relations advice certainly can be beneficial. It is important to recall, however, that public relations efforts only provide visibility and exposure whereas advertising will also awaken an interest in utilizing the practitioner's services. Still, many clinicians find advertising to be distasteful, expensive, and often of little value, but the use of publicity can viewed as both ethical and valuable. The central theme of such a campaign would be to highlight your uniqueness as a psychotherapist. It is important to stress those of the services you offer—such as forensic evaluations, child psychotherapy, or group therapy—that are not likely to be offered by many of your colleagues.

Both the written and electronic media can provide wide exposure to a practitioner if handled effectively. Probably the only thing more destructive to a new or developing private practice other than no reputation in the community is a negative reputation. By informing the science and health reporters on local newspapers and at television and radio stations of one's expertise and availability, one can become known in the community by being called upon to provide commentary in a wide range of topics that have news value as well as relevance to mental health. For example, many practitioners are interviewed during the Christmas season about the potentially adverse effects of the holidays upon the functioning of certain people, such as those prone to depression. This is an opportunity to bring yourself and your skills into focus in a potentially valuable way.

Many practitioners also maintain some contact with academia even though they are in full-time private practice. Those in part-time private practices can augment their income and expand their name recognition by teaching an occasional course, either at the university level or in a community college. Again, the most obvious aspect of teaching in terms of developing a private practice is that you become known by a group of individuals who may be sensitive to mental health issues and in a position to refer either themselves or acquaintances to you for professional services later on. By becoming familiar with the academics in the community, one may be invited to present guest lectures in one's area of specialization, again increasing one's exposure and name recognition.

Putting yourself in front of an audience serves the same purpose, whether it be a small group of concerned parents at an elementary school or a group of high-level managers attending a strategic planning meeting. The guiding principle in terms of developing a referral base is broad and comprehensive exposure. The objective is to get as many people to know about you and your work as possible. Invitations to speak, especially during the early years of one's practice, generally will pay dividends down the road. Even though the group listening to the presentation may not utilize your services directly, they become part of an informed group of possible referrers.

Expanding one's network of professional allegiances is also an essential aspect of developing a solid referral base. Professional entertainment is a simple and direct way to establish your visibility within the community. Many group practices, as well as individuals, hold annual open houses or receptions, not only to thank those who have referred in the past, but to reiterate the message that they remain available for future referrals. When moving into a new office or adding an associate, an ideal opportunity exists to invite colleagues and associates to enjoy your hospitality and to underscore your interest in maintaining professional relationships. Journal and book discussion groups, informal case conferences, and study groups will all benefit the private practitioner by keeping channels of communication and referral open.

Active participation in local, regional, state, and even national professional organizations can also serve as a vehicle for broader professional exposure. Political action committees are gaining wider acceptance among the professions as vehicles to influence the political process, which, in large part, controls the practice and professions of psychotherapy. By becoming involved in such an organization, practitioners are afforded not only the opportunity to have a hand in controlling their professional destinies but also the chance to meet a wide cross section of people who may be able to refer clients over time.

An easily overlooked aspect of developing a referral base is the simple introduction of yourself to other professionals in your community, and especially within the demographic vicinity of your office. After sending a professional announcement and perhaps a letter of introduction, telephone calls and informal meetings with physicians, dentists, attorneys, teachers, principals, members of the clergy, operaters of day-care centers, hospital administrators, and other "natural gatekeepers" can prove to be extremely valuable in gaining a professional foothold. The meetings can be brief but should include a description of your qualifications, experience, and commitment to provide high-quality services. Again, one need not be circumspect in terms of the point of the professional visit. Practitioners who are direct, concise, and modest in their representations are likely to remain the resources utilized by these gatekeepers when someone in need of assistance crosses their threshold.

Schools, colleges, and other educational facilities can provide excellent referral sources (Thomas, 1972). Counseling centers on most high school and college campuses will generally maintain a list of professionals in the community who will accept low-fee or sliding-fee-scale clients. However, it is unlikely that people working in such a setting will choose to refer to you until they have the opportunity to know you and trust your credibility. It becomes a practicel necessity for practitioners to get out of their offices and into the offices of other professionals who are in the position of providing referrals. When seeing a child or family, schedule an appointment with the child's teacher or school principal (if this is appropriate) and establish a communication link. Let the person from whom you expect to receive referrals get to know you and put the "name with the face." Keep in mind that a solid referral base is predicated on a network of relationships and a history of satisfied clients. Although some people will give a referee a list of three or four possible service providers, it is more likely that most will refer someone to your office because they know you and believe you do good work. Take great care not to disappoint the referrer's expectations.

Speaking engagements will keep your name, face, and reputation before the public, thus building up the base of people who know of you and your practice. Community groups, churches, synagogues, parent-teacher associations, and various political task forces all can serve as an arena for you in which to share information with "take-home value" with the audience, and also to give them an opportunity to evaluate you as a service provider.

The private practice that will flourish regardless of changes in third-party payment schedules, the growth of HMOs, or demographic changes in the community will be the practice that is based on referrals from satisfied clients. A simple sign in your waiting room indicating that your practice grows as a result of clients' giving your name to others can be invaluable. This can be done in a dignified and professional manner but the message needs to be transmitted; your current patients need to be aware that you are willing to accept new clients and that you would appreciate the opportunity to be of service.

The objective of a new practitioner in the community is obviously to fill the appointment book as quickly as possible. Within the limits of your competency, it would appear prudent to accept a full range of patients, some of whom may not be able to pay your regular and customary fee. Whereas a certain amount of *pro bono* work is ethically indicated and personally valuable, it will also serve as a vehicle to continue to develop a network of affiliations, associations, and awareness of you as a service provider. After the appointment book is full, you can begin the rather pleasant task of shaping your practice so as to fill more of your personal and professional objectives. This obviously will take months, and even years, to accomplish completely, but the initial objective is to begin providing service to the community so that the community becomes aware of you.

Remember that many potential clients work a regular nine-to-five day and will find it very inconvenient to come to your office at midmorning or midafternoon on a regular basis. In communities where there is a large number of potential providers, accessibility and availability become important factors in developing a referral base. Clients in need of professional services are not likely to tolerate a significant disruption in their workday nor to appreciate being placed on a waiting list. Thus, it will be advantageous for you to have both early-morning and early-evening appointments available, at least until you have acquired a roster of clients who are able to keep appointments during the regular business day. Some degree of creativity and flexibility is valuable in this regard. For example, some psychotherapists may choose to begin their day very early in the morning and end at midafternoon. Others begin seeing clients and patients at approximately the noon hour and work into the evening. A major factor for developing a referral base is conveying the idea that you are available and ready to be of assistance to someone in need.

You should be realistic and set limits on the type and number of clients you can work with effectively. Be clear with your referral sources by noting those individuals with whom you prefer not to work. It is important to make it clear that in an emergency, of course, you would be willing to see someone, at least initially, so that you can make the appropriate referral to another psychotherapist. Recalling that the only thing worse than no reputation is a bad reputation in the community, attempt to resist the illusion that you are able to work with anyone who comes in for help (Thomas, 1972). Certain people and certain types of problems can trigger so much emotion and anxiety in a psychotherapist that both the psychotherapist and the client will find it futile to attempt to work together. It is preferable to offer a referral to someone who is more willing to work with this person, or is more capable of doing so, than to struggle through the case yourself.

Educating other professionals as to the value and potential benefit of psychotherapy is an important element in establishing a solid referral base from which to draw. Many highly sophisticated professionals still view psychotherapy as part science and part art at best, and witchcraft or voodoo at worst (Kolb, 1987). Attorneys and other professionals whose job it is to help people with difficulties other than psychological ones may need to learn that psychotherapy can be a benefit to them as they seek a solution to a client's problems. Marital disputes, divorces and dissolutions, child-custody cases, personal injury cases, disability evaluations, and criminal defense cases all offer an opportunity for the psychotherapist to be of assistance. Attorneys, as natural gatekeepers, may encounter literally hundreds of new clients each year during the course of their work. Recognizing that a psychotherapist can help, in terms of both winning a case and helping the client, can be valuable for the attorney (and thus the practitioner).

Private as well as public schools can also serve as a valuable source of referrals. Be sure to introduce yourself to the teachers and school principal, and also to the school nurse, classroom aides, and clerical personnel. Each of these persons may be in a position to pass your name on to a parent who is having difficulty with a child. School psychologists often are inundated with evaluations to be conducted during the normal course of their work. By providing an opportunity to do a complete evaluation quickly and comprehensively (Webb, 1962), additional insights and understanding of the child's learning or behavioral problems can be gained quickly. Your worth as a resource to potential referrers will thus grow.

A private practice is a dynamic, evolving process. It is essential that the practitioner continue to direct some energy toward the maintenance and growth of the referral base. Communication and availability again are the central elements of maintaining a private practice. One must reiterate to colleagues and other professionals one's continuing availability and willingness to see new clients. By routinely sending short notes to referring colleagues, one can continue to bring this point home. Obviously, a brief "thank you" letter should be sent immediately after the first consultation with a newly referred client. This should also be done at the termination of treatment (you will need to obtain the patient's permission to communicate this information). In a dignified and professional way, you can also indicate your willingness to see other clients with similar difficulties.

Keep in mind that the referral process is a two-way street. Other professionals who refer to you can reasonably expect that you will refer clients to them when the need for their services arises. This may not happen frequently but it can be an invaluable way of establishing professional trust and confidence in your referral base. Thus, when establishing a new referral source, if appropriate, indicate your willingness to refer clients to the referral source when the need arises. Many professionals who refer to you are in the same position as you are in terms of wanting to develop a successful private practice.

There really is little mystique to a solid referral-based private practice. Those who refer to you simply must know who you are and what you do, and have faith that you will do it to your best ability. A private practice has to be nurtured and developed. As referral sources retire or move away, the private practitioner must pursue new avenues of business development. You never really know where your next client will come from. It becomes vital that many members of the community become aware of your work and feel comfortable in sending others to you for professional assistance. Visibility in the development of a positive, confident professional reputation in the community will serve as the core building block for the successful long-term private practice.

It may be important in reviewing the mythology associated with developing a referral base not to attempt to reinvent the wheel. Mental-health-service providers have been successful in changing economic, sociological, and political climates in maintaining the steady and consistent flow of clients into their consulting rooms. With planning, effort, organization, and consistency, a private practitioner, contrary to some current speculation (Cummings, 1987), should be able to remain alive and well for the foreseeable future. Attainment of this goal is certainly going to become more challenging with the increasing number of providers arriving on the scene and the decreasing number of consumers seeking their services. However, it still appears to be an acocmplishable task.

REFERENCES

Bernstein Research (1986). The future of health care delivery in America, 1985–1986/Standard and Poors Corporation, Standard OTC stock reports.

Cummings, N. (1987). On the future of professional psychology. Keynote Address, California State Psychological Association Annual Meeting, Coronado, Calif.

Fields, F.K. (1982). *Psychology and professional practice,* Stamford, Connecticut: Quorum Books, 1982.

Goodstein, L.D. (1986). Personal communication.

Kolb, M. (1987). "The future of mental health benefits in CHAMPUS programs. Presented to a joint meeting of the Academy of San Diego Psychologists and the Society of Psychiatric Physicians, San Diego.

Koocher, G.P. (1977). Advertising for psychologists: Pride and prejudice or sense and sensibility? *Professional Psychology, 8.*

Council for the National Register of Health Service Providers in Psychology (1987). *Register Report, The Newsletter for Psychologist Health Service Providers, 13* (2).

Sales, B.D. (1983). *The professional psychologist's handbook,* New York: Plenum Press.

Thomas, C.C. (1972). *Practical problems of a private psychotherapy practice,* Springfield: Thomas Co.

Webb, W.B. (1962). *The profession of psychology,* New York: University of Florida Press.

C H A P T E R
12

DEVELOPMENT OF REFERRAL RESOURCES

David Brinks, Ph.D.

INTRODUCTION

One of the first questions raised when considering establishing a private practice, whether full or part time, involves concern about where the clients are, and if they will utilize one's services. Certainly this is a legitimate and valid concern. While some therapists will initiate a practice by "sticking a toe into the water," beginning on a part-time basis and possibly with even a very small time commitment while remaining in a salaried position elsewhere, many others will not have income independent of their practice, and will be "diving" in with more at stake. Some will sublet a fully furnished and equipped office from another practitioner on a part-time basis, with very little outlay for setting up an office. Others will commit themselves to an office or a suite through a lease, invest in furniture, a telephone system, answering service, copy service, along with clerical, reception and billing service or personnel, all of which reflect a far greater economic and time investment and risk factor. Insuring a source of clients — being confident of a viable, functional referral base — is essential. Few will be in a position to carry the expenses of a fully equipped office for the two to three years often reported that is needed to establish a practice, let alone provide an income for self and family, without a referral source.

It is fair to assume that a therapist gets referrals because he or she has a unique quality that stands out in the mind of the person who is making the referral. This uniqueness may or may not be related to competence. The uniqueness may be the geographical location of one's office, the fee charged, or with whom one had lunch recently. No matter how one gets referrals, the issue of generating them is of ongoing concern in both beginning and maintaining a practice.

Where do referrals come from? In a 1981 survey of clinical social workers (Kelly & Alexander, 1985), 84 percent of the respondents (part-time private practitioners) indicated informal referral sources including former clients, word of mouth, friends and students, whereas only 41 percent of the respondents cited professional individuals as a referral source. Professional individuals included other therapists, clergy, attorneys, and social workers. Other sources of referral for these respondents included the medical profession (32 percent), social service and community organizations (21 percent) and the yellow pages (12 percent). Other research (Woodard, 1984) shows over 50 percent of referrals for psychologists coming from current or former patients and their families and friends.

Sturdivant (1987) supports the concept of a broad-based referral network: "how many referral sources you have is more important than how many referrals you receive from any one of them." He lists as the primary referral sources consumers who use your service, self-referrals and referrals from friends and former and current clients. This is consistent with research data cited above.

Sturdivant (1987b) also discusses the necessity of developing an effective marketing plan for generating better quality referrals, for expanding one's referral network, and for maintaining and servicing one's existing network. Part of the strategy in developing such a referral base involves effectively saying, in a variety of ways and formats, what you can do, then doing what you say, and communicating both in ways and places where it can be heard by others. Disseminating clear and accurate information in ways, places and times that people can hear will go far in eliminating barriers and generating referrals. People have to know that you want referrals.

This chapter will examine a variety of ways to generate clients, with detail sufficient for the practitioner to select and implement methods seen as most appropriate for one's individual circumstances.

GENERATING CLIENTS
THROUGH THE MASS MEDIA

The American Psychological Association Code of Ethics (1979) expanded the scope of advertising, and at the same time established limits. For example, quoting clients' laudatory statements, making appeals to fears, statements likely to create false or unjustified expectations of favorable results, all exceed limits established by the APA. Since that time, practitioners have increasingly expanded yellow page advertising, and have experimented with ads of various types and kinds, from classified to block to feature stories to press releases announcing upcoming events, and including public service announcements (PSAs).

Despite possible dislike for and embarrassment at using them, advertisements may help get a practice started in a new community. One approach that may help therapists in designing, constructing and using ads includes aiming at a particular type of client, i.e., adolescents, single parents, or couples, with a view toward filling an appointment book with the type of person you wish to serve without waiting for word of mouth. Another consideration is to stipulate your expertise. In addition, ads might be useful to help one get established quickly in a new geographic area, or when one's practice needs a shot in the arm. Things that can't be put into ads include self-aggrandizing statements, references to past performances, guarantees of therapy outcomes, appeals to fear and use of names or affiliations that may be misleading.

The major mass media sources include TV, radio and newspapers. Not to be overlooked are local and community newspapers, as well as throw-aways. Major newspapers will usually take classified or block advertisements for which you pay. The biggest challenge here is to comply with professional ethics and use discretion when marketing yourself. These same papers may be receptive to Public Service Announcements (PSAs), to press releases on seminars, workshops or other special events, such as the appearance in the community of a prominent speaker. To increase the probability of success with this approach there are specific ways to catch the attention of the newspaper editor who will make the decision about which requests to get into print. Local and community papers are often more receptive to such information if the event is to be held within the community served by the paper. They may also like human interest articles, such as how a person copes with the trauma of a disaster such as an earthquake or plane crash, or how to combat the pressures and stresses of major holidays. Letters to the editor regarding some community, political, or other event that is of wide appeal to the readership is another way of getting one's name before both the editor and the public.

It may be helpful to contact the city editor directly, provide him or her with a copy of your brochure or a reprint of an article you have published, and discuss briefly your special interests, bearing in mind the editor's busy schedule, and the fact that he or she is more interested in capturing attention of readers than in furthering your entrepreneurial interests. Human interest reporters and talk show hosts, in addition to city editors, may be interested in receiving a letter from you outlining your credentials, your areas of special interest and expertise, and topics about which you could speak effectively. A letter asking for an in-person interview to discuss being a resource and news source meets some of your needs for exposure and the potential for meeting some needs of the interviewer/editorial writer as well.

Keeping these editorial contacts current by sending them your periodic newsletters will provide them a regular source of information on timely topics as well as remind them of your service. Give them permission to reprint material you provide, giving credit to you and complete information about how you can be contacted.

Shery (1984) advertises the availability of prepared ads for generating self-referrals through the media. Prepared ads such as these may have the advantage of being readily available to you without having to create your own. They will probably also minimize the risk of exceeding legal and ethical concerns regarding this kind of advertising.

Many of the guidelines for getting one's name into the press apply also for TV and radio exposure. Richards (1987a) presents a format along with specific suggestions for getting free media exposure, including a sample letter to the station manager, and guidelines for PSAs, press releases, with a sample of each.

When there is a response from the media to your contact, it is imperative to be available for an interview. This may concern some phase of mental health and psychotherapy, or address a socially relevant issue, such as spouse abuse/child abuse, biofeedback, hypnosis, or some other topic on which you, of course, are an expert.

Hendrickson & Fraze (1986) raise a question about self-solicitation of clients by pursuing exposure through the mass media, and suggest that one should respond only if approached. Offering one's self to the media, however, when done within the bounds of professionalism, seems to be a legitimate and potentially effective way to generate referrals through the resulting exposure. Woodard (1984) reports that self-referral increased substantially through a high visibility media relations program, and supports the idea of an aggressive public awareness campaign. One way to get exposure from the media is simply to call local TV and radio stations, identify the producer, and introduce yourself. Be prepared to talk about how people deal with change and events that may be current—a particular holiday, school transition, or natural disaster.

It is useful to keep several prints of a glossy photo readily available to accompany a press release, or to give an organization that is sponsoring a speech or presentation by you, and encouraging that organization to do a press release.

REACHING CLIENTS
THROUGH THE YELLOW PAGES

When setting up in private practice and installing telephone service, one is almost always confronted with decisions regarding directory listings. Should one list in the yellow pages in addition to the white pages, and, if so, how? By single line name or by ad? By name or by specialty? By individual name and/or group name? With red ink or black? Under "Psychologist" or under some other heading? Under some other heading in addition to, or instead of? A single line name of the practitioner is less likely to produce self-referrals than an "ad" for some specialty or the name of a group. A name only listing in the yellow pages does not mean much to a person who does not know how to select a therapist or where to begin, and who is often, if not usually confused and overwhelmed by the endless columns of names. This writer experienced a dramatic upswing in self-referrals from yellow pages when he placed a specialization listing instead of the usual listing of his name. At best, the name listing seems to be useful in locating an individual whose name is already known. That in itself may be valuable enough to pay extra for multiple entries.

To list under "Psychologists," or under "Marriage Counselors," may present another decision, depending upon the nature of one's specialties and the kind of clientele one is seeking. Richards (1987) gives specific guidelines for developing a yellow page ad including the size of the ad, the name of the group, legal and ethical issues around listing services provided by you or the group.

Do's and don'ts in designing yellow page ads to attract new clients are also discussed by Browning & Browning (1986). They make a strong case for the use of in-column trademark listings over extra display ads on the free yellow page listings. They discuss issues of credibility, the name of one's practice, red-ink option for ads, the use of a Logo, listings that draw the most attention, and why yellow page listings are the most preferred marketing tool, if done correctly.

In general, guidelines for yellow page advertising operate on the premise that a single listing is better than none, as oftentimes people (referral sources) will use the yellow pages to look up addresses and phone numbers by name. Additional suggestions include researching the kinds of yellow page advertising that works in one's own location, without serious attention to the claims of ad salespeople. Other areas for decision include the section(s) in which to list, the use of display ads, cost concerns, the use of headlines, interfacing with your telephone system, and the concern over what colleagues will think.

Psychotherapy Finances (1984) elaborates on advertising issues and in a later issue addresses seven specific questions regarding getting the most for one's advertising dollar, including turning telephone calls into office visits. The use of private yellow page directories such as those published by the military, by special interest groups within the community such as religious organizations, and by community, commercial or business groups, is discussed by Browning & Browning (1986).

In a survey of doctoral level psychologists (Inman, 1983) it was shown that 7 percent of the responding psychologists reported yellow pages as very important, 16 percent as moderately important, and 77 percent as of little importance. In sharp contrast, the most important source of referrals for private practitioners was one's own patients, current and former (88 percent of the responding psychologists reported this, while another 26 percent reported patients as moderately important, for a total of 94 percent of the respondents). No discussion was presented of the many variables involved in yellow page advertising which may have affected these findings.

It is suggested that careful thought be given to if and how to utilize yellow pages, with reference to how other mental health practitioners in the geographic area advertise their services. Any use of yellow page directories should probably be designed as an advertising source rather than a simple listing. Consult also with the publishers of the directory, being careful here to separate professional advice from sales pitches. Be aware that this kind of advertising can be quite expensive, minimally $50 to $75 per month, and easily up to several hundred dollars, depending upon the size of the ad.

REACHING CLIENTS THROUGH THE MAIL AND THE USE OF MAILING LISTS

Another way to gain and maintain exposure for one's name is through the use of mailings to previous, current and potential consumers and to viable referral sources. This will require constantly building and updating of one's mailing lists to community organizations and agencies, mental health and related agencies, related professionals, and to individuals. The yellow page directories, with its different categories of agencies and professions, along with community directories provided by the Chamber of Commerce and the Visitor's Bureau, can provide invaluable sources. Professional directories can also be extremely useful for specific groups, for example, attorneys or ministerial associations. These are usually available through the city or regional associations or from the specific group. Individual lists can be generated from recent workshop participants, people who call or write for information, and people who attend lectures or other presentations. This is easily facilitated when registration is required, thereby providing you with names and addresses. These lists can be expanded by getting new names of interested people from current workshop participants, or inviting attendees at a speech or other presentation to provide names and addresses of people who may be interested in receiving copies of handouts used, announcements of future workshops, a copy of your brochure, or other information, such as your periodic newsletter. It is helpful to have a form readily available for people to provide complete and correct information on names and addresses. Along with any such mailing one should enclose two business cards, one for the recipient to keep and one to pass on to someone else.

Enclosing a brochure, newsletter, and/or cards in every piece of mail leaving your office is another way to make the mail do double duty for you. Any mailings should be of decent quality; they speak for you before you have a chance to speak for yourself. It may be difficult to overcome a negative first impression created by cheap-looking materials. Exercise care in using computer generated addresses and correspondence so that a personal touch is present to whatever extent is appropriate. Handwritten materials are discouraged, even for envelope addresses, as they lack the professional appearance one would expect of a first class organization.

The concept of a periodic newsletter emanating from one's office has received considerable attention in the literature on private practice. The use of a periodic newsletter reportedly reaps rewards in terms of new referrals and self-referral returns (for tune-ups) that substantially offset the expense of printing, publishing, and mailing. These newsletters can also be distributed to the media, often resulting in invitations for interviews or presentations. This chain of events greatly expands one's visibility, and increases the probability of yet further exposure and more referrals. This writer made numerous TV and radio appearances and granted several radio and newspaper interviews, as the result of periodic mailings of press releases announcing upcoming workshops, and enclosing brochures with a cover letter. It should also be mentioned that he had done his homework by attending media-conducted workshops on the preparation of press releases prior to mailing his first one.

Subscribing to one of several services providing prepared newsletters which would go out on one's own letterhead can save a great amount of time that would go into generating quality letters. Prepared letters are available through Growth and Leadership Consultants (1451 Grant Rd., Suite 102, Mountain View, CA 94040, 415–966–1144) and from Human Services, Inc. (4514 Travis, Suite 305, Dallas, TX 95205, toll free 1–800–873–2034).

Clarke (1985) discusses in detail the use of the mails specifically to generate and maintain a physician referral base. While many view a physician referral base with little optimism, the concepts presented by Clarke (1985) can be adapted to almost any professional group one sees as a viable and potential referral source. These professional groups, in addition to physicians, may include attorneys, particularly domestic relations attorneys for custody evaluations, and defense attorneys for serving as expert witnesses; dentists; for one with special offerings in pain or anxiety control; clergy; special educational groups such as school psychologists, school counselors, and administrators. Professional services such as Vocational Rehabilitation, SSI (Disability Evaluations), insurance companies for Employee Benefits (EBI) where assessment is often required as part of determining insurance benefits, and adoption agencies, particularly public ones, can all be strategized utilizing and/or adapting Clarke's model.

THE USE OF A BROCHURE
FOR REACHING CLIENT REFERRALS

Should one invest the time and money in designing and printing a brochure? What should and should not be included in a brochure? What are some of the benefits of a brochure? What kind of distribution should a brochure have? How can one assess his or her needs for a brochure? The bottom line answer to the above questions is "if it will generate referrals." Browning and Browning (1986) discuss these and other questions, along with providing specific suggestions for designing a brochure that brings in referrals. They provide concrete examples of comparisons between ineffective and effective brochures, including the technical aspects of design, format, and printing. The importance of this is stressed, as "you never get a second chance to make a first impression." The importance of professionalism and attractiveness of any brochure articulating your focus cannot overemphasized.

Equally important is that one follow closely the ethical guidelines of the profession, and any professional organizations to which one belongs, in deciding the contents of a brochure, or any printed material representing one's practice. Any promotional literature must be an accurate representation of what one does with no false claims. Facts can be stated interestingly. For example, pose a question and then provide the answer. Whatever is printed should represent excellence and quality.

Ways in which products of this quality can be utilized include being displayed and available to office clients and included in all office mailings of billings and correspondence. Carry some in your briefcase at all times for those unexpected contacts and networking opportunities on airplane flights or business or civic meetings. Collecting business cards at parties, meetings, on flights, or any other opportunity, and following up with a mailing of a brochure and/or your newsletter is another way to get one's name out there where it can generate referrals. One should always have a supply of these brochures at any out-of-office speech, workshop, seminar he or she does, and announce they will be available in the back of the room after the meeting, or make some arrangements for their distribution.

REACHING CLIENTS
IN BUSINESS AND INDUSTRY

Tapping the vast populations employed in business and industry has been the fantasy of many therapists. They see a large pool of referrals, but often are stymied when it comes to determining how to generate referrals from the population. Typical sources of contact include the personnel director, the Director of the Employee Assistance Program (EAP), if one exists, or the Director of Human Services or Human Resources, and union officials. Often referrals are made by persons in those positions for personal or social problems when job performance is affected. The rise of EAPs has resulted in many businesses and industries establishing their own "internal" EAP, where time-limited services are offered and then referrals are made to outside agencies or practitioners, oftentimes with third party payments (insurance coverage). Other EAP arrangements sometimes include an external arrangement, one in which the corporation or business has contracted with an independent agency external to the business to provide time-limited mental health consultative services to its employees.

Many of the same essentials apply in accepting an EAP referral as in accepting a referral from any other source. These include appropriate acknowledgement to the referrer, respect of confidentiality to the supervisor or employer, and clarity prior to accepting a referral about expectations regarding feedback. Keeping the referral source knowledgeable about your location, services, fees and providing this referral source copies of promotional literature (brochures, newsletters, announcements of upcoming workshops and presentations) and the occasional business lunch are important considerations.

An alternative to establishing oneself as a referral resource for therapeutic work is to become involved as a business consultant. It is viable to skillfully apply the concepts of family systems therapy, for example, to staff relation issues in the business setting. To do this requires that one be adept at making these applications, and that one be clear, articulate and charismatic in presenting oneself in defining and describing one's product (which is you and your service). It is essential that one know what he or she is doing, and move with confidence in doing it. Issues related to establishing oneself as a business consultant, as well as qualifications for being a therapist, include: having some business experience in order to understand the business culture; training in family therapy, as troubled business relations seem to have dynamics parallel to troubled family relationships; therapy skills enabling one to enhance an interpersonal relationship perspective as compared with a typical straightline causality mode of thinking so common to business; and specialized training and/or expertise in organizational development work.

Contacting management consulting firms, legal and accounting firms, and business associations like the National Family Business Council, may lead directly to referrals or inclusion on published lists of resources available to members. Speaking to local business groups is an effective way to attract referrals by demonstrating your specialized knowledge.

For more information on working with business, write to: OD Network, 1011 Park Avenue, Plainfield, New Jersey 07060. International Certified Consultants maintains a certification program; write to Ed Bartec, P.O. Box 1625, Station B, Nashville, Tennessee 37235.

Group training, individual therapy and other ways to get referrals from the Federal Government may be of special interrest to psychotherapists who practice near areas of large federal employment. While federal agencies cannot pay for psychotherapy, they often have insurance coverage which provides third party payments to private practitioners. An agency's employee coordinator (Employee Counseling Service Coordinator, Drug & Alcohol Abuse Coordinator, or a similar title) will be an appropriate contact for getting one's name on the list of psychotherapists available for referral.

If your interest is in providing training in a group setting, with the objective of developing a more effective employee, the Federal Office of Personnel Management in Washington, D.C. can provide information. The thousands of civilian federal employees across the country provide ready sources of referrals, if one can get access to them.

TELEPHONE SERVICES
AS A MEANS OF GENERATING REFERRALS

Separate from the use of the telephone directory yellow pages is the use of the telephone to provide various kinds of tape recorded message services. These have the potential for generating significant client referrals. Included in this category are services such as "Psychline," "Client-eze," "Tel-Med," and other tape system services, in which the caller can request to listen to a prepared tape message on any of a number of clinical topics. The developers of those systems report significant success in the development and success of their practices, as well as providing a worthwhile public service, with this strategy. Information on these systems can be obtained from the following addresses:

> Dr. Michael Shery
> Associated Psychotherapists of Colorado
> 1140 Pearl Street
> Boulder, Colorado 80302
> (303) 442–7192

> Lawrence R. Weathers, Ph.D. (Re: Client-eze tapes)
> W. 227 24th Ave.
> Spokane, Washington 99203
> (509) 838–8473

> Tel-Med (Re: Tel-Med tapes)
> 952 S. Mt. Vernon
> Colton, California 92324
> (714) 825–6034

Other telephone services which have been tried and are currently used by some include counseling by telephone, actually providing direct services by the therapist over the telephone. One must very carefully evaluate ethical and legal considerations for this approach to marketing and generating referrals and the commercialization of professional services.

TELEPHONE SYSTEMS AND REFERRALS:
RESOLVING TECHNOLOGICAL REALITIES

A potential source of trouble in generating client referrals may be inadequate telephone service for one's office. It is imperative that sufficient lines be available to handle one's telephone traffic. There are several ways to insure that lines are available so referrals can reach one's office without getting busy signals or, worse yet, no response. Reserving one line exclusively for incoming calls, staggering staff schedules so the therapists do not tie up the available lines every hour on the hour, are two options.

There has been considerable debate over whether an answering machine or an answering service is preferable. There are problems with each—yet many practitioners will, in reality, not have the financial underwriting necessary to support a full time person in the office to answer the telephone, so a decision regarding machine vs. service will be necessary. In addition, one will have to be concerned about telephone accessibility while in session or when away from the office. The use of an answering service seems to have more merit than the use of a machine. The human being on the receiving end of a call as compared with a taped message can mean a lot to a distraught caller whose frustration can be exacerbated by reaching a machine instead of a person. A human voice, even a minimum wage worker at an answering service, is probably more welcome than a taped message. In addition, answering service staff can be trained in ways of responding to callers, can be given specific instructions regarding therapist availability on special occasions (vacations, while out of office at conferences or away for an evening), and can be given instructions for emergency coverage and referral. At any rate, establishing oneself as a therapist means being available (different people have varying definitions of availability) so being accessible to clients is essential. Accessibility by phone is equally essential in establishing and maintaining a referral source. The person making a referral will want to know how the referral is going to be received and treated, and will base their assessment of your level of professionalism in part on their experience with your telephone system.

Clarke (1985) presents a detailed plan for using telephone contacts to establish and maintain a physician referral base. This model can be adapted to virtually any group viewed as a potential referral source.

REACHING CLIENTS
THROUGH THE COMMUNITY

The community is where people—your potential clients—live, work, and function. Potential referral sources live, work, and function there also. Reaching both potential clients and potential referral sources through community visibility is the key to building a private practice. Approaches include giving speeches and presentations, and conducting seminars and workshops. Appearing before groups is an essential ingredient of community visibility. Making these appearances on a courtesy basis, without remuneration, may pay off in free exposure and public relations value. It is not at all uncommon to have a self-referral weeks and even months following a presentation. Sometimes a referral will come because someone who heard you referred a friend or family member.

The list of available communiuty agencies and potential resources available to the practitioner as possible referral sources is virtually endless. Yellow page directories, business directories, convention and visitors bureau directories, speakers bureaus, the Better Business Bureau, and service club directories are several places to start identifying potential groups. The Chamber of Commerce can also provide lists of potential groups. If one has contacts in the educational community, appearing as a guest speaker in a class, whether public schools, community colleges, or upper division or graduate level, may lead to referrals. Private schools and technical training institutes may be receptive to presentations on topics such as test-taking anxiety, test-taking skills, dealing with phobias, study skills and habits, or how to achieve academic success.

Teaching a course through a community college, university, or community-based alternative education program may not provide many dollars directly, but the self-referrals from the classroom contact, and the "free" publicity through the course description in bulletin and flyers, can pay off tremendously. Doing a guest presentation in someone else's class is another way to go. This writer has received several long-term referrals from such appearances, including some people not in the class, but referred by a class member.

Service clubs and other organizations often looking for speakers include Kiwanis, Rotary, PTA, YMCA, boys or girls clubs, Boy or Girl Scouts, labor unions, Junior Forum, newcomers clubs, church singles groups, sorority/fraternity alumnae groups, police and sheriff's departments, probation, juvenile justice system, free clinics, telephone hot lines, fraternal organizations, community mental health centers, adolescent residential/treatment programs, and self-help groups (Parents Without Partners, Parents Anonymous). There are some very real limits on speaking to some self-help groups, such as AA, which believes that therapists should keep out of the picture and not destroy the self-help image.

Hendrickson & Fraze (1986) discuss offering workshops that would benefit the legal/judicial systems, i.e., workshops for those with drunk-driving charges. The American Psychological Association (1986) discusses strategies for impacting the courts, both civil and criminal, to serve as an expert witness, to assess sanity and fitness to stand trial, to enter a plea, to be sentenced, or to be executed. Civil court involvement may involve competency petitions for purposes of guardianship, disability determinations, expert witness and testimony in medical and mental health malpractice litigation, divorce proceedings, or child custody evaluations. The latter may include comprehensive evaluation of all immediate family members as well as some extended family members. Many states have crime victims' compensation funds that provide for psychological services to individuals who are victims of crimes. The State Attorney General's office, or the State's attorney in the local county of residence would be a place to access information.

Once some potential groups have been identified, bearing in mind your own expertise, select one or two speech topics, and write a letter outlining these topics to each organization, offering to speak to them. Tailor each letter specifically to the organization you are writing. Follow up with a telephone call to be sure the letter reached the appropriate person, and to determine which topic has the greatest appeal. In the letter or in the follow-up call, offer to meet in their office to talk, to meet with the Board of Directors, with the staff, or with whomever is appropriate. Tell them you are available for speeches, lectures, panels, or workshops on specified topics. Enclose a brochure, newsletter, and business cards.

In this discussion, it is imperative that you have the name of the director or administrator of any agency contacted, with some information about that person and the position. It is useful to develop a card file or some other means of systematizing agency information, including name, address, telephone number, contact person, dates, and nature of contacts. It is also necessary to show your ability to produce—to speak effectively and articulately on your fields of expertise and the agreed upon topic, and that you are able to articulate your offerings, specialization, and limitations. Be prepared to address issues such as type of therapy offered, approaches to treatment, fees, business arrangements, confidentiality, hospitalization, medication, and follow-up procedures. These kinds of presentations are seen as a key to generating referrals. Here are some tips for enhancing effectiveness and success in presentations (Browning & Browning, 1986):

1. Be personal. Make an effort to speak to people individually, rather than as a group.

2. Try to make eye contact with as many people as possible.

3. When appropriate, use your own life experience to illustrate a point.

4. Use vivid anecdotes and analogies to help create mental pictures that captivate an audience.

5. Be concrete. Give one good example to support each point.

6. Use an outline. This will make your speech more informal and natural than if you read a presentation word for word.

7. Project enthusiasm.

8. Handout brochures, newsletters and the like.

9. Use audio or visual aids (lecture no more than 70 percent of your allotted time).

10. End a presentation with group involvement; have a question and answer period, use a questionnaire, role playing, or a demonstration.

Richards (1987) presents an excellent discussion of the specifics of planning and conducting workshops for the community, including details of Public Service Announcements, and the preparation and use of handouts. Conducting workshops provides an opportunity for the public to have a sample of your work. It is a way to promote oneself ethically and in a quality fashion. If people like the sample they may want more and refer themselves, or refer others.

This writer's experience has been that workshops often produce a high frequency of immediate self-referrals. Also, it is not unusual for self or other referrals to come weeks or even months after a workshop.

Let it be said that any such workshop must be first class. It must be mentally stimulating and interesting, and emotionally touching. Attention must be given to the participants, so watch the tempo, pacing, and balance of didactic and participation/experiential. A very real benefit of conducting workshops is that it provides an opportunity for diversity and variety for the therapist, and can indeed be good therapy itself. Usually the fees provide a little extra income as well.

If talking to groups, conducting workshops or seminars, or giving presentations before groups is not for you, perhaps talking with individuals is more palatable. There is often opportunity to share the kinds of things one does with individuals—at social events, business or professional events, or even while traveling. While it would be totally inappropriate to talk about clients or in any way violate a professional confidence, it is possible to talk about situations and how you have helped people cope with them. You can also discuss what you are learning to do, by describing your own participation in training workshops.

Cookerly and McClaren (1982) present several pointers for successful speaking which, while aimed primarily at speaking before groups, have applicability to personal contact as well. These include relating to one's work, the use of humor, making specific application for the listeners, being clear and forthright about the "advertisement," how to get connected for the speakers' circuit, having a list of credentials available for the host, and providing news releases covering your speech to the neighborhood paper. Doing it well, with excellence, means preparation and rehearsal, plus the use of handouts and brochures. Browning & Browning (1986) present a number of case studies showing how therapists attract new referrals and build upon a growing clientele.

In reality, being an effective therapist does not necessarily guarantee being an effective speaker or presenter to either large groups or individuals. One may wish to consider bringing in an "expert" from outside the community to do the speaking. There may be a friend, colleague, or other relationship upon which you can prevail, perhaps by paying expenses, or by sharing registration receipts. Sponsoring and featuring such an expert can lead to increased visibility, networking, and referrals.

REACHING CLIENTS
THROUGH THE PROFESSIONS

Specific professional groups that may have referral potential include physicians, dentists, nurses, school psychologists and counselors, clergy, and attorneys. Social service and professional agencies include vocational rehabilitation, family services, mediation services, employee assistance programs, SSI, PPOs, HMOs, EBI, and the academic community, as well as other therapists. Networking through these and others can often lead to valuable contacts and potential referrals. These professionals are likely to have access to a number of potential clients, and may be in a position to repeatedly refer clients to you.

Physicians

Establishing a viable referral base among physicians is probably wrought with more misperceptions than many other professional referral sources. Physicians tend to be difficult to reach. Potential opportunities for establishing contact may be with one's own physician, the physician of one's spouse or children, or a client's physician with whom you have been able to consult or for some reason establish a contact. Perhaps discussion can revolve around the physician's interest in receiving referrals from you. Establishing a basis for reciprocal referrals may prove beneficial for all persons concerned. Clarke (1985) presents a very comprehensive and detailed model for establishing a physician referral base, including forms and letters.

Making oneself available to local medical societies, for hospital staff meetings, to family practice residency programs, and to nurses associations will increase visibility, contribute to networking, and establish you in the mind of those in the medical profession as an available resource. Previous discussion regarding effective presentation of one's specialties pertain here as well.

Whether one is targeting physicians, clergy, or attorneys, establishing networks by capitalizing on the informality of meetings and other functions is extremely important. For example, one might get acquainted with physicians or attorneys through one's religious affiliation or through one's social circles. Attending events with someone you know who is a member of a professional group who will introduce you to other professionals can facilitate entry as well as provide networking opportunities.

To successfully cultivate medical referrals it is necessary to be well integrated into the medical community. This can be done through regular contact with physicians, being active on a hospital staff, and participating professionally, not only locally but on a statewide and national basis as well. As a part of a small group of professionals who see each other regularly, whether your own profession or a related field, others will become familiar with you and your work. Serving on committees and volunteering for task forces or community service will aid in this attempt to enter a professional circle. Further development of professional referral resources can be facilitated through reciprocity: "How can I assist you in your needs?"

Making contact with all other professionals in your building, both letting them know about your work and learning about theirs, can establish reciprocal referral networking. Provide these people with a brochure, a newsletter, and one of your business cards. In addition to their commitment and concern for competent, professional help for their patients or clients, they may also want some recognition, appreciation, and possibly reciprocity.

The Clergy

Wright (1984) contends that clergy are a potentially strong, yet underutilized, referral source. As reasons for a low referral rate, he cites perceived differences in values (psychotherapists often see religion as detrimental to an individual's mental health), lack of awareness of resources, the stigma attached to mental health resources by some, and financial concerns. Other reasons include pejorative notions by the psychiatric community about some members of the clergy, and the fact that clergy see the referral process as a one-way street; clergy seldom receive consultation reports from professionals to whom they give referrals.

In some communities clergy are inundated with contacts by therapists soliciting referrals. A common response seems to be one of resistance to allocating time out of busy schedules to a practitioner unknown to them. This is especially true if there are known, trusted and respected therapists within the congregation. A "testimonial" or referral by another clergy known to you can be extremely helpful.

Receiving and providing service to referrals from within one's own congregation may present some unique situations and challenges, as religious groups often have social events and informal occasions where one is more likely to encounter clients directly. Learning how to handle these situations, dealing with one's own comfort/discomfort, is necessary. Providing free services, per one's specialties, is viable for religious organizations. Speaking engagements, workshops, or seminars on topics of relevance and interest, such as suicide, grief/death, marriage/divorce, particularly with sensitivity to and respect for the religious tenets of the group, may be well received and may produce referrals.

Attorneys

Private practitioners may find the civil and criminal justice system a viable market, particularly if one conducts evaluations to determine competency to stand trial. These kinds of services are usually paid for directly by the court or by the defendant's attorney. Psychologists can function in divorce proceedings and child custody evaluations, which may include comprehensive evaluations of all immediate family members as well as some of the extended family members involved. Other areas in which a psychologist can be involved include testifying as an expert witness in medical and mental health malpractice litigation, in competency petitions for purposes of guardianship, and in disability determination. Attorneys also use psychologists to assist in dealing with clients who are experiencing a psychological disorder. Not to be overlooked is the psychologist's work with victims of crimes. The State Attorney General's office usually has funding available for these services. In some cases, an individual's insurance will provide reimbursement.

In developing the legal system as a referral source one should have specialized training in forensics, and should consider the harsh realities of testifying as an expert witness. Functioning in someone else's arena can be quite different from functioning in one's own professional space.

Other Mental Health Practitioners

One probably won't get referrals from practitioners with the same specialties who live and work in the same geographical area. It will probably pay off more to get to know professionals who don't do what you do, who don't have the same areas of expertise as you do, or who are geographically distant enough to not see you as a competitor. Professionals are more likely to refer to one with a specialty different from his or her own. At the same time, identification with other practitioners (psychiatric, social work) may have a positive referral value.

People who live in another locale will occasionally have an opportunity to refer someone in, or moving to, your area. The message? Network—at regional, state and national levels, through meetings, and conventions. Get listed in state and national directories. Become a member of professional organizations—locally, regionally, and nationally. Hold offices, get known, and get to know others outside your own geographical area. Recently, within the period of one week, this writer received a referral from Alaska, and was asked to make a referral for someone in the Los Angeles area. There have been other recent requests for referrals in three other states.

Mediation

This may be of interest, either for direct involvement as a mediator, as part of a mediation-therapy team, or simply as a referral resource. Family mediation is an expansion of divorce mediation, with training courses for membership in the Academy of Family Mediators. For further information write: The Academy of Family Mediators, Mary Thode, Executive Director, P.O. Box 4686, Greenwich, Connecticut 06830.

Dramatic developments with the last 10 years have included the emergence of Preferred Provider Organizations (PPOs) and Employee Assistance Programs (EAPs), along with Health Maintenance Organizations (HMOs). There are variations in the way each of these groups is organized, and in how a private practitioner can become affiliated for purposes of establishing a client base. Detailed and persistent research will be required to determine if such affiliation is right for you. Further information on PPOs can be obtained from AMCRA, 5410 Grosvenor Lane, Suite 210, Bethesda, Maryland 20814. Information about EAPs can be obtained from ALMACA, 1800 North Kent St., Suite 908, Arlington, Virginia 22209; and the National Council on Alcoholism, 12 West 21st Street, New York, New York 10010.

Rehabilitation

Most states provide evaluation and limited treatment services for individuals who are unable to work due to mental/emotional impairment, or due to physical disability with psychological concomitant. It may be necessary for psychologists to contact the state agency conducting the program and apply to become a vendor of services. A patient being seen by a psychologist and who does not have the resources to pay because of unemployment may be eligible through Vocational Rehabilitation. Insurance companies may pay for evaluation of auto injury or other cases through Employee Benefits Insurance. The Federal Social Security Disability Program (SSI) and the Federal Workers Compensation Program (FECA) reimburse psychologists for evaluations. Contact EBI, Vocational Rehabilitation, Social Security, or Workers Compensation office through your local telephone directory for further information.

ISSUES IN REFERRAL

Facilitating The Referral

Probably few therapists know with any degree of accuracy what percent of attempted referrals are successful. Potential referral sources may appreciate being told how you wish a referral to be made, in order to increase success in making the referral. One approach to aiding the referral process may be to provide the potential referral source several copies of any form you may use for a referral, along with a cover letter explaining how to use the form (Hendrickson & Fraze, 7).

In addition, follow-up any meeting or contact with a potential referral source with a letter of appreciation for their time, even if you are not optimistic about this contact developing into a viable source. Any attempt at contact, such as a call not being returned in response to a message you left, or an appointment cancelled or missed, should also be followed up with a letter acknowledging your attempt and a brief statement of your services. Brochures, newsletters, or reprints of publications could also be included, along with several business cards. That person's need or interest may change at some point in the future, and you may be just the referral needed.

When a referral is successfully made, i.e., the client makes an appointment and appears for it, immediate acknowledgement is appropriate. This may take the form of an individualized letter to the referrer, or a form letter, or a pre-printed card with matching envelope. After a professional/therapeutic relationship has been established it is essential to obtain a release of information signature from the client/patient before sending a letter to the referral source. This is necessary because the content of such a letter will probably address clinical issues, as compared with the mere acknowledgement and statement of appreciation which usually characterizes the initial response. The following suggestions are provided by Hendrickson & Fraze (1986) for the contents of such a letter. The letter should be brief and inform the referring person that the appointment was kept, the name of the therapist who will be seeing the client/patient, future expectations regarding frequency and regularity of appointments, an indication that a letter of progress will be sent in the future (if this is one's plan), and an expression of appreciation for the referral.

Use Of Current Clients

"If your clients know you want to reach more people they are often very happy to help. You just have to let them know what they can do." (Cookerly & McClaren, 17) Some would challenge, raise questions about, and in some cases flat out disagree with the appropriateness of this strategy. Each practitioner will have to resolve this issue for him or herself. Professionalism must be adhered to.

Receiving/Making Referrals
Through The Agency Of Your Employment

Often people in practice on a part-time basis may have an opportunity to refer to themselves through their place of employment, or to receive referrals from co-workers. Others may be in a position to receive referrals through agencies with whom they consult, as a result of their consultative activities. Educators may have an opportunity to accept students as clients. These situations may initially appear to present good sources of clients. A closer examination may present issues of boundaries and of duality of relationships, plus of confidentiality and conflict of interest. Kelley & Alexander (1985) discuss ethical concerns of generating and receiving referrals through an agency for which the practitioner may also work. Related issues include determining if one's agency affiliation should be listed in practice information sources. When agency affiliation exists, whether employment or consultative, agency and board approval, in writing, should probably be obtained.

Solo Or Group Practice

A multi-disciplinary group practice is viewed by many as providing more opportunities for internal referral than a same-specialty group, and obviously a different referral potential than a solo practice. For example, one person may see a couple for relationship problems. Their children are having school problems so you refer to the child specialist in the same group. One child has clinical problems so you refer to your psychodiagnostician. Another has weight problems so a referral is made to the hypnosis specialist for weight control, or to the eating disorders person in the group. These specialists, in turn, refer to you for marriage/relationship problems, your specialty.

A real bonus is the opportunity for impromptu consultation and collaboration in a group setting. This can help one avoid the isolation that is often reported by solo practitioners.

Professionalism and Professional Development

A therapist in private practice must be wholly and clearly accountable to one's self for his or her practice development. If something works in the development of the practice, and referrals are successful, the credit is due. Conversely, when things don't work the practitioner must also assume responsibility and accountability.

In addition to issues of generating referrals, related issues which contribute to practice success, both through the professional and business aspects of the practice, are case load review, creative thinking time, quality time with one's family and/or personal support network, R & R, staying in touch with the professional community and colleagues through lunch or local meetings, and sharpening one's business savvy.

The would-be successful private practitioner must become good at making a consistent, positive and professional impression. An honest, outgoing, confident, straightforward (but never overstated) approach seems to work best. It is important to be in a position to meet the public and potential referral sources.

Viewing professional, social, and community events as opportunities to network, it is important to convey an attitude of success and professionalism at all times. With little effort, one can learn to capitalize on one's own, as well as one's spouse/partner's, events as opportunities for networking. Issues of attitude, motivation, dress and personal/professional/business organization, are discussed in greater detail by Jantz (1986).

Generalist Or Specialist?

Another issue many practitioners will face is the extent to which one should present oneself as a specialist. A concern, especially as one attempts to get established in the world of private practice, is that clients may be missed if there is an impression that his or her particular problem is not included among your areas of specialty. Admittedly, there is a possibility of someone self de-selecting. Examination of many yellow page directory listings will reveal some practitioners who announce to the world that they can do everything for everyone; they do it all. Such people probably get the fewest referrals, as they raise questions of credibility, both with potential consumers as well as with potential referral sources.

It is more believable to all readers to have one or two specialties. Articulate and present specialization realistically, in terms that are acceptable to the public: your potential clients. Specialties should be easily identifiable and relevant, not excessively limiting.

Convenience

Being available to clients at their convenience, not yours, may help generate referrals. Atypical hours, such as late evening, early morning, or weekends, may be valuable for clients who work, who are frequently out of town, and may possibly be functional and attractive for the therapist who is fully employed and starting a part-time practice. Having an accessible location is important, as is providing clear, easy-to-follow directions. Calling clients/patients a day ahead of scheduled appointments as a reminder may reduce no-show rates. You may consider not using your title if you leave a message (just leave first and last name), "I'm calling to confirm my meeting...," or "to remind _____ of our meeting tomorrow," or "to let _____ know I'm still planning to get together tomorrow." It may be important to the client that the nature of this appointment not be known in the work place and in some cases even at their home.

SUMMARY

This chapter has addressed a variety of topics related to generating referrals for one's private practice. The overall message is that a variety of populations, approaches and strategies exist, and that it is possible to utilize a variety of approaches and strategies to successfully establish referral sources. Implicit throughout is the idea that if a private practice is left to happen, it probably won't. But it can be made to happen. Implicit also is the importance of quality—doing whatever one does well, and doing it right. There is no room for anything else.

REFERENCES

Browning, C., & Browning, B. (1986). *Private Practice Handbook* (3rd Edition). Duncliffs International: Los Alamitos, CA.

Clarke, C. (1985). *How to build a physician referral base.* Referral Base Publications.

Cookerly, J., & McClaren, K. (1982). *How to increase your private practice power.* The Center for Counseling and Developmental Services, Inc.: Fort Worth, TX.

Hendrickson, D., & Fraze, J. (1986). *How to establish your own independent practice* (5th Edition). Accelerated Development, Inc.: Muncie, IN.

Inman, D., and Bascue, L. (1983). Referral sources of psychologists in private practice. *Psychological Reports,* 52, 865–866.

Jantz, G. (1986). *From ground zero: A creative private-practice handbook.* The Center for Counseling and Health Resources: Edmonds, WA.

Kelley, P., & Alexander, P. (1985). Part-time private practice: Practical and ethical considerations. *Social Work,* May–June: 254–258.

Marketing psychological services: A practitioner's guide. American Psychological Association: Washington, DC, 1986.

Psychotherapy Finances. 11(7)3–5, July 1984.

Psychotherapy Finances. 12(11)4, November 1985.

Richards, D. D. (1987a). Getting free radio exposure. *Private Practice News,* September, 1(9)13–14.

Richards, D. (1987b). Getting your name in print. *Private Practice News,* August, 1(8)10–23.

Richards, D. (1987c). The yellow pages—an essential part of your marketing approach. *Private Practice News,* May, 1(5)1–4.

Richards, D. (1987d). Using free presentations to attract prospective clients. *Private Practice News,* September 1(9)8–10.

Shery, M. (1984). *150 more patients a year with four simple ads.* Marketing Program, Associated Psychotherapists of Colorado, 2111 30th Street, Suite E, Boulder, CO 80301, (3)3 442–7382.

Sturdivant, S. (1987a). Building a referral network. *Private Practice News,* May, 1(5)5–7.

Sturdivant, S. (1987b). Marketing principles for counselors. *Private practice News,* June, 1(6)11–12.

Woodard, B. (1984). Offering free preventive mental health information as a means of generating patient self-referrals. *Marketing For Mental Health Services.* The Haworth Press: 83–90.

Wright, P. (1984). The counseling activities and referral practices of Canadian clergy in British Columbia. *Journal of Psychology and Theology,* 12(4): 294–304.

13

REFERRAL BY SPECIALTY

Richard N. Gevirtz, Ph.D.

Increasingly, psychologists are developing specialized areas of expertise. As this trend continues to gain momentum, information on promoting referrals for clients with problems in a specialty area is of interest to experienced and new practitioners alike. The present chapter examines the general principles in gaining referrals by specialty and uses one specific area (behavioral medicine) as an example.

DECIDING ON A SPECIALTY

The trend toward specialization in psychology has been discussed widely. Although arguments exist that the specialization movement will not best promote psychology, most practitioners are moving toward an identity beyond that of "general practitioner." This has the effect of opening new markets where psychologists have not been traditionally recognized. For this reason, most early specialists have had to pave their own way in getting referrals.

Most private practitioners begin choosing a specialty in graduate school but few do this as a formal process. In fact, the actual identity as a specialist is rarely made as a conscious decision, but evolves. One might take a neuropsychology sequence in graduate school but only become interested when completing a rotation on an internship. Or one might find that he or she is seeing a predominance of clients with eating disorders, and after further reading, professional workshops, and so on, begin to identify oneself as an eating-disorders specialist.

There are two important points to keep in mind when considering specialization: secure training that is appropriate for your field and acknowledge your ability to serve clients in that clinical area.

At one extreme we have all seen practitioners with limited training or experience simply declare themselves experts in biofeedback, neuropsychology, eating disorders, child therapy, chemical dependency, or some other special area. This is professionally and ethically unwarranted and these individuals should be gently confronted (as per American Psychological Association (APA) ethical guidelines). At the other extreme are practitioners with a great deal of experience, many workshops, extensive reading, and so forth, who do not feel qualified because they did not do postdoctoral studies at Stanford, Harvard, Yale or some other prestigious institution. Many in this group have a great deal to offer but have not felt justified in promoting themselves. A bit of advice: get an adequate amount of training and experience but then do not discount yourself. Some of the biggest research names in every specialty are ineffective clinicians. Clients do not care about your reputation in professional societies. They want caring, skilled professionals who are themselves good people. You may be the best possible clinician for your clients.

CHOOSING REFERRAL SOURCES

For those who do move toward specialization, it is crucial that you identify possible referral sources and begin a strategy to make yourself known to them.

Do not identify referral sources on the basis of theory. Find out where the referrals *actually* come from. Consider the example of a colleague who did postdoctoral work in cardiovascular health psychology and set up a practice in that specialty. He reasoned that since there were a million people in his city, at least 16 percent, or 160,000, were hypertensive. If only 1 percent of the hypertensives in his city were referred, he would be swamped. One year later he had received only two referrals for hypertension (one of which was full fee). In actuality, cardiologists and general practitioners do not often refer hypertensives to private practitioners.

To obtain accurate information concerning referral sources, call similar specialists in several other cities and ask precisely where their referrals come from. Here it pays to be assertive and to obtain concrete information, not generalities. For example, a colleague might say, "I get most of my child custody cases from lawyers." He or she might not say that the three target referring lawyers are friends or relatives. Try to pin down the kind of *networks* that really produce referrals. Almost all referrals do come from networking.

FORMULATING A MARKET STRATEGY

Professional Sources

Once you have a realistic idea of where the professional referral sources exist, begin a slow, persistent campaign to make yourself known to these sources. Solid, measured opinions and gentle persuasion from personal contacts generally will work better for you than a hard sell.

Most professionals (M.D.'s, lawyers, other mental health professionals) have much more allegiance to their clients than to you. They want the best person for their clients. Your expertise will not be communicated by a slick brochure and five-color business cards. Instead, the impression that you really care about people, are very competent in what you do, are well organized, and are thorough in your work speaks strongly. Try to find or develop a forum to meet these referral sources at which your best personal traits can shine through.

The General Public

1. Group presentations and community service. In most specialties, ample opportunities exist to speak to the general public. It is important to be pa-

tient in this endeavor. Most practitioners report that there is a fairly low initial return on their time. However, over time, name recognition increases and a critical mass is achieved. Referral sources hear about you a few times and decide to investigate. Keep active in any community service outlet for your interest. It is a good thing to do, in and of itself, and it will eventually pay off.

2. Media. When seeking print or electronic media exposure, here are some hints to keep in mind:

- Phone in ideas for articles or stories but always follow up with a written article,
- Present yourself as quotable and entertaining; avoid scientific jargon at first.
- Try to find clients with whom you were successful and who are willing to do testimonials for the story or interview (identities can be easily protected.
- Seek to make contacts with specific reporters.
- If you appear on a call-in show, ask a friend to call in one question that you want asked. Plan to stay after the show if more calls keep coming.
- Most reporters will privately forward your address or phone number to inquiries after the show.
- Ask for a readback to check for inaccuracies and misquotes. Do not ask to edit the article, however, as most media personnel will not comply and will see it as a "pushy" request.

PROFESSIONAL IDENTITY

Keep yourself active in professional societies that deal with your specialty. If none exist, start a local chapter (AABT, AAMFT, AAPB, state society, etc.). It is your ethical duty to keep up with the literature in your field. Beyond this, it establishes you as one of the identified specialists in this area. Newspapers, magazines, television programs, and radio stations seek experts through these networks. Often, university-based psychologists make referrals in this way. Identify yourself as a scientist/practitioner within psychology and use this as a strength.

Behavioral Medicine as an Example of These Principles

The general principles described can be illustrated through my own specialty, behavioral medicine. In talking to specialists in other areas, I have discovered a general commonality in overall goals and strategies. It is my hope that the following examples presented below can be of use to professionals in behavioral medicine and as a model for those in other clinical areas.

Health psychology or behavioral medicine has become the fastest growing subspecialty area in psychology. Division 38 (Health Psychology) of the APA has experienced rapid growth in the past five years. Many experts estimate a bright future for practitioners in this area (Matarazzo, 1980, 1982).

Referrals in behavioral medicine, as in most areas, can be divided into two components: (1) referrals from the lay public, and (2) referrals from other health-care professionals. Much can be done to increase the psychologist's visibility in both areas.

The Public at Large

The public is largely unaware of available services within behavioral medicine. Furthermore, many procedures with substantial scientific support are badly misunderstood by the average person. In addition, in the popular press behavior therapy is often associated with tyrannical control of behavior, biofeedback with altered states of consciousness, and relaxation training with meditation and religion. There still exists a "sixties" audience that wants to hear mind-over-matter parables, but this group comprises a small minority of the general public. In short, there is a critical need to correct common misinformation about the field.

When communicating with the public, practitioners often seek out friendly audiences. This has the effect of creating a separate "culture" for the acceptance of these services. In fact, it is really the larger population, from business people to engineers, who should be educated by behavioral medicine parctitioners. Successful practitioners must address this group.

Efforts to promote a behavioral medicine specialty should be targeted to these "tougher" audiences. In doing this, the psychologist must present himself or herself as a credible and critical model. To illustrate, the following is an example of a question from the audience: "Doctor, isn't it true that all illness is psychological?"

Possible responses: "Some people think that most illness is psychological." "All illness has a psychological component."

Better response (showing critical thinking skills): "No. Much of illness is not greatly affected by psychological factors. Here are the disorders for which we have solid scientific evidence to support this view. . . ."

The point is that some members of the audience would love to hear a simplistic, uncritical response, but in the long run, your reputation as a serious health-care professional will be better served by presenting yourself as a "tough-minded" health-care professional.

The corollary is that when you make statements about biofeedback for the treatment of neuromuscular disorders or in-vivo desensitization for agoraphobia, they are more likely to be believed. The attitude shift that seems to occur is, "I always thought that biofeedback was for people who wore love beads, but it is really now seen as an accepted treatment." This promotes the field as a whole, as well as you, the individual practitioner.

Audience Possibilities

Audiences love to see demonstrations. Even very simple devices can be great attention getters. Develop a slide or overhead show that emphasizes a few important ideas and *do not* say too much. Again, establish yourself as a credible source and stay away from a hard sell.

The opportunities to get your message across are numerous. Business groups are always looking for free talks on stress. Hospital auxiliaries usually need speakers, as do government groups and social service agencies, among others. If you have expertise in biofeedback (BCIA certification is helpful), always use it in your title.

Several biofeedback manufacturers offer press kits to assist you in approaching your local paper to do a human-interest or health-focus article on behavioral medicine. The reporters will usually not respond to direct offers from you, but will quickly follow up a lead from another professional. Involve yourself in networks, so that the health reporter hears of you, and then have material ready.

Usually, reporters need the interview "yesterday," so it is imperative that you guide the direction of the content as to what will be said. Directly ask what quotes might be used. Health professionals, especially psychologists and psychiatrists, are often misquoted. Be careful to speak in short, quotable sentences. For television, you can be sure that only 30-second blips will be used. The challenge is to get across the complexity of a disorder such as irritable bowel syndrome in 30 seconds. Typically, the professional talks to the interviewer for 15 minutes, carefully clarifying a point, only to hear an unrepresentative 30-second quote on the evening news health closeup. To avoid this, you must educate the reporter adequately.

If you have an opportunity to have a reporter participate in a sample treatment protocol, by all means take advantage of this. The resulting article will probably be worth its weight in gold.

Professional Referral Sources

Most referrals in behavioral medicine come from other health-care professionals, other psychologists, physicians, mental-health counselors, dentists, and attorneys. The challenge here is to get not just any referral, but an appropriate referral.

Much of what was stated above is applicable here. It is not effective to visit other health professionals to solicit referrals. Ask yourself if you would refer a client to anyone who took you to lunch and plied you with business cards.

Your referral sources generally want to send clients only to competent professionals. Your job, then, is to let other professionals become aware of your expertise.

Referrals are made by proximity. If you are perceived as competent or better, and are also in sight, you will get the referral. This means that attending medical grand rounds, professional-interest meetings, social clubs, and so on will help build your practice, if you persist long enough to be seen as a solid professional.

Do not try to make a "splash," but show your true colors whenever possible. In the end, you will be selected over a flashier alternative. Be prepared to stay at it for several years, though, if you expect this strategy to work. In this realm, as in most things in life, patience is the primary virtue.

Psychologists are unique among health-care professionals in having training in experimental research. Promote this perspective. You can still offer clinical insight, but label it as such. If you are seen as a likable and effective psychotherapist who is also a critical thinker, referrals will come your way.

It is often difficult to maintain a cognitive behavioral perspective in the face of pressure to offer psychodynamic interpretations for every patient who has not responded to traditional medical treatment. It is more effective, however, to touch only lightly on any theoretical perspective and to emphasize your concrete treatment plans.

For example, if a chronic-headache patient is sent by a neurologist who includes a critical analysis of the self-destructive nature of this patient, avoid arguing about the dynamics. Instead, outline a treatment plan that will overcome the pitfalls that the neurologist sees. If you begin to launch into a diatribe against object relations, you may lose this referral source.

Remember that many psychiatrists are actively promoting the superficiality of behavior medicine treatment modalities to their medical colleagues. While not always popular among medical specialties, psychiatry does influence the average physician's perspective. Its influence, then, must be recognized, respected, and, where appropriate, challenged.

A valuable role that psychologists can play in this context is as a liaison between medical personnel with limited time and the patient who wants more information. You might spend the better part of an hour visit clarifying the various treatments being used. When this happens, be sure to report back to your medical colleagues so that they can appreciate this valuable service. Often patients rate this clarification and explanation role as the most important service rendered.

Special Issues Within Common Disorders for Behavioral Medicine

Headaches   Headaches are one of the most common medical complaints, comprising a large proportion of all medical referrals, and especially neurology consultations (Leviton, 1978). Medical treatments have not been completely satisfactory, and a great deal of iatrogenic disease has been reported (primarily through medication misuse) (Bakal, 1982).

Behavioral techniques, such as biofeedback and relaxation training, and cognitive/behavioral therapies have been shown to be successful in the treatment of both muscle contraction and vascular headaches (Bakal, 1982).

Despite a formidable database, however, behavioral techniques are only now gaining acceptance among medical personnel. More scientific evidence will probably be needed to overcome the "snake-oil" reputation that all non-pharmacological treatments seem to share. With increased credibility, however, the treatment of headaches by behavioral medicine specialists will represent a real growth area.

In generating referrals for treating headaches, it is necessary that you convince medical and dental professionals that you offer something other than long-term psychotherapy. Most physicians and dentists have established referral targets for their patients who ask for, or seem to need, psychotherapy. To change their pattern, you must present a model for short-term treatment that makes sense to the referral source.

In providing this model, there are several issues to consider. You must have a coherent model for treatment and also be able to present it to the referring party (e.g. see Bakal, 1982). It is essential that you are competent and familiar with whatever treatment model you promote. Furthermore, you must understand a fair amount of the medical literature in this area. I recommend reading the journal *Headache* occasionally.

Be warned that many medical practitioners have coherent biomedical explanations for at least vascular headaches. They generally get good results from prophylactic propranalol and see no reason to switch. To change this mind-set, you must present the case for cost-effective treatment. As a start, you will probably get a "hopeless" case. If you can help, this will raise your "stock" dramatically. If not, try to get a more typical case, but perhaps someone who will not or cannot take drugs.

Most referrals for headaches will come from neurologists, with family practice specialists and dentists accounting for most other referrals. Neurologists see a large number of headache patients. If they referred even 10 percent of those diagnosed as having muscle contraction, vascular, or mixed headaches, this would represent a substantial referral source. For this reason, neurologists should be your primary target for referrals.

Be aware that there are many barriers to cross with neurological specialists. First and foremost is lack of up-to-date knowledge. Most neurologists do not have a current working knowledge of headache that differs from their medical school training—an unfortunate characteristic that must be kept in mind. As mentioned earlier, you must take every chance to present a sound coherent model that explains the mind/body linkage. This linkage may or may not be recognized by the medical professional. In-service lectures, case presentations, informal presentations, and the like can be used to accomplish this.

Once you get a referral, use a follow-up letter as a way of reinforcing your expertise and professionalism. This letter can be quite extensive and include explanations of EMG scans, cognitive techniques, relaxation training, and charting of symptoms. Use your training in data collection to impress the neurologist. For instance, neurologists rarely have patients chart headaches. Most psychologists with behavioral training recognize the value of this type of data. Use this knowledge to your advantage.

Patience is again required since recognition of behavioral techniques for headache is only slowly growing in medical literature.

Dental Disorders   Dental problems such as temperomandibular (TM) disorders (temperomandibular joint syndrome [TMJ] and myofascial pain disorders [MPD]), bruxism, and dental phobias make up another potential market for behavioral medicine practitioners.

Once again, specialized knowledge is required for competent care. More than most other areas of care, this problem demands an interdisciplinary focus. Almost every referral will be receiving dental care, orthodontic treatment, or physical therapy, or all three. First and foremost, therefore, you must understand the whole picture.

It is increasingly recognized by dentists that psychological factors play a role in TM disorders. With more scientific studies currently under way, this state of affairs will undoubtedly favor the inclusion of the psychologist while beginning to exclude dental treatments such as equilibration, which have little support in controlled trials.

Gaining referrals in this area requires contact with dental practitioners—which means talks, grand rounds, study groups, and formal contacts. Not every dentist will have a large number of referrable patients, so a great many contacts are necessary.

Once again, you must dispel the image of long-term therapeutic analysis in favor of shorter-term treatments. Difficult-to-treat patients are often labeled as "neurotic," "depressed," or "psychotic" by medical, and especially dental, professionals. You must maintain a balance here. If you do extensive assessment of each client, you run the risk of being perceived as an exorbitantly expensive "extra" treatment. Furthermore, there is little evidence of the utility of this type of assessment (Laskin, 1983). On the other hand, you must convince the referring dentist that you have taken his or her perception seriously.

Again, letters to referral sources can be used to educate them. It is especially useful to include a diagnostic muscle scan using EMG readings. In addition, the psychologist's role in the treatment team can be delineated here. These concepts seem to create a degree of acceptance among all concerned parties.

Dental Phobias Between 6 and 14 percent of the population do not see dentists because of their fear of dental procedures. With the current oversupply of dentists in most areas of the United States, there should be no shortage of dentists who are willing to work with you to reach out to people who are letting their teeth go to ruin because of phobic reactions. Here you must market to the general public and other dentists. By offering an understanding climate, many phobics can be persuaded to at least explore an in-vivo desensitization procedure. This approach, while promising, has only been tried in a few settings, to my knowledge.

Gastrointestinal Disorders Several gastrointestinal disorders have been shown to be effectively treated with behavioral methods. Treatment for fecal and urinary incontinence has been especially well established but requires specialized equipment and expertise.

Irritable bowel syndrome (IBS), however, offers the behavioral medicine practitioners in private practice a possible market. IBS patients represent a large proportion of all visits to gastroenterologists. Furthermore, because physicians cannot do much to help these patients, they are often only too happy to make a referral.

It is critical in dealing with referring physicians that you make it clear that you know the differences between inflammatory bowel disorders (ulcerative colitis and Crohn's disease) and IBS. Nothing creates a negative attitude toward psychologists as much as claims that disorders with obvious physical etiology are largely psychological. IBS, on the other hand, is clearly seen as having at least some psychological or emotional overlay, and often is viewed as completely psychological.

In IBS, the challenge comes in getting the client to see the role of a psychologist, since this implies that the disorder is "all in his or her head." An alliance with the physician can overcome this obstacle. This means that a comprehensive program is presented to the client by the physician that includes many components, one of which is biofeedback, behavioral training, or stress counseling (see Latimer, 1983).

Overall, most IBS patients are receiving inadequate care. The behavioral medicine treatment package seems to be the best available at the present time. However, this message has not gone out forcefully enough. To get referrals, you must find a way to educate gastroenterologists and other physicians.

Cardiovascular Disorders A large number of cardiovascular disorders have been shown to be amenable to behavioral treatment. The two disorders with the greatest potential for private practice clinicians are hypertension and coronary heart disease.

Hypertension With perhaps 60 million hypertensive Americans, half of whom are undiagnosed, and very poor treatment compliance for pharmaco-logical treatment, this disorder represents a massive market. Of the 30 or so million people who know they are hypertensive, only half are being treated, and perhaps half of these maintain adequate adherence. Several federal government reports have recommended life-style and behavioral treatments as the first line of defense.

Despite blue-ribbon recommendations, most practitioners report few refer-rals for hypertension. There are several reasons for this. First, physicians need to see causal mechanisms to believe in most treatments. Since, at present, we do not really know why behavioral interventions work, we must ask the refer-ring source to place faith in mind-over-body theories. Second, modern medicine has effective, well-researched medication to deal with this serious, silent illness. This makes it difficult to refer. Most physicians simply jump to the next logical step and prescribe, first, diuretics and then, if needed, vaso-active drugs. Third, most patients do not want to bother with any treatment that is not effortless. It takes quite a pep talk to get someone with no overt symptoms to consider an expensive and potentially embarrassing course of treatment when a pill will probably work.

Despite these and other barriers, many forces are operating that should eventually lead to a much wider clientele for behavioral treatment of hyper-tension. Many people are searching for nonpharmacological solutions to health problems and usually hear about biofeedback or other self-regulation measures. Many others cannot tolerate medications and are health conscious enough to pursue different avenues. In addition, better data that should at least partially support behavioral techniques are becoming available.

To obtain referrals for hypertension, it appears best to try to cater to special cases at first. These might include pilots or other highly trained personnel who cannot take medication. Another group to approach are any credible sources within the holistic health movement. In addition, women with pregnancy-induced hypertension who cannot take most medications have shown good results with behavioral techniques. The strategy here is to gain some credi-bility by working with unusual clients and strive for a slowly changing consciousness.

Most private clinicians do not find cardiologists a good referral source for hypertension, but instead look to internists and family-practice specialists.

Coronary Heart Disease   Coronary heart disease (CHD) also represents a massive potential for behavioral medicine. Here, again, a general attitude change will be necessary to put psychologists in the mainstream of CHD treat-ment. The Type A concept has certainly attracted a lot of attention, but with the current generation of realistic data, it remains to be seen what part psychosocial factors will play in mainstream treatment. One point to keep in mind here is that psychosocial stress (broadly defined) certainly is involved in CHD. This is widely accepted by the public, and to a lesser extent by the medical establishment. If no more is claimed than that stress management might also be useful for people with other high-risk factors or for people in-terested in reducing potential risk factors, a growing market should emerge. I have found it beneficial to soft-pedal Type A interventions, but this may not be true for others.

Cardiac Rehabilitation   Behavioral techniques are becoming associated with cardiac rehabilitation in many medical settings as well. Often, coronary patients are released for aftercare to private practitioners. Along with dealing with the weighty problems of someone who almost died, one might be able also to use relaxation training, and so forth. This would probably we welcomed by the attending physician as helpful.

THIRD-PARTY PAYERS

Progress has been made recently with regard to third-party payments. At least one aspect of behavioral medicine, biofeedback, is being accepted as a medical procedure with 80 percent coverage. This varies widely, but there is an apparent recognition of biofeedback for physical disorders and stress. Be sure to use your BCIA or state certification number, if you have one.

If behavioral medicine is not covered, it is probably wise to begin trying to "educating" the payer by sending materials and documentation, and asking clients to petition. Eventually, recognition may come and make your efforts worthwile.

Many psychologists simply bill behavioral medicine procedures as psychotherapy. This works, but has two disadvantages. First, it does not document, for the field, an efficient and cost-effective intervention, so that progress in education is slowed. Second, most coverage of psychotherapy is poor, making for more out-of-pocket expense for the client. For these reasons, it is recommended that the private clinician make a concerted effort to lobby third-party sources for specific coverage

SUMMARY

This chapter has attempted to delineate some general principles that may be useful in generating referrals for psychologists in specialty areas. It has discussed activities directed toward the general public, other mental-health professionals, and other professional referral sources. Behavioral medicine was used as an example to illustrate these points.

REFERENCES

Bakal, C.F. (1982). *The psychobiology of chronic headache.* New York: Springer.

Laskin, D., et al. (1983). *The president's conference on the examination, diagnosis and management of temporomandibular disorders.* Chicago: American Dental Association.

Latimer, P.R. (1983). *Functional gastrointestinal disorders: A behavioral approach.* New York: Springer.

Leviton, A. (1978). Epidemiology of headache. In *Advances in Neurology: Vol. 19.* New York: Raven Press.

Matarazzo, J.D. (1980). Behavioral health and behavioral medicine: Frontiers for a new health psychology. *American Psychologist, 35,* 807–817.

Matarazzo, J.D. (1982). Behavioral health's challenge to academic, scientific, and professional psychology. *American Psychologist, 37,* 1–14.

S E C T I O N

E

**Marketing and
Advertising**

CHAPTER
14

USING MARKETING AS A TOOL FOR PRACTICE DEVELOPMENT

Grace Conlee

It is important to understand what marketing truly is—what it can do for practice development and how the marketing process works to achieve your own goals and objectives. In the competitive health-care market today, the term "marketing" is used with abandon, often in reference to selling one's self or services.

My introduction to marketing came in 1977 when I was the director of public relations for an investor-owned private psychiatric hospital. By following the guidelines of the industry definition of marketing, we became very successful. According to that definition, marketing is "assessing the public's needs and wants and tailoring one's services or product lines to fill that unmet need." It has been quoted in numerous publications and at marketing seminars. I cannot tell you its origin, but I first encountered it in a 1974 book entitled *Marketing Healthcare,* by Robin MacStravick.

What we achieved at the hospital through market research, program development, and strategic planning as it relates to this definition has become the basis for my company's special focus on health-care marketing.

In the marketing and public relations industry, the terminology most commonly used today is "marketing communications." This chapter is dedicated to helping readers understand how marketing concepts, strategies, and communications tools can be used effectively to help develop their private practice.

For the past three years, I have been conducting marketing workshops for physicians, psychologists, hospitals, and specialty health-care organizations. From these workshops comes the foundation of a written marketing plan with short- and long-term goals and objectives. This process can be effectively applied to your practice.

I cannot stress enough the need for a written plan. All good intentions fall by the wayside without one. In many instances, the assistance of a professional consultant may be in order to help you develop such a comprehensive plan.

How do you find a qualified health-care marketing professional? Call your local hospital's marketing or public relations director and ask for a referral of two or three firms or independent consultants. Professional associations such as the Association for Healthcare Marketing and Public Relations, whose members are hospital and agency public relations and marketing professionals; the American Marketing Association's Healthcare Division; and the Public Relations Society of America are good resources.

When interviewing potential candidates, ask to see a sample copy of a written marketing plan. I carry a "blind" copy, with revealing information about the client deleted, to business development meetings. Content and style will vary, but there are some basics that should be included. Whether you hire a professional or undertake the project yourself, there are key elements to be included in the written marketing plan.

KEY ELEMENTS OF A WRITTEN MARKETING PLAN

Step 1. The Importance of a Mission Statement

It is important to show what business you are in, what services you deliver and to whom, how the practice is perceived by others, and, most important, how your practice differs from all the rest. That point of difference can set your practice apart and provide the basis for a successful marketing program. What are the strengths and weaknesses of the key participants in the practice? What kind of "focus" can be forged by the unique education, experiences, and strengths of the professional or group? This focus can become the mission statement.

As an example, we will use one group of mental-health professionals who had a built-in specialty. There are three psychologists and two marriage, family, and child counselors in the practice. In the group are members with experience in working with learning disabilities because of their teaching backgrounds, one with strengths in testing and evaluation, and a member who had been a pediatric nurse early in her career. This group can play on these collective strengths and position itself as the area specialists who work with families whose children and teenagers have academic, behavioral, or emotional problems.

The group's mission statement should reflect these strengths and might read: "The Harbortown Psychology Center is dedicated to improving school, peer, and family relationships of children with social, academic, and behavioral difficulties. Treating the family as a unit and focusing on the child's physical, psychosocial, and academic needs, HPC's staff of mental-health professionals believe in an integrated and cooperative approach involving the family and school in the child's treatment."

Another mission statement: "Southern California Orthotics and Prosthetics is dedicated to providing innovative, high-quality orthotic and prosthetic devices and aftercare service for disabled and injured individuals. SCOP's mission is to deliver efficient, dependable, and timely service to the physicians, physical therapists, and hospital rehabilitation centers requesting such services."

Once this important first step has been taken, it is time to go on to the next step.

2. Setting Goals and Objectives

Before you write a plan, it is important to set goals and objectives. These should be attainable, realistic, and measurable.

What are your broad goals? Where do you hope to find your practice in one, three, and five years? You may wish to become recognized as a specialist in a given area and position your practice accordingly. If you are in a new practice, your goals may be to reach a maximum number of patients by the end of a two-year period, but want steady growth leading you to that number during the interim. The objectives are the specific outcomes from each specific goal.

As an example, we will use Harbortown Psychology Center again. One of its goals is to increase the number of families seen for therapy.

The objective may be to become recognized as the specialty center for families whose children's academic difficulties are affecting their social and family relationships. To achieve this goal, the group members provide informal consultations with school counselors, and speak at Parent-Teacher Association and community group meetings. They provide positive parenting seminars in local pediatricians' offices and work with classroom teachers.

A more established practice may choose to emphasize one aspect of the practice in order to change the existing patient mix by case or reimbursement. For example, you may wish to increase the numbver of couples you see and decrease the number of adolescents.

I counsel my clients to coordinate their marketing and business plans. Ideally, the business manager, if there is one, should take part in the planning process because he or she will need to budget for the activities conducted to achieve the results that will help the group reach the goals set for growth and income.

Step 3. Targeting Markets: Internal Auditing, Research, and Analysis

It is important to point out here that, from a marketing perspective, "targeted markets" are most generally synonymous with *referral sources.* Two other chapters of this handbook are dedicated to referral sources. This chapter attempts to give you the means to reach these referral sources that are the life blood of every practice.

Internal Audit   To assess your existing patient base, I recommend conducting an internal audit of patient records. Unfortunately, most mental-health practitioners do not keep patient records in the same manner as do physical-health practitioners. However, it is essential to do so.

Develop a patient-trackng form for new patients, similar to the example illustrated in Table 1, to develop a profile of your existing patient base. After compiling three to six months of new patient information, you will be able to tell, in percentages, where your current referrals are coming from, the type of case you handle most, and other pertinent demographics such as each patient's age and gender and where they live and work.

Continue to use it for all new referrals to assess the effectiveness of your marketing activities as they are implemented. This tool will provide you with important information in the future. I recommend including the names of all callers, whether they become patients or not. Every inquiry should be considered a referral. If the call does not result in an office visit, there may be a problem with the way the receptionist handles the call, for example.

For readers who are relatively new to private practice, an internal audit may

NEW PATIENT SOURCING STATISTICS FORM FOR   198

DATE: NAME	AGE	SEX	REFERRED BY:	ZIP CODE	DIAGNOSIS/TX

CODES: A

B

TABLE 14.1

not be in order. But if you keep this statistics-gathering mechanism faithfully, you will be way ahead of the long-time practitioner who must go back and reconstruct this vital information.

The data extrapolated from this process should give you a patient profile and valuable referral information. For example, who refers to your practice? Do you, through professional networking, represent a large number of referrals? Do referrals come from colleagues, clinics, hospital emergency rooms, school counselors, social service agencies, or patients and their families? What percentage come from other health-care professionals or came as a result of a lecture you delivered to a parent group? How many result from yellow-pages advertising? This information will provide statistics that paint a picture of your practice for use in developing marketing strategies

Research When you have a good handle on where your referrals come from, the next step is to assess potential referral sources not yet tapped. You must also assess the external market forces that may affect your planning.

What are the factors you need to take into consideration when researching your service area? What is the service area and does limiting yourself to it restrict or enhance your chances of success?

A service area is the geographic area emanating from your office as the center and extending to a point from which a potential patient can reach the office in a reasonable length of travel time. In most metropolitan cities, that is 20–30 minutes by car. If the population density of that service area is heavy, you will have a greater pool of patients from which to draw. But there may also be more competition. Your patient sourcing statistics will tell you what percentage of your patients live or work in your service area. From this you can determine whether distance and travel time are an issue for your patients, and if proximity to work is more important than closeness to home.

In this busy world of working people, it may be that potential patients prefer to have a therapist close to their place of work rather than to their home. This information can be used to develop a marketing strategy aimed at people in the workplace in your service area.

What are the demographics of your service area? External forces include economic factors, ethnic balance, population density, and location. These external forces may determine the direction your practice should take.

How well is your practice doing in its market environment? How is your product priced, are your services perceived as specialized, and is your office accessible? What about the decor of the office? Is your staff perceived as friendly and helpful? Have you ever asked your patients how they feel about these issues?

What is the competition? Is the area saturated with competitors? Is there a noticeable absence of a particular type of service that could benefit the marketplace?

The next step is to collect information in your research related to these external areas:

- Economic — income levels, occupational mix, unemployment rates
- Geographic — region, county size, density, climate
- Demographics — age, sex, family size, family life cycle
- Social factors — education levels, religion, race, social class
- Psychographics — life-styles, values, attitudes

The local chamber of commerce or economic development offices are good resources for this type of information. They keep the data updated annually.

Understanding these market influences and how they affect your practice will help you in developing your marketing strategies

Analysis Analyze the research data you have collected from internal and external resources. Look closely at your existing patient base. How were they referred to your office, what type of patients do you see most, and are they the most profitable by reimbursement, for example? Who has referred the largest number of patients and why?

What services are in abundance in your service area? Where are the deficiencies? Is there an unmet need that you are capable of filling?

Are your service area's demographics conducive to your type of practice? Are your prices too high for the economic level of the area? Your research may have revealed that the large manufacturing plant in your area is going to relocate to another city, displacing many long-time employees. Is there an opportunity here for you to provide a service for the personnel department of that factory? The practice can provide transitional counseling for employees being retired early and unexpectedly, for example. Match the strengths of your practice to areas where you see a need or an opportunity.

The secrets of successful marketing are no longer a mystery when you understand these key steps in creating a strategic marketing plan for practice development. Now that you have formulated your plan, it is time to write one.

Step 4. Writing the Marketing Communications Plan

With internal and external research completed, you will be ready to integrate these data with your goals and mission statement to form the marketing strategies to reach your targeted audiences. These strategies will be outlined in the written marketing communications plan. The marketing communications plan should include the following elements:

1. Mission statement—who we are, what services we deliver.
2. Goals and objectives—long and short range.
3. Targeted markets—identifying groups we are trying to reach.
4. Marketing communications strategies—use of advertising, promotion, media, direct mail, community and public relations, collateral materials, and so forth to reach each of these markets.
5. Budget.
6. Review and evaluation.

Marketing Communications Tools We have already reviewed the first three elements of the written plan. Marketing communications, as stated previously, is a set of tools used to deliver a specific message to targeted audiences. These tools come in a variety of styles, approaches, and costs. Communications are essential and ongoing communications are particularly effective.

It is my professional opinion that marketing communications for healthcare professionals should be a simple process. First, target the audience, and second, tailor your message to appeal to that audience.

Use of the media to carry your message to the general public, sending a periodically published newsletter or communique to selected recipients, mailing brochures or other "sales" pieces to selected groups, and using advertising as a message to elicit a direct response are very common practices. Videotaped messages are becoming popular and are effective teaching tools for patients, colleagues, and referral sources. All of these tools can help deliver specific messages to the chosen groups of individuals who are your targeted markets. Used strategically, they become powerful tools.

The following outlines how these strategies can be used.

Media Relations   Media relations is the use of news releases, interviews, features, and appearances on radio and television to tell your story to the general public. When a mental-health professional becomes known as an "expert" in any given field, it generally is a result of a great deal of media attention to his or her subject matter, whether or not the "expert" designation is deserved. Reporters are traditionally looking for newsworthy subject matter, sources they can rely on for accurate information, ease of access (not often true for the busy psychologist), and credibility, meaning good academic and professional credentials.

Unfortunately, representatives of the media can be manipulated by clever "press agents." But in general, they are fair and looking for original material. Do not expect that because you want your name in print or on the air the local reporter or editor will agree. Save your media release for events of merit, such as new approaches to treatment, research-oriented material, grand openings, or new staff appointments.

It is better to make a few good contacts in the media and get to know them than it is to inundate them with superfluous releases.

A good way to do this is to subscribe to a clipping service. It can cost about $40.00 a month, but will be less expensive than hiring the services of a public relations consultant. Most clipping services will read all daily, weekly, and monthly publications in your city or county. For this fee they will clip articles you request on given subjects, such as mental-health and children, government-sponsored social service programs, or the homeless mentally ill, and mail them to you on a weekly basis.

In addition to keeping you well informed, this approach gives you the benefit of knowing what has already been printed, in which areas specific reporters are interested, and the basis for formulating letters to the editor in response to these articles. A personal note of comment to the reporter who wrote the article can be used to establish a relationship. After two or three notes to a particular reporter, he or she may call on you as a quotable source for a similar article in the future. Subsequent releases to the paper will be looked upon in a more favorable light as a result of this relationship.

Keep in mind when you do submit news releases to print media that most medical reporters are not interested in mental-health stories unless they have a scientific angle. Many medical reporters in metropolitan newspapers are extremely political and look for controversy or political angles. Family, life-style, and health sections are your best bet for placing story ideas.

Radio talk shows are generally a good format for interviews and listener call-in participation. Letters of inquiry to the show's producer are the way to get appearances on these shows. Television is a more difficult medium because of its needs for visual stories.

Such special events as taking charge of a booth at a health fair, presenting educational forums and symposia, and holding an open house for professional colleagues and referral sources are another form of practice development. The goal is to present yourself in as many positive and educational forums as possible.

Speakers bureaus can give professionals the platform to present series of lectures to professional and community groups. These groups might include Parent-Teachers' Associations, women's groups, Rotary, Chamber of Commerce, and health-care provider groups such as a specialty section of the local medical society. The members of the practice can form their own speakers bureau and promote it with the groups mentioned here.

Collateral materials are printed materials such as brochures, patient-education materials, and newsletters. These tools, if used well, can go a long way toward getting your message across to a number of different audiences.

If your practice has a unique focus, a brochure can be used to communicate complete information to target groups.

Newsletters are an excellent form of ongoing communications. Specialty practices, such as PMS clinics, learning disabilities centers, and child and family psychology centers, can use newsletters in a most effective manner. For a small or solo practice, the use of an occasional 'letter" to referral sources discussing timely topics can work as well. The consistency of the message, as well as the content, creates the impact.

Direct mail could be used on occasion, if targeted to the right audience. Because it is quite expensive, I am reluctant to recommend this tool for the majority of health-care professionals. Although direct mail is expensive for small groups, it is growing in popularity, and when it targets professionals already interested in what you have to say, I think it can be effective.

Advertising is covered in another chapter of this handbook, but it is also a tool for marketing communications, and a key element of any written plan. My personal feeling is that the jury is still out on the effectiveness of advertising in health care. In southern California, where my firm is located, general and specialty hospitals are spending enormous sums of money on paid advertising. Private health-care providers are following suit. Plastic surgeons and otolaryngologists (ear, nose, and throat specialists, now promoting themselves as head and neck surgeons) are battling it out in upscale magazines for the elective cosmetic surgery market, for example. If advertising is not effective in health care, it may be the message, and not the medium, that is at fault. There are occasions where advertising is appropriate, such as announcing one-time special events, grand openings, and so on. Yellow pages are one form of effective advertising and should be part of any marketing budget.

The increasing popularity of "advi-torials," the paid ads that look like editorial copy, is an indication of the difficulty in placing specific stories with the press through media relations. Again, competition for health headlines and feature stories to tout some aspect of treatment is forcing providers to use such ads to project the third-party endorsement readers associate with what they see in print or on television or hear on the radio.

Step 5. Establishing a Marketing Budget

At this point, it is important to evaluate the dollar value of a new patient in order to establish a marketing budget. The saying "It takes money to make money" is especially true today because of the competitive nature of the health-care industry. The industry standard for establishing a marketing budget is based on monthly income and differentiates between new and established practices. Recommended percentages of monthly income are as follows.

3–5 percent to remain at current level of patients
5–7 percent to expand and increase the patient base
7–10 percent to enter the market with a new practice

Let us examine the value of a patient to assist you in developing a budget. As an example, I will use a counseling session I held with a marriage, family, and child counselor, who had been a half-time staff social worker at a psychiatric hospital and in private practice the other half. She was leaving the hospital to go into full-time private practice and needed some marketing advice. One of her main concerns was an impending yellow-pages advertisement expense she had incurred as part of a coalition of MFCCs who placed a group "referral" type ad in two suburban yellow-pages directories. Her cost was just under $550.

To determine if this expense was justified, I asked her the following questions—which can be applied to your own practice.

1. How many referrals from these listings resulted in appointments?
   Answer: 11
2. How many times do you see a typical patient?
   Answer: 12–15
3. What is your hourly rate?
   Answer: $65

The 11 referrals that became patients, multiplied by 12 sessions at $65 per session, resulted in $8,580 in revenue; 15 times the original investment. Needless to say, she decided to subscribe to another year of yellow-pages ads.

The value of a new patient to health-care professionals varies from region to region throughout the United States, but this formula can be used to determine a new patient's dollar value to your practice. The added probability of that patient's becoming a referral source is high, and further increases the patient's value to you. This is a good reason to spend part of your marketing budget to solidify that patient's loyalty to you. The least expensive referrals to obtain come from your current patients.

Step 6. Evaluation and Assessment

Keeping statistics is the only sure way of measuring the effectiveness of your marketing campaign. Knowing if your referral sources responded to the communications plan aimed at them will be told on the bottom line of your patient sourcing statistics forms.

Earlier in this chapter, we stressed the importance of keeping statistics. After six months of a concentrated program, you should begin to see tangible results that, it is hoped, will match the short-term goals established in the beginning of this process.

Marketing communications is a *process* that will take commitment and the investment of your time, energy, and dollars to ensure its success. Without a means to measure the results and justify your investment, the process will be of no value.

If you find the results from your efforts to be less than hoped for, do not give up. If particular activities proved more effective, concentrate more efforts on that area. If some activities did not work, alter them in some way for another three months or discontinue them altogether.

Evaluation needs to be done quarterly. The benefit of this process should appear on the bottom line of your tax return in one year.

When your practice becomes busier, or has a shift in the desired patient mix, do not put marketing on the back burner. The second best time to be aggressive in your marketing activities is when the practice is doing well.

REFERENCES

Periodicals

Healthcare Marketing Report, Atlanta, GA. Beverly L. Seitz (Ed.).
Physicians Marketing, published by American Health Consultants, Atlanta, GA.
Health Marketing, Pat Mages (Ed.), published by HealthMark, Cleveland, TN.

Texts

MacStravick, R.E. (1974). *Marketing healthcare.* Germantown, PA: Aspen Systems.
Winston, W.J. (1983). *Marketing the group practice — Practical methods for the health care practitioner.* New York: Haworth Press.

CHAPTER

15

PUBLIC RELATIONS

Jo Clare Sullivan and Donald J. Viglione

WHAT IS PUBLICITY?

Whether it is a television story on teen suicide, a radio talk show on psychological development, or a review of drug rehabilitation centers in your local newspaper, the media provide consumers with a wealth of daily information. Dedicated to keeping consumers entertained and informed, the media—newspapers, radio, and television networks and the people they employ—work hard to gather factual information that may be of interest to their readers. You can help the media do their job, and increase your exposure to consumers, by engaging in an active publicity program.

Publicity is a term that public relations professionals use to describe the process of promoting a story or news item to the media. Often, people confuse advertising and publicity because they both involve providing a message for publication. However, with advertising, you create a specific message, and purchase advertising space in which to present it on a specific date. With publicity, you develop a specific message, and then provide it to the reporter or editor of your target medium, for example, a newspaper. In turn, the reporter or editor decides when your message might best serve the readership. In some cases, the editor or reporter may deem your message worthy of an entire story and contact you for more information, or may combine it and run it with other stories. In other cases, it may be decided that your message is of no interest to the readers and so it will not be used. If your message is eventually used, you are not "charged" for this free exposure of your name.

Some special publications and smaller newspapers comingle advertising and editorial functions by guaranteeing you free space for an article if you purchase a separate ad to run elsewhere in the paper. We agree with most public relations professionals who consider this to be paid publicity and treat it as advertising; consequently, we will not address this practice in this chapter. Such "publicity" is most frequently found in real estate or special supplement sections of the newspaper.

ETHICAL ISSUES

Publicity is handled like advertising according to the American Psychological Association (APA) ethical guidelines and is addressed under APA's

Principle 4—Public Statements (American Psychological Association, 1985). It is important to note that unethical practices may be legal, so that the APA guidelines are more restrictive than are the applicable laws and regulations. Accordingly, the APA considers misrepresentation, exaggeration, direct solicitation of clients, and testimonials by clients as unethical.

Furthermore, psychologists, through their publicity, are responsible for assisting the public in making informed decisions. Any publicity that impedes this goal would be unethical; for example, claims of unique talents and skills or appeals to the public's fears. It is a good idea to review the ethical principles to assure that your publicity conforms to them. During the past 10 years, these guidelines and interpretations have been liberalized as marketing one's services has become more important because of increased competition and the development of more varied services. In another light, publicity serves an important educational function and increases the ability of potential clients to make informed judgments.

HOW PUBLICITY CAN HELP YOU

Ideally, with repeated favorable exposure in the local media, publicity helps increase consumer awareness of your name and the services you provide. Over time, this awareness should have a cumulative effect and translate into increased demand for your services.

For example, let us say that over a two-month period, your local newspaper runs short news items about your local office opening in a new building; later it mentions a seminar you are sponsoring in its community events column; and several weeks later you are quoted in a feature story about new techniques in family therapy. The next time a pediatrician recommends you, along with two other professionals, the patient is more likely to contact you because he or she recognizes your name from the media.

TYPES OF PUBLICITY

Knowing the media is an important first step in learning how to obtain publicity for yourself and your events. Do some research. First, find out what publications and radio and television programs exist in your area. In addition to the daily newspaper, are there weekly, community, or special interest publications? What about publications in neighboring communities? Second, see if these publications have a special section or column dedicated to mental health.

In the next few paragraphs, we describe the characteristics of each of the media available to you. In the print media, there are all sizes and varieties of publications, but to get you started, we list the most common.

Most medium to large cities have at least one daily newspaper. Daily papers vary in size depending on their advertising revenues. However, they all usually have several sections, including sections on business, sports and life-style, and city and national news. Each section may have its own editor, who assigns reporters to gather stories and prioritizes articles based on the interests of the readers. You should become acquainted with the editors of the sections that would carry your story.

For example, you would probably find family counseling stories in a "lifestyle" or general city section of the paper, and so, if you were to have a story idea about psychology, you would present it to the editor of one of these sections. Better yet, if you noticed that one reporter has been designated as a medical writer, you would present your ideas to this person.

Most often, though, if you have general news items, send them to the city section. If you have news of a community event, send it to the writer of the community events column, and do so well in advance of the deadline for that column. For the specific names of newspapers and periodicals, as well as other publications and the call letters of television and radio stations in your area, consult a local media guide. These guides are often published locally by public relations associations, such as the Los Angeles Publicity Club. Nationally, a publication called *Bacon's* contains media information for various areas around the United States.

An inexpensive way to compile a media list is to just start by writing your own. Include the names of the editor or reporters, the publication's name and address, whether it is a weekly or daily, and deadline information and telephone number. When you have a news item or story idea on a local or national issue of current interest, you send it to all those on your list who might be interested in your idea.

PRESS RELEASES

Press releases are an effective tool for creating awareness about your practice, specialty areas, and new services. Using the local media to carry your message is not only cost-efficient (it is free except for your labor), but it also adds credibility to what you are saying. Getting "a little ink" in the local newspaper is not too difficult as long as you follow a few guidelines.

First, think of a newsworthy angle. If you are planning an event or just looking for a way to increase name recognition for your office, try using a timely theme or idea that not only will interest potential referral sources and patients but also the media. Consider current topics in the news, local or national, or problems that are beginning to emerge. For example, anorexia nervosa and child abuse are two topics that have been attracting public attention. Seasonal issues, such as those related to the Christmas holidays or returning to school in the fall, are also timely.

Second, plan ahead. Scheduling is essential to getting your message in print. A great story does not help the city editor when it arrives an hour after deadline. To get the most out of your publicity efforts, allow yourself plenty of time.

The following are just a few examples of the types of news releases you can prepare: new staff, new or additional offices, new services, promotions, staff and faculty appointments, seminars, special events, free services, community activities, sponsorships, donations.

You may also wish to increase your relationship with your local paper by delivering these releases personally to the reporter. This may seem time consuming, but if things work well, you may be the first person that the editor calls for information or a quote.

Promotions

Creating community awareness through a seminar or other promotion can be a successful way to increase name recognition and to educate the public about available treatments for problems in living. There are a variety of ways to get community and media attention without great expense.

In planning any promotion, you should have specific objectives in mind, for example: (1) increasing awareness among public agencies, potential patients, medical doctors, or others; (2) establishing yourself as an expert in an appropriate area; and (3) increasing awareness of your services with potential clients.

Plan an event around whatever objectives and audience you have in mind. Also, keep your target market in mind when selecting dates and times. For example, the first day of school is not a good day for a family-oriented event and evenings are not the best time for an event geared to attract seniors.

When deciding on a theme or idea for your event, think of something that will appeal not only to your clients, but also to the media. Keep photo possibilities in mind. It is easy to come up with imaginative ideas to help build name, services, and expertise awareness and to get media coverage. Here are a few suggestions.

1. Donate to or promote community programs to build favorable awareness.

2. Provide a donation to a local community organization and stage an interesting·photo for publicity.

3. Donate to a hospital (children's ward); show a child accepting the donation on behalf of the hospital.

4. Contribute to a youth orchestra, choir, or the like. Invite a local senior choir or other musical group to perform and make a contribution to the group in lieu of payment for the performance. Have a local art school or museum choose the winners of first, second, and third prizes. Along these lines, Adopt-A-School programs are available in some areas of the country.

It is important for you to get name recognition in these endeavors. Businesses can display pictures, certificates, or plaques concerning these promotions, but most of the time, such displays are inappropriate in psychologists' offices. Accordingly, you should encourage the organization or agency that you are supporting to publish or post your name.

Guidelines for Press Releases

Newspaper reporters follow a standard format, called AP (Associated Press) style. The closer you can fit a release to their standards and requirements, the less editing they will have to do and the better impression you will make. The essential aspects of the format are as follows:

1. Your releases should be on your office letterhead.

2. A contact name and phone number should be included on the release in case the reporter has follow-up questions.

3. The release should be double-spaced to allow room for editors' marks. Allow plenty of room at the top of the first page for additional editing.

4. The headline and dateline should be in all capital letters. A dateline appears at the beginning of a news article or press release, indicating where the story originated (e.g., LOS ANGELES – CLINICAL PSYCHOLOGY ASSOCIATES).

5. The date the release was sent should appear.

6. Photos accompanying news releases should be high-quality, black-and-white glossy prints, preferably 5 by 7 or 8 by 10.

7. A caption should be attached to the photo, identifying the subject matter and again including a contact name, phone number, and date.

8. A "#" sign (the number symbol) should appear at the end of the release, indicating that it is the end.

9. If two or more pages are required, the word "–more–" should be centered at the bottom of each page to indicate that more pages follow. The top of each subsequent page should include a "slug line" (all capitals) on the upper left side and the page number, usually written as 2-2-2-2 on the upper right.

The slug line should be an abbreviated headline – that is, CLINICAL PSYCHOLOGY ASSOCIATES, PARENTING SEMINAR.

10.The numbers one through nine should be spelled out. Use numerals for 10 and higher.

11.When a month is used with a specific date, in most cases the name of the month should be abbreviated, except for March, April, May, June, and July.

12.When listing a numbered address, use the abbreviations St., Ave., Blvd. (123 Main St.).

13.On the first reference to a person, include the full name and title. On subsequent references, use the last name only.

14.The press release should be as brief as possible. Shorter releases have a better likelihood of being run. Also, the most important information should appear at the beginning of the release. When editors shorten stories, they usually cut from the bottom up.

Additional Tips

There are a number of additional tips to keep in mind.

Never "double plant" a story – that is, give the same release to two different reporters at the same paper. Reporters do not always know what their co-workers are writing and it can cause embarrassment for yourself and annoyances for the reporters. Also, your working relationship with reporters and editors is quite important.

Avoid calling a newspaper to see whether it received the release or will run the story. Remember, since publicity is free, it is up to the editor's discretion to use the release. Most papers are sent hundreds of press releases daily. If a paper does accept your story, it may take weeks before you actually see it appear.

Newspapers want newsworthy stories. Be factual and objective in your release. Avoid self-serving statements. Read your local and community papers to see what type of news they run. You may find something that applies to what you are doing.

Photography Guidelines

If you plan to include a photo with a press release, it is important that you understand a few basic guidelines regarding publicity photography. Few editors still use standard ribbon-cutting and ground-breaking shots. Where possible, get more action-oriented photos if you want to see them in the local newspaper. Use your imagination. If you are taking group shots, be sure to limit the group size to six people per photo. Identifying more than six people in a caption is confusing and often an editor just will not bother to run the photo at all. Photos that feature children, political and community leaders, or local celebrities are often noticed by the press. Take advantage of any of these subjects. As a rule of thumb, try to avoid profile shots. You should be able to see both eyes of everyone in the picture. For publicity photos, always use black-and-white print film and at least a 35 mm format.

DEVELOPING A MEDIA LIST

Although the distribution of your press releases will be limited to your community and nearby areas, it is still important to maintain a current media list for those papers. It will save you time and make the distribution of your press releases much easier.

Computerized mailing lists are helpful but refrain from using impersonal mailing labels. The list should include community newspapers (daily or weekly) and radio stations. Most television stations serve large metropolitan areas. However, if there is an independent station in your community, list it as well. On the list, include the name, address, and phone number of each publication and station. The telephone directory may be a good source of these. Become familiar with the publication, for example, its special columns and sections on community events, people, promotions, and so forth.

Appealing to the target person on a more personal level is always advisable. Call the paper for the names of the reporters responsible for these areas, and include their names on your media list. If you are personally delivering a release to the paper, you will know to whom to give it. If you are mailing it, using the reporter's name is a much more personal approach. Update the list periodically, at least quarterly. Make sure the names and publications are current.

Include trade association journals on your media list, as well as the chapter newsletters for local psychological associations. Promoting yourself to your peers is a good way to generate referrals.

RELEASE SAMPLES

Here are some examples of releases you may want to send.

1. New personnel, faculty appointments, recognitions.
2. A new or additional office or a relocation.
3. New services you offer, new ventures (exclusive rights to serve a hospital or company).
4. Seminars and promotions.
5. Community involvement/sponsorships. It is a good idea to coordinate publicity with the community group involved. The group may have already planned to do its own publicity.
6. Media advisory. A media advisory may be used whe you want to invite a reporter to attend an event. This would be especially appropriate with educational seminars. The reporter may be interested in doing a consumer-oriented story based on what was learned at the seminar. (Reporters should always be allowed to attend seminars at no charge.) In preparing a media advisory, simply list the who, what, where, when, and any other additional information that may pique the reporters' interest.

The following are typical releases in the recommended format.

NEW VENTURES

> Contact: Mary Smith
> 457-1111
> June 19, 1987

CLINICAL PSYCHOLOGY ASSOCIATES
TO PROVIDE PSYCHOLOGICAL SERVICES

YOUR CITY—Mountain View Hospital has selected Clinical Psychology Associates as the exclusive provider of psychological testing service for its new adolescent facilities.

Mountain View Hospital is located in the northwest portion of Your City.

According to Mary Smith, spokesperson for Clinical Psychology Associates, the new adolescent psychiatric facility houses 45 beds.

Clinical Psychology Associates is located at 123 Main St.

# # #

SEMINAR

Contact: Mary Smith
457-1111
June 19, 1987

CLINICAL PSYCHOLOGY ASSOCIATES TO HOST SEMINAR

YOUR CITY—CLINICAL PSYCHOLOGY ASSOCIATES will sponsor a parenting seminar from 7 p.m. to 8 p.m., Monday, Nov. 5, at the group's office, located at 123 Main St.

"The seminar will provide parents with information on dealing with adolescents: helping to understand them, to communicate better, and to set limits on them," said Mary Smith, CLINICAL PSYCHOLOGY ASSO-CITATES spokesperson.

Guest speaker will be Bill Lander, a licensed clinical psychologist who specializes in treating adolescents and their families.

–more–

CLINICAL PSYCHOLOGY ASSOCIATES HOSTS SEMINAR   2-2-2-2

The seminar is free and seating is limited. Refreshments will be served. Reservations may be made by calling CLINICAL PSYCHOLOGY ASSO-CIATES at 457-1111.

# # #

COMMUNITY SPONSORSHIPS

Contact: Mary Smith
457-1111
June 19, 1987

CLINICAL PSYCHOLOGY ASSOCIATES SPONSOR TOY DRIVE

CLINICAL PSYCHOLOGY ASSOCIATES will sponsor a holiday toy drive for local needy children, announced Mary Smith, spokesperson.

Toy drop-off boxes will be set up at both of Your City Boys and Girls Club offices, located at 321 Main St. and 567 Fifth Ave.

"We encourage the residents of Your City to drop off a new toy at one of our offices," Smith said. "In addition, CLINICAL PSYCHOLOGY ASSO-CIATES will match a toy for every toy we receive."

The toy drive runs from Nov. 15 through Dec. 23. All toys collected will be donated to the Home for Orphaned Children.

PHOTO CAPTION—to accompany release
(to be taped to bottom of photo)

Contact: Mary Smith   June 19, 1987
          457-1111

TOYS FOR THE NEEDY—Mary Smith (left, spokesperson for CLINICAL
PSYCHOLOGY ASSOCIATES, and John Doe (right), manager of Your City
Boys/Girls Clubs, set up drop-off boxes for a holiday toy drive that the
Clinical Psychology group is sponsoring.

# # #

REFERENCES

American Psychological Association. (1985). *Directory of the American Psychological Association.* Washington, DC: Author.

Bacon's Publishing Co., Inc. (1988). *Bacon's Publicity Checker.* Chicago: Bacon's Publishing Co., Inc.

Carlson, L. (1982). *Publicity and promotion handbook: A complete guide for small business.* New York: Von Nostrand Reinhold.

French, C., Powell, E., & Angione, H. (1980). *Style book: The Associated Press style book and libel manual.* New York: Associated Press.

Klein, T., & Danzig, F. (1985). *Publicity: How to make the media work for you.* New York: Scribner.

Part
Two

Financial and Economic Management

Reuben Silver, Ph.D.
Editor

S E C T I O N

A

**Start-Up
Costs**

▼▼▼

C H A P T E R
16

SPACE AND OFFICE EQUIPMENT

Carroll L. Meek, Ph.D.

There is little doubt that an office reflects something about the therapist who is willing to work there. Individuals entering the therapist's office for the first time are drawing many conclusions about the type of person who has arranged the working space. Psychotherapies differ a great deal. The philosophies about office atmosphere (if considered at all), therefore, are also going to reflect the types of therapy provided. Therapists have often felt that they, personally, are the focal point when greeting a potential patient. Maybe they are, but I believe that *everything* is being scrutinized when a person enters the office space for the first time — including the environment.

Some therapies stoutly maintain and advocate that the therapist and the environment should be as "anonymous" as possible, a "blank slate," as it were, where the patient projects only himself or herself into the atmosphere. Even if this were possible, patients would still make those projections whether the office was austere or rich — a valuable source of therapy information.

Most patients enter therapy for the first time or with a new therapist with a certain degree of trepidation or fear. A comfortable atmosphere that demonstrates to them that the therapist has taken into account these forbidding sets of feelings conveys warmth and caring. Comfort in one's physical surroundings has already been demonstrated to be a way to alleviate stress. Therefore, it seems logical that efforts on the part of the therapist to reduce the stress of the therapy situation itself (i.e., to provide a positive and relaxing atmosphere) indicates that there is congruence in practice with stress-reduction theory, in general.

Individuals are afraid of a stilted or stifling approach to therapy. Given options, most will choose a creative therapist who, by example, is going to help each person develop his or her own brand of individuality and creativity. The personality of the therapist is shown by the way he or she deals with his or her own self-expression. The office should be a matter of personal taste and will (wittingly or unwittingly) reflect many aspects of the personality of the therapist. Therefore, it seems logical that one might capitalize on an intentional approach. What do you want your office space to reflect about you?

EXPENSES

In starting an independent practice, expenses are probably going to be a consideration. Evaluating one's budget will automatically eliminate some aspects of luxury in an office. I strongly believe that a living-room atmosphere is much more comfortable for patients than an office atmosphere, so it is certainly possible that some of your office accents can be taken from your own home or apartment. With costs in mind, shop around. Determine the "must have" and the "wait until later" items. Office furnishings can be added almost indefinitely, and if you take this option, you will find that your patients will catch on and will look for new things as your office takes shape over the months and years.

OFFICE SPACE

Although selecting office space and location is not a consideration of this chapter, it is important — especially if you can locate one in a well-traveled and well-known part of the town in which you live and which has a good reputation with a professional climate. Assuming you have found a space that is going to meet these requirements, the task is to furnish it with the above elements in mind.

Evaluate your space. What does it need? If you are frivolous, you will want to incorporate an atmosphere for your own personal comfort, as well as your patients'. A few moments must be spent in determining what you want to convey about yourself as a therapist. Since most people will be calling on the telephone to make appointments (a few may stop by), what they see when they arrive will determine or cement perceptions about you. Right from the beginning, they will be drawing conclusions about whether they are going to pursue therapy with you. The decision has not yet been made.

Now, given that you have considered all of the costs involved in developing an independent practice, it is important to determine whether you want to accomplish this endeavor in an extravagant or in a strict, down-to-earth fashion. Keep in mind, as you pursue your requirements, that an office that looks like it has been there for a long time will serve your purpose much better than stingy, economically impoverished surroundings that seem to have an air of "desperation" — this type of atmosphere may cause a certain degree of mistrust in your potential patients. You may wish to splurge on some items and be more frugal with others.

Examine Your Space

Take measurements of your space. Scrutinize it. Although many people are distrustful of their ability to fill space successfully and to make the best possible use of it, visualizing how equipment and furnishings will fit together will help you to make wiser decisions.

Make a Grid of Your Space

In creating your grid, each square should represent one foot. When you find office furnishings, you can calculate (on the grid) how much space the object of your desire is going to occupy. The grid will help you locate trouble spots and empty areas. Sometimes there is a temptation to pick something that is truly awe-inspiring in the executive realm of office furniture, but when it is in your office, you might find that the huge executive desk that looked rather small in the store will fill too much space in your area. It might overwhelm and intimidate rather than demonstrate competence and efficiency. It might also rule out other furnishings that would make your patients far more comfortable than a desk with a great deal of surface space that will either be empty or cluttered, but will not suit your needs in therapy.

Allow for Oversights

Some furniture might not fit well in the designated area. Colors might not go well together. Take into account the paint or paneling on the walls and the wall-to-wall carpeting, if there is any. Will the store allow a trial in your office, to see how things go together? Borrowing cushions or fabric samples from the couches or chairs of your choice is a simple way of determining whether those items will look attractive in the area.

Shop Around

Prepare a cost sheet. Check with several different outlets. Look at catalogs and mail-order outlets. Even if you do not want to obtain furniture by mail order, these sources can give you ideas of comparative costs and of what is available, and thus may save you time. You might consider buying items at local stores as those merchants might be more accommodating in taking items back in exchange for something more suitable or if something goes wrong. Also, stores sometimes will give you sizable discounts for purchases of several items at the same time.

What to Look For

Look for quality. Look for items that will have a long period of usefulness. Sturdy items will withstand the wear and tear a business must endure. It has already been mentioned that sturdiness serves the function of looking as though you have been in practice for awhile; it will also serve you better and longer. In addition, patients seem to be much more careful with obviously valuable furnishings than with things that can undoubtedly withstand much less wear and tear. This is a paradox of human nature. Also look for items that require low upkeep — choose practical tweeds that will not show dirt or spills and fabrics that will repel signs of use.

Style and Coherence

Sometimes choosing many pieces from one line of furnishings will add a dimension that will help tie all of your pieces together in a coherent fashion. Mixing in some antique pieces can add to the feeling of permanence, but they must fit with the overall impression you are trying to create. My predecessor had an antique washstand in her office, which made me look around for its accompanying chamber pot or shower—a lovely item for a bed-and-breakfast establishment, but not an office.

Most of the furniture in my office is a very thick oak in Danish modern style (with the exception of some of the antique pieces, which are also oak, and the curio cabinet, which is made of plywood but does not look like it). The modern pieces were purchased from an unfinished-furniture store, which had them finished with the stain of my choice. I chose a teak finish that darkened the oak and made the furnishings look much older than they were. Since the oak took on a darkened tone, this permitted me to add a square antique desk, an old oak rocking chair, a Crusader chair, and a black gun cabinet, which I had the dealer make into the curio cabinet. The curio cabinet is only a foot square but nearly reaches the ceiling. It proved to be the pivotal piece that tied all of the pieces together even though it was an afterthought—a luxurious touch, not a necessity. However, it ultimately served a utilitarian purpose when the drawers in the base became the storage place for children's toys.

EQUIPMENT

Your Desk

Do you want a desk? Is your office large enough to accommodate one? If so, what do you want to put in it? Do you want it to be a workspace or a storage area? Many people have expressed appreciation of the fact that the therapy area does not "house" a desk or other office equipment. Do people feel intimidated when you separate yourself from them with your desk? I think most people do not like artificial barriers between themselves and the therapist. Therefore, I divided my office in such a manner that the desk is visible, but not in the therapy area itself (see Figure 1). Look for a desk that houses the materials you want to put into it without overwhelming the therapy area.

Worktable

If you choose to have a worktable, this may hold your telephone, typewriter, computer equipment, or whatever else you may need. My desk and worktable are both accessible from the same swivel chair, and the table seems to double the work capacity and area. The worktable has a large amount of storage because it has a shelf underneath that can accommodate bulky items like stationary boxes and office forms. My telephone and billing records are also on this table, so everything I need regarding patients' records is immediately accessible when information is requested of me over the phone. I had this desk made to my specifications and in the same style as the rest of the furniture in my office by the person who finished the original furnishings.

Chairs

Determine how many people you are going to be likely to be working with at one time in therapy. Many people like the overstuffed, cozy, curl-up kind of chair, but many do not. A sofa can also be very useful. A few straight-backed chairs might be necessary and these can be moved around more easily to accommodate extra visitors. As already mentioned, there is a rocking chair in my office, which people can elect to sit in, although I generally take that chair for myself. With the slouching chairs provided, however, it is important to have some that will not make clients who have back problems uncomfortable. Since the rocking chair is straight-backed and easy to get out of, some people request it.

In arranging your seating, be aware that people will want options as to where to sit (i.e., some will want to sit near you and some will want as much distance from you as possible). Some may ask you where you usually sit so they can more adequately estimate the amount of distance they will need. Do you want, in addition, some folding chairs that you can store in a closet for unexpected or larger groups of people?

Do not forget a desk chair for yourself. This chair can double as an extra for emergencies when needed. Also, if you have a waiting area, will you need chairs there, as well?

Cushions, large and small, can be useful. When stacked, they can serve as floor seating or extra chair space. When scattered, they can serve as accents and many people will opt to lean on them or bunch them behind their backs.

Lighting

Your office may be equipped with fluorescent lighting. Keep in mind that many people are "allergic" to these bright lights. You may want to provide them with the option of indirect lighting. Being able to change the atmosphere in your office can be very helpful and many people will ask for a change in lighting. Some prefer a more intimate atmosphere provided by the indirect lighting, while some may be intimidated or fearful of it — or feel that you are artificially introducing a feeling of intimacy for which they are not ready. If you decide to provide these options, however, you may want to look at table or floor lamps, so the overheads can be turned off during therapy sessions if desired. As with the rest of your office furnishings, lamps should fit in with the decor you have chosen. If you have opted for sturdy furnishings, the lamps also should be heavy.

Answering Machine

Cutting personnel costs and the use of a telephone answering machine in private practice have been addressed in another volume (Meek, 1986). I chose to cut secretarial costs and utilized the extra funds to provide accents for my office. Depending on your locale, you may want to increase your patients' anonymity by utilizing such a device yourself. There is nothing else I value so highly as my answering machine. One must evaluate advantages of a service such as this, as well as the disadvantages. Some patients like dealing with a receptionist or live answering service; however, some will like dealing directly with you at all times with no intermediary — even if only by machine.

Telephone

Check with your telephone company about the options available. I chose to purchase my own telephone with options that seemed useful for my purposes. It will be important to shop around for a telephone with the features you would like to have. The telephone is a business expense you cannot do without and should be calculated into your start-up costs. Some telephone companies require a deposit at the outset but some will waive it if you have maintained a home telephone service in the area for a long time. Do not overlook the expense involved in maintaining a yellow-page listing—also extremely important. Although businesses vary according to likely sources of referral, many people look for therapists in the yellow pages and this will be an important resource for you. The phone company may ask for you to pay the entire cost of the yellow-page listing initially, but you might be able to negotiate to have the costs apportioned on a monthly, rather than yearly, basis. If you choose to have more than one yellow-page listing, you may be offered a discount for these additional advertisements.

The telephone company may also have additional services available. It might be well worth your time to meet with one of its representatives to discuss the possibilities. If there is more than one person in your practice, you may wish to have more than one line available. In some areas, there is an option called "call waiting." A signal alerts you when another call is coming in. You must then "immediately," but temporarily, disconnect your caller and take the other call. At the time I accepted telephone service, the hook-up for call waiting was provided at no additional charge. However, I soon found the service a nuisance and that it had far more disadvantages than advantages. You cannot disconnect a tearful caller "immediately." If I did not do so, the other caller would hear the regular ring (no busy signal) and hang up. In this way, the first caller felt intruded upon and the second was no longer there when I answered. I chose to let the second caller get a busy signal, not possible with call waiting, which at least gave hope that I was there.

Filing Space

Unfortunately, filing space has a tendency to fill itself up much more quickly than one might expect. It is important to have locked file storage of your patients' records, even if you work alone. When your patients see that their records are safely secured, they feel more confident. When taking your office measurements, be sure to include room for files and find a space for them that is not intrusive. Lateral files seem to protrude less into the office space than the old-fashioned type.

Filing cabinets can be as expensive or as inexpensive as you need. Determine whether it is really necessary to purchase expensive fireproof storage. Some file cabinets also contain a small safe, an index drawer, and two file drawers. I chose this type of cabinet as well as a four-drawer lateral file. They are both metal and in a color that blends in well with the rest of the office. I did not opt for fireproof storage cabinets.

Typewriter or Computer

I have two electronic typewriters with very limited storage capacity—one in my office and one at home. My personal preference is to do office work at home—reports and billing—so the most sophisticated typewriter is there. Since I do my own billing and report writing, the typewriter with a small amount of storage seems quite adequate for my needs. It permits me to store therapy codes, and to do the billing in a couple of hours. If you have expertise in computers (or a desire to learn), you may want to evaluate your need for such equipment. I have colleagues who do everything with their computers and all of their records and documents are stored therein. Whether you need one or not must be carefully evaluated in my estimation. I have not found the need for one since I am an expert typist and it does not take me very long to compose reports—sometimes a one-trial effort is all that is needed. You must examine your own experience and the work requirements to determine your need. Computer-made forms and statements may not be of very much help if they lack the polish that typeset forms might convey. If you do not have any expertise with either type of equipment and want to have a secretarial service, receptionist, or bookkeeper prepare your reports and billing, then this is another expense that must be anticipated.

Calculator

What kind of calculator do you want or need? Do you require storage capacity and a printout tape? Do you want a simple adding machine? If so, do you want one with batteries or the solar type? For the most part, as with other office equipment, calculators can be a minor or major expense, as you choose. I have found that the small solar calculator, which costs under $10, suits my needs. I did not need a printed tape.

Storage Cabinets and Bookcases

People are reassured by bookcases in a therapist's office. They will examine the books on the shelves and may identify some that are of interest to them. You will need a space to store patient handouts, billing forms, stationery, and so on. Therefore, look into the kinds of cabinet(s) or bookcases that will serve your needs. Some bookcases also contain fold-out desks. I have found that this type of bookcase is quite useful to house forms I routinely hand out to patients. The storage cabinet in which I store many of my office forms and stationery also doubles as a curio shelf—being a back-bar type. The back-bar has doors underneath that hide a storage area for cleaning supplies, tissues, light bulbs, tea, coffee, paper cups, and the like. Storage space should be provided for your journals and other research materials. Shelving in a closet may be the most inexpensive option for this purpose.

Tables

If you have decided to provide table lamps, then you might include end tables in your office. Also, a coffee table is a necessary "living room" accent.

Do you need a writing surface for testing? Will your desk or worktable serve this purpose? Is there an unobtrusive place for a permanent testing area? If not, do you want a fold-up table that can be used as needed and stored out of sight otherwise?

Carpets

Is your office already carpeted? If so, is it a carpet you can live with? Does it help with sound reduction? Does it tie your office together? My office had wall-to-wall carpeting in a black/white/orange tweed in a tightly looped weave. I could not live with it — neither could my patients. This was, therefore, an area in which I indulged myself with a great deal of extravagance. I chose a very thick Indian carpet that almost covers the entire therapy area. It is extremely durable and attractive. It not only hides the unattractive and distracting wall-to-wall carpeting, but it helps coordinate the entire therapy area. I also chose a smaller Persian carpet for the "office" side of my office, which covers the existing carpet in that area.

Soundproofing

Can people outside hear conversation taking place inside your office? If so, will you need to invest in office insulation or a different door? Will you need a sound system of some kind outside your office door? If you have chairs in your waiting area, such a system can be installed quite easily by attaching the speaker underneath one of these chairs. My radio/tape deck is inside my office and can be regulated from there, although the sounds outside of the office are not heard inside at all. A sound system will be appreciated by some and scorned by others, as many clients will wish to have quiet before meeting with you — a time to themselves to think about what they wish to accomplish during the therapy hour. However, with the explanation that it ensures their privacy, most people are willing to accept or tolerate the intrusion.

Door Bell

Since I work alone, I needed to have a device that would allow patients to let me know when they had arrived for their therapy hour. It also served to signal the patient I am with that someone else is waiting. Patients are instructed by a sign to ring the bell at the appointed time, and this has been quite effective, although teenagers who cannot wait to signal their arrival generally do so as soon as they hit the door. You may need to consider using such a device if you have decided that you will not be hiring a receptionist. Some colleagues of mine installed a light switch, which people turn on at the time of their appointment to light a bulb inside the therapy office; it is considered less intrusive. However, I have found it helpful for someone or something to intrude at the end of the hour. It seems to serve as a second motion that the time is up. The first signal is my chiming clock.

Timepieces

You may want a clock outside of your office. Since there is a pharmacy next door to me, patients use that clock or their own watches to determine when to ring the bell for their appointment. Inside my office I have a large digital clock that can be seen by individuals during therapy and I also have a chiming clock that chimes every half-hour. I have found these items to be indispensable. Having a chiming clock helps people regulate the course of their therapy hour.

Power Bars

You will find that you will receive, on the average, a yearly inspection by members of the local fire department. They will look for hazards and you will welcome their arrival as they can readily pinpoint likely areas of trouble. Extension cords and adapters allowing you to plug several items into one outlet are considered "no-no's" and you will be encouraged to alleviate the offense(s) within 24 hours. Power bars with circuit breakers in them can help you with this problem and they are approved by the fire department. Also, you can regulate the equipment that you want turned on at the same time each morning by one flick of a switch rather than by chasing around to turn on all of the items that need to be turned on. I have three power bars in my office—one is on all the time, another is turned on in the mornings, and the other is turned on only when needed (the video equipment). Several items are merely plugged into the wall because they are not in a congested location and there were outlets to accommodate them safely.

Wastebaskets

Oddly enough, the fire department was concerned with my lovely rattan wastebasket. It seems that, in our area, fire codes indicate that business establishments should utilize metal containers for waste. The rattan basket was retired to the top of one of my bookcases, and rather than the U.S. Army standard office wastebasket, I chose a brass and copper planter that is like a round bucket with a handle. It met the fire code requirement, and is a decorative object was well. It matches other planters in my office, as well as the brass table lamps.

Special Equipment

Each therapist must evaluate any specialties that might be offered in practice. Special equipment might be a major or minor expense, depending upon the therapies offered. Therapists must actively scrutinize their training and areas of expertise and, in my estimation, offer only those services with which they feel most comfortable. In private practice, I believe there is a very strong temptation to offer too many services, rather than relying on other professionals who have specialized in areas in which the practicing therapist may be less well qualified. Avoid the temptation to be a Jack- or Jill-of-all-trades. I routinely refer and avoid areas in which I feel I am less well qualified or for which I harbor a dislike.

Thus, it is important to make some decisions regarding the types of services you are going to offer. If working with children, play materials might be a necessity—including dolls, minifamilies, drawing equipment, and games. You also might want to consider making some of the items yourself. Sewing stores usually carry small panels of fabric that represent the fronts and backs of dolls; when sewn together, complete families, scenes, and so on can be created to be used in therapy with children. The flannel board can be created at minimal cost (flannel wrapped around fiber board and stapled to the back) and is a joy to children. Figures are cut from magazines and books, and flannel glued to their backs; when pressed onto the flannel board, they remain in position. Entire scenes can be created and therapists can develop a mammoth collection of possibilities. The cost is practically nothing.

Individuals who offer biofeedback will need to determine the types of tools necessary to provide an effective service. Testing equipment and scoring expenses may also need to be taken into account. Video equipment will include a camera (available in color or black and white), VCR, television monitor, remote control, and videotapes. The monitor should be easily seen but be unobtrusive. One might also wish to invest in a tape recorder if this is likely to be useful in one's practice. These items must be evaluated in terms of what they will actually add to your practice and how they will justify the expenses involved. If you do not plan to specialize at the outset, it might be helpful to take a wait-and-see attitude to determine the need for electronic or other equipment.

Plants

Plants are an inexpensive item, generally, and can give an office a lived-in appearance. Some of mine are 15 years old and have become extremely impressive, incompassing a large area, including the ceiling and walls. I have encountered only one individual who was allergic to plants and only one who was phobic about them. Plants seem to be well worth the investment. If you know nothing about them, look for specimens that survive well in adverse conditions (i.e., the typical office environment), that do not need a great deal of light, and that are likely to be unattractive to plant-destroying pests. Unfortunately, you have to bypass exotic plants in favor of the practical, but plants are a worthwhile addition to your office environment. Among plants that are likely to survive the hostile atmosphere of the office are African violets (placed by a north window or under a table lamp), philodendron, devil's ivy, Christmas cactus, hoya, and rubber plants. Stay away from ferns unless you have a very humid atmosphere—they tend to shed leaves. Asparagus ferns are predictably devoured by mites within weeks, regardless of the care you give them. Stay away from ivies, too, for the same reason. A few flowering plants of the exotic class might be a cheerful choice for the office coffee table, but they must be regarded as "throwaways"; their ability to survive for a long time in the office is quite limited. I treat myself now and then to one of these grocery-store specials.

Mailbox

Where will the postal service put your mail? Can your carrier get into your waiting area? If so, a mailbox outside your office door will be the best choice. If the letter carrier is barred from entry, then an outside mailbox will have to do. If inside, it will also be useful for patients who wish to drop things off for you — borrowed materials or payments. If outside, a waterproof mailbox of the commercial variety might be your best choice. My mailbox is oak, made in the same style as most of my office furnishings, by the person who made my worktable. It is four inches wide and a foot and a half deep with a slot approximately one inch wide. It will accommodate a week's worth of mail, it is locked by a small padlock and bolted to one of my waiting room chairs (on the floor), which is also bolted to the floor. You may need to notify the postal service of your existence. It is helpful to introduce yourself — I made a telephone call and told them my name, business, and location.

Signs

You will need to have a sign on the outer entrance, and probably inside as well, near your office door. My signs are painted in a beige weatherproof paint on a dark-stained wood. Neon signs are eschewed in my professional area and I believe are still not condoned by professional associations. My signs state:

Carroll L. Meek, Ph.D.
Counseling Psychologist
Licensed
National Register of Health
    Service Providers in Psychology
Counseling and Consultation
(Individual, Couple, Child, and
    Adolescent Therapy)

Accents

Although your personality will already be indicated by selection of furniture style and colors, accents provide an endless variety of ways in which you might choose to "tell" people about who you are. Clients are typically a bit unnerved when first arriving at your office, and items there can make them feel comfortable and "at home." I have gone to a great deal of effort to create a living-room atmosphere in my office, because I have found that it works well for me. I strongly believe that a sterile environment is intimidating or depressing to most people and I would much rather overwhelm them with comfort and a cozy atmosphere. Since I have mixed antiques and solid Danish-oak furniture, my office has a medieval feeling. Therefore, it seemed obvious to me to add some castlelike items to it. Some of the things you might like to consider are paintings, wall hangings, bric-a-brac, and toss or throw pillows.

I have found that adults are tickled by the fact that many of the items in my office are parodies of their "expectations" about therapy, which to many people are overwhelming and sources of fear — until they are confronted with something that will bring a smile to their lips. So I have included such things as peacock feathers, a crystal ball, Aladdin's lamp, Excalibur, a wizard's staff, a real hour glass, a basket of polished rocks, a kaleidoscope, music boxes, a jumping Jack, vases, crystals, and a unicorn mobile. For children, all of this provides a little relief and a different atmosphere from that of most doctors' offices. People like to fiddle with something so Mexican "worry" stones are nice to have around, too.

Since one of my hobbies is creating needlepoint tapestries, I have also utilized the opportunity to put a couple of these on my walls. The pictures and paintings I have chosen have a dreamlike, mystical quality. Something in this office seems to appeal to almost everyone, although one woman who is generally critical wrote on her First-Session Evaluation Form (Meek & Editors, 1985) that the "office seemed a little too eccentric." When I burst out laughing and said that that was the most charitable evaluation of my office I had ever seen, since it was "decidedly eccentric — not a 'little' eccentric," this produced a new twist.

Some visitors have wanted to know how people manage to work in a space with so many distractions. Oddly enough, I have never found that to be a problem, although some clients have expressed regrets that they did not have the time to spend there to study it thoroughly. I have noticed, however, chair changes — statements of "I want to get a different view" — but those changes have generally coincided with improvements in therapy and have resulted in changes of chairs that moved clients closer to me, not further away.

I must also say, for animal lovers everywhere, that I work with a Maltese dog in my office. My first, Tiffany, was my constant cotherapist for 11 years. When she died, the loneliness of that office without my companion was more than I could bear, and I acquired a distant relative of hers within a week. My current patients were told that we were going to be breaking in a new puppy, Katrina, and all greeted her arrival with relief and enthusiasm. At this writing, she is three years old, has been attending sessions since she was four months old, and is doing extremely well. The experiences of having a dog or puppy as a cotherapist is really the subject of another chapter, but you might consider it. It has been the most important asset to me I can possibly imagine, not to mention to my patients. Studies are now demonstrating that blood pressure and tension go down in the presence of an animal. I have found that a nonevaluative being like my Maltese has been a reassuring addition to my office.

GENERAL COMMENTS

As you can tell, I have not skimped on my office decor or budget, nor with my stationery and office forms. Whether or not you have just opened your doors, people want to have some certainty that you are likely to be there for awhile and that you are not a fly-by-night snake-oil salesperson. I must admit, however, that my first patient arrived when I had boxes stacked all around, my philodendron snaking all over the floor (not yet pinned to the walls and ceiling), and my hair up in the untidy manner of someone "just moving in." When I tried to schedule an appointment with her, she said that if I were not "busy," she would like to see me at once. That is just what we did.

I am assuming that money is an object to those who are attempting to establish a private enterprise of any kind. I also assume that one is going to have limited resources. Therefore, it will be important to you to establish your priorities in order to serve your public in as civilized a manner as possible. Basically, people are looking for a competent therapist they feel they can relate to in terms of their presenting problems. Therefore, just as my stacks of boxes and disarrayed hair can attest, if you meet their expectations as a person, they will stick with you. Your office is the cocoon in which they will work with you, and each person will be struggling with the decision about whether *you* will be the one who is going to be able to work best with him or her. Your office is not only likely to be a haven, but a positive inspiration, as well.

LAST STEPS

Survey your office again. Determine what you will need. Examine your budget and how much money you have to spend for each item. Decide what you want to do to express your personality—now is the time to make any therapy "statements" you want to make. Make a grid of your office, with each square representing a square foot. When shopping, sketch the items, in their proportional sizes, onto your grid. Visualize how all of the items are going to go together. Start with the basics and add as your finances allow. Keep in mind that there are likely to be some things that you will overlook that will be necessary to your functioning as a therapist, so provide funds for these. Will you automatically reach for a stapler and find it is not there, or for some scissors, or paper clips? How about weighing letters that might be a little too heavy for the one-ounce rate? How about a coffee pot or a kettle for hot water? Will you serve your patients tea or coffee (with and without caffeine)? Do you want a minirefrigerator? What kinds of extras will make your life as a therapist as comfortable as possible?

Go through this chapter again. Underline items mentioned that you need to consider for your office. After that, code in (N) necessary, (D) desired, (W) wait, and (N/U) no use in terms of your needs. First, concentrate on the necessary, then progress to the desired. You might catalog items with index cards to help you keep track of different items, stores, prices, measurements, and so on. The index cards can be arranged in order of purchases that must be made immediately and those which can wait.

MY OFFICE

Figure 1 is a diagram of the furnishings chosen for my office. Since the room I occupy is only 14 by 18 square feet, I found that space was important in terms of making the most adequate use of it. As you can see, I divided the

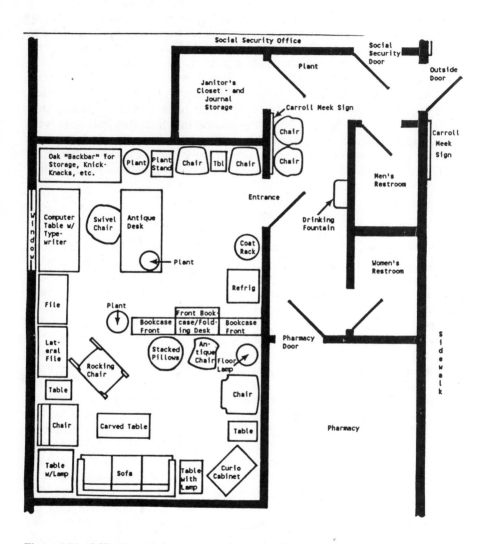

Figure 16-1. Office layout. Source: Freudenberger, H.J., Lewin, M.H., Meek, C.L. & Ritt, L.G. (1986). The private practice of psychology: Four variations. In P.A. Keller & L.G. Ritt (Eds.), *Innovations in clinical practice: A source book* (Vol. 5). Sarasota, Fla: Professional Resource Exchange, Inc., p. 239. Drawing by Aachen Designers, Gainesville, Fla. Reprinted with permission.

room into two areas using bookcases (three units) to separate the therapy from the office area. The division of the area created the illusion of two separate rooms rather than one.

REFERENCES

Freudenberger, H.J., Lewin, M.H., Meek, C.L., & Ritt, L.G. (1986). The private practice of psychology: Four variations. In P.A. Keller & L.G. Ritt (Eds.), *Innovations in clinical practice: A source book* (Vol. 5), pp. 233.244. Sarasota, FL: Professional Resource Exchange.

Meek, C.L., & Editors (1985). A collection of office forms. In P.A. Keller & L.G. Ritt (Eds.), *Innovations in clinical practice: A source book* (Vol. 4), pp. 345–357. Sarasota, FL: Professional Resource Exchange.

Meek, C.L. (1986). Guidelines for using an answering machine in your practice. In P.A. Keller & L.G. Ritt (Eds.), *Innovations in clinical practice: A source book* (Vol. 5), pp. 271–276. Sarasota, FL: Professional Resource Exchange.

17

INSURANCE AND OTHER START-UP COSTS

Frederick J. Smith, Ph.D.

The costs of setting up a private-practice office go far beyond the leasing of space and purchasing of furniture and equipment. Just as a home is more than a residence filled with furniture and appliances, so too, a private-practice office is more than a space containing a telephone, desk, chair, and couch. For both esthetic and functional reasons, a home needs to be decorated — and so does an office. The structure, its contents, and its owner need to be insured against loss and liability. The list of additional considerations can be extensive and more expensive than one might think (as anyone who has set up a house knows!). The purpose of this chapter is twofold: to catalog the things that need to be considered and to provide a sense of the costs involved.

INSURANCE

Malpractice

The recent crisis in liability insurance has received extensive media coverage. The effects of the crisis have been widespread; municipalities have been forced to reduce insurance coverage to levels they fear leave them vulnerable; school systems have had to curtail programs and activities for lack of affordable coverage; and recreational enterprises, such as ski areas, have closed because of exorbitant premiums or the complete unavailability of insurance from any source. Professional malpractice insurance has followed a similar course.

Malpractice insurance premiums have risen tremendously for all mental-health professionals. For psychologists, rates increased 1000 percent for the period 1983–1986. For psychiatrists, rates have increased 100 percent during the same period. Social workers have seen a smaller increase (38 percent), but the trend is still upward. Worse, leaders in these fields predict sizable increases in premiums for some time to come.

In terms of dollar amount, psychiatrists pay the largest premiums. For 1986, annual premiums ranged from $1,200 to $8,700 for $1 million/$3 million liability limits, depending on the geographical location of the practice. Psychologists faced a $585 annual premium for similar coverage for 1986 (regardless of location). Social workers paid $58 for similar limits for 1986. Obviously, malpractice insurance constitutes a much larger overhead cost for some professionals than others, but for all, it is an issue to be considered when establishing an independent private practice.

Because of the rise in liability insurance costs, some insurance carriers offer "claims made" types of insurance policies instead of "occurrence" types of insurance. So-called claims-made insurance is cheaper because it only covers claims against the insured during the policy period. On the other hand, occurrence-type policies cover the insured against claims of liability while the policy *was* in effect, although the claim itself may not be made until years later. In the case of claims-made insurance, once coverage has lapsed, a claim made will not be covered, although it may be for an event that occurred while the policy was in effect. In order to be insured against such claims, one must maintain the claims-made type of insurance long past the time when one stops practicing. For example, if one had practiced during the period 1975–1980 and had occurrence-type liability insurance, then a claim initiated in 1985 regarding an event that occurred in 1978 would be covered, though no insurance had been past the year 1980. In claims-made types of policies, only claims initiated during the period 1975–1980 regarding events occurring during that period would be covered. In order to maintain coverage, one would have to maintain the insurance policy right through 1985.

The above example is hardly farfetched. Recently, claims have been initiated as long as 15 years after the alleged event. It would appear that for all practical purposes there is no statute of limitations on malpractice or, for that matter, on other forms of liability. Once a claims-made policy has been purchased, it may have to be maintained for many years in order to have any real coverage against a tort liability suit. Though claims-made insurance may be cheaper in the short run, it will be much more costly in the long run.

Group policies, such as those sponsored by national professional organizations are generally less expensive than individually written policies. However, in certain locales, it may be cheaper to purchase an individual policy. Consult a local independent insurance broker who deals in commercial insurance and has had experience in writing these types of policies. Be sure to compare coverages of different policies, as well as prices.

Business Owner's Insurance

This form of insurance is the commercial equivalent of the familiar homeowners insurance policy. It covers loss of property as a result of fire (and other natural perils like wind or ice) or theft; bodily injuries; property damage; medical costs; and personal injury (liability other than professional liability). Premiums vary with the limits of coverage specified. A typical comprehensive policy is shown in the following.

Loss Covered	*Liability Limit*	
Business personal property	$ 21,400	
Exterior sign	300	
Comprehensive business liability:		
Bodily injury	1,000,000	
Property damage	1,000,000	
Fire legal liability	1,000,000	
Premises medical payment	5,000	each person
Personal injury and advertising injury	1,000,000	

In choosing policy limits of coverage, be aware that *increases* in policy limits cost little as compared with the basic policy premium. If, for instance, the insurance company's basic policy (the level of coverage below which the company will simply not write a policy) is for $500,000 personal injury liability and the premium is $100 per year, coverage could be doubled, even quadrupled, for a relatively small increase in annual premium (e.g., $1 million policy limit for $128 yearly or $2 million for $136 yearly).

Another consideration in choosing policy limits for business property is whether to insure for replacement value or actual cash value. Actual cash value is defined as the purchase price less depreciation to the time of the loss. Unless the property were relatively new, one would receive less than the purchase price if a loss were sustained. Although replacement-value insurance is generally more costly, it takes replacement cost into account with no deduction for depreciation. In the event of a catastrophic loss (e.g., the entire contents of one's office destroyed by fire), replacement-value insurance can seem like a real bargain. It should be noted that over time the premiums for replacement-value coverage will be higher than for actual cash-value coverage since the policy limits will not decrease (as they would with actual cash-value insurance as the property ages and drops in value), but actually will increase as the replacement costs increase with inflation.

Premiums for business owner's insurance range from less than $100 per year to several hundred dollars yearly depending on the coverage and the geographical location of the property. One final note: by all means, *read* the policy. Policyholders rarely do so until a financial loss is sustained. Every policy has exclusions. Once a loss has occurred, it is too late to discover that the property that was lost was excluded (e.g., the new personal computer that was installed last week) or that the cause of the loss was excluded (e.g., wind-driven rain and flood are covered perils but water leaking through the roof behind ice dams frozen on the eaves is not).

Worker's Compensation Insurance and Employee Disability Insurance

A majority of states require by law that all employees be provided with Worker's Compensation insurance to cover loss of income and medical and rehabilitative expenses resulting from work-related accidents and occupational diseases. Premiums vary with the type of work performed by the employee (e.g., operating a forklift is inherently riskier than typing) and the size of the payroll (i.e., the larger the payroll, the higher the insurance premium will be). No options exist as to the type of coverage purchased as these details are set by law. In addition to Worker's Compensation insurance, some states require the provision of employee disability insurance. Again, coverage is dictated by law and premiums vary with the type of work performed and the size of the payroll. Any independent insurance broker or agency handling business and commercial lines of insurance can provide information on the types of employee insurance required in a given area plus a quotation on approximate costs.

The costs of employing staff go far beyond the salaries or wages they are paid. In addition, the employer must purchase the forms of insurance described above and pay part of FICA (Social Security). These benefits typically run from 12 to 15 percent of the size of the payroll. Moreover, pension plans established on behalf of the employer may be obliged to cover employees as well (e.g., Keogh pension plans require employees to be covered under certain circumstances). Obviously, any medical, dental, or life insurance plans that are provided as part of an employee's benefits increase the employee benefit costs even further. The entire benefit package could easily add 20 to 30 percent to the wages or salaries paid. Because of this, it may be less costly to purchase office services separately, rather than to hire staff (i.e., telephone reception from an answering service, typing from a typing service, billing from a billing service, etc.).

Income Protective Plans

Disability income insurance plans provide benefits when one is partially or totally unable to work owing to illness, disease, or injury. Obviously, the extent to which one depends on private-practice income will determine the degree of importance of such insurance to a particular practitioner. Someone engaged in a small, part-time private practice and whose primary source of income includes a typical array of benefits, including annual leave, sick leave, and Worker's Compensation, may choose to forgo such a policy altogether. Conversely, someone in full-time practice with no other source of income should consider such a policy to be essential.

Premiums vary with the insured's age, with the face value of the benefit paid, with the length of time the benefits are paid, and particularly with the time between occurrence of disability and first payment (e.g., 30 days, 60 days, 90 days). Premium costs range in the area of several hundred dollars annually.

Another approach to disability income protection involves groups or consortiums of practitioners organized to provide a system of cross-coverage for each other in the event of disability. This type of arrangement may be viewed as self-insurance. The following is an example of an arrangement taken from a partnership agreement of a group of four clinicians:

> Article XVII (Disability): In the event of physical or mental disability of any of the parties, remaining parties shall provide services and coverage for the clients of the disabled party. Continuity of care for the disabled party's clients will be accomplished by assignment to each remaining party of specific clients or tasks, as determined by mutual agreement. Fees collected during the disability period will be credited as follows:
> - During the first three months, 100 percent to the disabled party.
> - During the fourth, fifth, and sixth months, 50 percent to the disabled party and 50 percent to the party who personally performed the services.
> - After six months, 100 percent to the party performing the services.

Such arrangements work particularly well in conjunction with disability insurance, since the latter always involve grace periods (e.g., 30, 60, 90 days) before benefits begin to be paid.

PRINTING

A full array of printed materials for a new practice may include the following:

> Letterheads (in two sizes, 8½ by 11½, 5½ by 8½)
> Billheads
> Statements
> Envelopes, plain (in sizes to accommodate the aboved)
> Envelopes, window (for statements and billheads)
> Business cards
> Appointment cards
> Announcement cards
> Special forms (for the clinical record)

The cost of even minimum quantities of these items could total several hundred dollars. There are various ways to economize.

1. Purchase multipurpose forms. Business cards and appointment cards can be printed back to back on the same stock, resulting in a dual-purpose item. Statements may be typed on letterhead, thus eliminating the need for separate forms. Eliminate announcement cards entirely. The consensus of practitioners who receive them is that they are worthless.

2. Order from one of the national specialty printers who cater to the professions. Compared with a local printer, they supply excellent-quality goods at the lowest possible prices, as much as 50 percent less in many cases. Their only disadvantage is the time to delivery (usually two to three weeks). If you can afford to wait, the savings are worthwhile.

DECORATING

If the services of an interior decorator have been used in selecting office furniture, then one may wish to allow the decorator to handle the entire decorating task. In that way, one is assured that walls, floors, and windows will coordinate with the furniture selected. Otherwise, the following remarks will serve to outline the issues involved in office decorating.

Wall Treatment

A fresh coat of paint is obviously the least expensive way of dealing with office walls. Wallpaper and paneling are costlier, in terms both of materials and the labor to install them. However, they do allow for the creation of much different atmospheres than does paint. To economize, consider papering or paneling only one or two walls and painting the rest. As for comparable costs, paint can be purchased for $10 to $20 per gallon, paper from $7 and up per roll, and paneling for $10 and up per sheet. One gallon of paint will cover 400 square feet, one roll of paper will cover 26 square feet, and one sheet of paneling (4 feet by 8 feet) will cover 30 square feet (taking into account losses due to cutting around doorways and windows). Cost of labor for painters and paperhangers may be figured at $10 to $20 per hour as a rough estimate. In most locales, contractors who specialize in small-scale commercial and residential work will readily supply estimates for labor.

Floor Treatment

Hard floors (wood, tile, or sheet goods) are durable and easy to maintain, but create a harsh atmosphere for an office. Unless hygienic issues are of primary importance, as in a physician's examining room, consider covering hard floors with carpeting or rugs to add a sense of warmth and comfort.

Certain clinical situations (e.g., group therapy, play therapy) may require the practitioner to limit sound transmission as much as possible. Since typical office walls and ceilings are acoustically "hard," carpeting and rugs may become a crucial choice in absorbing sound and limiting unwanted sound transmission. As a rough rule of thumb, one can figure that carpeting or rugs will cost a minimum of $1.50 per square foot (labor to install wall-to-wall carpeting is not included in this figure).

Wallpaper, paneling, and wall-to-wall carpeting, once installed, constitute improvements to property. They become part of the property itself and belong to the property owner. Because of this and the expense involved, it may be preferable to negotiate with the lessor to make such alterations to property as a condition of accepting the lease.

Window Treatment

Controlling light transmission is the primary function of window coverings. Obviously, shades and blinds do this more efficiently and effectively than do most curtains and drapes. Some consider the latter, however, as offering some versatility from a decorative standpoint. However, all types of window coverings can be used both functionally and decoratively. Costs vary widely and increase when an item is custom-made. Figure a minimum cost of $2 per square foot of window area covered.

Plants

Plants add immeasurably to the atmosphere of an office. The few plants needed for an individual office may be purchased at any local greenhouse at nominal cost. However, if an entire suite of offices is being supplied with plants, the overall cost can be quite high. In that case, one might consider one of the "rent-a-plant" services available in many areas. The plants are guaranteed, service and maintenance are part of the package, and monthly costs are far more affordable than a one-time, up-front outlay of perhaps several hundred dollars.

Magazines

The ubiquitous waiting-room magazine is a must, even for the client whose wait is brief. Subscriptions for weekly publications run approximately $27 per year as a minimum, while monthly publications cost approximately $17 per year.

As for the types of publications best suited for waiting rooms, those with the greatest appeal are the ones that can be scanned or read quickly. Weekly news magazines are a good choice, as are the weekly "people" magazines (i.e., those that feature brief vignettes of people in the news). The articles in such magazines can be read in five minutes or less; pictures and captions can be scanned rapidly. Magazines that feature longer articles are a poor choice. To the extent that clients are observed to be "reading" them, they are typically browsing instead (e.g., looking at the pictures in *National Geographic,* reading cartoons in *The New Yorker*).

OFFICE-SPACE MODIFICATIONS

A practice involving assessment and treatment of individual adolescent or adult clients may require no special office features. Most offices can be used "as is" when leased. However, the needs of specialty practices may require structural alterations before the space is usable. For example, playrooms or examination rooms may require the addition of a sink and associated plumbing. Special soundproofing, double doors, special wiring or electrical shielding to accommodate computers or biofeedback equipment, and alterations in architecture to accommodate audio and video recording devices are but a few examples of other kinds of modifications that may be required.

Estimates of the cost of such alterations can be obtained from local general contractors who specialize in renovations and additions to basic structures. Since some alterations can cost hundreds, or even thousands, of dollars, one should consider the following way of minimizing out-of-pocket expenses during start-up. Most lessors of commercial property are agreeable to making modifications to basic structures as long as the costs can be recouped and the resulting modifications do not make the property undesirable to subsequent lessees. The lessor may require a longer-term lease and some increase in rent to cover the costs of these changes, but the advantage to the lessee is obvious —it spreads these costs over the entire term of the lease.

ANSWERING SERVICES; ANSWERING MACHINES

Answering machines and services are a necessary evil. All practitioners have them and everyone seems to complain about them. Each offers certain advantages and disadvantages, which should be carefully considered before making a choice.

Machines are less expensive in the long run, ranging in initial cost from less than $100 to approximately $300. An answering service will run several hundred dollars a year. The specific cost of each will depend on the features desired. Machines offering such features as voice-activated recording, beeperless remote playback, variable outgoing messages, time and day stamping, and built-in phone will cost more than the basic model. Similarly, answering services featuring computerized storage of all messages and beeper-paging are more costly than those that record messages as hand-written notes and page by telephone.

The major advantage of an answering service over an answering machine is the capacity of the operator to function proactively. Experienced operators are more than simply message recorders and relayers. They can make judgments about a caller's distress and decide, if it seems warranted, to be very persistent in tracking down a clinician or using alternative means to deal with the situation. The following example illustrates the point.

> Late one Saturday morning the answering service contacted Dr. S. saying that a very distraught patient was calling from a phone booth. When he called the number he had been given, he got a wrong number. He called the answering service back to check the number and found that he had recorded it correctly. Assuming that he must have misdialed, he called the number again, but once again he did not reach the distraught caller.
>
> Minutes later the answering service called to relay the correct number. Presuming that they may have incorrectly recorded the number from the caller, two operators at the service began dialing combinations of the last four digits of the number they had with various three-digit exchange numbers for the local area. Within a few minutes, they had reached the caller at the phone booth where she was waiting for Dr. S. to return her call.
>
> Both Dr. S. and the caller were thankful for the operators' quick thinking, sense of responsibility, and initiative. In discussing the episode later with the operators, they explained that they had taken the actions they did because they felt that the caller might be suicidal. They were correct — she had been.

Check with colleagues in the area before selecting an answering service. Find out which services they use and their opinions about their quality. Also check with the services themselves to find out the type of clientele they serve. Answering services tend to cater to different types of commercial enterprises. Those that serve building contractors, printers, office machine suppliers, and the like are used to dealing with the customers of such enterprises. Those that cater to professionals, on the other hand, are used to taking calls from patients and clients. The operators acquire styles of handling callers, and those who deal with patients on a regular basis are more likely to respond to such calls in an appropriate and effective manner.

SIGNS

A simple, laminated, engraved, 2- by 10-inch plastic strip displaying a practitioner's name, appropriate for office door or desk, may be purchased for as little as $10. At the other extreme, an exterior sign displaying several names, including a free-standing frame and the cost of installation, may cost several hundred dollars. Costs vary with size, material (e.g., bronze versus plastic), labor (e.g., engraving versus painting), and type (i.e., interior signs are generally less expensive than exterior signs).

In selecting signs, keep in mind that their primary function is to direct the public to the location of one's office. Other considerations, such as decor, often influence choice, resulting in money wasted on an inadequate sign. For example, in designing exterior signs, the tendency is to select lettering sizes too small to be seen at a distance. Clients approaching the office in automobiles need to be able to read the sign at a greater distance than pedestrians on foot. Similarly, a brass nameplate elegantly engraved in script may look handsome on the office door, but will be of no value to those attempting to locate the office if it cannot be read without good lighting from more than three feet away.

DEPOSITS

Utilities routinely charge deposits in the amount of one or more months' expected charges for newly established businesses. Whereas electricity and heating may be included in the rent, telephone service is not. Even if the practitioner owns his or her own telephones and interior wiring, the local telephone service company will require a deposit. Though these deposits may be returned after a year or so, they tie up several hundred dollars in escrow at a time when the availability of working capital is crucial.

JANITORIAL SERVICES

Ideally, the lease agreement will include janitorial services. If it does not, then making arrangements with the same janitorial service that cleans the rest of the building is the simplest and perhaps least expensive choice. The costs of cleaning services vary with the extent and frequency of services performed and the size of the area being cleaned. Vacuuming floors twice weekly, emptying waste receptacles daily, dusting all horizontal surfaces once weekly, and washing interior and exterior window surfaces twice yearly is a reasonable minimum schedule. Obviously, periodic washing of walls and shampooing of carpets will add to the expense, but should be considered, if not as part of a regular cleaning schedule, then certainly on an as-needed basis.

SUPPLIES

Accounting Forms

One's accountant should be consulted regarding the appropriate forms and format for receipts, disbursements, payroll, and so forth. There are commercial publishers who provide entire sets of such forms, bound in the same ledger, designed specifically for professional offices. In any case, expect to pay $15 to $50 for an initial set of books.

Sundries

Consider the following list of office supplies. Prices are minimal, obtained from a recent catalog of a large-volume office supply dealer in a medium-size metropolitan area.

Item	Unit	Price
Manilla folders	box (100)	$ 10.65
File guides	set (27)	7.75
Adhesive labels	roll (100)	3.91
Rotary file, small	each	26.00
Typewriter ribbons	box (6)	14.10
Liquid paper	bottle	1.39
Scissors	pair	8.15
Dictionary	each	11.00
Paper, plain bond	ream	6.75
Cellophane tape	roll	1.02
Stapler	each	15.00
Rubber bands	box	1.47
Paper clips	box	4.75
Ballpoint pens	box (12)	3.48
Pencils	box (12)	2.64
	Total	$118.06

Even minimum quantities of these essentials add up to a considerable total price. As for ongoing supplies of these items, purchasing larger quantities results in lower prices; and the best prices are generally found at large office-supply dealers that cater to local commercial establishments (as opposed to the retail office-supply store often found in local shopping malls).

Be aware of wholesale dealers who call from faraway cities asking to speak to the "office manager" and announcing "rock bottom" sale prices on ballpoint pens or copier paper. Often these prices are no lower than can be found locally. Moreover, even if prices are lower, the sale items are probably so-called "loss leaders" designed to attract new business. The items and prices given in the full catalogs from these long-distance wholesalers usually are not particularly attractive, delivery will take longer than from a local supplier, and returns can be a major source of annoyance and frustration. The lowest possible price is not necessarily the most important consideration.

INITIAL ADVERTISING

Many practitioners question the value of initial advertising as a way of generating referrals. It might best be considered as a way of informing the public and one's colleagues of a new address and telephone number rather than as a way to stimulate business.

Advertising rates vary with the size of the advertisement, the circulation of the newspaper, and the days of the week on which the advertisement appears, with weekends being more expensive than weekdays.

MAINTENANCE CONTRACTS

Most new equipment is covered by a warranty, which typically includes parts and labor to repair the equipment for one year from the date of purchase. Maintenance agreements or contracts do one of two things: they either extend the basic warranty for parts and labor beyond the original warranty period, or they add features to the basic warranty (e.g., a guarantee that a technician will arrive to begin repairs within four hours of notification).

A maintenance contract can be compared to a health-insurance policy. On the one hand, it is a form of insurance against a costly overhaul of expensive equipment. On the other hand, assuming that some maintenance and repair are likely to be needed in the life of all machines (like some health care is likely to be required during a person's life), the maintenance agreement is a form of prepayment of costs that are inevitable. Nevertheless, the primary value of a maintenance agreement may lie more in its other features than in its core "parts and labor" warranty. For instance, if a piece of equipment (e.g., a telephone) is crucial to the operation of the practice, then guaranteed repair response times are very important. If temporary unavailability of the equipment (e.g., a typewriter) while it is under repair would seriously hamper operations, then the "loaner" feature of some maintenance contracts is important.

Avoiding breakdown in the first place (like maintaining good health) is the least expensive maintenance strategy in the long run. To that end, the most valuable feature of some maintenance agreements is preventative maintenance (PM). Regular, routine inspection, adjustment, cleaning, and lubrication are crucial to the continued operation of some types of equipment, especially electromechanical devices that are in frequent or constant use (e.g., copiers). For these types of equipment, PM can avoid costly overhauls and annoying down time. Other types of equipment (e.g., electronic devices such as hand-held calculators) require no PM.

The costs of maintenance contracts can be high — $168 per year, for example, for a typewriter that originally cost $850, $320 per year for a copier worth $2,800. The decision to purchae them involves a calculation of the risk of loss (of time, of money to repair or replace the item, of use of a critical device) as compared with their cost. If the item of equipment in question is not critical and is not likely to break down (i.e., is new or in good repair), or is constructed in such a way that repairs can be made quickly and easily (e.g., the repair of many primarily electronic devices involves the replacement of modules), then foregoing the purchase of a maintenance contract may seem to be the wise and economical choice. If such an item needs repair, the repair is paid for "out of pocket" in the expectation that, in the long run, to do so will be cheaper than purchasing a maintenance contract. Conversely, if the likelihood of repair is high, as with a used piece of equipment, the out-of-pocket strategy may be more costly in the long run than the price of a maintenance contract.

In any case, the details of a maintenance contract should be studied before any commitment is made. Moreover, the reputation of the firm providing the service should be investigated. A maintenance agreement is only as good as the people providing the service.

SUMMARY

The total cost of starting a practice varies with the choices made. Nevertheless, one should expect the cost of items discussed in this chapter to total at least $3,000. When added to the cost of leasing or buying space and equipment, the overall cost may well be $10,000 to start a practice.

The availability of sufficient capital to start and maintain a practice until it becomes profitable is the one factor that makes running a practice like operating any other small business. And since insufficient capital is the major reason why 90 percent of all new small businesses fail within two years of opening, it behooves the practitioner to be sure that enough money is available. Unlike many small businesses, most practices begin as part-time enterprises. In that regard, the practitioner may rely on another source of income while the practice grows, and that the practice does not turn a profit for awhile is not a major concern. If it pays for itself, that is, if income covers ongoing overhead costs, the practitioner may be satisfied. However, until profits cover not only ongoing overhead costs, but also the original start-up costs of establishing the practice, the enterprise cannot be called a financial success. Being aware of the amount of capital that is required to get to that point is a crucial aspect of planning.

▲   ▲   ▲

Part II Financial and Economic Management
(continued)

S E C T I O N

B

**Fee
Schedules**

▼ ▼ ▼

18

BASIC INCOME MANAGEMENT

Mark H. Lewin, Ph.D.

Psychology is a science, but the practice of psychology is a business.

High-quality services are important to every profession, but alone they are insufficient to ensure that a practice remains viable. Thus, although Diplomate status (e.g., the credentials of superior competence offered by the American Board of Professional Psychology and the American Board of Psychiatry and Neurology) is a valuable quality-control device, practitioners must be good business managers in order to establish and maintain practices within their communities.

Basic income management is one key to sustaining a personally fulfilling, community-oriented human service business. Cash flow is an esoteric term for a very simple concept. Cash flows through a business in two ways: in and out. Cash flowing in includes:

1. Revenue from professional services.

2. Money from sales of products (books, tapes, and other therapeutic or service aids; payment for articles written or talks presented, etc.).

3. Interest from bank accounts or loans, dividends from securities, and capital infusions by practitioners or others.

Cash flowing out includes all operating expenses. In human service practices, these expenses typically include:

- The practitioner's salary or draw and FICA (Social Security) payments.
- Secretarial wages and FICA payments.
- State and federal taxes.
- Unemployment insurance.
- Office rent.
- Office cleaning and maintenance.
- Office supplies.
- Professional services.
- Profession memberships, books, and journals.
- Continuing education and convention expenses.
- Postage.
- Telephone.
- Utilities.

- Travel expenses.
- Insurance: professional liability; medical; income protection; comprehensive fire, theft, and office liability; life.
- Professional services (legal, accounting, etc.).
- Pension payments.
- Miscellaneous other expenses (gifts, business lunches, charitable contributions, etc.).

OFFERING THE COMMUNITY NEEDED SERVICES IS NOT ENOUGH

Some practitioners correctly perceive unmet needs in their communities and incorrectly assume that merely by offering quality services, cash will flow in and cover their expenses. They usually learn the dangers of mistaking need for demand. Demand is the happy match of a "needed" service with clients and the available funds to pay for it.

Case Study One

(From an August 19, 1986, article in the Rochester, N.Y., *Times-Union.* Names of professionals have been altered, and minor changes made to improve readability.)

Six months ago — on a cold February afternoon — psychologist John Angler walked into a McDonald's Restaurant with his partner, psychiatrist Patti Grinder, ordered coffee, sat down, and cried.

Just months after Angler had given up a $100,000-plus income to become "a medical pioneer" in head-injury rehabilitation, it appeared that his dream was falling apart.

He had a good stream of patients coming to his new offices and testimonials of praise from patients, and their families were coming in, too.

Despite that, Angler's hope of establishing his own clinic and the pair's desire to break free of the constraints of traditional medicine — the bureaucracy-clogged environment of large hospitals — were sinking fast. A tangle of debt, personnel problems, and personality conflicts was closing in. "Why," Angler asked, "can it be this hard? Why do I have to go through this?"

Today, thanks in large part to a financial bailout by investors, Angler's business and his dream remain alive — but he is not yet out of the woods.

Angler's is a story of a medical man — an extremely confident 33-year-old — lost for a time in a business world he was not trained to understand.

In Angler's mind, there is no question that there is a need for his service. Traditional hospitals are not yet offering intensive, long-term rehabilitation services for people saved through recent advances in neurosurgery. At the same time, Angler saw government regulation of medical services changing to encourage replacing high-cost hospital care of patients with lower-cost treatments offered to patients who remain at home and visit outpatient clinics.

"I figured that would work well with the head-injured," Angler said. "Patients could live at home with the support of their families and come to my clinic during the day."

In early 1985, Angler and Grinder decided it was time to gear their operation to what they hoped would become a model for opening other outpatient centers around the country. They met with financial advisers, took on a business partner, persuaded a bank to grant a $100,000 start-up loan, mortgaged everything they owned, and eventually expanded the office to 6,000 square feet. They soon had about 22 full- and part-time employees.

Angler was confident. He talked of "hypergrowth" with his financial adviser. But the new year had hardly begun when Angler found out that despite what looked like a healthy patient load, he was almost bankrupt. His 22 employees were costing him about $5,500 a week, but, for a variety of reasons, money was not coming in. Payroll was running like a taxi meter. Some bills had never been sent out, and thousands of dollars in useless equipment had been purchased.

"I still have $12,000 in useless phone equipment sitting in storage," he said.

In addition, some insurance companies had not yet agreed that such outpatient head-injury rehabilitation was a service for which they would pay.

Turning the business around was not simple. "We had creditors breathing down our necks," Angler said. Banks were not the answer. They had already gone out on a limb and were not about to go farther.

Their accountant convinced them that the only way out from under was to sell a portion of their business to investors. A deal was eventually made: 49 percent of the business for $200,000.

That money, Angler hoped, would get creditors off his back and buy him time he needed to get patients' payments rolling in. Through February and March, while awaiting the influx of money, Angler and Grinder looked for ways to make ends meet.

"We went right down the list. Anything not absolutely necessary was gone." Including the cleaning service. "We were doctors by day, cleaners by night," Angler said.

For 14 weeks, neither Angler nor Grinder received a paycheck, but somehow they were able to scrounge up enough money to pay their employees each week and fight off rumors circulating through the medical community that their clinic was about to die.

The money soon arrived and the immediate heat was off. Angler moved to stabilize the business. Though it was head-injury rehabilitation that fired his entrepreneurial spirit, that service has proved difficult because insurance companies have been slow to recognize it as a service for which they will pay.

As a result, Angler has added a back-injury clinic and pediatric neurological services to the arsenal. The additions, he said, will eventually diversify services and improve the company's cash flow.

But the future of the company, Angler admits, rests on his ability to convince New York State and insurance companies that these new rehabilitation services for the head injured are necessary and, at about $200 a day, worth the expense.

Angler's lobbying effort, though, may be lengthy and it is not certain he has the time. Getting state recognition for a new service can be a two-year process.

Angler already has spent about $80,000 on legal advice in setting up the business and filling out state applications to prove there is a need for this new service. Without that state approval, it is not certain that insurance companies will consider head-injury rehabilitation as a benefit to offer their thousands of local customers.

"If I don't get them, I can't stay in business," Angler said. "It's that simple. I'll move to California, and set up private practice. There's my license on the wall."*

Analysis of the Case study

What lessons can be learned from this case study?

1. Business planning and basic income management are not merely abstract academic concepts. Ignoring them invites disaster. Avoiding proactive study of the realities of the marketplace, with associated strategic planning, organizing, directing, and controlling the total business operation, can sink a professional service operation.

Success is a function of testing your assumptions before committing major time and money to a project. Make sure there is a ready market—a market ready to pay for the services you will offer. One upstate New York group, for example, developed a well-formulated program to prepare people in their 50s for their retirement years. Before launching it, they went to several of the area's large employers and discovered that (a) everyone thought it was "a good thing," but (b) no one was ready to fund it. The companies' commitment to their retirees did not include financially supporting that type of proactive planning. Another group tried to sell "wellness training"; their market research determined that there were more internal (corporate) and external competitors (other consultants) than they had known about and that the market potential was weak. Creativity in new service development should be encouraged, but it is not wise to mortgage the homestead until much homework assures you that the odds and timing are right.

2. Check your cash-flow estimates. Do not overextend yourself. Do not overbuy; do not purchase expensive computer, telephone, or other equipment until you need it, and do not accept large payroll expenses until you can be assured that your income will be sufficient to carry them.

3. Remember that good intentions and high-quality services are not enough to make a dream come true. In short, to find personal and professional fulfillment in a little or big business, we must manage.

MANAGING: WHAT DOES IT REALLY MEAN OPERATIONALLY?

The practitioner is a businessperson. Each is the president and general manager of his or her own firm. And each is responsible for the following.

Planning and Budgeting

This involves selecting from among alternate courses of long- and short-range action, as well as priority setting and establishing obvjectives, policies, and procedures. It also includes building a budget based on specific assumptions and educated guesses about income and expenses.

Controlling

Controlling means monitoring the practice so that events conform to plans. It requires the establishment of measurable goals and contingency plans to correct for difficulties as they arise. Use the profit and loss statement, the balance sheet, and cash flow as management tools. Ensure follow-through.

Organizing

Organizing is ensuring that plans are carried out and specific objectives reached by establishing specific action plans with deadline dates.

Staffing

Staffing involves specifying support needs (secretarial, accounting, legal, management, additional psychological services, etc.), recruiting personnel, and selecting them and training them.

Directing

Directing is the process of guiding and supervising the staff, working with them to establish specific objectives, establishing a system of accountability, and motivating the staff and leading it to achieve goals.

Each practitioner is also the major, and sometimes the only, personal producer or income generator in the firm. Managers in large firms may spend the lion's share of their time managing while others produce income for the company. Independent practitioners must produce to exist, but must manage themselves while they produce.

Let us look at another case history to demonstrate the value of managing, and the dangers of not managing, a practice.

Case Study Two *

Dr. Arthur Brown's practice grew nicely. He enjoyed his mix of psychotherapy and psychodiagnostic work and derived much pleasure from the supervision and consulting he did at a rural community mental-health center about 30 miles south of his city. He deciced that he could now afford a secretary and he asked some friends if they knew of anyone who was available. He interviewed a few women and learned that he had given no thought to the specifics of what he expected his secretary to do. He hired an attractive woman who was a pleasant receptionist and a fair

---

* In December 1986, approximately two years after starting their business with the strong support of their investors, a major insurer, Blue Choice, "granted approval to pay for the services of neurorehab." In addition, it endorsed Dr. Angler's organization as the preferred provider in the area. If that endorsemenet had been obtained prior to starting the clinic's operation, many basic income management problems would have been obviated. One hurdle is now passed, but many more remain. For example, other insurers still need to approve the service and the possibility of strong competition from area hospitals still remains. The business aspects of practice development are as great as the professional challenges.

typist. She, however, had a strong need for affiliation. She soon became lonely and unhappy in the solitary job setting of her office. She left.

Brown then hired another woman, who spoke well and appeared to be well organized. She had previously worked for a law firm. She understood the concept of confidentiality, and she reported that she preferred working in a one-person office. At first he was pleased with her, then he began to note some paranoid ideation. He mentioned the change to a lawyer friend, who laughed and said, "And you're the psychologist." His secretary had a long history of idiosyncratic and oftentimes bizarre behavior; she was well known and *persona non grata* in the legal community where she had held several jobs. Why hadn't he checked references?

But Art Brown was a good learner. He had learned a little more about himself and about the employee-selection procedure. The next time around he took the hiring task more seriously. He defined the types of responsibilities he expected the secretary to assume, he developed a series of selection interview questions, and he called previous employers to verify the basic data and obtain references. He discovered that new governmental regulations severely restricted the sharing of specific judgments about a previous employee's performance, but he also discovered that his systematic search enabled him to select a winner.

Little by little, Art's secretary took over more and more responsibilities. She handled his banking, organized his records, and established a "tickler file" to ensure his follow-up on numerous matters. She also began to schedule appointments for him. He had previously spent much time talking with referrers or potential clients before setting a time to meet with them. He was thrilled with the time savings that accrued.

His practice was growing very profitable, but he was spending more time report writing than he had previously, and he was enjoying his work less. After a year had gone by, he began to realize what had happened. He had lost control of his practice. He was very busy, but he had never given any conscious thought to specifying plans and directions in which he wanted to go. His professional life was being directed by others. Several community gatekeepers valued his diagnostic work. They kept a steady flow of clients coming his way. His secretary booked them as she had been instructed to. As a result, so much time was filled in with diagnostic work that it began to crowd out opportunities for therapy and for "marketing" visits to people and settings that could broaden his work opportunities.

Recognizing this, he decided to define the type of practice he wanted, specify specific action plans to achieve it, and develop a means of monitoring his practice on a monthly, quarterly, and annual basis to ensure that results conformed to his plans. For example, he decided to limit himself to four diagnostic evaluations per week. He scheduled appointments further ahead than he had ever done before, and he established a system whereby he could fill in canceled appointments from those on his waiting list. He had become a manager who was able to control his practice as well as the personal satisfactions derived from it.

THE TOOLS OF MONEY MANAGEMENT

Budgeting

A carefully considered budget, including a cash-flow forecast, is an essential tool when determining the amount of money that will be needed to keep

---

*From: Lewin (1978).

a practice alive. Initial forecasts are likely to be far different from actual results, but the longer a practitioner has been in business, the closer the estimate should be to the actual results. Indeed, my group practice's estimated expenses for 1986 (established in December 1985) differed by less than 1 percent from the actual year end results. That, however, was my 19th year of practice—and a time of low inflation. My estimate of cash receipts was less accurate, as it has always been. I opt to make a conservative estimate of income in order to maximize the probability that all bills will be paid promptly and that I will find no unpleasant surprises in accounts payable. That policy may not be a good accounting practice, but it meets my psychological needs. That is important, too.

Cash Flow

Client (patient) fees are the major source of cash inflow for most practices. Stable, long-term psychotherapy practices and those with long-term consultantships can budget more easily than those dependent upon diagnostic referrals, forensic work, "incidental" industrial consltations, short-term counseling, career assessments, new and not yet widely accepted services, or other types of "piece work" professional activities. Historical results are an excellent basis for making projections when all things are equal. Unfortunately, that is not always the case.

Numerous factors must be considered if forecasts are to be accurate: increased competition; decreased demand due to population shifts (the closing of a military base or a major area employer, etc.); the story of health maintenance organizations (HMO) and preferred provider organizations (PPO) that limit the free market of potential clients; the retirement, death, or changing referral patterns of key referral sources; economic downturns in the local economy; and other socioeconomig and political factors.

This type of analysis also highlights the need to take corrective action. Practitioners who proactively note trends and position themselves to weather the storms of change are likely to emerge stronger. The following are examples of ways to implement proactive strategies.

1. Develop relationships with the general managers and human resources staffs of companies planning large layoffs or shutdowns. This can lead to referrals for individual and family therapy and stress management, consultation regarding career retraining, outplacement counseling, counseling of managers about how to deal with their feelings about laying off long-term associates, and the like.

2. Develop special skills not offered by HMO or PPO practitioners. This can lead to referrals for such work as child and family custody evaluations, forensic assignments, biofeedback, pain-control therapy, divorce mediation, divorce adjustment counseling, counseling of individuals with brain damage and with their families, substance-abuse counseling, counseling and problem solving with family members in family-owned businesses, and so on.

3. Seek contacts and a referral base in underserviced communities within an hour's drive from your home. These part-time practices often grow rapidly.

4. Develop new sources of referral. Lawyers, accountants, the clergy, directors of community organizations, and personnel managers are often under-

utilized gatekeepers of referral.

5. Gain greater visibility via radio, television, and newspaper coverage; developing a practice newsletter and other forms of public relations can also strengthen your competitive position.

Another method of increasing receipts is to raise your fees. Many business-people dread the idea and fear that it will alienate their clientele. It may drive away some clients and some prospective clients, but it need not. A careful study of competitive rates in your community can give you a good idea of where your rates lie. The benefits of using you and your services, however, may well enable you to expect and obtain a premium. You may also be willing to lose 10 percent of your business if you can achieve a 10 percent fee increase. This can enable your income to remain stable while giving you more time for professional development activities — or to be spent in other ways. There is much folklore about how much one can raise rates for current and new clients. My experience, however, suggests that the practitioner's comfort level with the change is the most important variable in successfully changing fee levels.

Estimating Cash Receipts

Estimating cash receipts is not the same as estimating billings. Most practitioners discover that not everyone pays — and that even those who do pay may not pay promptly. Many practitioners now expect payment at the time of service. That avoids any collection problem but it probably reduces the number of clients served. Indeed, some potential clients who would pay are likely to be forced to seek another professional who will agree to wait until a divorce is final, a personal injury suit settled, a year-end bonus is received, or the messiah arrives. It is helpful to estimate the lag in payments when constructing a budget. Your landlord, the telephone company, and other suppliers are less interested in your accounts receivable (what you are owed) than in receiving prompt payment of their bills.

A cash-flow worksheet can help you plan your professional and personal activities. It will permit you to estimate how much money you will have at any particular time. It can enable you to pinpoint areas that need attention before danger points are reached. It will enable you to estimate how much cash will flow into and out of your practice and when those flows will occur. The best guide for this estimate is the historical pattern of receipts and payables.

Chart I. Monthly Receipts by Category of Payers

Months	JN	FB	MR	AP	MA	JU	JY	AU	ST	OC	NO	DE	Total
Individuals:													
Blue Cross:													
insurer A:													
Insurer B:													
State Agency A:													
State Agency B:													
Other A:													
Other B:													
TOTAL:													

Chart II. Monthly Receipts: Estimated vs Actual

Estimated/Actual Receipts 19____

Months	JN	FB	MR	AP	MA	JU	JY	AU	ST	OC	NO	DE	Total
Individuals: est.													
actual													
Blue Cross: est.													
actual													
Insurer A: est.													
actual													
Insurer B: est.													
actual													
State Agency A: est.													
actual													
State Agency B: est.													
actual													
Other A: est.													
actual													
Other B: est.													
actual													
TOTAL:													

Cash Receipts Analysis

A historical review of income by month and/or by type of client can enable you to determine whether or not there are seasonal variations in your practice's income. Some practitioners, dependent upon third-party payers, may discover that a state agency characteristically slows payments toward certain phases of its fiscal year or during periods of high vacation time usage. Others may find that certain insurance companies review treatment claims and delay payments of some of them. Still other practitioners may note peaks and valleys within their own billings and receipts. This information can help you estimate your cash receipts more accurately. It can also enable you to take action to rearrange your professional and personal lives in line with your desired objectives.

A simple chart (Chart I) can help graphically depict cycles in your receipts.

If you see a need for improvement in your billing and collections procedures, you can sit down and specify action plans to overcome the barriers. Among plans to consider are the following.

1. Develop specific payment policies and communicate them in writing to your staff and your clients. Discuss your fee structure with your clients early in the relationship. Then adhere to them and expect your associates and your clients to do so, too. Develop specific policies and forms that need to be completed for the exceptions that may arise. (For example, have clients sign a contract to make payments on a regular basis or to assume responsibility for payments if spouses or third-party payers decline to do so.)

2. Learn as much as you can about third-party payers and their reimbursement policies. Complete their forms in the way they expect; this cuts down on slow payments and on denials of payments that have been requested for nonreimbursible services.

3. Review your accounts receivable at least monthly. This will enable you to note aging accounts and make efforts to collect them. Develop procedures

for communicating increasing concern about aging accounts. Do it in a businesslike and nonabrasive way.

4. Gather complete information about your clients during their first visit. The client's full name, address, place of work, telephone number, spouse's name and place of work, insurance coverage, and date of birth are all important data to have in completing insurance forms and using other third-party

Chart III. Cash Outflow Analysis

Estimated Fixed and Variable Monthly Payments

Item	Estimated Expenses					
	Jan.	Feb.	March	April	May	June
Salary/"draw" of practitioner						
FICA (Social Security)						
Secretarial and other wages						
Secretarial FICA						
State and federal taxes						
Unemployment insurance						
Office rent						
Office cleaning/maintenance						
Office supplies (pens, paper, stationery, typewriter ribbons, photocopying, etc.)						
Professional supplies						
Professional memberships, books, and journals						
Continuing education/convention expenses						
Postage						
Telephone						
Utilities						
Travel expenses						
Professional liability insurance						
Medical insurance						
Income protection insurance						
Comprehensive fire, theft, office liability insurance						
Life insurance						
Professional insurance (legal and accounting)						
Pension payments						
Depreciation on furniture/office equipment						
Miscellaneous (gifts, business lunches, charity, allowance for uncollectables, etc.)						
TOTAL						

means of collecting monies due. Help clients determine the limits of their insurance coverage; this can avoid unpleasant surprises after treatment has begun.

5. Encourage (some practitioners insist on) payment at the time of service.

Cash Outflow

A historical review of your expenses can be an invaluable tool in avoiding financial surprises — and shocks. Most practices have both fixed and variable expenses, and many outflow items (insurance premiums, legal and accounting fees, taxes, major charitable gifts, continuing education and convention expenses, pension payments, etc.) become due just once or twice a year. Forecasting your cash flow and noting the balance between receipts and expenses, therefore, can be helpful in managing one's life and work.

Charts III and IV can be used to forecast expenses. Combined with the data in Charts I and II, a monthly liquidity report (Chart V) can be developed. It is merely an efficient way of helping you determine the profitability of your practice and the extent of the reserves you are likely to have at your disposal.

This knowledge of your financial resources can help you determine how prepared you are to deal with emergencies. It can serve as a Distant Early Warning (DEW-line) system. It can help you decide what types of actions, if any, are needed to maintain the viability of your professional practice.

For instance, a sharp increase in accounts receivable aged over 90 days should lead to problem solving to collect those monies and establish a system to make sure the situation never becomes damaging. Similarly, a sharp decrease in cash on hand can lead to efforts to speed the process of billing and eliciting payments — and of slowing down the process of accounts payable. It can also lead to analyzing the flow of referrals from your key referral sources and determining if there are needs to (1) refresh and renew their awareness of your availability, (2) seek new referral sources, (3) establish a line of credit with a bank, or (4) develop other remedial efforts.

Saving Money

Most practitioners, especially after several good years — or after working as employees in organizations that do not focus attention on the costs of running the business, fail to give careful thought to ways of increasing their income by taking steps to save money. Some of these steps are as follows:

1. Learning to process insurance claims quickly and accurately. This saves administrative time and brings dollars in so they can work for you.

2. Taking cash discounts whenever they are available. These often include 2 percent for payment within 10 days of receiving the bill.

3. Bargaining when purchasing goods and services. Often one can obtain free a one-year service contract or a significant discount on a purchase merely by asking for it.

4. Making volume purchases. These can be a bargain if you are sure you can use the quantity within a reasonable period of time.

Chart IV. Cash Outflow Analysis — Estimated vs Actual

Estimated/Actual 19____

Item	Expenses
Salary/"draw" of practitioner est.	
actual	
FICA (Social Security) est.	
actual	
Secretarial and other wages est.	
actual	
Secretarial FICA est.	
actual	
State and federal taxes est.	
actual	
Unemployment insurance est.	
actual	
Office rent est.	
actual	
Office cleaning/ maintenance est.	
actual	
Office supplies (pens, paper, stationery, typewriter ribbons, photocopying, etc.) est.	
actual	
Professional supplies est.	
actual	
Professional memberships, books, and journals est.	
actual	
Continuing education/ convention expenses est.	
actual	
Postage est.	
actual	
Telephone est.	
actual	
Utilities est.	
actual	
Travel expenses est.	
actual	
Professional liability insurance est.	
actual	
Medical insurance est.	
actual	
Income protection insurance est.	
actual	

Chart IV. Cash Outflow Analysis — Estimated vs. Actual

Comprehensive fire, theft,
   office liability insurance   est.
                              actual

            Life insurance   est.
                              actual

Professional insurance
   (legal and accounting)   est.
                              actual

         Pension payments   est.
                              actual

Depreciation on furniture/
         office equipment   est.
                              actual

   Miscellaneous (gifts,
business lunches, charity,
   allowance for uncollec-
            tables, etc.)   est.
                              actual   _____

            TOTAL

5. Leasing to avoid large money outlays for equipment that may quickly become obsolete.

6. Using temporary help or free-lance workers rather than full-time employees when your needs may not be permanent. The higher per-hour cost may be well worth the money saved if you pay people only when they are actually needed.

7. Utilizing management. Since time is the only commodity that service deliverers sell, more efficient use of it permits them to meet the needs of more clients and to earn more money while doing so.

8. Avoiding nonessential outlays. The first case history in this chapter noted that the practitioner had bought several thousand dollars of telephone equipment that was not used. Many others have unused or underutilized computers, biofeedback equipment, and fancy furniture and gadgetry that can-

Chart V. Liquidity Report

	Current Month	Next Month Forecast Actual
Cash on hand (and in bank)	_____	_____
Accounts receivable:	_____	_____
30 days	_____	_____
60 days	_____	_____
90 days	_____	_____
over 90 days	_____	_____

not be cost justified. Items that improve the quality of one's work life have value, but savings will accrue when nonessential purchases are curtailed.

9. Bartering. The value of the items received must be recorded for income tax purposes, but it often makes things easier for both the practitioner and client when products or services are bartered for the practitioner's services.

10. Investing surplus cash, including the prompt banking of checks. This can earn money. Placing money in money market funds, certificates of deposit, Treasury bills, or other such investments earns money that would otherwise be lost if it were placed in non-interest-bearing business checking accounts.

REFERENCES

Cash flow/cash management, *Small Business Reporter* (1982, 1984). San Francisco, CA: Bank of America NT and SA.

Head-injured patients (1986). *Blue Choice Provider News,* Rocheste, NY.

Lavin, C. (1986). The painful making of an entrepreneur, *Times-Union,* Rochester, NY.

Lewin, M.H. (1979). Establishing and maintaining a successful professional practice, Rochester, NY: Professional Development Institute.

Psychotherapy Finances: Managing Your Practice and Your Money. A monthly newsletter (which includes an annual fee survey report) published by Ridgewood Finance Institute, Inc., Box 609, Ridgewood, NJ 07451.

Thirty ways to improve your billing and collections. Procom special report. Procom (publisher of a monthly practice management newsletter), 5799 Tall Oaks Road, Madison, WI 53711.

U.S. Small Business Administration. Publishes many helpful booklets and, through SCORE, offers free consultation. See U.S. government in telephone book.

FEE SCHEDULING AND MONITORING

Mathilda B. Canter, Ph.D., and Herbert J. Freudenberger, Ph.D.

FEE SETTING IN INDEPENDENT PRACTICE

Traditionally, health-service providers have had difficulty in reconciling social conscience, altruism, and other wishes to help with practical needs to pay their bills, human wishes to provide well for self and family, and even needs to demonstrate the success that is so often measured financially in our world.

For the professional in independent practice, decisions regarding fees are extremely important, and require considerable thought and self-awareness. One must ask oneself such questions as: How do I feel about money? In what way is the fee reflected in transference and countertransference issues that manifest themselves in treatment? What are the fee practices of male and female therapists? Are they different? One needs to ask further: How do I go about collecting money from my clients? How much am I worth, or are my services worth, in dollars and cents? Am I comfortable with a profession that happens to be a business, or am I running a business that happens to be a profession? How much should I charge for what? Should I use a sliding scale for fee setting? Should I bill for payment, or insist on payment at each session? How do I feel about *pro bono* work? About people who do not pay their bills? About using collection agencies or "lawyer letters" to force payment? What do I do about insurance and copayments? What about preferred provider organizations? The questions are myriad, but we shall try, in this chapter, to cover the basic dilemmas and considerations to be dealt with concerning fees in independent practice.

In the following sections, we first discuss fee/policy setting, then address the communication of such matters to clients, and finally consider collection issues and the psychodynamics of the meanng of money in therapy.

DECISION MAKING ABOUT FEES

For the professional working in a clinic or agency, where fees are set by some administrator or agency board and collected by someone other than the professional service provider, or where the practitioner works in a free clinic, Freudenberger (1973, 1974) agrees with Eissler (1974), who suggests: "A person may have little money, and he may indeed be deprived of a great deal; nevertheless this does not necessarily mean that he has the outlook of the poor. The psychology of the poor is characterized by an outlook on life in which what is essential is that the possiblity of choices is almost completely by necessities that are imposed by the outside world, which in turn affects the involvement and outcome of free psychotherapy."

For persons in independent practice, the setting of fees is a very complex and critical part of their responsibility is to themselves and to their clients. Before your shingle is hung, it is important to draw up a list of the professional services you feel competent to offer and are willing to provide. You may be surprised at how many different categories of fees you need to establish.

TYPES OF FEES

Obviously, the therapist must set therapy fees. But some of the categories require careful thought and important decisions: How much should I charge for initial visits—if at all? For individual therapy? Couples? Families? Group? And for some of these services, will I offer a 30-minute session? A 45- or 50-minute hour? A 90-minute session? And at what rates? And what about psychological testing, consultations, supervision, and forensic work such as consultation with attorneys, record reveiwing, depositions, and court appearances? You may know what to charge for a full battery of psychodiagnostic tests, but what about a Wechsler alone? A Rorschach? An MMPI or a Strong Campbell? The breakdown of functions is important, and can avoid embarrassment and the setting of "off-the-top-of-the head" fees that may not be equitable.

DECISION FACTORS

Arriving at appropriate fees is often a complex process. In the course of treatment, many fee-related problems and resistances may occur that, along with many óther variables, must be considered in reaching yur decisions.

Professional Self-Worth / Attitudes Regarding Money

It is essential to confront the frequently uncomfortable issue of what you think you are "worth." Unless you feel at ease with the fees you are asking, you will have elements introduced into your therapy or other services that may well dilute your effectiveness. This is particularly true for the psychotherapist in independent practice. Often one finds that psychotherapists disavow the importance of money, claiming that they are really functioning as professionals, and that professionals are not "in business." But it is important to point out that the independent practitioner *is* in business—in the business of being a professional—and that therapists who are uncomfortable with money issues really need to do some self-exploration. You might ask yourself what money means to you, and what it meant to your parents. How was money handled by your parents in their home? What feelings about money were present? Were money issues handled secretly or openly, easily or fraught with tension? Were your parents poor? Were they affluent? How was money given to you? Also, how early in life did you begin to work for money? Do you enjoy your work and seek satisfaction in it other than monetary compensation?

As Fruedenberger (1987) suggested, is money one of the components that might promote impairment in psychologists? We must also be aware of the therapist who operates as a "superior being," fostering dependency in his or her clients by being very "liberal" about fees and the payment of fees. You must examine yourself, as such exploration may help you to come to terms with yourself as a practitioner, and prevent destructive transference and countertransference issues from impeding your effectiveness. It is critical that you come to the conclusion that you are worth what you charge, that you deserve the compensation, and that your fees seem appropriate to you. And it is important that you consider parity with other professional disciplines whose practitioners' training and competence you equal.

In addition to the working through of money attitudes and self-worth, you should consider the level of your training and credentialing and the breadth and depth of your experience — all of which reflect on the value of your services and should be involved in any decision about fees.

Time

Time is of the essence in setting fees, as the skills professionals offer frequently involve low-volume factors that greatly affect income potential. We have addressed the various types of services that go into the creation of a fee schedule, but there is another type of service — one that relates to time — that should be considered. Practitioners need to think through the way in which they wish to handle such services as telephone calls from clients, calls to or from other professionals (e.g. school personnel, or lawyers), reports, correspondence, reading of patients' journals, and filling out insurance forms. Experienced practitioners know that such activities consume significant amounts of professional time. Some take a lesson from attorneys and keep a timer running when they are not "in session" but are providing services. Some prefer not to charge separately for such "extracurricular" time, considering that these activities and services are expected as an extension of the primary services rendered, and take them into consideration in the initial fee-setting process. While rationales can be provided for either system, each practitioner should adopt one method and establish fees accordingly.

Practice Costs / Budgetary Requirements

The calculation of fixed office expenses such as rent or mortgage payments, insurance, secretarial and other services, telephone, and supplies and equipment can be helpful in making decisions regarding the fee levels that you choose to set. And, of course, personal levels of income necessary to "manage" or to live in the style you consider appropriate may also come into the decision-making process. Although they should not, and probably could not, determine attainable fees, such considerations may help to temper idealism with reality, if impracticality tends to be a problem for you.

The Marketplace

It is necessary to know what the reasonable and customary fees are in your community, as well as the patterns of service provision and the degree of competition you face. Obviously, any fee setting must be done within the bounds of a reasonable expectation that you will find markets for the services you are ready to provide. Whatever your worth and needs, if competent services are available elsewhere at significantly lower cost, other factors being equal, you will not be able to develop a viable practice. You will need to reflect on how to market yourself in the future. [Freudenberger (1985) suggests that the issues of inflation, stagflation or recessions, and a declining patient population certainly will affect your fee-setting practices.)] Inman and Bascue (1983) found that "patients are currently the most important source of referrals for health service psychologists in private practice. This also suggests that young and new practitioners might need to concentrate on developing a variety of alternative referral sources."

While it is important not to risk violating antitrust laws, it certainly appears reasonable to make inquiries regarding the range of fees charged by colleagues whose work and judgment you respect.

SETTING OFFICE POLICIES REGARDING FEES

Sliding Scales

For some, the use of a sliding scale that sets fees for service according to family size and income, ranging from zero to full fee, is a comfortable and practical way to temper idealism and function professionally. Many social service agencies and other nonprofit organizations use a sliding scale of fees, and would willingly share their scale with you, to help you get an idea of what is available in your community.

Some do not use a rigid sliding scale, but negotiate fees on an individual basis, depending on the patient's income, with no "customary" fee. Others set a standard fee, but reserve the right to reduce fees in unusual instances.

Reduced Fees

Some practitioners do not consider a reduction of fees appropriate. For others, the reduction of fees to accommodate clients who fall on hard times, or people with whom they wish to work but who cannot afford their standard fees, is an acceptable option. However, there are philosophical and countertransference issues that must be addressed. For those professionals who see the cutting of fees as a devaluation of their services and therefore detrimental to therapy, the option is obviously not viable. For some, resentment may develop, with a negative countertransference that has decidedly nontherapeutic effects. It is essential that service providers be comfortable with the ways in which they establish and implement fee agreements. As DiBella (1980) suggested, "Part of fee setting is deciding on sliding-scale issues, which is fraught with potential traps. For example, after accepting a fee for less than he feels he is worth, the physician often finds his benevolence becoming resentment or condescension."

A funny example occurred with a colleague's patient who spoke of "Waiting for Godot" in his therapy and the colleague commented, "Yes, I've been meaning to speak with you about the dough [money] you owe me." The patient was quite upset and commented, "I was not talking of money, I was talking of the play 'Waiting for Godot.' Here a bit of countertransference was translated into resentment about a lowered fee and money owed to the therapist.

Perhaps you become aware that a client has had a decrease in income and think that you might wish to lower your fee in the middle of therapy. Or perhaps you have cut your fee on the basis of the patient's stated ability to pay, and there comes a time when you find yourself questioning the appropriateness of the agreed-upon amount. You may hear the patient talking about large expenditures, which generates in you some indignation that there is money for certain luxuries but not to pay your full fee. Or perhaps for other reasons it appears that the patient has not been truthful regarding income. In any of these instances, it is important to address the issues with the individual and renegotiate. As Keith-Speigel and Koocher (1985) indicated, "Many clients may be vulnerable to potential abuse because of emotional dependency, social naiveté, psychosis or other psychopathological conditions, and the psychologist should not take advantage of these factors."

INSURANCE AND FEES

Because of the increasing utilization of insurance coverage by clients, it is particularly important to examine the setting of fees in the context of that coverage. It must be clearly understood that the charges made to insurance companies must be accurate and must reflect the *reasonable and customary* fees you charge in your practice. Some practitioners, who reduce fees for patients who are having financial difficulties, believe that it is proper to bill the insurance company for their usual fee and either "forgive" or reduce the client copayment. This is *not* acceptable practice. Insurance covers a *percentage* of the fee, rather than a flat amount, and the policy holder is expected to pay his or her share. If, for example, you bill the insurance company $75 for a psychotherapy session and the insurance company pays 80 percent ($60 in this instance), your client is expected to pay the other 20 percent ($15). If you waive that copayment, the insurance company would consider $60 as your fee and be responsible for only 80 percent of $60, or $48. Legally and ethically, the practitioner must hold the client responsible for the full copayment. Of course, the practitioner may make whatever temporal arrangements seem appropriate for the ultimate collection or writeoff of the balance due.

CANCELLATION POLICIES

It is very important to establish a policy, which you believe is appropriate, regarding the cancellation or missing of appointments. Because a late cancellation or "no show" potentially represents an income loss that may be a significant percentage of the practitioner's daily income, a charge is frequently levied. This may range from a percentage — usually 50 percent — of the full fee to the full fee itself. Whatever policy is set, it should be with the awareness that insurance companies generally do not pay for treatment that has not actually been rendered.

Some practitioners offer a telephone session to the individual who is unable to be present physically in the office but can communicate in this way.

PROFESSIONAL COURTESY

In many professions, the giving of professional courtesy has been traditional. It is important to identify a comfort level for yourself in this regard. While some *pro bono* work is considered a part of a practitioner's responsibility, it is often the professional who comes for treatment who is best able to pay. Since treatment involves large blocks of ongoing professional time, it seems reasonable for therapists to levy charges on those patients. Both authors see many professional colleagues in their practices. Giving professional courtesy, therefore, would present significant cash-flow problems. One of the authors noted, some years ago, that as her practice included more and more therapists, she was feeling increasingly honored as her income decreased.

Freudenberger (1984, 1985) firmly believes that in view of the many transference and countertransference issues that will emerge during the treatment of the health professional, it is essential to evaluate the reasons for giving professional courtesy. One needs to look at the presenting symptoms and the reasons for seeking treatment. "Usually, the healer-helper has a difficult time viewing himself/herself in the role of patient. He fears a loss of dignity, a loss of power, a loss of self-esteem." It is therefore essential that a clear policy of payment and parity of payment be established during the first or, at the latest, the second visit.

A policy that works for some is to give no professional courtesy unless it is a financial hardship for the individual to pay the standard fee, in which case as much of a reduction as necesary is acceptable. Such reductions frequently are made for graduate students or for colleagues just beginning a practice. Some practitioners do not charge for the initial consultation. Others do. Whatever the policy adopted, the practitioner must consider it appropriate so that it does not interfere with the services being provided.

RAISING FEES

From time to time, practitioners will choose to raise their fees. On those occasions, some policy decisions are necesary. Those providing services by the unit may need only to announce their increases. However, therapists need to have a policy regarding the client who is in the midst of treatment. Some therapists believe that once they have contracted to render services at a particular fee, increases are inappropriate except in very unusual circumstances. Some beleive that no patient's fees should ever be raised once therapy has begun because patients, in a sense, are "captive." Others believe that therapists, like barbers, publishers, and pediatricians, are entitled to increase their fees as their own expenses rise. DiBella (1987) suggests that the raising of fees "forces the therapist and patient to see the therapist as interested in money or selling time for money, and as aggressive enough to be demanding more from the patient. This might clash with the therapist's wish to be a benevolent healer and friend, who might then avoid legitimate fee raises." The overall impression is that therapists need to deal with this issue on an individual basis, taking into account the phase of therapy and the psychodynamics of the client.

FEE SPLITTING

Fee splitting is a practice that involves the "kicking back" of part of the fee one earns in payment for the referral. It has long been considered unethical. However, the Federal Trade Comission has recently expressed concern regarding the possible anti-trust implications of restricting this practice. The outcome of the negotiations between the Federal Trade Commission and the American Psychological Association are not yet determined as of this writing. But the American Psychological Association has discontinued adjudicating fee splitting cases while awaiting the results of the negotiations. Should fee splitting become "legitimized," there are some practitioners who would not agree with that philosophy and choose not to engage in the practice anyway. Others might accept the option.

There is one category of financial arrangement that raises questions in many practitioners regarding possible fee splitting. When a practitioner rents office space and services from another practitioner, the amount paid to the latter is frequently based on the number of clients seen, and may be stipulated as a percentage of the fees earned. Is this fee splitting? We do not believe that it is, even if the patients have been referred by the rent collector, provided the percentage is based on the costs of the space, including the number of hours it is used, the cost of telephone, service and clerical support, and the use of equipment and supplies. If the charge can be justified by these expenses plus a reasonable profit, this arrangement does not constitute fee splitting.

COMMUNICATING ABOUT FEES

General Considerations

For your own protection, as well as for the protection of your clients and your professional relationships with them, it is essential that information about fees and fee-related policies be given very clearly, and that fees be fully discussed early in the therapeutic relationship, preferably before services are rendered. The many complaints to state credentialing boards about fees relate to the reluctance of many therapists to talk about fees, to people's lack of understanding of those fees, and to the failure of the professional practitioner to communicate clearly and openly concerning fees and fee-related issues. The needs of the distressed individual coming for help and emotional support and the need of the therapist to be caring do not relieve the practitioner from the obligation to address the issue of fees.

The first client contact is frequently via the telephone. If there is a charge for the first contact, then that fee should be agreed upon during the conversation, and the indivudual informed that payment is expected at the time of the first session. It is recommended that it be explained to the caller that fees will be discussed during the face-to-face meeting.

Certainly, there are times when a financial discussion is not at all appropriate during a first session. For example, you might deliberately avoid discussing fees with severely depressed or suicidal patients who come in so disturbed they are not capable of concentrating on fee-related matters. Or you might deliberately postpone such discussion with schizoid or borderline persons whose object relatedness is so poorly developed or evolved that they are unable to relate to you or your fees at that point. Such persons might perceive a discussion of fees as evidence that your sole concern in offering treatment is financial, and that care, concern, and a genuine desire to help are negligible. With such individuals, the therapist must be alert to the appropriate timing for a discussion and seize the opportunity as soon as possible.

Generally, however, the most appropriate time to discuss fees and other office policies is during the initial session. Practitioners should have worked through their own issues around money and fees for service, and should be able to address with comfort such issues as the patients' feelings about the fees and their ability to pay. Some may say they can afford services because they wish to work with you when in reality the fee is beyond their capacity to pay. It is the practitioner's responsibility to assess the patient's financial ability to meet the fee schedule.

Among matters to be addressed at the initial session or shortly therafter as therapeutically feasible, are fees per session; duration and frequency of sessions, cancellation policies; insurance arrangements; interest charges, if any; credit-card charge options, if available; billing procedures, if any; and methods of payment. Money issues consistently arise during the course of treatment and need to be dealt with appropriately in order to ascertain whether the particular individual may be resisting or progressing in treatment.

Pay attention to the way in which the patient reacts, especially during the initial sessions, to the issue of money. Does the patient become childlike, excessively dependent, suspicious, or unrealistic about his or her self-concept and the ability to pay your fee? The ways in which patients respond to money-related issues are excellent topics for future discussions.

Fees and Referrals

In the initial interview, the frequency of therapeutic sessions needs to be discussed. The client's expectations and financial situation, and the therapist's orientation and beliefs regarding the most effective frequency, must be considered. At times, scheduling problems dictate fewer sessions that might be most desirable. Therapists may refuse to start work with individuals who, for example, say they can come in only biweekly or monthly, because they do not believe that the work will be sufficiently productive.

If finances are the issue, the therapist is responsible for advising the individual of the availability of less costly services in the community and making the appropriate referrals. Of course, some therapists may choose to reduce the fee, or arrange for a long-term payment plan, if they can do so without imperiling therapeutic effectiveness. However, the therapist needs to be very much aware that the extension of credit may become complicated during the course of treatment, because "if the patient and therapist fail to distinguish, emotionally, between subjective aspects of their transaction in the introduction of this parameter, it is most likely that the procedure will adversely affect treatment" (Hofling & Rosenbaum, 1980).

Insurance Matters

The utilization or nonutilization of insurance to pay for treatment/services should be addressed at the start of the professional relationship. If, for example, the client chooses not to use available coverage for reasons of privacy or fear of vocational consequences, it is important that the client agree to and be able to afford the fee. Such an understanding reduces the probability that nonreimbursement from a third party will become a recurring issue during treatment.

Should the patient elect to use insurance coverage, the practitioner should clearly present expectations regarding the handling of this matter. It is important to communicate that the bill is the responsibility of the client, and that if, for example, the insurance does not cover as expected, the client will be expected to pay the entire amount. Where insurance is used, the practitioner must decide whether he or she (or staff) will take the responsiblity for filing insurance forms or the client will be expected to do so. If fees are charged for the filing of claims or reports, these should be clearly stipulated. Halbert (1987) indicated that the therapist needs to ascertain whether the insurance coverage is the patient's, the spouse's, or, in the case of an adolescent, a parent's. Halbert notes "The complexity of the insurance forms that must be filled out by the therapist varies from the most simple, requiring only name, dates of treatment, and the diagnosis, to those asking for detailed, personal information about the patient. Depending on the unconscious conflicts of the individual patient, the psychological significance and emotional ramifications of the insurance may assume major importance in the therapy and may even compromise the patient's treatability."

Cancellation Policies

As indicated above, cancellation policies vary from practitioner to practitioner. Many make no charge if given 24 hours' notice, on the assumption that they have the opportunity to fill that hour with another client. It is common to charge for broken appointments or late cancellations. Obviously, if this happens frequently, the therapist needs to consider the matter within the therapeutic context—to examine the reasons behind the frequent disruptions of the schedule and to deal with the material generated. One of the authors tends not to charge for occasional missed appointments where an illness or unforeseeable event interfered, but may make a charge, in consultation with the patient, if there is going to be a prolonged period of disruption of therapy.

That charge is levied to reserve the time slot for the patient, who must see it as a fair cost.

Both authors explain to their patients, at the start of therapy, as part of the general communication regarding fee mechanics, that they charge the full fee if 24 hours of notice is not given. They make it clear that it has nothing to do with the reason for not keeping the appointment — that they do not sit in judgment and decide that it was not the patient's fault so there is no fee, or that the fee is levied as a punishment for being "bad." Rather, they point out that they need to be paid for their time, and the principle of the theater ticket is invoked: if they do not have time to "resell" a ticket to a seat in their consulting room for that date and time, the ticket remains the patient's responsibility. They also add that should they fill the hours, despite short notice, they do *not* charge, as they do not need to be paid twice for their time. They explain that if the patient is using insurance, most companies do not pay for services not actually rendered, and therefore the entire fee will have to be the patient's respnsibility.

Additionally, they offer the patient the opportunity to use the time with them on the telephone if, for example, he or she cannot make the trip to the office for whatever reason (e.g., an accident, illness, or inclement weather). The time, it is explained, is the patient's to use, and they would rather he or she use it than not use it. They also make a point of noting in the patient's file that the 24-hour notice and insurance questions were addressed. They always ask the patient if he or she has any problems with the policy, or any questions to ask, and they discuss whatever needs to be discussed. In all of their years of practice, both psychologists have never experienced a backlash of this policy. One of the reasons is that they do not invoke the policy unless it has been discussed. If there is any question about whether the patient has been informed, the charge is not levied, but is discussed, and therapy proceeds.

Vacations

Therapists and patients, too, are entitled to take vacations. It is critical that the therapist notify patients at least four to six weeks in advance about anticipated long absences. If communication in the initial sessions has been quite complete, it may be anticipated that the patients, too, are aware of the desirability of their communicating to the therapist as early as possible any plans they may have that would involve their not keeping regularly scheduled appointments. In the case of the therapist's vacation, early anouncements tend to allow for working through of any feelings of abandonment on the part of the patient, permit patients to schedule their vacations when the therapist will be away, if they so desire, and preclude negative feelings on the part of the therapist who might have been helped by earlier knowledge of a patient's expectation of nonappearance.

SPECIAL ARRANGEMENTS

Children / Adolescents

When someone other than the client is responsible for the bills, a special situation arises. In working with children and adolescents in particular, it is usually the parent(s) who pay. At times, when an adolescent is being treated, a parent refuses to pay once the desired behavior change has been achieved, often because of feelings of inadequacy based on the therapist's ability to change the adolescent's behavior, which the parent was unable to do. It is important for the therapist to discuss fees with both the parents and the adolescent, initially, and sometimes even to have them all sign a contract stipulating all of the payment expectations and conditions, including charges for consultations and missed appointments.

It seems inappropriate to charge continually for sessions that the adolescent misses without notifying the parent of that fact. One way to deal with such a situation is to ask the adolescent to make a partial payment toward the fee that is being charged to the parent. This tactic may elicit from the adolescent a more serious commitment to the treatment process.

Spouses

While in the past the practice was much more common than it is today, it is still frequently the case that one spouse, often the male, will pay for a spouse's treatment. Once again, the client may change behavior and attitudes in the course of therapy, and the spouse may not welcome that change and may not wish to pay the bills. Appropriate discussion with the couple concerning treatment expectations and the method of payment may remedy the problem. In many instances, of course, a spouse does not wish to have his or her partner involved, and confidentiality principles preclude such discussion.

INTEREST CHARGES

Many believe that it is "unprofessional" to charge interest. Neither of the authors do. However, it is an option that may be discussed when the buildup of a balance is anticipated because of the collection agreement proposed. One colleague indicated to us that she is now charging interest for balances beyond one month. She believes that it has significantly increased her income. It is interesting to note that once you indicate your desire for prompt payment, new bills are moved from the "bottom of the pile" of unpaid bills to the top.

One of the options available in setting fees in the initial collection agreement is to arrange for a patient to pay a regular monthly payment that may be lower than the monthly bill incurred, and permit a balance to build, with the understanding that after therapy is terminated, the payments will continue until the bill has been paid in full. One of the authors does make such an arrangement, at times, and stipulates that there will be no interest charged on that balance. Once that stipulation has been made, of course, one does not have the right, ethically, to change the rule. Others may agree to regular partial payments, but charge interest. If this is done, it is essential that the client receive a full explanation of the costs involved, percentages and so on.

THE BILL

If you adopt a system of monthly billing, your bill should include the following:

- Balance due from prior months, if any.
- Dates, place, type of service, with charge for each service.
- Credits for any payments received during the month.
- Balance currently due.

In addition, if your client will be using insurance coverage and be submitting the bills to the insurance company for reimbursement, your bill should include in addition to the above:

- The diagnosis (now generally ICD-9CM code).
- The CPT-4 code for each service.
- Your Social Security or tax ID number.

Computer software is now available for billing purposes which you may choose to utilize. There are also pegboard and other billing systems that tie billing into the recording of daily office activity. The accountant whom you use for your office accounts can be of great help in making decisions about the system that is best for you.

A self-addressed return envelope might be included with your bill.

KEEPING TABS ON COLLECTING

Many practitioners dislike the financial aspects of a practice, and tend to forget about them until a cash-flow problem arises. But for therapeutic reasons, it is important for the practitioner to be aware of the status of patients' bills in those instances where cash payments are not the *modus operandi*. We recommend that the practitioner review, on a monthly basis, all client ledger sheets. If the bill has not been paid according to the terms of the agreement, the issue must be discussed so that a satisfactory resolution is developed that permits the therapeutic process to continue constructively. If secretaries handle the billing, they should provide the practitioner with a list of noncomplying clients. The practitioner then can decide which situations require his or her personal attention.

ADJUSTING COLLECTION POLICIES

Occasionally during the course of therapy, the initial agreement concerning fees needs to be reexamined. A fee that was reasonable at the beginning of treatment may not be so for the patient who experiences a sharp drop in income. The agreed-upon fee may become a burden to the patient when the frequency of sessions needs to be increased. Under those conditions, some therapists negotiate a new contract. For example, one of the authors provides clients in such circumstances with two options: one is to pay at the initially agreed-upon rate, and let the balance build. Payments are increased when the patient is able to meet them. At the end of treatment, payments continue until the debt is paid. This method can work well with therapists who do not charge interest, and for patients and therapists who can "live with" a mounting debt. For those who would be distressed by owing money, a lower fee is offered. What is important is that the therapist be aware of the patient's situation, only make offers that are acceptable, and not jeopardize the therapeutic needs of the patient. In those instances where neither option is acceptable to the patient, remaining with the status quo or making referrals to sliding-scale agencies or other service providers should be considered.

COLLECTION PROBLEMS

Most clients fulfill their financial responsibilities without problems. But there are times when patients do not pay as they had agreed to do, and although some therapists find it extremely difficult to broach the subject of a mounting bill, the problem must be discussed.

Following Up on Bills

If a patient terminates and a bill is not paid as promised, numerous options are available. Often a reminder telephone call (from you or your secretary) is all that is necessary. A follow-up call, if needed, may be made to negotiate a satisfactory payment plan, whether it involves regular partial payments of a stipulated amount or a commitment to pay by a designated date.

A series of notes or calls increasingly firm in nature may be successful in eliciting the payment due. Bills that reflect "aging," the number of days or months that a bill has been outstanding, can help to emphasize the long-overdue nature of accounts.

The following is a representative list of five graduated notes that might be sent with your bills.

1. "Second billing. Please respond."
2. "Your attention to this overdue account would be appreciated very much."
3. "Payment on this account has not been received. Is there a problem? Please contact this office regarding this bill."
4. "We have been very patient. Please remit, so that we do not have to take further action."
5. "This bill is long outstanding, and you have not chosen to contact us regarding it. Unless we hear from you by_____[stipulate a date 10 days hence] we shall turn this account over for collection to a collection agent/to our attorney for collection/we shall take you to small claims court."

The options stipulated in note no.5 are discussed in the following.

Learning About Collection Techniques

It is suggested that you, or your secretary, attend one of the many collections seminars given in cities across the country. Local collection agencies frequently sponsor such seminars, or know when they will be given in your community and whom to contact regarding attendance. These can be very productive, offering information regarding proper and improper collection techniques and many ways of avoiding collection problems and facilitating collections.

The U.S. Government publishes an invaluable pamphlet called "Fair Debt Collection," which can be acquired for 50 cents (as of this writing) by ordering #409M from the Consumer Information Catalogue, Consumer Information Center, Pueblo, CO 81109.

When All Else Fails

When telephone calls and letters of increasing firmness do not result in payment, then what? You may turn an account over to a collection agency, which will charge you a percentage of your bill, the exact figures generally depending on the age of the account. You can turn the account over to a collections attorney, with whom you have discussed fees and the options the attorney may exercise. You can take the client to a small claims court if the bill is under $500–$600 (the exact ceiling is set by each state). Or you can write off the bill. Before selecting any of these options, it is important to be aware of your feelings about them and the risks that are involved.

It is not uncommon for malpractice suits and complaints to state regulatory boards to be filed by people who are pressed for payment. Knowing your patients will permit you to make an informed decision concerning the risks involved in choosing a particular collection option. It is a mistake to believe that the only factor in assuming risk is the legitimacy of billing.

If you choose to pursue collection, it is important to have some sort of guideline that makes sense to you. For example, one of the authors will not turn an account over for collection unless the individual makes absolutely no response to repeated billings, suggesting no intention to acknowledge the charge incurred, let alone to pay it.

Collection Agencies / Attorneys

If you decide to use a collection agency or a collections attorney, it may be helpful to check with colleagues in your area and to talk to a number of agencies and attorneys, so that you get a good idea of the range of fees and can be sure that you select an agent experienced in working on professional accounts. Collection agencies will do what they can to contact the individual and start payment. Generally, the payments are made to the agency, which then remits to the practitioner the agreed-upon percentage. Some agencies provide practitioners with a printed agency form, which is sent to the patient. If payment is generated by receipt of the form, as sometimes happens, the collection agency does not claim a fee. Sometimes the collection agency determines that no payment is likely because of the individual's financial situation. If the recommendation is to write off the account, there should be no charge to you. If court action is to be undertaken, there should be prior consultation with the practitioner. It is interesting to note that one of the authors, in all her years of practice, has had only one occasion on which she permitted a collection agency to take a patient to court. Although no interest had been charged the patient, the judge, in ordering payment, assessed the patient what he considered to be fair interest charges, which she paid, along with the balance of her bill.

If you choose a collections attorney, you will need to discuss the kinds of services you wish performed. Usually, an attorney will start with a letter to your client, with an allusion to court action if the bill is not paid. Whether or not you wish to have the attorney take the case to court is something for you to decide. But you need to be clear about the fees that the attorney will charge you for the services you wish to have rendered.

Small Claims Court

While the small claims court option can be exercised with considerable success, it is important to be aware that this option generally takes a significant amount of professional time, and in some instances would not be an economically sound choice. On the other hand, economics do not necessarily determine our choices.

CLOSING REMARKS

Money has an overdetermined value for many individuals. It may symbolize their sense of worth and value, it may serve to validate their sense of power, or it may speak to their acquisitive needs. It may also express itself in work addiction, in a pursuit of self-esteem, which in turn may lead to personal and professional burnout (Freudenberger, 1980, 1985).

Money and fees are one of the last strongholds of therapy that we find uncomfortable to discuss. If not properly handled in treatment, the matter may promote dissatisfaction, conflict, tension, or an ethical malpractice suit.

Fees and their collection provide the practitioner with the structural support needed to furnish services and fulfill professional potential. If proper thought and care go into policy making and implementation as described, the practitioner can be free to practice without the problems and disruptions that can come out of disorganized and careless fee-related decisions.

The practitioner has a great deal of leeway in the selection of operatng principles regarding the handling of money in practice. Within the legal and ethical limits provided, the guiding principle must be the comfort and conviction of the practitioner and the ultimate well-being of the patient.

REFERENCES

DiBella, G.A.W. (1980). Mastering money issues that complicate treatment: The last taboo. *American Journal of Psychotherapy, 12*(4). 510-522.

DiBella, G.A.W. (1987). Money issues that complicate treatment. In D.W. Kroeger (Ed.), *The last taboo, money as symbol and reality in psychotherapy and psychoanalysis,* New York: Brunner/Mazel.

Eissler, K.R. (1974). On some theroretical and technical problems regarding the payment of fees for psychoanalytic treatment. *International Review of Psych-Analysis, 1*(73), 73-101.

Freudenberger, H.J. (1973). The psychologist in a free clinic setting: An alternative model in health care. *Psychotherapy: Theory, Research and Practice, 10*(1), 52-61.

Freudenberger, H.J. (1974). *The free clinic handbook. Journal of Social Issues, 30*(1), 1-203.

Freudenberger, H.J. (1984). Impaired clinicians coping with burnout, *Innovations in clinical practice: A source book.* Sarasota, FL: Professional Resource Exchange.

Freudenberger, H.J. (1985). How to market ourselves in the future. *Psychotherapy in Private Practice, 3*(3)., 33-37.

Freudenberger, H.J. (1986). The health professional in treatment: Symptoms, dynamics and treatment issues, In C.D. Scott, & J. Hank, (Eds.), *Heal thyself: The health of health care professionals.* New York: Brunner/Mazel.

Freudenberger, H.J. (1987). Chemical abuse among psychologists: Symptoms, causes and treatment issues. In R.R. Kilburg, P.E. Nathan & R.W. Thoresun (Eds.), *Professionals in distress* (pp.135-152). Washington, D.C.: American Psychological Assoication.

Freudenberger, H.J., and Richelson, G. (1980). *Burnout: How to beat the high cost of success.* New York: Bantam Books.

Freudenberger, H.J. & North, G. (1986). *Women's burnout: How to spot it, how to reverse it and how to prevent it.* New York: Penguin Books.

Goldensohn, S.S. (1986). Transference, countertransference and other therapeutic issues in a health maintenance organization (HMO). In D.W. Kroeger (Ed.), *The last taboo money as symbol and reality in psychotherapy and psychoanalysis.* New York: Brunner/Mazel.

Halpert, E. (1986). The meaning and effects of insurance in psychotherapy and psychoanalysis, In D. Krueger (Ed.), *The last taboo: money as symbol and reality in psychotherapy and psychoanalysis.* New York: Brunner/Mazel.

Hoffling, C.K. & Rosenbaum, M. (1980). The extension of credit ot patients in psychoanalysis and psychotherapy. *Bulletin of the Menninger Clinic, 44*(4). 327-344.

Inman, D.J. & Bascue, L.O. (1983). Referral sources of psychologists in private practice. *Psychological Reports, 52,* 895-866.

Keith-Spiegel, P., & Koocher, G. (1985). *Ethics in psychology.* New York: Random House.

C H A P T E R
20

THIRD-PARTY PAYMENTS

Howard M. Cohen, Ph.D.

"While nothing is more uncertain than the duration of a single life, nothing is more certain than the average duration of a thousand lives" (Boorstin, 1974). That statement, made in the middle of the 19th century by Elizur Wright, a reformer, abolitionist, and zealous crusader who has been referred to as the "Father of Life Insurance," is not apt to be disputed by today's psychological statisticians. It underscores the actuarial basis for insurance that has a long history in Western civilization.

Insurance began with the protection of maritime risks in ancient times and progressed through the protection of widows and children through life insurance, to casualty insurance, and then to the protection of the aged. How difficult it is for many in contemporary times to realize that insurance arrived, particularly in the United States, as a substitute for the protection and help that previously had been provided by family, neighbors, religious congregations, and the general community (Boorstin, 1974). With the advance of technology, specialization, and geographical mobility, the traditional supports of an earlier age have often become inaccessible. It should come as no surprise, therefore, that an aspect so fundamental to our lives as protection of health, of necessity, must be provided by insurance, a fiscal intermediary, or a third-party payer.

Since the advent of Medicare and Medicaid, third-party payment, either through government or private expenditure, has made health care available to the great majority of residents of the United States. The questions that must be asked in general have to do with accessibility, quality, and reimbursement levels. It would appear vital to the mental-health professions to think in terms of how insurance fits into the broad health picture and, more specifically, of the impact that third-party payment has for the practitioner.

This chapter summarizes the current available types of third-party mental-health benefits, issues that arise from third-party payment, and the directions that mental-health plans and benefits may take in the future.

TYPES OF THIRD-PARTY COVERAGE

Although most residents of the United States, particularly since the enactment of Medicaid and Medicare, are covered by private or government benefits, there are vast differences among the types and amounts of benefits available. As Flynn (1985) suggests, mental health historically has not been financially underwritten as well as has general medical-care services. There has been a lingering unfamiliarity with what were thought to be potential costs of these programs and what appeared to be controversial measurements of cost-effectiveness. Nevertheless, government and employers in general have come to realize that the cost to productivity of not providing mental and substance-abuse benefits may be too devastating to disregard. As such, a wide variety of insurance programs with mental-health benefits currently exist and new ones will be coming on line.

As recently as 1986, 18 states had some form of mandated mental health benefits (Taft, 1986), while 29 states required that any potential insurance group be informed that such benefits were available. A number of states, including New York, are now reviewing the possibility of seeking mandated benefits legislation. This is always considered with an eye to cost. Government is ever alert to the possibility that additional mandated coverage, be it eyeglasses, dental prostheses, or psychotherapy, will increase the cost of premiums, which has the potential of driving employers out of a state and making it difficult to attract new employers to that state. The effect of premiums is made clear by the fact that, in 1983, "total public and private expenditures for health care in the United States accounted for over forty percent of total employee benefit expenditures" (Arnould & Van Vorst, 1984).

In any event, whenever a state-mandated minimum mental-health benefit is enacted into law, it usually is written into contracts as a ceiling of benefits rather than a floor. To put it in other terms, whatever a law mandates as minimum benefits, whether it be days of hospitalization or outpatient psychotherapy, generally becomes the maximum benefit in the plan. It is left to the competitive marketplace to provide higher levels of care at lesser cost to the subscriber. For example, if a $700 minimum is required by law or regulation for outpatient psychotherapy, that often becomes the maximum allowable under a negotiated policy.

A typical method of cost containment that is incorporated into plans that seek to prevent overutilization, but at the same time encourage patient involvement and commitment to the tratment process, is to impose, customarily, a 20 to 50 percent copayment feature (after the deductible is met). Other examples are annual, as well as lifetime, caps on dollar amounts of benefits.

Inpatient Benefits

Most mental-health policies that provide inpatient benefits allow for 30 days of treatment, including the broad range of diagnostic and treatment services rendered by practitioners. Some policies restrict these benefits to a psychiatric hospital, but more often than not the benefits apply for care in a psychiatric ward of a general hospital.

What should not be overlooked is that third-party payment by the government or public sector has long been involved in care at military, Veterans Administration, Public Health, state, county, and municipal hospitals. The fiscal intermediary has had a long tradition prior to office practice.

Practitioners who are not physicians should b e aware that staff privileges are important in hospitals, and that if such services are not accessible to patients, there may be denial of benefits to the facility. It is important that those on the staff become familiar with accreditation standards, reimbursemenmt schedules, and requirements for services by third-party payers involved.

Outpatient Benefits — Private Sector

A variety of government and private third-party benefits programs exist

Alcohol Treatment   Many states have mandated or make available options for the treatment of alcohol and drug abuse. New York's most recent law on alcoholism and alcohol abuse,[1] for example, mandates treatment in centers certified by the Division of Alcohol and Substance Abuse. The regulations allow for 60 visits, 20 of which may be for family members, and five of those 20 for family members even if the alleged alcoholic is not undergoing treatment.

No-Fault Insurance   No-fault insurance is for the treatment of personal injury as a result of a motor vehicle accident. This form of third-party payment usually allows for services by any appropriate licensed provider, and usually prohibits any provider from setting a fee in excess of what is set forth in the schedule of fees and services promulgated by the states. The fee schedule is revised frequently and amended annually. State professional associations should be in contact with their respective insurance departments to make known the range of customary services providced by practitioners and what are current fair and equitable fees.

In the event of an automobile accident, patients submit the provider's bills to their insurance carrier. Any exception to the fee schedule, usually because of an unusual procedure, must receive prior approval, and any violation of the schedule will be reported to the state's insurance departments. In states with freedom of choice (FOC) laws, practitioners, such as psychologists, are viewed as independent providers. An example of a no-fault insurance is the New York State law.

Worker's Compensation   A program similar to no-fault insurance but pertaining to inujury occurring in the workplace is worker's compensation. In some states, only physicians are considered independent providers.

Practitioners, such as psychologists, should have their professional associations protest to the appropriate state agency the denial of benefits to employees and the increases in costs that the restriction imposes on the worker's compensation programs.

Outpatient Benefits — Public Sector

Until the amendment to the Social Security laws in 1965, which provided for Medicaid and Medicare programs, state and local government provided more support for health than did the federal government (Gibson, 1983).

Medicaid   Medicaid is the joint federal-state health program for low-income people, administered by the state under federal guidelines. The usual federal share of state Medicaid dollars is based upon a formula involving the per-capita income in each state. Federal support varies from approximately 50 to 78 percent, with the poorer states and those having higher unemployment rates receiving the greater share of federal monies.

Mental-health benefits and fees vary from state to state, but more often than not are considerably below marketplace fees and with noticeable differentials between professions. States have a number of options within the guidelines and may experiment with different approaches. Naturally, states and localities are concerned about costs. In one instance, the city of New York (New York City, 1984), with the approval of the state of New York, obtained a variance that denied access of Medicaid enrollees to psychological providers. New York City insisted that it was in compliance with the law since Medicaid recipients could have access to psychologists at municipal clinics. It was only through the efforts of the New York State Psychological Association (Cohen, 1985) that the variance, which had been in place for years, was removed.

For psychologists to become providers, they must register with the state regulatory agency that administers the program. Social workers and nurses are generally not registered as independent providers. Often there is mandated consultation with, or certification of necessity of treatment by, a physician. In such cases, efforts are being made to remove that provision, which makes the program more costly, with no benefit to the patient.

Medicare   Medicare is the federal health-care program for the elderly. The current status of outpatient psychotherapy is an allowance of $250 per year, with a $250, or 50 percent, copayment when treatment is rendered by a psychiatrist. Other mental-health practitioners are not recognized in this program as psychotherapy providers. The only exception is when the psychologist provides psychotherapy within the framework of a health maintenance organization (HMO). Psychological examinations, however, are permitted within both the usual office practice and HMOs, at a fee limited to $150.

The exclusion of nonphysician providers by law and of psychiatric providers by economics leaves a substantial segment of our population, perhaps that segment with the greatest need, without the benefit of mental-health support. This will be discussed further later in this chapter.

Supplementary Security Income (SSI)   SSI is a federal program, administered by the state for the aged, the disabled, and the blind. Each state designates a lead agency for the regulation of the program, which, in addition to furnishing monthly payments, makes available to the claimants disability evaluations and vocational rehabilitation. The state must abide by the criteria for mental impairment established by the Social Security laws and regulations. Psychologists and psychiatrists are responsible for the determination of the presence and severity of mental impairment. Traditional psychological assessment procedures, including tests and interviews, are administered, with fees usually derived from the workers' compensation schedules.

Crime Victims' Compensation   With the increasing public concerns regarding the effects of crimes on their victims, states are moving into areas of assistance to those who have sustained some type of injury as a result of having been a victim of a crime. A New York State law (the New York State Crime Victims Compensation law), a model of this type, created a Crime Victims Board to which a claimant who has suffered financial difficulty can apply and may be entitled to compensation in the form of direct monetary aid, occupational rehabilitation, and/or counseling services. The counseling or psychotherapy services are available only to those who have suffered severe trauma, such as the family of a homicide victim or a person who has been raped. Although financial loss is a criterion for compensation, an exception is made for those who were victims of sexual crimes and others who had incurred their injuries while acting as a Good Samaritan.

Diagnostic and psychotherapeutic services may be sought by the claimant from practicing psychologists, and these services are reimbursable at fees set by the Crime Victims Board.

Civilian Health and Medical Program of the Uniformed Services (CHAMPUS) CHAMPUS, a federal program for the dependents of armed forces personnel, provides for a broad range of mental-health services. Psychiatrists, psychologists, and social workers are recognized under this program.

PROFESSIONAL ISSUES AND THIRD-PARTY PAYMENT

With the transition of fee-for-service paid directly by the patient to the intervention of the fiscal intermediary has come controversy and turbulence that often have created a roiling of the psychotherapeutic waters. Chief among the complaints of both practitioners and their patients was the concern regarding confidentiality and the subsidiary problems of informed consent, the extent of information necessary to furnish to a third-party payer, routing of claims, the exchange of information through insurance companies and government agencies, peer review, and so on. Additional but somewhat separate issues derive from the self-insured groups, the denial of insurance, and the responsibilities both of providers and the third-party payers.

Confidentiality and Access to Private Communications

The nature of mental-health practice, be it assessment or treatment, requires a confidentiality of communication between the clinician and patient. Those elements of practice have become canons of state and national ethical codes, as well as having been written into law and regulation in forms of confidentiality and privileged communication statutes in the varying jurisdictions (DeKraai & Salies, 1981; Toronto, 1986). With rare exceptions, the concept of privileged communication, in some states, takes precedence over the admissibility of evidence, and consequently justice—that is, practitioners may not disclose, even in a court of law, information obtained from patients.

Enter the third-party payer. Here we are not dealing with risk to the public, but with a government or private third-party payer who has agreed contractually to provide benefits for a class of disorders when the need for treatment has been established and appropriate treatment rendered by licensees, acting within the scope of their licenses. The requirement to determine if there is compliance with the contract in the above terms is not merely due to the third-party payer's administration of the program, but is insisted upon by the union or employer that represents the individual patient. This need to determine if there is compliance with the contract is not so different from the action of a school board, which wants to make sure that a teacher is qualified and is teaching the expected curriculum for the fifth grade.

It is similar, and yet quite different, because in the instance of the third-party payment for psychological services, it affects what heretofore had been confidential and privileged.

Justification of Claims When a union or employer, public or private, signs an agreement with an insurance company to provide specific benefits, that third-party payer must have some information to determine whether the diagnosis or treatment is covered by the contract. Not to do that would violate the contract, and would conceivably result in increasing costs, higher premiums, and the possibility of future exclusion of mental-health benefits.

Thus it becomes necessary for the practitioner to provide the minimum information necessary to justify the beneficiary's claim. There is generally no law or regulation that states how much information the provider must supply, but there should be some indication of diagnosis, symptoms, type of treatment, functional impairment, goals, change of condition, and so on. The data supplied, which should be sufficient to justify the claim, need not be lengthy or reveal intricate details of the patient's life. That type of information has been provided in hospitals and university training programs, has been exchanged with colleagues for training and consultation purposes for decades, and, except for concerns of confidentiality, would not be an issue.

Some questions raised by patients and practitioners quite rightly and naturally are: How is the material protected? Could patients lose their jobs were the information to find its way into the wrong hands? Will the person be denied other insurance?

Generally, there is no law or regulation requiring third-party payers to keep confidential the information they receive. Nevertheless, health insurance companies provide protection through encoding, limited access, and locked files in the medical departments. It is not in the interest of insurance companies to breach confidentiality, and there is very little evidence that this occurs. However, professional associations should work toward enacting legislation that would limit access to patient information and protect confidentiality.

Routing of Claims Routing of claims is a process that lends itself to breaches of confidentiality, and perhaps more so than the information provided directly to third-party payers. In most jurisdictions, employees file claims with the personnel office (sometimes via the manager), which submits them to the insurance company. Therein lies the possibility that people who know the patients can learn the diagnosis and the nature of the problems. Most enlightened companies, unions, and public employers voluntarily allow their members or employees to submit claims directly to the insurance company. Those who have no need to know should have no access to information. The problem would be eased were laws enacted providing for direct routing of claims.

In any case, patients should understand that if they are to receive benefits, the practitioner will have to provide appropriate information on the insurance form. (The insurance contract so mandates.) Accordingly, the practitioner should request a dated informed consent from the patient regarding that procedure.

Although the entrance of the third-party payer on the scene has undoubtedly complicated a very private professional relationship, there has been an easing of the financial burden of treatrment for the patient and an exponential increase in the number of people who now have access to psychological treatment.

The ever-increasing availability of mental-health benefits through third-party payments remains in the shakedown phase, with issues of confidentiality and access to information a consideration that is being faced in a variety of ways, for example, clauses in contracts specifying limits in access, better routing, less frequent reports, which should be limited to the most necessary information. Through these types of fine-tuning and imaginative approaches, more streamlined mental-health packages will evolve that will lessen the concerns of patients regarding confidentiality.

Employee Retirement Income Security Act of 1974 (ERISA)   This federal law has exacerbated the confidentiality issue and has undercut the FOC laws enacted by the states.

The law states, "The provisions of [ERISA] shall supersede any and all state laws insofar as they may now or hereafter relate to any employee benefit plan [covered by ERISA]."[2] In short, this law permits any group (union, employee, etc.) to become self-insured, and in that manner to be out from under the umbrella of state insurance laws and regulations. To become self-insured requires that the group itself assume the risk of health costs rather than pay premiums to an insurance company, or assume the financial risks and contract out to an insurance company the administration of the program.

Since insurance is mainly regulated by the states, the various mandates and protections provided in the different state jurisdictions are evaded, or if followed, are done so only by voluntary compliance. One need not mention the apparent cost savings and the incentive to reduce benefits through this means of third-party payment. Undoubtedly, some of the major employers in the country who are self-insured provide benefits similar to those in the customary insurance plan, but in the main, self-insured programs are less apt to provide benefits such as are mandated in the heavily regulated states. And it is estimated that approximately 40 to 50 percent of policies now written are of the self-insured variety.

How has this affected the practitioner?

Confidentiality   The concern of the lack of laws regarding confidential mental-health files has been exacerbated by the processing of claims by the patients' own personnel offices or unions. The possibility of breaches of confidentiality under these circumstances is dangerous and can seriously impair a therapeutic relationship. This author attended one meeting with a vice-president of a major corporation, who, when informed of psychology's concerns, replied, "It is most important for us to know about the mental conditions of our employees, for their behavior not only reflects on the reputation of this company, but we are indeed liable for their activities while on the job." Were that view to become prevalent, the effect on psychotherapy would be profound.

FOC   Since self-insured groups are exempt from FOC state laws, their contracts may exclude coverage for practitioners, such as psychologists, even in plans where mental-health benefits are offered. The group can elect to honor FOC or disregard it, with impunity.

In this instance, state insurance departments, which are charged with protecting the public; private insurance companies, which stand to lose a good share of the underwriting of contracts; and providers all share a common interest in having the Congress review and amend ERISA.

In the meantime, if practitioners or patients in a state with FOC laws are denied reimbursement, the first order of business is to determine whether the group to which the patients are subscribers is self-insured. If that is the case, the practitioners should enlist the aid of their state professional association to use its informational resources to persuade the self-insured group that it is to the advantage of the group and its members to adhere to FOC laws.

Denial of Life and Disability Insurance

A problem related to the issue of confidentiality is the denial of insurance contracts to individuals who have been treated for a mental disorder. Many states, such as New York, have insurance laws that read, "No individual or entity shall refuse to issue or review, or shall cancel any policy of insurance, because of any past treatment for a mental disability of the insured."

However, the caveat is that if the third-party payer can demonstrate that denial is based on "sound underwriting and actuarial principles reasonably related to actual or anticipated loss experience",[4] the policy may be denied. However, the burden of proof is on the company, not on the applicant for the policy.

Again, this issue should be brought to the attention of state insurance departments by practitioners, patients, and state professional associations. There is no evidence that supports a general underwriting rule of denying benefits to those who have been treated for an emotional problem.

Practitioners' Responsibilities

Reports   It has always been incumbent upon a health provider to furnish reports of a patient's condition and treatment to whomever that patient designates as the recipient of the report (see, for example, New York State Rules of Unprofessional Conduct[5]). Thus that request by a patient for the practitioner to send a treatment report to the third-party payer, after appropriate informed consent, is no different from any other similar request the patient may make. Practitioners are bound to comply with that request, which involves no breach of contract or violation of confidentiality provided that the information to justify treatment is minimal and appropriate.

It is advisable, however, that in the initial meeting with the patient, after the ground rules and form of payment have been discussed, mention is made of third-party payment and its requirements for submission of reports.

Although completion of forms takes time, they focus both the clinician and patient on goals and treatment plans. Yet the practitioner's time is valuable, but there currently is no means of transferring the charge for form completion to the third-party payer. However, practitioners should include a reasonable charge for that time in their fee schedule, just as is done with other office overhead.

Unkept Appointments   A missed visit is costly to the practitioner, but it would be fraudulent to list that visit as a treatment session on an insurance form. Reimbursement is for a service provided, and although it could be argued that the service was available and scheduled, and it was through no fault of the practitioner that it did not take place, it cannot assumed to be a treatment session. One can indicate on the claim form or statement that the appointment was unkept and legitimately charge for it, as would be done with the self-paying patient, but it must be left to the insurer to determine if it will allow benefits for the session. The guideline is: Be forthright in billing, and if you question a decision, contact the company.

Lending One's License   Practitioners may not lend their license to an unlicensed individual for billing purposes. The individual practitioner in most states is not entitled to supervise another unlicensed individual who is providing services to an insurance subscriber. Insurance plans usually cover benefits only when rendered by a properly licensed person. Practitioners who lend their licenses jeopardize those licenses. Practitioners should never indicate that they are providing treatment when that is not the case. Not only does that place the license at risk, but benefits are likely to be denied the patient and the practitioner could face criminal prosecution.

DIRECTION FOR THE FUTURE

Over 98 percent of the population of the United States are covered by health benefits. Unfortunately, mental disorders are not as well covered as are physical illnesses. And outpatient mental-health care is generally less adequately reimbursed than is inpatient treatment. Nevertheless, with the increasing recognition of financial loss resulting from emotional or substance-abuse problems, a greater share of the health dollar is being assigned to mental-health benefits.

There is every reason to believe that there will be reconsideration by those states that have not enacted mandated benefits. We can expect to see expanded benefits, greater availability of services to the aged, and substance-abuse treatment laws, as well as expansion of benefits under HMOs. All of this appears to be in the public interest and merits the endorsement of practitioners.

It would be misleading and unrealistic, however, for any professional to believe that, when fiscal intermediaries intervene between the provider and the patient, some efforts of cost and quality control will not be part of any enlargement of benefits. With the advent of Medicaid, Medicare, and particularly CHAMPUS, quality and utilization reviews were required. Indeed, the CHAMPUS mental-health program would not have been endorsed by the Congress if a precise peer-review process had not been set in place. The quality and utilization reviews and peer-review programs have expanded to other commercial and governmental programs and there is no reason to believe that any new programs that evolve will not have provisions for review. This is consistent with the "good profession" monitoring its own people and assuring competency and quality of care.

There is certainly apt to be greater emphasis on prospective review for third-party payment. Companies and government agencies are likely to want to approve a treatment approach after an initial number of visits, and prior to subsequent visits. This practice is in contrast to providing benefits after the fact.

We can expect to see various experimental benefit packages. Medicaid will attempt to implement minimum and variable copayment features. Some employers will provide their employees with annual lump-sum health benefits in dollar amounts, any part of which is not used may be retained by the employee. The financial incentive for not overutilizing is obvious. But what are the implications for underutilizing by those in genuine need? These are but examples of new approaches that can be expected to undergo try-out periods.

In effect, third-party payment, in its variety of forms, has become the customary manner of reimbursing mental-health services. It has permitted such services to be within the reach of most people. The design of these programs and packages will continue to adapt to the needs of our society and it is up to all concerned to ensure a good fit to quality standards of practice. Indeed, third-party payments have been a means of promoting human welfare, safeguarding the interests of the public, and attempting to maintain standards of competency of service.

REFERENCES

Arnould, R.J., & Van Vorst, C.B. (1984). Supply response to market and regulatory forces in health care. In Meyer, J.A. (Ed.), *Incentives vs. controls in health policy: Broadening the debate.* Washington, DC: American Enterprise Institute for Public Policy Research.

Boorstin, D.J. (1974). *The Americans: The democratic experience.* New York: Vintage Books, p. 175.

Cohen, H.M. (1975). *Insurance update.* Bulletin. New York: New York State Psychological Association.

DeKraai, M.B., & Salies, B.D. (1980). Privileged communications of psychologists. Mimeographed. American Psychological Association.

Flynn, T.J. (1985). Issues and trends in the organization and financing of mental health benefits. Mimeographed. Washington, DC: American Enterprise Institute.

Gibson, R. (1983). Quiet revolution in Medicaid in market reforms. In Meyer, J.A. (Ed.), *Current issues, new directions, strategic decisions.* Washington, DC: American Enterprise Institute for Public Policy Research.

New York City will try to keep Medicaid variance. (1984). *New York State Psychologist, 35,* 5-6.

Taft, N.B. (1986). Major state laws on group insurance benefit mandates and offers. Mimeographed.

Taranto, R.G. (1986). The psychiatrist-patient privilege and third-party payers: Commonwealth v. Kobrin. *Law, Medicine, and Health Care, 14*(1), 25-29.

FOOTNOTES

1. 52.24 of Title 11 of the Official Compilation of Codes, Rules and Regulations (Regulation No. 62).

2. Automobile Insurance Reform Act (Chapter 892 of the Laws of 1977) (11 NYCRR 68).

3. 29 U.S. Code, 1144(a), 1974 Employer Retirement Security Act, Sec. 514(a).

4. New York State Insurance Law. Sect. 2608(a)(b).

5. New York State Rules of Unprofessional Conduct (Board of Regents). Sect. 29.2(1)(b).

CHAPTER
21

COLLECTIONS

Carmi Harari, Ed.D.

C onsciousness about collection of fees is basic to the private practice of psychotherapy. Therapists should be aware of the significance of the financial aspects, which, along with other matters, should be made explicit in the verbal contract established between the psychotherapist and the client or patient. Collection of fees provides all or part of the psychotherapist's income and is a significant barometer of a working therapeutic relationship.

The collection of fees and related issues needs to be considered from three standpoints: the practical issues; the therapeutic issues; and the ethical, moral, and legal issues.

PRACTICAL ISSUES

As a very young psychologist and beginning psychotherapist, I was so pleased to have patients place their confidence in me that, after arranging the fee to be paid, I sometimes did not pay careful attention to its collection. In later years, I was to describe philosophically my expensive early course in "money management," by which I meant such things as unpaid accrued bills, ineffectual efforts to collect payments, or at times committing myself to payment arrangements that later proved to be antitherapeutic in their effect. The influence on my income was a significant stimulus to rapid learning. The question of the fee-for-services sometimes arises in making the first consultation appointment or needs to be addressed at the initial consultation session. Establishment of the fee involves placing oneself within the general fee range current in a geographical area as well as knowing where one falls on the scale of personal experience and seniority. Obviously, the fee must take into account the client's ability to pay and the therapist's financial requirements.

It is essential that the therapist be comfortable with the fee established. When this comfort does not exist, one could predict that technical problems will arise and interfere with the therapeutic process. The collection of fees involves such issues as how, when, and by whom the fee is to be paid. Is payment to be by the session, week, or month? Will it be paid by check or in cash? Will it be paid by the client, spouse, friend, lover, or parent, or charged to a corporate account? Is the patient covered for outpatient psychotherapy by insurance? Patients are not always certain of their coverage and psychotherapy is not included in many health insurance policies. I often ask prospective patients who inquire about whether insurance is accepted to check the extent of their coverage, either on their written policy or with their employee benefits officer.

Recently, several people have phoned for appointments in the mistaken belief that they were fully covered. In many cases, they did not confirm their first appointment when they learned that coverage for psychotherapy was either very limited or not covered by their policy and that they were responsible for their own payments. In some instances where I did ask them to check their policies complications have arisen concerning their entitlement to coverage, to the detriment of the therapy and an unclear financial contract. Clarification in advance of insurance coverage might decrease the number of completed referrals but might help ensure that those accepted enter therapy with a clear sense of their financial obligation. In instances where psychotherapy coverage is clear, and my assessment of client responsibility permits, I will accept an arrangement in which payment for therapy follows reimbursement by the insurance carrier. In all such instances, I make clear the patient's responsibility for payment should the insurer disqualify the insured.

Assignment of fees to be paid directly by the insurer to the psychologist appears undesirable to me, as do other forms of payment by others, because it separates payment responsibility from the ongoing relationship with the client. I prefer, and generally seek, to have the adult client take direct responsibility for payment even when the funds will come from another person or entity. An exception arises in the case of minors, who are not personally responsible financially for their treatment. Acceptance of participant provider fees paid by insurance companies at a generally lower rate than prevailing fees requires individual judgment and depends very much on the individual therapist's requirements and resources—which means that relatively new therapists may agree to their lower fees in order to fill hours and develop their practice. The slow payment to the provider typical in many instances can be remedied in part by prompt billing with close attention to all required items on the forms.

A recent situation may serve to illustrate some hazards involved in accepting insurance reimbursement without verifying the nature of the coverage. A police officer and his wife consulted me for marital therapy. My assumption that police coverage for psychotherapy is generally adequate proved to be mistaken on two counts. Neither of the couple had paid for and enrolled for psychotherapy benefits under their general health insurance. Upon their agreement to enroll for such coverage, I continued therapy with them. They then informed me that they would discontinue treatment when they reached the limit of their coverage. Regular monthly billing brought no response until, six months after ending therapy, they sent me an insurance company check for approximately one-third of the billing on a per-session basis, with an indication that that was the maximum benefit to which they were entitled. After several notes and calls from my office, the remaining balance has still not been fully paid some 12 months after terminating therapy. In retrospect, the options before me included not going ahead with the sessions after the initial consultation until the true nature of their coverage was verified, or arranging, if they would agree, for full payment by them with insurance company reimbursement to go to them directly.

Questions of financial responsibility for missed appointment, lateness, vacations, and legal holidays need to be clearly articulated in advance. I find, however, it to be too oppressive to deal with all contingencies beforehand and leave some to be dealt with when particular events arise. At such times, I generally set policy for the next occasion and do not require that the single instance be paid for. It must be said that my general guideline is that the patient is responsible for all scheduled sessions. I require 24 to 48 hours' notice for a needed change of appointment but will make a change on shorter notice if we can arrive at a mutually agreeable time. In general, I do not find patients abusing the agreed-upon schedule of appointments, but on occasion it needs to be dealt with as an issue in therapy when such abuse appears excessive. I plan my working year on a 10-month basis, whereas some therapists count on 11 months, and I leave patients the option of meeting or not in July and August, depending on my availability.

Patients covered by insurance often require a monthly bill, which appears on my letterhead, and includes my name, address, license number, patient's name, diagnosis, dates of service, and charges. Some noninsured patients request monthly bills for their own records; others do not. In a few cases, patients ask for a year-end list of sessions and charges for tax or other purposes. For various contingencies that may arise, it is desirable to have a record book or card file in which basic information is listed, including the patient's address, home and work telephone numbers, the diagnosis according to the third edition of the *Diagnostic and Statistical Manual of Mental Disorders* in words and numbers (or the current standard diagnosis), and a record of fees and payments. The question of often arises as to whether a fixed-fee or sliding scale is preferable. I generally maintain a fairly narrow range of regular fees and always carry some low-cost individuals who require my services and are of particular interest to me. I try to find other appropriate resources for those whom I do not accept in treatment. I belong to several referral panels — my psychoanalytic organization and two psychology societies, one regional and one local — and I accept occasional referrals at low fees, particularly when we can meet during unfilled hours. I regard it as a matter of professional responsibility to be able to provide service for persons unable to pay standard fees. Recently, a young high-school student phoned for an appointment and offered to pay $5, which I accepted. I believe that all patients should make some payment from their own resources to whatever extent is possible.

At times I have accepted patients at lower-than-usual fees for particular periods, for example, graduate students in psychology, social work, or law, sometimes with arrangements for the accrued balance to be paid at some later date or after graduation. My experience with such arrangements has been generally favorable.

When some designated person other than the therapist, secretary, receptionist, or office manager accepts fees and makes appointments, it is crucial that the therapist keep close to each situation and can relate these transactions to the ongoing work. Such matters as cancellations, changes, and makeup sessions require that a clear contract be established with regard to financial responsibility. When I start treatment with a new person, I establish the regularity of appointments as to one, two, or more per week, as well as our responsibility to each other for the time and the financial responsibility for the appointment times specifically set aside for the patient. One cannot stress too much the importance of keeping careful records of service, fees, payments, and balance due.

Fee increases sometimes become necessary in periods of inflation, in order to keep up with the general economy. It requires great care and individual consideration of special circumstances and must be taken up with the patient with sufficient lead time. I generally make changes either on the approximate anniversary of beginning treatment, in September after a vacation break, or as of January 1, with at least one month's notice. Patients usually agree but sometimes may bring up special circumstances that require consideration or delay. At times some patients, because of changed economic circumstances owing to a loss or reduction of income, request a reduction of their fee, usually for a particular period or contingency, such as returning to work or finding a job.

THERAPEUTIC ISSUES

The pattern of payments may provide signals about the therapeutic process. Although rare, there have been a few individuals who have paid me at the beginning of a session as though not to maintain any commitment or obligation beyond one session. This is certainly not the only possible interpretation. Other payment phenomena that bear looking at are checks that are unsigned or undated, have the wrong date or amount, or show a discrepancy between amounts given in words and in figures. What does an over- or under-payment mean? The answers to and working out of these questions are to be found only in the therapeutic process.

Most patients who pay by check have their checks ready at the end of the session. In some instances, patients fumble for their checkbook and pen and begin to write their check at the end of the session. I generally ask these patients to complete their checks in the waiting room and leave them for me so that I can begin my next session, which permits me to keep my sessions to the allotted times. With some people, time must be allowed at the end of the session for scheduling and payment. The dynamics of seeking extra time can become part of a diagnostic appraisal of the therapeutic relationship. Some patients have reacted with anger at the suggestion that payment or discussion of appointments properly falls within the scheduled appointment time.

Although accounts should not be allowed to become delinquent, some may do so for various reasons. It is essential to devise a workable plan with the patient and seek to reduce the arrears in a regular and consistent manner as quickly as possible. One may have to review other options, such as a loan to reduce or eliminate the arrears, and current payments must be kept up to date. Motivational issues and attitudes toward therapy and the therapist need to be explored, and this may provide important insights into underlying causes of the problem. I have found that a greater percentage of built-up arrears in my practice have occurred when other significant persons in the patient's life are responsible for payment. Nonpayment or delayed payment may reflect relationship issues between the two, or even a not-so-unconscious reaction to changes in the patient's attitude and behavior. This suggests yet another reason for developing a therapeutic contract initially in which funds for therapy are made available to the adult patient and are independent of the relationship with the person responsible for payment.

Delinquent accounts of patients who terminate therapy present a different problem. Regular monthly billing, together with a reminder note with an invitation to telephone if there is some "problem" in relation to paying the bill, is often helpful. If necessary, a telephone call to the former patient by the therapist may secure an agreement for one or several periodic payments. When these methods do not bring results, there is often anger and the thought may arise of using a professional debt-collection agency or legal action. It is difficult to predict or control how the employees of collection agencies will behave toward the debtor. Inasmuch as they represent you in the community, you will need to judge whether you wish to continue your own efforts for collection or turn it over to the agency. Fees of 30 to 50 percent contingent on collection are common. It may be important to evaluate your anger and to recognize your own role in creating or permitting the problem to develop. Sometimes an appropriately worded letter from your attorney may help to resolve the situation with your former patient. In extreme situations, you may wish to consider taking legal action for collection of an unpaid bill. Consultation with your attorney and working on either a fee-for-service basis or on a contingency basis may prove appropriate. Contingency fees are higher, especially if the risk that the court or legal action may not be successful is great.

Some patients who refuse to pay may accuse you of neglect or some other failing. A recent experience of mine is illustrative. A colleague of long standing referred to me a woman with multiple severe medical problems and a history of highly disturbed relationships. At our first consultation session, she expressed anger at the referring psychologist for not accepting her for treatment. She was critical of my voice and my manner and of the appearance of my office. She exploded several times but, after discussion, agreed to continue with me. Several subsequent sessions found her storming out angrily over what she called my "inattention." Another time I found her pounding on my office door while I was in a session. She insisted that I had made an appointment with her rather than with the patient I was with. A brief discussion in an effort to show her that she was in error was futile and she left, but did telephone to say that she would keep her next appointment. She kept the appointment, but again took affront and stormed out. Billing for three unpaid sessions has brought no response.

Questions sometimes arise about charging for patients' phone calls. I regard this somewhat similarly to changing appointments and tend to deal with such matters on an individual basis. That is to say, I make a subjective evaluation of whether the calls are excessive or within the norm. In general, I receive few phone calls from patients other than technical ones to change an appointment or ask for a statement. Anxious individuals sometimes require the reassurance of a few minutes of talk on the telephone with me. When I judge that the frequency or duration of calls is excessive, I let my patient know that I will keep track of and bill for calls at the end of the month on the basis of 10-minute units at the regular session fee. I have not had to invoke this often, and when I have, it has either greatly reduced the number and duration of calls or it has become clear that the calls are a necessary aspect of the ongoing therapy at a particular time. It is important to note that when I receive such a call, I arrange for the patient to call me back at a time convenient to me.

I sometimes schedule phone sessions with patients whose work or some special situation takes them out of town for one or more sessions. I have had occasion to conduct phone sessions for several months with a patient on a temporary work assignment in Alaska, and somewhat more frequently between California and New York with patients whose work takes them to both coasts. Regular billing at the end of the month takes care of these sessions, with the patient carrying the telephone charges. In a few other instances, because of illness of the patient, a new baby, or an injury, I have also conducted telephone sessions. These are typically for one or two sessions at most.

Some prospective patients offer to pay for therapy by providing some service for the therapist such as clerical or secretarial work or carpentry, or an artist may offer paintings. Such arrangements complicate the always complex and often difficult relationship between therapist and patient by introducing another reality with potential for misinterpretation or feelings of exploitation by the patient. It may be important for the therapist to think through why such a barter arrangement might seem attractive or appropriate. The issue of having to appraise the worth of your patient's work in money terms may create difficulties. I recommend against such arrangements. I have been solicited by brokers who offered to place me on a list that they circulate of individuals prepared to exchange professional services for other services of value. It might prove more helpful to prospective psychotherapy patients to sell their services elsewhere and use the proceeds to pay for psychotherapy.

Ethical, Moral, and Legal Issues

Important issues of an ethical, moral, and legal nature may arise. Fee splitting raises the possibility of inappropriate referrals or providing unnecessary services and is a direct violation of the *Ethical Principles of Psychologists* (American Psychological Association, 1981). Charging for services not provided, although rare, may constitute a criminal offense. Patients may request insurance billing for more sessions or at a higher cost to cover the deductible part of their insurance policy. Others may ask that bills be prepared for services within a covered period rather than for the actual period. All such forms of collusion, aside from being unethical, are likely to have very negative effects on the treatment relationship; moreover, they would constitute fraud, which could lead to criminal prosecution and the loss of one's license. The negative therapeutic effect may be found in the nature of the unethical and immoral relationship, which can spread to other areas of the therapeutic work. It must be regarded as a booby trap waiting to explode.

In the course of practicing psychotherapy, one may learn from patients not only about aspects of their personal financial situations, but also about hidden assets. It is very important not to react to such information to any greater degree than one would to any other "information" revealed in therapy and to be able to treat it as simply part of the flow of therapeutic material.

Obviously, it must be held in confidence and not be exploited. Therapists must evaluate carefully their own financial requirements and appropriate charges and resist any temptation to reap financial gain from such knowledge. Another area of potential exploitation may arise in relation to financial or economic information, and similarly needs to be guarded against.

A final word. Many of the areas discussed in this chapter have been based on 40 years of experience and represent a distillation of my direct and indirect experience, as well as the experiences of colleagues, students, and supervisees. While the volume of which this is a part will fill a very valuable place as a professional resource, no book and no one person has all the answers. The importance of meeting with peers and colleagues and reviewing specific issues within our professional organizations cannot be overemphasized.

REFERENCE

American Psychological Association. (1981). *Ethical principles of psychologists* (revised). Washington, DC: Author.

C H A P T E R
22

DIVERSIFICATION IN CLINICAL PRACTICE:
Primary- and Tertiary-Care Considerations

David B. Adams, Ph.D.

S pecialization and subspecialization within the professions have undergone an evolutionary process. This evolution is the result of recognition by both the consuming public and the practicing professional that there is a need for differentiation of services. Specialization permits the targeted treatment of the patient's specific problems by the clinician, and is a concept that has proved viable in the marketplace.

All professions initially follow a common evolutionary path of the generalist model. Subsequent skills and applications are refined, and the circumscribed disciplinary boundaries and limitations of specialty areas are created.

Refining and limiting services may narrow the provider's responsibility and assist the consumer in appropriate decision making. In some cases, however, it may seem little more than a sophisticated marketing strategy.

While the implications are that the consumer, in this case the patient, will benefit from the careful restriction of service availability, the risks to the public are not necessarily minimized by a professional's definition of the limited practice. Additionally, the financial success of a practitioner is not guaranteed by the mere adherence to a specialist professional model. This chapter addresses clinical, ethical, and economic issues in the building of the subspecialty practice and the creation of a diversified model.

The licensing of a single profession cuts across social and political concerns. When a discipline reaches a certain level of skill development and application, licensure is sought by government to ensure the public welfare; by society to ensure professional accountability; and by the provider to define territorial boundaries for the viability and ultimate survival of the professional group. Thus, restriction of access to the professions is a goal shared by many, although each group may be responding on the basis of its special interest.

The government's motivation to activate effective licensing statutes is the conviction that restricted access to skill application serves the public good. In recent years, this has required not only an initially convincing presentation, but continued accountability from the licensed group (Fox, 1986).

The license to practice, having once been an assured definition of professional identity, is now greatly offset by the large number of groups seeking and achieving licensure. Specialization is designed to allow distinction from the throngs seeking legislative clout and protection.

The sunset legislation (Act. 11.61; *Legislative Review of Regulatory Functions:* "The Regulatory Sunset Act") is intended to ensure controlled access to the status of a licensed profession. This not only serves the interest of the profession, but protects the consumer as well. When professional psychology achieved licensed status in the United States, for example, one state, followed by the next, began dealing with the implementation of sunset legislation. This made psychology ultimately responsible for proving its own worth even during its infancy. Continuation of licensure has proved formidable to maintain, and has placed psychology at a considerable disadvantage when compared with other, more aged, professions.

GENERIC LICENSURE AND SPECIALIZATION

Most professions have been permitted a protracted history of service delivery before fractionation and subspecialization of the field have become issues. Mental health's developmental period has emerged from a diverse interdisciplinary unfolding. Thus, the field has been characterized by self-scrutiny and territorial imperatives, perhaps far too early in the maturational process. There has been insufficient time to establish an effective professional role model for specialization. The specialty model, however, may be adapted from the elder professions of medicine and law.

The generic license for the practice of law and that for the practice of medicine and surgery are attached to professions in which the beginning generalist model later fell into disfavor. The practitioners of medicine and law found that professional practice was more easily defined, and limits of responsibility better managed, when practice was limited to specific and predefined boundaries. The public also became more selective, if not more experienced, shoppers for professional services. At least conceptually, the individual learns when to seek out a pediatrician or a gynecologist, a divorce attorney or a tax attorney. These choices now are commonplace.

One of the benefits of limiting services to one area is that the specialist is afforded the luxury of knowing more and more about less and less. Specialization not only defines limits of responsibility, but also suggests increased expertise compared with general practitioners who may manage identical cases. Specialization and subspecialization thus have economic, legal, and personal security facets. These are created by refining the definition of the market share, limiting culpability by restricting activity, and even permitting the professional the luxury of not engaging in those occupational tasks that are sometimes unrewarding or threatening.

PROFESSIONAL LIFE-STYLE AND PRACTICE DECISIONS

The Florida "Sick Doctor Statute"[1] defined the process for evaluating the impaired physician, and was evidence of global realization that professional practice carried as many liabilities as advantages, especially in the arena of health-service delivery. The statute stated that no hospital staff bylaws could include questioning a physician's fitness to practice before the physician's clinical judgment and skills became openly impaired.

This action was the result of the provider's having been placed in a conflictual role characterized by long work hours, inordinately high social expectations, legal consequences, and escalating competition. Retreat from the family had become pathognomonic of medical practice and immersion in the world of compromised competency. Drug and alcohol abuse and diffusely expressed dysphoria became more prevalent.

Concurrently, in the idealistic 1960s American society seemed to want a return to the use of a primary physician. To this physician would be brought the preponderance of medical problems; what could not be managed within his or her own practice could be triaged among the subspecialties.

During that same period, other fields were changing as well. Psychology had become steeped in humanistic theory; family systems and cognition were being added back to the black box of behaviorism. Clinical psychology, which had not been practiced long enough or had a sufficient database to become specialty oriented, easily became entrenched in the generalist-practitioner model. Only in the 1980s have yellow-pages listings of mental-health professionals become liberally sprinkled with "practice limited to" and "specializing in" assertions.

In the last two decades, much data have been gathered about the viability of a general (or family practice) structure, and the true versus perceived demand for specialty practices. Despite pockets of limited access to health care in some rural settings, the production of health-care providers is perceived to be in excess of likely future demand. In urban hospitals, generalist practitioners have had their clinical privileges sharply curtailed.

Compounded by the impact of health maintenance organizations and changes in insurance laws, the concept of the general practitioner of any profession meeting an entire family's needs may not be applicable in today's market. Thus, specialists with tightly circumscribed practice emphases appear increasingly abundant.

In psychology, for example, practices have arisen with exclusive emphasis upon treatment of phobias, treatment of sexual dysfunction, modification of addictive behaviors, rehabilitation for brain injury, management of chronic pain, and treatment of eating disorders. Again, practice boundaries confine the clinical material with which the practitioner is expected to keep current. Although limiting the size of the population serviced, specialization permits a viable means of practice building, since it enables specific and targeted marketing strategies.

The specialty practice also permits a degree of identity formation less easily established and maintained in a general practice. Specialization and subspecialization (e.g., child psychoanalysis) provides a ready definition of the practice to prospective patients.

DIVERSIFICATION—CLINICAL SKILL VERSUS PATIENT POPULATION

There are some specific advantages to the general practice model. Diversity offsets tendencies toward professional boredom and fatigue, which can lead to the possibility of an impaired clinician. An unrewarding practice can contribute to an adjustment disorder characterized by depression and its attendant feelings of helplessness, emptiness, and diminished self-regard. General practice increases the market access and enables the clinician, especially the new clinician, seemingly to anticipate greater patient flow, generate revenue, and obviate financial insecurity. However, the generalist model may be too loosely defined to allow an unestablished individual to define an area of expertise and thus stand out from the competition. Specialization, with its circumscribed clinical applications and confined patient population, not only delineates territorial expectancies, but it also offers specificity. Specialty practices permit the opportunity for treatment of only those behaviors and patient groups in which the clinician is most interested and with which he or she feels most comfortable.

Specialization, therefore, can be conceptualized in at least two different ways: along lines of clinical skill and application and along lines of patient population served.

As an example, chronic-pain treatment centers may differ in their specific approaches, but the complaints and the patient populations are assumed to be homogeneous. Pediatric neurology may resemble to an extent its adult counterpart, but the unique stage of neurological development and impact of treatment outcomes for children may differentiate this specialty area. The treatment of anorexia nervosa and bulimia nervosa, involving predominantly female patients with a significant behavioral component, may differ from general practice along dimensions of both skill and population.

Clinicians either may choose their clinical skill area (e.g., psychodiagnostic assessment) and/or have specific interest in a population (e.g., acutely psychotic patients or noncompliant diabetics). In mental health, establishing a practice that is marketed to referral sources (be they other providers or other facilities) as an exclusively diagnostic facility is specialization along a skill domain. The practice may be organized around a setting (e.g., industrial-organizational-managerial training) or around a process (e.g., disability determination).

This orientation choice enables referral sources to form conceptual boundaries for a given practice. Referral sources are often in a quandary as to whether "this is the type of patient you see" or "this is the type of problem you handle," or even if "this may be something in (or outside of) your area."

Referring professionals naturally gravitate toward the practice that makes them most comfortable with the way in which their referrals are received. The referring agents often accurately feel that they maintain ultimate responsibility for the patient since the referral implies endorsement. They need positive outcomes from these referrals, thereby increasing the probability that they will recognize the need for specialized referral when it arises, and be comfortable referring to a less traditional practice model.

Diversification of the general practice over time could include the movement into forensic assessment for municipal and federal courts or neuropsychological assessment for worker's compensation cases or health and liability insurers, or movement into human resources for the measurement of job performance potential or managerial skill acquisition. The practitioner who has chosen a generalist model need not restrict activity; indeed, that practice may demand one or more areas of emphasis for economic survival.

Specialization within a specific population may include such choices as exclusive treatment of particular age groups, cases involving particular diagnostic entities, or patients in specific vocations or settings or having exposure to similar stimuli, such as families of alcoholics, sexually molested children, or high-technology line staff workers. Diversification of that practice, in turn, generally begins at the level of involvement with clinical material that relates to the core of the practice.

Psychologists who offer divorce mediation and marital therapies, for example, often find themselves exposed to the option of involvement with child-custody decisions. Alternatively, demand may increase for sexual therapies. Marketing to family court settings and attorneys specializing in such cases may enable movement into those areas.

THE MARKETING OF THE PRACTITIONER

This step assumes, in all cases of impending practice diversification, that the requisite knowledge base has been obtained through continuing education programs. Additionally, one must be cognizant of the ever-changing direction from which referrals may arise. Gynecologists and urologists may be the new referral base for mental-health professionals as sexual therapies are incorporated into the diversifying practice. It is increasingly essential that one not only recognize, but develop the ability to reach, these changing sources of referrals. Observation of impending and declining trends becomes essential.

The marketing process, whether it occurs in the legal, industrial, or medical arena, requires its own level of sophistication. Many clinicians cannot market themselves.

"Marketing is the analysis, planning, implementation and control of carefully formulated programs designed to bring about voluntary exchanges of values with target markets for the purpose of achieving organizational objectives. It relies heavily on designing the organization's offering in terms of the target market's needs and desires, and on using effective pricing, communication, and distribution to inform, motivate and service the markets" (Kotler & Bloom, 1984).

Until the last decade, the commercial marketing of the professions was deemed inappropriate, if not unethical. Prior to 1979, professional associations such as the American Medical Association were unified in their contention that advertising was inappropriate in the professional community, meeting neither the need of the profession nor the need of the public (Bloom, 1977).

However, careful marketing can help to assuage consumer uncertainty about professional services. Even after the successful completion of psychotherapy, for instance, the patient is free to question the necessity of the process or the vissisitudes of the transference–countertransferrence phenomenon. Marketing is continuous.

Patient (consumer) education plays a larger role in the marketing of health care than in the marketing of goods. The consumer is uncertain about health services. The professional's choice of clinical procedure from an armamentarium of available approaches may be central to resolving this uncertainty or obviating it from the onset.

Most psychotherapists, for example, are aware that patients recently have been encouraged to interview their doctors before committing to treatment. The doctor–patient relationship is, obviously, pivotal. But frequently, even (if not especially) the patient who has seen a number of therapists may not be capable of making an informed decision. Sometimes, previous exposure to the competition may complicate the process of seeking further treatment.

Most professional fields have traditionally responded to competition by attempting to fortify the uniqueness of their offerings, although communication of that uniqueness may be difficult to achieve. Psychology has, in recent years, attempted to redefine a market sector by modifying the image of the patient or altering the stance of the provider (Adams, 1986). This has been done by attempting to reconceptualize either the patient or the doctor role. One of the first, and perhaps least effective, examples of the effort was the introduction in psychology of the term "client" referring to a patient, in the hope of mitigating the person's sense of helplessness or anger at being stigmatized. Concurrently, calling oneself a "counselor" as opposed to psychologist is an attempt to soften the impact of seeking treatment.

The market niche, however, appears to be unmodified by these attempts. Simply, patients may wish to be patients and may want to see doctors. Attempts at redirection can potentially drive the patient to other providers.

Psychology's market niche has found itself defined, not by the profession's conceptual efforts, but by the expanded marketing undertaken by organized medicine.

EXAMPLE OF TREND DIVERSIFICATION

Specialization as a marketing vehicle is promoted by the relatively recent and rapidly expanding impact of big business on the health-care industry. This growth has occurred so quickly that nonprofessional ownership of health care may become the industry's own "metastatic" disease.

To put it succinctly, if it is a viable, marketable commodity, whether it be enamel bonding of teeth, child-custody determination, or chronic-pain management, business concerns wish to foster the belief that their organization, clinic, hospital, or service-delivery system *specializes* in the management of that issue. Many problems, such as eating disorders, have a short history of economic emphasis and are especially vulnerable to such media exploitation, because of the public's combination of dread and ignorance regarding the disorder.

The market for specific services has led the health-care corporations to choose specialty practices based on trends in the delivery system, rather than necessarily enduring needs. For the purposes of illustration, the changes in psychology's delivery system will demonstrate this changing market.

Two current examples in industrial settings are the issues of outplacement and employee-assistance programs (EAPs). Although both involve primarily psychological functions, most programs in each category are administered and implemented with only cursory attention paid to psychology. Both areas represent rich, albeit time-specific, opportunities for the practicing/consulting clinician.

Many clinicians who made early career affiliations with industrial/organizational psychology engaged in professional applications such as managerial training seminars. The last five years have seen a marked growth in EAPs and the outplacement process. The former is designed to intervene at a staff level with problems affecting worker productivity. Outplacement, however, is for manager-level executives, and has become the term attached to a company's use of a third party in the discharging of the employee. Firing an employee never has a purely positive outcome. An aggrieved, emotionally labile employee makes for poor relations in the industrial community and is a potential source of litigation for the employer.

Companies recently saw the wisdom in paying a third party to find a new position for an employee who was to be discharged. The fee typically is not insubstantial. The service varies among outplacement companies, but is usually constructed around a support group, resumé-writing assistance, job-interview assistance, and some minimal diagnostic assessment. It is psychological work handled by nonpsychologists.

Again, the EAP programs, while ideally suited to the clinical repertoire of mental-health professionals, tend to be administered and staffed by nonprofessionals. The EAP is often designed around a per capita fee, where the employer pays a specific fee per employee on an annual basis and the service is available to all employees. The EAP has tended to be a marketing strategy of counseling availability without the standards of care demanded of licensed practitioners. Although some of these programs have been efficiently and effectively managed, it is possible to sell EAP programs in bulk since industry's payment for services is almost guaranteed to be in excess of utilization.

These EAP service programs thus may be sold at greater than actual resource ability to meet peak demand, since this "peak" will probably not occur. The likelihood that industry will yield to a more cost-contained examination of such service shopping is high.

Similarly, outplacement has been chiefly the domain of business consultant groups, former industry executives, and the occasional industrial psychologist. As with any trend in human services marketing, the range of the quality of service is wide, and quality of care, when care is given, is difficult to assess.

Little doubt exists that a discharged employee, especially one at a managerial level, is likely to be experiencing acute trauma, and worrying about the management of family, financial obligations, and future career. Without psychologists directly involved in outplacement, the fired manager and family are unlikely to have their psychological needs diagnosed, much less treated. Despite the trend nature of industrial concerns, the potential for the diversifying psychologist to benefit is high.

Entrance into the area is not only competitive, but requires a nonclinical (i.e., business) sophistication in an arena that has strong, though unrecognized, clinical implications. The acquisition of business skills is just one more area that must be considered in order to survive in today's market.

PROPRIETORSHIP OF CLINICAL SKILLS IN PSYCHOLOGY

As described earlier, specialization follows a natural evolutionary path as a profession develops an increasing wealth of data and tools with which to accomplish tasks. The mental-health field has needed clinical ammunition with which to transcend its position as a neonate among the health-care professions. The tools and their sophistication are increasing logarithmically. They consist not only of advanced psychometric procedures and devices of increasing refinement, but also of computers to assist in data analysis and synthesis, biobehavioral devices such as clinical biofeedback, and psychopharmacologic agents.

It is important to note that psychology has been for decades at the forefront of the creation of such tools, and potentially in increasing their effectiveness and ultimate functional utility in health-care delivery. "Psychologists have played a leading role in the investigating and developing of treatment approaches for" a variety of clinical conditions in which psychophysiology is involved in the etiology and/or in the amelioration of the disorder (Simon et al., 1986).

Even a cursory review of instrumentation, both diagnostic and therapeutic, reflects the role of psychologists in the design and refinement of procedures and devices, from the early identification of proneness to a disease to the management of disorders and conditions that affect behavior. Divisions of the American Psychological Association (APA) and stand-alone proprietary organizations of psychologists have been created to deal with research, training, and application in these emerging fields. These have ranged from APA's Division of Psychopharmacology and Computers in Psychology to the broader-based Biofeedback Society of America.

In the preponderance of cases, the people involved in the research, development, and empirical refinement of both devices and procedures are excluded from clinical application. Despite this restriction imposed by proprietorship over clinical devices, in many settings psychologists function as inpatient care directors, ultimately recommend which medication is likely to be the most effective on the basis of test results, and are the key clinicians in head-injury settings, chronic-pain programs, and phobia treatment facilities.

Simply, psychologists are permitted to design physical procedures but have sanctions placed on their use of them. This, in turn, affects "the public's evaluations of psychology along with what the public understands about the field" (Wood et al., 1986). This evaluation determines the marketability of the field and its ultimate survival; ". . . it is doubtful that the public has ever had a reasonable understanding of the nature of the field" (Benjamin, 1986).

The lines between procedures performed by psychologists, the public's understanding of the field and its services, and the ultimate survival of the field for its own sake and that of human welfare are direct and unquestionable. The restriction of psychology from the use of physical procedures creates a marketing dilemma. The separation of psychology from the procedures it has helped to design becomes a replay of mind–body dualism, implying that two professions of distinct domain must exist to manage two forms of human suffering, the physical and the psychological, which one must then also perceive as distinct. To do so is to ignore the impact of the biopsychosocial model, and to ignore a potentially rich area of practice specialization.

MENTAL HEALTH IN THE MARKETPLACE

Not only does the restriction of specialization come from sanctions on the use of physical procedures, but competition for psychology comes from two sources: paraprofessional groups and the allied health groups. Alternatively, this can be dichotomized chiefly into the unlicensed groups and the licensed providers. When examining the field of market availability, all groups claiming similar domains must be considered competitors; effective competitors, therefore, must be considered predators. Competition in the marketplace is, and was meant to be, a complex series of aggressive, protective, and proactive behaviors designed to maintain and expand the domain. Therefore, it is useful to envision competition as a challenge to grow, rather than as a threat to existence.

PHYSICAL INTERVENTIONS AS MARKETING SOLUTIONS

The marketing of psychology, as with the marketing of any professional service, has many problems that are germane only to the professions and rarely exist in traditional product markets. For example, the professional has third-party accountability: restraining a violent patient may meet the demands of the moment and the safety of the environment, but it may sharply contrast with the needs of the family, the admitting physician, or the hospital.

In the purchase and consumption of tangible goods, the consumer is little concerned with the issue of prior experience. In the marketing and subsequent sales of professional services, the patient wants to know if the clinician has had previous experience with similar services. Does the doctor who is delivering psychotherapeutic or psychopharmacologic services to the chronic-pain patient, the doctor who is employing transcutaneous electrical nerve stimulators, know about the neurophysiology of this pain sensation? Is the doctor dealing with this child's encopresis (lack of bowel control) fully aware of its etiology and permitted to utilize rectal electromyographic feedback technology? Higher levels of quality control are demanded in human service delivery where health and welfare are dependent variables.

A case (Fox, 1986) has been made for abandoning psychology's traditional passive stance with regard to blocked access to the delivery of physical interventions in the care of patients. The field must decide whether its educational foundation provides the appropriate structure from which all forms of intervention logically extend. Is an education founded in psychology, upon which biological education is then added, inherently inferior to an education that begins at the biological, and for which psychological research and practice have been demonstrated to be an afterthought? The market access accorded the profession hangs on that very decision.

THE DEMAND FOR MARKET VIABILITY

The marketing of a profession has philosophical implications and sociological impact. Professions in an idealized democracy have an obligation to strive toward the goal of meeting society's needs and demands. This is the philanthropic focus of marketing. The pragmatic aspect of marketing relates to financial considerations: the profession must be maintained in a state of economic viability in order that it may survive and, it is hoped, thrive.

An adaptive stance, however, is the nominal position, one that states that before a profession can meet the needs and demands of its society, it must develop durability in the marketplace, survival before service, and profit from technological advances before concern for contributing to them.

In order for a profession to become durable, it must reach its intended market and be profitably utilized. This is the goal of marketing a profession, whether it be general practice or the most closely defined subspecialty. Ultimately, the ability to branch out into different fields of specialization will depend upon the ability to market in an ever-more-competitive environment. In order to convince the public that specialty areas such as physical intervention are viable, clinicians must see themselves in expanded roles of leadership and believe in their own capacity to fill those roles competently.

REFERENCES

Adams, D.B. (1986). The issues of images: Professional and public. *Independent Practitioner, 6*(2), 27-29.

Benjamin, L.T. (1986). Why don't they understand us? A history of psychology's public image. *American Psychologist, 41,* 941-946.

Bloom, P. (1977). Advertising in the professions: The critical issues. *Journal of Marketing,* 103-110, July.

Fox, R. (1986). Further thoughts on psychologists' prescribing drugs: A response to Brandsma and Frey. *Georgia Psychologist, 39*(2), 24-28.

Kotler, P., & Bloom, N. (1984). *Marketing professional services.* Englewood Cliffs, NJ: Prentice-Hall.

Simon, N., Bogacki, D., Favell, J., Lovass, I., Risley, T., Surwit, R., & Wiens, A. (1984). Psychologists' use of physical procedures and interventions. *Psychologists' use of physical procedures task force report* (Draft), 1-23, March.

Wood, W., Jones, M., & Benjamin, L.T. (1986). Surveying psychology's public image. *American Psychologist, 41,* 947-953.

FOOTNOTE

1. Sec. 2, 69-205, Laws of Florida (Florida Medical Practice Act); Florida Statute 458-1201 (i)V ("Sick Doctor Statute"), passed in 1969 and added to the medical practice act.

C H A P T E R
23

THE ROLE OF FEES IN PSYCHOTHERAPY AND PSYCHOANALYSIS

Robert C. Lane, Ph.D., and James W. Hull, Ph.D.

The whole complex matter of money is rarely treated in a satisfactory or sufficient manner.—Eissler (1974)

Payment or nonpayment may represent different things on different levels to different patients, or to the same patient at different times.—Allen (1971)

We can learn a great deal about our patients if we scrutinize how they regard and handle money; the same is true for ourselves as therapists.— Krueger (1986)

This chapter is based on the assumption that the question of fees and payment represents a crucial aspect of the psychotherapeutic process. Payment of the fee may be seen as a concrete embodiment of the transactional aspect of psychotherapy—it represents one form of the exchange or barter that consititutes a core dimension of the treatment process. Because of this, the manner in which the fee is handled or not handled by the therapist may be expected to have pervasive and profound effects on therapy. In this chapter, we review the literature on fees from several different vantage points. We begin by reviewing theoretical discussions of the role of payment in psychotherapy, then discuss different possible fee arrangements the therapist can make with his or her patient. Next we consider the effects of modifications in usual fee practices, and the symbolic meanings that payment can acquire. In the final section, we take up special topics related to fees, including third-party payment, health maintenance organizations (HMOs) and treatment of the wealthy.

THEORETICAL VIEWS

A number of different theoretical views have been advanced regarding the role of fees in psychotherapy. Freud (1913) felt that the fee was primarily for the benefit of the analyst, a means of insuring self-preservation and security, as well as enhancing power. He wrote, "It is more responsible to acknowledge one's actual needs and claims than acting the part of the disinterested philanthropist." In this context he stated that analysts should not be afraid of charging a high fee because they have at their disposal an effective method of treatment, and argued that an adequate fee will assure the analyst's comfort, eliminating the deleterious effect of outside influences and concerns on the analyst's concentration.

Some authors have stressed that the fee is a necessary and intrinsic part of the treatment process. Menninger (1958) and others (Davids, 1964; Haak, 1957; Kukie, 1950; Menninger & Holtzmann, 1973) have argued that payment of the fee must involve a sacrifice for the patient, if the therapeutic process is to be meaningful. A high fee is seen as a necessary motivational factor so that treatment does not become a "matter of indifference."

A different version of this view that the fee is an intrinsic part of treatment has been presented by Langs (1973, 1976) and his followers Ranay (1986) and Halpert (1972, 1973, 1985, 1986). These authors argue that the fee is a crucial part of the frame of psychotherapy, which is the vehicle for the therapeutic change. Modifications in standard fee arrangements are viewed as a sign of therapist countertransference difficulties that usually interfere with the objectivity of treatment. In the case of modifications rooted in the external conditions of the patient's life, such as when the patient suddenly loses his or her job, the effect can be to take the focus away from exploring the patient's intrapsychic world, which is the primary analytic task. Raney (1986), feels that violations of the frame in regard to fee arrangements are "essentially uninterpretable," and although things may seem to be resolved at the level of the patients's manifest content, analysis of unconscious derivatives tells a different story. In discussing fees, these authors stress the analysis of derivatives resulting from such breaks in the frame.

A final view holds that the fee should be for services rendered. One spokesperson for this approach has been Fromm-Reichmann (1950), who argues that analysts are not exempt from the general standard in our society that there should be no payment if services are not delivered. Hence she feels it is indefensible for psychotherapists to charge for missed sessions, a point of view that differs substantially from that of Freud and other classical analysts.

In reviewing these various theoretical approaches, we find ourselves most in agreement with the position of Langs and Halpert, although with some qualifications. We agree that the fee constitutes a crucial part of the frame of psychotherapy. In our own work, however, we allow for occasional modifications rooted in reality considerations, and we do not believe that these are "essentially uninterpretable," as Raney holds. We feel that such a "tempered version" of Langs' and Halpert's position is consistent with Freud's concern with providing for the analyst's own security, but has the additional advantage of addressing the interpersonal–interactional aspect of the fee question. We have serious doubts about the position advocated by Menninger, feeling that at times it can provide a rationale for expression of the therapist's anger. Similarly, we have concerns about the fee-for-service principle, feeling that it creates too great a disturbance in the psychotherapeutic frame and intereferes with the patient's sense of possessing in an hour of the therapist's time.

FEE ARRANGEMENTS

A therapist's view regarding the role of fees in psychotherapy will have numerous implications for what arrangements he or she makes with patients, as well as how he or she attempts to resolve the payment issues that inevitably arise during the course of treatment. Schonbar (1986) has differentiated between rigid and flexible approaches to payment. One example of a rigid approach is Freud's (1913) principle of "leasing" an hour to patients: "A certain hour of my available working day is appointed to each patient; it is his and he is libel for it, even if he does not make use of it." This policy is a natural consequence of Freud's view discussed above that fees are primarily for the protection of the analyst's own security. A rigid fee arrangement also is integral to Langs' view that the fee constitutes a crucial part of the psychoanalytic frame, and modifications around fee, including the use of insurance, interfere with the objectivity of the therapeutic process. Langs advocates not accepting the patient's insurance, and not changing a fee once it is set. Menninger's view that payment of the fee must involve a sacrifice for the patient also can lead to a rigid payment approach. He advocates setting a fee somewhat higher than the patient can comfortably afford, and not discussing the rationale concerning the fee with patients.

A more flexible approach is implied by Fromm-Reichmann in her view that the fee is for services rendered. Adoption of such a policy means that the therapist must develop his or her own guidelines for the decisions that must be made — for example — what justifies a higher or lower fee, when should fees be increased, and by how much?

Another example of a flexible approach to payment is that presented by Blanck and Blanck (1974), who argue for a fee policy that takes into account the level of ego integration the patient has achieved. These authors feel that patients with well-structured egos may be able to withstand the frustration implicit in a transitional approach, and for such patients, a rigorous policy may be in order. However, more disturbed patients may require a flexible approach, involving setting fee requirements slightly ahead of what the patient can fulfill, "without insisting on immediate compliance." They feel that this has the advantage of providing the patient with "tolerable doses of frustration" that will maximize ego growth. The Blancks feel that too rigid a fee policy, for example, demanding that the patient take his or her vacation at the same time as the analyst, leads to a situation of indenture, which can nip emerging autonomy in the bud. This can be especially harmful for narcissistic patients. Eissler (1974) makes a related point when he argues that fee modifications may be necessary to keep severely schizoidal or depressed patients in treatment. Jacobs (1986) discusses this principle in regard to delinquents and other patients with ego boundary deficits.

Schonbar (1986) argues for a policy of "rational flexibility": "What I do about these fee issues depends in large part on what I see as their message and meaning, and I try to embed my decision on what I understand is going on, so that the major thrust of whatever I decide is therapeutic in intent rather than simply business oriented or countertransferential."

Finally, mention should be made of Jacobs' (1986) recommendations regarding the process of setting the fee. He stresses the importance of an overall "atmosphere of safety" in which fee issues can come up naturally and be resolved in a mutually acceptable manner. Actual decisions may vary from time to time and patient to patient, depending on the particular wish, defense, or transference resistance that is operating at the time. Jacobs cautions especially against prematurely setting the fee: "The setting of the fee before meanings can be fully explored may imply to both the therapist and patient that the subject is somewhat outside the province of full analytic inquiry, especially in those instances in which the patient readily agrees to pay the fee proposed by the therapist." Also important are the recommendations regarding fees in the American Psychoanalytic Assocation's "Guides on Professional Conduct for Psychoanalysts," which are summarized by Michaels (1969). With regard to fee setting, these guidelines state that the following factors should be taken into consideration: the experience and professional standing of the therapist, the patient's ability to pay, and the prevailing rates charged for comparable time and service in the community. It is recommended that individuals in need of psychotherapeutic services who cannot afford either usual or reduced fees be referred to low-cost services, and it is clearly stated that a fee that is too high or will create a family financial crisis is unjustifiable. Frequency and sequence of visits should depend exclusively on the patient's psychological condition, and financial considerations should not determine these decisions.

Our own view is that Freud's principle of leasing an hour can provide a solid framework for the various fee arrangements that are set up with individual patients. As mentioned above, we temper this policy with some degree of flexibility around the acceptance of insurance and fee adjustments, particularly in response to pressing considerations, such as loss of a job or other financial setbacks. Finally, we feel that the modifications and adjustments suggested by Blanck and Blanck are especially important, and that a therapist's willingness to make fee arrangements that are appropriate to the patient's developmental level may be crucial in helping severely disturbed patients remain in treatment.

EFFECTS OF MODIFICATIONS AROUND FEES

Much of the literature on fees addresses the effects of modifications in payment on the psychotherapeutic process. Schonbar (1986) makes the point that there has been little empirical work on this topic, but many therapists believe in the likelihood of negative outcomes when fees are modified, and this belief is used to justify a more rigid policy.

Freud (1913) argued against the idea of providing free treatment, both because it involves a great cost to the analyst who is giving up a significant part of his or her income, and because such treatment increases the level of the resistance and secondary gain for remaining ill. He felt that free treatment frequently led to increased mistrust, resentment, dependency, and other forms of negative transference.

Langs and his followers have devoted much attention to the negative effects of frame disturbances involving fee modification. They argue that if the overall frame is secure, there will be almost no references to fee in the patient's associations. However, when there is a deviation around fee, constituting a break in the frame, this will show up in derivatives. Modifications acquire different meanings for different patients, and these meanings may change over time. A low fee may be taken as a symbol of the patient's diminshed value to the analyst. The patient may feel indignant or intruded upon when the modification includes reporting to a third-party payer such as an insurance company. In this situation, patients also may feel guilty, that they are getting something for nothing, stealing, or being manipulative. Finally, the patient may interpret a lowered fee as a sign that the analyst is unwilling to accept the patient's aggression, or is as hypocritical about money as the rest of society.

A number of other writers have discussed the negative consequences that can result from fee modifications. Nash and Cavenar (1976) found in a study of five cases in a Veterans Administration setting that free treatment tended to interfere with therapeutic progress. They speculated that their patients might have felt too guilty to improve, or that the therapists might have felt too deprived to treat. They also noted that particular problems arose with patients with overt sexual-identity problems who tended to assume that the analyst wanted sexual favors in return for a reduced fee. Blanck and Blanck (1974) have argued that fees can be a reflection of the therapist's self-esteem, and an inadequate fee can denigrate both the therapist and the therapy. Too low a fee also tends to prevent the growth of the patient's self-esteem and to encourage fantasies of being a favored child. Finally, DiBella (1986) discussed other complications that can result from modifications around fees. He argued that there is a direct correlation between neglect of money issues and poor management with regard to other features of treatment, a point also made by Chessick (1968) and Schwartz and Wolff (1969). Other countertransference problems can include denigration of the patient, withdrawal on the part of the therapist, a delayed response to phone calls, or cutting the hours short. Too high a fee may conflict with the therapist's need to be benevolent.

In contrast to the above authors, a number of studies reviewed by Schonbar (1985) suggest that payment of a fee is not necessary for therapeutic progress to occur, and that free treatment does not necessarily lead to less gain. Lorand and Console (1958) felt that no special problems arose in a free clinic that were different from those that would routinely appear in a private practice setting. Lievano (1967) in a study of 20 outpatients, found no relation between payment and outcome. Glasser and Duggan (1969) and Chodoff (1972) also found few differences in practice in a free clinic. Paris (1962–63), Liptzen (1977), and Markson (1977) argued that in Canada, where comprehensive health insurance is normal, the lack of a fee is seen as less disruptive than in the United States, where payment is expected. However, Paris points out that problems still arise in the Canadian system, especially with regard to missed sessions and the necessity to present an insurance card. Mintz (1971) and Schofield (1971) point out that the relation between sacrifice and outcome that Menninger hypothesized has never been empirically demonstrated. Herron and Stikowski (1986) also found that the therapeutic value of paying a fee had never been proved or disproved by empirical research. Other writers, such as Bruch (1974), Chessick (1969), Fromm-Reichmann (1950), and Paolino (1981) have failed to report damage resulting from a flexible fee policy.

Finally, several surveys should be mentioned. Hofling and Rosenbaum (1986) surveyed 157 psychoanalysts and psychotherapists. They found that 78% had extended credit to their patients in whole or in part, with an understanding that they would be repaid. On the average, credit had been extended to three different patients for each therapist. Of the 322 patients to which fee credit was extended, two-thirds had repaid the amount in full, with only a small percentage making no effort at repayment. Nearly half of those patients to whom credit had been extended showed neither a clearly favorable nor unfavorable response. Of those responses that were reported, most were positive. Lasky (1984) reported on the conflicts concerning fees exierienced by 60 psychoanalysts and psychotherapists. She found that two-thirds reported some degree of intrapsychic conflict, with ambivalence particularly acute among female therapists, who tended to be very aware of the conflicting demands of work and family, gratifying the patient's needs, and providing for their own financial security. Her findings agreed with those of Goldklank (1982), who reported that female therapists were much more likely to feel locked into a caretaking role and to put the needs of patients first. With regard to sex differences, Burnside (1986) found that female therapists tend to be paid significantly less, regardless of setting, degree, or specialization, and also are more likely to see patients at reduced fees.

In spite of the mixed findings from empirical studies, we concur with Langs that fee modifications constitute significant disruptions of the treatment frame that acquire different meanings to different patients. Instead of refraining from all modifications, however, we feel the therapist should be realistic and make whatever arrangements are most appropriate, and then strive to understand with the patient the transference and countertransference meanings that ensue. If patient and therapist can successfully explore the different meanings that these modifications acquire, the overall work of the treatment can proceed, and in some cases will be enhanced, as the unraveling of conflicted feelings about money reveals dynamics that had been hidden. Finally, although we do not endorse free treatment, we do feel that therapists should contribute some portion of their time to low-cost treatment, especially with regard to candidates in training, but here again the anaylsis of transference and countertransference meanings is crucial.

THE SYMBOLIC MEANING OF FEES

Psychotherapy fees can acquire a number of different symbolic meanings for patients and therapists. Payment of the fee may come to represent a variety of inner issues for both parties, depending on the therapist's orientation, the dynamics of the patient and the therapist, the patient's level of ego development, and the stage of therapy (Allen, 1971; Tulipan, 1986).

Fuqua (1986) and Blanck and Blanck (1974) have summarized the classical psychoanalytic view of money as an anal product. Resistances concerning money and payment are seen as a manifestation of character difficulties rooted in the anal stage of development. Fuqua states, "Money represents anal meanings unconsciously, and it tends to be handled with the pleasure and need to control, retain and release that originally obtained toward one's bowel products." The tasks of the anal stage include learning to say No and to employ the aggressive drive in the service of separation and identity formation, and struggles around payment may provide a vehicle for expressing these conflicts.

Several other authors have commented on the way in which money issues may represent conflicts around aggression and separation-individuation. Langs (1973) has pointed out that the fee offers one means by which the patient can really frustrate or harm the analyst. Borneman (1976) points out that all money belongs to somebody and taking is a form of aggression on the part of the therapist. In a related view, Haak (1957) has argued that paying a fee can help to counteract the patient's guilt for attacking the analyst. He feels that lowering the fee may inhibit the patient's aggression, and may be rooted in the analyst's guilt, masochism, or fear of being greedy.

Gedo (1962) has discussed how the unpaid bill may come to function as a transitional phenomenon, serving to deny in fantasy the patient's separateness from the analyst. In this regard, Hilles (1971) discussed the treatment of a patient severely in arrears. She tried to deal "experimentally with the issue of nonpayment through interpretation, rather than as a reality problem which required an immediate realistic solution." In time she found that for this patient, payment meant giving up a negative identity with respect to the mother, surrendering a last barrier against merging. In this context, nonpayment also functioned as a way of holding onto the therapist because of the large investment already made, consistent with Gedo's thesis. Other symbolic meanings that money and fees can acquire have been discussed by Allen (1971): The fee "may represent the giving or withholding of milk or nourishment, gifts or swearing, a vehicle for control, a phallus, power, or a bribe." Schwartz and Wolff (1969) point out that patients may have the fantasy that the therapist is a prostitute because he or she takes money for love.

A number of different countertransferential meanings of fees and problems concerning fees may be identified. The therapist's attitude toward payment is influenced by his or her theoretical orientation, as well as past training or the lack thereof regarding the handling of fees. Also important are the therapist's own early object relationships, particularly as these involved conflicts related to money, and the role of money in his or her own treatment. In addition, the therapist's reactions are influenced by the transference-countertransference dynamics active in the treatment at that moment, which will vary from patient to patient, and relevant circumstances from the therapist's own life. It is certain that some of the symbolic meanings described are as relevant to the therapist as to the patient; for example, money may provide the therapist with a means of expressing aggression toward the patient as a defense against unconscious wishes to merge, or an experience of transitional relatedness, allowing him or her to deny separateness from the patient. We have found little discussion of such symbolic meanings for the therapist in our review of the literature. Instead, most work on this topic documents the frequency of therapist countertransference difficulties in handling the fee, without exploring personal meanings for the therapist. For example, Fingert (1952) discussed how a lower fee may represent neurotic acting out, especially for beginning therapists. Pasternak and Treiger (1976) documented the "extraordinary departures from usual practice" residents engage in around payment issues. Buckley, Karasu, and Charles (1976) found that avoidance of fee setting is one of the 10 most frequent mistakes reported by supervisors. Finally, Meyers (1976) found in a study of 20 psychiatric residents that all had had patients in arrears at one time or another, that 19 of the 20 preferred fees to be collected by the receptionist, and that all overestimated by two or three times the average amount that their patients were paying. A number of authors (Di Bella, 1986; Jacobs, 1986; Pasternak & Treiger, 1976) have made the point that psychotherapy training usually fails to address adequately issues of payment, and that this neglect extends to supervision.

We feel that unraveling the symbolic meanings attached to money and payment constitutes the most important work that therapist and patient can engage in with regard to the fee. The literature provides vivid examples of the many symbolic meanings that may exist at different levels of psychological development for both patient and therapist, and the manner in which these may shift over the course of treatment. We feel that as long as these overlapping and interrelated meanings are carefully attended to and understood by both patient and therapist, the problems caused by particular modifications may be resolved and the overall work of treatment enhanced, since money issues then become another avenue for exploring the patient's unconscious conflicts.

THIRD-PARTY PAYMENT, HMOs, AND THE WEALTHY

Schonbar (1956) makes the point that no studies of third-party payment separate the confounding effects of reporting, diagnosis, and confidentiality breeches from payment factors alone. Gray (1972) has argued that insurance coverage has little adverse effect on the conduct of otherwise adequate analyses, provided that the contract remains between the doctor and the patient. Similarly, Chadoff (1986) has argued that the possible deleterious effects of third-party payment are no longer a live issue, and that third-party influences have been incorporated into the treatment situation without disruptive effects on outcome. Scharfstein (1978) reported that insurance support improved the condition of some patients, when assessed in terms of relapse rate, hospitalization, and self-reports of satisfaction. However, Langs (1976) has argued strongly that the violations of confidentiality inherent in third-party payment are too disruptive of the bipersonal field to allow analysis to be carried on effectively.

Halpert's (1972, 1973, 1985, 1986) position is somewhat between these two extremes. He suggests that insurance does not have to become the primary focus of treatment, but can become a focus for resistance and lead to important opportunities for the interpretation of conflict. He feels that the dynamic meanings around insurance parallel the meanings around money in the noninsured patient, but insurance makes it harder to analyze these issues by facilitating a distancing and isolation of feeling and thought. Halpert points out that completing insurance forms requires the analyst to act rather than speak. Also, the insurance company, unlike the analyst, gratifies transference wishes. These conditions lead to a number of common unconscious fantasies, including fantasies of theft, robbery, and collusion, particularly with regard to the question of assigning diagnoses, which may lead the patient to feel that the analyst is corrupt. Patients also may experience intrusiveness and exposure in relation to insurance coverage, which may acquire primal scene or other primitive sexual meanings. For example, the insurance company may be experienced as an excited child peering into the parents' bedroom, with the filling out of the forms unconsciously representing intercourse, impregnation, or sexual submission, and the form itself symbolizing the patient's or the analyst's body. Other common fantasies involve the need for control and protection against castration or the depletion of body contents. Halpert argues that some patients may be unanalyzable under these conditions; for example, the anal-obsessive patient whose treatment is completely reimbursed may feel in such danger of being raped that analysis cannot proceed.

Goldensohn (1986) has discussed issues related to HMOs and the manner in which prepaid group-practice plans and the socioeconomic status of their clientele influence transference–countertransference dynamics. With regard to transference, he feels that upper-middle-class patients tend to believe that "expensive is better," and since HMOs are inexpensive, patients may feel they are receiving treatment of lesser quality. In spite of such negative expectations, Goldensohn feels that these patients often are helped in HMO settings. Lower-class and poor patients tend to feel that free treatment is not worth anything, and they may experience shame and guilt in going to an HMO. Therapy with such clients may be more focused on symptoms and concrete reality problems, with a more interpersonal orientation, carried out on an intermittent basis. Self-image may be enhanced in such clients as a result of the increased attention. With regard to countertransference issues, Goldensohn says that the lower salary in HMOs may lead to morale problems among therapists. Also, because therapists do not have to concern themselves with billing, they may not adequately address money issues in the treatment. The lack of a fee-for-service removes the therapist's incentive to practice in the most efficient manner. At times, therapists may wish to please authority figures by seeing more patients, and they may experience conflicts among representing the interest of the plan, the patient's interest in feeling better, and their own needs and perspectives.

Finally, several authors have discussed the special problems that arise in treating the wealthy patient. Olsson (1986) identifies the following as major dynamic issues mentioned in the literature on the wealthy: (1) extreme narcissism; (2) sociopathy; (3) maternal deprivation and anaclitic depression; (4) paternal deprivation; (5) impaired identity formation; (6) geographical mobility or elusiveness; (7) weakened family structure; and (8) special problem dynamics involving fees. He points out how the therapist's envy of such patients can lead to special treatment or to contempt as a reaction formation. He conceptualizes these treatments along the lines of what one would expect from narcissistic personalities generally, with a focus on idealization, devaluation, and merger fantasies. Stone (1972) cites depression, narcissistic character disorder, and sociopathy as the most frequently encountered diagnoses among children of the superrich. He describes a multigenerational pattern of lack of emotional responsiveness, with wives turning to their husbands as parent surrogates. The rich, in their quest for "the best," can become obstructionistic and threaten to control the treatment. They are not awed by psychiatric practitioners, whom they tend to regard as "impotent charlatans or unscrupulous shamans." Stone notes that such patients are prone to "hospitalitis," partly because the cost of a lengthy stay is no obstacle. Wahl (1974) has pointed out how the wealthy, like any minority, have a strong suspicion of outsiders. Countertransference problems he noted included a tendency to treat the patient like a friend, or to gossip and drop names. Therapists also may tend to act chivalrous, involving a merger with the patient in fantasy. Finally, Weintraub (1964) has discussed the strong influences on the hospital staff that VIP patients may exert.

Our own position on the question of insurance coverage is similar to that of Halpert. We feel that more troublesome issues are raised by third-party coverage than writers such as Chadoff suggest, but we are not as pessimistic about the deleterious effects as is Langs. Therapists need to be realistic, recognizing that the majority of practice these days will involve some insurance coverage. In our view, the key once again lies with the analysis of those unconscious meanings that arise, and in this effort Halpert's ideas are particularly useful. Our position with regard to HMOs and treatment of the wealthy is similar. Short-term problem-focused psychotherapy in the context of an HMO is increasingly common and accepted, while the special problems of treating the wealthy remain for most therapists an infrequent challenge. In both cases, we feel that the first task is to understand the inner meanings these special circumstances acquire for patient and therapist, and that such understanding will be a key to allowing the therapeutic process to continue to unfold.

SUMMARY

In the literature on fees, a number of broad themes can be identified. There is general consensus that questions of payment constitute a core dimension of the psychotherapeutic process, a dimension that is all too often neglected. This neglect originates in a number of factors, including the taboo attached to money in our society, the particular discomforts patient and therapist feel with regard to payment, and a widespread lack of instruction about payment in the training of psychotherapists. This neglect also is reflected in the relative dearth of empirical studies on fees and payment.

Various theoretical positions have been advanced regarding the role of payment in therapy, including the view that the fee is primarily for the therapist's benefit, that it is a necessary and intrinsic part of the therapeutic process, or that it represents payment for services rendered. Different fee arrangements have been described, rooted partly in these theoretical perspectives. A major focus of the literature has been the effects of modifications in fee arrangements. There is a consensus that such modifications are very common, but little agreement about the consequences and sparse empirical support for any one view.

A number of writers in this field have addressed the personal and symbolic meanings that fees can acquire for both therapist and patient. One point upon which most authors do agree is that questions of payment often provide a direct look at the central transferential responses of patients and countertransferential responses of therapists. With the recent increase in alternate forms of payment such as insurance and HMOs, and the special problems that these arrangements imply, it becomes even more important for practitioners to focus on the meaning of the ongoing exchange or barter with patients that occurs when the fee is paid.

REFERENCES

Allen, A. (1971). The fee as a therapeutic tool. *Psychoanalytic Quarterly, 40,* 132–140.

Blanck, G. & Blanck, R. (1974). *Ego psychology: Theory and practice.* New York: Columbia University Press.

Borneman, E. (1976). *The psychoanalysis of money.* New York: Urizen Books.

Bruch, H. (1974). *Learning psychotherapy.* Cambridge, MA: Harvard University Press.

Buckley, P., Karasu, T., & Charles, E. (1979). Common mistakes in psychotherapy. *American Journal of Psychiatry, 136,* 1578–1580.

Burnside, M. (1986). Fee practices of male and female therapists. In D. Krueger (Ed.), *The last taboo: Money as symbol and reality in psychotherapy and psychoanalysis.* New York: Brunner/Mazel.

Chessick, R. (1980). Ethical and psychodynamic aspects of payment for psychotherapy. *Voices, 3,* 26–31.

Chessick, R. (1969). *How psychotherapy heals.* New York: Science House.

Chodoff, P. (1972). The effect of third party payment on the practice of psychiatry. *American Journal of Psychiatry, 129,* 540–545.

Chodoff, P. (1986). The effect of third party payment on the practice of psychotherapy. In D. Krueger (Ed.), *The last taboo: Money as symbol and reality in psychotherapy and psychoanalysis.* New York: Brunner/Mazel.

Davids, A. (1964). The relation of cognitive-dissonance theory to an aspect of psychotherapeutic practice. *American Psychologist, 19,* 329.

DiBella, G. (1986). Money issues that complicate treatment. In D. Krueger (Ed.), *The last taboo: Money as symbol and reality in psychotherapy and psychoanalysis.* New York: Brunner/Mazel.

Eissler, K. (1974). On some theoretical and technical problems regarding the payment of fees for psychoanalytical treatment. *International Review of Psychoanalysis, 1,* 73–101.

Fingert, A. (1952). Comments on the psychoanalytic significance of the fee. *Bulletin of the Menninger Clinic, 16,* 98–104.

Freud, S. (1913). On beginning the treatment. Further recommendations on the technique of psychoanalysis I. In J. Strachey (Ed.), *The standard edition of the complete psychological works of Sigmund Freud* (Vol. 12). London: Hogarth Press, 1958.

Fromm-Reichmann, F. (1950). *Principles of intensive psychotherapy.* Chicago: University of Chicago Press.

Fuqua, P. (1986). Classical psychoanalytic views of money. In D. Krueger (Ed.), *The last taboo: Money as symbol and reality in psychotherapy and psychoanalysis.* New York: Brunner/Mazel.

Gedo, J. (1962). A note on nonpayment of psychiatric fees. *International Journal of Psychoanalysis, 44,* 368–371.

Glasser, M. & Duggan, T. (1969). Prepaid psychiatric experience with UAW members. *American Journal of Psychiatry, 126,* 675–681.

Goldensohn, S. (1986). Transference, countertransference and other therapeutic issues in a health maintenance organization (HMO). In D. Krueger (Ed.), *The last taboo: Money as symbol and reality in psychotherapy and psychoanalysis.* New York: Brunner/Mazel.

Goldklank, S. (1982). *My family made me do it: The influence of family or origin process on family therapists' occupational choice.* Unpublished doctoral dissertation, Adelphi University, Institute of Advanced Psychological Studies, Garden City, NY.

Gray, S. (1973). Does insurance affect psychoanalytic practice? *Bulletin of the Philadelphia Association of Psychoanalysis, 23,* 101–110.

Haak, N. (1957). Comments on the analytic situation. *International Journal of Psychoanalysis, 38,* 183.

Halpert, E. (1972). The effect of insurance on psychoanalytic treatment. *Journal of the American Psychoanalytical Association, 20,* 122–133.

Halpert, E. (1973). A meaning of insurance in psychotherapy. *International Journal of Psychoanalytic Psychotherapy, 1,* 62–68.

Halpert, E. (1985). Insurance. *Journal of the American Psychoanalytic Association, 33,* 937–949.

Halpert, E. (1986). The meaning and effects of insurance in psychoanalysis and psychotherapy. In D. Krueger (Ed.), *The last taboo: Money as symbol and reality in psychotherapy and psychoanalysis.* New York: Brunner/Mazel.

Herron, W., & Sitkowski, S. (1986). Effect of fees on psychotherapy: What is the evidence? *Professional Psychology: Research and Practice, 17,* 347–351.

Hilles, L. (1971). The clinical management of the nonpayment patient: A case study. *Bulletin of the Menninger Clinic, 35,* 98–112.

Hofling, C. & Rosenbaum, M. (1956). The extension of credit to patients in psychoanalysis and psychotherapy. In D. Krueger (Ed.), *The last taboo: Money as symbol and reality in psychotherapy and psychoanalysis.* New York: Brunner/Mazel.

Jacobs, D. (1986). On negotiating fees with psychotherapy and psychoanalytic patients. In D. Krueger (Ed.), *The last taboo: Money as symbol and reality in psychotherapy and psychoanalysis.* New York: Brunner/Mazel.

Krueger, D. (1986). *The last taboo: Money as symbol and reality in psychotherapy and psychoanalysis.* New York: Brunner/Mazel.

Kubie, L. (1950). *Practical and theoretical aspects of psychoanalysis.* New York: International Universities Press.

Langs, R. (1973). *The technique of psychoanalytic psychotherapy* (Vol. I). New York: Jason Aronson.

Langs, R. (1976). *The bipersonal field.* New York: Jason Aronson.

Lasky, E. (1984). Psychoanalysts and psychotherapists conflicts about setting fees. *Psychoanalytic Psychology, 1,* 289–300.

Lievano, J. (1987). Observations about payment of psychotherapy fees. *Psychiatric Quarterly, 41,* 324–328.

Liptzen, B. (1977). The effects of national health insurance on Canadian psychiatry: The Ontario experience. *American Journal of Psychiatry, 134,* 248–252.

Lorand, S., & Console, W. (1958). Therapeutic results in psychoanalytic treatment without fee. *International Journal of Psychoanalysis, 39,* 59–65.

Markson, E. (1977). The impact of national health insurance on the practice of psychiatry: The Canadian experience: The clinical practice of psychotherapy. Unpublished paper presented at the American Psychiatric Association, Toronto, Canada.

Menninger, K. (1958). *Theory of psychoanalytic technique.* New York: Basic Books.

Menninger, K., & Holzmann, P. (1973). *Theory of psychoanalytic technique.* New York: Basic Books.

Meyers, B. (1976). Attitudes of psychiatric residents toward payment of psychotherapy fees. *American Journal of Psychiatry, 133,* 1460–1462.

Michaels, J. (1969). Guides on professional conduct for psychoanalysts. *Journal of the American Psychoanalytic Association, 17,* 291–311.

Mintz, L. (1971). Patient fees and psychotherapeutic transactions. *Journal of Consulting and Clinical Psychology, 36,* 1–8.

Nash, J., & Cavenar. (1976). Free psychotherapy: An inquiry into resistance. *American Journal of Psychiatry, 133,* 1066–1069.

Olsson, P., (1986). Complexities in the psychology and psychotherapy of the phenomenally wealthy. In D. Krueger (Ed.), *The last taboo: Money as symbol and reality in psychotherapy and psychoanalysis.* New York: Brunner/Mazel.

Paolino, T. (1981). *Psychoanalytic psychotherapy.* New York: Brunner/Mazel.

Paris, J. (1982–83). Frame disturbances in no-fee psychotherapy. *International Journal of Psychoanalytic Psychotherapy, 9,* 133–146.

Pasternak, S., & Treiger, P. (1976). Psychotherapy fees and residency training. *American Journal of Psychiatry, 133,* 1064–1066.

Raney, J. (1986). The effect of fees on the course and outcome of psychotherapy and psychoanalysis. In D. Krueger (Ed.), *Money as symbol and reality in psychotherapy and psychoanalysis.* New York: Brunner/Mazel.

Scharfstein, S. (1978). Third party payors: To pay or not to pay. *American Journal of Psychiatry, 135,* 1185–1188.

Schofield, W. (1971). Psychotherapy: The unknown versus the untold. *Journal of Consulting and Clinical Psychology, 36,* 9–11.

Schonbar, R. (1986). The fee as a focus of transference and countertransference in treatment. In D. Krueger (Ed.), *The last taboo: Money as symbol and reality in psychotherapy and psychoanalysis.* New York: Brunner/Mazel.

Schwartz, E., & Wolff, A. (1969). Money matters. *International Mental Health Research Newsletter, 11,* 4–7.

Stone, M. (1972). Treating the wealthy and their children. *International Journal of Child Psychotherapy, 1,* 15–46.

Tulipan, A. (1986). Fee policy as an extension of the therapist's style and orientation. In D. Krueger (Ed.), *The last taboo: Money as symbol and reality in psychotherapy and psychoanalysis.* New York: Brunner/Mazel.

Wahl, C. (1974). Psychoanalysis of the rich, the famous and the influential. *Contemporary Psychoanalysis, 10,* 171–85.

Weintraub, W. (1964). The VIP syndrome: A clinical study in hospital psychiatry. *Journal of Nerves and Mental Disease, 138,* 181–193.

SECTION

C

Income Expansion

C H A P T E R
24

TECHNIQUES FOR EXPANSION

James K. Morrison, Ph.D.

It would seem inevitable that, with an estimated half-million people now earning their living providing some form of counseling (Department of Health and Human Services, 1982), we would in recent years witness a proliferation of books that provide useful information to private practitioners on developing the private practice of psychotherapy (Browning, 1982; Cookerly & McClaren, 1982; Hendrickson, Janney, & Fraze, 1978; Keller & Ritt, 1983; Levin, 1983; Lewin, 1978). The importance of expanding one's income is highlighted by a survey by the Division of Clinical and Professional Psychology of the California State Psychological Association in the early 1970s in which practicing clinicians ranked the economics of private practice high on their list of priorities with which they wanted their profession to deal (Zemlich, 1983). More recently, a market research study in 1980 by the Psycheconomics Committee of the same California State Psychological Association confirmed the high clinican interest in the money aspect of private practice.

The purpose of this chapter is to explain how one can expand a private practice once it has been established for at least one year. Although previous chapters have touched upon some of the issues concerning expanding a practice simply by addressng how to set up a clinical practice, this chapter will view those issues within the context of how one can further expand income once one is already established.

Since the individuality of each clinical practice would seem to preclude a description of solutions to every problem, most of the topics covered will serve the purpose of simply raising a wide variety of questions the readers might ask themselves when pondering whether there is a need or desire to increase a practice's income. It is perhaps best in this situation to force readers to do the work by simply making them consider each topic within the context of their practice and personality, since any attempt to advise practitioners on developing income depends on too many variables (e.g., present expertise, interest in new areas, desire to work with other clinicans in a group practice, willingness to "hustle" a bit, being a risk taker, location of practice, type of client population, need for certain problem-solving skills, and countless others).

The following techniques would seem to be important ones in any decision to expand a practice. The questions relevant to those techniques will allow the clinical practitioner to consider seriously the multivaried factors involved in increasing business income.

LOCATION

Perhaps one of the most important questions concerning expanding a practice is whether you are in the right place to do what you want to do. Those therapists with an acute business sense will always ask where the money in their area is. If you did not ask this question when you first established a practice — possibly because you simply located where you could find an office, where you were known, or where your home was — then you need to ask after the first year or so whether or not you wish to expand your income.

If you want to charge fees comparable to those of successful medical practitioners, then you must consider an upper-middle-class or, preferably, an upper-class neighborhood, where clients can pay your fees, and where they tend to be more reliable in keeping their appointments and in making payments. Such a clientele also more easily understands the concept of paying for an uncalled appointment that is not kept.

Finding the right location may involve the unwanted burden of moving and all that that entails. But if you want to do away with a sliding-scale fee schedule, which may reduce your potential income by 20 to 40 percent, then you have to serve a population that can afford your full fee.

The discovery of a locale for your office that will increase your income will probably carry with it the added benefit of having the type of clients whom you will find intellectually stimulating, and who have more potential to respond to insight-oriented psychotherapy (for those therapists so inclined). Pro bono work is not difficult to work into your caseload for those of you wise enough to realize that we all need to keep contact with a wide diversity of people and problems.

Other questions to ask related to a good location, at least for the comfort of your well-paying clients, are: Is there adequate parking at your new office site? Is your office fairly easily accessible by car? Is the building comfortable and attractive enought to justify your fees? Can you furnish the office to make it comfortable and pleasant for your clientele? Are there restrooms? Is the parking lot well lit at night?

CLIENT POPULATION

Once you have selected a location, that decision locks you in, as long as you stay there, to greater exposure to a particular population. That is why this topic is so closely intertwined with the previous one.

Should you limit your clientele to a certain sex (e.g., some women psychotherapists seem to do that when they advertise that they specialize in "women's issues")? Should you limit your clients to one age group (e.g., adults)? Or to one type of problem (e.g., anxiety)? The answer is "no" to all of the above if you really want to expand your established practice.

Prochaska, Nash, and Norcross (1986) concluded from their national survey of full-time practitioners that "full-time practitioners may not be able to afford — literally and figuratively — stringent client modality, or theory selection" (p.64). If you specialized when you opened your practice, you have probably limited your income. Of course, if you now want to work with a wide variety of clients (both sexes, all ages, and most problems), you may have to obtain more training, but that should be no problem these days because of the plethora of workshops available on any topic or skill you can imagine. For example, if after five years of practice you realize that there is a real market for self-hypnosis, you can sign up for a series of workshops and training courses to learn that skill.

MARKETING AND ADVERTSING

If you have already tried to expand your income, you have probably already gained some experience in marketing and advertising. As you must have heard many times before, a basic hurdle you must overcome is to recognize that you are in a business and you are in it to make money (Zemlich, 1983), among other things.

As Zemlich (1983) has said: "Practice promotion requires selling yourself to others who have the potential to make referrals. It is important that you learn to 'package yourself' and learn to get the information about yourself into the right hands" (p.5). I, for example, in my early practice did not feel very comfortable with any advertising other than a yellow-pages name listing. However, I learned that listing in the yellow pages (probably still the best advertising for psychotherapists) my speciality areas and the fact that I work with clients of either sex and all ages helps clients to select me rather than others who just list a name.

Marketing is simply asking what the consumer wants and needs and then determining how you can respond to that need (Freudenberger, 1985). You do not have to be a hustler, although some practitioners are afraid that marketing implies this. I can adhere to *all* of my ethical principles and still feel comfortable with marketing. For example, in the years to come (2,005 and after), there is probably going to be a large group of baby boomers who will be retiring and may need retirement counseling. Since that generation has always consulted counselors, the market may be huge in the near future for services of a psychological nature.

Whether you like it or not, the consumer will increasingly dictate the type of health-care services you provide (Freudenberger, 1985). Therefore, to expand your practice properly in the future, you may have to work out lucrative relationships with health maintenance organizations (HMOs) and similar groups; and to do more consulting with them than you wanted to do in the past.

Marketing principles may also dictate that you make renewed efforts to form working relationships with physicians who are usually isolated from people in the mental-health professions and certainly from psychotherapists (Zayas-Bazan & Tapp, 1983). Lunching periodically with physicians in your area could lead to a greatly expanded practice if they get to know you well enough to entrust their patients to you.

Barker (1983) has aptly stated that "the 1980s are simultaneously the best of times and the worst of times" for the private practice of psychotherapy. While the public is spending a lot of money on therapy (more than two million Americans annually see private practitioners; see Department of Health and Human Services, 1981), there are so many practitioners seeking a shrinking number of available clients that things are changing. More and more people are going to HMOs. What do you do? You adapt. You become creative. You advertise before all the rest do. You talk to HMOs about referrals. You look for new markets. You develop new skills. Remember that there are now over 25,000 psychiatrists, 30,000 psychologists, 45,000 social workers, 30,000 nurses, and countless others providing psychotherapy services (Department of Health and Human Services, 1981).

SELF-PROMOTION

Do you promote yourself in the best possible way to clients and prospective clients? Some changes in this area can also lead to more clients and more income. Ask yourself the following questions. If you answer "no" or "not really" to many of these questions, then perhaps you should consider your image in the community.

Do you dress in such a way that all your clients would feel proud to refer others to you? Are you polite and friendly in the way you greet clients in the waiting room or office? Are you always well-groomed? Are you emphatically a consumer-oriented therapist (Morrison, 1984)? Do you sometimes answer telephone calls directly, or at least return them within the hour? Have you worked out fee collecting in a way that does not promote resentment, except perhaps among the 10 percent who give everyone a problem? Is your office neat, comfortable, and pleasant? Do you project the right amount of warmth and professionalism when you speak in public? Do people who work in the the same building (if there are others) find you the type of person they might want to see for counseling? Do you answer requests for information from doctors and agencies promptly? If you have an answering service, how sure are you that those who take the calls are polite, warm, patient, and understanding to callers? If you have an answering machine, how does your voice sound to others? (I have been frequently told that people want to see me just because of my friendly, warm, but professional-sounding voice on a message tape.) You may have some work to do after answering these questions. But your income will increase in proportion to the changes you make.

A CONSUMER-ORIENTED APPROACH

Freudenberger (1985) has stated emphatically: "Whether we like it or not, more and more the consumer will dictate the type of health care services we provide in the future" (p.37). In a detailed article (Morrison, 1979), I have spoken of a "consumer-oriented approach to psychotherapy." I believe this approach to be one of the reasons why I have been successful in full-time private practice despite all the "gloom and doom" written about such a practice in recent years. A consumer-oriented approach to psychotherapy brings into sharper focus the perspective and the role of the client as consumer of therapy. With some exceptions (Strupp, 1975; Strupp, Fox & Lessler, 1969), the more common approach in psychotherapy appears to be a focus more on the therapist's perspective of the client's problems than on the client's view of these same problems.

As clarified in detail elsewhere (Morrison, 1984a), a therapist may want to consider promoting a better image, and thus a better business, by following some of these consumer-oriented steps:

(1) Explain the therapeutic approach thoroughly.
(2) Specify credentials.
(3) Make confidentiality contracts with clients.
(4) Draw up treatment contracts.
(5) Form feedback groups of former clients to advise on one's practice.
(6) Conduct outcome research on one's therapy so one can feed back the results to new clients.
(7) Demystify the therapeutic process to reduce clients' dependence on therapists.

If clients feel you are taking such steps to protect them, they will not hesitate to refer to you members of their family and close friends. They know you will take good care of them. One survey (Tryon, 1983) has shown that clients are most frequently referred by *other* clients.

FEE INCREASES

I cannot think of a faster way to expand your practice income than through fee increases. I believe it is imperative to become knowledgeable about the current fees in your area so that you will not be timid about raising your fees. Unless you feel you are less competent than the average practitioner, why should you not charge as much as others in your profession? Raising a fee from $75 to $80 for a 45-minute session instantly increases your income almost 7 percent. Of course, I believe it is only fair to prepare your clients for this fee change, but few, if any, will change their minds about therapy because of the higher fee.

You must be careful, however, not to price yourself out of the market. If 20 percent of your clients call you because of an ad in the yellow pages or in a newspaper, you will lose some prospective business since such clients often call more than one therapist to compare fees and may choose the therapist with the lowest fee. However, clients referred by friends, physicians, or agencies will usually not do that, unless, of course, they have been given several names.

It is important to get used to the idea that all you have to do in a good location is to charge what you feel you deserve (even a fee as high as any in the area) and clients, referred by people they trust, will pay it. I am not suggesting that you rip off a client, but if, for example, as a psychologist you provide the same service (e.g., individual psychotherapy) to a client as a psychiatrist, you should be paid the same fee. Probably you should increase your fee $5 a year in most years — in some years by $10 — just to keep up with inflation. If you do not, you had better find a new location and clientele or you may be less than successful as a businessperson.

IMPROVING YOUR COLLECTION SYSTEM

Another quick way to increase income is to establish a more effective method of collecting fees. The best method, if you can get away with it without reducing the number of sessions a client is able to see you, is to ask for payment at the end of each session. With some insurance plans, of course, you must wait for direct payment and thus cannot collect on the day the service is provided. But, where possible, wise and business-oriented therapists will collect fees as soon as they can. What about special arrangements? What about the clients you agree to see even though they cannot pay as they go? What if they do not respond to your monthly billing? How do you collect? Expanding your income depends on fast, efficient methods of collecting those unpaid bills.

First, forget about using a lawyer who charges a flat fee to seek judgment against the client. You can pay the lawyer more than you are trying to collect. And, from my experience, you still will not actually collect your money.

Second, you can use a reliable collection agency connected with a lawyer's office, which charges you 33 percent or 50 percent (depending on whether it only sends letters or also writes up judgments) of the fee to be collected. I have had excellent success with such an agency and, after I send three letters with no response, I remit the appropriate information to the collection agency and save myself the hassle of trying to collect further. Good businesses operate the same way. In a study of my own practice (Morrison, 1985) I found that my uncollected fees amount to 1.3 percent of my total fees charged, an excellent collection percentage for any business. I believe that the advice offered above has something to do with that low rate.

CONSULTATION

Many psychotherapists find that they can quickly expand their private practice income by doing consultation work with industry, HMOs, mental-health clinics, insurance companies, and a wide assortment of other agencies and organizations. In fact, the resourceful psychotherapist of the future may need such fee-for-service work in order to compensate for a shrinking market shared by a plethora of mental-health providers. But you will have to sell yourself and your services. If you have alcohol and drug counseling as specialty areas, you may be in demand by large organizations who want their employees to "kick their habit" as it would save them a lot of money by not having to fire experienced, trained workers.

More and more companies are likely to discover that they can establish their own HMOs and save a great deal on insurance. If you help them to set up their psychological services, there may be a lucrative reward for such consultation.

If you keep alert to the future trends in services, you may find ways to offer your skills. But remember, simply sending out your "curriculum vitae" is not enough — no matter how intriguing your cover letter. You will want to talk to the right person in the organization and it may take some investigating to find out who that person is.

Consultation can pay large dividends in some areas and you can make large strides to expand your income when you discover and develop certain key relationships. Be patient at first; do not start charging fees until you have spent some "free time" talking over your ideas with such organizations.

FORMATION OF GROUPS

Those psychotherapists who never offered group therapy in their early practice may want to consider this possibility as a way of developing income. Usually, groups entail some evening work but you generally can, even with a low fee, make more money in a 45-minute group session than you can in a 45-minute individual session. You might take advantage of this by scheduling three or four group sessions a week.

It is difficult to begin group counseling early in your practice because the community is not really aware of your presence and your willingness to see people in groups may not be as popular as in their heyday in the late 1960s and 1970s. There now is a demand for a greater variety of groups, such as those that focus on specific problems, including weight reduction; AIDS; victims of abuse; death of parents, spouses, or children; and self-help skills learning.

WORKSHOPS

Once you develop a specialty skill (e.g., clinical hypnosis, biofeedback, grieving techniques), all you have to do is get into the workshop business in order to further your income. It helps to have an academic position so that you can use the university facilities to present workshops and do the preworkshop mailngs that are necessary. However, you could also make the acquaintance of other workshhop leaders who might be willing to pay you to do workshops with them.

Workshops at first take more time than the time is worth in terms of money, but once you have put together a format that generates participants' enthusiasm, the profit margin becomes greater. If the workshop becomes popular, the fees for the workshop can also be increased. Soon you will find that the profit margin can be fairly large.

If you have a secretary or other assistants who can do the mailings, make hotel arrangements, and so on, it will save you valuable time and make the whole process cost-effective. If you do not have such help, then you may not want to consider going on the workshop circuit.

INSURANCE

Some psychotherapists are so caught up in the idea of receiving payment at each session that they actively discourage more than six to eight sessions with those clients who really need more work. If those clients who have good insurance coverage can be charged at each session only the deductible plus whatever percentage of the fee the insurance will not cover, and if you will wait for insurance reimbursement, the delay in total payment will be well compensated for by a doubling or tripling of needed sessions. Such a practice certainly expands income. However, some insurance plans may entail such a long wait (four to six months) for reimbusement or hold back a percentage of the fee to the end of the year that one may want to make an exception here.

OBSERVING TRENDS

An alert practitioner will keep up with trends in services by keeping up with his or her reading (e.g., state psychological bulletins, *APA Monitor, Psychotherapy in Private Practice,*). If you feel that a need for a particular service will arise, prepare for it now. Get some training and start planning.

It would help a practitioner to scan available statistics periodically for his or her area with regard to population growth or decline, average income of residents, age categories of the largest percentage of people there, number of married and unmarried persons, and other data that help to guide you in designing new services to fill a growing need. Astute observations and conclusions will make sure you can continually increase your business income for some time to come.

DEVELOPING PSYCHOLOGICAL TESTING SERVICES

One clinical psycholgist I know marketed the service of providing psychological testing of clients with computerized analysis of the results. He sold the idea to a number of psychotherapists and physicians in the area and greatly increased his income and contacts.

You might also want to consider doing psychological testing to fill in some of your empty hours. If you have some expertise in this area, it would be worthwhile to increase your income by offering this service, at least until your available hours are full.

CONTACT WITH PEERS

One possible way of generating other ways to increase your business is to maintain contact with your peers, although this is not always an easy thing to do in private practice, especially if you are a solo practitioner. But arranging lunches with peers, or even forming a private practice discussion group, will frequently suggest ways of generating income that you had overlooked. Such contact may also give you more courage to raise your fees, at least when you find out that the others have done so. Thus, this last way of increasing income may suggest new methods I have not considered in this chapter.

CONCLUSION

In this chapter, I have tried to outline many of the possible ways in which clinicians in private practice might expand their income once they have become established for at least a year. I have frequently emphasized that one should study the current and projected needs of the client, and that a consumer-oriented approach to clients is not only an ethical way to go, but also a lucrative one. In a recent survey (Bascue & Inman, 1984), both clinical and counseling psycholgists clearly rated clients as the most important referral source. If that is the case, the practitioner who truly wishes to increase the money made from private practice must take excellent care of his or her clients as that is the best marketing device of all.

I do not claim to have exhausted all the possible ways of expanding one's profits, but perhaps some of my recommendations have generated other, even more creative, ideas on your part. I have always been a great believer in a clinican doing things his or her own way, whether in therapy or in the business of private practice. Some practitioners find it too abhorrent to hustle, but, as described earlier, there are many alternatives that will work to increase income. Just never stop thinking about ever new and creative ways of conducting your business.

REFERENCES

Barker, R.L. (1983). Supply side economics in private psycotherapy practice. *Psychotherapy in Private Practice, 1,* 71-81.

Bascue, L.O., & Inman, D.J. (1984). A comparison of private practice activities and clinical and counseling psychologists. *Psychotherapy in Private Practice, 2,*67-73.

Browning, C.H. (1982). *Private practice handbook: The tools, tactics and techniques for successful practice development* (2nd ed.). Los Alamitos, CA: Durcliff.

Cookerly, J.R., & McClaren, K. (1982). *How to increase your private practice power.* Fort Worth, TX: Center for Counseling and Developmental Services.

Department of Health and Human Services. (1981). *Health resources statistics,* 1979-80 edition. Washington, D.C.: Government Printing Office.

Department of Health and Human Services. (1982). *Health resources studies (report on health personnel in the United States),* Washington, D.C.: Government Printing Office.

Freudenerger, H.J. (1985). How to market ourselves in the future. *Psychotherapy in Private Practice, 3,* 33-37.

Hendrickson, D.E., Janney, S.P., & Fraze, J.E. (1978). *How to establish your own private practice.* Muncie, IN: Contemporary Press, 1978.

Keller, P.A., & Ritt, L.G. (Eds.) (1984). *Innovations in clinical practice: A source book* (Vol. III). Sarasota, Fl: Professional Resources Exchange.

Levin, A.M. (1983). *The private practice of psychotherapy.* New York: Free Press.

Lewin, M.H. (1978). *Establishing and maintaining a successsful professional practice.* Rochester, NY: Professional Development Institute.

Morrison, J.K. (1978). The client as consumer and evaluator of community mental health services. *American Journal of Community Psychology, 6,* 147-155.

Morrison, J.K. (1979). A consumer-oriented approach to psychotherapy. *Psychotherapy: Theory, Research and Practice, 16,* 381-384.

Morrison, J.K. (1983). Tracking referrals for psychotherapy in private practice. *Psychotherapy in Private Practice, 1,* 9-14.

Morrison, J.K. (1984a). Eight steps toward protecting the psychotherapy client from "consumer fraud." In J. Harriman (Ed.), *Does psychotherapy really help people?* (pp.144-153.) Springfield, Ill: Charles C. Thomas.

Morrison, J.K. (1984b). A consumer approach to clinical practice. In P.A. Keller & L.G. Ritt (Eds.), *Innovations in clinical practice: A source book* (Vol.III). (pp.213-220.) Sarasota, Fl: Professional Resources Exchange.

Morrsion, J.K. (1985). Settling "delinquent" accounts in private practice: A five-year review of the data. *Psychotherapy in Private Practice, 3,* 23-27.

Prochaska, J.O., Nash, J.M., & Norcross, J.C. (1986). Independent psychological practice: A a national survey of full-time practitioners. *Psychotherapy in Private Practice, 4,* 57-66.

Strupp, H.H. (1975). On failing one's patient. *Psychotherapy: Theory, Research and Practice, 12,* 39-41.

Strupp, H.H., Fox, R.E., & Lessler, K. (1969). *Patients view their psychotherapy.*Baltimore: Johns Hopkins Press.

Tryon, G.S. (1983). How full-time practitioners market their services: A national survey. *Psychotherapy in Private Practice, 1,* 91-100.

Zaya-Bazan, C., & Tapp, J.T. (1983). The psychologist in the medical community: Developing the medical referral. *Psychotherapy in Private Practice, 1,* 51-56.

Zemlich, M.J. (1983). Psych-economics: The business of psychology. *Psychotherapy in Private Practice, 1,* 1-7.

C H A P T E R
25

SELF-HELP AND PRIVATE PRACTITIONERS: WHAT DO WE NEED TO KNOW?

Peggy Watkins-Ferrell, M.A.,
and Leonard A. Jason, Ph.D.

Perhaps it is a bit unusual for a chapter on self-help to be included in a book entitled *The Encyclopedic Handbook of Private Practice.* Without doubt, many private practitioners might legitimately have reservations about some aspects of the self-help movement, and might ask such questions as: What exactly is the self-help movement all about? Is it possible that some people could be, at minimum, provided help based on unsubstantiated principles and, at worst, provided treatment that is ethically questionable? Could these groups, with their sometimes skeptical attitude toward traditional psychotherapy, be deterring people from obtaining help from trained professionals, whose techniques are based on principles that are more empirically sound? Many have heard of myths promulgated by these groups—such as once an alcoholic, always one—but we know from research that some alcoholics can become controlled drinkers. With these types of concerns, is it not natural for at least some mental-health professionals to have doubts about this vast, unregulated, and unlicensed alternative mental-health-delivery system? In this chapter, we explore some of these concerns and questions regarding self-help groups, looking at both the benefits and limitations of the self-help movement. Additionally, we emphasize throughout how mental-health professionals and self-helpers may be able to work together to develop a more integrated and comprehensive mental-health-delivery system.

A GROWING MOVEMENT

First, we need to examine the recent growth of the self-help movement and provide some insights as to exactly what self-help is. Over the past 10 years, self-help groups have become an increasingly important source of help for people struggling with various issues and life crises. There has been a burgeoning growth in the numbers of various self-help groups; Gartner and Riessman (1982) report that there are approximately 500,000 groups in the United States, involving more than 15 million people. In fact, the groups are increasing at such a rapid pace that it is almost impossible to keep track of them (Borman, 1986). The 1986 *Self-Help Directory,* which covers the Chicago metropolitan area alone, lists more than 1,100 groups for 270 problems. The compilers of this directory report that this is double the number that they were able to locate approximately two years ago (Borman, 1986).

There is also an increasing number of self-help centers and clearinghouses. Currently, 30 or more centers across the United States and Canada perform various activities, including compiling information, publishing directories, providing referral by telephone, and conducting training sessions (Borman, 1986). The self-help movement has also been quite active in many other parts of the world, including the United Kingdom, Australia, West Germany, Holland, Poland, and Sweden (Katz, 1984). Furthermore, over the past decade, self-help has increasingly been discussed in the scientific literature. It is clear that self-help groups are here to stay and thus professionals need information regarding this growing movement in the field of mental health.

WHAT IS SELF-HELP?

Many definitions of self-help/mutual aid have been put forth. These definitions typically characterize self-help as a group activity and thus rule out solitary self-help activity. Spiegel (1982) states: "Self-help and mutual support groups comprise those voluntary associations of individuals with a common problem, stigma, or life situation which involves no professional control, although there may be professional involvement of a consultative kind, and in which there is no financial profit. Such groups usually engage in a combination of mutual help to members and to the public and political activity" (p. 99). As noted by Gartner and Riessman (1977), the following characteristics can generally be applied to most self-help groups:

1. The groups involve face-to-face interactions.
2. The groups originate spontaneously in that the participants organize the group.
3. The group members are fairly equal in power and the leadership role typically rotates among the members.
4. The group members agree on and engage in some type of constructive action toward shared goals.
5. The members typically start in a position of powerlessness.
6. The group provides a reference group for the members.

Other defining characteristics include a strong emphasis on the helper-therapy principle (e.g., those who help are helped the most) and reliance on the indigenous knowledge of the group members (Riessman, 1985).

We would like to highlight a number of features that serve to distinguish self-help groups from most typical professional therapy groups:

1. There is no fee.
2. There is nonprofessional leadership that typically rotates.
3. Group meetings follow a regular set agenda each week.

4. Group members are placed in both the role of helper and helpee.

5. Group members have a common issue and act as role models for each other.

6. Group members frequently interact outside of group meetings.

TYPES OF SELF-HELP GROUPS

Within these defining characteristics, there exist a wide variety of mutual-aid groups that address a broad spectrum of conditions and issues. Some groups engage in political activity whereas other, such as Alcoholics Anonymous (AA), steer clear of this type of activity. Various writers have attempted to categorize self-help groups. Levy (1976) presents a typology of self-help groups based upon their purposes and composition. His typology consists of four types of mutual-aid groups:

1. Groups defined by their purpose to eliminate or control some problematic behavior. An example of such a group would be Overeaters Anonymous (OA).

2. Groups composed of individuals who "share a common status or predicament that entails some degree of stress." The purpose of these groups is the reduction of this stress through mutual support and the sharing of coping strategies and advice. In general, there is no attempt to change their status, but instead the group focuses on how to continue with life in spite of the situation (e.g., widowhood).

3. Mutual-aid groups that are survival oriented. These groups consist of individuals whom society has labeled deviant or who are discriminated against because of their life-style, race, sex, sexual orientation, and so on. The groups tend to focus on helping members maintain or enhance their self-esteem and frequently work toward improving their situation through political activities. Examples of such groups would be women's groups, senior citizens' groups, or gay liberation groups.

4. Mutual-aid groups formed around such goals as pursuing personal growth or self-actualization. In these groups, there is no defined condition that connects the group members. An example would be informal experientially oriented groups.

THE EXTENT OF PROFESSIONAL INVOLVEMENT

Another important feature that distinguishes self-help groups is the degree of professional involvement in the groups. Some groups, such as AA, have no professional involvement and make it very clear that none is wanted. Other groups, such as Parents Anonymous (PA), have a great deal of professional involvement. For example, each chapter of PA is required to have a volunteer professional sponsor. A sponsor attends the weekly meetings, acts as a consultant, is a resource to the parent chairperson, and presents a positive role model of a professional who can make referrals. The sponsor often also acts as a liaison with other agencies in the community that deal with issues of family violence and thus provides credibility for the program in the community at large. However, PA also makes it very clear that the professional sponsor serves the group rather than controlling it, and a professional sponsor can be asked to leave at any time if the group members decide that this is in their best interest. Most self-help groups fall somewhere between these two extremes, with some professional involvement. Many professionals have even been instrumental in starting self-help groups (e.g., Recovery) or act as periodic consultants.

As will be discussed in more detail later, there are possible dangers when mental-health professionals become involved with self-help groups, but there are also dangers when professionals do not become involved. Some groups welcome professional involvement; others do not. The fact that some self-help groups exclude professional involvement does not necessarily mean that these groups are not doing good things or that they are not helpful to their members, but such groups may not be the ones to which we would most comfortably make a referral. Many self-help groups are willing to talk with professionals concerning their objectives and often have literature to share regarding the group's philosophy. As professionals, we may want to approach self-help groups and obtain information so that we can feel secure in making a referral for a particular client. The most serious problems might result when referrals are made blindly to groups we know nothing about. If you were treating a client and a problem arose that you felt you were not professionally able to treat, you might make a referral to a specialist, to whom you had either talked directly or about whom had heard good things in the mental-health community. You probably would not make a referral to a therapist whom you knew nothing about. One could naturally ask why a similar situation should not be valid for referrals to self-help groups. If you knew the type of helping that goes on in the self-help group to which you are making a referral, you probably would be more confident that your client would receive good care. The process of making referrals to and receiving referrals from self-help groups will be discussed in more detail in a later section.

DOES SELF-HELP WORK?

The topic of what makes self-help/mutual aid work has also received a great deal of attention in recent years. The vast majority of groups make no attempt to assess their own effectiveness, and we consider this a major problem and a significant avenue for us to explore in the coming years. Active members often say that they "know" that their group works, and consequently they do not see any reason or need for systematic evaluation. However, although we as professionals may also believe that psychotherapy works, and may receive confirmatory feedback from clients, we strive to evaluate our work in a more stringent, data-based fashion. We believe that the success of the self-help movement is to some extent going to be based on the willingness of groups to begin to take a close look at the groups' effectiveness. For example, we need answers to many critical questions, including: How many people do not return after the first meeting? What type of people benefit from self-help groups, and what type of people do not? Why do people drop out? What type of people might benefit from a combination of a self-help group and individual therapy?

Levy (1976) presents a number of behavioral and cognitive processes that are believed to play a role in the operation of self-help groups. These processes are based on observations of group meetings, interviews with group members, questionnaires, and a review of the popular and scientific literature. The processes he postulates include:

1. Providing social reinforcement for the development of healthy behaviors and the elimination of problem behaviors (e.g., praise, applause).
2. Affording training, indoctrination, and support in the use of self-control behaviors.
3. Modeling positive behavior, coping strategies, and behavior-change techniques.
4. Providing members with examples of actions they can take to alter their social environment.
5. Providing members with a rationale for their condition and for the group's way of coping with or changing it.
6. Providing normative information and advice.
7. Expanding the repertoire of alternative perceptions and actions for coping with the problem.
8. Increasing the ability to discriminate events.
9. Supporting changes in attitudes.
10. Reducing a feeling of isolation.
11. Developing an alternative culture and social structure.

Reissman (1985) sees one of the most important processes of self-help groups as that of empowering its members. The process of being able to help oneself and help others creates a feeling of being able to control some aspects of one's life. When self-helpers discuss their groups, feelings of energy, excitement, and empowerment often become evident. People meet and share with others who are in the same boat and who understand what it is like to be there. Self-report data are typically quite favorable, with members reporting that their group is very helpful. For example, one member of an OA group shared her feeling that it was "such a relief coming into OA and finding out that I was not the only person in the world who hid food." She continued by saying, "I can get on the phone and call someone and say this has been a terrible day and people understand." One member of a Tough Love group in sharing the feelings she has about her group stated, "You get in there and there is this sense of camaraderie and other people who have these same problems and you feel good." A member of a widows' group asserted, "It was such an eye opener and such a release to tell all these things that I had inside to other people and have them listen—the marvelous thing about the groups is that people listen—they don't shut you off."

In general, the literature reports many claims that self-help groups are beneficial to their members, but the lack of rigorous research to support such reports is disturbing. However, we would like to add that from the literature and from our contact with dozens of groups, it appears that the majority of self-help groups are generally not harmful to their members because they involve no coercion. That is, if a person does not like the group, that person can just opt not to attend another meeting, and this frequently happens. We believe, however, that an overly optimistic view is also inappropriate. There are probably groups in different communities that are led by marginal people, where control, inappropriate advice, and other cultlike processes are operating. But we must be careful not to condemn an entire self-help movement because of several potentially harmful groups, just as we do not dismiss the field of psychotherapy when we hear about the inappropriate activities of some of our peers. Once again, this illustrates the importance of professionals' becoming familiar with the self-help groups in their communities in order to identify those groups with which appropriate contact and cross-referrals might be made.

PROFESSIONALS' ATTITUDES REGARDING SELF-HELP

As noted earlier, there has been a tremendous increase in professional interest in the self-help movement. Levy (1978) conducted a national survey regarding the attitudes and referral patterns of outpatient mental-health facilities in relation to self-help groups. Overall, the evaluations were quite positive, with 46.7 percent agreeing that self-help groups have an important or very important role in a comprehensive mental-health-care delivery system. Furthermore, approximately 48 percent of the agencies reported that they make either frequent or occasional referrals to self-help groups. However, only 30.7 percent of the respondents reported that the probability was high that their agencies would be willing to explore and work toward a comprehensive mental-health-care delivery system that integrated their activities with those of self-help groups. A recent survey of social workers indicated that 88 percent rated their attitude toward self-help groups as positive or very positive, whereas only 3 percent indicated that their attitude was negative (Toseland & Hacker, 1985). However, 60 percent of the social workers surveyed believed that self-help groups are biased against professional help and discourage group members from seeking additional help when it may be needed.

These surveys may shed some light on the gulf that often seems to exist between self-helpers and professionals. They suggest that, overall, professionals have positive attitudes toward self-help, but are reluctant to become involved more directly with this movement. This may be due to the frequent suggestions that self-help groups are antiprofessional. While this is certainly true in some instances, most recent findings suggest that self-help groups welcome professional involvement, as long as the professionals do not attempt to control or take over the group (Toseland & Hacker, 1985). There may be deeper, more personal issues that are also involved in the rift between professionals and self-helpers. Some of the groups (e.g., AA) were formed as a direct response to the inadequacies or the ineffectiveness of the professional caregiving system. Thus, some group members or leaders may have experienced frustrating interactions with professionals in the past. Furthermore, when someone who has little or no training develops an approach that is reported at least to be as effective as ours, we naturally may react less than favorably. Sometimes we might feel in competition with self-help groups for clients. Especially during economic downturns, people may favor less expensive help, and self-help groups are a viable option. We may harbor a hidden fear that if self-help is an alternative, and one that might be very attractive from a financial point of view, then we might need to expend even more resources on marketing and developing referral sources in order to maintain a share of the available clients.

While recognizing these concerns, we truly believe that both professional and self-help approaches are needed and that self-help will not replace therapy. We believe that it is more a matter of fit. For example, one individual might benefit the most from self-help, another from individual therapy, and another from a combination of the two approaches. Furthermore, especially in the area of the addictions (e.g., obesity, smoking, alcoholism), the combination of the two approaches might revolutionize the way we view and treat these problems. We know that as professionals we are able to have an impact on these behaviors while we are in contact with the client, but that relapse rates tend to be high. Although there are many problems with defining specific rates, relapse rates for the addictions are assumed to range from 50 percent to as high as 90 percent (Brownell, Marlatt, Lichtenstein, & Wilson, 1986). Research has suggested that social support may be an important variable in the prevention of relapse in the area of the addictions (Brownell et al., 1986). Consequently, it seems to make sense that a combination of therapy with the supportive long-term environment of a self-help group might help to eliminate these high relapse rates. For example, a client struggling to maintain newly learned eating patterns could be channeled into a self-help group that could provide the long-term support that is typically necessary, but not always financially feasible through psychotherapy. Furthermore, as connections are developed between professionals and self-help groups, a cross-referral system could be developed in which professionals receive referrals from the groups as well as make referrals to them.

COLLABORATION BETWEEN PROFESSIONALS AND SELF-HELPERS

It is important to recognize that the self-help movement has not been entirely a grass-roots movement, supported only by indigenous self-help group members (Borman, 1986). During the past 50 years, some professionals have encouraged the movement and have played important roles in the development of such groups as Recovery, Inc., and PA (Borman, 1986). It seems clear that professionals will continue to interact with self-help groups in various ways. For this reason, it is important to examine what roles professionals have played and what effect their involvement has on self-help groups. Only through critical examination of this process can the professional community come to understand how to collaborate most effectively with self-help groups. This type of information could also be included in the training of mental-health professionals, along with practicum experiences that involve collaborative efforts with self-help groups. In this way, future mental-health professionals would be more prepared for the adoption of appropriate collaborative roles that would benefit both self-help groups and the professional community. The remainder of this chapter will explore the interface between self-helpers and professionals, with an emphasis on appropriate roles for professionals.

The first important point to recognize is that when professionals work with self-help groups, they need to break away from the typical therapist–client model. In other words, instead of viewing the self-help group as the client and the professional as the therapist, both parties should be viewed as having areas of knowledge and expertise to offer and share in the development of a collaborative partnership. Chutis (1983) presents four features of self-help groups that help to illustrate the point. The first feature is that the decision-making authority lies with the self-help group and not with the mental-health professional. Second, Chutis points out that intrapsychic dynamics are not the focus of self-help groups and are not valued by the groups. Instead, the groups emphasize helping behaviors, coping skills, and problem-solving approaches, and consequently the professional working with self-help groups needs to stay with this focus. Varying from it would create the danger of replicating professional services as opposed to offering a new type of service. Professionals must be careful not to tamper with the methods of helping utilized in self-help groups in order to prevent altering the effective ingredients of self-help. It should not be our goal to turn self-help groups into a type of psychotherapy group, but instead to enhance the natural methods of helping that occur in self-help groups. Third, self-help groups value the expertise that comes from the day-to-day experiencing of a problem or situation, more so than expertise gained from academic credentials.

The final point Chutis makes is that while self-help group members possess a number of natural helping qualities, they do not necessarily have the skills required to address issues involving group processes or maintenance of the group over an extended period of time. She suggests that the professional skills that can be the most effective and accepted by self-help group members are community organization, group work, communications, public relations, and fund raising.

Chutis (1983) also describes more specifically how professionals at mental-health centers can collaborate in the development and maintenance of self-help groups. The first prerequisite is to gain agency support for such groups. Without agency support, this type of collaboration would be extremely difficult. It should be recognized that gaining agency support can be a lengthy, time-consuming, and sometimes difficult process. At first, agencies may see little reason to support self-help groups and may view this activity as a low priority. Agencies may need to be helped to see the potential benefits for the agency, such as the development of a cross-referral system and publicity for the agency as a whole in the community. Chutis goes on to describe various roles professionals can play in the development of a self-help group. These include providing organizational advice to the group, helping with publicity, helping the group to gain legitimacy in the community, coleading a group, and generally being a consultant to the group in such areas as resources, group process, leadership, and helping skills.

These activities suggest roles for professionals that are very different from the typical roles mental-health professionals engage in and for which they are trained. Community organizing, generating publicity, and fund raising are not part of the typical training curriculum for most mental-health professionals. Additionally, these features suggest the need for a true collaboration in which professionals enter into a relationship characterized by reciprocal learning. It seems to make sense that professionals have skills that could be beneficial to self-help groups, but it seems to be also true that professionals could learn a great deal from self-help groups about natural helping and normal ways of coping with transitions and life crises.

Others have also written about various roles professionals might take in their interactions with self-help groups. Gartner and Riessman (1982) recommend an increasingly strong relationship between professionals and self-help groups. They suggest that professionals can bring to self-help groups the values of a systematic approach, particular skills such as public relations or process skills, and access to resources. Hedrick (1985) also suggests a role for professionals that focuses on giving assistance in such areas as organizing and maintaining groups. Hedrick discusses another role in which professionals make referrals and distribute information about self-help. She suggests that one effective method of distributing information is by including presentations on self-help groups at regional and national professional meetings and educational seminars, and by including references to these groups in publications. She recommends that professionals provide guidance in conducting meetings and workshops, publishing directories and newsletters, raising funds, and coordinating activities.

Hedrick makes the critically important distinction between a professional performing such activities for a group and a professional helping with such activities. The first would be an inappropriate role whereas the second would be an appropriate collaborative role. The distinction between these roles can become extremely subtle in that, as professionals, we may unwittingly alter the group process just by being present. Group members may tend to place the professional in a leadership role or may act differently with a professional present. It seems to be crucial for professionals to constantly be aware of the tendency to take over an activity instead of staying within the true spirit of a collaborative model. A final suggestion Hedrick discusses is the potential for building coalitions of members and supporters of self-help groups who are interested in working together to attain self-help goals and to provide each other support in the process. Jason et al.'s (1988a) description of the emergence of the Inner City Self-Help Center in Chicago is an excellent example of what can be accomplished, as well as of the difficulties that may be encountered when self-helpers and professionals collaborate in the development of self-help groups.

Gottlieb (1983) presents the argument that mental-health consultation as it is typically practiced is an inappropriate form of collaboration with mutual-help groups. For example, teaching active listening skills to self-helpers might alter their natural helping styles and consequently might undermine some of the effective ingredients of the self-help movement. He suggests that mental-health professionals share other skills, such as their background in basic research, evaluative research, problem solving, and program planning. He recommends that professionals become directly involved in the development of self-help groups by identifying and bringing together individuals in similar stressful situations and helping to develop a general model to be followed at group meetings. He also suggests that professionals refer clients to appropriate self-help groups in the community. Gottlieb reports that workshops have been conducted with medical students on the utilization of self-help groups as additional treatment resources. Professionals can make an effort to familiarize themselves with the self-help groups that exist in their community. Often this type of information can be obtained through self-help clearinghouses. Members of self-help groups should not be approached as solely potential clients, but also as collaborators who have knowledge to offer.

COLLABORATIVE EXAMPLES

Jason (1985) presents an innovative example of how professionals might collaborate with self-help groups in delivering mental-health services through the media. A project is described in which self-help groups were given the radio time for one hour a week. During the first half-hour, the process of self-help was demonstrated by three self-help group members; calls were taken from the audience for the remainder of the show. A mental-health professional acted as moderator, introducing the concept of the show, informing the audience about the issues each group dealt with, and setting up conditions that would facilitate the self-help process in the studio environment. The same mental-health professional functioned as a researcher, collecting data on the effect of the show. Additionally, a panel of mental-health professionals evaluated the content of the broadcasts and indicated that no incorrect, harmful, or unethical information was given to the audience callers by the self-help members. The mental-health professional in this example can be seen in a number of valuable collaborative roles, including that of providing assistance in achieving credibility for the concept of self-help by promoting and hosting this type of programming, providing widespread publicity for the groups that appeared on the show, and adding to the body of scientific literature on the process of self-help, thereby bringing self-help to the attention of mental-health professionals. A media program such as this could also be quite useful to private practitioners who wish to familiarize themselves with the self-help groups in the community. By listening to the broadcast, professionals could gain a good understanding of how various groups operate and whether a particular group might be a good fit for a particular client.

Jason et al. (1988b) also present an example of how a mental-health professional can act as a facilitator in connecting various types of natural support systems. Consultation on the self-help approach and the availability of self-help groups in the community for various problems was provided to a number of religious leaders. Jason et al. (1988b) report that following consultation to clergy members, an increase in various activities related to self-help groups was reported. These activities included referring members of church congregations to self-help groups, publicizing self-help groups, and even starting groups. This project seems to provide strong support for the role of mental-health professionals in providing community gatekeepers, such as clergy, with information about self-help, including what groups are active in the gatekeeper's community. In a similar vein, a mental-health professional who has had extensive experience with numerous self-help groups could act as a consultant to other mental-health professionals who are interested in utilizing self-help groups as an adjunct to therapy for some of their clients.

CONDUCTING RESEARCH
FOR SELF-HELP GROUPS

Lavoie (1984) suggests that an appropriate role for mental-health professionals collaborating with self-help groups is that of a researcher, because the vast majority of self-help groups do not perceive research as a way to help the group. Therefore, she proposes an action-research model in which research is designed to be of benefit to the group as well as to add to the scientific literature. She suggests that this type of research could provide possible solutions to problems faced by self-help groups, and could help to determine the effective elements operating in a self-help group. This type of research could also begin to answer questions about the appropriate roles for professionals in self-help organizations. Self-help groups may not have the necessary research skills or resources to evaluate their organizations effectively. Through this type of collaboration, mental-health professionals who possess research skills can help self-help groups to examine their strengths and weaknesses, and also add to the scientific literature on self-help.

A group of researchers has been extensively studying GROW International, a mutual-help organization for individuals with a history of emotional or psychiatric problems (Rappaport et al., 1985). These researchers report continuously making an attempt not to put themselves in the role of experts, and also not to put the GROW members in the role of subjects. Instead, attempts to foster a "resource collaborator" model in which both parties had a role in determining the research approach were implemented. One very interesting aspect of this research has examined the impact of professional involvement on the social climate and behavior in GROW groups (Toro et al., 1986). Because of a lack of leadership, some of the GROW groups were led by professionals. Consequently, the researchers were able to compare professionally led groups with groups with indigenous leadership on measures of perceived social climate and actual observed behavior among group members. Results indicated that the use of professional leaders can have an effect on both the perceived social climate and the members' actual behavior. Members of professionally led groups tended to perceive the group as less encouraging of free action and expression. These members also perceived their leader as more controlling. Another interesting finding is that the professional leaders showed more directive sorts of behaviors, and more often requested members to provide personal information, but at the same time provided less personal information about themselves. The authors state that generally it seemed as if the professionals were more controlling during the meetings, perhaps discouraging informal and less "deep" behaviors in their group members. The authors conclude that the involvement of professionals as leaders can change the nature of self-help groups. They go on to suggest that professionals might want to consider this carefully in the formation of collaborative relationships, especially recognizing that professionals might hinder some of the effective components of the self-help approach.

Research such as this is critically important to the decisions of whether and how professionals should collaborate with self-help groups. As Gartner and Riessman (1984) suggest, with collaboration comes the danger of co-opting and professionalizing self-help. This seems to be especially true when professionals act as leaders or coleaders of self-help groups. Actually, it can be questioned whether a professionally led group can be classified as self-help in the true sense of the definition. However, it may also be important to examine how other professional and self-help group collaborations affect the self-help approach. It certainly seems possible that if a professional acts as a consultant to a self-help group, the approach may be altered in some way. The critical question is whether this consultation has a positive or negative effect on the functioning of the group. Sometimes we are too quick to assume that our help is of benefit to others. We need to consider that the effective ingredients in self-help groups may be qualitatively different from the types of processes that are characteristic of traditional psychotherapy such as advice giving. Collaboration with self-help groups also needs to work toward fostering independence, especially if one of the effective ingredients in self-help is the empowerment of group members.

MAKING AND RECEIVING REFERRALS

At this time, probably one of the most important collaborator roles for professionals is that of making referrals and receiving referrals from self-help groups. Many members of self-help groups are also in some type of therapy, and we believe that the two can operate in harmony. Sometimes, as professionals, we see little motivation to cultivate and enter into collaborative relationships with self-help groups. We often have limited time and energy and must be selective in choosing our activities. To engage in a new and unfamiliar activity with little visible financial reward may not be a high priority for us. However, we strongly believe that the potential for numerous cross-referral systems exists that could benefit mental-health professionals, self-helpers, and their clients. For example, professionals who specialize in eating disorders may want to form a relationship with a local self-help group in order both to make referrals to this group and to cultivate a relationship in which the group makes referrals to the professional. In this way, the professional expands his or her practice, the self-help group gains members, and ultimately the client benefits from receiving support from two valuable sources.

Typically, professionals can contact self-help groups directly if they are interested in obtaining information about a particular group. Self-help clearinghouses are often able to provide some of this information, as well as the name and telephone number of a person the professional can contact to find out how the group operates. Professionals can talk with clients whom they have referred to self-help groups regarding the nature of the groups. Perhaps one of the most critical variables is the fit between the group and the individual. A recent media program, developed by the second author, aired on the local news and focused on issues of nutrition and weight loss. As part of this programming, mental-health professionals helped to channel individuals into self-help groups that would best suit their eating-related problems. In implementing this project, the investigators learned that there are a variety of weight-loss self-help groups (e.g., OA, Take Off Pounds Sensibly, Weight Watchers); one person might fit in very well with the group philosophy of OA with its references to help from a higher power, whereas another might benefit more from Take Off Pounds Sensibly. Furthermore, different chapters of the same self-help organization sometimes differ, with one chapter catering to the needs of older, married women, for example, and another to younger, single women. As we become more familiar with self-help groups through research, practical experience, and word of mouth, we will be better able to channel people into groups that best meet their needs.

The following questions relate to qualities of self-help groups that professionals may want to look for when determining whether to make a referral to a particular group:

1. Is the "group leader" willing to speak with you on the telephone, or perhaps even to meet with you in person?
2. Does the group have written literature that it would be willing to share with you?
3. Would it be possible to speak with other members of the group?
4. Does the group have a regular format that is followed at each meeting?
5. How are newcomers welcomed into the group?
6. Does the group make any attempt to evaluate its own effectiveness?
7. What type of people seem to get the most out of their group and what type are less successful with the group?
8. Are people allowed to leave the group whenever they wish?
9. Are there any guidelines for crisis situations (e.g., when a group member shares with the group that he or she is contemplating suicide)?

We believe that these types of questions can be extremely helpful when making a decision regarding a referral.

CONCLUSION

At this point in time, professionals should remain somewhat careful in their interactions with self-help groups. Supportive activities such as referring clients, providing space for groups to meet, disseminating publicity, developing new leadership, or similar actions are appropriate and valuable activities for professionals. Until further research is conducted that delineates the effective ingredients in self-help, however, perhaps it is best that professionals not tamper with the indigenous self-help approach. Furthermore, all collaborations, no matter how minor, need to be carefully assessed. It is possible that even a supportive action such as providing meeting space could alter the self-help process, depending on the environment of this space. For example, meetings held in a community mental-health center might create a different group social climate than those held in a church. Perhaps most damaging are those instances when professionals convey to self-helpers that the professionals know best how the self-help groups should be run. These concerns are not intended to suggest that professionals should stay away from self-help groups, but instead to highlight the importance of recognizing that collaboration may create both positive and negative consequences. Professionals need to recognize this and strive to learn how best to maximize the positives while minimizing the negatives.

The same can be said with regard to self-helpers. They must recognize and be willing to evaluate the possibility that their approach might not be best for every individual and that some group members might need additional help. Although not documented to date in the literature, it is conceivable that some self-help groups might do damage to clients (e.g., by suggesting biological, genetic, or spiritual explanations for behavior problems that are more parsimoniously understood as learned), and this possibility needs to be considered when working with self-help groups. Should the movement be regulated? At this point, this might create more damage than benefit, although just as movies are rated for viewers, perhaps one day citizen groups will also develop rating systems for groups, to better inform consumers of the types of helping the groups provide.

Some self-help groups need to be more open to research and involvement with the professional community in general. Self-helpers also need to be willing to reach out and work collaboratively. It is vital that both self-helpers and professionals strive to maximize the fit between the individual client and the therapeutic approach, rather than getting caught up in maximizing their own needs. Only through collaboration can we best serve those in need of help and maximize the benefits of the professional caregiving system and the self-help movement.

We have looked at both the positives and the negatives of the growing self-help movement. In a vein similar to the field of psychotherapy, it has the potential for abuses as well as for great benefits. We have also examined the numerous avenues through which professionals and self-helpers can interact collaboratively. We believe that collaboration conducted in a true mutually cooperative spirit can hold many benefits for both the professional and self-help communities.

REFERENCES

Borman, L.D. (1986). Self-help/mutual aid groups: Strategies for prevention. In H.M. Raff (Ed.), *Directory of self help mutual aid groups* (pp. 1–7). Chicago: The Self-Help Center.

Brownell, K.D., Marlatt, G.A., Lichtenstein, E., & Wilson, G.T. (1986). Understanding and preventing relapse. *American Psychologist, 41*(7), 765–782.

Chutis, L. (1983). Special roles of mental health professionals in self-help group development. In R. Hess & J. Hermalin (Eds.), *Innovations in prevention* (pp. 65–73). New York: Haworth Press.

Gartner, A., & Reissman F. (1977). *Self-help in the human services.* San Francisco: Jossey-Bass.

Gartner, A.J., & Reissman, F. (1982). Self-help and mental health. *Hospital and Community Psychiatry, 33*(8), 631–635.

Gartner, A.J., & Reissman, F. (1984). *The self-help revolution.* New York: Human Sciences Press.

Gottlieb, B.H. (1983). Opportunities for collaboration with informal support systems. In S. Cooper & W.F. Hodges (Eds.), *The mental health consultation field* (pp. 181–203). New York: Human Sciences Press.

Hedrick, H.L. (1985). Expanded roles in holistic prevention for allied health professionals. *Journal of Allied Health, 14*(4), 455–461.

Jason, L.A. (1985). Using the media to foster self-help groups. *Professional Psychology: Research and Practice, 16*(3), 455–464.

Jason, L.A., Goodman, D., Thomas, N., Iacono, G., Tabon, D., & Todd-Baxter, A. (1988b). Clergy's knowledge of self-help groups in a large metropolitan area. *Journal of Psychology and Theology, 16,* 34–40.

Jason, L.A., Tabon, D., Tait, E., Iacono, G., Goodman, D., Watkins-Farrell, P., & Huggins, G. (1988a). The emergence of the Inner City Self-Help Center. *Journal of Community Psychology, 16,* 287–295.

Katz, A. (1984). Self-help groups: An international perspective. In A. Gartner & F. Riessman (Eds.), *The self-help revolution* (pp. 233–242). New York: Human Sciences Press.

Lavoie, F. (1984). Action research: A new model of interaction between the professional and self-help groups. In A. Gartner & F. Riessman (Eds.), *The self-help revolution* (pp. 173–182). New York: Human Sciences Press.

Levy, L.H. (1976). Self-help groups: Types and psychological processes. *The Journal of Applied Behavioral Science, 12,* 310–322.

Levy, L.H. (1978). Self-help groups viewed by mental health professionals: A survey and comments. *American Journal of Community Psychology, 6*(4), 305–313.

Rappaport, J., Seidman, E., Toro, P.A., McFadden, L.S., Reischl, T.M., Roberts, L.J., Salem, D.A., Stein, C.H., & Zimmerman, M.A. (1985). Collaborative research with a mutual help organization. *Social Policy, 15,* 12–24.

Riessman, F. (1985). New dimensions in self-help. *Social Policy, 15,* 2–4.

Spiegel, D. (1982). Self-help and mutual-support groups: A synthesis of the recent literature. In D.E. Biegel & A.J. Naparstek (Eds.), *Community support systems and mental health: Practice, policy, and research* (pp. 98–117). New York: Springer Publishing.

Toro, P.A., Reischl, T.M., Zimmerman, M.A., Rappaport, J., Seidman, E., Luke, D.A., & Roberts, L.J. (1986). *The impact of professional involvement on social climate and behavior in mutual help groups.* Unpublished manuscript.

Toseland, R.W., & Hacker, L. (1985). Social workers' use of self-help groups as a resource for clients. *Social Work, 30*(3), 232–237.

26

PROFESSIONAL SPECIALIZATION: GROUP PSYCHOTHERAPY

Max Rosenbaum, Ph.D.

The idea of developing skills in group therapy is often attractive to the clinician. Generally, the therapist will make more money by working with groups of patients—but will work much harder than in the practice of individual therapy. Any group therapist who leaves a group session refreshed and ebullient has not been doing his or her job. Group therapy is draining and demands a lot of the therapist. On the other hand, it is enormously challenging and emotionally gratifying. It challenges the therapist because it enables the professional to reach a larger patient population. It gratifies the idealism that should have been part of the attraction to clinical practice. The therapist is able to see more patients, and the individual patient, during his or her growth, is able to have a positive effect on a network of family and friends. However, group therapists must be clear as to the structure and practice of group therapy lest they become discouraged and give it up. In the following, I discuss important factors concerning group treatment and the patient–therapist relationship.

The treatment of emotionally troubled patients in groups is now an accepted part of psychotherapy. Since World War II, in the United States, as well as in many other countries, shortages of mental-health personnel have intensified the effort to find economical and shorter forms of psychotherapy. After the war, because of the limited availability of psychiatrists, psychologists, social workers, and nurses were encouraged to become skilled in group psychotherapy. Psychologists, because of their research training, studied group processes. Social workers extended the concepts of group psychotherapy to the treatment of married couples and families. Nurses began to introduce group techniques into general hospitals. Later, pastoral counselors began to train in group psychotherapy and became active in bringing group approaches to many religious communities. They then set up clinics and counseling centers as extensions of religious settings. Currently, there are many disciplines involved in the practice of group psychotherapy and there is a great deal of cross-fertilization as each of the mental-health disciplines brings to the field a different point of view—one that is not wedded to the traditional medical view of pathology and the overconcern with pathology in psychiatry. If there is one obvious stress in group psychotherapy in any of the mental-health disciplines, it is the stress on what is right with people as opposed to what is wrong.

A more basic appeal of group psychotherapy relates to what is happening in the American culture, as well as many other cultures of the world. As the traditional networks of human relationships have been dissolved with the tremendous mobility of the American population, there has been an increase in the loneliness of many people and a growing sense of isolation. Large urban settings reinforce the sense of loneliness. A positive factor in the urban setting is that the anonymity of the individual makes the idea of group treatment less threatening as there is much less chance that the person will meet someone he or she already knows. Resistance to group treatment becomes intensified in more rural and less sparsely settled areas where people have much contact outside of the group.

The methods of group psychotherapy are suitable for adults, adolescents, children, and the elderly. In addition, the small, interacting, nontherapeutic group is effective in many different settings. It often serves to enhance communication, to lessen rivalries, to help to establish a more equitable distribution of workload and responsibilities, and to help group participants join together to work toward a particular institution's goal. The trained group psychotherapist, while not working to achieve a psychotherapeutic result, can by virtue of training aid in the effective functioning of people in educational settings. It is important to remember that group psychotherapy, and an extension of its techniques, enables the practitioner to use skills in all types of settings, with all age groups, and with all types of emotional distress. If the therapist who leads the group is not properly trained and experienced, group treatment will not be effective, the patients will not benefit, and the therapist will become disillusioned. It is important to differentiate between the desire of people to come together, which may be an admirable goal, and a group that is therapeutic in nature and focuses on personality and behavioral changes. Whatever the age group, and whether play therapy is used as with children, or activity therapy as with adolescents, or discussion as with adults, the essential characteristics of the therapy process remain the same.

There are settings in which the overeager therapist takes on a task without considering the milieu in which group psychotherapy is to be practiced. In institutional settings with homogeneous populations, the administrative staff often puts pressure on the psychotherapist to treat groups of people without proper consideration of the selection process. In certain settings, education, advice, suggestion, or some type of guidance is equated with psychotherapy. While all of these may help with an individual's emotional distress, they should not be confused with psychotherapy whose aim is to effect such changes within the personality structure, whatever the degree of changes. A woman in her 50s in the process of divorce, facing a single life after 27 years of marriage, is referred for group therapy. Actually, she is searching for a peer group with which to share her fears about being single, and while her difficulty in facing her new life situation should be explored, she may be unwilling to move to any level other than a supportive hand-holding experience. The referral source, her family physician, although well meaning, intends for this patient to use the group as a socializing experience. This admirable goal may have nothing to do with the goals of the group psychotherapist. The group setting is often seen as a panacea for whatever ails the distressed individual. An executive who is fired from a job without adequate outplacement may need job counseling, but this is not group psychotherapy. If the discharge is related to the person's inability to relate to other workers, that is an entirely different matter. But if industry decides on a retrenchment in personnel and the executive is a victim of economics, we are in an area that is *not* group psychotherapy.

Some practitioners, in an effort to expand the base of professional referrals, serve as consultants to industry—which may or may not result in referrals. Unions are often suspicious as to the loyalty of the professional who is paid by industry. In some situations, the chief executive officer insists upon the right to get feedback from the professional who is paid as a consultant and is counseling employees. It is a very thin line that must be carefully negotiated. My experience has been to maintain a professional contact outside of the industrial setting. If one is employed as a consultant, it is more prudent to refer to other professionals so that there is no pressure to report to the executive level of the company that pays the consulting fee. Many industries employ social workers in what is called employee assistance programs (EAPs). These workers are often sources of referrals, but they may request feedback that is more in the industry's interest than in that of the employee. Obviously, if an employee has a tendency to commit arson and is working in a chemical plant, this is a matter of community concern. But how much can be shared with the referring EAP worker is questionable. If the employee made direct contact with the professional, it is unethical to reveal confidences. There are many employees who are conflicted about going to a referral source that has contact with an EAP program. This is the downside of maintaining contact with an industry referral source.

None of what I have described is intended to downgrade the idea of professional consultation and referral in industrial settings where employees are experiencing personal problems that may impair satisfactory work performance. My own experience is that EAP professionals try to do counseling in-house. While it is often stressed that records are treated with complete confidentiality and do not become part of the employee's personnel file, only long-term experience will prove whether EAP programs have an autonomy within the industrial setting that pays for the service. Again, my own experience has been that I have been called upon when the situation has become so deteriorated that more expert and experienced help is required.

I have stressed the importance of the psychotherapist defining what kind of population is to be worked with in a professional practice lest the referral source become disillusioned with the group psychotherapy. The very word *group* often sets off a chain of events where the referral source has a distorted idea of group psychotherapy and confuses it with a socialization experience. This may happen when a psychotherapist who practices individual treatment looks for a setting in which the patient can meet other people. The clinician who is developing a referral network is often unwilling to turn away referrals and so accepts a patient for group treatment who is really seeking socialization. While there are controversies as to which patients are acceptable for group therapy, my own experience over many years of practice has taught me to be less bound by diagnostic formulations and more open to meeting with the new patient and getting a sense of what the patient is looking for in psychotherapy. In this way, there is an openness about the first meeting with the patient and the clinician acquires enough data that an accurate assessment can be made as to the suitability of group psychotherapy for the patient. There are, as a result of the consultation, enough data to report back to the referral source if group treatment is not appropriate. In the development of a professional practice, the referral source becomes clear as to which patients may be appropriate for group treatment, and when in doubt may encourage the patient to accept the idea of a consultation in order to ascertain group suitability. This must be handled with sensitivity since every patient will react to the group psychotherapist's first consultation as a screening device. If the patient is told that he or she is not suitable for the group, the patient may experience rejection, related possibly to earlier experiences of being rejected. Some patients react with eagerness to the idea of a group, but this is a rare situation. For the most part, although patients express a desire for group treatment, they react to placement in a group as a rejection by the therapist, largely because they feel that the therapist is to be shared with other patients—a recreation of sharing the parent with other siblings.

A patient, no matter how eager to begin, is not ready for the group after the initial consultation. This has to be clarified for both the patient and the referral source, especially if the referral source is a practitioner who has worked with the patient in individual therapy. Some group therapists believe that you can begin a group "cold," but that is undesirable. A group therapist should see a patient at least four to six times to establish a relationship and set the therapeutic climate in motion. Some psychotherapists rely largely on diagnostic criteria and deemphasize preparation. Others suggest a trial period, a kind of test prescription. I do not agree with either of these approaches. Diagnosis may be more a function of the therapist's need to categorize the patient. A trial period leaves the door open for a speedy departure and encourages the prospective patient to believe that "this isn't what I need."

Unlike the individual therapist, the group therapist's intent is to prepare the patient for a group. Everything that is done in the individual meetings is in preparation for the therapy group. The patient, prepared for a confidential personal interview, has been failed by the original family. Even if patients know this, they have not fully accepted the trauma. If the original group—the family—has failed the patient, why should the patient accept the idea of a therapy group and face the possibility of a repetition of past hurts and traumas? Some patients, referred for group therapy, feel that they have been rejected by the original referring therapist. They are embittered and bring the anger to the group therapist. Many secretly hope for a one-to-one relationship with the therapist. On occasion the group therapist is overenthusiastic about group treatment so that the patient comes to believe that it is a panacea for living and a refuge from whatever ails the world at large. Sometimes the patient, almost in a spirit of resignation, will state, "I'll join a group because I need friends badly," or "The group will teach me how to live better." These are worthwhile desires but the patient is giving the group a social purpose and denying the full meaning of the group and its therapeutic possibilities. The type of resigned group acceptance that has been described always proves to be an obstacle to group treatment.

Many patients consider a recommendation for group therapy as settling for second best. No matter what they have been told by others about the efficacy of such treatment, they fear a loss of individuality in the group and believe that only the omnipotent and magical therapist can effect a cure. Often a patient will say when a group is suggested: "What can they do for me, these people? They are as screwed up as I am." But because the group therapist believes in the group, there is no straying from the presentation of the group as an important curative force. This is the message that the patient comes to believe. If the therapist is skeptical, the patient will be doubtful and resistant in group treatment.

Each patient, no matter how much individual therapy he or she has had, needs individual preparation with the group therapist. In hospital settings, patients are arbitrarily assigned to groups for therapy. In private practice, the patient must have a transference pattern develop where there is belief in the group therapist, even if the belief is minimal.

While I have noted the minimum amount of time necessary to set up a therapeutic attitude, there is no stipulated time set for each patient before group entry. Some patients may be seen intensively for 10 meetings over a space of three weeks. Others may have to be seen weekly or several times a week for a year. Those patients who have been referred for group treatment as a socializing experience generally lack sufficient motivation for intensive work. They are often resentful of themselves and others. If three of these people are placed in a group by a novice group therapist, all present will become discouraged. Both patient and group therapist may give up the group method. It is unrealistic to suggest that a fixed schedule of visits will be effective for the preparation of the patient. Different patients evoke different responses in the therapist. Current research has validated the importance of the resonance between therapist and patient (Strupp & Binder, 1984). This resonance is even more critical when the patient is being prepared for a group as there will be no further individual visits after the patient has entered the group.

Some therapists routinely practice combined therapy, where the patient is seen both individually and in group treatment. Patients with fragile ego structures may need the routine visits with the therapist on an individual basis, but many therapists have found that this practice dilutes the intensity of the group experience as the patient feels that significant material can be saved for individual meetings and not shared with the group. Sometimes the use of combined therapy is more to alleviate the anxiety of the therapist who is concerned about maintaining a one-to-one relationship. The therapist may not be fully convinced of the effectiveness of group therapy. Along the same lines, some therapists will only work with patients after the patients have undergone psychological testing. While diagnostic tests may be helpful in some instances, they are rarely helpful in predicting group participation, behavior, and outcome. What the tests do is set up a stress situation where the patient's cooperation, interest, or compliance may give clues as to what his or her group participation will be like. The patient who is detached during the psychological testing procedure may be the same during the group. But here, again, the stimulus of other group members may elicit responses that are not to be found when one examines test results.

Whatever the referral source, the first step in work with the patient is history taking, diagnosis and prognosis, and determination of group suitability. The novice group therapist, it is hoped, has prepared the referral source for the first steps that will be taken with the patient during the first consultation. During that initial consultation, if the therapist is satisfied that the patient may be suitable for a group, the transference, which is dormant, will be activated. Patients perceive therapists as parent figures or significant adults, and if the referral source has been enthusiastic about the group therapist, the positive transference will be brought to the initial consultation in spite of the patient's fears. It is during the first visits that the therapist communicates an interest and concern that inspire in the patient a feeling that the therapist is an ally. This has been described by some workers as the therapeutic alliance. But whatever the description, the patient's knowledge that the group therapist is truly concerned will enable the patient to sustain entry into the group although experiencing fear or a desire to flee. It is during the preparatory phase that patients often become resistant and noncooperative. Patients may return to the original referral source and complain about the group therapist. There are some patients who appear to move easily into the group, but these often prove to be compliant patients who hope to please the group therapist and so become the preferred patients.

After the therapist and patient agree that group therapy is appropriate, the therapist may have second thoughts about the wisdom of the clinical decision. The patient may begin to exhibit behavior that would contradict immediate group placement. An example of such behavior is acute anxiety, where the group is expected to be a sounding board without any feedback or interaction. For the most part, this behavior is resistance to group treatment and a desire to maintain the one-to-one-relationship. The patient may request detailed information about other group members but all these requests should be denied with the simple comment: "I don't want to color your perceptions. I will not tell group members in advance about you and will not tell you about group members. It will begin as a new experience for all concerned." The new patient *is* told that the group is not similar to other groups that exist in society—that there is no exact way to believe and that the patient is to enter the group and be whatever he or she is. The patient is always reminded that the group will benefit all its members and that regular attendance and participation are critical if the therapy is to be effective.

The issue of regular attendance and participation is directly related to the payment that the therapist intends to receive but there is a form of emotional payment that is rarely noted by practicing clinicians. This payment is the gratification of working with another human being during a growth process. In individual therapy, certain concessions may be made concerning time and scheduling of appointments. Both therapist and patient have some latitude, such as rescheduling an appointment or increasing the frequency of visits if the patient has to leave therapy for reasons not related to resistance. But once the group psychotherapist commits to a scheduled time and place for group meetings, there is no possibility of changing the schedule without disturbing other group members. The patient is responsible for the payment of the fee whether or not he or she attends, which may lead to an "empty chair" group where patients make the financial commitment but simply do not show up for meetings. The reasons for absence often sound reasonable, and since the group therapist is reimbursed whether or not the patient is present, there is a tendency to go along with the resistance and not to question what is going on. Other group members notice this very quickly and the group begins to lose its effectiveness. Through years of practice, I have never felt comfortable with accepting a payment for an absence that may mask resistance. I request the patient to explain any absence from the group. Sometimes, such absences are unavoidable and I do not feel comfortable being paid for a missed group meeting. Other therapists feel that time has been put aside for the meeting and the session should be paid for whatever the reason. I accept this as a valid procedure, but it is not right for me; each group therapist will have to make that policy decision. I do make it very clear that as group therapist, I have set aside the time and expect to be reimbursed. While the resistance mechanisms are not encouraged, I do note that there may be circumstances where the patient will have to be absent, and these absences will be discussed as part of therapy.

What has been described applies to adult patients. When the patient population is composed of children or adolescents, the group therapist will have to set a standard fee payment schedule regardless of the child or adolescent's attendance. There are simply too many conceivable excuses when one works with children and adolescents — from common childhood diseases to participating in basketball practice. It is important that the group therapist not collude with resistance, but it is equally important that the professional be adequately reimbursed for scheduling a therapy group.

The administration of a therapy group is difficult, and generally quite tedious as well as frustrating. Most professionals, when they have to charge for a professional service, become very anxious. If the therapist is inexperienced and not quite certain as to the value of the therapy, or is ambivalent about his or her own competency, the question of billing becomes intertwined with that of the therapist's self-worth. When the therapist becomes too directive or controlling about fees and administration, the patient senses a loss of empathy and may withdraw from therapy. The therapist does set the time and place for meeting. Experience has indicated that once a time is set, it is difficult to change it. The patient, often feeling unworthy, is asked to join a therapy group, and at the same time is asked to give of himself or herself by the payment of money. In individual therapy, the payment of the fee and its dynamic meaning are often avoided by sending monthly statements through the mail or having a secretary handle the billing. In the group, patients very quickly discuss the fee and what each is paying. The patient tests the therapist and equates the fee with love. A question frequently asked by the patients is: "Would you see me if I could not pay you?" The patient rarely understands that it is the time that is being paid for, not the interest and concern the therapist brings to the meeting. And even when it is explained, the distrustful patient is not sure.

The fee for group psychotherapy is dictated by the community setting and finances of each patient, as well as by the patient's earning capacity. The group therapist must be clear that group therapy is not second-best treatment. The clear decision is then made as to what the time spent with a group of patients is worth to the therapist. If the therapist spends an hour and a half and wants to be reimbursed $80, he or she may decide to divide the $80 by the six patients in the group, a little more than $13 per patient. Or the therapist may feel that work with a group is more difficult and want to be reimbursed $90. In this case, each group member would pay $15. Since a very active and involved group may run a little longer, or group members may want to speak with the therapist after the session, it is wiser to set aside two hours. The therapist then calculates what each patient is to pay proportionately for the group meeting. Almost without exception, group members will calculate what the group therapist is earning, and may express resentment toward the "exorbitantly paid" group leader. None of these comments are to be deflected but patients are to be encouraged to express resentment, something that is rarely done in individual therapy where a patient does not have the support of other group members. It is easier for the group therapist to charge each group member the same fee. This limits rivalries and objections, an important point as an inexperienced group psychotherapist can feel overwhelmed by the pressure and criticism of group members, especially if the therapist feels unsure of what is going on. It is upsetting for a novice group therapist to be faced with the combined anger of group members who attack the therapist for supposed avarice and greed. All such attacks should be explored but the meetings should not disintegrate into a discussion of psychotherapy economics. If the patient's resentments toward group treatment have been dealt with in the preparatory individual sessions, no matter how briefly, the issue of payment will have come up early in therapy. To repeat, the issue of fee must always be addressed psychodynamically.

After some time has passed and the group therapist forms a second group, the idea of graduated fees is conceivable. Or the group therapist may decide to raise the fee (this is generally done with difficulty), or waive or lower fees. Some of my foreign colleagues, practicing in countries where there is rampant inflation, have grown accustomed to establishing fees based on an inflation index. In the individual preparatory sessions, the patient may be told that there are group members who pay more or less, depending on their finances. It is not necessary to go into detail as to how the therapist arrives at the fee structure, but it is important that the therapist be clear as to what the fee is and how it is to be collected. Some therapists mail billing statements and others distribute them to patients, either monthly, weekly, or at the end of each group meeting. Working-class patients prefer to pay weekly or at the end of a session. Some therapists encourage patients to leave payment on the therapist's desk; others ask that payment be made directly. The more personal the payment, the more important is the therapy for both patient and therapist. The patient is often uneasy about paying the therapist for the professional service. The impersonal payment keeps the aura of benign charity or a benign parent and perpetuates an unreal transaction. Many therapists, unsure of their worth, mail bills or turn the task over to a secretary or receptionist, as if often done in a clinic. The fact is that the therapist must earn a living and is supported by the patients' payments. This payment does not detract from the therapist's commitment. The patient is reacted to as someone who pays for a service, not as an object of pity or charity. If one handles fee payment in an indirect manner, the therapeutic process will become confused, and will ultimately strengthen the patient's resistance to change. Direct payment is authentic and validates the patient as a person.

To repeat, the practice of group psychotherapy in private practice is financially rewarding. But unless group therapists believe in the process, a process in which they are asked to expend more of themselves, they are not justified in making more money. Because the group therapist earns more money working with a group of patients, there are occasions where patients feel that they may ask for a waiver of the fee or a delay in payment. The rationale of the patient is clear — the therapist is able to extend this privilege. Essentially, as in individual therapy, the therapist is asked to be a bank and to wait for payment of the money owed. Unlike with individual therapy, the money owed may mount up rather quickly. One senior therapist, who prided himself on his liberal political views, permitted group members to owe him over a period of time. When he attempted to collect payment, he encountered enormous resistance. The position of the patients was that this psychiatrist, by his acceptance of their behavior, had encouraged them to become indebted, and now they were angry and resistant to payment. I would conclude from this and similar experiences that, like the parent who must set limits in child rearing, the group therapist must also be clear as to the responsibilities of leadership.

REFERRALS

Ultimately, the best referral source is the ex-patient who has had a satisfactory result. There is no referral source that is better than the "satisfied customer." Many therapists keep in contact with ex-patients, either at holiday time with greeting cards or through a newsletter. Patients like to be informed as to what the "doctor" is doing in his or her professional life, and ex-patients are very interested, and often quite excited, when they hear or read about some professional activity of the person who once treated them. In smaller communities, the professional should belong to community groups and establish high visibility. Referrals often come from sources that are totally unexpected. Recently, I was contacted by a letter carrier who, in delivering my mail, realized that I am a mental-health professional and decided to ask me for a consultation. The local pharmacy, even in an age of supermarket drug stores, is in constant contact with the community and is an excellent source of referrals.

The practice of group psychotherapy is one part of the therapist's skills. It is important that while the skill is recognized, the group therapist is not seen by the referral community as exclusively engaged in the practice of group therapy. This type of perception will lead to a very unbalanced practice and deny the group therapist the experiences of working with individuals, couples, and families. While special expertise in working with groups should be publicized, it should not be stated as an exclusive skill.

Speculations about the future of group psychotherapy in the United States are mixed. Because of the plethora of minimally trained people who tout themselves as experts in group treatment, carefully trained group psychotherapists should be careful to delineate their skills and training. A listing simply as practicing group psychotherapy is very likely to cast the practitioner with those people who are self-described psychotherapists. It is important to ally oneself early in a professional career with the existing professional organization(s) that require standards of proficiency and competency. Such membership is of importance both to the patient and to the referral source.

It is helpful in the building of a practice to speak to different professional groups that are part of the health professions. In this way, people will come to recognize the particular skill of the practitioner, which is valuable as long as it is not perceived as an exclusive skill.

When the professional who practices group psychotherapy becomes visible to colleagues from different geographic areas, it is a form of "networking." Other professionals get to know you personally, have a sense of what you do and who you are, and have more confidence in making a referral rather than consulting a directory of qualified professionals. Two major aspects of a professional's background that influence the consumer—in this case, the patient—are compassion—Do you show understanding and concern for the person in distress?—and whether there is a "fit" between patient and therapist. Colleagues, like the consumer patient, will also note the compassion and compatibility of a practitioner to whom they want to refer. Attendance at professional meetings not only serves to keep clinical skills active and up to date, but also maintains the network of referrals from colleagues.

Training in group psychotherapy is now available in many countries. Most local societies offer supplementary training and invite senior professionals to lecture to the society membership. There are regional training institutes, and postdoctoral university programs offer group therapy training. The American Group Psychotherapy Association holds a brief training institute before its annual conference for those people who want additional training. Institutes have also been sponsored by the International Association for Group Psychotherapy. Such programs afford the opportunity to witness different types of group psychotherapy as practiced in different parts of the world. It is very important that practicing professionals keep abreast of what is going on in group psychotherapy, and national and international conferences are good places in which to learn and to share clinical experiences.

Over the past decade, there has been a lack of enthusiasm in the United States concerning the practice of group psychotherapy, but this does not appear to be the case in Latin America or Europe. It is conceivable that the too easy grouping of individuals to discuss emotional problems, and the fact that groups are often led by people with minimal training, has disenchanted many referral sources. However, the trained professional should not fear this situation, but rather regard it as a challenge.

Many group psychotherapists, as they practice, want to expand their skills. Often they move into the study and practice of family therapy. Since the family is the original group, this makes sense, and is, in addition, a source of emotional gratification to the psychotherapist.

REFERENCES

Azima, F.J.C., & Richmond, L. (1986). *Adolescents in groups.* Madison, CT: International Universities Press.

Mullan, H., & Rosenbaum, M. (1982). *Group psychotherapy: Theory and practice* (rev. ed.). New York: Free Press.

Riester, A.E., & Kraft, I.A. (1987). *Child group psychotherapy: Future tense.* Madison, CT: International Universities Press.

Rosenbaum, M. (1982). *Ethics and values in psychotherapy.* New York: Free Press.

Rosenbaum, M. & Berger, M.M. (1982). *Group psychotherapy and group function* (rev. ed.). New York: Basic Books.

Rosenbaum, M., & Snadowsky, A. (1976). *The intensive group experience.* New York: Free Press.

Strupp, H., & Binder, J. (1984). *Psychotherapy in a new key.* New York: Basic Books.

C H A P T E R
27

EXPANSION THROUGH MOVEMENTS:
New Opportunities for Private Practice in Hospitals and Health-Care Settings

Michael F. Enright, Ph.D.

P sychologists and other mental-health professionals have enjoyed increased freedom and autonomy over the past two decades as private practitioners of psychological care. Recent surveys suggest that this trend is continuing and that many mental-health professionals see private practice as the most desirable modality (Tyron, 1983). Changes in both federal law and the willingness nationally on the part of the insurance industry to underwrite the cost of mental-health service have signaled a need for private practitioners to expand their referral base to ensure viability in the changing economy. Clearly, if private mental-health practitioners ignore the shifts in the marketplace, their personal incomes are likely to decrease.

The following fictitious story is an example of what is happening across the country. Dr. Osborne, a 45-year-old psychologist in private practice in New York City, has, for some years, been enjoying a relatively steady rate of referrals for psychotherapy. He sees his patients two to three times a week and has enjoyed the luxury of being able to turn away an occasional patient because his schedule is too full. Over the past six months, however, Dr. Osborne has noticed that he has been receiving fewer and fewer referrals. His concern has grown as he has become aware that he had first two, and then four, and now six free hours during the week, and that his accounts receivable have dropped off markedly for the first time since he became a private practitioner. Forced to investigate the cause of this change in his practice, Dr. Osborne has discovered that two private psychiatiric hospitals have opened their doors within a 10-block radius of his office. He further discovers that the hospitals refer only to members of their medical staff and are involved in a competitive marketing policy.

This chapter will focus on the current opportunities open to psychologists in private practice, in hospitals, and in health care. Concurrently, it is presented as a model for clinical social workers, nurse practitioners, and other specialty-trained mental-health professionals. The need for psychologists in hosptials and health care comes at an opportune time in the profession. The number of health care providers in psychology more than doubled between 1974 and 1985 (Dorken, Stapp, & Vanden Bos, 1986). There are a variety of emerging trends in heath-care reimbursement that proved bountiful opportunities for private mental health-care practitioners. Included in these are the development of the individual provider association (IPAs), joint partnership venture under elaborate and creative corporate sturctures, affiliation with employee assistance programs (EAPs), and the emerging area of hospital practice.

Traditionally, psychologists have been involved in the practice of delivering service in hospital settings. Hospitals and health clinics continue to be the site of internship training for the majority of applied psychologists (Eggert, Laughlin, Hutell, et al., 1987). As a result of recent profound changes in American medicine, psycholgists can take advantage of a variety of new and exciting opportunities in hospitals and health care. These changes have come about, ironically, because of the success enjoyed by medical practitioners over the past 20–30 years. Unfortunately, this success has not eluded the attention of several sectors of American society. The first group interested in the success of modern medicine represents "for profit" business interests. The early 1970s heralded a tremedous growth in health for profit and changed the course of American medicine in its wake. The second group that has decided to cash in on the success of American medicine comprises trial lawyers, who see wealthy physicians and large malpractice insurance policies as fertile ground for personal-injury awards. Because of the current medico-legal environment, hospitals no longer can afford to ignore the psychological and emotional needs of their pateints. Keernan, Pasnau, and Richardson (1981) reported a $900,000 settlement paid by a hosptial that overlooked the psychological and neurological needs of patients seen in the emergency room. In this increasingly litigious health-care environment, hospital administrators are becoming more aware of the emotional and psychological needs of the patients being served in their facilities.

As the cost of health care reached 11 percent of the Gross National Product in the early 1980s, the federal government acted to control these costs. Although it was aimed at cost control, this was the most far-reaching action curtailing medical success. Finally, the most profound change accompanying the monetary success of medical practitioners may be that many physicians have lost touch with the reason they chose to go into medicine in the first place, and they now run their practices with the same cold aloofness used in making business decisions. Increasingly, the focus of medicine is on expensive technical procedures, sometimes at the cost of understanding the psychological needs and fears of the people being treated. Consider the following statement by Ransom Arthur (1985), an M.D.:

> The modern demands for managerial efficency and maximally profitable use of resources, regulatory pressure with its insistence on standardized procedures, and the sheer weight of technological equipment with its own implied imperative all work to change the mood of the traditional medical consultation and to limit severely the time for conversation with the patient. It will be very hard for physicians to break through these obstacles and have extended initmate converasations with even a few patients. Of course, in some rural practices and among those who can afford truly personalized care, open communications will continue. People in large ciites who are enrolled in full scale medical care organizations may have to learn to accept care that is standardized and instrumentally correct but, at the very least, impersonal. Perhaps the public will rebel against this approach...it may be that trust between physician and the patient will be irrelevant to life in the 21st century society. (p. 113)

As medical technology is successful in eliminating the most dreaded and contagious diseases by treatment and prevention, modern medicine has increasingly concerned itself with trauma, sports injuries, and stress-related illnesses. This shift away from an expertise in the treatment and contol of infectious diseases toward understanding the patient's emotional and psycholgical response to shock and injury, motivation for recovery, and habit responses places psychology and psychological treatment at the forefront of medical practice (Richards, 1987). This development has occurred at a time when many leaders in psychiatry have embraced a biological model for understanding human behavior and relinquished their posture of expertise in psycholgical understanding of human health.

Because artificial barriers exist in many states and jurisdictions that prohibit nonmedical health-care providers from having full medical staff privileges, legislation has been enacted in California and Georgia that guarantees psychologists access to the medical staff of hospitals as full and equal participants. Further, recent action taken by the District of Columbia has given additional recognition to psychologists and other nonmedical health-care providers as independent health-care agents, prohibiting hospitals from restricting mental-health practice in their facilities or restricting membership on the medical staff (Tanney, 1983).

HISTORICAL PERSPECTIVE

In the early part of this century, psychologists began applying the principles of psychological theory to the task of alleviating the suffering of patients. The interface for this application of theoretical constructs was the hospital. In the 1920s and 1930s, psychologists began taking on the role of psychological diagnostician, in both public mental-health facilites and private psychiatric hospitals. It was in this context that psychologist's expertise in the assessment of individual psychopathology came to be respected and requested by those members of the medical community responsible for the treatment of mental illness.

Psychologists took a large step forward during World War II, moving out of the limited position of diagnostician and into the role of psychotherapeutic agent. This was the first time that non-psychiatrically trained physicians were given access to psychological practitioners on a large scale. As primary-care physicians and surgeons were faced with the overwhemlming task of meeting the psycholgocal needs of the war casualties, psychologists were asked not only to assess pathology, but also to begin to develop interventions based on sound psycholgical principles for military personnel suffering from "shell shock" and post traumatic distress. After the war, many of these psychologists remained in the Veterans' Administration (VA) to develop what became the core of clinical training through the VA hospitals. The VA health-care system continues to be on the leading edge of psycholgy's emergence as an autonomous health-care profession and has presented innovative models for the delivery of psycholgical services outside of the traditional psychiatirc ward. (Schenkenberg, Petersen, Wood, et al. 1981).

Since the late 1950s, psychologists have demostrated their desire to act independently by developing private practices on a fee-for-service basis. Many psychologists set up private practice on a part-time basis to complement their work as either hospital employees, clinical professors in academic settings, or adminstrators in community mental-health and other social programs, and later expanded their hours to full-time private practice.

The fictitious example of Dr. Arnold Isaacson of Pacific Palisades, Calif., is typical of a private practitioner in the 1960s. Dr. Isaacson, who held an academic position at the University of California at Los Angeles as a clinical psychology faculty member, began to see patients privately as a way to continue having access to clinical practice with the intent of enhancing his ability to teach. However, after several years, finding that the rewards of private practice were more desirable than those in the university, he became a full-time practitioner in solo practice with an office attached to his home. Dr. Isaacson saw eight patients a day and took Thursday afternoons off to continue to lecture at the university. He had no experience with providing services in any environment outside of his office and enjoyed a relatively trouble-free practice through the 1960s and into the 1970s. As freedom-of-choice legislation was passed, Dr. Isaacson noticed that having parity with psychiatrists in the outpatient arena increased his income initially, but soon his professional time became encumbered by the clerical demands of third-party payers. Finally, the aggravations and vicissitudes of the peer review system caused Dr. Isaacson to discontinue any involvement in assisting his patients in making insurance claims. To remain solvent, he found he had to join the staff of a nearby hospital and become part of a closed-panel preferred provider organization (PPO). Dr. Isaacson's story is an example of a successful practitioner who finds himself having to reevaluate the delivery of his services to meet the changes in the marketplace.

The last 30 years have had a profound effect on psycholgical practitioners. Psychologists have discovered that not only are they capable of taking the sole repsonsibility for treating those in their charge, but they also actually prefer to work without the supervision of an authority figure. Private practicing psychologists in outpatient settings find themsleves in circumstances not unlike that of surgeons, in which they must make critical decisions in what coud be life or death situations (and often with less control than the physician in the surgical theater). It is no surprise that psychologists in private practice come to a hospital ward expecting nothing less than full control and responsibility for the care of their patients and reject the artificial restraints placed on their practice by psychiatrists and other members of the medical community.

Psychologists are becoming increasingly intolerant of the parochial system that demads that they give over responsibility for the people in their care to physicians simply because a patient needs the restrictive, controlled, or specialized environment of a hospital. This breach in the continuity of care at a time when the patient is most vulnerable and in need of the continuing support of the primary therapist has caused many psycholgists to reconsider their nonaffiliation with a hospital. In fact, some psychologists have found themselves forced to refer to a psychiatrist when their patient is hospitalized. It is not uncommon for referring psychologists to find that they are allowed to see their patients only during visiting hours while they are in the hospital, or in some cases not at all. It is no wonder that many psychologists are exploring ways to secure a passport into the previously foreign territory of the hospital.

NEW HEALTH-CARE DELIVERY SYSTEMS

Recent changes in the way health care is delivered in the United States have both placed limitations on and created opportunities for the private practitioner. These changes have taken place in the private as well as public sectors and are at the center of an understanding of how a psychologist can effectively work in health-care institutions.

In the private sector, two changes in the delivery of health care—the health maintenance organization (HMO) and the PPO—make it imperative that psychologists have medical staff membership in order to take advantage of the opportunities available to them.

The develpment of HMOs has been viewed as anathema to private practice and psychologists since these organizations demand that psychologists assume the role of employees in a primarily medical corporate structure. Most HMOs are owned by either physician-dominated or physician-controlled corporations. In some of these business arrangements, medical staff members who work with the corporation are allowed to purchase shares in the corporation, after a probationary period, thereby gaining a voice in policy decisions. Most HMOs limit medical staff membership to physicians and prohibit psychologists from joining the staff. Without medical staff membership, psychologists are effectively barred from having a meaningful role in the organizations.

HMOs were created to promote health and, ostensibly, to reduce health-care costs. An HMO is a corporation established to put health-care facilities and personnel in locations accessible to subscribers. Subscribers pay premiums in return for health care when it is needed. The advantage to subscribers is that if they have regular checkups and expedient health care, they will avoid many of the more costly procedures resulting from neglect, and the inability to pay for preventive care. In the contract, however, subscribers forfeit the right to chose specific health-care providers and have no option whatsoever to choose a private practicing psychologist or mental-health-care professional. All health care in HMOs is directed through a physician "gatekeeper," who is charged with making the assessment and referral for consultation. Psychologists, social workers, and other specialty counselors are employed by the corporation and receive referrals only at the direction of the physician gatekeeper. Consequently, mental-health care in HMOs is necessarily short-term and goal oriented. Mental-health services are in-house, provided by employees, and rarely contracted out to private practitioners.

The other recently emerged private-sector program that has affected the viability of private practicing psychologists is the PPO. It is a panel of professional health-care providers who contract with an agency or agencies to provide health care at a given fee scale. This fee scale is often below the usual and customary charges in the community, region, or state. The theory behind the PPO is that it reduces health-care costs and has advantages for both providers and subscribers. It is advantageous to the providers because participation in the plan guarantees a large pool of patients, making up for the reduction in fees. It is advantageous to subscribers because it reduces the cost of health care. It is not, however, advantageous to any health-care provider who is not on the panel, since subscribers can only utitilze panel members for health-care services. PPO membership has been limited in many areas to medical staff members only. Psychologists have had limited success in setting up psychological PPOs. The established and growing PPOs are owned and operated by physician-dominated corporations. This model is problematic for psychologists and other health-care providers, not because it limits involvement to employees only, as in the HMO, but because organized medicine has worked to prohibit private practitioners who are not physicians from being included on the PPO panels.

There are several new generations of the PPO phenomenon, including the independent provider corporation (IPC), which is a corporation made up of one or mode medical staffs (once again excluding nonmedical staff members) developed to market the services of the IPC members and to bid for contracts with third-party payers; and the physician health organization (PHO), essentially created to do the same. The threat from HMOs and PPOs to private practitioners is growing. American Medical International (AMI), a large, for-profit health-care corporation, has developed many PPOs in selected hospitals across the country. Humana Hospitals have 800,000 enrolled in a PPO and expect to have four million enrollees by the year 1990 (Health Industrial Complex, 1986). In a 1983 survey, the California Hospital Association found that 30 percent of its 535 member hospitals had already contracted with or were in the process of developing, PPOs (Dorkin, Stapp, & Vander Bos, 1986). Clearly, medical staff membership is crucial to the survival of the private practitioner for inclusion on PPO panels and in contracting relationships with HMOs.

The current trend in American health care toward corporate competition and the develpment of HMOs and PPOs is also of concern to the medical community. Brant Mittler, M.D., a San Antonio, Texas, cardiologist and member of an alliance called Physicians Who Care, was quoted in the *Wall Street Journal* (Mittler, 1986) as saying, "We are worried that when doctors become hired hands in giant corporations, they will worry more about saving dollars than saving lives." The same article reported on a movement within the medical community to develp an organization called Independent Doctors of America, and another group entitled Committee to Save Private Patient Care, both aimed at fighting the trend of removing physicians from control of their practice. Perhaps physicians have more reason to worry in this regard than do private practicing psychologists. Until recently, only fee-for-service physicians could be full members of the American Medical Association. The trememdous revolution in the competition for the health-care dollar by private industry makes it easy to predict that by the turn of the century fewer than 25 percent of physicians will be in private practice.

The public sector has also taken action that has caused far-reaching changes in health care. The federal government is responsible for two of these changes. The first was the attempt by Congress to control the rising costs of health care in the Medicare program by developing the prospective payment program* through the change in the reimbursement process to diagnostically related groups (DRGs). The Congress chose to adopt the prospective payment program in the face of enormous health costs. Lynn May, past associate administrator of the Health Care Financing Administration, reported in 1982 that the total cost for Medicare and Medicaid in 1976 was $6 billion. The federal government was spending $6 billion a month only six years later, in 1982 (May, 1982). In the past, hospitals have been reimbursed for the cost of hospitalization based on the length of time the patient stayed in the hospital. With the change to DRGs, the hospitals are reimbursed solely according to the criteria established for the diagnosis. This means, for example, that if a person is hospitalized with a diagnosis that allows for 10 days of care and is only treated for eight days, the hospital actually stands to profit on the hospitalization. However, if the patient stays more than 10 days, then the hospital accumulates a greater debt with every day the patient remains hospitalized.

The second important development in the public sector occured when the Social Security Administration changed its regulations in 1984 to include psychologists as medical experts in the assessment of psychiatirc disabilities*. This change in Social Security policy marks a landmark in the assessment of the psychological functioning and well-being of millions of disabled citizens in this country. Early reports from psychologists who are medical advisors reveal a rather shocking profile of disabled citizens whose cases are up for appeal. Review of the records of the disabled suggests that many of thse patients were first seen by physicians in hospitals; their psychological and emotional needs were, in many cases, overlooked; and their conditions were treated either solely or primarily with medical interventions. The case studies of these patients show a developing pattern of failed medical and surgical intervention at the expense of psychological needs. Because hospitals are the initial point of contact for these patients, it is important that psychologists take the lead in early diagnosis and treatment of this high-risk group. A systematic research project has been suggested to explore the concern that many of these patients might never have been on the federal disability roles had their psychological needs been diagnosed and met early in their treatment.

FUTURE TRENDS

Private practitioners who stay abreast of the rapidly changing health-care delivery system not only ensure their viability, but also facilitate success in their practices.

Increasingly, hospitals are owned by large, for-profit (proprietary), health-care corporations. It can be estimated, if current trends continue, that by the turn of the century hospitals and health care in the United States will be dominated by 5 to 10 large health-care corporations. These corporations must be accountable to their investors and, therefore, must provide health care that is expedient and appropriate. The movement away from the dominant control of hospitals by the medical establishment to the corporation further opens up possibilities for psychologists in private practice. Innovative pscyhologists who have specific treatments programs are already beginning to contract with corporations in the management of pain and the control of unhealthy and self-defeating habits, such as smoking, overeating, and alcoholism. Psychological interventions are increasingly demanded in every area of health care, including, but not limited to, general hospitals, psychiatric hospitals, hospices, nursing homes, rehabilitation hospitals, chemical-dependency residency programs, institutions for the developmentally disabled, and out-patient clinics (both surgical and medical centers). In the hospital, psychologists are becoming more and more specialized. The most notable development in this area is the emergence of pediatric psychology, which is a combination of developmental, clinical, and medical psychology, and stands as a psychological specialty side by side with the medical specialty of pediatrics.

The psychologist of the future must be prepared to deal with large cor-porate entities on an individual and, more important, contractual level. Prac-titioners may find that only through affiliation with PPOs or other groups of practitioners will they be able to survive. Private practitioners have a choice of becoming partners with medical practitioners or being employed by them. Affiliation with medical practitioners will be extremely important in the future.

HOW TO ENHANCE YOUR PRACTICE

The change in payment for Medicare patients to the prospective payment program (which will likely be adopted by insurance companies) has motivated hospital administrators to make sure that hospitalized patients are treated and released expediently. This situation opens several opportunities for psychologists. Since hospitals are reimbursed for the number of patients rather than the number of patient days, psychologists who can make referrals to a hospital and fill hospital beds have been warmly received by hospital ad-ministrators. In this regard, the control of only one medical bed by a practi-tioner can mean having access to a sizable amount of money in real dollars. Another opportunity for psychologists is outside the psychiatric/psychological ward in the general hospital. Psychological consultations that assist hospital medical staffs and administrators in making accurate diagnoses save hospitals more expensive laboratory tests and technological procedures and are welcom-ed by hospital administrators, who stand to lose income from the limitations of the DRGs.

Since the early 1970s, organized psychiatry has been acutely aware of the need for psychological consultation on medical and surgical wards. In order to meet this need, psychiatrists have attempted to evolve from psychosomatic medicine to a subspecialty of consultation-liaison psychiatry. Several hospital-based centers in the United States have attempted to develp model consultation-liaison programs in psychiatry; the leaders in this movement are James Strain, M.D., at Mount Sinai Hospital in New York City, and Robert Pasnau, M.D., at the University of California at Los Angeles.

Interestingly, the success of psychiatrists working in a consultation-liaison model is questionable. The following is a quotation from the 1986 president of the American Psychiatric Association (Pasnau, 1982):

Consultation-liaison psychiatry is at the crossroads. In light of many apparently conflicting goals and pressures from within and outside psychiatry, consultation-liaison psychiatry can expect to continue to sputter along without firm financial support from the departments of psychiatry in the general hospital, whether it will lose its teaching emphasis and return to the old-fashioned consultation model, or be supplanted by behavioral medicine and lose its identity remain unanswered questions. If it meets the research, fiscal and political changes, finds a way to make peace with psychologists and other behavioral scientists, develops a close collaboration with nursing, continues to enjoy the support of departments of psychiatry, and transforms the consultation model into a more comprehensive consultation liaison model, the future of liaison psychiatry will be bright indeed. (p. 995).

From the vice-president of the American Psychiatric Association comes support of the fact that organized psychiatry is very much aware of the options available to psychologists in and around hospitals (Fink, 1986).

Two recent trends now make it more important than ever for psychiatrists to unify. The first is the explosion in the number of clinical psychologists, who have captured more and more of the available patients. The second is the dangerous trend toward giving psychologists hospital staff appointments with admission privileges. Under the formula that a psychologist plus a general physician equals a psychiatrist, psychologists can effectively intrude upon a hospital, the one area of psychiatry that up to now has been sacrosanct. (p. 816)

Psychologists who can work with primary-care physicians and surgeons to enhance the quality of hospital treatment and thereby reduce the number of patient days in the hospital will find growing opportunities and acceptance, not only on the part of hospital administrators, but by nonpsychiatrically trained physicians, as well.

The most formidable obstacle to the success of consultation-liaison psychiatry has been the difficulty of being reimbursed for psychiatric services. Consultation-liaison is expensive work because it demands that the practitioner visit the patient on the ward rather than waiting for the patient to come to the private office. Time must also be spent working with the treatment team, which consists of the attending physician, nursing staff, and other support personnel. Further, the practitioner must review the patient's chart and all other pertinent documents. Finally, the consultation-liaison practitioner must overcome the attitude in medicine and among third-party payers that medical procedures such as surgery, physical examinations, and laboratory investigations are more important than psychological assessment and care and, therefore, deserve higher payment than "talk treatment." Private psychologists entering the general hospital as consultation-liaison specialists must be aware of psychiatry's difficulties. These obstacles can be managed, and perhaps overcome, by following these guidelines:

1. Establish relationships in advance with nursing personnel to facilitate communication and teamwork.

2. Establish contracts with hospital administrations for consultation in specific area of service, (i.e., emergency service, pain management, surgical service, and so on.).

3. Make rounds at the same time as the attending physician to facilitate communication and joint decision making.

4. Educate and instruct attending physicians in appropriate referrals to reduce confusion and needlessly lost time.

5. Develop a team approach with the attending physician to reduce resistance on the part of the patient.

6. Identify all costs to the patient for services before proceeding, and receive informed consent from the patient.

7. Use Current Procdural Terminology codes (CPT-4) to reduce confusion with third-party payers, and clearly outline the nature of your involvement on the ward.

8. Identify specifically all bills to patients as being separate from the hospital bill and the bills of other medical providers.

There remains one final word of caution for practitioners interested in consultation-liaison work. It takes time to establish working professional relationships with attending physicians and nursing staffs in hospitals. Time spent in the initial phases of developing a relationship is best thought of as lost to the process; there is little chance of being reimbursed for this activity. Practitioners should be careful that they do not get caught up in "giving away" their valuable professional advice over the long term. At a recent continuing education workshop on hospital practice, one of the participants reported working for two years at no fee on a primary-care unit of the hospital with which she was affiliated. After checking with hospital personnel, she discovered that they had assumed she was charging the hospital for her time. Her apparent need to be helpful and her lack of familiarity with the above guidelines threatened her ability to continue as a liaison specialist. The involvement of nonphysicians in health care is not uniformly viewed as a threat by organized psychiatry. Some leaders in the psychiatric community have even looked forward to closer professional relationships. According to Pasnau (1982, p. 994): "Increasingly, clinical psychologists who have been trained along with psychiatric residents in consultation-liaison methods are finding professional satisfaction and careers in performing liaison activities in general hospital settings, together with psychiatrists in a collegial relationship."

Among the many unique opportunities for psychologists in health care in the 1980s have been those outside of the traditional setting in a major metropolitan area. There are 1401 small hospitals (with six to 49 beds each) in the United States, many of them in rural areas (American Hospital Association, 1986). These hospitals tend to be traditional general (or medical-surgical) hospitals with no psychiatric ward and, in many cases, no psychiatrist. Enright (1985) points out that the need for consultation on the emotional and psychological symptoms of patients in these hospitals can be greater than in large cities. Further, many of these hospitals act as first-line psychological receiving centers for the community and need qualified mental-health personnel. Because of a larger number of psychologists than psychiatrists in rural areas, and because many psychologists have been willing to move to such areas, affiliation with small hospitals is often available to them, and, in many cases, they are welcomed by their physician colleagues who are in need of psychological consultation. For example, in Wyoming there are approximately

100 licensed psychologist for a population of close to 400,000. There are, however, only a few psychiatrists. Wyoming is ranked 51st in the nation with 2.5 psychiatrists per 100,000 population (*Economic Fact Book*, 1983). There are 26 small hospitals in Wyoming that provide triage in emergency psychological intervention in the communities where they are located. Psychologists have developed positive relationships with community physicians, who are often interested in working with doctoral-level colleagues, and who are predisposed toward consulting psychologists. Part of this positive attitude may stem from the fact that they do not see psychologists as members of their profession and so do not feel threatened that they might attempt to compete for their patients.

Another area that presents an opportunity for private practitioners is in specialty hospitals. Psychologists across the country are finding a warm reception in women's hospitals, where they work with obstetricians and gynecologists in the care of infertility patients, the development and implementation of childbirth preparation classes, and the treatment of women who have various special needs related to pregnancy or sterility. Treating physicians, as well as nursing staffs, often respond positively to psychologists who can assist them in developing techniques and programs for meeting the needs of patients in this population. This opportunity obviously also exists in specialized facilities treating persons suffering chemical dependencies.

Another at-risk population that is in desperate need of psychological consultation is patients in nursing homes. As the mean age of the U.S. population gradually increases, specific treatments and services for geriatric patients are taking on a greater importance. Psychologists should take the initiative to clarify the appropriateness of psychological intervention for members of the nursing-home community, especially in view of the fact that many of these patients reveive only cursory psychological care and, in many cases, psychopharmacological intervention in the place of sound psychological planning. One comprehensive study (Bovner, Kafonek, Filipp, et al., 1986) found that 94 percent of the residents in an intermediate-care nursing home suffered from a major psychiatric disorder. An Institute of Medicine report (1986) summarized the task well:

> Depression, demoralization and social isolation have been measured and associated with social functioning, physical health status, premature mortality, and activity levels. Thus greater attention should be paid to the mental health aspects of care, including appropriate assessment and management techniques for mental and behavioral problems. ... (p. 381)

At the very least, nursing-home residents are in need of thorough psychological evaluations. Psychiatrists in private practice have only begun to tap the potential of this growing population. And psychological protocol only recently has been develped to assess the neurological functioning of geriatric patients in nursing homes, their attitudes toward the nursing home and life in general, the functioning of their families, and, most important, the effects of medications and combinations of medications prescribed for these patients.

There is a great deal of confusion on the part of psychologists who are not aware that they can be paid their ususal and customary fees by charging for psychological assessments under Part B of Medicare. (These charges can be made without the supervision of a physician, if they are for "diagnositic services" rather than for psychotherapeutic interventions.)

Visionary psychologists who are willing to take responsibility for their own actions and who prefer to work as independent agents have the ability to develop the ultimate psychological treatment program in conjunction with health-care facilities. There are two environments in which such a program cna be developed—the psychological ward in a general hospital or a free-standing psychological hospital.

The experience of psychologists in California, where recent legislation has greatly improved opportunities for practice, confirms that psycologists with courage and foresight can develop a total package of psychological health care by contracting with a hospital or health-care management group to provide services on a psychological ward. Pioneering arrangements have been made by a group of psychologists who are responsible for the total care of the patient, both on the ward as an inpatient and in the psychologist's office as an outpatient.

In the psychological hospital concept, an individual psychologist or a group of practicing psychologists own and maintain a psychological free-standing inpatient unit where the psychologist has full control over the care and treatment of patients who are hospitalized. Once again, after discharge from the hospital, these patients are seen in the outpatient offices of the same psychological group to ensure continuity of care.

SUMMARY

Whether mental-health providers like it or not, mental health is rapidly moving into the mainstream of American health care. This change demands that professional mental-health providers make adjustments in the way they practice in order to stay competitive in today's marketplace. The tide of change brings with it opportunities in hospitals and health care that have been, until recently, open only to physicians. For professionals who are willing to seize the opportunities before them, the future is bright indeed.

REFERENCES

American Hospital Assoication, (1986). *Hospital statistics,* Chicago.

Arthur, R.J. (1985). Public perceptions of medicine. *New England Journal of Medicine, 312,* (17), 1130.

Dorken, H., Stapp, J., & Vanden Bos, G.R. (1986). Licensed psychologists: A decade of major growth. In: H. Dorken (Eds), *Professional psychology in transition.* (pp.3-19). San Francisco; Jossey-Bass.

Economic fact book for psychiatry. (1983) Washington, DC: American Psychiatric Press.

Eggert, M.A., Laughlin, P.R., Hutell, R.R., Stedman, J.M., Solway, K.S., & Carrington, C.H. (1987). The psychology internship marketplace today. *Professional psychology: Research and Practice. 18* (2), 165-171.

Enright, M.F. (1985). The psychologist in Medical arts practice and small hospitals. *Psychotherapy in Private Practice. 3,* (1), 9-21.

Fink, P.J. (1986). Dealing with psychiatry's stigma. *Hospital and Community Psychiatry. 37* (8), 814-818.

Institute of Medicine. (1986). *Improving the quality of care in nursing homes.* Washington, DC: National Academy Press.

Keernan, C.V., Pasnau, R.O., & Richardson, M. (1981). Medical behaviorial explosion affects hospital operation policy. *Hospitals. 55*, 56-59.

May, L. (1982). Remarks before Public Policy Forum, Divisions 12 and 38, American Psychological Association, Washington, DC.

Mittler, B. (1986). *The Wall Street Journal,* June 26, p. 10.

Pasnau, R.O. (1982). Consultation-liaison psychiatry at the crossroads: The search for a definition for the 1980's. *Hospital and Community Psychiatry, 33,* 989-995.

Richards, S.A. (1987). Health care in the 80's and beyond. *Psychotherapy in Private Practice. 5* (1), 39-45.

Rovner, B.W., Kafonek, S., Filipp, L., Lucas, M.J. & Folstein, M.F. (1986). Prevalence of mental illness in a community nursing home. *American Journal of Psychiatry, 143* (11), 1446-1449.

Schenkenberg, T., Peterson, D., Wood, D., DaBell, R. (1981). Psychological consultation/liaison in a medical and neurological setting: Physician's appraisal. *Professional Psychology, 12* (3), 309-317.

Tanney, M.F. (1983). Hospital privileges for psychologists: A legislative model. *American Psychologist. 38,* 1232-1237.

The Health Industrial complex. (1986). *Register Reports, 25* (13) 1-15.

Tyron, G. (1981). Full-time private practie in the United States: Results of a national survey. *Professional Psychology, 14* 685-696.

C H A P T E R
28

EMPLOYEE ASSITANCE PROGRAMS

Robert Wishnoff, Ed.D.

THE HISTORY BEHIND THE CONCEPT

The forerunner of the employee assistance program (EAP) was the occupational alcohol program (OAP), which began when some large corporate employers recognized that recovering alcoholics could become effective and productive workers. Some of the recovering individuals helped establish in-house Alcoholics Anonymous groups, which were the real beginnings of worksite alcohol recovery programs.

There was a problem with the OAP concept. For one thing, the supervisor was forced to play diagnostician, a difficult and possibly dangerous role. However, since intervention techniques proved valuable, a shift in a approach occurred that would be more acceptable and useful to the employee. Work performance became the vehicle by which employees with alcohol problems recognized their difficulties.

As with any good idea, improvements, refinements, and specialization lead to a more useful outcome. Through the success of the OAP, the broad-brush (any type of problem) EAP began to be considered the most useful approach. This approach is now the standard used by most major employers, and small and medium-sized businesses have begun to offer EAP services to their employees in growing numbers.

As more people began to recognize the pervasive effects of alcohol abuse, and that the disease had elements beyond those just affecting the abuser, the expansion of OAP services was viewed as inevitable. EAPs initially developed in the 1970s. In the beginning, they were set up and staffed by recovering alcoholics and others with firsthand knowledge of the disease. But with an increasing need to provide services, a variety of professionals, including psychologists, physicians, social workers, and other mental-health professionals, entered the field. Companies recognized the valuable role that professionals could play in providing the needed services. Professionals also began to recognize their need to better understand the etiology and treatment of alcoholism and drug abuse.

Within the growing ranks of EAP service provides, conflicts developed among the new professional groups in this infant service business. Turf issues, training, educational backgrounds, and personal and professional experience all contributed to an active dialogue in a new professional association, the Association of Labor Management Adminstrators and Consultants on Alcoholism (ALMACA).

During the past 15 years, EAPs have obviously gone through a number of changes as the professional in them have grown to understand each other better. The field is now made up of professionals from many disciplines. Social workers probably are the leading group. Schools of social work have devleoped graduate specialities in EAPs and in industrial/ occupational social work. Certified alcohol counselors, substance-abuse specialists, personnel specialists, guidance counselors, and other interested groups now also provide this service.

WHAT'S AHEAD?

The planning process in developing services in this area needs to be well defined. In the following sections, we will explore two ways to work in the EAP environment. We will discuss the entrepreneurial role as an EAP consultant, either as a solo practitioner or as part of an established practice, and will also cover the professional's opportunity as a service provider to an existing EAP. In this capacity, the professional will serve in an evaluative and treatment role, and in this way will work with the EAP providers as an important resource. In either role, clinicans can expand their income potential.

DEVELOPING YOUR OWN EAP CONSULTING PRACTICE

Personal and Professional Preparation

With the beginning of the maturation of EAPs, informal seminars and formal courses leading to certificaiton have become available. It is certainly advanteageous to find the better offerings. ALMACA has begun a certification process that promises to become the most visible and respected credentail. Along with the certification, a clear understanding of the theory and practice will be gained. With this information, you will learn how to enter the field in a way that coincides with your position and interests.

Professional Associations and Societies

ALMACA, the largest and most visible of the associations, serves its members and the public in many ways. From an information-retrieval services to lobbying, membership can provide many opportunities; networking may be the most advantageous.

ALMACA is composed of national, regional, and, in many cases, local groups. Check with the national association for more information about groups in your area. Write to ALMACA at 1800 North Kent Street, Arlington, VA 22209, or call (703) 522-6272.

A newer group is the North American Congress on Employee Assistance Progams (NAC/EAP). This gorup seems to be more oriented toward professional development. NAC/EAP has conducted a high-level institute each summer for the past few yeas. It can be contacted at 2145 Crooks Road, Suite 103, Troy, MI 48084; (313) 543-9580.

Membership in either or both of thse organizations will help in developing and maintaining broad knowledge of the professional activities within the EAP field. During the past few years, EAP programs have begun to surface at national conventions, such as those of the American Psychological Association, the National Association of Social Workers, and the Aemrican Public Health Association. As more professionals enter the field, presentations will be given at more national conferences. Both researchers and practitioners will be anxious to share their knowledge.

Professional Literature

As with most profesional groups and associations, the journals and other publications of the EAP organizations are a source of revenue. Moreover, journals and newsletters offer timely news and features that can aid any professional in keeping up with the latest ideas in the field. ALMACA has been publishing the *ALMACAN* for 17 years. The *EAP Digest* is probably the most widely circulated magazine-type professional publication available in the field. It is published by Performance Resource Press. Both of thse journals provide a well-balanced and current perspective of EAP issues.

In addition to these two standard bearers, other professional journals feature more specialized articles in the fields of counseling and industrial psychology, occupational social work, public health, alcohol and substance abuse, and human resources and personnel management. Through the ALMACA information-retrieval service, many of the best articles on file can be reviewed.

Professional Issues

As in many professions, conflicts, jealousies, and competition are realistic isues to confront. Conflicts of interest surface for those clincians doing EAP consultations, assessment and referral, and ongoing treatment.

Such activities can be legitimate, but others may not see it this way. It is important to recognize your professional colleagues' position so that difficulties may be avoided. Depending on your location, the competition and jealousy issues may be negligible or serious.

Becuse operating an EAP is more business related than the traditional professional practice, a more visible presence in your community will be evident. Recognizing this from the beginning will be helpful in responding to colleagues' concerns about ethics, competition, and advertising problems. Some of these issues are highly charged. The basis of the problems lies in the questions of who makes how much money. As in any profession, when it comes to financial issues, unfortuante jealousies appear. Because professionals from many diverse backgroiunds are involved in EAP work, the normal lines of communication sometimes are not as clear. Therefore, rumors, stories, and myths may arise in the field.

On the positive side, in the EAP profession today, practitioners will be supportive and helpful, even if it is in a competitive environment. The real professionals will recognize that the more healthy competition available, the more the market will be aware and ready to purchase their services.

BUSINESS DEVELOPMENT AND PLAN

Community Business Awareness

The professional EAP provider, ragardless of discipline, is a business person. As a business person, recognizing what is going on in your community, which is really your market, is of critical importance.

Market research that you can do alone or with the help of a marketing consultant may help you understand what your business plan may look like.

Getting feedback from Chamber of Commerce officials and other business leaders may help you begin to make the most important contacts you will need in selling your services.

The Market Place

Depending on your geographical location, you may find a highly competitive market for your services or no others in the EAP business. This fact may help you decide the type of service you wish to provide.

In a competitive market, you may consider being a treatment resource rather than becoming another EAP consultant. If you really want to be a consultant, then segmenting your market and trying a target group of businesses may be your best plan.

Marketing and Public Relations

Starting an EAP is like beginning any other business; the more established your plan is, the better will be the outcome. As part of your plan, a certain amount of your budget needs to go for advertising and public relations. Your plan and expertise will determine your need to hire professionals in those fields.

The use of an advertising agency or public relations person will automatically put you in touch with other business leaders. These professionals can best advise where and how to get your EAP known. If you do it alone, try to make contact with the business editors at local newspapers and television stations.

The best advertising often can be accomplished at no cost, although it requires some effort on your part. But financially speaking, you are your most important asset. You must consider your own personality and ability to sell yourself. If you do not see yourself as a salesperson, then stop here, or get a partner whose talents lie in this area.

Tools of the Trade

Although it may seem easy to provide client EAP services, you must get all the details organized if the job is to be professional. Many of these details not only will help you to succeed, but may even help protect you if a problem should develop. First, setting your fee will be important. The amount charged will depend on whether or not your have competition, the services you offer, and your market. A survey of your local professional associations can be very useful in positioning you financially.

Consultation with an attorney is important. Have a contract or agreement in standard form ready to be signed when you succeed in selling your program. A standard form should be adequate for most businesses, but at times it may require more specific legal consideration.

Forming relationships with professional providers in your community can result in a number of important outcomes. Initially, referral agreements between you and treatment providers will be useful. They help establish a relationship among the service providers and yourself. Vital information is specified in these agreements. Fees, hours of operation, insurance eleigibility, specialities, and the like will all be clearly identified.

The referral agreements may help in the communication of professional and confidential information. In many instances, release-of-information requests will be required, especially in alcohol- and substance-abuse cases. In addition to a standard release form, specific forms are needed for these problems.

Along with the information flow that the referral agreements provide, the contacts with key community professionals will serve a public relations and marketing function. They may be able to open up new doors for you as a professional. They will soon realize that as your EAP expands, so will their referrals from you. Soon a synergistic relationship is achieved. Everyone benefits, and the relationship will assure continued good will among the professionals, even in small communities.

To better educate community resources, as well as provide for management training, an "EAP Supervisor's Training Manual" should be developed. An important part of the EAP is having supervisors make timely referrals to the program when eveidence is clear that a worker is having a problem. Helping supervisors with this process is essential to the long-term succes of the EAP.

The supervisory training needs to be defined, developed, and in operation when the EAP begins. When marketing your program to potential customers, or explaining your role to professional resources, the manual and other training materials should be reviewed.

Along with these training materials, other educational seminar packages may also be helpful, both in marketing your services and in delivering your product. Topics may vary among consultants and EAPs, but some standard topics currently are stress management, budget and other financial issues (retirement, single-parent economics), assertiveness, and wellness.

You may rely on the expertise of other staff people in conducting these seminars or you may lead them yourself. Large EAPs frequently have a specific training professional. You may find that you can use your professional colleagues in this role, either as paid consultants, or as voluntary contributors in return for referral consideration.

Having consider all these important details, the major elements of operation will have been covered. One final consideration is to check on both your malpractice insurance and liability insurance. Some companies may require a "hold harmless clause" in your contract, which may require special attention by you and your insurance agent in examining your business and professional liability insurance. Although there have not been many lawsuits in the profession, this does not mean that you are immune. As part of the details of your business planning, make sure you check out as many eventualities as possible.

Open for Business

Depending on the type of services you offer, you will need to consider your hours of operation and office procedures. For many EAP providers, a 24-hour availability is not unusual. If you are in a competitive market, this around-the-clock setup will probably be standard. If it is not, it may be your competitive edge. Obviously, you will not be in the office all the time. At times, you will be with clients doing assessment work, or at a company doing marketing or training.

The staff you employ is important. The receptionist/secretary may be critical to your success. This person will provide the personal touch needed to make client callers feel comfortable in making appointments or to help prospective corporate clients get needed business information more quickly.

If a receptionist is not going to answer your telephone during normal business hours, make sure that you have a professional answering service. Today, in the service-oriented EAP center, paging equipment and cellular phones are becoming standard. If you are offering prompt, professional services, you need to be easily reachable at all times. There is nothing worse for your credibilty than to offer this crisis service and not be responsive — in which case, you might even be considered negligent.

In addition to the answering service, a one-person program will need professional backup coverage. This need not be an EAP person specifically, although having the person be fully attuned to your system of operation is important. Your professional backup will need to be able to handle a crisis situation, to do assessments, and to make referrals. Such an arrangement will be important not only for your clients, but for your own personal and professional sanity as well. Everyone needs to get away sometime and backup coverage will allow you to do it more comfortably.

Corporate Relations As in any business, reports will need to be generated from your statistical records. Standard reports may be issued for most companies from your normal record-keeping process. Your corporate clients will look for user information to help justify the program or to make improvements in visible areas. Good record keeping will help you cost out your service, keep track of your time, and, most importantly, translate the confidential work you do into meaningful data so that your corporate clients can review the program results.

In some instances, different corporate clients will want specific types of data recorded. If known in advance, you can easily incorporate this requirement into your intake sheets and statistical records. There are a number of software packages available that could ease your record-keeping worries and make report generating much simpler. In a small EAP center or in a large one, a computer can be a real asset.

Maintaining consistent contact with your participating corporate clients will help ensure continual program support and possible expansion. Such helpful services, beyond your utilization reports, could include informative newsletters, service-expansion updates, a clipping service with reprints of relevant articles, and periodic seminars, luncheons, or other business gatherings. All of these can help develop and maintain the type of service image you want to present for future EAP expansion.

Clients — Direct Service

From the clinician's perspective, the assessment and referral process may be the most frustrating. The training and experience of most providers are in the treatment area. Passing clients off to others may seem strange to those who have been in private practice. An issue raised earlier about referral versus treatment is an important consideration. It is necessary that you make your position clear to employees coming into your office for assistance. The last thing your clients need is confusion about the assessment, referral, and treatment process. During employee orientation programs at the onset of the EAP, they will have been told about the process the program uses in this respect. Because employees or their dependents may not always remember that they have been given this information, it is always helpful to clarify the process issues early.

It is also important to inform clients about your follow-up practices. You may track them differently according to whether they are management referrals or self-referrals. The type of problem diagnosed will also imply a different tracking system. Part of your follow-up system may be made easier with good cooperative relationships among your referral resources.

All businesses have limitations. Recognizing what they are early on may help alleviate problems before they arise. Do not market services you cannot deliver and do not offer services beyond the scope of the EAP if you have not described these in your agreement or contract. Many EAP providers have found themselves doing more than they bargained for and are not getting paid for it.

Evaluation

If your record-keeping system is adequate, evaluating certain facets of the program will be made easier. A specific research and evaluation program may be designed if your interests lie in this area. However, little scientific research has been done with EAPs. The major reason is that research and evaluation have not been profitable in the private sector. The academic community only recently has been focusing on EAP programs and developing the kind of research useful for the professional and business community.

Your own program evaluation is important in terms of your service delivery and clients' satisfaction. Understanding that people resolved their problems and translating the change into positive work performance behavior are of greatest corporate interest. Programatically, questioning client users of your service and referral services could give you important feedback that will be beneficial for further program development.

Loose Ends

The relatively brief history, but continuous development of the EAP profession certainly has made for an interesting and exciting business venture. I have pointed out the nuances that allow individual practitioners to explore their own professional boundaries and to create programs based on their skills and community needs. The result will be either an EAP consulting practice for one person or a multifaceted group that will encompass many professionals delivering services in unique ways.

My perspective calls for the new professional EAP provider to build upon a solid foundation, based on the critical elements established during the EAP movement's 15-year history. Using the basic structures presented, as well as your own ideas, will contribute to your plan for services.

Of course, these concepts may be more than you are willing to undertake at this point — which is fine for now, because too many have entered the field ill prepared and not ready to succeed with this fast-paced approach to intervening in human problems.

If you want to expand your professional practice and your income potential and to work with the EAP professionals, another way is possible. The following section will orient you to a direct provider approach to service delivery. You will find a model to work from so that a positive partnership between our practice and the EAP providers will be soundly established.

WORKING WITH EAPS

Offering your clinical treatment services to EAP consultants in your community could be a lucrative and stimulating expansion concept. The most aggressive clinicians may want better to understand the clinical needs and business expectations of the EAP consultants. Developing a clear understanding of the EAP operation will give you a definite advantage in working with the professionals in the EAP field. For the part-time clinician who wishes to do more, EAP counseling may be the easisest and most consistent source of referrals and profit.

Working Relationships

Most EAP providers have real and special needs when they seek to hire clinicians in the referral process. Two primary concerns are your clinical specialty interests and your availability for consultations.

If you are interested in working very closely with an EAP, try to develop a specialty relationship with one. The EAP wants a relationship with a professional who will assume a great responsiblity with the clients. The clinician needs to realize that success with clients helps to ensure new referrals and to enhance the EAP's credibility. Clinical providers need to be licensed in order to be eligible for insurance reimbursement, but in some cases the insurance requirements are not as critical.

Belonging to health maintenance organizations (HMO) and preferred provider organizations (PPO) groups may also enhance your availability for direct service delivery. Participating with third-party carriers can help in the referral process and benefit the financial aspects of the client–clincian relationship.

As a licensed mental-health provider, you understand the importance of confidentiality. Within the EAP process, confidentiality becomes even more apparent because it is a paramount concern in the workplace EAP environment. Keep this issue in mind when scheduling appointments with people referred from an EAP. No one wants to run into a co-worker at the therapist's office.

Leaving the office to market their services may be a new endeavor for many professionals. EAP consultants would prefer to get to know their referral resources, and so for this reason going to the EAP is important. Schedule a time to go to the EAP office, meet the staff members, and provide them with all the details of your practice.

Services

You may want to discuss your expertise at furnishing other services for the EAP. Beyond your specific counseling skills, testing, workshops, and seminars may be very helpful adjuncts to the program.

An important issue to consider is your fees. If you develop a good business relationship with an EAP, you may want to consider a special fee structure. This will enhance your referral possibilities and position you in a positive way with the EAP provider. Although a special EAP fee is not a necessity, it is becoming more of an acceptable business practice in this day of preferred provider agreements. If such a fee is not in your best interest, consider a sliding-scale system to be used when appropriate with a key EAP referral. In certain instances, someone may benefit from your services, but may not be able to afford them, even with insurance.

Your hours of operation are again of prime importance to the EAP. If you are interested in making this relationship grow, find out what the needs are of the EAP. For example, after-work appointments are a necessity, as many employees cannot afford to lose time from work.

Evening and Saturday availability is important to the EAP provider. These time slots are especially valuable when working with marital and family therapy cases because of the inconvenience of having two or more people leave work or school to be present for an appointment. Many people also work on a variety of shifts and schedules, so flexibility in scheduling treatment is an important option an EAP provider looks for in the professional referral community.

If you have been in private practice, you probably have had backup coverage for emergency situtations. Many EAPs have the resources to handle crises situations. However, it is helpful to let the EAP know when you are away or otherwise unable to accept referrals.

If all goes well, your practice and the EAP will work well together and both will grow. The basic need of the EAP is service. The EAP will look for timely opportunities, flexible hours and fees, and a high-quality professional work. Some clinical providers wonder about working with different EAPs but, this does not pose a conflict as long as confidentiality remains intact and and special business relationships are treated in a proprietary manner. The only client conflict that might arise would be if the clinical provider were to offer competing EAP services. For some clincians, this is how they moved from a clinician role into the EAP consulting field. If you become interested in making such a change acting as a referral source to an EAP, just let the EAP know. Perhaps a joint venture could be developed, rather than two good people competing.

SUMMARY

The decision either to become an EAP consultant or to be a clincial provider to existing EAPs could lead to income expansion and personal growth and success. A number of considerations, both professional and personal, have been pointed out to guide you in a clearer direction. It is essential that in any new venture you anticipate mistakes and hazards, recognizing them as learning experiences. In the EAP field, because it is relatively new, each new step will provide important information for you and the profession. Expansion and growth of all types, especially financial, are almost certain if sound professional service is developed.

C H A P T E R
29

VOCATIONAL REHABILITATION

Patricia M. Dvonch, Ph.D.

During the past year, this private-sector rehabilitation counselor has engaged in tasks that include diagnostic initial interviews; medical management; vocational evaluation; job-skills transfer; job assessment and analysis; employer, physician, therapist, and attorney visits; and coordination of medical report information with vocational and functional capacity data to complete a vocational rehabilitation evaluation for a client's Social Security Disability Insurance (SSDI) benefits appeal. The counselor has also conferred with and submitted monthly, written reports to insurers of Workers' Compensation and long-term disability (LTD) benefits programs; completed testing and assessment for vocational rehabilitation recommendations and planning; and explored job alternatives, job possibilities with a client's former employer, and job modifications, and developed resumés. In addition, the counselor has attended workshops, talked with colleagues and claims representatives, found information in texts and brochures, and sought experts to become knowledgeable about the rules and regulations of the Workers' Compensation laws; read and reread the SSDI benefits regulations and policies; and learned to approach and to talk, on a peer level, with client attorneys and treating physicians, to encourage cooperation and assistance in drawing up vocational rehabilitation plans that assist clients and are critical to a successful return to work plan.

One might ask on what basis this person engaged in all of these varying activities, and what training, education, and experience were necessary to provide this counselor with the knowledge, skills, information, and confidence to become involved in the tasks and functions of a private-sector rehabilitation provider. The response might be that, in this particular situation, the counselor has a master's degree and a doctoral degree in rehabilitation counseling; experience as a vocational rehabilitation counselor in a large city hospital; consultant experience in diverse clinics and on research studies (e.g., orthopedics, rheumatic diseases, spinal cord injury); many years of teaching graduate students in a rehabilitation counselor education program in a large, private university; and, finally, 10 years of providing testimony as a vocational expert for the Social Security Administration/Office of Hearings and Appeals. This counselor, alternatively, might possess a master's degree in rehabilitation counseling; be a certified rehabilitation counselor (CRC); have five to 10 years of employment as a rehabilitation counselor/evaluator in several private, not-for-profit, comprehensive rehabilitation agencies; or have worked in agencies that serve clients with physical, sensory, and mental disabilities.

WHAT IS PRIVATE-SECTOR REHABILITATION?

Upon reviewing the above account, many familiar — and some unfamiliar — components are readily noted by the traditional vocationsl rehabilitation counselor who is employed in the public state/federal or private not-for-profit sector. Vocational rehabilitation in the private not-for-profit sector is a fairly recent phenomenon, with a history of 10–15 years at most as a burgeoning new field, though vocational rehabilitation counselors have been self-employed as private consultants, as career counselors, and as vocational experts with the federal government for many years. Schwartz (1986) notes that "for 50 years (1920–1970) virtually all vocational rehabilitation services were provided by public agencies." Federal mandates and appropriations, designed to assist handicapped Americans to enter or return to work, literally created and shaped the field. During this period, the economic and social benefits of restoring disabled citizens to gainful and productive employment activities were well established and documented. Changes occurred when, in 1973, the Federal Rehabilitation Act (1) mandated service accountability in the Individual Written Rehabilitation Plan (IWRP), (2) eliminated the word "vocational," (3) established that a service priority be given the most severely disabled, and (4) recognized independent living as an acceptable and significant outcome.

This hallmark legislation served to open the door for services to be offered in the private sector (Matkin, 1985). The public sector found itself faced with providing services over a longer period and consequently with an expenditure of more funds per capita for each more severely disabled client. A result of modified delivery focus and insufficient funds to provide necessary services for those clients with less severe handicaps, in part, persuaded these individuals and their insurance providers to seek vocational assistance elsewhere. The private sector performed "private rehab" because it understood the goal of return to *previous* level, not *optimal* level. For public divisions of vocational rehabilitation (DVR), "optimal" may be appropriate. But it is not the responsibility of the insurance contract.

An added impetus to the growth of private-sector rehabilitation came in 1975, when California became the first state to mandate vocational rehabilitation services as part of its Worker's Compensation statutes. Rising costs of industrially injured claimants for medical expenses and payment of lost wages, in excess of $22.5 billion in 1982, compelled a number of companies to look at possible ways in which to contain costs as well as have more control over the vocational rehabilitation of injured workers. Many insurance companies require vocational rehabilitation to preinjury level, whereas their experience with state rehabilitation counselors showed placement of injured workers into two-year training programs to assist them toward their optimal potential, which is the state/federal policy. The insurer's obligation to continue compensation payments until training programs are ompleted was another impetus to employing private-sector rehabilitation firms to oversee medical management and return injured employees to work. It appears that these efforts have been successful in reducing costs in both areas (Weed & Field, 1986).

Employers, alarmed at the realization that health-care and disability costs have become a significant expense of doing business, are utilizing in-house rehabilitation staff and contracting with private rehabilitation firms as part of their strategy to contain these costs. Early identification at the workplace of disability and related problems, facilitation of returning to work, and modification of jobs, when necessary, are a few of the ways to enable disabled/injured workers to continue being productive employees (Tate, Habeck, & Galvin, 1986). Only in the 1980s, and initially researched and tested in Finland, Sweden, and Australia, has the conceptual base for efficient industry-based disability management programs been effectively set up to screen employees in need of job reassignment, make ergonomic changes in job sites, and provide educational programs addressing low back pain, stress, and cardiac rehabilitation. Among U.S. companies that have become increasingly involved in developing and conducting disability management approaches are Xerox, 3M Corporation, Herman Miller, Inc., Steelcase, Inc., and Control Data. This approach requires collaboration among industry management, labor, and the individual worker. Effective communication and coordination and the use of a multidisciplinary team are very important (Tate et al., 1986).

WHY CHOOSE PRIVATE-SECTOR REHABILITATION?

Individual professionals choose private-sector vocational rehabilitation for a variety of reasons: to be independent, as a "respite from the stifling bureaucracy" of the public system, or to earn a better salary. Hayes (1987) notes that they do so because corporate salaries are considerably higher than those in the "helping professions," and the corporate community (insurers, industry, attorneys), are comfortable paying an hourly rate commensurate with that for professionals in the world of commerce; they wish to work with disabled persons who appear to be more interested in or have a better chance to return to work, because they have been members of the work force; and they hope to deliver services to clients in a more creative and quicker way, using vendors with less vested interest in prolonged evaluation and unnecessary services. Finally, they want to expand their professional horizons into an arena that offers more and more diversity where populations in need of services continue to be newly identified, thus offering the opportunity to provide quality, timely, and cost-effective medical/rehabilitation management and vocational rehabilitation services to injured and ill workers through insurers, corporations, and attorneys. Rehabilitation counseling professionals add yet another reason: to seek recognition of the skills and knowledge that they can provide. As Hayes (1987) points out, many established counselors and rehabilitation educators contract as consultants with attorneys, physicians, or economists to augment their income, to broaden their skill base, to keep skills current, to experience the rewards of the client–counselor relationship, and "to do what I teach."

WHAT TRAINING, EDUCATION, AND
WORK EXPERIENCE ARE REQUIRED?

Private practice for vocational rehabilitation counselors has a variety of meanings for the practitioner. For that reason, practice in this field is very attractive to a broad range of individuals with diverse educations, training, and experience. Rehabilitation counselors, nurses, job developers and specialists, and occupational therapists are among those most frequently encountered. Rehabilitation nurses have been active in private-sector rehabilitation for longer than other professionals. They were situated in corporate industry in medical departments, and had some understanding of medical terminology and the effect of disease and injuries on the work of the employee. Nurses perceive their role as primarily that of service planner and coordinator (Matkin, 1982). Rehabilitation nurses frequently provide services in catastrophic case management (CCM), the goal of which is to provide the best care at the best cost. CCM is designed as a more patient-oriented, holistic approach and generally takes place early in rehabilitation service. It is life-care planning; as it looks beyond acute needs, the rehabilitation nurse requires knowledge of evaluation, education, therapeutic equipment, drugs, medical care, and maintenance needs. In addition, the provider must have access to information regarding costs, upkeep, implementation, and change over a sustained period of time.

Providers of private-sector vocational rehabilitation are, ideally, professionals trained, educated, and experienced in the field of vocational rehabilitation counseling. They are persons with knowledge of the principles, practices, and philosophy of this 65-year-old profession, which was created out of a need to return wounded World War I veterans to the workplace. Realistically, the special skills and knowledge of the rehabilitation nurse could contribute needed expertise for private practice.

Lynch and Martin (1982) looked at private-sector rehabilitation providers' education level, area of specialization, and knowledge, skills, and information thought to be important to private-practice counselors. Of 147 study participants, 95 percent held at least a bachelor's degree, 64 percent held masters' degrees, and 14 percent held doctoral degrees. Major fields of study represented were rehabilitation counseling, 53 percent; psychology, 25 percent; and nursing, 11 percent. Sixty-four percent were CRCs and 85 percent had at least five years of work experience in rehabilitation — 42 percent in private for-profit rehabilitation firms, 19 percent as private consultants, and 16 percent with insurance companies; some 89 percent of the study participants served clients with physical disabilities. A study, reported by Matkin (1982), found that well over half (61 percent) of the persons currently practicing in the private rehabilitation sector have at least a master's degree, approximately 37 percent are CRCs, and 25 percent are registered nurses. Seventy-one percent have between one and five years of work experience in the private sector, and over half (56 percent) work with a maximum caseload of 11 to 30 clients a month (Matkin, 1985).

For those persons who have graduated from accredited rehabilitation couseling education programs, the knowledge and skills they possess typically are grounded in educational curricula that have remained basically unchanged since the mid-1950s (Matkin, 1985). Lynch and Martin (1982) cited 10 knowledge areas as most important for the private-sector provider: functional capacity assessment, employment and skill-transfer knowledge, job-placement and job-seeking skill techniques, interpersonal communication and writing skills, and job analysis/modification and job-development techniques. Written and verbal communication skills training is a part of most graduate-level education, and is crucial in the development of a private rehabilitation practice. Practitioners generally just utilize verbal communication ability in establishing trust, rapport, and respect with clients, family members, and treatment team providers and vendors. Private-practice providers must develop an ability to write, gather, synthesize, and report information to different audiences. A need frequently expressed by private-sector managers (administrators) is that counselors change from clinical to corporate English expression. The private-sector practitioner must present as one who is comfortable and knowledgeable in both the language and dress of the corporate community, one who must be at ease when developing business relationships with insurance claims representatives, attorneys, client employers, and union and corporate managers. Verbal and written communication encompasses other roles as well: the marketing and developing of new accounts, the training of staff, and acting as a consultation resource to corporate management, economists, and attorneys. It has been reported that companies contracting for private-sector rehabilitation counselors look for the master's degree in rehabilitation counseling and for the CRC as requirements. Providers and employers agree that three to five years of rehabilitation experience are a prerequisite to successful performance.

Buyers and providers of private rehabilitation find other competencies essential to successful practice. High on the list are human resource management, industrial and organizational psychology, marketing strategies, and labor market economics. Add to these knowledge of the disability benefit system, Workers' Compensation laws, SSDI regulations, and LTD policies and contracts to assure an adequate level of professionalism.

Job placement as a goal for clients with disabilities has been the *raison d'être* of the rehabilitation counseling process since its beginnings in the 1920s. About 1975, the federal government through the Rehabilitation Services Administration mandated that RSA-funded rehabilitation counselor education programs emphasize this concept in course offerings and clinical practice assignments. A number of these programs have responded to this task, and many of the same universities have taken the lead in developing curricula that address the need to understand business and industry better. For example, New York University's graduate program offers a sequence of courses in the Graduate School of Business Administration and major corporations provide internship sites; Michigan State University's rehabilitation counseling program has a cooperative agreement with the School of Labor and Industrial Relations that permits students to enroll in elective courses, such as personnel management, employee relations, and organizational development. Drake University's program for placement specialists includes courses in marketing and management (Habeck & Ellien, 1986).

IN WHAT SETTINGS IS PRIVATE-SECTOR
REHABILITATION PRACTICED?

Insurance companies are the largest employer of the private-sector practitioner. The rehabilitation specialist is instrumental in coordinating benefits programs, and in implementing and monitoring the services provided to assist the injured insured in reaching medical and physical stabilization, through appropriate treatment, therapy, and training, with a goal of return to work; benefits and goals may differ depending on the type of insurance (e.g., LTD and Workers' Compensation). With LTD, the specialist may guide the injured worker in an application for SSDI benefits.

Corporate industry employs rehabilitation counselors/specialists in disability management programs, employee assistance programs (EAPs), human resource management, and counseling and personnel departments. These professionals provide numerous services to workers with a goal of intervention in the personal and economic costs of injury and disability. Services may include transfer of workers to less stressful or less physically demanding jobs; job modification, career guidance, and personal, job-related, and retirement counseling; presentation of disability awareness programs; and the holding of workshops to inform management and staff of the effects of affirmative action laws on corporate practices and policy.

Private-sector rehabilitation firms are private, fee-for-services providers of quality, timely, and cost-effective rehabilitation management and vocational rehabilitation services to insurance carriers, claimants, and other referral sources. Project goals to referring insurance companies and to referred individuals are professional services in the areas of rehabilitation management, resource coordination, vocational assessment and recommendations, plan implementation, job development, and selective job placement. Other programs and services include CCM, Social Security eligibility evaluation and claim assistance, and disability management planning.

Medical settings include at least 500 health maintenance organization (HMOs) and comprehensive medical rehabilitation centers (CMRCs), throughout the country. The latter concentrate exclusively on rehabilitation programs for head injury, stroke, spinal cord injury, neuromuscular disabilities, and so on. They are interdisciplinary in concept, offer a vast array of challenges, are fast paced, and serve a high volume of clients (Kaplan, 1986).

Private consulting (self-employed) is another option. Private-sector rehabilitation typically comes about from one's own on-the-job experience and as a response to industry, insurer, and private rehabilitation firm needs. Consultants to these sources generally go in to review, set up, monitor, or evaluate a particular program. Increasingly, however, opportunities for rehabilitation counselors to contribute to the American legal system have also opened up, notably within the past 10 years. In this context, the professional is generally called a vocational expert (VE) when called upon to testify before an administrative law judge (ALJ) in the Federal Social Security Administration's Hearings and Appeals Court. In this capacity, the VE assesses and provides objective testimony as to the effect a claimant's disability has on that individual's capacity to perform work, and whether jobs are available in the area or national economy. The professional may act as an expert witness, defined by Blau as "any person who, by nature of her or his training or experience in a science, a trade, or an art, has information that is not likely to be known by the average juror. An expert may be called to provide testimony in the course of any adversary hearing, which may be a civil trial or a criminal court" (Krieshok, 1987). Blau continues, "Anyone associated with mental health or rehabilitation can expect to be called to court. . .they can make a significant contribution to human welfare because the crowding of the court dockets is. . .among the 10 most serious social problems in America." Early settlement is a frequent outcome of their involvement. The rehabilitation counselor might also testify in cases of personal-injury litigation, in loss of salary and tenure, and in child-custody and marital-dissolution cases. Information is provided to educate a jury, but the jury makes the ultimate decision.

Stressful and troubling considerations of an ethical and philosophical nature, as well as practical problems of time, schedule, and collection of fees, are inherent in expert witness consulting. The effective consultant is one who recognizes, assesses, and learns to handle the issues and problems in order to enjoy the rewards and satisfactions in practive (Shawhan, 1985). With the exception of industrial, insurance, and medical settings, any other of the above settings requires that the private-sector rehabilitation practitioner learn about the fundamentals of setting up her or his own business. Hayes (1987) assesses the advice of experts on establishing a private practice and suggests that business practices and guidance on legal and tax matters are crucial to future financial success. Record keeping, the legal implications of fees, handling and collecting of accounts, malpractice-suit and personal-injury representation, tax matters, pension plans, and employee benefits are all matters to be discussed with an attorney. An accountant offering advice on taxes, financing, bookkeeping, and various financial systems is also a necessary adjunct to the private-practice entrepreneur.

HOW DOES ONE ENTER THE FIELD?

A first step to entering the field is to become aware of it. Make inquiries about its purposes, practices, and policies, and the qualifications and experience required. What are the working conditions, job tenure, salary, and benefits? Are there opportunities for promotion and growth? Do these factors differ in the various settings, such as private rehabilitation firms, industry, or insurance companies? The curious professional must carry out an intensive self-appraisal as well: Are my education, training, and experience appropriate to the demands? What are my career goals? What are my immediate and long-range personal, social, and professional needs and goals?

The applicant's personal characteristics and traits must be considered and measured in relation to basic facts of private practice. Do I like to work independently and alone or do I need the collegial and social atmosphere and stimulation found in an office? Am I organized? Can I plan appropriately to meet the organization's need for the monthly client progress reports and billable hour quotas necessary to earn my salary? Am I a pragmatist in assessing what is a business charge and what is my own overinvolvement or obsession in thinking through a problem, and thus my personal expense? Am I comfortable in juggling and making decisions that satisfy the requirements of the insurer, the attorney, the physician, and so on and the expressed wishes and needs of a client? Do I consider "return to previous job level" sufficient, or do I believe that the client's optimal potential should be attained? These are just a few of the many considerations one must confront and resolve. As more and more private not-for-profit rehabilitation agencies and state/federal OVRs develop their own Workers' Compensation units as a part of their overall operation and services, the interested counselor has an opportunity to "test the waters" of private-sector rehabilitation without facing some of the potential hazards of "going private."

JOB TITLES AND PROFESSIONAL BACKGROUND—EFFECT ON PRACTICE

The private-sector practitioner answers to the titles of rehabilitation counselor/consultant/specialist, vocational counselor/consultant/specialist, marketing consultant/specialist, case management supervisor, vice-president, or president. All are titles encountered in private practice. The comparatively new arena of private-sector rehabilitation is open and attractive to a broad spectrum of professionals. Lay counselor, psychologist, nurse, evaluator, special educator, physical or occupational therapist, economist, personnel counselor, attorney, or insurance provider—any of these professionals may elect to become private-sector practitioners. Each enters the field with her or his own area of expertise, training, experience, philosophy, and ethics. Each, we are certain, believes she or he will succeed. Why then are there failures? Why do we hear industry and insurance managers cite costly, ineffective service from some private-rehabilitation providers? Insurers contend that providers are too client oriented, request too many costly services, and, fail to have the client return to work. Further complaints point to a lack of follow-through, and add that honest up-front opinion in regard to the client is not forthcoming.

Concerned leaders suggest numerous causes for such complaints, including lack of knowledge of good business practices, insurance and benefit systems, and appropriate qualifications for personnel. It is incumbent on management in rehabilitation firms to have financial and business management skills and marketing experience. Managers need to know corporate disability policy, and the goals of a company; they need to ask if the company's need is for medical case management or job placement services. What are the union rules and regulations and needs? The firm's counselors, consultants, and specialists must possess excellent clinical and rehabilitation process skills, have good ideas, and do creative planning with clients for return to work. In an increasingly competitive marketplace, private rehabilitation providers need to understand the effect of corporate culture on the rehabilitation process and practice. Does industry support return-to-work efforts? Does the company employ people with disabilities? Is there a strong commitment to human resource development? If the company uses an insurer, are rehabilitation benefits provided? What are they? Does the company communicate the benefits of rehabilitation and reemployment to injured employees?

Success of rehabilitation lies in and depends on the timeliness of referrals.

The degree of rehabilitation success drops drastically when referral is delayed. Important factors in establishing referral eligibility/determination are age, diagnosis, skills, family support, and employment motivation (Hayes, 1987). Thus, cooperation with and understanding of company policy are essential for good practice outcome.

WHAT ARE THE USUAL TASKS AND FUNCTIONS OF PROFESSIONALS IN PRIVATE-PRACTICE REHABILITATION? OR WALKING THROUGH AN AVERAGE DAY

The private-practice rehabilitation professional will encounter, uniquely, most facets of family, employment, allied health, legal, and corporate dynamics. Each requires a different approach and different content. All will offer help only to the extent that they perceive and concur that help is offered in return. For example, the counselor should take the following steps.

Client   Visit the client and conduct an initial diagnostic interview, marked by an intensive demographic inquiry. This must include the person's age, family status, education, additional training, work experience, hobbies and interests, as well as personal observations of the interviewer, medical data, and names of any treating physicians, therapists, and attorneys.

Family   Meet family members to explain the role and objectives of the firm, to gain family support and cooperation in medical/rehabilitation management, and to carry out vocational planning for the client's return to work.

Physician   Contact by telephone and letter to gain cooperation and assistance in establishing diagnosis, treatment plan, prognosis, and probable medical outcome, and evaluate functional capacity and work-release date. Medical/rehabilitation management is the foundation for vocational planning: we cannot proceed with safety and viability without proper medical treatment and functional knowledge (Jasper, 1987).

Allied Health (PT, OT, Speech)   Either by visit or by letter, obtain reports on treatment goals and client progress to enhance the client's return to work.

Psychotherapist   Obtain a report on treatment goals for realistic and expeditious vocational planning and job exploration.

Attorney   Establish collaborative working relationship to further the goals of the client. These may include Workers' Compensation claim, SSDI benefits claim, and third-party suits.

Employer (Boss, Supervisor, Personnel)   Contact in vocational planning to assess options for return to same job or for a modified or different job with same employer. Also, observe job being carried out and analyze tasks performed and obtain work references to provide client with proof of performance as a valued worker should a future job search become necessary.

Insurer   Provide data and written reports on all aspects of work with a client, and obtain authorization to proceed with plan, to contact physician, attorney, and so on, and to maintain accountability.

In addition to these contacts, the counselor will be engaged at one time or another in analysis of clients' jobs, and the transferability of skills to alternative light-duty, sedentary jobs. The counselor will develop job resumés, assist in job-seeking skill training, conduct labor market surveys, search for transportation for client travel to treatment appointments, and coordinate medical and vocational data and process material for clients at SSDI claim hearings. Written monthly reports to the insurer include medical and vocational planning updates, client concerns, vocational testing results, interpretations and recommendations, a summary, and recommendations for continued services and planning activities with the client.

Students ask: Is private practice an arena one should consider upon graduation, or does it require some traditional agency experience and supervision? If one carefully considers the above roster of tasks and functions, it is obvious that a great deal of experience is necessary to enter the private-practice arena.

SIMILARITIES AND DIFFERENCES IN PUBLIC- AND PRIVATE-SECTOR REHABILITATION PRACTICE

Weed and Field (1986) identified "a revolution of sorts underway" over the past 15 years, when they examined the literature concerning similarities and differences in public- and private-sector rehabilitation practice. An increase in private-sector opportunities and an accompanying decline in public-sector jobs was but one indication of change; this has affected university programs, professional associations (a rise in National Association of Rehabilitation Professionals in the Private Sector (NARPPS) membership and a corresponding decline in National Rehabilitation Counseling Association (NRCA) membership), business, insurance companies, and state agencies, as well as people in training and persons who may be employed in the public sector.

Although strain and frustration with the state/federal system may have been the impetus for many to move into private practice, it is clear from field studies that injured workers tend to be difficult clients. Generous benefits, from a number of sources, and the possibility of receiving great financial settlements or continued long-term benefit payments often contribute to clients' reluctance to engage in return-to-work planning. The objective of private-sector rehabilitation in some ways is quite different from that of the public sector in that transfer of skills — not advanced education or training — is the most cost-effective means of returning the injured worker to gainful employment.

There are probably more similarities than differences — notably, education and training in the rehabilitation process, which are basic to both arenas. The Council on Rehabilitation Education (CORE) has adjusted its standards to encompass rehabilitation counseling in both settings (Weed & Field, 1986). Universities, too, are following this lead and placing greater emphasis on business practices, organizational culture, and policy structure of the corporate community.

A sampling of the ways in which differences occur in structure and setting; in policy; and in tasks and functions is given in the table.

Area	Public Sector	Private Sector
Funding base	State/federal matching dollars	Providers expected to maintain or exceed the daily, weekly, and monthly billable casework quotas agreed upon
Type of client	Broad spectrum of disabling conditions	Primarily industrially injured
Services solution	Optimal; may include long evaluation and training	Goal is return to former job level or preinjury wage
Setting	Usually a large bureaucratic organization	Comparatively smaller organization
Client solution	Client comes to counselor	Counselor goes to client
Professional training	Usually vocational rehabilitation counseling	Diverse backgrounds, including VRC, nurse, job-development specialists, OT, and PT therapists
Caseload	Often 100 or more	20–30 for a full-time counselor
Medical management monitoring	Usually none	Frequent service provision
Job-placement activities	Less active	Required objective in most instances

In the past five years, state/federal and not-for-profit agencies have developed Workers' Compensation units offering in-house services either free or at fees less than the private sector. While this competition with the private sector can be viewed as adversarial, it may also work to the benefit of the client; with the prospect of better and less costly service provision by both public and private providers. It is true that in private-sector practice one has the ability to work with a client without the encumbrances of the state/federal system, which may limit the scope of services and often results in a slower response to client needs.

Other key concepts undergirding the practice of private rehabilitation include the following.

1. *Cost-effectiveness and efficiency.* Private practice is cost-effective in providing service for a safe and appropriate return to work for the injured worker.

2. *Accountability.* Companies and insurers contract with private-sector firms to cut costs and get claimants back to work in a limited period of time. There is a time/management factor and cases can and must proceed fast and effectively. Each telephone call, each visit, each letter, and each monthly report must move the case one step closer to closure.

3 *Thoroughness in planning.* Contact with all treatment providers, physicians, the employer, the attorney, and the claims representative is required, and all activities are identified and coordinate in a multifaceted approach to effect a viable vocational rehabilitation plan.

4. *Placement record.* In private practice, the rate is one placement with every four clients; in the public sector, this figure is one placement for every eight clients served (Jasper, 1987).

5. *Client's trust.* The client's trust is an essential component, where enthusiasm and action toward return to work can arouse a sense of urgency in the client, who may fear recurrence of or addiitional injury; failure to be able to function in a new type of job; and loss of benefits, with little or no understanding of her or his benefit coverage (OPTIONS, Associates, Inc., staff, 1987).

ETHICAL CHALLENGES TO A NEW REHABILITATION PRACTICE ARENA

"Going private" implies a prerequisite set of skills and personal characteristics that are not easily defined. Shawhan (1985) examines qualities necessary for the private practitioner. He offers as a key concept an orientation of "caring *about,* not *for,* the individual; that is, we must care about the needs of, and respect, this person, for her or his interests and abilities. This concept is rooted not in charity or pity, but in the value, dignity, and capacity we see in the individual. Shawhan goes on to say that we must evaluate, not judge, to determine significance or worth by careful appraisal, rather than becoming preoccupied with weaknesses and problems. What can the individual do? What are the transferable skills? What is the family support? Is the client motivated to return to work? What modifications can be made? What job openings exist? What products or services can be provided? Shawhan calls this an expective rehabilitation orientation; that is, we expect positives in ourselves and in our clients. "Our industry and professional training are based on the worth and dignity of the individual, the value of meaningful work, and the capacity of our free enterprise system.

As we move into the world of commerce and industry, where cost effectiveness and profit are the motivating factors, our integrity and rehabilitation philosophy emerge as critical to both the practitioner and the client. This situation presents practical and ethical challenges to the profession, as more and more private-sector practitioners take positions with corporations as "in-house" counselors or disability management specialists who work with the injured/chronically ill employee, as consultants to attorneys in personal injury and other lawsuits, with employment agencies, and with insurance companies. In all cases, the private-sector rehabilitation counselor receives payment directly from the source, which then may feel the counselor is more responsive to the source's needs (Weed & Field, 1986).

The private sector is in the process of developing a unique profession. The NARPPS reports approximately 1,500 private rehabilitation companies in 1985 in the United State. These firms range from one-person, private-sector providers to large state, regional, national, and international operations. It behooves the profession to respond to the needs of each of these potential employers/vendors, and yet maintain its basic, essential, ethical and moral philosophy of rehabilitation. NARPPS and the Insurance Rehabilitation Study Group are taking leadership roles in addressing the critical issues and questions of: professional conduct; service-delivery standards; education, training, and experience; advocacy; testimony; confidentiality; business practice; and professional certification (Schwartz, 1986). More and more frequently, graduates of rehabilitation counselor education programs are considering private-sector rehabilitation as a viable career. Private practice appears to satisfy a need to assist persons with disabilities, and at the same time offers a life-style commensurate with that of friends and colleagues with careers in management, the stock market, law, engineering, and the like that provide the potential for high income and membership in the corporate community.

Questions begin to arise in the first months of practice. Private-sector practitioners soon come up against hard decisions; they feel compelled to take sides — does the employer (insurance company, etc.) have the best interests of the client in mind? The counselor has chosen a profession with a philosophy based on helping people reach their own goals. The new practitioner is now in conflict: a client says, "actualize my work potential," and the claims representative says, "preinjury level job placement." How does one integrate the "profit motive" and the "service motive" (Taylor, 1985)?

Taylor addresses these dilemmas in two ways: (1) by describing the unique characteristics of private-sector rehabilitation that have produced uncertainty about ethical behavior among its practitioners, and (2) by providing specific ethical guidelines for the private-sector practitioner. It is highly probable that, as with any new entrepreneurial venture, the field attracts persons who are not qualified. Other motives and goals emerge that are in conflict with those held by the professional group itself (Taylor, 1985). Rehabilitation counselors have been certified since 1975, and some dozen or so states include them under a "Licensed Counselor" title, which protects the consumer. On the whole however, private-sector rehabilitation is still an open field, a free-enterprise system that lacks the controls valued by the practitioners themselves — the ethical standards learned in university programs and the belief that profits can be earned in an ethical way. The skepticism of some practitioners of public-sector rehabilitation concerning the private sector stems from the latter's profit orientation. Not only is there a basic philosophical struggle with the profit principle, but there also exists a crusading spirit to introduce rehabilitation into the mainstream to provide valuable human services to a larger, needful audience, a service for which private industry is willing to pay and which can only be good for the profession.

Competency, objectivity in relation to others, and confidence in oneself as a counselor, are the strengths that will provide a base that results in provision of services in the client's best interests. Taylor asserts that in any profession it is desirable for its practitioners to behave consistently and positively, which concurs with Shawhan's "expectant" rehabilitation philosophy, as discussed previously. Taylor sees as the goal of service adjustment between the disabled person and the environment, recognition of one's individuality and rights, and responsibility for one's behavior. He holds that productive activity, maximum vocational independence, and employment are important psychological benefits for injured workers. To assure the success of these goals, it is necessary to take a position on standards of practice to assist each member of the profession in deciding what action to take when a situation of conflict arises in her or his work. Clarification of the counselor's responsibilities gives the professional some assurance that members' practices will not be detrimental to the general functions and purposes of the profession. A code of ethics must be formulated to guarantee society that our services meet the social codes and moral expectations of the community.

In essence, the Code of Ethics statements of NRCA (1972) and NARPPS (1981) provide private-sector rehabilitation with a set of guidelines for ethical professional practice. However, there are issues specific to the private sector that Taylor reviews as follows:

• *Profit motive.* Hard and efficient work will produce more income (profit). The outcome depends on our own efforts. The potential conflict: Will it plealse the insurer and yet work in the client's best interests?

• *Competition.* There exists competition with one another, not only in the marketplace, but in the courtroom. These situations challenge objectivity.

• *Litigation.* Workers' Compensation is fraught with legal concerns and the counselor is faced with practical problems — such as the attorney's interference with the counselor's work with the client. Which side is one on?

• *Vested interests.* States, insurance adjusters, and employers seek different ends. One protects the rights of individuals; another wants minimum cost and successful closure. The attorney wants the maximum from the client's disability and the counselor wants the client's maximum ability. The pressures interfere with the quality of services.

• *Rehabilitation goal.* The goal is different in the private sector than in the public sector, as it is established by the benefit system; that is, a return to suitable employment as quickly as possible.

• *Diversity of practitioners.* In training and background, "qualified" means different things in different states and situations. Do all agree on advocacy for clients, on the importance of confidentiality, and so on?

• *Outlaw image.* Private-sector practitioners have been accused by traditional counselors of being less than professional, less dedicated. Counselors often believe the "bad press" is attributable to the unprofessional conduct of some firms and practitioners. Taylor's thesis contends that with a strong commitment and competency, a counselor can work ethically in any setting. To obviate the notion that private rehabilitation is or may be a different profession, Taylor makes a neat distinction, observing that the private sector is an "arena," another place to practice rehabilitation counseling, and thus has produced these ethical dilemmas that clash with basic philosophical precepts of rehabilitation (1985). Private-sector rehabilitation must guard against vulnerability, not compromise rehabilitation efforts.

The business of rehabilitation is now *big* business and needs to be managed well. Is the rehabilitation professional trained to do this or will we see business people or insurance companies running rehabilitation firms? IRA, Crawford, and Constitution Rehabilitation are firms owned by insurance companies. How do we ensure the survival of the rehabilitation practitioner who has much to offer the private-sector field? Perhaps managers of private rehabilitation firms can cooperate in setting enforceable industry-wide policies to help resolve the conflicts and dilemmas faced by private-sector practitioners. They can establish the groundwork to deal with issues of rehabilitation goals, competition, unfair marketing practices, and the like created by a rapidly growing and highly competitive service industry that significantly affects the lives of most disabled people (Taylor, 1985).

TRENDS

When speaking with leaders and administrators in private-sector rehabilitation, one hears of opportunities — of expanding services, of greater visibility, of a more educated public. Jasper (1987) cites a decided change taking place in service and treatment intervention in the early stages of disability. Where 15 years ago it was almost exclusively the province of Workers' Compensation, today it is a holistic disability management programs approach. Disability management programs are found in hospitals, clinics, corporations, and insurance companies. Such early and expanded services to newly injured or ill workers can serve ultimately only to upgrade Workers' Compensation practices. In CCM and LTD cases, a trend toward more frequent use of rehabilitation nurses, and the utilization of early work and physical-capacity evaluation has been noted by Banks (1987) and by Edgecombe (1987). Such services, according to these sources, are valuable not only to the employer, but also to judges in personal-injury and spousal-support court cases, in return-to-work potential, in most earnings, and in the value of a spouse's contribution to the marriage in determining a settlement.

Work-capacity evaluation is fast becoming an important resource, which utilizes the concepts and practices developed in sports medicine, and where rehabilitation counselors, evaluators, physical and occupational therapists, and nurses work in a team approach. These exciting trends increase the involvement of the employer, the client, and the family, and the prospect is to see the client and her or his family become their own consumers. The benefits of early rehabilitation will be realized in every aspect of individual, physical, and psychological health; in family situations; in work; and in social areas. When compared with the loss in psychological, financial, and physical function, these changes can mean timely, cost-effective resolution and return to work for the client. The field is diversifying and expanding, Anderson (1987) suggests, especially as Workers' Compensation moves away from mandating rehabilitation services, as has occurred in several states, to recognition of the cost-effective benefits to corporations and insurers. Another arena in which the use of private rehabilitation providers is gaining is as expert witnesses in legal situations. Again, Edgecombe states, work-capacity evaluation is providing "more work than people can handle."

Negative aspects as accrue to any growing industry are noted in the move of large corporations to buy out private rehabilitation firms and then to utilize these services (in-house) for all of their disabled workers. Additionally, there exists a tendency to employ poorly qualified people as rehabilitation counselors. Pirating of clients, as firms hire personnel from competitive companies, is another unprofessional device that undermines and diminishes the fine work and services that private-sector rehabilitation can provide to the consumer.

Adherence to high professional standards and to excellence in practice and in marketing programs is essential for the field. Private- and public-sector rehabilitation providers, university educators, and professional organizations are well advised to confront these concerns, and one another, to establish sound, clear, ethical behavior, with the ultimate goal of providing the injured worker with the services to which she or he is entitled.

REFERENCES

Anderson, M. (1987). Vector, Westminister, CA. Personal communication.

Banks, J. (1987). Work Recovery Center, Tucson, AZ. Personal communication.

Edgecombe, J. (1987). Personal communication.

Field, T. (1987). University of Georgia, Athens. Personal communication.

Habeck, R., & Ellien V. (1986). Implications of worksite practice for rehabilitation counselor education and training. *Journal of Applied Rehabilitation Counseling,* *17*(3), 49–54.

Hayes, L. (1987). Opening a private practice: The pitfalls and rewards. *Guidepost.* AACD. *30*(5), 1–5.

Jasper, K. (1987). OPTIONS Associates, Quincy, MA. Personal communication.

Kaplan, S. (1986). Rehabilitation counseling in medical settings: Career opportunities. *Journal of Applied Rehabilitation Counseling, 17*(2),43–44.

Krieshok, T. (1987). Psychologists and counselors in the legal system: A dialogue with Theodore Blau. *Journal of Counseling and Development, 66,* 69–72.

Lynch, R., & Martin, T. (1982 Aug.–Sept.). Rehabilitation counseling in the private sector: A training needs survey. *Journal of Rehabilitation.* pp. 51–53, 73.

Matkin, R. (1985). The state of private sector rehabilitation. In L. Taylor et al. (Eds.), *Handbook of private sector rehabilitation.* New York: Springer Publishing Co.

OPTIONS Associates, Inc., Staff (Nov. 1987). Personal communication.

Shawhan, C. (1985). Getting professional training and preparation. In L. Taylor et al. (Eds.), *Handbook of private sector rehabilitation.* New York: Springer Publishing Co.

Schwartz, G. (1986). Selected criteria and performance standards for employers to use in contracting with private sector rehabilitation firms. AT&T Project, in progress.

Tate, D., Habeck, R., & Galvin, D. (1986). Disability management: Origins, concepts, and principles for practice. *Journal of Applied Rehabilitation Counseling, 17*(3), 5–12.

Taylor, L.J. (1985). Being an ethical professional in private sector rehabilitation. In Taylor et al. (Eds.), *Handbook of private-sector rehabilitation.* New York: Springer Publishing Co.

Weed, R., & Field, T. (1986). The differences and similarities betwen public and private sector vocational rehabilitation: A literature review. *Journal of Applied Rehabilitation Counseling, 17*(2), 11–16.

C H A P T E R
30

TEACHING

David Clayson, Ph.D.

This chapter will deal with some of the ways in which teaching can be used for income expansion. For many private practitioners, teaching is a memorable aspect of their own years of training and presents a particularly attractive way of generating income. It can offer personal benefits that range from interactions with young people and the collegiality of peers that characterize association with traditional educational institutions to the peculiar satisfactions found in private entrepreneurship. By definition, teaching involves bringing out the latent capabilities of the learner (educating), an objective closely akin to the goals of private practice. Teaching may require devising formal or methodical approaches to developing skills (instructing), drilling students with a specific end in view (training), or disciplining individuals in what is hard to master (schooling). The strategies of teaching are many and, when identified with specific needs, can be put to highly practical use. This chapter will take a broad view of teaching activity. It will examine teaching in traditional settings, continuing educatiopn, consultation, and conferences.

SPECIALIZATION

It is of great importance that the practitioner who wishes to use teaching to enhance income develop an area of special expertise. Advanced preparation in something beyond basic generic education can provide a potentially important competitive advantage both within and beyond institutional settings. The number of possibilities for specialization is nearly limitless. The following is just a small sample of available options.

Childhood
    Language development/problems
    Emotional/motivational development
    Social behavior
    Parent–child/family relations
    Child abuse
    Physical/motor development
    Learning disabilities
Adolescence
Adulthood
Aging

Development of the
   Mentally retarded
   Physically handicapped
   Blind
   Deaf
Intra- and intergroup processes
Alcohol/drug use
Psychotherapy
   Behavioral/conditioning
   Group/family/couples
   Sex/marital
   Individual
   Sexual dysfunction

Traditional Settings

For many practitioners, membership on the part-time faculty of a university or college has particular appeal because it permits a continuation of both familiar, gratifying activity and learning. The system of higher education in the United States is vast. In 1987, there were 3,200 degree-granting colleges and universities in the country. These institutions employed 648,000 teachers, of whom approximately 207,000 (32 percent) were part-time (*National Faculty Directory,* 1987). In view of sharply rising costs, most institutions of higher learning are increasingly reluctant to commit scarce resources to tenured faculty. Consequently, the number of part-time positions can be expected to rise. The availability of part-time employment varies considerably, depending upon the institution and region and whether an urban or a rural setting. Because of his or her divided commitments, the practitioner/faculty member may face a variety of problems associated with being an "outsider" to an educational institution; yet, like other teachers, he or she may perform tasks that are essential to an institution's mission and maintenance needs.

Continuing Education

Continuing education courses—both in and outside formal educational settings—provide a second natural area of economic opportunity for the private practitioner. While financial and other resources may be uncertain at a given time, virtually all continuing educators are salient about the future of continuing education. Changes in human service professions are expected to result in a greater demand for continuing education and staff development. New instructional formats and task analyses will make it possible to deliver services more effectively and efficiently. The use of continuing education as a change in strategy is becoming better understood and is acquiring more legitimacy. Continuing edicators themselves are finding a common identity and increasing strength within their practice arena. Private practitioners who are prepared to provide teaching services often shift their attention from preprofessional education—the one-time preparation for beginning practice—to ongoing and continuous education for changing practice.

Some educators have emphasized the half-life of education in various professions (Lauffer, 1977, pp. 190–191). For example, the estimate of the half-life of medical knowledge is now considered to be five years. Human service professions are continually affected by new scientific discoveries and technological innovations. They are subject to fluctuations in the social environment surrounding their practices. These environments change so rapidly that earlier perceptions and established skills increasingly become passé in light of current concerns and conceptions. The implications for education in the human services is clear: a one-time infusion of knowledge and skill no longer will be acceptable, if indeed it ever was.

Continuing educators may be independent professionals who market their own services to mental-health agencies or who organize courses and work out seminars for individual consumers. Increasingly, however, these individuals have discovered the advantages of joining with others to establish consultation, research, service, or training firms. Educational activities can also emerge from interactions among practitioners, administrators, and educators who initially join together because of common intgerests. As such, this type of group may last for only a short time or may continue over many years. These groups develop as a source of learning where professionals can go for help with practice problems, to learn new skills or techniques, and to share information from formally organized and structured conferences they attend to address these issues. Such groups are often easily expanded to become economically viable groups for continuing education purposes.

Supervision and Tutoring

For practitioners who, by personal preference or though time constraints, prefer an essentially independent contribution to continuing education, supervision or tutoring is a frequent choice. In the role of supervisor, the practitioner may provide advanced instruction to individuals or groups for a range of professional skills (psychotherapy, psychodiagnostic evaluation, etc.). Just as the successful practitioner is developed over time on the basis of referrals from patients, so, too, success as a supervisor can develop from the referrals of supervisees.

Tutoring is a service that is rapidly gaining ground as the need for professionals to teach individuals or groups who are preparing for diplomate status, certification or licensing examinations, or a range of other qualifying tests increases. As always, the development of a reputation for effectiveness in such roles is of great importance.

Models for Group Instruction

In teaching groups of people, traditional models of instruction still predominate (although newer techniques have been used increasingly with considerable success). Traditional models have generally taken the form of seminars, workshops, institutes, symposia, and retreats. These can be defined as follows:

• *Seminar.* A meeting of a relatively small group of people in which information is provided by a leader and discussed by the group.

• *Workshop.* A seminar emphasizing free discussion and exchange of ideas and practical methods, skills, and principles. Such meetings are typically designed for adults already in the field.

• *Institute.* A meeting for formal instruction or a brief course of such meetings. Institutes can be structured in such a way as to provide credit or certification of attendance to participants.

• *Symposium.* A meeting at which several speakers deliver short addresses on a topic or related topics.

• *Retreat.* A period of group withdrawal (e.g., to a resort or camp) under a director/teacher. Any of the above instructional formats may be used in a retreat.

All of these meetings are intended to provide an occasion for the formal interchange of views.

Because continuing educators who are also practitioners tend to be closely attuned to the needs and interests of professionals in the field, they may be among the first to identify issues that concern the practitioner. They are in an ideal position to carry these concerns back to their colleagues. They are also ideally placed to understand the effectiveness of newer teaching techniques such as Tavistock-style meetings, T-groups, or sensitivity training. They may have more direct experience with systems change models, which might include such diverse educational approaches as awareness-raising workshops, problem-focused conferences, and public information campaigns.

CONSULTATION

A Form Of Continuing Education

Consultation can be thought of as a form of continuing education and teaching in the role of consultant is one of the most common ways of expanding income. Consulting can take many forms and take place in many settings. It can include contact with schools, community organizations, fraternal groups, self-help groups, and industry. Just as particular groups have special areas of educational need, so, too, do particular populations of people. It is known that every stage of human and group change involves stress. Lewin (1978) has identified neglected or not commonly considered areas that carry great promise for the extension of consultation services;

Precollege issues and problems (college-bound students)
Prework issues and problems (high-school and college graduates)
Prepromotion
Prejob change
Prefirings/layoffs
Predivorce
Preretirement
Retirement

Readmission to nursing homes
Health problems/abuse
Illness of a loved one
Vacation planning

The most common approach to becoming a consultant is through association with agencies that have developed a roster of local practitioners as a means of receiving help with specific problems. The consumer of a consultation service is often a subunit of a service organization, the total organization itself, a complex of service organizations or providers, or a local chapter or affiliate of a professional association. Typically, someone or some group within the unit recognizes a problem that needs to be addressed. This problem is generally defined in terms of poor and inefficient organizational performance, low morale, poor communication, or inappropriate management style.

Once the problem has been perceived, even if it is not identified fully, the consultant will generally become involved in the effort to define the problem operationally and to design a plan to overcome it. The consultant is frequently responsible for managing training or learning activities aimed at overcoming the identified problem. The employing agency or other organization becomes a consumer that may also perceive itself as the recipient of a service. The individual worker in the agency is often viewed as the target of change.

Two Common Models Of Consultation Service

Two common approaches to consultation service are the process model and the agency development model. Process consultation involves teaching courses on staff development. Dorn (1956) details the process in which, as an outside professional, the consultant facilitates the interaction of some natural group or system in achieving a more or less commonly defined task or goal. The emphasis is on improving the functioning of the work or task group. The client system is preexisting and continuing: the group teaching relationship of the consultant is viewed as temporary input into an ongoing operation. The consultant in a staff development program has already developed a program. The rationale for the process consultant is that the consultant remains in his or her area of expertise and, therefore, is able to provide the client with high-quality, specialized input in an area of specific need.

The objectives of the agency development model are complementary to, yet quite different from, the individually oriented training and development found in the process model. Rather than attempt to change groups of individuals to fit the organizatio or to provide multiple choices to the individual, agency development focuses more directly on changing the organization to fit its members. It utilizes course work and other means to effect changes in the way the organization is managed and the manner in which staff members relate to each other. The underlying assumption is that greater job satisfaction and better internal relations will ultimately increase effectiveness and efficiency.

In management terms, education for agency development draws on the "human relations school" for its orientation, in contrast to in-service training, which draws on the "scientific management school." Agency devlopment relies heavily on teaching approaches in which units within the agency (and sometimes the whole agency) are engaged in a collaborative process. This may be the most difficult form of staff development to conduct. It requires participation in decision making by various staff levels in the organization. The most common activities do not look like traditional training but include group problem solving, team building, and the development of new communication channels.

Consultation With Schools

Consultation with schools is the most common form of consultation activity for practitioners. In working with teachers and administrators in a school system, the consultant often has the unique opportunity to teach, and sometimes to demonstrate, mental-health principles to teachers. He or she can communicate to teachers the fact that human feelings can be talked about without shame, making judgments, or blaming individuals or labeling them as "bad." Consultants, by their attentiveness to and concern and respect for their professional colleagues, demonstrate their relationship to the teacher as a colleague whose problems, with their attendant mixed feelings, are of mutual concern. A consultant's encouragement of verbal expression of the teacher's feelings about his or her work is greatly enhanced by the consultant's progressively clarifying that he or she is not there to analyze the teacher's personal problems.

Consultants can demonstrate in many ways that their jobs as experts in interpersonal relations are to help teachers understand themselves in terms of the jobs they are doing, and in particular to help them to become consciously aware of their feelings about particular problems they are facing. Because consultants are "outside" the system, the tasks they perform in a school setting may be not fully understood or appreciated at first. Many of their actions may be suspect. They have to be justified. And justification comes only from a consultant's own successful practice or the successful practice of others in similar positions. Because the practices of consultants, even within the same profession, are extremely varied, few agreed-upon models for consultation/practice exist. Standardized patterns are only now in the process of evolution.

In recent years, a number of federal and state regulations have been enacted requiring schools to deliver psychological services and instruction. The major impetus to these regulations is Public Law 94-142, called the Education for All Handicapped Children Act of 1975 (Pressman, 1979). Regulations apply to the area of special education and serve children diagnosed as suspected of having difficulty regarding emotional disturbance, retardation, learning disabilities, neurological problems, and other problems that interfere with learning. Regulations often mandate that these children receive clinical services or education under the auspices of the school. Many schools contract with clinical psychologists and other health professionals to provide both clinical services and instruction to students on and off school campuses.

Special Problems And Issues For The
Practitioner/Consultant

Many newcomers to the consulting relationship naively or arrogantly approach work with consultees as if they were "patients" who are simply being seen in a different setting. Inevitably, the relationship deteriorates. Seasoned individuals, entering into such unfamiliar situations, immediately recognize their need to seek information and to learn with the task before they are prepared to instruct. Mental-health consultation requires the practitioner to have a much broader range of skills and capabilities than is required of individuals in private practice. Beyond financial gain, the restrictiveness of private practice and the narrower life it provides are frequently central reasons why private practitioners develop consulting relationships. Teaching in the role of a consultant requires considerably more flexibility and professional adaptability than needed in psychotherapy. Further, the usefulness of the consultant is constantly under review, as his or her cost-effectiveness will be of central concern to the employer.

Consultants will ultimately reduce their marketability by attempting to be overinclusive in the presentation of their skills. Potential clients will be concerned if they have difficulty identifying the consultant's area of expertise. It is generally unlikely that the consultant is an expert in a number of areas. Because potential clients often hire consultants on the basis of their reputation, many will avoid the risk of being disappointed by not hiring a consultant if they are at all concerned about the individual's expertise. Thus, for example, the private practitioner who offers courses on staff development needs to be specific about areas of specialization. Instead of saying "family counseling," the practitioner would better say "behavioral approach to family counseling." Rather than indicate "career development," the consultant should indicate "midlife career development." Practitioners who wish to become consultants must always ask themselves, "What can I teach that is different or better than what others teach?" And, "Will other professionals have any interest in such a program?" Most important, "Who would be interested enough in such a course to commit part of their budget to it?"

Private practitioners who seek to learn consultation methods must generally unlearn some of their ways of thinking about and working with people. Consultees are collaborators, not patients; they are clients, not counselees. The personal psychopathology of individuals taught in the consultation role is generally not the object of discussion. Thus, the satisfaction and rewards of consultation efforts are not always the same in the individual practice of psychotherapy. Consultees may matter of factly accept the improvement of their work, sometimes not being aware of how they have been helped. When they are aware, they may not acknowledge it to the consultant. Thus, since the usual ways of gauging one's effectiveness and usefulness may be missing, in critical moments it is often difficult for the consultant to refrain from using the tried-and-true methods of individual psychotherapy.

One of the most difficult problems confronting consultants is that of dealing with the omnipotence and omniscience that are often ascribed to them by agency executives and groups as they look to them to apply their expertise to a wide variety of community phenomena. Executives can become acutely disappointed when they discover that the consultant's ideas are not very new or that they require careful collaborative assessment, including that of the role of the educator. The executive's manifest disenchantment with the magic of the mental-health specialist may be a difficult factor with which to deal, especially when expressed in a group situation. Consultants must be prepared, then, to be perceived as experts who can make things right, in much the same way that parents are so perceived by children.

Many factors determine the behavior of people toward consultants. Indeed, client responses are influenced by their stereotyped view of the role and status of the mental health professional. Consultants who understand that previous experience molds the attitudes of clients will enhance the work of the group.

Transference Phenomena And Perception As An Intruder

Transference phenomena have been explored by Berlin (1977), who has observed that, if not understood, they may lead to certain unconscious expectations of the consultant, which may result in a sense of bewilderment, anger, disappointment, unrealistic self-expectation, and, most of all, ineffective teaching. In the consultation setting, invitations to form alliances, to join rebellions, or to support the status quo may occur without any overt stimulation by the consultant, and may reflect both current power struggles and group process and old parent–child and sibling relationships.

Awareness of transference phenomena may enable consultants to understand how and why individual members of the group react to them as they do and why their comments are used by others in defensive or aggressive ways. They must come to understand individual needs and pressures, the hierarchical problems in the group, the status needs of various members, the power struggles, the sibling rivalries in which they are participants, and the behind-the-scenes manipulations. They must also become aware of how their presence and comments may be used to fulfill both individual and group needs.

Consultants should recognize that they may be regarded as intruders who will analyze and dissect the individuals and the group, and find some hidden troubles. This aspect of a transference situation must be understood. Sometimes consultants are expected to understand situations without information having been made explicit, as if they are benign, nonhostile, accepting, and understanding persons who do not assign blame or assess fault. They must demonstrate that they are indeed collaborators and that their understanding of human beings as individuals and in groups is used only in the service of the common work. Within this context, consultants need to be alert to the undue weight often given to their comments and to the fact that some of their innocent and defensive remarks will be misconstrued, taken out of context, and repeated to them in moments of impasse in a way that they never intended them to be used.

The Importance Of Sociological Factors

Consultants should be responsive to the social ecology of the setting in which they function. Researchers such as Plog (1977) have explored problems that can arise when consultants do not look beyond the personal psychology of the individuals they are teaching. Consultants must constantly be aware of the variety of social forces at work in a given setting. Rather than condemn their negative influence, they must learn to work with these realities toward improved final outcomes for the individuals being taught.

Thus, greater sensitivity on the part of consultants to the sociology of the situation and their keener assessment of possible options for those involved can contribute imensely to their overall usefulness. For example, the consultant can assist the school superintendent to walk the delicate line that exists in working with contentious parent groups or the welfare agency to deal more effectively with its own ponderous bureaucracy. Because of their deeper awareness of the problems of both management and employees, consultants generally develop a greater respect for the "establishment." Their work with administrators, executives, and others in positions of responsibility provides an understanding of the problems faced by these individuals and the risks that they face in all courses of action they take. The consultant is generally more willing to side with management and support its efforts to achieve certain goals because he or she understands the implications of alternative courses of action.

CONFERENCES

Objectives Of Conferences

Conferences are a particularly effective way to apply teaching techniques for income enhancement. Lauffer (1977, pp. 34–35) has suggested that conferences generally attempt to accomplish one or more of the following four objectives: information dissemination, problem solving and decision making, information exchange, and fact finding. At information-giving conferences, it is up to the participant to decide whether or not to use the knowledge given for action or problem solving after the conference. The problem-solving or decision-making conference is designed to seek group agreement or action on some problem, issue, or policy. The convener expects that decisions will be made or that problems will be solved at the meeting. The hoped-for outcome could be a plan of action strategy to be used by the participant. When the objectives of the conference are modest, success tends to be greater than when they are complex or ambitious.

The information-exchange conference provides participants with an opportunity to gain and share information with each other rather than to get it exclusively from a convener or outside source. The convener's objective is to provide a setting for an atmosphere conducive to comparisons of notes among participants. The focus of an information-exchange conference is generally on the work participants do, the problems they share, or the approaches they find useful in solving problems. The fact-finding conference elicits information and opinions from participants to be used as a basis for future planning. It differs also in that information is not necessarily secured for use by its participants. Information generated may be directed at policy groups and others that may need it to make more effective decisions in allocating resources.

The No-Fee Conference And Volunteer Service

One of the most important and effective ways in which private practitioners can introduce themselves and their expertise to the community is by conducting conferences in community settings for no fee. On such occasions, the consumer will be introduced to the skills and potential usefulness of the practitioner without obligation and with the positive sense that always accompanies something given complimentarily. A number of organizations are available for presentations and conferences, if these are considered to be of basic interest and relevant to the particular population involved. If successful, the "halo" effect of such conferences can well extend far beyond a specific occasion or group. Acquiring a reputation as an expert, innovator, resource, facilitator, and approachable professional can go a long way toward establishing a practitioner as an individual who would be a better choice than someone else for the kind of teaching role involved in such conferences.

Beyond good citizenship, the same public-relations benefits accrue from volunteer service on committees of various local organizations. These can be extremely useful in establishing a practitioner's special skills in the community. One might consider the following types of organizations as particularly useful for volunteer service: the Association for Retarded Citizens, Big Brothers, church groups, fraternal organizations, private clubs, parents' associations, school boards, and self-help groups.

The Importance Of Preparation

A significant amount of time, energy, and preparation must be devoted to the development and organization of a course. Practitioners who intend to present their programs to others should have a reasonably good idea of how the material will be received. The most effective way to determine this is through trial runs in different settings. For example, consider a staff development course. The practitioner presenting this type of course should be entertaining as well as informative. Creative case histories, anecdotes, and exercises that will be well received by audiences need to be developed. It is always advantageous to have an option or two available in the event that something does not work as well as expected. The successful course will give clients more than they expected, promote informal learning before they complete the course, and — very important — result in the convener learning from the clients.

A not uncommon phenomenon is for the enthusiasm about a staff development program to disappear after the course has been completed. Thus, it is important for the conference developer to promote informal learning in various activities after the course has ended. These activities might include "brainstorming" sessions during the course, references to be used in teacher meetings, and encouragement for the class to meet again on its own in the future.

Conference Organization And Planning

To begin with, the convener should be familiar with the proposed conference site. Resorts or hotels that permit all activities of the conference are preferred. If the conference is going to be presented on a regular basis (for example, annually), it is best to afford equal access to people from various regions by rotating the site geographically in accordance with the facilities available. All expenses, including those of preconference planning, should be budgeted as reimbursable expenses via the conference registration fee.

In general, the ratio of expenses to projected registration income should be amortized at 75 percent just to break even. For example, if 100 registrants are expected, the registration fee sufficient to cover expenses should be established on the basis of 75 registrants. This ratio produces a 25 percent reserved contingency in the event that inclement weather, an energy crisis, unexpected expenses, or other emergencies preclude antitipated attendance or revenues. The profit margin must be established above this ratio. Consideration should be given to establishing a lower registration fee for spouses, guests, and so on. The following provides some idea of the preparation that goes into a conference (see Jax, 1981).

The educational experience may begin before the actual start of the conference or the convening of its participants. This is especially true when there has been careful planning for those for whom the conference is intended. The

Conference Organization and Planning Schedule

2 years in advance	Select site, dates; reserve meeting rooms.
10–12 months in advance	Select conference theme.
3–6 months in advance	Set planning budget and honoraria limits (if any).
3–6 months in advance	Formalize speakers'/presenters' agreements; make meal arrangements.
60–90 days in advance	Distribute conference announcements and registration information. Notice should appear in professional newsletters (e.g., *APA Monitor,* state or local publications).
30 days in advance	Send ads to printer. Arrange for speaker/presenter equipment.
10 days before	Preregistration deadline. Verify meal counts. Assign spaces for sessions. Assemble registration packets.
30–60 days after	Write thank-you letters to exhibitors. Pay conference bills.

convener can elicit input from expected conference participants in advance of their attendance through questionnaires that ask about facts, attitudes, interests, and definitions of problems. Interviews and preconference meetings can also be utilized.

Conferences held in populated areas can generally rely on traditional public-relations techniques. In rural area, experience shows that sending out an array of messages and brochures is generally futile. What is needed is one or two people from those areas to pick up a new bit of information from a colleague who has attended a conference or to come to a training program outside their area. They will soon pass the word and the spread effect will very often lead to opportunities for new conferences in outlying areas.

Conference Evaluation

To improve and to further develop teaching programs, conveners need specific feedback. Organizers must realize that their programs are in continual need of improvement and updating. Courses must be examined from all aspects, and a determination made regarding whether the participants' needs are being met. This assessment should be made before the next course is given, not after it. Above all, the convener must realize that a satisfied previous client will be the best recommendation for the next client.

Answers to the following types of questions generally provide the most useful information for future planning.

1. Which sessions did you attend?
2. Will the content of each session be useful to you in your work?
3. Was the material presented in an interesting manner?
4. Do you feel the presenters were competent to present their topics?
5. If audio/visuals were utilized by the presenter, do you feel that they detracted from or enhanced the presentation?
6. Was there enough variety among the topics offered?
7. How do you feel about the conference length?
8. Overall, how would you rate the quality of the conference?

CONCLUSION

This chapter has dealt with ways in which teaching might be utilized for income expansion. Potential rewards vary widely for this activity and, for the most part, can be expected to increase as the practitioner shifts away from organizations and structures that are created by others toward greater independence and increased entrepreneurship. Thus, the financial gain to be found within the familiar framework of institutional settings will be the most limited.

Continuing education opportunities—notably those organized apart from institutions—can offer much greater financial incentives. Supervision, tutoring, and cosponsorship of seminars, workshops, institutes, symposia, and retreats have proved to have financial potential. But the greatest possibilities for economic gain may be found in consultantships and the organization of conferences. Time constraints and the pull (often powerful) to one type of teaching over another are very important factors to consider in making professional choices. Beyond these, the extent to which teaching will play a meaningful role in expanding a practitioner's income will be determined by the practitioner's capacity for, and pleasure in, independent effort and a degree of risk taking.

REFERENCES

Berlin, I.N. (1977). Some lessons learned in 25 years of mental health consultation to schools. In S.C. Plog and P.I. Ahmed (Eds.), *Principles and techniques of mental health consultation* (p. 31). New York, London: Plenum Medical Book Company.

Dorn, F.J. (1986). The road to workshop consultation: Some directions for the new traveler. *American Mental Health Counselors Association Journal, 8*(2), 53.

Jax, J.J. (Ed.). 1981). *Blueprint for success. A manual for conventions, seminars and workshops.* Madison, WI. Wisconsin Library Association.

Lauffer, A. (1977). *The practice of continuing education in the human services.* New York: McGraw-Hill Book Co.

Lewin, M.H. (1978). *Establishing and maintaining a successful professional practice* (pp. 136–39). Rochester, NY: Professional Development Institute.

National faculty directory (7th ed.. Vol. 1, p. 8). (1987). Detroit, MI: Gale Research Co.

Plog, S.C., & Ahmed, P.I. (Eds.) (1977). *Principles and techniques of mental health consultation* (p. 5). New York, London: Plenum Medical Book Co.

Pressman, R.M. (1979). *Private practice. A handbook for the independent mental health practitioner* (p. 128). New York: Gardner Press.

SECTION

D

Economic Issues

▼ ▼ ▼

C H A P T E R
31

NATIONAL HEALTH INSURANCE

Rogers H. Wright, Ph.D.

N ational health insurance (NHI) and a national health service plan (NHSP) appear to be ideas whose time has gone. The concept of a universal health plan first became widely apparent in the late 1930s during a period of profound social reform, but the late 1980s hears little reference to the broad scope of care originally envisioned. Obviously, something discouraged the implementation of the concept; events of such dramatic impact that the enthusiasms initially provoked by concepts of NHI and NHSP have so waned in intensity that an informal survey by this writer in 1987 could determine not a single prominent member of Congress who expressed an intent to introduce such legislation into the Congress. Further, nationally prominent advocates, such as Senator Edward Kennedy (1987), have clearly moved away from supporting a national health insurance plan as part of their foreseeable future political agenda.

Dr. Patrick DeLeon, psychologist/legislative assistant to Sen. Daniel Inouye, recently noted in a personal communication that the national health agenda has generally been concluded by the federal Congress, and further that only the details of such a program remained to be completed by state legislatures.

Before the 1980s, and given the enthusiasm generated by concepts of universal health coverage, enactment of such legislation appeared to be almost inevitable. The decades between 1940 and 1980 saw England (and other European countries) adopt "cradle to grave" health service plans — plans representing ambitious implementations of a national health service agenda. However, during much of this period, cultural attitudes toward statism in the United States were such that the only governmentally provided health benefits were those accorded to "wards of the government" (e.g., health services provided by the Indian Medical Service, services to Veterans, and services — such as they were, and are — to the poor and indigent). This culture's commitment to individual responsibility was epitomized in the health field by the feeling that consumers are responsible for their own health care. In fact, the only nationally successful health plan was initiated by physician groups (who formed the Blue Cross/Blue Shield prepaid insurance plans covering some of the cost of inpatient and outpatient care). Coverage by "the Blues" was relatively expensive, and in those early days was restricted to a relatively small percentage of the population. A survey of representative literature of the period reveals almost no discussion of any national health plan.

World War II accelerated the growth of federal responsibility for health-care delivery because large numbers of the American consuming public were exposed to governmentally provided health care, a government responsibility carried into the postwar era in the form of "veteran benefits." However, by 1965, concerns about the economics of health-care delivery (particularly for the elderly) and changing American attitudes relative to personal responsibility resulted in the passage of companion legislation—Medicare and Medicaid—that covered the young of indigent parents and the elderly; this legislation based on a "fee for service" model was enacted despite the massed opposition of health-care providers.

Medicare and Medicaid are actually amendments to the Social Security Act, federal legislation from the late 1930s establishing a national retirement income program on an actuarial base. The health-care amendments were also presumably actuarially based, and, as earlier noted, followed the private sector fee-for-service model (with payments being made by the government agency to private health-care providers). Concurrently, the health-care insurance industry aggressively merchandized health-care coverage (largely to employers), an operation that was so successful that by the early 1970s it was repeatedly estimated that upward of 85 percent of the U.S. population were covered by some form of prepaid health insurance; that is, either through the Medicare/Medicaid program or through employer-provided health insurance plans. Individual health insurance was also available on a prepayment basis, but the cost to the individual was such that a relatively small percentage of the population opted for individual coverage.

The continuing escalation of health-care costs occasioned widespread concern about access to adequate health services and made employer-provided health insurance an increasingly popular item with workers. To many employees first entering the job market or changing jobs, the potential employer's health benefits program was frequently more important than the same company's deferred compensation or pension plan—an ironic state of affairs that only recently has been given a long second thought by many employees. The elaboration of Medicare/Medicaid coverage, the proliferation of employer-supported insurance programs, and broad social programs, such as the federally sponsored "Great Society/War on Poverty" initiatives, coalesced into a conception of a "right" to health care, a conception virtually unheard of a few decades ago.

Mental-health services followed the same general pattern during this period; that is, there was increasing acceptance and utilization of mental-health services of all kinds accompanied by employer-supported prepaid insurance plans covering mental-health benefits. Although the Social Security/Medicare/Medicaid programs had (and continue to have) mental-health coverage, the covered mental-health benefits are minimal, the preponderant myth being that mental-health problems are not prominent among the very young or the elderly. The private sector began to offer broad mental-health coverage, initially for inpatient service; then extending as the consumption of mental-health benefits increased, to more elaborate coverage for outpatient mental-health services.

Through the decades of the 1960s and 1970s, and with the Democratic party taking the leadership at both the national and state level, much was heard about the desirability of enacting some form of national health insurance, including mental-health coverage (Kiesler, Cummings, & Vanden Bos, 1979). State and federal legislatures systematically broadened the nature and extent of coverage, and new providers in both the physical-medicine and mental-health areas were statutorily recognized. The same time span saw greater state and federal support for increasing or expanding training facilities and service-delivery centers such as hospitals and community mental-health centers. Developments in the mental-health field followed the same pattern; for example, one major health-care underwriter (Prudential) actually aggressively merchandized a so-called "high option" mental-health benefit providing the insured with almost unlimited coverage for the consumption of mental-health services.

However, despite the widespread conception of health care as an individual right, NHI/NHSP covering the full population was never enacted, even though similar legislation was implemented by countries as disparate as Britain, West Germany, Norway, Denmark, Sweden, Switzerland, Italy, Greece, and Japan. Given widely popular acceptance of the concept of prepayment/government responsibility for health care, the United States' failure to enact universal NHI/NHSP appears to reflect the interaction of a number of factors.

DETERRENTS TO NHI/NHSP

It is tempting to speculate that the very magnitude of coverage available through Medicare/Medicaid programs, individual and employer-provided prepayment plans, and the like, precluded the necessity of legislating an ambitious universal health plan, and it does appear likely that the extensiveness of such available coverage has mitigated, to some degree, the urgency with which Congress has viewed the issue. Nevertheless, broad areas of exposure potentially affecting large numbers of people remain uncovered; thus, to explain the waning enthusiasm for NHI/NHSP as diminished need overlooks a blatant economic, social, and political reality. At the risk of oversimplification, it can be said that one of the primary deterrents to the enactment of further universal health programs in the United States has been the fact that the cost of such programs is staggering and has consistently been underestimated (Shalowicz, 1987).

From the standpoint of the insured-consumer, the history of Medicare from its onset has been one of steadily increasing premiums and declining benefits. The continued erosion of covered services (in an effort to cope with increasing costs) has resulted in a situation in which inpatient services have been severely limited and coinsurance responsibilities for both inpatient and outpatient service weigh very heavily on retired persons with fixed incomes. The early, enthusiastic vision of a national health plan for the aged, ensuring adequate medical services at a moderate fee, has proved largely illusory. Elders with the economic means to subscribe find that their broad range of health needs is covered only if they privately purchase one of the Medicare supplemental insurance plans. Existing gaps in inpatient coverage are so substantial that the Reagan administration in 1987 proposed an ambitious supplemental program to be paid for by the individual consumer at a cost variously estimated as ranging from $500 to $2,000 per year. However, even with the most comprehensive of supplemental plans, the elderly are still vulnerable in some of their areas of greatest need. For example, few of the supplemental plans cover extended-care facilities such as long-term convalescent centers or nursing homes for the physically or mentally infirm elderly.

The consequence of underestimating consumption in Medicare/Medicaid has been cost overruns, which, when the government is the third-party subsidizer, can be addressed by additional ("emergency") appropriations, by denying claims, or by a process called "passing through." Hospital administrators, professional associations, and health insurer associations have repeatedly charged that Medicare and Medicaid consistently have failed to pay fully for services consumed, either by inadequately proscribed reimbursement or by arbitrarily refusing to pay hospital and provider charges. The result (cost-shifting) has been that substantial amounts of the cost for service to the Medicare/Medicaid populations have passed through to the private sector in t.ie form of higher charges for private services. The escalating cost of the service to the private sector has widened the gap between Medicare/Medicaid services and the private sector, in turn confronting legislators with the necessity for ever-increasing appropriations for Medicare/Medicaid.

Another significant factor in what has been termed the inflationary explosion of health-care cost has been the long-term and cumulative effects of governmental involvement in other aspects of health delivery. Ambitious governmental programs such as the Hill-Burton Act (a program that encouraged the construction of inpatient facilities) have cumulatively resulted in excessive numbers of hospitals. Health Insurance Association of American (HIAA) surveys of such inpatient facilities conducted in the late 1970s and early 1980s found that in many areas of the country occupancy rates ranged from 50 to 70 percent (in situations where the economics of inpatient care demanded 80 to 85 percent occupancy for economic viability).

Concurrent with support for increasing numbers of health-care facilities were governmental training grants, specific tuitional grants, and stipends for student health-care providers. The unforeseen consequence has been an explosion of health-care facilities and providers that has resulted, in many areas, in an excess of health-care capacity. Facilities and providers must deliver services in order to survive. As more service is consumed, more services are designed to be consumed, and the increased consumption occasions greater cost to the third-party agency subsidizing the service program. The built-in inflationary spiral brought about by the underestimation of cost and the consequent cost shifting to the private sector, compounded by the public's increasing demand for health services and ever-larger numbers of practitioners to provide those services, have created an apparently unending upward spiral of health-care costs, an upward spiral that was augmented by worldwide inflation in the late 1970s and early 1980s.

Another factor chilling enthusiasms for enactment of NHI or NHSP has been the experience of those countries in which such plans have operated. A recent survey of worldwide experience conducted by United Press International (UPI) (Denningan, 1987) summarizes the degradation of health-care delivery that apparently is an almost universal attendant to national health plans. The findings of the survey suggest that the national health program in Denmark is trying to resolve the issue of whether it is better to perform live-saving liver and heart transplants or to treat approximately twice that number of patients with thigh-bone fractures. The UPI survey further reported that, although in Sweden adequate health-care standards are maintained, the system is so clogged by bureaucracy that patients may wait years for so-called "elective surgery" (e.g., a hip-joint replacement) despite the fact that the national health plan accounts for approximately 10 percent of the country's Gross National Product.

The national health plan in England reports much of the same degradation; that is, "shoddy hospitals, shortages of beds and equipment, long lines in waiting rooms, and often years of delay in the treatment of painful, if nonfatal, ailments." The cost to the Britain economy is reportedly 11 percent of the national budget. Equipment scarcities result in "hospitals increasingly turn[ing] to public charity to buy modern scanners and other equipment because the state cannot provide all they need." The UPI survey found that in Norway "overall quality [of delivered care] is high, but public spending cuts have created a shortage of personnel and forced hositals to shut entire wards," while in Italy and Greece, "delays of months and years are common, even for patients needing serious surgery, hospitals are overcrowded, patients in some are in 'camp' beds in the corridors and nonemergency cases have to wait several months for surgery or even x-rays." In Japan with two national health programs, the survey reported that "the Japanese hospitals are considered unsanitary. . . ." Complaints of poor service and long delays at increasing cost have not been lost on the U.S. Congress, especially as it struggles with historic budget deficits.

In the United States, costs of the Medicaid/Medicare program have resulted in the development of a concept of diagnostically related groups (DRGs) wherein a national standard of care for a given diagnostic entity is prescribed by governmental regulation. A recent 1986 Health Care Financing Administration (HCFA) report suggests that hospitals servicing substantial Medicare/Medicaid patients have a significantly higher mortality rate than do other hospitals in the same locations.

These same concerns with utilization and cost have encouraged the development of health maintenance organizations (HMOs) and preferred provider organizations (PPO's), which contract on a capitated basis for the provision of service. The net effect of the DRGs, capitated care, and so forth has frequently been discharge from inpatient facilities "quicker but sicker," and, in both inpatient and outpatient settings, increasing limitations on relevant service, conflict of interest, and excessive or questionable use of professional service review mechanisms, all allegedly in the interest of containing cost (Duerksen, 1986).

The consequent decline in the quantity and quality of available physical-health care as a response to widespread third-party containment efforts and planning has its parallel in mental-health-service delivery. Though, as earlier noted, mental-health benefits in governmentally sponsored programs such as Medicare and Medicaid were never substantial, in the private sector, third-party coverage of such benefits was at one time quite extensive. Typically, such mental-health coverage featured low deductibles and favorable coinsurance (most commonly 80/20), and the coverage was only infrequently "capped" as to either the amount of care consumed (for a given unit of time) of the dollars expended for care in the covered period. As earlier noted, the Prudential Insurance Company was still merchandizing a high-option mental-health benefit as late as the early 1980s. In the early years of this decade, Senator Kennedy was widely quoted as having been persuaded that it was possible to cover psychoanalysis (as such) under third-party benefit programs.

Regrettably during this earlier period, understanding of the traditional mental-health-service transaction was minimal and actuarial evaluations of utilization were naive. The consequence was again a substantial underestimate of cost and a level of utilization far in excess of expectations. The response again paralleled occurrences in physical-health-care delivery; namely, increasing limitations on both the range and extent of benefit coverage. At present, it is almost impossible to find a federal governmental program (CHAMPUS excluded) that does not so severely limit the mental-health benefit as to render it, at best, palliative or supportive, and, at worst, merely symbolic (e.g., in some Medicaid programs, nonphysician mental-health providers are limited to a maximum of two visits per month).

The CHAMPUS program covering a highly at-risk population (the dependents of military personnel) is constantly concerned with what is described as excessive mental-health-service utilization (i.e., mental-health claims in excess of 30 percent) — a not necessarily excessive utilization in such a highly at-risk population. CHAMPUS agency management has also developed extensive utilization review mechanisms, which, at best, are excessively frequent, intrusive, and often unnecessarily violative of patient confidence, and are questionably cost-effective in restricting consumption.

In the private sector, the predominant current pattern of coverage is almost universally a substantial deductible with 50/50 coinsurance, and, more frequently than not, an annual cap of $500 to $1,000 and/or a cap on the number of visits in the covered period. Many such third-party coverages further intrude into the treatment process by limiting consumption of the benefit to some periodic schedule, such as once a week. Coverage for inpatient care has also been severely limited; for example, CHAMPUS programs, except in the most unusual circumstance, are limited to no more than 30 days, restrictions that are rapidly being emulated in the private sector.

These restrictions on benefits have had a profound effect on both the kind and nature of mental-health services. Specifically, and almost without exception, mental-health benefit programs stress the use of medication — at times, to the point where chemotherapeutic intervention is widely perceived as the treatment of choice. Another specific effect of such restricted benefit packages in psychotherapy is a heavy emphasis on short-term, supportive interventions, frequently at the expense of long-term, intensive types of psychotherapy. Concurrently, such sensitivity to cost containment has also encouraged the utilization of progressively lower levels of credentialed personnel, and many company-sponsored mental-health programs feature service delivery by "counselors," all too frequently individuals lacking experience in or minimally trained in mental-health-service delivery. In many employee assistance programs (EAPs), the "counselor's" competence is frequently limited to having experienced the same or a similar psychological difficulty that is currently in a state of arrest or remission. This is especially likely to be the case in many EAP substance-abuse programs.

CURRENT STATUS

Given the apparently uncontrollable acceleration of cost and the U.S. public's apparent disenchantment with highly institutionalized governmental care programs, it is not surprising that Congress is unwilling to enact legislation expanding the Medicare/Medicaid concept to cover the population at large. Nor is it particularly confounding that there seems to be no widespread enthusiasm for some kind of national health insurance, a fact attested to by the total absence of legislation that would establish either of these programs. Current thinking seems to favor continued shifting of the cost of health-care programs to the private sector (Freudenheim, 1986) while maintaining some variation or combination of fee-for-service or prepaid capitated programs. Although some economists question the long-term economic viability of the model, currently HMOs and PPOs seem to have little difficulty recruiting service provider personnel, perhaps in part reflecting widespread practitioner apprehension about the ultimate form of the nation's health-delivery service or the current glut of health-service providers of all disciplines. However, students are already aware of diminishing employment opportunities in the health-care job market, an awareness reflected in substantial reductions in the number of candidates for medical schools, clinical psychology training programs, and the like. The long-range effect of these factors may be a reduction in the oversupply of providers and a consequent ultimate difficulty in recruiting sufficient staff for HMO/PPO organizations. As noted earlier, Senator Kennedy has introduced legislation mandating employers to provide extended mental-health benefits that would cover the bulk of the American population.

Regardless of the funding mechanism, and whether the delivery system is public, private, or a combination thereof, it is reasonable to expect (1) continued efforts to control cost and (2) continuing diminution of the quality and quantity of health care available. The future for mental-health-care providers under such funding mechanisms seems even more grim. Dr. Nicholas Cummings (1987), former president of the American Psychological Association and researcher in mental-health-care economics and short-term interventions, has warned his psychological colleagues that less costly mental-health-care interventions must be found. According to Dr. Cummings, failure to reduce costs will result in clinical psychology losing its role as a significant force in the mental-health-care delivery system by the end of the decade. Another well-established trend (as noted earlier) is the delivery of mental-health services by less highly credentialed mental-health personnel. Studies conducted in California indicate that well before the end of the decade, credentialed marriage and child counselors (MFCCs) trained at the master's-degree level will significantly exceed the combined numbers of board-certified psychiatrists and credentialed, doctoral-level clinical psychologists.

With the burden of health care borne mainly by employers and employer groups, third-party payers are increasingly actively involving themselves in the health-delivery system. This involvement is most prominently manifested in self-insurance programs managed by third-party administrators, through corporate insurance departments making heavy use of third-party or employee-benefit risk management, and through utilization review consultants. In the mental-health field as earlier noted, much of the service delivery is through company-operated EAPs (DiBlase, 1987), a fairly recent phenomenon developed primarily as an employer response to substance abuse among employees. Initially, EAPs were frequently directed and staffed by drug, alcohol, and substance-abuse counselors, many of whom lacked formal training or credentials. Now many such programs are directed by marriage and family counselors, as noted above, credentialed generally at the master's level. As a demonstrated resource within the company for dealing with all kinds of employee difficulties, such EAPs, often acting in concert with the benefits management program, began to enhance their utility by providing increasingly broader ranges of mental health services. Some employers require their workers, before using their mental-health benefits, to consult with the EAP, which determines the type of treatment. For example, in the NCR program, a model for that approach, EAP personnel decide on the type of treatment — short term, crisis intervention, or palliative/supportive short-term "counseling" — and whether it will be supplied by in-house staff. Inasmuch as these departments meter large amounts of health-care delivery of all kinds (especially mental-health care), they are obviously in a position to have substantial economic impact in negotiating with HMOs/PPOs, independent providers, and small groups of practitioners in the community. Significant discounts are clearly expected to be a prominent feature of such negotiations. One troubling aspect of this new development is the conflict-of-interest position in which the EAP personnel are likely to find themselves. One wonders if the decision between short- and long-term counseling will be determined primarily by perceived health-care needs or by the company's concern with health-care costs.

SUMMARY

In light of a history of uncontrolled cost, huge budgetary deficits, excessive bureaucracy, declines in both quantity and quality of care, and attempts to shift the costs to the private sector, it seems unlikely that the Congress will soon attempt enactment of a universal, federal national health insurance or service plan.

REFERENCES

Cummings, N. (1987 March). Invited address. California State Psychological Association Convention.

Dennigan, M. (1987 Feb. 22). America ponders national health plan as others tally flaws. *San Diego Union,* p.C5.

DiBlase, D. (1987 March 9). NCR offers new program for mental health coverage. Benefit beat. *Business Insurance,* p.3.

Duerksen, S. (1986 Dec. 3) Health group advises doctors: Less care means more profits. *San Diego Tribune.*

Freudenheim, M. (1986 Oct. 7). Mental health costs soaring. *New York Times,* p.40.

National Health Care Financing Administration. (1986). Scope of work for PRO contract. Office of Medical Review, Health Standards and Quality Bureau. Washington, DC: author.

Kennedy delays health care bill. (1987 March 9). *Business Insurance,* p.2.

Kiesler, C. A., Cummings, N. A., & VandenBos, G. R. (1979). *Psychology and national health insurance.* Washington DC: American Psychoogical Association.

Shalowicz, D. (1987 March 23). Researcher questions Kennedy proposal. *Business Insurance,* p.47.

C H A P T E R
32

PROFESSIONAL INCORPORATION

J. G. Benedict, Ph.D.

I f you are considering incorporating your practice, this process and its potential outcomes will deserve considerable attention.

For many practitioners who incorporated in the mid-1970s, a byword for them now may be, "Those were the good old days." What used to be a considerable advantage for the self-employed private practitioner has now been so significantly affected by tax-law changes that it has been almost completely eroded. Nevertheless, for some there may still remain some advantages to the process of incorporation. Electing to establish a corporation, however, requires a careful consideration of the various advantages and disadvantages.

I shall present the advantages that existed before the changes in the tax laws and then discuss the current situation. Readers can evaluate the future desirability of incorporation. Please note that this account is based on my own personal experience with incorporation rather than on a base of legal or corporate expertise.

In preparing this material, I realized that the laws regarding professional incorporation differ considerably from state to state. Moreover, nationally they have been changing gradually over the past 18 years. Anyone considering forming a professional corporation should attend to rule 1: *Consult a tax attorney in your state!* This should be done before any further consideration is given to the idea. It could preclude further consideration of incorporation and save time and energy.

A review of the advantages that originally made the professional corporation attractive may be useful history. It not only helps to appreciate the professional corporation's current status, but it also will provide a helpful structure for considering some of the business decisions that are involved in a private practice. Many who incorporated in the mid-1970s thought it was a great opportunity for gaining tax benefits and practice flexibility. Those who are still incorporated, however, may wish to reevaluate and reconsider whether to continue with their corporation in light of current tax revisions. The concept was a good one in its time; however, its advantages seem to have largely disappeared.

The general advantage of the professional corporation (PC) was that it enabled private practitioners, such as physicians, psychologists, lawyers, accountants, and musicians, to have some of the same tax benefits that were then available to corporate executives in the United States, but not to the unincorporated professional practitioner.

The Internal Revenue Service (IRS), on August 8, 1969, reached the decision that ". . . in response to recent decisions of the Federal Courts, it is conceding that organizations of doctors, lawyers, and other professional people organized under state professional association acts will, generally, be treated as corporations for tax pusposes" (Eaton, 1986, pp. 1–4). Furthermore, the Tax Reform Act of 1969, jokingly referred to by some as the "Lawyers' and Accountants' Relief Act of 1969," contained provisions that directly and indirectly increased the attractiveness of the professional service corporation as a disciplined format for the business aspects of a professional practice. Although the Tax Reform Act of 1974 further expanded the HRF-10 (Keogh) pension plans for the sole proprietor, the PC remained more attractive as a retirement plan.

Additional statutory changes were necessary for practitioners to incorporate. State legislatures had to specify the nature of such entities by passing practice acts and by defining *licensed* practitioners who could incorporate. Most states now have such statutes in force. However, since the statutes vary from state to state, it is important to consult a locally practicing tax attorney before establishing a PC. If you are planning to conduct your practice in more than one state, seek legal advice.

The major advantages of corporate status seem to derive from two characteristics of the corporate structure: (1) the corporation as a disciplined format for doing business, and (2) the practitioner as both owner and employee. Partnerships and sole proprietorships do not have the same inherent degree of discipline in their structure or accounting methods. Moreover, the corporation has an identity separate from the individuals in it, and yet it can function in many ways as if it were an individual. That fact, for the professionals, can have significant implications for the actual service delivery and taxes. Some of the tax and operational benefits result from the fact that the practitioner is both the owner-employer and an employee of the corporation. This creates tax benefits and enables the professional person to preserve capital by reducing needless outflow, a benefit not available to the unincorporated individual.

DeBruyn (1976) has taken the formal tax literature and explained it in relatively easily understood language. The factors that emerge from his discussion are (1) retirement plan factors, (2) other tax factors, and (3) nontax factors (i.e., the effect of corporate characteristics on the practice of a particular profession).

BENEFITS OF BEING INCORPORATED

Retirement Benefits

Significant benefits were realized at the outset of the establishment of PCs. There had been stringent limitations on the amounts that individuals could set aside for their retirement programs before the establishment of the Keogh Act (HR-10) in 1962. Contributions that were then limited to $1,250 were increased to a $2,500 limit in 1966, and to $7,500 in 1974 (Tax Reform Act of 1974). The actual percentage of a person's salary that could be contributed in 1962 was 10 percent, which was increased to 15 percent in 1974 as a result of that tax reform act. This reform enabled the self-employed plans to compete more effectively with the retirement plans possible under the PCs. With the higher established maximum contribution and the increased percentage contribution, the gap between the nonincorporated plans and the retirement benefits of the PC continued to close.

Still, the advantage remained with the corporate retirement plan. The desirability of using the corporate retirement plan increased as the net income of the individual exceeded $37,500. The maximum HR-10 limit was a $7,500 contribution; however, the maximum under the PC retirement plan was established as the lesser of 25 percent of compensation or $25,000. The actual amount of one's net profit had to be at least $125,000 in order to set aside the maximum retirement contribution of $25,000 and still permit a salary of $100,000. As one's net earnings increased from $37,500 to $125,000, the amount of retirement set aside increased from $7,500 to $25,000.

Although the disparity between professionals and their corporate executive counterparts had at least partially been dealt with by the increased amount that the self-employed could contribute to a retirement plan (HR-10), the corporate executive retained a benefits edge. Companies remained relatively unlimited as to the amounts that they could set aside on behalf of their executives' retirement programs.

Two other advantages were Social Security integration and delayed investing.

Social Security integration essentially means that Social Security contributions (FICA) are calculated into the compensation of all employees in such a way as to meet a part of the requirements for the corporation's contributions to that employee's retirement program. The net effect is to permit more than one tier of retirement benefits for different employment levels. DeBruyn (1976) explained that by combining FICA with certain percentage levels of compensation, the FICA payments would meet the requirement of nondiscriminatory contribution to retirement without increasing the actual cash contribution required of the professional. He has also provided a more detailed explanation of the way in which that works.

The delayed vesting issues are also quite complicated and the reader is referred to DeBruyn for further details. Essentially, however, this strategy enables the PC to limit vesting in the retirement plan to those employees who are going to be actively contributing to the retirement funds for a reasonable period of time and to assure proper recovery of their nonvested interest if they should leave the corporation before retirement.

A further restriction that can be placed on the retirement program is to limit participation to full-time employees. By restricting the corporate employees to less than half-time, the corporation can reduce its required contributions to only the FICA contributions. This neither increases the costliness of operation nor complicates the management of the retirement plans.

Where one employee is shared by more than one PC, or two separate business entities, care must be taken to prevent that part-time person acquiring the status of a full-time, shared employee. DeBruyn discusses several ways to set up the plan and operate it within the rules of the IRS and still not have the part-time employee participate in the retirement program of the corporation.

Employees who are less than half-time need not be included in the corporate retirement program so long as their hours of service to the corporation can be shown to be less than 1,000 hrs. per year. In the case of a shared, part-time staff employee, care must be taken to make sure that, in the eyes of the IRS, the employee is not a full-time employee. Despite the fact that the employee's salary is paid by two or more practitioners, the IRS has determined in past cases that a mutual employee, such as a secretary, is a full-time employee despite being paid with two separate half-time checks. One way to avoid this problem is to have such a staff person be a part-time employee of the corporation of one business entity and have the office needs and space provided by one of the office-sharing entities. The other entities are then in a clearly contractual position with part-time staff members.

Employee Protection Costs

For professional employees, the protections afforded by the various corporate programs are essentially those they would provide for themselves in a solo practice—malpractice insurance, disability protection, health insurance, and so on. When the corporation furnishes various benefits, however, such benefits usually have to be provided for all staff persons. In addition to extra costs for retirement programs and employee taxes, additional liability protection, health insurance protection, unemployment insurance, and worker's compensation must be afforded.

Another benefit of the PC retirement plan was that it was more flexible than the Keogh plan. That situation has changed substantially because individual retirement accounts (IRAs) and Keogh plans currently permit the investor to direct the investment activities of the self-employed plan despite the fact that the funds are monitored and kept by a bank or some other approved financial entity, not by an individual.

A significant feature was that the corporate plan could also lend funds to plan participants, so long as there was no discrimination against groups of borrowers. Such was not possible under the HR-10 plans. While one could borrow no more than one's vested amount, one could essentially contribute further to one's fund by the amount of interest paid to the fund. Of course, the downside risk was and is that the amount borrowed could be lost to the fund if the borrower defaulted.

Distribution Of Funds

At the time of my incorporation, the method of payout of the accumulated funds in the retirement program was an important consideration; that is, how to manage the distribution of funds to a vested employee at the time of retirement or if the practice were not to continue. The corporate employee's funds could be distributed without special tax penalty before age 59½ if the employee terminated employment or the corporation dissolved. The Keogh plans, on the other hand, still require a penalty for early withdrawal.

Another aspect of the distribution problem was that a large lump-sum distribution could be taxed as regular income. A special income-averaging provision enabled that lump-sum to be taxed as if it had been distributed over the ensuing 10 years, thereby reducing the taxation rate to a reasonable level rather than having the amount treated as one year's salary and taxed at the maximum level.

A third aspect related to estate planning. With the Keogh or other personally arranged retirement plans, the accumulated money, on the death of the individual, would be considered part of the professional's estate. Under the corporate plan, the funds to be distributed would be excluded from the employee's estate, thereby reducing the estate tax. As DeBruyn noted, however, the tax advantage may be offset by the increased income tax that might have to be paid out as a result of the distribution to all the beneficiaries.

Many fringe benefits were realized as a result of corporate status. Both the self-employed and the corporate professional had retirement programs available. The PC could, however, provide medical expense reimbursement plans, wage-continuation plans, health and accident plans, and tax-free death benefits up to $5,000, which are unavailable to the unincorporated professional.

Medical Benefits

Corporate employees have long had the opportunity to receive medical care at the company clinic or at the expense of the company. Now, with the professionals in the status of owner-employees, they are able to avail themselves of the same advantages. Professionals are then on a par with the company executives who not only had health-care benefits, but also were afforded numerous recreational perks. It was possible for the individual, private practicing professional to have some of the same benefits under the PC that all the employees of most companies could have under their company's health plans.

The corporate medical benefit can often go far beyond the benefits of the insurance coverage alone. It can cover both the cost of the health insurance and the deductible or participating coinsurance required of the employee. That essentially means free health care, or if the professional is providing the funds, at least it uses pretax dollars that are going to the deferral of health costs.

For the PC employee, all medical bills for the key personnel could be directly paid by the PC which would then be reimbursed for the covered benefits by the health-care insurance carried by the corporation for the professional. Since it is logical that the best interest of the corporate entity is served by insuring the health of the principal professionals, full coverage by the PC is a defensible expense and has been so accepted by the IRS.

Wage-Continuation Plans

There are essentially two general wage-continuation plans. One is the unemployment insurance provision that can be maintained for all corporate employees. Since these are corporate expenses, they are paid for by pretax dollars; the professional as a qualified person in some states can also elect not to pay for such unemployment protection, an option that is not recommended for financial reasons.

A second income-protection plan is insurance for loss of income due to disability. The corporation, again, could provide employees with this type of benefit. This plan, which is also an insurance issue, will be covered in the next section.

Insurance Benefits

The types of insurance that could be purchased by the incorporated practitioner far exceeded those that the unincorporated practitioner could provide in himself or herself with pretax dollars. As a key employee of the corporation, the interests of the corporation are best served by having the professional employee's health and earning capability adequately insured. The future of the corporation is better assured if its principals are insured and the corporation is protected against income loss.

It was also possible to use the various insurance products as a part of the pension plan of the corporation. A policy within the pension plan becomes a property of the pension plan and subject to special rules affecting contributions to and investment decisions within that pension program. More recently, however, insurance packages have been sufficiently changed and improved that it is less attractive to have the insurance products within the pension plan. One reason is that the tax-deferred earnings from insurance annuity policies are too low to bother sheltering that income inside the plan. It is best to maximize the tax-deferred earnings within the pension investment portfolio.

In most instances where insurance benefits are paid for by the corporation, some portion of the corporately paid premium must be reported as supplementary income to the insured employee. That portion must be reported as ordinary income on the professional's personal tax return and is taxed accordingly. The nonincome portion of the premium is, however, paid for from pretax dollars and is not reportable by the professional.

Another use of the various insurance products relates to issues concerning other professionals in the practice. It is desirable to insure individual professional employees/participants for an amount sufficient to cover various expenses that could result at the closing of that person's practice because of death or incapacitation. Such insurance would reimburse the surviving professional persons for the costs of closing the practice and the handling of insurance reports for patients whose therapist's practice has ended. This particular use of insurance also can provide the professional's surviving family members with the benefits of the residual value of the practice in the form of receivables, and so on. It is possible, as well, to provide protection of corporate practice by exchanging insurance coverage between the licensed practitioner outside the PC and the principal or principals within. Accompanying this mutual insurance with a buy–sell agreement can assure surviving patients with continuation of service and also implement collection efforts on receivables.

Such policy arrangements often have more favorable tax consequences than personal life insurance. For example, the corporation can own the policy but name a family member as a beneficiary. There is a $50,000 limit on the amount of this insurance that can be maintained by the corporation. If this amount is exceeded, the premium for the additional insurance must be reported as regular income by the employee.

The PC could also provide an additional benefit—tax-free death benefits up to $5,000. These benefits are funded either by a nominal term policy or out of cash surplus on hand and before any settlement of a deceased's estatge, including stock shares and other corporate funds.

Expense Coverage

Although the business expenses that one can charge off for tax purposes are essentially the same for the PC as they are for self-employed individuals, it is my opinion that the handling of those expenses is made easier. Payment of routine operating expenses by the PC from its operating funds makes it possible for many expenses to be covered with pretax dollars.

There are expenses for the corporation that become indirect benefits for the employees. The corporation can, for example, provide all employees with paper, pencils, postage, and so on, as a fringe benefit. These items cannot be too large, however, without their needing to be reported as additional income.

At one time, it was possible to have the PC own a vehicle for use by an employee for business-related travel. This usage was not tightly monitored, and detailed records were not stringently required. The employee was required nominally to reimburse the PC for personal use of the "company car," in much the same way as with other companies that provide their employees with vehicles. The depreciation of that vehicle's value could be sheltered within corporate depreciation allowances, thus creating a substantial tax savings. The IRS closed that loophole in 1985 with increased documentation requirements and the requirement that the use of the vehicle had to be reflected as additional compensation.

Cash Protection   The advantage of a cash-protection program was primarily based on the fact that the corporation could retain up to $150,000 in assets without additional tax consequences. On the surface, this appeared to allow the practitioner to accrue a reserve of pretax operating capital, derived from profits, and on which the minimum tax of 15 percent for corporate profits would apply through December 31, 1987. With the tax revisions of the 1987 Congress including increased rates for personal service corporations, these benefits have all but disappeared. The profits are now taxed at the higher corporate rates at the time of their accrual and again in the future when they are paid out to the practitioner in the form of either salary or dividends. Accordingly, the corporation is better off not reporting a profit. If all earnings are consumed by corporate expenses, including salaries, the corporate tax is lessened and double taxation averted.

Tax Credits

Investment tax credits seemed more applicable to the equipment holdings of the professional corporation than to the other possible business formats for the practice. The depreciation rates, the listing of expenses of many supplies as corporate operating costs, and the carrying over of the tax credits from year to year to offset profits seemed to favor the corporation.

OTHER TAX BENEFITS

Since corporate employees are covered by tax-free worker's compensation and unemployment protection, they benefit by not having to provide these benefits from after-tax dollars. The unemployment protection is available only within the constraints of state laws, and sometimes is available only on request. If utilized, such state unemployment compensation would supplement unemployment benefits or disability income protection otherwise provided by some sort of insurance program. The corporation's share of the FICA is a deductible operating expense, and as such is another tax benefit.

Another significant tax benefit has been that the corporation could select a fiscal year other than the calendar year. By so doing, the payment of salaries could be adjusted beneficially to raise or lower income within the personal tax year of the employee-professional. For example, if the corporation had realized a profit and the professional were to be paid a bonus, it could be timed to make maximum use of tax losses or rates at year's end. That is, the employee–professional could receive the bonus in his or her tax year of choice, the one with the most allowable offsetting deductions.

Some would also regard the corporate tax withholding to be a benefit rather than having to file quarterly tax estimates.

NONTAX FEATURES

Operational Benefits

Limitation of personal liability is another operational benefit of the PC. This derives from the basic nature of the corporation: it can function essentially as an individual, separate from the individuals within, yet having some of the rights of an individual, such as legal powers and privileges, but also liabilities. This protects the individuals within the corporation from legal responsibility for the functioning of the corporation, protects the assets of the individuals within the corporation from the financial obligations of the corporation, and permits the body of the corporation to do business as if it were an individual. This protection does not affect the need for quality service or compliance with state laws. It may, however, limit malpractice liability of other stockholders, and limit other types of financial liability.

While certain circumstances exist wherein the corporate veil may be pierced and personal responsibility established, there are many other situations where personal suit could be instituted but the corporate veil would provide protection not available to the sole proprietor.

The PC permits the professional practice to be conducted with more flexibility. Some of the actual services being performed in the name of the corporation may be delivered by various individuals in the corporation. Treatment services in the psychological PC, just like legal services in the attorney's PC, might be partly carried out by another provider to increase office efficiency but not interfere with the service responsibility of the professional person. This particular feature greatly enhances the efficiency of the practicing professional person, and yet does not interfere with the lines of responsibility to and the care of the client's needs.

POTENTIAL DISADVANTAGES

Added Operating Costs

Running a company is more costly than conducting a sole proprietorship or partnership because of the increased cost of attorneys' fees for the maintenance of the corporate records and the paperwork for the retirement programs, especially as these are amended constantly.

The preparation of payroll, the paperwork to be done in conjunction with unemployment insurance, worker's compensation, and the various withholding taxes are added accounting and bookkeeping requirements for the PC.

The corporate tax preparation at year's end is more complicated and costly even though payroll and accounting services can be used for much of this work. Sole proprietorship requires only the filing of a Schedule C in the tax return and single-entry bookkeeping. The corporate return requires double-entry bookkeeping to produce a balance sheet for the assessment of the performance of the business. The latter is a more costly and yet more disciplined system for stating your business condition.

Maintaining a corporation requires at least an annual meeting of the board of directors, at which the attorney and the accountant for the corporation are present. This represents an additional cost of operation. (The PC can, however, pay for a dinner for the board of directors and at least add some oral gratification to an otherwise mundane activity.)

There are a variety of technical checks that have to be made to assure compliance with the specific statutes regarding corporations, and procedural changes have to be made because tax revisions continue to be made in Congress. Similarly, the changing ERISA requirements for the retirement programs demand that you stay closely in touch with the consulting attorney to assure full compliance. Attorney fees, therefore, become a significant budget item.

While the direct cost of FICA to the professional is reduced because of employee status, the total FICA contribution increases to 15.02 percent when the professional's personal contribution (7.51 percent) and the corporation's contribution 7.51 percent) are added together. The individual rate otherwise is 13.02 percent, or 2 percent less. The difference is expected to disappear according to legislative mandate by 1990.

The disadvantage of having to file a separate tax return for the corporation, rather than the single return that is required for the unincorporated practitioner, is a small but costly annoyance.

The amount of money that can be kept in the corporation ($150,000) does not increase with the number of professionals among the stockholders of the corporation. Obviously, that benefit is progressively eroded as the number of professionals increases.

An additional cost of operation is the potential contribution for and maintenance of a retirement program for the nonprofessional, and, quite likely, non-income-producing employees. If the staff members are "rented" from an agency, or if they are contract employees for a limited number of hours per week (under 20), the corporation is not required to maintain a retirement program for them. It is also opitional whether FICA be paid for contract employees. I have always done so as part of their total compensation.

To some extent, these additional costs can be built in as a supplement to the income of the staff person. For the most part, however, the additional costs simply accrue as additional overhead expense for the corporate practice.

CURRENT STATUS

The appeal of incorporation has, as was noted above, been substantially eroded by the various tax reform initiatives that have been enacted since the passage of the 1969 enabling legislation. The amount of professional income required to make incorporation feasible has risen considerably. The figure that was advised by DeBruyn (1976) was a minimum of $65,000–$75,000. On the basis of that figure alone and the figure that inflation would now dictate, the amount that now would be suggested might exceed $200,000 in gross income. Not many practices in the United States would justify incorporation on the basis of this set of criteria alone.

There is some current sentiment that the consideration of a Subchapter S corporation may be more beneficial to the practicing professional than the professional service corporation.

The current status of the various advantages and benefits discussed is as follows:

1. *Retirement plans.* These have not changed essentially within the PC; however, the HR-10 (Keogh) plans have been changed both as to flexibility and contribution limits. Accordingly, there is virtually no difference in their actual parameters.

2. *Tax factors.*

a. Medical benefits. These have been significantly restricted by the new tax reform.

b. Wage-continuation plans. These plans remain intact. The pretax dollar may still apply to this type of assurance of income in the corporation's best interest. Worker's compensation and unemployment insurance are still company-provided.

c. Dividends-received deduction. This benefit has been reduced from 85 percent to 80 percent and continues to require the corporation to hold the stock more than 45 days (Silverstein, 1987, pp. 341–342).

d. Social Security. This remains a partial contribution by the PC.

e. Cash protection. This appears not to have changed, the $150,000 cash reserve limit remaining in effect. The disadvantage comes from the fact that the tax rate reduction places corporate taxation and personal tax rates very close to each other. The net effect is the double taxation that occurs when tax is paid on corporation profit and then again by the employee on salary or dividends.

f. Deferred compensation. This benefit has been totally eliminated. The retirement plans remain in effect.

g. Corporate insurance benefits. The buy–sell protection is still possible. Key-employee insurance remains allowable.

h. Distribution of retirement funds. Changes made in this retirement benefit related mainly to the elimination of the capital gains deduction. Dividends and accrual continue untaxed, but the distributed proceeds will be treated as ordinary income, making the deferral less attractive.

If You Decide To Proceed

On adding up the pros and cons, there appear to be fewer and fewer reasons to consider professional incorporation. A few tax advantages exist, but hardly enough to offset the additional accounting and legal expenses unless the corporate income exceeds the $150,000 level (this is only a rough estimate of the lower limit).

To decide whether or not to discontinue, one must first look at the cost of continuing operation and then at the cost of dismantling. There is not that much continuing difference in the cost of operating a corporation versus a partnership or solo practice. The more costly tax returns, accounting fees, and legal fees are offset by the enhanced quality of the practice that results from business discipline. Wage-continuation plans and other insurance benefits would be given up if one were to discontinue corporate operation.

Dismantling costs would result from converting the retirement plan to an HR-10 plan, from the changing of the employee status to proprietor status, and from the legal dissolution. Unless another corporation were formed, one would have to begin filing quarterly tax estimates and no longer pay taxes through monthly withholding.

There are probably only three reasons to consider for establishing a professional corporation at this time: to limit practice liability, to benefit from the corporate veil, and to avail oneself of the corporate structure as the more desirable way to do business.

Whether your next move is to incorporate or to consider abolishing a professional corporation, the careful counsel of a tax attorney is a must.

If you do plan to incorporate, practice limitations, tax benefits and consequences, and legal protection resulting from corporate status can vary from state to state. Limitations may exist regarding insurance coverage for patients and may be greatly affected by unique statutes of specific states.

As an example of the latter situation, the peer review statutes in some states may restrict the process to individual practitioners and not group practitioners. It may be a different matter if statutes concerning corporate operations were to conflict with laws affecting individual practice. For example, New Jersey and, to a different degree, New York have statutes affecting peer review that could have possible conflicting consequences for the PC.

Your attorney should be expected to help you decide, along with your accountant, where the financial cutoff point may be for your particular situation. The cost of the legal preparation, the cost of disestablishing the corporation if you should ever need to, and the added operating costs the corporate structure would bring are all items to consider.

Clearly, an attorney will be needed to set up a retirement program properly. Meeting the demands of ERISA requirements will prove costly unless the attorney you select has a model program that can be adapted to your needs. An attorney who has the necessary model structure as well as experience with professional corporations is a good choice. When all is said and done: *Question your sanity.*

If you have a PC, it is probably better that you keep it in case tax rates go up again and make the differential tax rates favorable. If you are not incorporated, it probably is not a good idea to do so at this time.

REFERENCES

Eaton, B.C. (1986). *Professional corporations and associations,* Vol. 17 (Rev.). New York: M. Bender & Co.

DeBruyn, J. (1976). Incorporating the professional. *The Colorado Lawyer,* 1–16, Jan.

Silverstein, L.L. (Ed.) (1987). *Tax management portfolios: The Tax Reform Act of 1986.* Vol. II, *Detailed analysis.* Washington, DC: Bureau of National Affairs.

C H A P T E R
33

THE SALE AND PURCHASE OF A PRIVATE HEALTH-SERVICE-PROVIDER PSYCHOLOGY PRACTICE

Robert D. Weitz, Ph.D., and
Richard M. Samuels, Ph.D.

THE SALE

by Robert D. Weitz

At this time, little factual information is available regarding the selling and purchase of a private health-service-provider psychology practice. This chapter is based on the ideas and experiences of the coauthors, who apparently were the first psychologists in the United States involved in such a transaction.

There are a number of reasons why practitioners may wish to sell their psychology practices. Some may need to move to another area because of personal or family problems; others may have lost their interest (burnout) in the field and seek a change in occupation. Perhaps the majority who wish to sell their practices are seeking retirement. Regardless of the reasons for selling, it is important that the seller have an established postsale plan to avoid a disruptive and disturbing period of social accommodation.

After the sale, if the practitioner moves to another state with plans to establish another practice or to seek a position with a mental-health agency, the subject of licensure or certification becomes highly important. This matter, obviously, needs to be resolved before the geographical move, if a new practice or position is planned.

Selling The Practice

It is elementary to note that if we attempt to sell an object or a service, that product must have an intrinsic value to the purchaser. What, then, must be the characteristics of a psychology practitioner facility to merit salability? What must be the characteristics of the practice to offer reasonable assurance to the purchaser that the investment is sound?

First, the practice must be a recognized service in the community. Next, the practitioner should be personally well known in the community and recognized as an individual associated with the mental-health field. Further, there should be a well-established source of client referral. And finally, there must be established contacts with schools, mental-health agencies, businesses, and so on.

What was there about my practice that caused me to believe it could be sold? To begin with, I was the first practicing psychologist in the state of New Jersey and among the first in the entire country. In addition to my own services, I maintained a staff of three part-time psychologists and a secretary. My work was primarily concerned with psychological testing and psychotherapy, but I also served as consultant to a number of public and private agencies, including police departments, court systems, rehabilitation services, schools, adoption agencies, and mental-health facilities. These relationships provided a steady stream of referrals. In addition, referrals were regularly forthcoming from professionals in other fields, including medical doctors, dentists, lawyers, optometrists, and podiatrists. Relationships with these agencies and professionals had been established over a period of many years. Last, but by no means least, there were regular referrals from hundreds of clients who were known to the office from past years.

As for the worth of a psychology practice, no well-defined guidelines have been established to determine the value of a given practice. Accordingly, I, as the seller, will detail what I did in my endeavor to arrive at a sale price for my practice—a practice conducted for over 30 years.

I initially attempted to search the available psychology information resources but with no success. I then inquired of several colleagues in various parts of the country, but they, too, had no information to offer regarding the sale of a psychology practice. Accordingly, to establish some guidelines, I contacted several medical doctors, dentists, and lawyers, some of whom had sold a practice and some who could provide information to determine how a selling price might be reached. In all, I had little to go on in my effort to determine the price to charge for my practice and so had to establish my own guidelines. I did this with the aid of my accountant. It was decided that the selling price would be fixed at the average of the gross annual income for the three years immediately preceding the anticipated date of sale.

During the years following the sale of my practice, and particularly after publication of my article "I Sold My Private Practice" (Weitz, 1983), I have received numerous telephone calls and written inquiries concerning the value of a practice. These inquiries came from widows of deceased psychologists, individuals in the process of ending a partnership, and psychologists who were seeking to sell or purchase a practice. Further, I have been involved as an expert witness in cases where one psychologist sued another because of a contract dispute.

Following the decision to sell and having arrived at a selling price, how does one go about locating a buyer? Obviously, the first approach is by word of mouth—advising your colleagues of your decision to sell. Through colleagues, it is likely that a number of leads to prospective purchasers will develop. Further, advertising in both local and national printed media may prove helpful. With regard to national advertising, however, the seller needs to be cautious. I learned from my experience that the advertisement may attract unqualified individuals (con artists), who seek to profit by becoming involved with the seller. Some want to gain a partnership and others, who have false hopes of being licensed, attempt to use the seller to gain a license through the back door. In the final analysis, it is more than likely that the sale will be realized through the seller's personal endeavor to locate a buyer.

Following is an account regarding the sale of my practice.

> During the spring of 1973, I attended a sex therapy workshop conducted by the N.J. College of Medicine and Dentistry. One presentation was made by a young man—a staff psychologist in the Division of Obstetrics and Gynecology. His command of the subject, his obvious self-confidence and his generally personable manner made a strong impression upon me. Here was the person who could readily replace me. Upon the conclusion of his presentation, I introduced myself and congratulated him. During the discussion which followed, I learned that he was interested in private practice and had started to build a practice in another part of the state. I told him of my desire to sell my practice and of my belief that he would do well as my successor. He was interested. Meetings followed involving lawyers, accountants and our respective wives. Within two months an agreement was reached and the sales contract was signed. (p. 102)

In the selection of a buyer, there are a number of significant considerations of importance to the seller, including (1) the education and training of the prospective buyer, (2) the likelihood that the buyer's personality will be appropriate to the practice, (3) the social and emotional stability of the buyer, and (4) the ability of the purchaser to handle the financial responsibilities of the transaction.

With respect to the matter of contract, details of individual arrangements obviously differ. As one example of a contract, the following details the provisions made in the contract with the purchaser of my practice, Dr. Samuels.

1. The sales price was established at the average level of the gross income covering the three years 1972 through 1975.

2. The purchaser would make an initial payment of 10 percent of the purchase price, with the balance to be paid in weekly installments, without interest, over a 10-year period, beginning January 1, 1976.

3. The purchaser would be covered by life insurance, with the seller as beneficiary, up to the financial limit of the balance due on the sale price, and the estate as beneficiary beyond that amount.

4. A partnership would be established for two years following the sale with financial arrangements as follows:

    a. For the first year, the purchaser would work at the practice three days a week, whereas the seller would continue on a full-time basis. Both parties would share equally regarding expenses and income.

    b. For the second year of the partnership, the seller would work at the practice for two days a week and the buyer would work on a full-time basis. Both parties would continue to share equally in expenses and income.

5. At the end of the second year, the partnership would automatically be dissolved, with the buyer assuming full ownership and management of the practice.

6. It was the seller's responsibility to introduce the buyer to as many referral sources as possible and to introduce him to the community at large.

7. At the conclusion of the partnership, the seller's name would remain on the stationery as a consultant.

Concerning the established payment plan, of major significance was the matter of taxes related to the sale. By establishing an installment payment plan, I, as the seller, was able to save considerably as compared with the tax responsibility had full payment been made at the time of the sale.

With regard to the matter of life insurance on the buyer with the seller named as beneficiary (a 10-year term policy was put into effect), I was assured of full payment in the event of the death of the purchaser. With each installment payment by the purchaser, that amount accrued to his estate.

With respect to the office participation during the two years of partnership, having the purchaser work three days a week at the office allowed him to continue his medical-school position, and sharing the net income provided him with a considerable increment in his yearly earnings. In addition, his presence resulted in a significant increase in the gross income for the office. I, on the other hand, was able to share the net office income in the second year of the agreement while being present at the office but two days a week. This allowed me an easy transition to my relocation in Florida. It did require, however, weekly commuting between Florida and New Jersey for 50 weeks during the second year of the partnership.

The success of the buyer in the maintenance and growth of the practice is obviously of mutual concern to the buyer and seller. Thus, in accordance with the contractual agreement, it is highly important that the seller aid the buyer in becoming known to the community. This requires personal introduction to other professionals, to members of business and professional groups, and to the administrators of educational institutions, legal agencies, police departments, and so on. In serving as a cotherapist, the buyer is gradually introduced to the current clientele.

As a final area of discussion, I shall deal with the question of the moral aspects involved in the sale of a health-service psychology practice. It is recognized that there are purists in the ranks of psychology who believe that the sale of a practice violates the confidentiality rights of the clients. There is no evidence in the "Ethical Principles of Psychologists" (American Psychological Association, 1981a) or in the "Specialty Guidelines for the Delivery of Services" (American Psychological Association, 1981b) to suggest that the sale of a practice is professionally immoral. In fact, there is evidence to the contrary; principle 2.3.5 of the "Specialty Guidelines for the Delivery of Services" states: "The records are the property of the psychologist or the facility in which the psychologist works and are therefore the responsibility of the psychologist annd subject to his or her control." Further, what more protection would a client need considering the fact that the care of the office records would be turned over to another professional psychologist who is bound by the same ethical principles and standards as the psychologist who sells the practice?

There are a number of factors that favor the preservation and maintenance of records by the purchaser of the practice. For example, over the years I have received requests from government agencies for the test results of a mentally retarded adult who was studied at the office during that individual's childhood years. Such requests usually arise when someone in the family is seeking financial assistance for the retarded individual. Another reason for the preservation of records is that, in a well-established practice, the psychologist will probably be called upon to provide services for the children of former clients.

To conclude, it is likely that most health-service psychological practices have a sale value and that, with adequate planning, a qualified purchaser will be found and an effective transfer of the practice accomplished.

THE PURCHASE

BY *Richard M. Samuels*

Choosing a career path is often fraught with uncertainties, and in my personal situation, the choices that were before me in 1973 seemed almost endless. The prospect of enjoying the academic life, and being in the forefront of the sexual revolution at the time appeared most promising and exciting. (We certainly could not foresee the devastation that the AIDS epidemic would wreak on this movement.)

Like many psychologists in a medical-school setting, I was maintaining a modest part-time practice, using several offices in different parts of the state, including my office at medical school. The thought of full-time private practice was tempered due to my (by no means unique) need to maintain an adequate income after leaving the security of my medical-school position.

The establishment of a private practice requires that much time be spent in the office to accommodate the needs of patients, some of whom can come only during the day, and others of whom can come only in the evenings. Additionally, public speaking appearances, consultancies, and the like truly require that a full-time commitment be made to the task.

Holding a full-time job while trying to develop a private practice is extremely difficult at best, and sometimes makes the task impossible to accomplish. It was fortuitous that I invited Dr. Weitz to attend a sex therapy workshop. Having met him only very briefly in his role as acting dean of the Organizing Council for the College of Professional Psychology (New Jersey), I was impressed by his dynamic personality and obvious enthusiasm for our profession. Thus, it took no coaxing to invite him at the suggestion of the senior medical school psychologist, and before very long, Dr. Weitz had approached me regarding the purchase of his practice.

He has described the details of our most satisfactory arrangements in the first part of this article. Over the years, numerous colleagues have contacted us regarding the potential sale or purchase of a practice and a number of guidelines have evolved from these conversations, as presented in the following.

The goals of the buyer are different from those of the seller. An ideal transaction for a seller would be to acquire a lump-sum payment for the practice and to retire upon receipt of the funds. The buyer, on the other hand, would prefer to spread payments over a long period of time and to establish a period of partnership with the seller, in order for an orderly transition to take place. Practically speaking, most buy-and-sell agreements fall between these two extremes.

While the financial value of the practice can be set, using gross revenue as a guideline, the real value of the practice depends on the nature of the referral sources cultivated by the seller, the age and personality of the seller, and, of course, the seller's reputation. If Bob had been a psychoanalyst and I a strict behaviorist, his referral sources would probably not be enthusiastic about sending their patients to me. Thus, it is important to look for a seller whose therapeutic orientation is at least similar to that of the buyer.

Personality styles are important, too. An outgoing, verbal, and assertive therapist develops a reputation for that particular therapeutic style. The individual buying the practice should have a personality consistent with that of the seller, and if the seller receives numerous referrals from pediatricians, for example, but the buyer prefers working with married couples, then those referral sources are not nearly as valuable as they at first may appear.

Perhaps most important to an orderly transition is the suggested one- or two-year period of partnership. During this time, the buyer of the practice would be introduced to the referral sources and the professional contacts evolved over the years by the seller. The transition of good will is as important as the amount of money generated by the practice at the time of sale.

It is also helpful if the buyer brings to the practice a new specialty or therapeutic modality. For example, if the buyer enters the practice with biofeedback equipment and has a specialty in sex therapy, whereas the seller had been primarily a child and forensic specialist, then two types of referral strains will be feeding the combined practice. This will increase the patient flow and create an expansion of the practice rather than simply a replacement of the therapist. When marketed correctly, the gradual withdrawal of the seller will have less of a negative impact on revenues than had these new services not been introduced.

A business partnership, like marriage, is something that must be given a great deal of consideration. In any business, friction between partners is deleterious. In a psychology practice, a personality conflict can be devastating. It is imperative that the buyer and seller familiarize themselves with each other, both professionally and personally. Time spent together (with spouses, if applicable) is crucial in helping to assess the degree of compatability. Patients can be very perceptive of any friction that may exist.

Purchase of a psychological practice can be an excellent investment for the buyer, but the buyer must be careful that he or she is compatible with the seller and that the financial arrangements for the purchase will not be burdensome. One must assess the personalities of the participants in the deal, and carefully examine the suitability of existing referral sources and the likelihood of their transfer to the buyer. The therapeutic styles of the therapists should also be similar, but benefits will be accrued if the buyer introduces a new specialty. The buyer should be prepared to spend extra time in order to meet the referral sources, agencies, and facilities that the seller has spent many years cultivating.

Buying a practice is similar to moving into someone else's home. You should feel comfortable with the existing arrangements and yet envision a future that will reflect your personality. So conducted, the purchase of a psychology practice can bring great rewards for all involved.

REFERENCES

American Psychological Association. (1981a). *Ethical principles of psychologists* (rev.). Washington, DC: Author.

American Psychological Association. (1981b). Specialty guidelines for the delivery of services. *American Psychologist, 36,* 639–681.

Weitz, Robert (1983). I sold my private practice. *Psychotherapy in Private Practice, 1,* 101–104.

34

INSURANCE

William E. Mariano, Esq.

INTRODUCTION

"Insurance" is legally defined as a contract whereby one undertakes to indemnify another against loss, damage, or liability arising from an unknown or contingent event that may occur in the future.

One purchases insurance to provide compensation to another when a wrong or injury has been determined as the responsibility of the insured. The most common example is automobile liability insurance. Insurance is also purchased as protection for oneself in case of an injury, accident, or the happening of a defined event. The best-known types of such insurance are fire, automobile-collision, and income-protection insurance.

Most important, insurance not only pays damages when one is found liable or to have erred, but also pays the cost of a legal defense, whether or not the suit is a frivolous one without merit or merely to contain and limit the loss.

TYPES OF INSURANCE

Every professional engaged in private practice needs insurance protection to pay damages and to provide a legal defense not only if the practitioner commits malpractice, but also as protection against acts of negligence. Practitioners are also advised to maintain indemnity-type insurance that will protect them in case of such personal loss as firm fire and against loss of income as a result of illness or fire.

In preparing an insurance package, the practitioner must consider:

1. The types of insurance coverage needed.
2. The types of policy available.
3. The scope of coverage available and, for indemnity coverage, the benefits provided.

The common forms of policy to consider are the following.

1. *Malpractice insurance.* This is insurance against accidental injuries to others arising out of the practice of one's profession. The coverage is very nar-

row in scope and pertains only to liability related to the performance of professional services.

2. *Liability or casualty insurance.* This policy insures against accidental injury to others not covered by malpractice insurance. It is the common tort or negligence coverage — "trip and fall" insurance — and protects the insured with respect to liability arising out of activity not actually involving the practice of one's profession.

3. *Commercial general liability insurance.* A broad form of business liability coverage, it protects one against liability for bodily injury arising out of one's operations within the United States, its territories and possessions, Puerto Rico, and Canada. Coverage is very broad and exclusions generally are confined to areas otherwise protected by public policy coverages, such as injury to employees and damage resulting from intentional acts and pollution. The standard policy adopted by the industry and generally available is the "claims-made" form.

4. *Personal catastrophe liability insurance.* This policy provides higher limits of coverage than those provided for in one's basic policy and also furnishes primary coverage in areas generally not protected. This insurance is designed to afford additional protection and to fill any gaps not covered under the basic standard liability policies.

5. *Legal liability coverage.* This policy indemnifies against occurrences for which one has legal liability but that are not covered by general accident or casualty policies or the commercial general liability policy. A common form of this coverage is water damage — coverage to insure legal liability for flooding another's property.

6. *Workers' compensation and disability insurance.* An employer is required to maintain this public policy insurance to indemnify a worker for injury incurred in the course of employment or to provide income in the event of protracted illness not related to employment. The employer is personally liable for the benefit if insurance is not maintained.

7. *Medical payments coverage.* This is a form of "no-fault" insurance coverage that will pay medical bills incurred by an injured person regardless of whether or not the person was at fault. Most homeowners' or tenants' liability insurance policies contain such a benefit in very limited amounts.

The types of insurance listed are generally referred to as liability or accident insurance. The coverage provided is designed to pay a person injured by any act of the insured practitioner.

INDEMNITY INSURANCE

The following categories of insurance coverage are generally referred to as "indemnity insurance" and are designed to pay the insured practitioner for any loss or injury to the insured. The difference is that this type of policy provides for indemnity against loss to the insured as opposed to providing indemnity against liability for injury to another.

The more common forms of insurance coverage available in the indemnity area are as follows:

1. *Fire insurance.* This type of insurance indemnifies the insured against all losses to houses, buildings, and furnishings. (Most such policies also cover the cost of cleanup.) Additional coverage may be required to insure against loss of valuable papers, such as patient records. This is an area of protection not to be overlooked, since, in the case of a profession, such loss can exceed the loss caused by damage to furniture and furnishings.

2. *Accident or disability income protection.* Such insurance provides the practitioner with protection if disabled and unable to continue to earn an income. A practitioner in the mental-health field must select this coverage carefully. It is best to try to obtain this coverage from one's professional association. Most policies require *total* disability before payment of benefit. It has not been unheard of for a carrier to deny benefit to the recovering heart-attack patient who has spoken to a patient on the telephone on the grounds that the practitioner is not totally and absolutely disabled.

Every type of insurance coverage has variations and must be studied in order to determine its overall applicability to each individual practitioner's areas of exposure.

Policy Forms

One characteristic of policies most important to understand is the difference between the claims-made and the "occurrence" form of policy. Malpractice coverage, while currently an occurrence-type policy, is generally being converted to a claims-made form by the insurance carriers. Few carriers continue to write anything but a claims-made commercial general liability policy.

A claims-made policy requires one to be insured with the company not only when the incident or accident occurs, but also when the claim is made or one is sued. An occurrence policy pays a claim if the coverage was in effect at the time the incident or accident transpired. An automobile insurance policy is an example of an occurrence policy.

Given the choice of coverage, an occurrence-type policy is to be preferred since, under a claims-made policy, you will be left without protection unless you continue to renew the policy. As long as you continue to renew with the company, it is obligated to protect you. However, once the policy is terminated for any reason, the company is no longer obligated to defend you or pay any judgment against you. The only way to obtain protection when you cancel or do not renew a claims-made policy is to buy "tail" or "extended reporting" coverage. This coverage only extends the period of time in which you have to make a report of an incident or claim. The actual incident or accident must still have happened during the period the original coverage was in effect. For every type of claim that can be asserted, there is a statute of limitations. Generally, for malpractice and negligence claims the statute is one and a half to three years. Thus, a lawsuit can be commenced within 15, 18 or 36 months after an event. A claims-policy is generally written for 12 months. If the claim is made in the 13th month and the policy has not been renewed or a tail purchased, you are uninsured and therefore unprotected.

PURCHASING
OF POLICIES

In purchasing any insurance, the practitioner is advised to study the policy and prepare a comparative list. One suggestion is to set up separate parallel columns indicating what each policy covers, what is excluded from coverage, and other areas where the practitioner feels coverage may be needed. For example, when you purchase casualty or liability insurance for your workspace, does it provide coverage if a patient with claustrophobia becomes stuck in the elevator? Even though your landlord may ultimately be liable and not you, does the policy provide and pay for legal defense? Does it protect you if another therapist renting space from you is overheard joking about the appearance of one of your patients whom the therapist saw in the waiting room?

The answer to these questions can only be determined by studying the language of the policy offered. While the above liability would be covered under most commercial general liability policies, it would not be included in the liability coverage provided as part of the common malpractice policy. It is sound advice to have all coverages reviewed by a professional insurance consultant or broker as it is unlikely, even with plain-language policies, that you will have sufficient knowledge to understand the coverage provided, and, what is most critical, to understand what coverage is lacking.

If the practitioner is renting office space to others as subtenants, utilizes independent contractors seeking patients in his or her office, or has any other space-utilization arrangement, he or she may become a landlord and additional or different insurance may be required. A landlord's liability policy may be advisable.

Many practitioners maintain offices in their home and have a homeowner's or apartment renter's liability policy. As a general rule, these policies do not provide coverage if a patient is injured while on or coming onto the premises. The basic standard homeowner's policy specifically excludes coverage for bodily injury or property damage arising out of business pursuits of an insured. Usually a rider is required to provide this coverage. Does the bodily injury coverage of the more common malpractice policy include such coverage? Probably not. The common malpractice policy limits coverage for bodily injury or property damage caused by an occurrence on the premised *used principally* in one's professional practice. Perhaps one's specific office area qualifies, but do the common areas used as one's residence or areas such as the sidewalk also qualify? The answer is that they probably do not as the principal use of the premises is as one's residence and the professional office use is only incidental.

Each practitioner's insurance needs are different. They must be thought out, analyzed, and discussed with a qualified insurance agent. In many instances, whether or not a particular area of activity or location is insured presents a gray area without a clear-cut answer. Disclosure to the carrier is important to ensure coverage and, if possible, the practitioner should obtain a written confirmation that the particular area of activity or concern is in fact insured under the coverage purchased.

MALPRACTICE INSURANCE
FOR THE PROFESSIONAL

Every professional practitioner must maintain malpractice insurance. One must maintain this insurance primarily because it is professionally responsible to provide this protection for one's patients in the event a mistake is made; one also must maintain it because we are all human and we do make mistakes. Finally, and most important, malpractice insurance pays for a legal defense against any claim asserted against the insured, even though it is without merit.

Malpractice insurance is designed to pay on your behalf any sums you become legally obligated to pay as damages because of any wrongful act or omission arising out of the performance of professional services. Coverage is also provided for liability incurred through the acts or omissions of any other person for whose actions you are legally responsible. Thus, it can cover acts and omissions of your employees, including those of clerical employees and of independent contractors seeing your patients.

Every malpractice policy's coverage and exclusions, however, must be reviewed in light of each practitioner's individual circumstances. A major exclusion of the basic malpractice policy is coverage for acts of "a managerial or administrative nature," except for "wrongful acts of the insured as a member of a formal accreditation or professional review board of a hospital or professional society, or professional licensing board." In each instance, when practitioners become active in any professional organization, they must determine whether or not they are covered by the above language. The words "accreditation" and "professional" review board have specific meanings. Activities beyond the scope of the defining language may not be covered. The language is broad enough to require practitioners to review their activities and determine whether or not any fall within the exception.

It is to be noted that the standard personal catastrophe liability insurance policy provides coverage for a person's acts or failure to act as an officer, trustee, or director of a not-for-profit corporation or association. This could provide coverage for one's activities with professional associates. Again, however, the practitioner must read the language of the policy very carefully with regard to the activities engaged in as the language used is not consistent in all policies.

All malpractice policies now contain an exclusion of coverage for, or special provisions relating to, sexual misconduct. The most common policy places a $25,000 cap on payments for damages when sexual misconduct is alleged (misconduct need not be proved) in the suit. The carrier is required to provide full legal defense up to the time a settlement is paid or proposed. The insured has the right to refuse settlement but then must pay all further costs of defense himself or herself.

ADDITIONAL COVERAGES

As indicated, there are other coverages any practitioner is advised to have. In addition to a homeowner's or tenant's liability policy, the private practitioner should carry a "personal catastrophe liability policy." This type of coverage is generally offered in conjunction with one's homeowner's or tenant's policy or is sponsored by alumni or professional groups.

Personal Catastrophe Liability

The personal catastrophe liability policy is designed to provide additional coverage above the limits of liability policies (it is sometimes referred to as an "excess" coverage policy) and to fill gaps or areas not covered by these policies and malpractice insurance. This type of policy is intended to be an all-exclusive coverage and provides protection for false arrest, detention, or imprisonment, as well as invasions of rights of privacy. The personal catastrophe liability policy specifically excludes coverage for business activities. Most important, most policies cover acts or omissions while serving as an officer, director, or trustee of a not-for-profit corporation.

Commercial Umbrella

Commercial umbrella policies are also available. They provide the same type of increased limit protection and fill the gaps for coverage not provided by the commercial general liability and malpractice policies.

Rental Property

The practitioner who rents space must be concerned with two other areas of coverage — liability resulting from damage to the building in which one rents or to another's property as a result of a fire or water damage due to one's negligence. While the standard commercial general liability policy will generally pay for damage to another person's property in that portion of the premises adjacent to you, it will not pay for damage to the portion of the building you occupy. Fire or water legal liability is therefore needed to pay for damage to the actual premises you are occupying. If the damage is caused by your negligence (e.g., leaving the coffee pot on overnight), you are liable to the landlord to rebuild your rented space as well as any other part of the building that is damaged. Legal liability fire coverage fills the gap left in the standard liability policy coverages.

Multiperil Policies

Many carriers also provide package or multiperil policies. Such a policy is often referred to as a special multiperil policy, comprehensive business policy, business owner's policy, or professional office package. Packaging policies in this manner generally reduces costs. However, each policy, whatever it is called, must be examined to determine whether it contains all the coverage needed and whether it is better to add coverage as riders to other basic policies, such as a homeowner's or tenant's policy.

CONCLUSION

Having determined the coverages required, you must determine the limits of coverage you should purchase. In today's world, coverage of $1 million is not considered too great. Generally, the cost of higher limits is nominal. The higher the limit of liability, the lower is the cost of the increment. In addition, cost savings can be obtained by using the personal catastrophe or commercial umbrella type of coverage.

In purchasing coverage, you must ascertain which policy limits apply "per occurrence" or which apply in the aggregate in any one policy year. If liabilities are aggregated, it means the policy will actually be obligated to pay a smaller total amount if several lawsuits are paid during a policy year than would be the case with a per-occurrence policy. The difference in this type of coverage should be reflected in premium cost.

The practitioner should examine carefully who in addition to himself or herself is the insured under each policy. If the practitioner is a professional corporation or association, he or she, as well as the corporation, should be named as insured. Are employees insured? Are members of the administrative staff or independent contractors insured? The common malpractice policy protects the insured for liability arising out of the acts of any other person for whose action the insured may be liable. This coverage is comprehensive and would appear to cover all situations. However, again note that the coverage is limited to liability arising solely out of the performance of professional services. If the incident does not arise out of the rendition of a professional service to the insured's patient, it is not covered. For example, your secretary, in helping a colleague in your office, prepares a report and sends it to the wrong person. This is not a professional service for one of your patients and so is not covered under the malpractice policy but by the commercial general liability policy.

Finally, it is important to practice risk management. You should discuss your business program and activities with your insurance agent and attorney. Many insurance companies, particularly if you purchase package coverage, will offer a professional risk-management review.

C H A P T E R
35

TAXES AND INVESTMENTS

Donald Robbins, C.P.A., Ph.D.,

This chapter focuses on two major issues: federal income taxation and investments. We shall explore the various legal forms a practitioner's practice may take and the federal income tax consequences of each. Major changes in federal income taxation have occurred because of the Tax Reform Act (TRA) of 1986 (Prentice-Hall Information Services, 1986), resulting in changes in strategies and considerations for the tax years 1987 and beyond. As a result, the practitioner should not generalize the information in this chapter to years prior to 1987. Further, the consideration of state (and local) income taxes is beyond the scope of this chapter, because of the varied laws found across the 50 states and the municipalities that have taxes on income. Many of the states do conform to the Internal Revenue Code (IRS) with minor changes. However, even among these states, most, to date, have not enacted all of the changes resulting from TRA 1986, or even the earlier Economic Recovery Tax Act of 1981 (Prentice-Hall Information Services, 1981)

After considering federal income tax issues, we turn to major issues relating to investments and capital accumulation. This chapter is meant to give the practitioner an overview of income tax and investment considerations. It is not meant to replace professional advice and consultation. I suspect that the practitioners reading this chapter would place severe limitations on how one could administer proper "self-help" for emotional disturbances without professional guidance. In the same light I would advise practitioners not to engage in self-help regarding taxation and investments without the appropriate professional consultants and advisors.

INCOME TAX CONSIDERATIONS

For the typical practitioner, the issues surrounding income taxation are very similar to those that confront any typical professional — for example, an accountant, attorney, physician, or psychologist. A private practice may take one of a number of business forms. You may operate as a sole proprietor or incorporate your practice. If you operate in conjunction with others, you may operate as a partnership or as a corporation with stockholders; a looser relationship may be in the form of an association of individuals or corporations.

Sole Proprietorship

A sole proprietorship is a business conducted by a single individual. In contrast to other legal entities, it is the simplest form of doing business and is typically subject to a minimum of government regulation. Before turning to issues of operating as a proprietor or as a corporation, let us consider two important questions: (1) whether the records should be maintained on a cash or accrual basis; and (2) general recordkeeping considerations.

A cash-basis taxpayer is one who reports income when it is collected and expenses when they are paid. An accrual-basis taxpayer, on the other hand, reports income when it is earned, and not necessarily collected (e.g., after seeing a patient, or at the least, after billing the patient). Expenses are reported as incurred rather than when paid. We will leave the theoretical issue of which method "truly reflects" income to those engaged in accounting theory. Rather we will consider the pragmatic issues involved in such a decision. Professionals, whether operating as sole proprietors or corporations may use the cash basis. Most corporations with gross revenues of over \$5 million cannot use the cash method. For the Internal Revenue Service (IRS), the overriding considerations are whether any major distortion of income occurs and whether there is consistency from year to year in whatever method is chosen. The traditional reason for choosing the cash basis is that it makes for easier record keeping. Basically, if you keep track of your receipts and expenditures, you have most of the relevant information. In addition, the cash-basis method is appealing because it also yields a net income figure that is, with only a few adjustments, similar to that derived from cash-flow considerations. All that is meant here by "cash-flow considerations" is simply what most business people mean when they ask their accountant, "How am I doing?" You start the week with S dollars; you receive R dollars in fees and spend E dollars on business expenses, leaving you with $S + R - E$ dollars at the end of the week. Your income for the week is $R - E$ dollars. That is the cash basis. For the accrual basis, there are further considerations. Specifically, you actually billed B dollars and collected C dollars of it; you also collected W dollars of prior-period billing, for a total cash received of $C + W = R$ dollars. Furthermore, you incurred I dollars of expenses, paid for J of these and also paid for V dollars of the prior-period expenses for a total of $J + V = E$ dollars spent. Thus, your accrual basis income for the week was $B - I$ dollars. Your cash flow was the difference between your receipts and your disbursements, namely, R (which is $C + W$) − E (which is $J + V$), as above. The different "income" arrived at by the two methods often leads to professionals wondering why, if they earned so much, they do not have many dollars. The use of the cash-basis method does not preclude your keeping records regarding how much is owed to you and how much you owe. In fact, you will want to maintain records that give you this information, so that your record-keeping requirements are, first, for the information you need in conducting your practice (that is your business after all!) and second, to satisfy whatever government regulations there may be (primarily, the IRS and state and local revenue services). Let us now turn to record-keeping considerations.

Basic Record Keeping   It should be noted at the outset that the primary reason for record keeping is to keep track of your business—your appointments, how much time you put in, your expenses, your income. Contrary to the oft-repeated phrase about "the government" forcing you to keep certain records, although in some instances this is true, your basic records are kept for you to determine how you are doing whether an income tax structure exists or not. Of course, given the federal income tax requirements, there are additional records required by the IRS. Since all practitioners must maintain some sort of appointment book, this book becomes your basic source of information for your record-keeping system. In addition to noting patient appointments, you should note professional meetings and consultations with colleagues, cash expenses, and generally time spent on a variety of business and professional activities. This basic "diary" may be very useful in trying to reconstruct or prove what you do with your time with regard to an IRS examination.

A separate checking account should be maintained by the sole proprietor that is separate from a personal checking account. To the extent possible, keep separate credit cards for the practice as well. The reason is bookkeeping simplicity. Why complicate things unnecessarily, especially in terms of separating personal from business expenditures, by keeping only one account? By having separate checking accounts, and being the only one with access to the business account, the determination of how your practice is doing financially is made considerably easier. The simplest possible system would be to use duplicates of statements sent to patients as your "receivables ledger" (i.e., the "what is owed to you ledger") filed in alphabetical order. Upon payment, the statement is marked paid, dated, and removed and placed in the alphabetical "paid" folder. Checks should be endorsed and deposited within 24 hours of rceipt, and entered in the checkbook supplied by your bank. Similarly, statements (or bills) sent to third parties (insurance companies) should be prepared in duplicate and filed in the same manner. If you send out many statements, you may wish to invest in a "one-write" system, so called because, through the use of carbon, you record the billing and prepare the invoice at one writing. You could also purchase two-part carbonized forms or simply photocopy the statements. The volume of work will determine which of the specific techniques you use.

To ease the end-of-the-month billing "crunch," you might consider staggering your billings. Specifically, you could prepare and mail approximately a fourth of your statements each week. It avoids using a single large block of time, and results in a much smoother cash-flow situation. The crunch mentioned above is not only the monthly billings that typically occur, but also the end-of-the-month bookkeeping routine that one should follow. At least once a month, or more frequently if desired (weekly), you should summarize your receipts for items paid in cash, referring to the notations you have made in your appointment book or diary to be sure to include cash expenses for which you could not (or did not) get a receipt. These receipts can be placed in an envelope and marked for the period. The expenses should be analyzed by category, and the totals recorded on the envelope and added to the expenses paid by check or charged.

A similar system is used for bills from vendors. When you receive a bill, it should be placed in an unpaid-bill folder; this folder may be separated by

Figure 35-1. **The flow of record-keeping events**

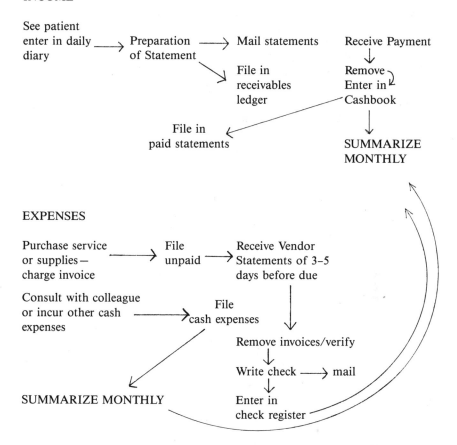

INCOME

EXPENSES

due date, and within each date, filed alphabetically. The bills should be paid three to five days prior to this due date. At that time, the paid bills are marked as such with the date and check number and removed and placed in an alaphabetical paid-bill folder. The date, check number, amount, and payee should be recorded in the checkbook register (the one supplied by your local bank). The checkbook register thus serves as another basic record-keeping instrument. At the end of each month, the information in the checkbook should be analyzed by category and recorded on a summary sheet so that monthly figures and year-to-date figures are shown separately. This summary also serves as a cash-flow statement; it tells you how much came in (and for what) and how many dollars went out (and for what); adding the beginning checkbook balance readily yields the closing checkbook balance. Figure 1 shows the flow of record-keeping events. Typical income and expense categories, income statement form, and cash-flow form are shown in Table 1.

A Note About Computers and Record Keeping The availability of relatively inexpensive microcomputers and appropriate programs (software) can make your record-keeping chores relatively painless. Most practitioners will require a device (or service) to prepare reports. A word processing program together with a microcomputer will meet these needs. In addition, the computer could then be used for some of your record keeping. Instead of recording deposits and checks written in the register supplied by your local bank, you could enter this information in your computer using a program specifically designed to track income and expenses. This will eliminate the monthly summarizing routine since almost all of these programs do this automatically. They also calculate the year-to-date figures, and often geenrate cash-flow statements and a variety of financial statements that you would never attempt unless you were a financial professional. It is clearly a time saver. If you do a reasonable amount of third-party billing, there are programs available that will streamline your billing proceures with the outcome, either

Table 35-1 **Typical Categories and Statements**

Income	Expenses	
Fees	Office supplies	Postage
Honorarium	Copying costs	Auto expenses
Royalties	Delivery/messenger	Parking/tolls
Testing fees	Office maintenance	Rent
Teaching	Equipment repairs	Utilities
Other	Tel/Tel. ans. service	Prof. fees
	Office equipment	Advertising
	Office furniture	Promotion
	Dues/subscriptions	Consultants
	Salary/wages	Payroll taxes
	Malpractice ins.	Gen. ins.
	Health ins.	Other fringes
	Wkmen Comp. ins.	Airfares
	Meals	Lodging
	Local Transportation	Entertainment
	Returned checks	Bank charges
	Seminars	Registr. fees
	Other Educ. expenses	Mtge. interest
	Other busin. interest	Pension exp.
	Licenses/permits	Computer exp.
	Other taxes	Other exp.

Income Statement
  Income
  Less: expenses
  Net operating income

Cash flow statement
  Net operating income
  Add: noncash items
  Less: Mortgage payments
        Loan payments
        Equipment and furniture
  Net cash excess (deficit)

a printed statement to send to the third party, or, if you purchase a "modem," an ability to bill the third party electronically; that is, trasmit the billing infor- mation over the telephone lines. For those not requiring third-party billing, you might consider purchasing a modem for your computer (a "modem" is simply a device that permits you to transmit and receive information over the telephone lines) so that you can do your banking electronically. The major reason for this is that when you enter the information about your checks writ- ten, it is transmitted to your bank (and can be paid when you specify); also, generally these systems permit up to 50 categories, so that you have your checkbook expenditures analyzed for you.

Taxes When operating as a sole proprietor, you are subject to self- employment as well as income taxes. If you were working for someone else or some other company, in addition to income tax withholding, Social Secur- ity taxes would be withheld from your salary. Your employer would match the amount of Social Security tax that was withheld. Being self-employed does not exempt you from the Social Security system, and, in this case, you must pay both the employee's and employer's share of Social Security. The self- employment tax rate is simply twice the Social Security rate deducted from one's wages. For 1987, the Social Security rate deducted from one's wage was 7.15 percent (on amounts up to $43,800); thus, the self-employment rate was 14.3 percent. However, for 1987 there was a special credit of 2 percent reduc- ing the self-employemnt tax rate to 12.3 percent. The maximum amounts taxed under Social Security are increased each year by statute based on increases in the consumer price index. The tax rates increased (under prior law) to 15.02 percent for 1988–89 and then will increase to 15.3 percent for 1990 and later. The amounts withheld from wages are at one-half of these rates. There is still a special 2 percent credit for self-employment taxes for 1988–89. Thereafter, the credit is replaced by a deduction equal to 50 percent of the taxes on self- employment income. This credit will put self-employed individuals on the same footing as wage earners, since employees are not taxed on the Social Security taxes paid by their employer (the 50 percent of the tax that the employer pays toward the Social Security).

Table 2 shows the income tax rates for 1988 and 1989 for married and un-

Table 35-2A. **Individual Income Tax Rates for 1988**

Married Filing Jointly			Single			Head of Household	
Taxable Income	Tax	% on Excess	Taxable Income	Tax	% on Excess	Tax	% on Excess
$ 0	$ 0	15%	$ 0	$ 0	15%	$ 0	15%
29,750	4,463	28	17,850	2,678	28	2,678	15
71,900	16,265	33	23,900	4,372	28	3,585	28
149,250	41,790	28	43,150	9,762	33	8,975	28
			61,650	15,867	33	14,155	33
			89,560	25,077	28	23,365	33
			123,790	34,661	28	34,661	28

Source: Department of the Treasury, Internal Revenue Service, Tax Reform Act of 1986, *Pocket Guide*, RC, SE Pub. 163 (7-87).

Table 35.2B. **Individual Income Tax Rates for 1989**

Married Filing Jointly			Single			Head of Household		
Taxable Income	Tax	% on Excess	Taxable Income	Tax	% on Excess	Taxable Income	Tax	% on Excess
$ 0	$ 0	15%	$ 0	$ 0	15%	$ 0	$ 0	15%
30,950	4,643	28	18,550	2,783	28	24,850	3,728	28
74,850	16,935	33	44,900	10,161	33	64,200	14,746	33
155,320	*	*	93,130	*	*	128,810	*	*

*Essentially a flat 28% and phase out of dependency exemptions.
Source: Department of the Treasury, Internal Revenue Service, Form 1040-ES, for 1989.

married taxpayers. The rates are based on taxable income. For purposes of this chapter, we will ignore itemized deductions (unless relevant) and deductions for personal exemptions as they are not related to business considerations. If you operate your practice as a sole proprietor, you will be required to use the same fiscal year for your business as you use for yourself. For almost all taxpayers this is the calendar year. Since you do not have any taxes withheld, you must file and pay estimated income and self-employment taxes. For 1989, you must pay one quarter of your estimated tax by April 15, 1989; June 15, 1989; October 15, 1989; and January 15, 1990. The estimated taxes paid must be at least 90 percent of your actual liability or there will be penalties to be paid. To avoid a penalty you should pay at least 100 percent of the prior year's tax liability or 90 percent of the current year's. The 90 percent requirement is part of TRA 1986, and the penalty is automatic, unless you have paid 100 percent of the prior year's tax liability as an estimate for the current year.

Some Special Considerations   Beginning January 1, 1987, you could deduct only 80 percent of bona fide business meals and entertainment. You no longer could deduct the cost of a "quiet business meal." That is, unless specific business is discussed during, directly preceding, or directly following the meal, no deduction is allowed. It is your responsibility to establish that the meal was directly related to or associated with the active conduct of your practice. Further, only 80 percent of these meals are deductible. The cost of meals while away from home overnight on business is also only 80% deductible, as are expenses associated with business entertainment. However, transportation expenses to and from the place of entertainment or meals are fully deductible. This is where your appointment book comes in. In it, you should note the amount spent, the time and place of the travel, entertainment, meals; the specific business purpose or matter discussed (not simply "goodwill"); and the business relationship to you of the person(s) involved. Travel expenses for attending a convention, seminar, or workshop related to your practice are deductible in full. However, if you are not an active participant in the business-related convention, no deduction will be allowed.

Some practitioners have an office in their home. The Tax Reform Act of 1986 limits the deduction for the home office in that the deduction cannot be greater than the taxpayer's net income from the business. As a result, you cannot generate a tax loss based on your use of your home as an office.

However, amounts disallowed may be carried forward to future years. The amounts that may be deductible for business travel on cruise ships or other luxury water transportation is limited. Self-employed individuals may now deduct as business expenses 25 percent of the amounts paid for health insurance.

When you purchase equipment used in your practice, rather than deduct it in the year paid, you generally must depreciate it over its so-called useful life. For most office machinery, this will be five years, while for office furniture and fixtures, it will be seven years. Office buildings will be depreciated over 27.5 years whereas for residential property the life is 31.5 years. The depreciation method can be the straight-line method (cost less salvage value divided by the number of years), which typically yields the same deduction each year, or a declining-balance method that yields higher deductions in the earlier year. Usually one half of a year's depreciation is allowed in the year of acquisition and sale or disposal. However, if more than 40 percent of the total property acquired during the year is placed in service during the last three months of the year, you are only permitted a one-fourth instead of one-half a deduction as noted above. There is also a so-called Section 179 deduction that allows, in lieu of depreciation, an expense deduction for property acquired up to the amount of $10,000 in any one year. However, this deduction cannot be greater than the taxable income from the business. As a result, you cannot generate a tax loss based upon this deduction, although the excess may be carried forward to future years. There are still available some tax credits, not deductions, which are directly deducted from your tax liability (within certain limits. Credits exist for rehabilitation of historic buildings, business energy and targeted jobs. The maximum tax that can be offset by these credits is $25,000 plus 75 percent of the tax over $25,000.

There are special rules regarding the deductibility of a self-employed person's automobile. Deductions must be based on the business use of the car. As a result, you must maintain either a separate car for business or mileage records indicating business and personal use. You then calculate the business portion (percent) and this percent of your total expenses is deductible. Depreciating a car is somewhat complicated. The useful life could be as little as three years; if the auto is a "luxury" car (it cost more than $12,800), it could be depreciated over six years. If the business use does not exceed 50% of the total use, then the car must be depreciated over six years using a straight-line (in contrast to an accelerated) method. If you lease a car, you may have to include an amount in income, based on tables derived by the IRS, which estimates a value for the use of the car. Income must be picked up only for so-called luxury cars (valued more than $11,250). Rather than deduct actual expenses, you could simply keep track of your mileage and deduct 24¢ per business mile for the first 15,000 miles and 11 cents per mile thereafter. Thus, keeping track of the time, place, mileage, and purpose of each business trip (plus tolls and parking) is all that would be necessary to secure these deductions. In addition to supplying information about automobiles, computers are considered "listed property." If you use listed property 50 percent or less in your practice, then you must use the straight-line method and you cannot use the Section 179 expense deduction.

Pension Plans   There are plans that can be set up to allow contributions to be made to a qualified plan and the income earned in the plan accumulates tax-free. A self-employed individual can set up a pension plan similar to corporate plans. The plans for self-employed individuals are typically called "Keogh" plans. It may be a defined-benefit plan under which contributions are designed to provide a specific amount at retirement. Alternatively, the plan could be a defined-contribution plan, where specific contributions, rather than a targeted benefit, are made. There are two types of defined-contribution plans, a money-purchase plan and a profit-sharing plan. In the money-purchase plan, the amount stated must be contributed every year. You must obtain a waiver from the IRS to skip or reduce a contribution. The limits are essentially the same for corporate plans so that similar considerations exist. The most positive argument for contributions to any pension plan is that the income grows tax-free over the years and becomes taxable only when received at retirement. There are rules governing early retirements, early withdrawals, and late withdrawals. If you receive any distribution before age 59½, there is a 10 percent excise-tax penalty, in addition to the tax to be paid. There are exceptions (death, disability, age 55 retirement if you receive periodic payments for life). You are required to take, at the least, a minimum distribution from a qualified plan by age 70½. The minimum distribution must be the equivalent of what you would receive if you purchased a life annuity. If the distribution is too small, there is a 50 percent penalty for the shortfall. If the pension is too large, there is a 15 percent excise-tax penalty. "Too large" is defined as more than $150,000 in any one year adjusted for changes in the consumer price index. For a lump-sum payment, you are allowed five times the annual rate before being subject to the excise tax. In order for a plan to qualify, you must cover all employees, as long as they work full time and are 21 years old. Plan participants become "vested," that is, have legal ownership of their account, according to a variety of schedules. When the principal has a large share, the plan is considered top heavy and is subject to a minimum contribution for employees and a faster vesting schedule.

Individual retirement accounts (IRA) have all but been eliminated as tax shelters for many middle-income taxpayers. If either spouse is covered by a qualified pension plan and the combined adjusted gross income is $50,000 or more, no deduction is allowed for an IRA ($35,000 for singles). Nondeductible IRA contributions may be made up to the lesser of earned income or $2,000 per individual. Although these amounts are not tax deductible, they do accumulate tax-free until withdrawn. One could also set up a simplified employee plan (SEP) which consists of an IRA for each employee that the employer contributes to.

The alternative minimum tax (AMT) has been changed so that taxpayers must pay much more attention to its applications. You start with your taxable income and add back certain itemized deductions, passive losses, excess depreciation, and certain tax preferences, which gives you alternative minimum taxable income. This amount is reduced by an exemption equal to $40,000 for married parents filing a joint return, $30,000 for single individuals, and $20,000 for married parents filing separately. The exemptions are phased out beginning at $150,000 for married persons filing jointly and is totally eliminated at $310,000. These values are $112,500 and $232,500, respectively, for single individuals. The AMT rate is 21 percent. If the AMT is greater than the regular tax, you pay the AMT.

Other Issues What if you employ your spouse and/or chldren? There must be a bona fide business relationship for you to employ them. If you have a pension plan, they can be covered by the plan. If your children are less than 18 years old, you do not pay or deduct Social Security taxes from their wages.

On Becoming a Corporation

The major advantage of using the corporate form for conducting a business is that it gives the owner(s) limited liability. Since the corporation is a separate legal entity, only the assets of the corporation are subject to creditor acquisition, while the non-corporate assets of the shareholders generally are free from corporate entanglements. However, in the case of professionals, it is unclear whether limited liability does exist even in a corporate form. Most states allow professionals to incorporate, although this does not necessarily free the shareholder professionals from personal liability. These are so-called "professional corporations" or "professional associations," hence the initials after one's name PC or PA. These professional corporations are often treated differently from regular, nonprofessional non-personal-service corporations. Based on TRA 1986 personal-service corporations must have a calendar year beginning January 1 as of 1988. Many in existence today have other than calendar years; that is, they were free to choose any 12-month period. The record-keeping requirements for a corporation are often greater than those required for a partnership or proprietorship. There are typically many more government regulatory agencies to which corporations must report. A separate checking account *must* be maintained, not merely to separate personal and business income and expenditures, but because the corporation is a separate legal entity and must be treated as such. If the shareholders mingled their own funds with those of the corporations, the IRS can ignore the corporate form and treat all of the transactions as attributed to the shareholders. This would seem to undo part of the reason for incorporating. However, the record-keeping comments made earlier with regard to a single proprietorship are relevant here as well. Although more information is required on corporate income tax returns, in contrast to the Schedule C the sole proprietor must file, this information should be available to a sole proprietor for business and not tax reasons. Nevertheless, there is more record keeping and reporting for corporations and fees for professional services for corporations are typically higher than for individuals. Another reason often given for incorporating is that the corporation has a perpetual "life," that is, even if shareholders die, the corporation continues in existence. In fact, it does so until a specific act of corporate liquidation occurs. Bringing new professionals into a practice may be easier with a corporate form since it will involve the sale or distribution of stock of the corporation. Otherwise, you would be changing from a sole proprietorship to a partnership, or from a partnership to yet another partnership. Given the additional record-keeping burden and higher fees, why incorporate? Are there any advantages from an income tax view? If you incorporate, you will be paid as an Officer of the corporation. Your salary will be subject to all federal, state, and local (if any) payroll taxes. Any income remaining in the corporation will be taxed at a corporate

Table 35-3. **Corporation Federal Income Tax Rates**

Taxable Income	Periods Before 7/1/87, %	Periods After 6/30/87, %
$ 0-$ 25,000	15	15
25,001– 50,000	18	15
50,001– 75,000	30	25
75,001– 100,000	40	34
100,001– 335,000	46	39
335,001– 1,000,000	46	34
1,000,001– 1,405,000	51	34
over $1,405,000	46	34

Source: Department of the Treasury, Internal Revenue Service. Tax Reform Act of 1986, *Pocket Guide*. RC SE Pub. 163 (7-87)

Table 35-4. **Federal Income Tax Liabilities for Various Business Entities; Net Income from Sole Proprietor $50,000**

	Sole Proprietor	C Corporation	
		Corporation	Officer
Fee	$100,000	$100,000	
Expenses	50,000	50,000	
Net income (individual)	50,000		
Pension	5,000	5,000	
Salary		35,000	$35,000
Payroll taxes		3,000	
Net income (corp.)		7,000	
Deductions and exemptions	10,000		10,000
Taxable income	35,000	7,000	25,000
FIT*	7,480	1,050	4,744
SET†	5,859		
Social Security§		2,630	2,630
Total tax burden	13,339	3,680	7,374
Add: corporate tax	—	—	3,680
Totals for comparison	13,339		11,054

*For ease of illustration, the following considerations govern: single taxpayer using 1988 rates; total itemized deduction and exemptions $10,000; FIT=calculated federal income taxes assuming no other income.

†SET=self-employment tax used 13.02 percent on maximum of $45,000 or $5,859 (1988 rates).

§Social Security=Social Security taxes paid. As a corporate officer, the amount of 7.51% of $35,000 is withheld and the same amount is paid for by the corporation.

Note 1. As a C corporation, if the maximum salary is drawn, $42,000, additional Social Security taxes of $526 are withheld and are matched by the corporation for a total of $1,052; an additional $2,160 of personal FIT is created while the corporation would have 0 FIT. As a result, the total tax burden is now $11,054+$1,052+$2,160–$1,050=$13,216.

Note 2. As an S corporation, the figures in Note 1 would hold unless the additional $7,000 (the corporate "income") was paid as a dividend rather than as salary. In this case, there would not be any additional Social Security taxes so that the total tax burden would be $13,216–$1,052=$12,164.

Table 35-5. **Federal Income Tax Liabilities for Various Business Entities; Net Income from Sole Proprietor $100,000**

	Sole Proprietor	C Corporation	
		Corporation	Officer
Fee	$150,000	$150,000	
Expenses	50,000	50,000	
Net income (individual)	100,000		
Pension	10,000	10,000	
Salary		70,000	$70,000
Payroll taxes		3,000	
Net income (corp.)		17,000	
Deductions and exemptions	10,000		10,000
Taxable income	80,000	17,000	60,000
FIT*	21,984	2,550	15,379
SET†	5,859		
Social Security§		3,380	3,380
Total tax burden	27,843	5,930	18,759
Add: corporate tax	—	—	5,930
Totals for comparison	27,843		24,689

*For ease of illustration, the following considerations govern: single taxpayer using 1988 rates; total itemized deduction and exemptions $10,000; FIT=calculated federal income taxes assuming no other income.

†SET=self-employment tax used 13.02 percent on maximum of $45,000 or $5,859 (1988 rates).

§Social Security=Social Security taxes paid. As a corporate officer, the amount of 7.51% of $45,000 (maximum amount) is withheld and the same amount is paid for by the corporation.

Note 1. As a C corporation, if the maximum salary is drawn, $87,000, an additional $5,667 of personal FIT is created while the corporation would have 0 FIT. As a result, the total tax burden is now $24,689+$5,667-$2,550=$27,806.

Note 2. As an S corporation, the figures in Note 1 would hold even if the additional $17,000 (the corporate "income") was paid as a dividend rather than as salary. This is because the $70,000 salary is already over the Social Security maximum of $45,000 for 1988.

level. The corporate tax rates are shown in Table 3 for 1987 and 1988. Tables 4, 5, and 6 illustrate the possible effects of incorporating a private practice that has a net income of $50,000, $100,000, and $200,000, respectively. These tables show that if taxable income remains in the corporation, the total federal income tax can be less in the corporate form in contrast to a sole proprietorship. On the other hand, if you draw the maximum possible salary, there is no difference of any significance.

If you wish the corporate form for non-income tax reasons, but do not like some of the corporate tax effects, is there a way to have both worlds? In fact, there is. A corporation that pays tax as one is called a C corporation. In 1958 (Faber & Holbrook, 1983), Congress passed legislation that permitted, under certain circumstances, a corporation to be taxed as if it were a partnership while retaining its corporate form. This legislation has undergone numerous changes and has led to the creation of S corporations. An S corporation is a legal corporation whose shareholders have elected to be taxed as if they were a partnership. The effect is that any corporate income, rather than being taxed at the corporate level, is passed through to the shareholders and they pay tax at their individual rates. Tables 4, 5, and 6 show the effects of the S corporation election. It is identical to the case where the maximum salary is drawn.

The requirements for an S corporation are as follows: it must have no more than 35 shareholders, it must have one class of stock, and it must be a domestic corporation (i.e., formed in the United States). If there are no differences between an S corporation and a C corporation with the maximum salary drawn, then why elect S corporation status? S corporations avoid certain issues, such as unreasonable compensation, excess accumulated earnings, and the corporate alternative minimum tax.

Disadvantages are that the shareholders pay tax on the income even if no

Table 35-6. Federal Income Tax Liabilities for Various Business Entities; Net Income from Sole Proprietor $200,000

| | Sole Proprietor | C Corporation | |
		Corporation	Officer
Fee	$250,000	$250,000	
Expenses	50,000	50,000	
Net income (individual)	200,000		
Pension	20,000	20,000	
Salary		150,000	$150,000
Payroll taxes		3,000	
Net income (corp.)		27,000	
Deductions and exemptions	10,000		10,000
Taxable income	170,000	27,000	140,000
FIT*	47,600	4,050	39,200
SET†	5,859		
Social Security§		3,380	3,380
Total tax burden	53,459	7,430	42,580
Add: corporate tax	—	—	7,430
Totals for comparison	53,459		50,010

*For ease of illustration, the following considerations govern: single taxpayer using 1988 rates; total itemized deduction and exemptions $10,000; FIT=calculated federal income taxes assuming no other income.
†SET=self-employment tax used 13.02 percent on maximum of $45,000 or $5,859 (1988 rates).
§Social Security=Social Security taxes paid. As a corporate officer, the amount of 7.51% of $45,000 (maximum for 1988) is withheld and the same amount is paid for by the corporation.

Note 1. As a C corporation, if the maximum salary is drawn, $177,000, an additional $7,560 of personal FIT is created while the corporation would have 0 FIT. As a result, the total tax burden is now $50,010+$7,560−$4,050=$53,520.

Note 2. As an S corporation, the figures in Note 1 would hold even if the additional $27,000 (the corporate "income") was paid as a dividend rather than as salary. This is because the salary of $150,000 is already over the Social Security limit of $45,000 for 1988.

cash was received; S corporation status is not recognized in many states, resulting in treatment as a C corporation for state income tax purposes, and the taxable year is restricted to a calendar year.

A critical decision point is whether you have to draw all of the corporation's profits as income for yourself. If you must, from an income tax point of view, there may not be any point in incorporating, much less electing S status. If there is a non-income tax reason for incorporating and you draw all of the income as salary, then it seems reasonable to elect S status. However, if you can leave funds in the corporation for expansion and the like, Tables 4, 5, and 6 show there is some immediate savings by electing the corporation form and being taxed as a C corporation. There is one more major difference between an S corporation and a C corporation. If the practice is sold, before TRA 1986 the usual sequence was a corporate liquidation followed by a sale. The tax would typically be at the shareholder level. Under the new tax law, there is a corporate capital gains tax and upon distribution to the shareholders, another tax on the individual level. However, if the corporation was an S corporation since inception, the tax would only be at the shareholder level. If the corporation converted from a C to an S corporation there is a 10-year period during which a capital gains tax could be assessed. However, one of the exemptions is for corporations valued at less than $10 million as long as they have fewer than 11 persons owning more than 50 percent of the stock *if* they elected S status for a taxable year beginning before January 1, 1989. Since S corporations must be on a calendar year, the election must have been good for calendar year 1988, and the election must be made on or before the 15th day of the third month of the elected year, namely, March 15, 1988. This exemption is only for certain kinds of assets so that the built-in gains tax may still apply in part. One must think very clearly in terms of potential long-term plans and the tax consequences before incorporating, and if incorporated, whether to be a C or an S corporation. After the completion of this chapter, a critically important tax bill was passed. Please refer to the note after the References for the essential components.

Additional tax considerations regarding proprietor versus a corporation. If you have an office in your home and you incorporate, you actually would be leasing the office space to the corporation. The amount should be what is considered an arms-length transaction. The charge would be rental expense to the corporation. On your personal return, you would report the rental income and the proportionate share of expenses attributed to the home office that you paid for personally. However, the TRA 1986 does not allow a deduction for the rental of a home office if your employer rents it. Since you are an officer-employee of the corporation, this provision would seem to apply to you. It would seem reasonable that you should be able to deduct the proportionate share of home expenses that are directly attributable to your business. There are also specific regulations regarding substantiation of certain expenses for shareholder-employees. However, if you maintain adequate records as a proprietor, the same practice should suffice for the shareholder-employee.

Most of the special topics for sole proprietors apply to corporations as well. The depreciation rules are the same. The value of the personal use of a company car is a taxable fringe benefit. It is subject to payroll tax witholding and must be reported on your W-2 form. Similar rules exist for leased cars. If an owner of more than 5% uses a company-leased car and the business use does not exceed 50 percent, then the corporation may have to add a one-time-only "inclusion amount" to its gross income. This happens particularly if it is a luxury car, defined here as an automobile that is valued at more than $11,250. You should also be aware of the corporation AMT. Basically, this is the corporation's taxable income plus accelerated depreciation plus tax preferences plus "book income adjustment." An exemption of $40,000 is subtracted and the balance is taxed at 20 percent — if the AMT is larger than the regular tax you pay it. The exemption is reduced by 25 cents for every $1 that alternative minimum taxable income exceeds $150,000. The investment tax credit (ITC) cannot reduce the AMT by more than 25 percent of AMT tax or 75 percent of the regular tax. "Book income adjustment" is defined as an increase by one half of the excess of pretax book income (the income of the corporation reported on financial statements) over the alternative minimum taxable income (AMTI). The major adjustment for a personal-service corporation is that depreciation is computed differently for the "regular tax" than for the alternative minimum tax. Generally, the "useful lives" are shorter for the regular tax, yielding small write-offs for the AMT and thus higher income.

For corporations there is a dividends received deduction of 80 percent of the dividends received from domestic corporations. Thus, you almost escape corporation tax on investments of dividend-paying corporations. If you have too much investment income, you could be subject to personal holding company rules. There is also for S corporations a limit on the amount of investment income. A corporation must also make estimated-tax payments and be exposed to penalties if less than 90 percent of tax is paid. Employee benefit plans are essentially the same for corporate and noncorporate plans.

Under the Tax Reform Act of 1984(6) (Prentice-Hall, 1984), loans from shareholders to corporations and vice-versa must carry market interest rates (unless less than $10,000). If they do not, then interest must be "imputed," treating it as if interest has been paid. To avoid these rules, you should simply pay interest at the current market rate on any outstanding liability.

Employment Taxes and Independent Contractors   Many practitioners use the services of people, often on a part-time basis. The question of whether they are employees or independent contractors often arises. If they are employees, you must withhold Social Security and possibly income taxes from the wages, as well as pay unemployment and disability taxes in some jurisdictions. There may even be workers' compensation coverage so that the additional cost for employees could be 10–15 percent of the salary or wages you are paying them. In addition, if you have a qualified pension plan, all full-time employees over 21 years of age generally must be covered. The common-law standards are used to determine the relationship. Individuals are employees if they perform services that are subject to the control of the employer, both as to what work must be done and how the work must be done. If the employer has the right to control only the result of the work and not the means of accomplishing the result, the individual, generally, is an independent contractor.

Typically, when you incorporate an existing practice, it is nontaxable under IRC section 351, as long as you follow a few rules. Only property (including money) can be transferred to a corporation on a tax-free basis. Therefore, you cannot transfer services for stock without incurring a tax liability for the income (the services). Immediately after the transfer, the transferors must own 80 percent or more of the stock. A problem arises for a cash-basis taxpayer (as most professionals are) if the unpaid bills (liabilities) are assumed by the corporation. The best procedure is to pay the liabilities as the proprietor and not transfer any unpaid liabilities.

The Partnership Form

This form of business entity generally provides the business with the benefits of complementary skills and potentially larger amounts of available capital. It avoids the potential double taxation of a corporation. The major disadvantage is unlimited liability and the fact that one partner's acts bind all of the other partners. Also, as the number of partners increase, the chances for disagreement increase. You should have a formal buy-sell agreement to cover disputes, sale, or death. Record keeping is essentially the same as for a corporation. Partnerships and S corporations are treated in almost an identical manner from a federal income tax view.

Association of Corporations

Sometimes a partnership is formed and the partners are professional corporations. The partnership typically hires the nonprofessional staff and administers the practices. Practitioners maintain their own pension and other plans through their own corporation. Whether employees can be excluded from pension and other fringe benefits through this device may be questionable. In any event, the partnership is treated as any other partnership from an income tax view.

Some practitioners have multiple positions—private practice, a university position, author, lecturer. How does one handle all of this? The issues are very similar to those with which we have been dealing. If you are an author and have royalty income, you would have to assign the rights to the property (i.e., the book and subsequent editions) to the corporation, not merely the income, if you wanted the income to be attributed to a corporation. The TRA 1986 includes a major change for authors. Specifically, the law provides that the costs incurred in producing a motion picture or researching and writing a book must be capitalized. This means that authors no longer can deduct expenses as they pay for them. Instead, the costs of researching and writing a specific book will be accumulated, and only when income begins to flow, will the expenses be deductible. Fortunately, the Technical and Miscellaneous Revenue Act of 1988 (TAMRA) specifically exempts costs of writers, artists and photographers in producing creative property from this provision. With a variety of positions, the question of the best form to conduct business will be largely determined by how much you can leave in the corporation. Thus, your needs have to be thought out carefully and explicitly, which brings us to investments. But before turning to investments, let us point out that the TRA 1986 has created three categories of income: active, earned income (which we have been dealing with until now); portfolio income (dividends, interest, capital gains); and passive income (income derived from activities that you do not actively participate in). It is assumed that real estate is a passive activity. There is a limited exception in cases where you do actively participate and your gross income is less than $100,000.

INVESTMENTS

In this section we discuss the major issues relating to investments. First, one must ask oneself the question, "Investment for what?" That is, you must specify a goal rather than some free-floating feeling that it seems like a good thing to do or that others you know do it. For the practitioner there are three major reasons: (1) college funds for children; (2) retirement; and (3) general capital accumulation.

College Funding

The TRA of 1986 dealt a fairly severe blow to those parents who are attempting to deal with the significantly rising costs of higher education by setting funds aside for the child at an early age. The taxation of unearned income for children under 14 years of age proceeds as follows; the first $500 is not taxed; the next $500 is taxed at the child's rate (typically the lowest possible rate, which is 15 percent for 1988). Anything over $1,000 will be taxed at the parents' *highest* rate. Children 14 years of age or older will be taxed at their own rates throughout. This rule is for unearned income only. Earned income is taxed at the child's rate. Recall that earned income consists of salary, wages, and professional fees. The child can offset earned income with the child's standard deduction, which is $3,000 for 1988. Bear in mind that $500 of it was used up against unearned income. Generally the child is no longer allowed a dependency exemption for itself. If children can perform meaningful work in an arms-length transaction, then it clearly pays to hire them and pay them. There are no Social Security taxes and the income is totally taxable to the children. The first $2,040 (after $500 is applied against unearned income) of fees and salaries were not taxed in 1988. The new law has forced a change in strategy. Once children under 14 years of age have more than $10–12,000 in their name, tax-sheltered investments need to be considered, for example, tax-exempt bonds; various forms of life insurance policies that accumulate tax-free; single-payment annuities, all of which attempt to postpone taxes on increases in value until the funds are used, presumably after the child attains the age of 14; grantor trusts (Clifford Trusts), which under prior law gave the income to the child while the parent/grantor retained the principal, may no longer be useful. Under current law, the income is taxed to the grantor. Typical income-shifting strategies (e.g. stock in an S corporation and family partnerships) can now only be used for children 14 years and older. Recently passed TAMRA, beginning January 1, 1990, allows interest on Series EE bonds to be exempt from tax if the bonds are used to finance your child's college education. The exemption is phased out for gross incomes between $60,000 and $90,000 (joint returns) and $40,000 and $55,000 (individual returns).

Retirement

The life expectancy is now 80–81 years for males and 81–82 for females. One contribution to your pension that should not be overlooked is Social Security. Another source is your pension from your practice. The final source is yourself. Here again the advice of a professional is invaluable in assisting you at attempting to realize your financial goals. Given the increased life expectancies, you must take into account an assumed inflation rate along with a pre- and postretirement budget in order to determine the annual income you will need to accomplish your financial goals for retirement. Given these figures, you can then determine how much capital needs to be accumulated to achieve these ends.

General Capital Accumulation

Here, too, you must also set some specific goals, so that the appropriate strategies would be adapted. You must also determine your own level of acceptance of risk. Your specific goals and your resources will determine, in part, the level of risk you should be taking. To the extent there are discretionary funds left, then your own risk tolerance must be determined.

We will now turn to a brief consideration of various investment instruments.

Taxable money-market accounts and large negotiable certificates of deposit have no particular tax advantages but are generally regarded as very secure investments. Instruments that have some tax advantages that are readily available are six-month bank certificate of deposits (CDs). As a cash-basis taxpayer, one defers income until the maturity date. Any certificate purchased after July 1 defers the tax to the following year. Some banks offer three- and nine-month CDs with more options.

The U.S. Treasury issues a variety of instruments. There are U.S. Treasury bills (T-bills), which are exempt from state and local income taxes. The minimum amount is $10,000, and with 3, 6 and 12-month maturities. These instruments are purchased at a discount and the discount is interest income. There are also U.S. Treasury notes that range in maturity from one to seven years, as well as U.S. Treasury bonds with five- to 30-year maturities. The minimum is usually $1,000. Interest is paid semiannually on these instruments. There are also series EE bonds, which are also purchased at a discount. Income can be deferred until maturity, which can be five years or more. At maturity, EE bonds can be rolled over into HH bonds and taxes can be defered until the HH bonds mature.

There are also a number of federally sponsored credit agencies, which as a group are known as the Federal Farm Credit Banks and the Federal Home Loan Banks. They issue obligations (minimum $5,000) for short-term as well as long-term maturities. The very-short-term obligations require a minimum of $50,000. The well-known "Fannie Mae"—or the Federal National Mortgage Association—is privately owned and has similar instruments. All of these obligations are exempt from state and local income taxes. The Government National Mortgage Association (GNMA, so-called "Ginnie Mae") is a wholly owned government corporation within the Department of Housing and Urban

Development. It buys mortgages from private lenders and issues "pass-through" securities that include both principal and interest in their monthly payments to investors. As a result, investors should reinvest part of the monthly payment, at least the principal portion. Unit investment trusts have been created that hold a few GNMA mortgage pools; also, GNMA mutual funds have been created that have a greater diversity than the unit trusts. The mutual funds, as do most mutual funds, carry a transaction cost.

Bonds of state and local government and U.S. territories and possessions (i.e., municipal bonds) are exempt from federal income taxes, and also from the state income taxes in the state of issue. The minimum is usually $5,000. There are also municipal bond funds or tax-free unit trusts that hold such instruments.

Zero-coupon CDs or zero-coupon Treasuries have relatively long-term maturities whose increase in value each year is taxable, but have underlying U.S. Treasuries or bank CDs. Interest is not paid until maturity although the annual increase in value is subject to federal income taxes. Then there are bonds issued by large private corporations that typically pay higher interest rates than that of government agencies. Of course, there are common stocks, mutual funds, and a variety of investment instruments tied to private corporations. All of the instruments discussed also have a "secondary market" — that is, they are traded publicly so that sales prior to maturity may be made and they provide opportunities for gain. Of course, these actions involve more risk than holding these securities to maturity.

There are also a variety of insurance-related products such as single-payment annuities, universal life insurance, and whole life insurance that one may investigate. Real estate investments are another area, although TRA 1986 eliminated the tax-shelter aspect. In fact, a good rule to follow is to consider investment on its economic merits. If there are some tax advantages, consider that as a bonus. One should not enter into an investment because of perceived tax advantages.

One final note regarding investments. The past decade has seen enormous increases in the value of personal residences. One result is that many people purchasing a home believe they are also making an investment that should increase in value, perhaps 5–10 percent per year. This thinking is obviously based on the experience of the past decade during which, in many areas, residential property has soared in value. It is my belief that one must separate investment goals and activities from one's personal residence. Your residence should be simply that, a place to live in that you enjoy for a variety of non-financial reasons. If, in addition, you earn a considerable amount of money when you sell it, consider it as a bonus. Those who assume that their residence will yield substantial equity and thus provide a substantial source of funds for retirement may find themselves significantly short of their goals when they actually attempt to sell their home.

REFERENCES

Faber, P.L., & Holbrook, M.E. (1983). *Subchapter S manual. A special break for small business corporations.* Englewood Cliffs, NJ: Prentice-Hall, Inc.

Economic Recovery Act of 1981. Englewood Cliffs, NJ: Prentice-Hall (1981).

Prentice-Hall Infomration Services (1984). Tax Reform Act of 1984. Englewood Cliffs, NJ: author.

Prentice-Hall Information Services (1986). Tax Reform Act of 1986. Paramus, NJ: author.

Prentice-Hall Information Services (1987). Proposed Tax Reform Act of 1987. Paramus, NJ: author.

Prentice-Hall Information Services (1987). Tax provisions of the Omnibus Budget Reconciliation Act of 1987. Paramus, NJ: author.

Prentice-Hall Information Services (1988). The Technical and Miscellaneous Revenue Act of 1988. Paramus, NJ.

Note: (On December 22, 1987, the Omnibus Budget Reconciliation Act (Prentice-Hall Information Services, 1987) was passed. This law contains provisions that will have an enormous impact on the taxation of personal service corporations. Beginning January 1, 1988, personal service corporations are taxed at a flat 34 percent. The definition of a personal-service corporation clearly includes a professional corporation so that this provision will have a major impact on those practitioners who are contemplating incorporation, as well as those already operating in the corporate form. The effect of a flat 34 percent rate (instead of one beginning at 15 percent on the examples shown in Tables 4, 5, and 6 will demonstrate the obvious. The corporate taxes would be increased by $1,330, $3,230, and $5,130 in Tables 4, 5, and 6, respectively. As a result, the total tax for comparison to the tax generated by operating as a sole proprietor becomes $12,384, $27,919, and $55,140, respectively for Tables 4, 5, and 6. It is clear that any tax savings in the corporate form has been eliminated. (In Table 4, the overall tax is still less in the corporate form because of the salary, which is well below the Social Security maximum so that savings on self-employment tax result.) It would appear that, if tax considerations are of major importance, the practitioner may not wish to incorporate. For those already operating in the corporate form, an election to S corporation status should be given very serious consideration.

▲ ▲ ▲

Part II Financial and Economic Management
(continued)

S E C T I O N

E

**Career
Management**

▼ ▼ ▼

36

POSTACADEMIC TRAINING: STAYING CURRENT AND SPECIALIZATION TRAINING

Robert H. Goldstein, Ph.D.

The really important things in life are those things you learn after you know it all.

Each of the major mental-health professions from which private practitioners emerge has evolved its own pattern of education and training. Psychology, psychiatry, social work, and nursing have all developed academic models for preparing mental-health practitioners that are based on some combination of didactic classroom exercises and practical, experiential exposure. In this chapter, we consider various forms of educational opportunities that are available to expand upon or to supplement this type of formal academic preparation. This survey of postacademic training will focus specifically on the current status of such training activities within the field of psychology, but the general issues raised and the conclusions drawn are equally applicable to the other mental-health specialties as well.

During the 20th century, psychology has evolved both as a field of scientific study and, increasingly, as the basis for one of the major helping professions. As the field has grown in complexity and sophistication, ongoing attention has been paid to the issue of how those who wish to enter the field should best be prepared to do so. Questions that have been the focus of consideration include such matters as what should be taught, where this teaching should take place and by whom, and when in the course of a budding psychologist's career all this should happen. A number of national conferences have, over the years, addressed these issues, and each of these has in turn had a major impact on the nature and focus of professional education. There is still some dispute as to whether psychologists educated at the master's level are adequately prepared to undertake clinical work, but the prevailing view appears to be that the doctoral level of education, extending over four to five years after the undergraduate degree, should be the basis for entry-level participation in the field.

The Boulder model (Raimy, 1950) of researcher/clinician established a pattern of graduate education that emphasized both aspects of psychology's heritage. A thorough grounding in the rigorous study of the scientific approach to human behavior was to be combined with extensive training in applied clinical activities. The yearlong internship was to be the culmination of education for professional practice. This Boulder model of training of the scientific researcher/clinician was the dominant theme in psychology training for some decades. The major locus of that training was the university department of psychology.

A recent shift to a more applied professional emphasis in graduate education has reflected the view that the field has matured to the point at which a sufficient body of information and skills has developed to permit education to focus primarily on the application of this corpus of knowledge. This has, in turn, been accompanied by the growth of educational programs in settings other than university graduate departments.

Almost all training models have acknowledged, however, that the time available within the typical doctoral-level training program is insufficient for full training in all the relevant areas of clinical activity. Even in the Boulder conference report it was recognized that professional levels of skill in the areas of psychodiagnosis and psychotherapy required additional time and supervised experience. Hence, further training, particularly in clinical areas, was seen to be necessary for a psychologist to be able to enter into the world of professional practice at a journeyman level of competence.

GOALS

The purpose of this additional training following completion of the regular academic program was, and to a considerable extent still is, intended to achieve several goals. Primary among these goals is the attainment of advanced levels of general clinical skill. Particularly for those whose careers will be devoted to training other psychologists, there is a need for a greater scope of clinical experience than can typically be achieved via an internship. The pattern of rewards and reinforcements for budding university department psychologists has usually led them to an early focus on research productivity and publications. One can see the ever-present possibility that the university clinical training programs could be conducted by psychologists who themselves had had limited experience with the realities of the clinical world. Indeed, this issue has been at times the source of some conflict between the academic departments and the clinical centers that provide practica or internships. Thus, a period of postdoctoral training can be seen as crucial for adequately preparing those who would train the next generation. Similarly, advanced general clinical training is crucial for psychologists who have sought careers in settings such as medical schools where they must clearly establish their professional competence in a way that would allow them to participate in the education of other general health-service providers and mental-health specialists.

A second purpose of postacademic education is the development or improvement of specialized skills, particularly in areas inadequately or not at all covered in the traditional comprehensive academic programs. Even a solid set of practicum and internship experiences may not provide much exposure to certain age groups or diagnostic populations, such as children, the aged, or the chronically psychotic. Furthermore, graduates of many training programs may be quite familiar with certain specific techniques of treatment or with a particular theoretical orientation, but may have relatively little knowledge of other methods or other points of view. Postacademic training serves, therefore, to deepen and focus clinical competencies in areas that require more intensive or more extensive preparation.

A third goal of advanced or postacademic training derives from the constantly changing and evolving nature of the field. New areas of activity and interest are emerging with what appears to be, at times, astonishing speed. Many of these areas, such as neuropsychology or health psychology, are young enough that psychologists who are not recent graduates may have had no significant exposure to training in these fields. The number of training programs with specific foci in some of these newer fields is still quite small, and opportunities for education are limited. Thus, postacademic education is a major vehicle for achieving professional competence in some of the more recently developed specialty areas.

Finally, in a field as dynamic and expanding as psychology, even the well-prepared professional can find his or her knowledge base moving toward obsolescence at a disconcertingly rapid pace. Both the practical demands of continuing education requirements and the ethical obligations to maintain one's professional skills at a level consistent with contemporary standards impel practicing psychologists to seek out sources of current information that can provide renewal or replacement of no-longer-relevant professional practices and techniques.

Given the various goals of postacademic education and the various motives that direct psychologists toward the achievement of these goals, it is not surprising to find that a substantial amount of psychology's educational resources is being devoted to training activities that follow or expand upon those provided by basic academic programs.

TRAINING SITES

A psychologist who wises to pursue a postacademic course of study will find that there are many places where this activity can be undertaken. Perhaps the most widely known of these are the formal programs of postdoctoral education, typically offered in the form of a fellowship, that are provided in a broad variety of clinical settings. Notices of the availability of such fellowships frequently appear in the monthly newspaper issued by the American Psychological Association (APA), the *APA Monitor,* and in the APA's official journal, *The American Psychologist.* However, the most comprehensive single compendium of information regarding fellowships is the annual directory published by the Association of Psychology Internship Centers (APIC) (Carrington, 1986–87). In addition to listing internships, the directory has, for some years, included a special section containing descriptions of postdoctoral programs. Detailed information regarding the content of the training programs, specialized aspects, stipend levels, and so on is presented in a well-organized and informative manner. For those interested in work with children, the *Directory of Internship Programs in Clinical, Child, and Pediatric Psychology* (Tuma, 1986–87) has been published on a frequently updated basis since 1976. As is the case with the APIC directory, this child-focused listing also contains detailed information regarding postdoctoral fellowship programs.

In the most recent APIC directory, some 69 separate, identifiable programs are described that are available in the United States, plus two programs located in Canada. These programs offer a total of approximately 215 fellowship positions. Of these, 185 (86 percent) carry some type of stipend; the rest are unfunded.

The directory of child training programs lists 23 centers that offer postdoctoral opportunities, and that provide a total of 49 positions. However, as 11 of these programs appear to be identical with listings in the APIC directory, the actual number of additional child fellowship sites would seem to be 12, and the number of additional fellowship slots available in the United States to be 38, with seven other positions available in Canada. This directory also includes a listing of 17 other postdoctoral internship positions, six of which are also listed in the APIC directory, and so the number of additional child postdoctoral internships seems to be 11. Thus, the grand total of formally listed postdoctoral positions available in the United States and Canada appears to be approximately 264. With approximately 2,000 new psychology doctorates currently being granted each year, opportunities for postdoctoral education appear to be available for fewer than 15 percent of those graduated.

There has obviously been considerable growth in the availability of postdoctoral opportunities, since the 1974 APIC directory listed only 14 programs offering a total of 46 positions, in addition to a number of opportunities that then existed at formal training sites. The training programs currently available in the United States are distributed among 32 different states, an apparently wide dispersion that is offset by the fact that four states (California, Massachusetts, New York, and Rhode Island) alone account for 125 slots, or about

Table 36-1
Types of Postdoctoral Training Programs
Listed in 1986-87 Training Directories

Area of Training	No. of Programs	No. of Training Positions
General clinical	31	108
Neuropsychology	11	25
Child and family	12	23
Health psychology/ behavioral medicine	11	23
Geropsychology	6	15
Adolescents	5	8
Mental retardation	2	5
Eating disorders	2	2
Rehabilitation	1	5
College mental health	1	1
Partial hospitalization	1	1
Forensic	1	1
Totals	84	209

one-half of the total number of positions offered. As is the case with regard to so many other health-care or educational resources, there appears to be an unbalanced concentration of facilities in a relatively small number of high-population areas.

The sources of funding available to support training programs appear to be quite varied. Information about this matter is not readily available, but it would appear that training grants, research support, and, in many instances, institutional funds derived from clinical revenues represent the primary mechanisms by which fellowship stipends are generated.

Table 1 presents a categorization of the type of training provided by the programs of the APIC and child listings.

It is clear that the majority of opportunities are for general clinical training, although within many of these a number of specialized experiences are provided. For example, some 20 of the 108 general fellowship positions are described as emphasizing psychotherapy, whereas 43 others offer a variety of specialty experiences. Some programs provide choices among a number of different specialities within a single setting. Fellowships with a focus on neuropsychology, child and family work, and health psychology/behavioral medicine make up the next most widely available types of programs. The remainder constitute a broad span of emphases on work with various clinical populations or types of treatment approaches.

The program emphases of the fellowship offerings described in the child directory reflect the ambiguity that exists with regard to the definition of the nature of that specialty. Fifty-seven percent of the programs describe themselves as being in pediatric psychology, 16 percent as being in child clinical psychology, and 36 percent as a combination of the two.

Table 36-2
Types of Postdoctoral Training Sites

	APIC Directory	*Child Directory*
Medical school	33	14
Private psychiatric hospital	11	4
VA center	7	
Private medical center	6	
Community mental-health center	4	
Public psychiatric hospital	4	1
Other mental-health center	2	
Military health center	2	
Psychology training center	2	
Child guidance center	1	1
University health service	1	
Totals	73	20

Postdoctoral programs are conducted by a wide variety of organizations and institutions. Table 2 lists the types of training sites for the programs listed in the APIC directory and in the child directory. While considerable diversity is evidcnt, it is also clear that a relatively small range of institutions provides the majority of postdoctoral programs. University medical schools and medical centers account for almost one-half of the total number of programs. Moreover, these medical centers also tend to have the largest number of training slots. It is clear that more than half of all psychology postdoctoral training in this country occurs in medical school settings. Private psychiatric hospitals and Veterans Administration (VA) centers represent the next largest source of such training. Among the child postdoctoral programs, of the 20 additional training sites that can be identified, 16 are either directly within or closely affiliated with schools of medicine.

The rapid growth in the numbers of psychologists in medical schools has been a significant phenomenon within the past 20 years. It is noteworthy that a substantial number of predoctoral internships are also provided in medical school settings. There may be some irony, moreover, in the fact that, while the fields of clinical psychology and medicine over several decades have been involved in many forms of political and economic competition, the two fields have become, in fact, active collaborators in the advanced training of psychologists. Indeed, many of these psychologists have moved on to assume faculty positions in the nation's medical schools.

CONTINUING EDUCATION

One of the major motivations for the pursuit of postacademic education is the requirement for some sort of continuing education (CE) activity, which 16 states have legislated as a condition of the maintenance of a psychologist's licensing or certification in that state. Fourteen of these states require CE activity for doctoral-level psychologists, and two states have established the requirement for master's-level psychologists, but not for doctoral-level professionals. Two states have imposed the requirement of CE credits for both doctoral- and master's-level psychologists. While this reflects a clear perception of the need for updating and refreshing one's professional knowledge, the fact that only a minority of states have defined CE as a necessity would suggest that it has not yet become a generally accepted orientation. None of the Canadian provinces has, as of this writing, apparently legislated such a requirement either.

Among the states that have statutory CE regulations, the nature of the educational requirement varies quite widely. The number of annual CE hours required ranges from 50 hours per year in two states to five hours per year in one state. The median number of annual required CE hours is 20.

One of the difficult issues in the CE area derives from the fact that it is far easier to establish a quantitative requirement of a certain number of annual education hours than it is to establish meaningful guidelines specifying the content of the CE experience. There are many forms such educational programming could take and, as one could imagine, they can range from the sophisticated and productive to the perfunctory and ineffectual.

The APA has, through its Office of Continuing Education, provided an invaluable service to both the professional community and state licensing authorities—a mechanism for the evaluation and approval of institutions and other organizations that offer CE programs. For the 1985–86 year, some 235 organizations had achieved the status of approved sponsor organizations. The significance of the sponsor-approved system is apparent in the fact that all of the states that have CE requirements accept participation in a program offered by an APA-approved sponsor as evidence of a bona fide professional experience.

These 235 approved sponsors provided approximately 1,600 CE activities during the 1985–86 year. It is estimated that more than 20,000 psychologists attended these activities. Obviously, this attendance figure may reflect the participation at more than one activity by any given psychologist.

The approval system is an ongoing one and reviews for renewal of approved status of a CE sponsor are conducted on a regular basis. The number of approved sponsors appears to be rising, with 30 or more new sponsor programs requesting review during each of the past several years. It should be noted that the current system reviews the sponsoring *organization,* but does not evaluate the quality of the individual programs offered by that organization. Given the number of offerings available, evaluation of each program would involve a substantial expenditure of time and effort, and one that would undoubtedly overtax the resources of the APA's CE office. It is reasonable to assume, however, that programs offered by approved sponsors would reflect the fact that the sponsoring organization has been judged as having the resources and capacity for producing professional-level educational experiences.

An updated listing of APA-approved sponsors appears with some regularity in the *APA Monitor.* Interested professionals may consult that listing to determine whether a CE sponsor has achieved APA CE approval.

In addition to APA's function in evaluating the sponsorship of CE programs, it provides, through its convention system, a setting in which important CE activity also takes place. Each year, a series of workshops and programs is offered in conjunction with the APA's national convention. These are generally conducted during the week immediately preceding the convention, thus enabling psychologists to set aside a single period of time within which a variety of professional activities may be scheduled.

During the three-year period 1984–86, approximately 30 workshop programs were conducted in conjunction with each annual convention, with a total attendance of between 700 and 950 per year. In 1987, the APA offered 25 different CE programs, almost all of them one-day sessions from four to eight hours in length. One two-day, 12-hour program was also provided. The average cost of these programs was just under $17.50 per CE credit hour, with a range of from $14.25 to $22.50 per hour. They are designed as relatively small workshops rather than as large lecture-type programs, with a median allowed enrollment of 30 participants and a range of 24 to 50.

Approximately 50 percent of those participating in such workshops had attended a CE program at APA in a previous year, which would suggest that the experience of prior attendance had been sufficiently reinforcing as to encourage subsequent enrollment. The value of these programs is further highlighted by the reports of attendees as to how important a role the availability of CE workshops was in their decision to attend the convention in the first place. In each of several years, just under 50 percent of those responding indicated that the CE workshop was a "very important" factor in their decision to attend the convention. Evaluation of the quality of the workshops has been consistently positive, even allowing for some not-unexpected variability in the degree to which the programs and the instructors have been viewed as providing what those in attendance had expected to receive. It would appear, then, that the APA-affiliated workshops are perceived as a useful mechanism for updating or expanding a psychologist's competencies.

The APA national program is supplemented by CE activities conducted in conjunction with the APA conventions by some of the regional psychological organizations. Also, the American Board of Professional Psychology for many years has sponsored a postgraduate institute that has offered a wide array of one- to three-day programs dealing with topics in the area of psychological assessment methods and treatment approaches, as well as with issues relating to specialized areas of application of psychological skills, such as work with forensic or child populations.

The various divisions of the APA also sponsor special educational programs. For example, Division 14, Industrial and Organizational Psychology, for over 30 years has conducted a variety of workshop programs on a broad range of topics that are relevant to the activities of psychologists working in that area. The *APA Monitor* is a major source of information concerning the extensive variety of specialized workshop programs that are regularly advertised in that publication.

In view of all this CE activity, it is reasonable to ask what the impact of the statutory CE requirements has been. One study of this question carried out among psychologists in Maryland (Brown, 1982) suggests that the introduction of CE requirements for psychologists in that state did not significantly increase the total amount of CE activity in the year following that requirement's initiation, compared with the year preceding it. However, there had been an increase in the number of hours devoted to CE activities during a four-year period before the CE requirement was established. It would appear that the availability of CE programs was a major factor in that increase. These researchers concluded that psychologists who are more involved in providing direct service are more likely to have enrolled in a formal course of the sort provided in an institute or workshop setting. Moreover, there was no indication that experienced or well-prepared psychologists were any less likely to enroll in such programs than were those who were less adequately prepared for clinical service and hence more in need of continued education. On the basis of their survey, the authors suggest that guidelines for CE requirements should be flexible and should reflect the type of activity that psychologists value rather than require specific types of educational content.

Another study of CE activities among psychologists, this time in Connecticut (Allen, Nelson, & Sheckley, 1987), confirmed some earlier observations that structured workshop programs are not the preferred vehicle for expanding or updating professional knowledge and skills. This survey revealed that the reading of books (an average of 10 per year) and opportunities for personal contacts with colleagues were more highly valued as CE sources than were formal convention-centered programs. Of note is the finding that the more experienced the practitioner, the more valuable and rewarding are books perceived. Less-experienced psychologists reportedly place greater value on personal contacts, particularly in settings supplying informal peer review, general intellectual stimulation and emotional support. Again, there appears to be a preference for activities that fit more effectively into widely varied professional routines and life-styles. To the extent that CE activities are self-directed (e.g., reading books), they become difficult to monitor or to incorporate in existing statutory CE requirements. It is somewhat paradoxical that the type of activities, such as formal workshops, that lend themselves easily to the meeting of regulatory requirements may not be the kinds of activities that professionals themselves see as most desirable, accessible, or beneficial. This dilemma represents an issue with which the profession will have to struggle for some time to come. Possibly newer technologies such as videotape materials may represent a solution to this problem, but the few efforts in this direction that have been attempted do not appear to have been very successful.

Professional practice in psychology is regulated in some manner by all 50 of the United States and eight Canadian provinces. In all but two states, Kansas and Wisconsin, formal granting of certification or licensure to a psychologist by the state board of psychology depends on satisfactory passage of a written examination designed to assess a candidate's knowledge of the field of psychology. Most states employ the nationally standardized Examination for Professional Practice in Psychology (EPPP) as part of the process of evaluating a psychologist's professional preparation. This examination is developed by the executive committee of the American Association of State Psychology Boards. In addition, many states supplement the EPPP with their own procedures, such as essay examinations or oral tests. Each state board may set its own passing-grade requirements on the EPPP, and implement a grading system for its own written or oral examination.

The existence of this examination requirement is a powerful stimulus, among those persons who wish to obtain state licensure or certification, to pursue a program of study and preparation for such an examination. Beginning in the mid-1970s, a substantial educational enterprise developed that assists candidates in confronting this examination hurdle. In recent years, over 5,000 individuals have sat for these state examinations. It is currently estimated that more than 60 percent of these candidates have had some contact with the examination review system.

There are currently three major examination-preparation enterprises, each of which advertises its services widely. Each offers both an intensive classroom program and an independent home-study course. The workshop programs are given at various locations around the country. All three services provide courses in New York City, two conduct programs in Los Angeles, two offer workshops in the Florida area, and one service currently conducts programs in nine other cities. The courses generally cover a wide range of content, and each provides a set of written textual material for enrollees. Special preparation for the essay examnination required by New York State is available through each service, and two of the three offer special preparation for the California oral examinations. There is some variation among the services with regard to the format of their review programs; some of them conduct a comprehensive survey within a single course and others offer individual instructional units for research and clinical areas separately. The full programs provide from 60 to 70 CE credit hours, at a cost of between $620 and $795. Home-study materials are available for between $365 and $375.

When this kind of review service first appeared, questions were raised regarding the ethics of what were sometimes called "cram" courses, but there is now a general consensus that they serve a useful purpose for the profession. There is little basis on which one can determine the value of the programs, however, since careful, controlled research on the relationship between examination preparation and performance is difficult to conduct. Nevertheless, the large number of psychologists who participate in such programs would suggest that examination candidates view the investment of time and money in a review program as worthwhile.

EFFECT ON CAREER

Having briefly surveyed the major varieties of postacademic education available in psychology currently, there remains the question of what effect the pursuit of such education has on a psychologist's career. In one sense, this question should really not be asked, as those entering a profession should understand that they have embarked on a lifelong course of learning, and that there is never a time when one's education is really completed. But from a practical perspective, it is fair to ask whether there is a tangible benefit to be derived from formal study beyond the professional degree.

The answer to this question is obvious with regard to the need for meeting statutory CE requirements. In order to continue to practice, one must continue to learn or, at the very least, to participate in those activities in which learning is possible. This is, in a sense, part of the cost of doing business.

Similarly, if the chance of passing a state licensing examination is increased by participation in a formal, postacademic course of study, then the benefit is obvious. Furthermore, the enhanced sense of personal competence that comes with staying current in one's field, or in acquiring new professional skills, can be highly reinforcing.

Aside from such considerations, however, it is difficult to identify an empirical basis for answering the practical question noted above. One study (Klesges, Sanchez, & Stanton, 1982) of the hiring process for academic clinical faculty positions indicated that among a sample of newly hired clinical faculty, 10 percent had had formal postdoctoral training. Another report (Ponterotto & Furlong, 1986) of a study of the hiring of academicians in counseling psychology departments revealed that 17 percent of psychologists appointed to faculty positions had pursued training at the postdoctoral level. A survey of clinical neuropsychology instructors in APA-approved internship sites revealed that 34 percent of the respondents had obtained some formal postdoctoral training in their specialty area (McCarrney, 1985).

In none of these studies was there any clear indication that having postdoctoral training was a particular advantage in obtaining an academic position. Nevertheless, it is the author's clear impression that having a year or two of postdoctoral training does make a candidate more attractive to a potential employer, particularly if teaching, supervisory, or significant administrative responsibilities are involved. Aside from whatever real advantages there are in increased knowledge and skill, the pursuit of postdoctoral training would indicate to an employer that the psychologist recognizes that there is more yet to be learned, and that attitude may well reflect something that is truly central to being a professional.

FUTURE DIRECTIONS

Finally, what can one say regarding the future of postdoctoral training? It is clear that over recent years there has been a major decline in governmental support for postacademic training of this type. National Institute of Mental Health and other funding for training programs has decreased sharply and, absent major shifts in the political atmosphere, it is unlikely that substantial federal support for fellowship stipends will soon reappear. It is possible, however, that training grants in specialized fields, such as work with children, the aged, minority populations, and physically ill patients, may continue in some form. Nevertheless, if postdoctoral training is to continue, it is clear that other mechanisms for supporting it will need to be identified.

An interesting recent development has been the report of the latest national conference on psychology internship training (Belar, 1987). It contains a recommendation that the internship should be extended to a two-year experience, one year of which would be postdissertation and essentially equivalent to a postdoctoral year. This recommendation recognizes that most states already require at least one year of postdegree supervised experience for purposes of licensure. It may be, therefore, that one of the original factors that had led to the development of postdoctoral training—the recognition that one year of internship was insufficient to fully prepare a student for entry into the profession—may be in the process of changing. If this does come about, it will, perhaps, confirm the wisdom of the original caveat in the Boulder document that training beyond what currently could be provided in graduate schools is necessary to produce a fully functioning professional psychologist.

REFERENCES

Allen, G., Nelson, W., & Sheckley, B. (1987). Continuing education activities of Connecticut psychologists. *Professional Psychology, 18,* 78–80.

Belar, C. (Ed.) (1987). *Proceedings: National Conference on Internship Training in Psychology.* Washington, DC: Association of Psychology Internship Centers.

Brown, R., Leichtman, S., Blass, T., & Fleisher, E. (1982). Mandated continuing education: Impact on Maryland's psychologists. *Professional Psychology, 13,* 404–411.

Carrington, C. (Ed.) (1986–87). *Directory of internship programs in professional psychology* (15th Ed.). Washington, DC: Association of Psychology Internship Centers.

Klesges, R., Sanchez, V., & Stanton, A. (1982). Obtaining employment in academia: The hiring process and characteristics of successful applicants. *Professional Psychology, 13,* 577–586.

McCarrney, R. (1985). Educational backgrounds of clinical neuropsychologists in APA-approved internship sites. *Professional Psychology, 16,* 773–780.

Ponterotto, J., & Furlong, M. (1986). A profile of recently employed academicians in APA-approved and non-approved counseling psychology programs. *Professional Psychology, 17,* 65–68.

Raimy, V. (Ed.) (1950). *Training in clinical psychology.* Englewood Cliffs, NJ: Prentice-Hall.

Tuma, J. (Ed.) (1986–87). *Directory: Internship programs in clinical child and pediatric psychology* (6th ed.). Baton Rouge, LA: Louisiana State University.

C H A P T E R
37

CAREER AS BUSINESS

Steven Walfish, Ph.D., and
Dale Lee Coovert, Ph.D.

According to the *Oxford English Dictionary* (OED), a "career" is a term derived from a succession of Latin and French words meaning "road-way" and "racetrack." These early forms of the word offer apt analogies for "career" in the modern sense, such that we often speak of one's "career track." Specifically, however, the definition most appropriate to the present discussion is "a course of professional life or employment, which affords opportunity for progress or advancement in the world."

Both etymologically and in an applied sense, "business" is "busy ness." Again turning to the *OED,* we find more than an entire page devoted to elaborating upon this simple definition. Inescapably, however, "business" means keeping busy. In a more specific sense, one not so clearly addressed in the standard English-language reference works, "business" suggests the establishment and maintenance of a functional legal and social entity, for the explicit or implicit purpose of generating income. While this definition may appear better suited to MacDonalds or Mr. Muffler than to mental health, the professional in private practice is, simply put, a business person whose products are mental-health services. We call our customers clients, or patients, but as is the case in the fast-food hamburger world, our businesses (i.e., practices) will thrive or fail as a direct function of these customers. Implications of this fact of life will be discussed in the following.

For increasing numbers of mental-health professionals who choose to pursue private practice as their career track, the career of mental-health-service provision becomes the business of mental-health-service provision. For many mental-health-service providers, such an approach to the delivery of their services may appear dangerously mercenary. While attitudes of delivering services in the public sector are changing to become more business oriented (Goplerud, Walfish, & Broskowski, 1985), it is imperative for economic survival that the private practitioner adopt such an attitude. However, economic success and the delivery of quality mental-health services within a humanistic framework are not mutually exclusive concepts.

This chapter will elaborate upon issues relating the business of private practice to the choice of such a pursuit (or roadway) as one's career track. We will discuss issues related to (1) the dreams vs. the realities of such a business; (2) emotional and practical decisions that lead one to this career path; (3) developing and maintaining this type of business; (4) how this business affects, and in many ways, limits the owner's personal life, and (5) career satisfaction with this business choice compared with other settings in which mental-health professionals may choose to earn a living.

THE RISE AND FALL OF IDEALISM

For many in the mental-health professions, the development of a full-time private practice is the culmination of a long-term dream. Upon entering graduate training, although many individuals aspire to a career in research or work in the public sector, the predominant desire is to "hang out one's shingle." For someone who wants to reap the rewards of several years of a costly, time-consuming and personally draining experience, this may represent the "light at the end of the tunnel" after overcoming numerous obstacles and surviving the bedlam and politics (Sumprer & Walfish, 1983) of graduate school.

However, while dreams and aspirations provide the necessary motivation, the realities of life in private practice often hit the neophyte mental-health professional, and this punch is usually not delivered in a very soft manner. In a very informative paper, Taylor (1978) discusses issues related to the demythologizing of private practice. He contends that fairy-tale conceptualizations concerning the private sector are widespread among peers working in other settings, among clients, and on the part of the general public.

While it may hold true for some, it is our belief that a private practice is not a glamorous endeavor but rather a very nice way to help human beings and to earn a living at the same time. As we will discuss below, many of the values that lead one to human-service work in the first place need to be resolved in order to reach a level of harmony in achieving each of these goals.

Bernay (1983) points out that, philosophically, we hold the notion, as health-care professionals and healers, that altruism, service, and poverty are synonymous. The emergent result of this belief, she argues, is a personality that is passive, long-suffering, nurturing but deprived, ethical, and proper. Further, these attitudes, according to Bernay, "lead us to conduct our practices more in the manner of a Mom and Pop store rather than as established professionals." On the other hand, Cantor (1983) contends that anyone who decides to enter private practice, and wants to do so successfully, has to be able to generate a self-image of an entrepreneur that is both acceptable and gratifying. The problem, as Cantor views it, is that because psychotherapy is perceived as being helpful and nurturing, accepting money directly from clients may lead to guilt engendered by role conflict.

The result is that the private practitioner must resolve the conflict about wanting to help people and to be altruistic (two basic values in an effective helping professional) while at the same time charging money for these *services*. Although at least one-third of private practitioners lower their fees in the face of a client's inability to pay the standard full fee (Tryon, 1983a), this

The authors would like to thank Gerard F. Sumprer for comments on an earlier draft of this manuscript.

dilemma persists. If this confict is not resolved, the result will be an unhappy, confused, angry, and probably ineffective therapist. Following cognitive theory, we view the notion that we should not take care of our own needs and that we can help people when our own needs are not met as an irrational belief.

The second major issue to be resolved in the development of a practice is that this mode of delivering mental-health services is actually a business, one in which the service provider is actually the owner. Businesses need customers to whom to deliver services, and need to generate profits in order to remain open.

It is not unusual for practitioners to become disenchanted with their practice as the details of business get in the way of being a mental-health-service provider. However, potential practitioners should be warned — and this is not usually discussed in "cocktail illusions" (Taylor, 1978) of what a practice will be like — that issues of charging and collecting fees for services rendered, haggling with insurance companies, competing with health maintenance organizations (HMOs) and preferred provider organizations (PPOs), marketing services, hiring and firing support personnel, having records subpoenaed, buying supplies, ensuring coverage while away on vacation, negotiating a lease for one's office, choosing the right health and disability insurance packages, and keeping accurate records (in case of audit by the Internal Revenue Service or becoming a defendant in a lawsuit) are not occasional nuisances but the everyday realities of running an effective (in terms of treatment and positive cash flow) practice. There is nothing glamorous about sending out fifth notices on overdue accounts with threats of turning over the account to a collection agency.

Bernay (1983) contends that as mental-health-serice providers, we deny our desire to earn money because we feel a lack of confidence in our own self-worth and in the value of our skills. We believe that this attitude is reinforced in two significant ways. The first is the graduate school training experience itself. Although there are exceptions, the atmosphere of most training programs is perceived as being especially noxious (Mahoney, 1974; Sumprer & Walfish, 1983) in terms of reducing one's self-concept both as a human being (as a result of being in a one-down powerless position) and as a mental-health-service provider (constantly being reminded that "while you say you know something, there is a whole lot more that you don't know"). Contrast this with the typical education in medical school in which the student is continually told what an "elite" individual he or she is and the socialization of the "deity complex" begins.

Second, graduate training (especially in psychology) emphasizes a thorough knowledge of research in the area of efficacy of assessment and treatment. What any good scholar of psychotherapy outcome research realizes is that the delivery of mental-health services is at best inexact. What types of clients benefit from what types of services and under what conditions are there questions in the mental-health arena that have yet to be resolved? The result of this view is an acute awareness of how much we do not know. Another dilemma to be resolved is the necessity to charge fees (not exactly low fees either in most cases) for delivering these inexact services. Taylor (1978) suggests that "demythologizing" private practice requires that one recognize and accept the limitations of psychotherapy.

EMOTIONAL TRANSITIONS LEADING TO A PRIVATE PRACTICE

But why choose private practice as a career path over other roadways, such as teaching, research, or work in the public sector? The issues leading to this choice are complex and will be explored in this and other sections of this chapter. However, suffice it to say that more and more mental-health professionals are making such a choice. Prochaska, Nash, and Norcross (1986) present data pointing to the dramatic increase in the percentage of mental-health professionals leaving public agencies and entering the private arena. The Division of the Independent Practice of Psychology (Division 42) is now the third largest division in the American Psychological Association (APA). The typical full-time private practitioner, according to its data, sees 27 clients per week. The typical part-time practitioner engages in 10 hours of client contact per week (Prochaska & Norcross, 1983). In another study by this research group (Norcross, Nash, & Prochaska, 1985), data are presented to suggest that almost half of the part-time practitioners would prefer to be engaged in full-time practice if given unlimited demand for their services. As such, it appears that a full-time practice may be the most desirable position for the mental-health-service provider.

Most people do not leave graduate school and immediately begin a full-time private practice. The typical scenario begins with acceptance of a full-time position in a private or public human service agency. There are many reasons for this choice, including: (1) lack of clinical expertise just after clinical training and the need to obtain further clinical experience, (2) licensure and supervision restrictions, (3) lack of referral contacts, and (4) the need for economic survival (which includes, in many cases, the payments of large student loans that financed graduate training). During this first year or two, the new professional may begin a part-time private practice in order to "test the waters." Developmentally, this period is an important time in that in these early years the individual may make a decision as to whether to maintain this full-time position concurrently with a part-time practice or to pursue a full-time practice.

Hauck (1983) gives the advice that if the mental-health professional wants a comfortable life and can deal with the guilt of having material benefits, then private practice is an ideal work setting. He goes on to describe the "ideal personality" of the private practitioner—one who has a need for independence, has a desire to be his or her own boss, and is comfortable with working long hours. Moreover, Taylor (1978) suggests that individual practitioners are literally forced by daily challenges to learn more, grow personally, and question yesterday's assumptions.

Many personal issues emerge that influence the decision to pursue full-time practice. After working for an agency for a few years, the professional may now feel that he or she can function adequately and competently without supervision. This *confidence* level may help spur him or her on to this transition. The need to be *independent* and to make one's own decisions, a need not often met when working through the bureaucratic channels in the agency, becomes quite appealing to those experiencing public agency burnout. *Financial needs* play a role in deciding to make this transition, in that normal developmental transitions (e.g., buying a home, having children, buying a new car) come into play. For many individuals, the development of a full-time private practice is the next step in a logical life progression.

PRACTICAL ISSUES LEADING TO A PRIVATE PRACTICE

The practical issues involved in having a full-time private practice as a career choice can be summed up in two words: *time* and *money.*

The typical mental-health-service provider works a structured 8:00 A.M. to 5:00 P.M. schedule, five days a week. On occasion, there will be some flexibility, such as working four 10-hour days, leaving one day a week for private practice of consultation, or working some evening hours in the clinic, which then allows flexible time during the week for pursuits outside of the organization. In private practice, time becomes a valuable resource. Individual practitioners can structure their week in any way that will meet their needs. For example, we know one couple who has opted for both choices. He is in full-time practice and she works at an agency. While she is getting ready to go to work in the morning, it is not unusual for him to go off to play racketball. Some practitioners do not see clients until 11:00 A.M.; others do not see them after 5:00 P.M. Practitioners typically have one day off per week from doing any type of clinical work. We know one practitioner who takes an entire week off each month, as a means of self-renewal and to avoid burnout. The point is that practitioners control their calendars, allowing for flexibility in child care and for accomplishing personal tasks without having to leave everything for the weekend.

Clearly, not everyone in private practice gets rich. The formula to achieving financial security in private practice has yet to be written, but will certainly contain such elements as (1) being willing to work long and hard hours, (2) having excellent communication skills, (3) having the spirit of an entrepreneur, (4) being extremely skilled (so people will want to purchase the service you are rendering), (5) being fair and ethical, (6) knowing the right people, and (6) being lucky. However, one thing is clear: the financial possibilities are greater for those in private practice than for those working for an institution.

Let us use psychologists as an example. The APA publishes figures on salaries of psychologists. In one report, Stapp and Fulcher (1981) present data on median salaries for psychologists by setting and years of experience. For comparison purposes, we will focus on an experience level of five to nine years and examine salary levels in four separate settings. These figures are presented in Table 1. As can be seen from these data, the typical university counseling center psychologist earns the least. Salaries are slightly higher for those working in public settings. This figure jumps approximately 40 percent for persons employed in private psychiatric hospitals. However, there is no comparison when these three settings are compared with a private practice. Private practitioners earn almost 50 percent more than those working in a private hospital and almost double those in the other three settings. To elaborate further on the financial possibilities of a private practice, there is typically an upper limit (which is relatively low) as to what one can earn in an agency setting. It is very unusual for psychologists working in an agency to earn $50,000 per year. This figure is not unusual in a private practice where earnings of $100,000 or more, while not the usual, are certainly not rare.

DEVELOPING YOUR BUSINESS

An axiom one inevitably hears when talking to business people is that there are three main ingredients necessary to establish a successful business: location, location, and location! Among mental-health professionals beginning in private practice, this tongue-in-cheek formula might be rewritten as referrals, referrals, and referrals!

According to a recent Delphi poll of Fellows of the APA's Division of Independent Practice (Walfish & Coovert, 1989), the most important consideration in establishing a private practice is referrals. Of the 32 responses to our request for recommendations for establishing a private practice, 44 percent were related directly or indirectly to seeking and maintaining referral sources. These covered a wide range of strategies, from volunteer work in various community agencies (to create visibility and a high profile) to simply getting the word out that one has opened a practice and is available to see clients. Many of the respondents in our survey agreed that teaching in a university, a clinical setting, or an adult education program would be helpful in generating referrals. Less well received was the suggestion that visibility might be gained through involvement in the media, especially television and radio.

There is, of course, much more to establishing a private practice than the "three R's." The most popular business strategy suggested by the panel of experts in our study was to develop a "genuine commitment to your client's welfare." This is a reflection of the essential merger of good business sense and sound ethics that must characterize the successful mental-health professional in private practice. Such a commitment also helps resolve the dilemma

Table 37-1. Salaries of Psychologists in Four Work Settings with Five to Nine Years of Experience

Work Setting	Sarary
University counseling center	$23,000
Public psychiatric hospital	$26,200
Private psychiatric hospital	$33,200
Private practice	$47,000

Data are abstracted from Stapp & Fulcher (1981).

discussed previously of delivering quality services for a fee in a way that is also humanistic. Two other strategies readily endorsed by our respondents concerned the quality of work done by the private practitioner: (1) Do not practice beyond your level of competence and training. (2) Perform at a superior level. Perhaps the most important conclusion that we drew from the results of our study was a commitment to excellence in the delivery of a quality product.

MAINTAINING YOUR BUSINESS

Maintaining a private practice requires a special balance of skills and attitudes. According to the respondents in our Delphi poll (Walfish & Coovert, 1989), the most important strategies for maintaining a successful practice are those related to training and continuing education, keeping a positive attitude about one's work and clientele, guarding against burnout, and doing quality work.

Training is an essential component in the foundation of any private practice in the mental-health arena. Again, the products that we sell are mental-health services; learning our product requires training. Our Delphi panel emphasized the importance of training in many forms. First, thorough and diversified clinical training was suggested, at both the graduate and post-graduate level. Continuing education, with a particular emphasis on updating old skills and adding new ones, was viewed as an important and essential endeavor by our panel. Along these lines, Taylor (1978) contends that individuals are literally forced by daily challenges to learn more, grow personally, and question yesterday's assumptions. Continuing education should be viewed as a commitment to both personal and economic survival for the private practitioner. Finally, our respondents emphasized the need to maintain a network of colleagues, for both social support and peer supervision on difficult cases.

Another area that was frequently addressed by our panel was the need to maintain a positive attitude. This included positive attitudes towards clients (who, as satisfied customers, become a key referral source) and toward your work. "Take your work seriously and be able to see the humor and nobility of it," wrote one respondent. Therapeutic skills are a necessary but not sufficient condition for positive behavior change to occur. The missing ingredients in this formula leading to a client's positive change are compassion, empathy, congruence, and a genuine caring for the human being you are trying to help.

A related area is protection against burnout. Such safeguards as personal psychotherapy and a support system of colleagues were offered as buffers against personal and professional burnout. One respondent made the important distinction between burnout and boredom, suggesting that the two may become easily confused.

Finally, our respondents emphasized the importance of quality work. As any honest business person knows, a quality product is the mainstay of any business. Further, it is our contention that the delivery of a quality product is not only an important business consideration, but, in the case of the mental-health private practitioner, an ethical responsibility as well.

"I NEVER PROMISED YOU A ROSE GARDEN"

The majority of our Delphi poll respondents (Walfish & Coovert, 1989) agreed that one of the most important tips for graduate students considering private practice as their career path is to "create, early on, a schedule that allows you ample time for family, recreation, and vigorous exercise." There is, however, a particular cost involved in time off.

Hauck (1983) elaborates on this point:

> In private practice the security that you have in the future will depend greatly on your own efforts. Your retirement plan will be one for which you will have to finance. Your medical program is one for which you will have to pay. You may have to pay for the fringe benefits of your employees as well. You will not get paid vacations working for yourself. Each day that you take off is lost income, to say nothing of the cost to you of your vacation.

Private practice, then, is a world in which there is no "free lunch." Every hour spent away from your practice is an hour not spent nurturing your practice and generating revenues. There is a fine line that separates the hard worker from the workaholic.

Such a dedication to one's work entails not only personal sacrifices, but to those practitioners who have families, sacrifices by all family members. The private practitioner is typically at the office a great deal of the time. However, when at home, no activity is immune to interruptions in the form of client emergencies. Unlike therapists in most agency settings, the private-practice psychotherapist has additional motivation (e.g., financial) to work odd hours to accommodate client schedules. Few successful practices are built on a strict 9-to-5 schedule.

Two studies have attempted to identify the disadvantages of choosing a private practice as a career track. Tryon (1983b) asked 160 full-time private practitioners to list the pleasures and displeasures of their work. Isolation, time pressures, and economic uncertainty were viewed as the major limitations, within this setting. Nash, Norcross, and Prochaska (1984) identified time pressures, economic uncertainty, caseload uncertainty, business aspects, and excessive workloads as the five dominant stressors in the private-practice setting. In addition, many respondents alluded to insurance companies and third-party reimbursers.

CAREER SATISFACTION

Perhaps the best reason for choosing private practice as a career path is that this is the work setting, at least among psychologists, that offers the greatest job and career satisfaction. Several studies will be presented below that help to elaborate on this point.

The question of career satisfaction among psychologists has been pursued from the vantage point of recent graduates (Walfish, Polifka, & Stenmark, 1985), longitudinally over a 25-year period (Kelly, Goldberg, Fiske, & Kilkowski, 1978), and from a cross section of psychotherapists (Prochaska & Norcross, 1983).

In the study of recent graduates (Walfish et al., 1985), almost all of the respondents indicated satisfaction with their choice of clinical psychology as a career. This is in contrast to earlier studies of older and more experienced clinicians.

The classic early study of Kelly and Goldberg (1959) found a significant dissatisfaction (36 percent) with the choice of clinical psychology as a career at a 10-year follow-up period. This same sample was once again surveyed after 25 years (Kelly, Goldberg, Fiske, & Kilkowski, 1978) and there was even greater dissatisfaction (46 percent) with the choice. What is interesting about these two studies was the relatively low number of individuals who were in a private-practice setting. However, upon close examination of those data it can be seen that the greatest satisfaction with the choice of clinical psychology as a career could be found in those engaged in full-time private practice.

Simono and Wachiowiak (1983) examined career-satisfaction issues in a sample of university counseling center psychologists. Those planning to leave this employment setting, most often for private practice, cited as their reasons for leaving (1) personal growth and change and (2) poor pay.

Boice and Myers (1986) conducted a study comparing the satisfaction of a sample of psychologists in private practice and one in a unversity academic setting. In contrast to academics, private practitioners tended to experience (1) fewer job-related stressors, (2) more positive physical health, and (3) more positive mental health. Those in the academic setting appeared especially concerned about (1) being "bogged down" in paperwork and committees, and (2) low salaries. Further, in terms of feeling accepted by their colleagues and profession, academics were more concerned than practitioners regarding (1) a lack of recognition, and (2) a concern over their colleague's misbehaviors. While graduate training in psychology tends to glorify the academic setting—there is a press for trainees to pursue teaching positions—Boice and Myers (1986) conclude from the results of their study that academia may be a less idyllic work site than traditionally supposed.

Prochaska and Norcross (1983a, 1983b) present data from a study they conducted with a national sample of psychotherapists. They found that private practice was the modal employment setting for those in the sample. Of special interest to the current discussion were the survey questions focusing upon career satisfaction. Ninety percent of the sample were either "quite satisfied" or "very satisfied" with their choice of psychology as a career. The percentage of therapists who were disastisfied with some aspect of their career choice was actually quite small (7 percent).

In this study, the researchers also made several comparisons between those in private practice settings and another sample of psychotherapists employed in the public sector. Of specific concern to the present discussion, the authors concluded that, compared with the public-sector therapists, independent practitioners appear to be more satisfied with their career choice.

As another measure of career satisfaction, these authors presented their subjects with the following question: "If I had my life to live over again (knowing what I know now), I would try to end up in...", and were presented with five alternatives. Those therapists in private practice were more likely than those in the public sector to make the same choice once again.

Nash et al. (1984) attempted to quantify specific aspects of satisfaction regarding the choice of independent practice as a career. Specifically, practitioners found professional independence, promoting patient growth, autonomy, professional success, and enjoyment of the work as the most satisfying components. Surprisingly, "high income" was not considered one of the primary satisfactions. Perhaps this was due to the "uncertainty" of income (as reported by Tryon, 1983) as one of the main stressors involved in this type of business.

IN CONCLUSION

In this chapter, we have tried to make the point that operating a business titled "Private Practice" as a career track in the mental-health field involves many complex practical and value decisions. Being able to merge one's values as a helping professional while at the same time accepting fees for doing so must be accomplished. Practical issues in being able to begin and maintain a successful practice must then be resolved. Also, we have not tried to paint a picture that is free from problems and stress. However, as can be seen from the data reviewed here, private practice may be the most satisfying of all work settings among which the mental-health-service provider can choose.

REFERENCES

Bernay, T. (1983). Making a practice: Overcoming passivity and masochism. *Psychotherapy In Private Practice, 1,* 25–29.

Boice, R., & Myers, P. (1986). Which setting is healthier and happier: Academe or private practice? Paper presented at the Annual Convention of the American Psychological Association, Washington, DC.

Cantor, D. (1983). Independent practice: Minding your own business. *Psychotherapy In Private Practice, 1,* 19–24.

Goplerud, E., Walfish, S., & Broskowski, A. (1985). Weathering the cuts: A Delphi survey on surviving cutbacks in community mental health. *Community Mental Health Journal, 21,* 14–27.

Hauck, P. (1983). The psychologist in independent practice. Unpublished manuscript. Available from S. Walfish upon request.

Kelly, E., & Goldberg, L. (1959). Correlates of later performance and specialization in psychology: A follow-up study of trainees assessed in the VA selection research project. *Psychological Monographs, 73* whole no. 482.

Kelly, E., Goldberg, L., Fiske, D., & Kilkowski, J. (1978). Twenty-five years later: A follow-up study of graduate students in clinical psychology assessed in the VA selection research project. *American Psychologist, 33,* 746–755.

Nash, J., Norcross, J., & Prochaska, J. (1984). Satisfactions and stresses of independent practice. *Psychotherapy In Private Practice, 2,* 39–48.

Prochaska, J., & Norcross, J. (1983a). Contemporary psychotherapists: A national survey of characteristics, practices, orientations, and attitudes. *Psychotherapy: Theory, Research and Practice, 20,* 161–173.

Prochaska, J., & Norcross, J. (1983b). Psychotherapists in independent practice: Some findings and issues. *Professional Psychology: Research and Practice, 14,* 869–881.

Prochaska, J., Nash, J., & Norcross, J. (1986). Independent psychological practice: A national survey of full-time practitioners. *Psychotherapy In Private Practice, 4,* 57–66.

Simono, R., & Wachiowiak, D. (1983). Career patterns in college counseling centers:

Counseling psychologists report on their past, present, and future. *Professional Psychology: Research and Practice, 14,* 142–148.

Stapp, J., & Fulcher, R. (1981). *Salaries in psychology: 1981.* Washington, DC: American Psychological Association.

Sumprer, G., & Walfish, S. (1983). The politics of graduate school. Unpublished manuscript. Available from S. Walfish upon request.

Taylor, R. (1978). Demythologizing private practice. *Professional Psychology,* 68–70.

Tryon, G. (1983a). Full-time private practice in the United States: Results of a national survey. *Professional Psychology: Research and Practice, 14,* 685–696.

Tryon, G. (1983b). The pleasures and displeasures of full-time private practice. *The Clinical Psychologist, 36,* 45–48.

Walfish, S., & Coovert, D. (1989). Developing and maintaining an independent practice. A Delphi poll. *Professional Psychology: Research and Practice, 20,* 54–55.

Walfish, S., Polifka, J., & Stenmark, D. (1985). Career satisfaction in clinical psychology. *Professional Psychology: Research and Practice, 16,* 576–580.

HEALTH-CARE DELIVERY
BY ORGANIZED PROVIDERS:
HMOs AND PPOs

A. Steven Frankel, Ph.D.

One of the most fundamental shifts in the fabric of our society has been taking place in recent years. Health care, which represents over 11 percent of the Gross National Product of this nation, is becoming "businessized" (Frankel, 1986, p. 263). The transition from a model of health-care delivery that places the professional in charge of deciding what to treat, in what way to treat, in what context (e.g., in- vs. outpatient) to treat, how long to treat, and how much to charge for treatment is rapidly giving way to models that involve mixtures of concepts such as "gatekeepers," second opinions, prior authorizations, managed care, quality assurance, peer review, professional standards review, utilization review, and cost containment.

Modest yellow-pages ads that conformed to professional society recommendations are being replaced by ads for "product lines," such as Mid-Life Institute, Center for Anxiety Management, Phobia Recovery Center, and Center for Teens Only (United Yellow Pages, 1987, p. 467). Print media, which rarely went beyond ads for improving one's memory through hypnosis, are now carrying ads for mental-health services such as "Busted," an ad showing a teenager in handcuffs and suggesting that antisocial behavior patterns may be the result of "adolescent depression"—a condition for which a certain hospital program has been developed. Or, for adults, a full-page magazine ad suggests that "Millions of Americans are still living in the Great Depression" (*L.A. Magazine,* 1987 July).

To understand these developments, one must look more closely at the issues of escalating health-care costs, as well as the increased value placed on entrepreneurial activity.

ESCALATING HEALTH-CARE COSTS

By now, it should be no secret to any health-care practitioner that health-care costs have grown far in excess of any of the usual measures. The *Register Reports* (1987a), for example, show that while the 1985-86 Consumer Price Index increased by 1.1 percent, the corresponding increase in health care was 7.7 percent, with physician fees at 7.8 percent and hospital rates at 7.7 percent.

Not only has this been true for health care in general, it has been true for mental health care as well. "Mental Health Costs Soaring" blares a headline in the *New York Times* (1986) section on business and health (p. 30). "'Psychiatric care is obviously out of control,' says Kenneth S. Abramowitz, a health-care analyst at Sanford C. Bernstein & Company." "Mr. Norton [a health-care specialist with William M. Mercer-Meidinger Inc., benefits consultants] said, 'Anywhere from one-third to one-half of the total costs of health benefits for adolescents is probably unnecessary'" (*New York Times,* 1986, p. 30).

Faced with these increases in costs, third-party payers—the people who write the checks for services, including insurance companies, corporations, self-insured trusts, and government agencies—have become increasingly concerned. After some years of grumbling and faltering attempts to ask providers to control costs themselves, they took matters into their own lobbyists' hands and attempted to rectify the situation by seeking legislative relief.

In 1982, the California legislature passed a series of bills that provided the occasion for the kinds of changes described above. Bills AB799 and AB3480 provided for businesses and insurance companies to negotiate fees with providers. Now, instead of paying for health-care costs at ever-increasing "usual and customary" rates, third-party payers were able to establish fee schedules for various health-care services and were able to shift some of the costs of health care back to the insureds by increasing deductibles, paying percentages of fees, and even capping or limiting the absolute amount of dollars available for certain types of services. Additionally, these laws provided for "third-party payers" to contract directly with providers for discounted services, and to provide incentives for their insureds to utilize these discounted services (Frankel, 1986, p. 262).

As third-party payers became more insistent on accountability and responsibility, they became increasingly interested in and open to approaches by the business community itself—people who spoke the same language, who used the same concepts, and whose way of dealing with problems reflected commonality of philosophy with those whose companies made up the vast bulk of insureds. Among the most aggressive responders to the call for businessization were the huge hospital ownership corporations, whose acquisitiveness and expansionism have led many of them into serious financial difficulties as the very cost-containment measures that they supported resulted in low hospital censuses and lost revenues (Frankel, 1986; *Register Reports,* 1987b, p. 14).

Insurance companies leaped into the sea of opportunity created by changing laws by offering health-care services themselves, while large health-care systems began to offer their services combined with insurance packages. As with so many areas of business in the 1980s, the entrepreneurial spirit was nurtured by changing laws, changing needs, and changing opportunities.

PROFESSIONAL HYBRIDS— HMOs AND PPOs

In addition to the hospital ownership and the insurance and medical service companies that rushed to capture as large a share as possible of the expanding health-care market, there has been an explosive growth of a variety of hybrid organizations—combinations of business people and professionals. As the National Health Lawyers Association "Introduction to Alternative Delivery Mechanisms" so aptly notes, "The entrepreneurial spirit, then, has permeated the health-care field, and cost containment and operational efficiency rank as major concerns among health attorneys, physicians, hospital administrators, insurance executives and other health professionals charged with the delivery of quality care at a minimum of financial excess" (Johnson, 1986, p. 3).

HMOs

"An HMO [health maintenance organization] is essentially a combination of a financing mechanism—prepayment—with a particular mode of delivery which employs management controls to ensure effective utilization of services by members" (Boochever, 1986, p. 5). As also noted in the November 1986 issue of *Register Reports* (p. 8), HMOs have the following characteristics:

1. An organized system of health care in a geographic area.
2. A set of basic health benefits specified by state or federal law and regulations (see Rolph, Rich, Ginsburg, Hosek, Keenan, & Gertler, 1986).
3. A voluntarily enrolled group of persons.
4. A predetermined and fixed payment made by or on behalf of the enrollees *without* regard to the amount of actual services.

The February 1987 *Register Reports* (p. 10) describes the four basic HMO structural models:

1. The *staff* model, in which providers are salaried employees of the HMO, who deliver services in HMO-owned facilities.
2. The *group* model, in which the HMO contracts with one or more groups of multispecialty providers who deliver services at their facilities.
3. The *independent practice association* (IPA) model, in which the HMO contracts with individual providers, through an association, to deliver services in the providers' own offices.
4. The *direct contract/network* model, in which the HMO contracts with the providers directly to deliver services to HMO members in the providers' own offices.

A Brief History of HMOs   While HMOs actually have been around since the late 1920s, they did not begin to grow significantly until the 1970s. To illustrate, there were approximately 30 HMOs serving 3 million enrollees in 1970; in 1986, there were 400 HMOs serving approximately 20 million enrollees. The February 1987 *Register Reports* (p. 1) presents data predicting that, by 1990, over 700 HMOs will serve almost 70 million enrollees (about 40 percent of the population).

As DeLeon, Uyeda, and Welch (1985) point out, despite organized medicine's intense opposition to the HMO concept, the Nixon administration's call for a "true health system" as opposed to a "sickness system" (Nixon, 1971) led to the Health Maintenance Organization Act of 1973 (PL93-222), preempting state law restrictions on HMOs and providing federal grants and loans for their support—including, as of 1981, federal loans for for-profit as well as for nonprofit HMOs (Boochever, 1986).

Despite the discontinuation of federal funding support in the early 1980s, the federal government clearly supports HMOs by offering a "qualified" status to those that meet certain criteria (see Boochever, 1986, p. 7). Qualified HMOs then receive a marketing advantage, as all employers of 25 or more persons *must* offer their employees an opportunity to enroll in one as an alternative to the company's existing health plan if a qualified HMO in the service area so requests or "mandates." "Moreover, if more than one HMO mandates such an employer, the employer must offer its employees one federally qualified HMO that is organized on either the IPA or Direct Contract/Network model as well as one organized on either the Staff or Group model" (Boochever, 1986, p. 7).

Problems with HMOs   While HMOs have grown incredibly over the past decade [e.g., overall growth from 1984–85 was 18.9 percent, with IPA models leading the pack at 28.6 percent growth, group model plans showing the least growth at 7.3 percent, and in the middle, staff models at 19.7 percent and network models at 16.9 percent (Baldwin, 1987, p. 46)], several problems have emerged. First, a 13-year Rand study of a Seattle HMO cited in the November 1986 issue of *Register Reports* (p. 8) indicates a 5 percent higher rate of enrollee dissatisfaction with the care offered by the HMO (15 percent dissatisfied) than with care offered in traditional programs, with complaints focusing on precisely those areas of care that provide the greatest cost savings for HMOs (long waits for appointments and reduced availability of hospital care and specialists).

A second problem for HMOs is that most of them actually lose money or fail to meet revenue estimates. Indeed, the "News Digest" of *Modern Healthcare* (1987a) reports that the smaller the HMO, the greater is the likelihood of losses, resulting in a falling out in the industry and increasing risk for professionals who affiliate with newer HMOs. The report refers to a "general malaise" of the HMO industry, and a tendency for greater diversification of product lines, including the development of preferred provider organizations (PPOs).

A third problem is the need to strengthen governmental oversight of HMOs as a result of charges of mismanagement of funds, and even charges of criminal wrongdoing (Baldwin, 1987).

Fourth, and most telling from the point of view of the fundamental purpose of HMOs, recent data suggest that HMOs may not be effective in controlling health-care costs in general (*Register Reports,* 1987, p. 4; DeLeon, Uyeda, & Welch, 1985), and hospital costs in particular (*Modern Healthcare,* 1987a, p. 26)!

Fifth, there are some serious problems relative to the role of nonphysician providers. As noted by DeLeon, Uyeda, and Welch (1985) and Tulkin and Frank (1985), HMOs utilize primary-care physicians as "gatekeepers" of care, so that patients must be referred to a specialist by the primary-care physician. Complaints that specialists in general are underutilized, and that nonphysicians such as psychologists, social workers, and marriage/family counselors, who often are hired as employees without the status offered to physicians, are generally excluded from the referral pool, or are underutilized "behavioral medicine specialists," are most frequently made. As Tulin and Frank note, despite the significant contributions by psychologists that their HMO system has acknowledged, and despite increasingly broad roles played by psychologists in their HMO (including hospital privileges, quite unusual for an HMO), "psychologists are not equals with HMO physicians. We do not share the profits, attend shareholders' meetings, or vote in the elections for the board of directors. Some of these inequities may change in the future, but for the present, psychologists working in HMOs must be willing to accept that they have an alliance with medicine but not a partnership" (p. 1127).

PPOs

Anthony (1986, p. 11), who calls PPOs "a major new product in the health insurance industry," defines a PPO as "a health-care financing and delivery program which provides financial incentives to consumers to utilize a select panel of preferred providers. Such providers typically include physicians and hospitals as well as home health, long-term care, laboratory and others. Payment for services is typically on a negotiated fee-for-services basis with discounts often accompanied by guarantees of increased volume and rapid turnaround of claims. The arrangement between purchasers and providers is solidified through contractual arrangements embodying the results of negotiations between the parties. Consumers are typically not locked into receiving services only from the preferred providers but receive financial incentives to do so."

Bindman and Hefele (1985), in further clarifying the distinction between PPOs and HMOs, offer the following principles (pp. 203–204):

1. More open than IPA-model HMOs in selection of providers by subscribers.

2. Providers are less at risk financially, as fee-for-service or cost-plus programs typical of PPOs do not have the risk of having to provide more services than a prepaid contract (capitated contract) would require in the case of an unanticipated demand for services. However, this should be qualified because many employers increasingly insist on some sort of risk sharing between themselves and providers.

3. Fewer restrictive laws for PPOs than HMOs, since HMOs are more like insurance programs, resulting in more restrictive insurance laws.

4. Utilization review mechanisms even tighter than those round in IPA-model HMOs, as the key to PPO success in the marketplace is cost control of high-quality services.

Brief History of PPOs   Unlike the history section for HMOs, which was brief to facilitate ease of acquiring information, the section on the history of PPOs is brief because they have only been around for a few years. Enabled by the California Legislature in 1982, a mere handful of PPOs existed a few years ago. The industry has grown so rapidly now that data reported in the November 1986 issue of *Register Reports* (p. 11) project that approximately 45 percent of the population will be served by PPOs in the 1990s. As reported above, HMOs that are beginning to show falloffs in enrollment are planning new PPO "products," as the primary patient complaints about HMOs are reduced significantly by PPOs. Large insurance companies have initiated PPOs, as have some of the large hospital ownership corporations.

Nonphysicians still find themselves in difficult positions with PPOs. In California, for example, state law requires that PPOs engage psychologist panel members "whenever possible," and most psychologists are dismayed at the number of PPOs that find it "not possible" to enroll them as panel providers. One reason that enrollment in a PPO may not be possible is that many PPOs require that providers be members of hospital staffs in order to be on the panel. When nonphysicians are barred from having admitting privileges at hospitals, it is difficult for them to be providers. This issue lies at the heart of the struggle for such privileges for many provider groups such as psychologists.

However, predominantly psychologist PPOs exist, at least in California and Massachusetts (Bindman & Hefele, 1985), and this writer is an equal partner with one other psychologist and two psychiatrists in a mental-health PPO (Frankel, 1988). Again, opportunities for entrepreneurial activity in the current health-care marketplace abound.

Caveats   Despite the current proliferation of PPOs, there are some clear causes for concern when it comes to participating as a provider. Michele Licht is an attorney who has been involved in the profession of psychology for some years. She has (Licht, 1984, pp. 27–28) prepared a list of concerns that all practitioners should address with any PPO before agreeing to be a participating provider. Her list is as follows:

1. Organizational form of the PPO. PPOs will be structured and organized in a variety of ways, but most commonly they will be sponsored by an insurance company, provider group, or entrepreneurial group. You should be concerned about the financial viability of the PPO, its potential for maintaining an adequate subscriber pool, its reputation, and other basic organizational traits.

2. Covered services. It is recommended that you request the PPO to provide you with a standard provider contract. Specifically, you will want to be aware of what benefits and exclusions the PPO will provide for psychological services and any deductibles or copayments that may be required. Knowing this information can help you avoid future problems, and you can also be useful in assisting a client in understanding available benefits.

3. Provider compensation schedule. Read the provider contract carefully to understand how you will be reimbursed for your services and what limitations, if any, will be placed on your reimbursement. If there is a payment schedule, *make sure you understand it.* Most provider contracts will ask you to accept a discount from your usual fee or from the usual or customary fee in your area as determined by the PPO.

You should also read the provider contract to determine whether you may bill the subscriber directly for noncovered services. Some PPO provider contracts require that the provider accept PPO reimbursement as payment in full and restrict any direct billing of subscribers, even for noncovered services. In addition, you should check the contract to see whether the PPO is required to pay you within a specified number of days.

4. Buy-in Fee. Many PPOs require that providers make a one-time payment to the PPO for the privilege of being a participating provider and being listed in a directory of plan providers. If there is a buy-in fee, you should carefully analyze the PPO's stability, and its ability to maintain an adequate patient pool, versus your investment in it.

5. Risk of loss. Some PPO contracts require that providers share in the risk of loss. For example, the PPO may withhold a percent of the provider's payment for a year. If the PPO has had a good year, it may return to the provider the amount withheld plus a share in the profits. If the PPO does not do well, the provider may be asked to take the withheld amount as a loss.

6. Utilization review. Make sure you understand exactly how the PPO's utilization review process will function. If there is a panel to review psychological services, what is the makeup of that panel? How frequently will reviews be conducted? Will there be an appeals process, and if so, what standards will be used in the review? On what basis may reviews be initiated?

7. Referral arrangements. Some PPO contracts require that their providers refer patients only to other PPO participating providers. Therefore, you may wish to review the list of other participating providers before signing on.

8. Provider directory. Some PPO contracts require that you permit your name and address to be given to PPO subscribers. This may include listing in a directory of PPO participating providers, which would most likely be to your advantage as a referral source. You may, however, want to request that the PPO give you an opportunity to review any materials using your name before they are distributed, to avoid the potential for ethical problems.

9. "Hold harmless" clauses. Some PPOs require that the provider carry all malpractice risks and hold the PPO completely harmless. This presents serious problems for providers. For example, if treatment is terminated prematurely because of a PPO determination, the PPO should share in any liability. However, a hold-harmless clause would make the provider *solely liable,* even though the PPO made the determination. Moreover, many liability policies exclude contractually assumed liability. Thus, you may not be covered at all under any policy carried by the PPO.

10. Professional insurance policy. Review your own professional insurance policy to make certain that there are no exclusions that may apply to your contracting with the PPO.

11. Contract hospitals. Find out which hospitals will be available for admission of PPO subscribers. Most PPOs limit admissions to hospitals that have contracted with the PPO. If you do not have privileges at the contracting hospitals, find out what arrangements will be made if a patient of yours requires hospitalization.

12. Continuity of care. Read the provider contract to determine what provision is made for continuing treatment of subscribers who are under active treatment, if and when the subscriber contract is terminated.

CONCLUSIONS

There is little doubt but that we are in the midst of a major revolution in health care, including mental health. Our way of defining ourselves, of offering our services, of seeing how our services fit into the broader scope of patterns of care, and our roles as professionals/business persons all are changing. Our standards for professional service delivery and our ethical canons will be sorely tested in the next decades. It is hoped that this introductory guide may offer some small degree of help in understanding and coping with these changes.

REFERENCES

Anthony, M. (1986). PPOs. In J. Johnson (Ed.,), *Introduction to alternative delivery mechanisms: HMOs, PPOs & CMPs*. Washington, DC: National Health Law Association.

Baldwin, M. (1987a). IPA–Model growth leads expansion. *Modern Healthcare, 17*(3), 46.

Baldwin, M. (1987b). Proposals beginning to surface to ensure better oversight of nation's HMO industry. *Modern Healthcare, 17*(14), 42.

Bindman, A.J., & Hefele, T.J. (1985). Preferred provider organizations. In P.A. Keller & L.G. Ritt (Eds.), *Innovations in clinical practice: A source book* (Vol. 4, pp. 203–214). Sarasota, FL: Professional Resource Exchange.

Boochever, S. (1986). Health maikntenance organizations. In J. Johnson (Ed.), *Introduction to alternative delivery mechanisms: HMOs, PPOs & CMPs*. Washington, DC: National Health Law Association.

DeLeon, P., Uyeda, M., & Welch, B. (1985). Psychology and HMOs: New partnership or new adversary. *American Psychologist, 40*(10), 1122–1124.

Frankel, A.S. (1982). Preferred providers, platitudes and panic: Standards of practice and the insurance industry. *Professional Psychologist, 6,* 27–30.

Frankel, A.S. (1986). Changes in health care delivery: A guide for the independent practitioner. In P.A. Keller and L.G. Ritt (Eds.), *Innovations in clinical practice: A source book* (Vol. 5, pp. 261–269). Sarasota, FL: Professional Resource Exchange.

Frankel, A.S. (1988). The Private psychiatric hospital as a crucible for innovative approaches to service delivery. *Psychotherapy, 25*(3), 429–433.

Johnson, J. (Ed.) (1986). *Introduction to alternative delivery mechanisms: HMOs, PPOs & CMPs*. Washington, DC: National Health Law Association.

Licht, M. (1984). PPOs: Everything you've always wanted to know but were afraid to ask. *Professional Psychologist, 6,* 27–29.

L.A. Magazine (1987 July). Ad for Charter Pacific Hospital.

Modern Healthcare (1987a) *17*(14), 28.

Modern Healthcare 1987b), *17*(9), 26.

New York Times (1986 Oct. 7). Business and health, p. 30.

Nixon, R. (1971). Special message to the Congress proposing a national health strategy. *Public papers of the Presidents of the United States* (pp. 170–186). Washington, DC: U.S. Government Printing Office.

Register Reports (1986), *13*(1).

Register Reports (1987a), *13*(2).

Register Reports (1987b), *13*(3).

Rolph, E.S., Rich, J.P., Ginsburg, P.B., Hosek, S.D., Keenan, K.M., & Gertler, G.B. (1986). *State laws and regulations governing preferred provider organizations*. Santa Monica, CA: Rand Corp.

Tulkin, S.R., & Frank, G.W. (1985). The changing role of psychologists in health maintenance organizations. *American Psychologist, 40*(10), 1125–1130.

United Yellow Pages (1987). *South Bay united* (p. 467). Beverly Hills, CA: United Publishers Corp.

Part
Three

Emotional Issues

George Stricker, Ph.D.
Editor

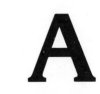

Part III Emotional Issues **(continued)**

S E C T I O N

A

**The Mystique
of Private
Practice**

39

PRIVATE PRACTICE: PROMISE AND REALITY

Sheila Coonerty, Ph.D.

W ithin the mental health profession, the concept of establishing a private practice often taps the deepest fantasies of therapists regarding the creative aspects of their work. If as therapists we are both scientists and artists, it is to our private work that many of us turn to discover and to create. In this way, private practice is often imagined as a haven from external pressures and realities, a place where therapists can hope to discover and fulfill their own promise. To invest an aspect of our work with such intense meaning inevitably leads to considerable potential for both satisfaction and disillusionment. If we are to approach our work realistically and avoid needless pressure on patients to fill our needs, it may be useful to explore the promises that draw us to private work as well as the realities that both fulfill and frustrate us along the way.

In 1929, Virginia Woolf, in her essay, *A Room of One's Own,* summed up the essential elements for a woman's being able to work creatively—money and a room of one's own. It was her thesis that financial security would allow a comfortable, relatively worryfree existence in which the mind could be turned to higher concerns. A room of one's own would allow the privacy, control, and autonomy necessary to nurture the creative process. These same two elements can be viewed as forming the core of the promise that private practice holds for mental health practitioners.

The promise of financial success, as well as of the resultant comfortable living when one is away from this often difficult work, is a universal attraction of a private practice. In contrast to the fixed and relatively low salaries associated with institutional positions, private practice is seen as having a potential for financial success limited only by one's ability to attract patients. With the hope for financial success also come the fantasy of prestige in the larger community and the independence of being one's own boss.

As to a room of one's own, the wish for the space, time, and freedom to be creative in one's work is a major draw of private practice. Such a metaphorical "room" holds promise of professional independence, personal flexibility in life-styles, and intellectual as well as emotional challenge and stimulation. It is in the promise of intensive private work that we invest our deepest fantasies and fears as to our ability to achieve a high level of success and creativity in our efforts to help others grow and change. Free from external constraints and pressures, we see ourselves fulfilling our potential as members of a helping profession.

The extent to which a private practice fulfills such promises can be a major determinant of our sense of satisfaction in our work. However, instant fulfillment is unlikely, as the process of developing as a private practitioner involves inevitable mistakes, disappointments, and frustrations. The promise involved, if it is to become reality, must be nurtured over time and grow with accumulated experience. Not everyone finds fulfillment in private practice nor is it likely that all aspects of one's practice will be equally fulfilling.

Having summarized the essential elements of the promise of private practice, we shall now examine more closely the specific promises encompassed in the overarching concepts of financial success and a room of one's own. Although this list is by no means comprehensive, major aspects of the promises and realities described here echo those in the mental health literature and were confirmed in a survey of those presently functioning as private practitioners. The most common of these promises and their accompanying realities will be described below.

IN-DEPTH CREATIVE WORK

Promise: Without external constraints, a private practice will leave one free to do more in-depth creative work.

After spending early training years working in hospitals and clinics, therapists often view a private practice as an opportunity to work freely, unshackled by the constraints of an institution. We imagine that the work would go more quickly and more easily if we were free to pursue it at our own pace without outside interference. In contemplating the start of a practice, therapists often dream of being able to do "real" therapy, somehow reaching to loftier ideals than is possible in a public setting.

Reality: It takes two to work both creatively and intensely.

It is often a stunning discovery to beginning private practitioners that patients are not always willing or able to work more freely or at a quicker pace than they do. Just as we feel we are getting somewhere, people stop coming or put up powerful resistances to joining in the work. Creative work in therapy, the joint act of discovery, depends on the ability of both partners in the venture to find the necessary safety and motivation to move forward. Although the so-called good, well-motivated, intelligent, and insightful patient may be somewhat more prevalent in private work, there is no shortage of serious disturbance or lack of motivation in the private sector.

Within certain reality constraints that will be discussed later, private practitioners have the option of choosing whom they treat and how; therefore, we can shape some of the characteristics of our practice. Free from the demand to work equally effectively with any and all patients, we often experience a sense of personal growth and freedom in developing our own styles and preferences.

As we do so, another reality emerges. While still limited by external concerns in our capacity to create and work intensively, we experience our own potential for creative energy as endless. As the chance to test our creative potential becomes a reality, we must also come to terms with the limits of our own ability to maintain a high level of intensity and creativity for therapeutic hour after therapeutic hour. Thus, it is not only the patients but also the therapist who find that limits exist in our capacity to function at such intensity over long periods of time.

JOB FLEXIBILITY

Promise: Private practice allows considerable job flexibility. One can decide when and how much to work at a given time.

The rigors of the work of psychotherapy are such that therapists often turn to private practice for relief from being "on" at the demand of a 9-to-5 work schedule. Control over the amount and timing of one's work is a powerful motivator for establishing oneself privately. In addition to deciding how much and when one wants to practice as a therapist, many practitioners look to broaden the scope of their work through teaching, research, and writing. Primarily, however, the fantasy is one of increased time for a private life to offset the difficulty of practicing as a psychotherapist.

Reality: Flexibility is an advantage to private practice, but it can carry a price.

There is in fact a great deal of potential for flexibility in making one's own work schedule in private practice. Limits to the fantasy of making one's own schedule do exist, however. These limits are largely those of reality concerns: how much flexibility can a therapist *afford,* financially as well as in terms of professional standing in the community. It is often forgotten by the beginning practitioner that the success of a private practice is linked to treating enough patients to become established in a community. It is also necessary to cultivate referral sources who will look to rely on our availability to accept patients as well as to our professional reputation among colleagues.

It comes as a surprise to many therapists beginning private work that referral sources and practices have an unpredictable rhythm that often seems beyond the therapist's control. Referrals do not come simply because we want them, nor do they stop coming when we begin to feel overworked. In addition, the prime hours for seeing patients may well be those a therapist would most like to spend at home with family and friends.

To establish a practice and cultivate referral sources, it is often necessary for a beginning private practitioner to work longer or more erratic hours and have less predictability and flexibility than exist in an institutional position. Such a sacrifice for a period of time is seen as an investment in future flexibility as one becomes established. Over time, the rhythms of the individual's practice become more apparent, leaving the practitioner less vulnerable to constant worries about financial and personal failure. However, practitioners may become so used to the long hours and cultivation of referral sources that the original aim of a more flexible life-style is forgotten. In contrast to institutional positions, where one's time is so often taken up with tasks other than psychotherapy, long hours of therapeutic work can lead to emotional burnout if not balanced with other pursuits.

PROFESSIONAL INDEPENDENCE

Promise: Private practice allows one to be professionally independent.

Many therapists, tired of constant intrusions on their life and work by institutional systems, also see private practice as an opportunity to be an entrepreneur. Chafing under systems-imposed limits and rules, we fantasize the world of private work as being one in which, as our own bosses, we make our own decisions for professionally appropriate reasons. The ability to work independently without having to adjust one's style and beliefs to those of an occasionally antagonistic system is appealing.

Reality: Although more independent than those in institutional settings, we struggle with the constraints of the external world in the form of third-party payments and interference of patients' job and family obligations. Also, independence can at times lead to isolation, professionally and personally.

Many practitioners in the private sector do feel that they have considerably greater freedom in decision making than they would have in the public sector. For many, the entrepreneurial nature of a private practice allows them to experiment and often to flourish. However, the reality of societal constraints and third-party payments must still be dealt with. The limits insurance companies *do* place on number of sessions, type of treatment, and amount of fees are a real constraint on the private practitioner. One must either strike a compromise between one's ideals of treatment or fees and the available funds or choose to treat the narrow segment of society that can afford to pay without insurance.

Despite such constraints, it still remains possible in private work to consider problems with external systems in terms of individual cases. Flexibility is always available to those whose business decisions affect no larger concerns than their own. However, clinicians often find themselves uncomfortable with just such a lack of externally imposed rules and tend to feel the need to establish their own structure as to what individual compromises they will accept. The fear is that to be without some standard personal "rules" in such an emotionally charged line of work is to leave oneself open to countertherapeutic countertransference reactions that may interfere with clear decision making. Most prevalent in those beginning private practice is the tendency to feel that concern with their own financial and time needs seems somehow selfish and inappropriate in the face of the suffering of those who come for help. It is often only after feeling "burned" by a patient that one is able to focus clearly on weighing equally one's own needs.

In working with children, the parents can often impose considerable restrictions and limits to what treatment they will support. With adults, the financial and personal constraints imposed by job and family may be considerable. In contrast to the systems-related constraints of the public sector, these often take on an intensely personal character that colors the entire course of treatment.

Another aspect of independent practice that is often a surprise is the degree of isolation involved in private work. Such isolation can be professionally wearing when one is dealing with assaultive, fragile, suicidal, or otherwise difficult patients. Gone is the easily available psychiatric consultation or second opinion of an institutional setting. Decisions can at times seem overwhelming, and the enormous personal responsibility can feel isolating.

A more personal form of isolation comes from spending the day seeing patients, subduing one's own needs and desires in the interest of treatment, and having little normal social interaction with the colleagues and support staff often taken for granted in institutional work. Each of us has a different level of tolerance for such isolation and must adjust his or her work accordingly. It is often the need for a less isolated existence that draws some to professional organizations or training institutes where they can develop ties with others in the field. For others, relief lies in cultivating family ties or other relationships well removed from the mental health field.

INTELLECTUAL CHALLENGE

Promise: Private practice will be intellectually challenging.

A parallel belief to that of one's ability to create in private practice is that such work will provide intellectual challenge and excitement. Intensive work with motivated patients promises that one will be pushed to the limits of what one knows and beyond. Exposure to many different kinds of patients is also seen as adding to the sense of challenge.

Reality: Private practice can be at times intensely challenging intellectually and at times boring and stultifying.

The sheer volume of work done over years of private practice assures that one will meet intellectual extremes of experience. For every sense of exciting challenge and adventure with a particular patient, there may be long periods of intellectual boredom and stultification with that patient or others. Revelations that were once puzzling and exciting may in time become mundane. A patient's necessary insistence on reworking what was once challenging material at times threatens to deaden the listener's skills. The intellectual challenge of private practice is indeed one of its great rewards. However, efforts must be made periodically to lift inevitable boredom and reignite excitement through sharing difficult material with colleagues or with the larger professional community. Often, those who supervise others in their field experience a reawakening of excitement in their own work.

EMOTIONAL STIMULATION

Promise: Private practice will be emotionally stimulating.

The opportunity to share in the process of so many life paths other than one's own promises considerable emotional excitement and stimulation. The extremely personal nature of the private interaction adds a promise of emotional depth to the work. It is hoped that such emotional rewards will balance the natural frustrations of therapeutic work.

Reality: The work is emotionally stimulating, at times beyhond what we feel we can bear.

Often unexpected for those beginning private practice is the intensity of their personal reactions to the need to be so consistently emotionally available. It is not uncommon to feel drained, sucked dry. It is often only after one has made commitments to certain demanding aspects of the work that the limits of what one can share emotionally become apparent. Some practitioners find that they have a high level of tolerance for their work's intruding at times into their private lives. Others find that they have little or no such tolerance, and react to such intrusions in intensely negative ways.

Over time, the private practitioner must learn to listen to his or her own limits, so as to pace the work and regulate the types of patients seen to best fit personal needs. It is *because* the work of a private practitioner can be so emotionally stimulating and satisfying that great care must be taken to guard one's own needs for emotional retreat, rather than succumbing to anger at the patient who unknowingly demands so much.

FINANCIAL SUCCESS

Promise: A private practice will allow financial success.

The relatively high hourly fee commanded in a private practice, in comparison with public sector salaries, often seems like an irresistible attraction. The beginning practitioner fantasizes days of intensive and satisfying work (in a well-decorated, comfortably large office suite shared with kindly colleagues) alternating with escapes to a personal life unencumbered by financial worries or needs. After years of struggle and sacrifices in graduate school, the siren call of a successful private practice seems irresistible.

Reality: Private practice is a small business. As such, it is subject to all of the vagaries, headaches, and insecurities of any other small business.

When asked to describe what surprised them most about beginning a private practice, most therapists unhesitatingly respond that no one warned them that they would have to be a businessperson. Many emphatically complain that professional training ignored this aspect of the work, much to their later detriment. Often, there is a wish to be able to function above such mundane concerns. This wish is summed up in the common protest: "But I am a *therapist*, not a businessman!"

There *is* potential for a comfortable, even high, level of financial success in the establishment of a private practice. However, such success depends on one's capacity and desire to function as a businessperson. From keeping records and setting and collecting fees to seeking referrals and deciding upon one's ethical stance in reference to low-income patients, the work is permeated with business concerns. Decisions must be made and compromises reached from the point of view of their financial effect. Some eventually choose to turn such aspects of their work over to business professionals; others decide to sacrifice possible higher profits for the personal comfort of a low-key business attitude. Whatever the decision, much is to be considered, and early in a private practice many mistakes can be made if financial aspects are not taken seriously.

Another difference for those used to working in the public sector is the uncertainty and insecurity of depending on patients for one's own financial welfare. No regular paycheck can be counted on to cover one's expenses. Private practices are subject to dramatic increases and drops, as well as to bad faith. Only time and experience can help one to discern patterns and thus adjust expectations. For some, the insecurity of financial concerns is an over-whelming and unwelcome intrusion on the therapeutic work. For others, greed at times overshadows therapeutic and ethical concerns.

When therapists fantasize about the promise of financial success, the lack of a regular paycheck is not taken into consideration initially. Neither is the cost of setting up and maintaining one's office and establishing professional contacts. On the positive side, those entering private practice rarely understand the tax advantages associated with being in business for oneself, and thus are often surprised to find the difference between one's gross and one's taxable income. There are others who, without the enforced discipline of automatic withholding, spend without consideration for the government's share. They are of course in for a rude awakening.

Despite the insecurities and difficulties of learning to manage a small business, many therapists express considerable satisfaction in their ability to master the necessary skills and, as a result, in watching their income rise and stabilize. With financial security often comes an increased ability to give oneself more wholeheartedly to the work at hand.

CONCLUSIONS

The promises and realities listed above are those most often seen as central to our fantasies about, and attraction to, private practice. For each individual, the motivations for and dreams about private practice vary. Through summarizing those that are most common to beginning practitioners, the author hopes that a framework can be established for viewing private work realistically. A realistic sense of the work ahead may make it easier for practitioners to resolve problems early on in their work and proceed to fulfill the promise of private practice in ways best suited to their own styles and needs.

Our initial reaction to the realities of a private practice is often one of increased anxiety, an increased sense of vulnerability and stress. Goals and assumptions about one's fitness for this work and potential for success are often reevaluated. Some leave the private sector and with disappointment or relief return to the public sector. Most ride out their initial difficulties, gradually adjusting their own needs and dreams to the realities of the work.

For some, a part-time private practice is the answer. A part-time practice can allow for increased financial security and stability, greater fulfillment of social needs, and a wider variety of professional work. In addition, part-time private practice may offer some increased control over the type of work done and patients seen privately. Those who choose part-time practice often do so initially out of a need for financial stability. Those who settle into a part-time practice often express great satisfaction with the variety and flexibility of combining two types of work while still noting increased financial security.

For others, the split between two jobs is seen as wearing. Their ultimate freedom is in a commitment to a full-time private practice. Since a full-time practice rarely extends past a 32-hour week, many feel that this ultimately leads to the greatest freedom and flexibility in life-style. In addition, a full-time practice may increase intellectual stimulation as financial necessity dictates that a broader range of patients be seen and interventions be used. The mastery of a variety of therapeutic skills can be experienced as extremely satisfying. Often, a full-time, successful private practice can lead to considerable financial rewards.

Over time, the promises of financial security and a room of one's own become increasingly a reality for those committed to private practice. With experience, each practitioner frames individual solutions to the problems of working privately. If the realities are accepted and dealt with accordingly, the sense of control over one's life and work as well as the level of professional satisfaction promise to be high. For those in early stages of establishing a private practice, it should be reassuring to note that many established practitioners report a strong sense of satisfaction in their work and a belief that over time early promises have indeed become the reality.

REFERENCE

Woolf, V. (1929). *A room of one's own.* New York: Harcourt, Brace, Jovanovich.

C H A P T E R
40

RISKS AND REWARDS OF INDEPENDENT PRACTICE

Herbert J. Freudenberger, Ph.D.,
and Theodore Kurtz, M.A.

It is unfortunate that an article of this type was not available during the authors' clinical graduate training. In our educational process we learned a good deal about psychopathology, diagnosis, psychological testing, and treatment. However, as we entered independent practice a few decades ago we did so with scant knowledge or understanding of the risks and rewards that lay ahead of us.

We are presently witnessing significant changes in the health care marketplace. Computers, insurance, and third-party reimbursement policies are increasingly being utilized in the service of reduction of health care costs. We face increased competition from many health care professionals, the rising financial costs that are needed to maintain a practice, and increased vulnerability and the potential threat of a malpractice suit.

The authors have between them over one-half century of independent practice experience. It is from this vantage point that we will describe and discuss the risks and rewards of independent practice.

ISSUES OF CLIMATE, TERRAIN, AND GEOGRAPHY

We find that the climate of independent practice has taken a dramatic shift over the past number of years. What used to be a balmy, sunny, and pleasant atmosphere has given way to an increasing number of turbulent and dangerous storms.

Twenty years ago when the office phone rang, more likely than not it was a call from a new patient, a current patient, or a colleague. Now, when the phone rings, it might also be an insurance company questioning your treatment report; an attorney representing a former client who claims that everything, including the weather, is your fault; a new patient telling you that his physician has told him that he needs "medical psychotherapy" instead of your "talking cure"; an HMO inviting you to join at one-third of your current fee; the same HMO suggesting that you ought to take up its offer if you want a practice at all; a corporation's benefit officer informing you that you are not one of their preferred providers and that your services will not be reimbursed; a colleague with empty hours looking for referrals; your landlord telling you that the buildiong has decided that professional offices no longer are congruent with the needs or image of the building; your cooperative board president informaing you of the latest assessment to fix the roof and elevator; or a call from a stockbroker in some distant city who is willing to give you the financial opportunity of your lifetime.

The terrain of independent practice has been hit by numerous earthquakes. The boundary lines we used to know have shifted. More of our patients are opting for short-term treatment. More of our patients are more disturbed, needy, draining, and demanding. Substance abusers, borderlines, and severe character disorders are now commonplace.

Freudenberger (1983) commented that in the last number of years

> many of our patients have come to us feeling empty; are the victims of violence; a battered child, a rape or incest victim. Our patients may be depressed, paranoid, express a loss of sense of self, deprived of significant affect relationships, suffer from an inability to be intimate or may be narcissistic. (p. 84)

Individual therapy is being supplemented or replaced by family therapy, group therapy, or conjoint therapy. More patients terminate prematurely and tend to seek symptom removal. More call to make an appointment and never show up. The terrain, once lush, is increasingly desertlike—with HMOs, PPOs, and IPAs each claiming to be the oasis of the future.

The terrain has become littered by an overwhelming abundance of choices. When we were in graduate school, we had the feeling that we could get our arms around a fair portion of the basic knowledge in our discipline. Now we are inundated by scores of different schools of therapy; dozens and dozens of conferences and workshops; and hundreds of books, articles, and journals; even the program of the American Psychological Association annual convention has taken on the breadth and scope of the Manhattan telephone book. It is understandable that we might feel overwhelmed.

Additionally, the geography of independent practice has changed. There used to be a few well-defined professions offering mental health services. Boundary lines once well defined have become more permeable and fluid. We now compete with a host of other professionals such as psychiatrists, marriage and family therapists, sex counselors, health educators, guidance counselors, alcohol counselors, social workers, school psychologists, lay analysts, and even some self-appointed experts, each clamoring for recognition and acknowledgement. The consumer, overwhelmed and confused, sometiems throws the baby out with the bath water.

EGO WOUNDS

Since the climate for the independent practitioner has become increasingly hostile, therapists who feel insecure, especially those in part-time practice, may need to brace themselves for an onslaught of various and sundry stresses. Most vulnerable are those therapists who are approval needy for gratifications that have been on the wane as the assault has been on the rise. The assault on the independent practitioner has taken many forms.

As you are well aware, premiums for malpractice insurance have increased geometrically in the past several years. This rise in premiums is a result of greatly increased litigation against mental health professionals. Many of you already may know of a colleague who has been sued. This is one of the more stressful events for an independently practicing professional. The thought of subpoenas, examinations before trial, prosecuting attorneys' cross-examinations, and the public scrutiny of one's work leaves many mature and seasoned therapists frightened, anxious, stressed, and burned out (Freudenberger, 1984).

Another set of harrassments comes from insurance carriers. Filling out time-consuming treatment reports and other requests for information often gives the therapist the feeling that the insurance company believes that he or she is mercenary and manipulative in attempting to keep people in treatment. Insurance carriers want to know what is wrong with the patient and how long it is going to take you to fix the problem — with the emphasis on how long and the implication of hurry up. With each visit to your mailbox may come another question and challenge to your integrity and professionalism.

Another ego wound occurs when our treatment fails. Some of our patients, despite our best efforts, do not improve. After months or years of effort, the patient still struggles with the same conflicts and anxieties. If we are caring professionals, we cannot help becoming frustrated. Our pride is wounded. We question our skills.

Other wounds occur when we work with difficult and resistant patients. We sometimes have to endure an onslaught of anger, invectives, and challenges. We are bombarded by the patient's difficulties, pathology, and turbulent transferences.

In the expression of transference on the part of the patient, the analyst seeks to "separate" his or her own ego, which is both a perceptive and an emotive faculty, into observing and experiencing selves. As Goldberg (1986) suggests, "Therapist reponses which are expressed affectively rather than transformed into cognitive concepts have generally been regarded as clinically inappropriate — a countertransferential reaction which mitigates effective analytic work." The continued consequences of emotive countertransference responses serve to promote the risk of poor perceptions, poor judgments, and actions on the part of the therapists that may be detrimental to both therapist and patient.

The therapist also needs to cope with stresses associated with his or her therapeutic role. Sustaining a delicate and sometimes precarious equilibrium between intimacy, objectivity, and countertransference feelings is often energy depleting.

Many patients are needy but difficult to feed. Our need to feed them may become thwarted, and our self-esteem may take a nosedive. Additionally, there are patients who have difficulty taking responsibility for their own lives. They view us as the omnipotent parent who will make all things better. Hopefully, we will not buy into that wish. The overall view, however, is that some days the work of independent practice is draining and exhausting.

Another wound can be explained through the derivation of the word "therapy." We are reminded that the word comes from the verb "to wait," as in one who waits on tables. Our purpose is to wait upon or to serve our patients. We listen to our patients in an attempt to discern their order—what it is that they need in order to be nurtured and to learn to nurture themselves. Yet, despite our efforts, many patients only pick at our psychic food, reject it, complain that it is not quite right, claim that our interpretations are either overcooked or undercooked or stale and not palatable, and then get up and leave the table, possibly without paying their bill.

Our need to be compassionate may cause other stresses. Our psychic restaurants are always open, and we are often called upon for special orders. We have difficulty saying no and protecting our own resources. As a consequence, we drain ourselves through excessive work and diligence and may suffer the consequences of professional impairment. Freudenberger (1984) describes this impairment as "physical and mental disability, debilitation through aging, drug abuse, alcoholism, depression, suicidal thoughts or a sexual involvement with clients" (p. 223).

Individuals enter the mental health profession for a variety of reasons that may contribute to subsequent problems. These motivations are multidetermined and may include achievement, personal growth, financial reward, status, self-awareness, and intellectual stimulation (Freudenberger & Robbins, 1979).

Over a prolonged period of time therapists, as a consequence of their need to feel superior, may create, as Marmor (1953) comments, "a sense of mystery resulting from a need to posture a sense of omnipotence." These feelings of superiority may lead to emotional detachment from patients or promote in patients a continued wish to gratify the therapist's needs to feel important. The alienation process and detachment within the therapist lead to serious impairment and difficulties in functioning in a practice setting.

Another ego wound is promoted by the emphasis on short-term psychotherapy. Many of us were trained to do long-term analytic therapy. We were reared to divide our therapy into phases—beginning, middle, end, and termination—with each phase lasting several months. We hoped to see analytic patients several times per week and to interpret transference phenomena carefully and precisely. We prided ourselves on our knowledge of dynamics and our skill in working through processes. The reality, in recent years, has been that many of our patients sign on only for short-term work. They come in to work on a problem or symptoms of whatever may be causing the most anxiety and malfunctioning.

In a relatively short period of time they get a handle on the symptom, and leave. These patients never quite take their coats off and thus deprive us of our need to become deeply and significantly involved. What used to be a several-course dinner has been replaced by a meal at a fast-food franchise. Our patients, signaling the tenor of the society, come to eat and run. They want to absorb their calories quickly and sometimes desire junk food therapy—not the substance filled with nutrients that we are so eager to provide. This requires a serious rethinking of whether our past training is applicable to today's world, and how much shifting is required in reorienting ourselves for today's marketplace.

As a result of this short-term emphasis, we need an ever-increasing number of referrals in order to fill our therapy time. We have found that a number of our colleagues increasingly have empty time in their schedules. Many experienced practitioners are underutilized and have been reduced to essentially part-time schedules. Some therapists have consolidated their sessions and now work only 3 or 4 days per week. Others are still "available" 5 or 6 days per week but have "breaks" of several hours each throughout the course of their work week. The part-time therapist is especially vulnerable to economic and case load uncertainties.

Recent research suggests that more experienced clinicians have a greater degree of comfort, flexibility, and confidence in stressful situations. Rice et al. (1972) suggest that experienced therapists have a more flexible, idiosyncratic, and differentiated style, and appear to be more sensitive to their own negative countertransference feelings, and thereby tend to reduce anxiety and discomfort as well as risks to themselves.

Increasingly, therapists must market themselves. The day when clinicians sat in their offices waiting for the phone to ring is coming to an end. All clinicians should take careful note of the trends in the marketing of professional services and need to think through and reflect on a marketing strategy tailored to their needs, their geographic location, and the kinds of patients who might be seeking their services.

ISOLATION

As Freudenberger (1986a) indicates, "Recent research has left little doubt that psychotherapists, almost without exception, find the practice of psychotherapy to be a very isolating experience." As Guy (1987) suggests, isolation may be physical; it may manifest itself in one's separation from one's colleagues, from the outside world, and from family and friends; and it may culminate in a psychic isolation wherein we are immune to portions of feelings within ourselves.

As Freudenberger and Robbins (1979) describe the isolation:

> By the very nature of analytic (psychotherapeutic) work, the therapist stands alone, separate and autonomous. The normal amount of social give and take that is commonly associated with most work situations is quite limited and often absent. In most work environments there is some opportunity for sharing and even some acting out without dire consequences. Relatedness for the analyst (therapist) is specifically limited to promoting the therapeutic process. To be sure, there is interpersonal contact, but it is a skewed one. There is intensity but at the same time there are limitations on the extent of mutuality. Under these controlled conditions, analytic work can be exciting and challenging, but also very lonely. (p. 288)

Within the framework of this lonely and isolating environment many things can go awry. Isolated therapists tend to overidentify with their patients as their work becomes their life. Increasingly, they look to their patients to gratify them. They tend to look upon their patients as their social contact and may live vicariously through them.

As previously indicated, isolation distorts judgment, and some therapists become grandiose and feel omnipotent in order to compensate for their felt loss of grasp in their own lives. This is fertile ground for therapeutic abuse and is counterproductive for both the therapists and their patients. It is also our belief that arrogant therapists are the ones most likely to get sued. Their mask of invincibility will most likely be uncovered in court. They may be able to deny and rationalize their behavior to themselves, but, when examined in the bright light of reality, the rationalizations will collapse upon themselves.

Isolation also tends to feed upon itself. Isolated clinicians become more withdrawn and passive. Their lack of a viable support system takes a toll on the psychic spirit. This malaise is fed by their difficulty in confiding openly to friends or family. They need to present a picture of control, and thus rob themselves of the genuine sharing of thoughts and feelings that would sustain them. Instead, they maintain a secretive posture and grow increasingly lonely. The rift between their public image and how they genuinely feel widens. Many isolated clinicians are trapped by the image they have worked so hard to create. In studies conducted by Bermak (1977) and Tryon (1983), they both found that isolation was the number one complaint among practitioners.

PERSONAL DISENCHANTMENTS
AND EXPECTATIONS

The personal disenchantments that occur may be a function of personal or financial reversals, failed relationships or marriages, loss of loved ones, illnesses, accidents, aging, or a feeling of cynicism and frustration with one's career (Freudenberger, 1986b). Guy et al. (1987) found that "75% of the psychotherapists surveyed nationwide reported that they had experienced one or more potential distressing episodes during the past three years of their life."

Therapists have a difficult time acknowledging that they are getting into difficulty. As Klauber (1983) indicated:

> The analyst's emotional task is always immensely difficult. The central problem of psychoanalytic identity, therefore, seems to me to lie in finding a balance between the years of training necessary for a student approaching mid-life or past it, to master a highly exacting conceptual system and technique. To this should be added the effect of the economic sanctions which are never wholly forgotten where analysts are dependent on private practice for their livelihood.

Additionally, therapists work under time pressure, always feeling a shortage of time because of emergencies, a patient's serious upset during a session, or the reality recognition that a major element of what we as therapists sell is time.

Along with these felt pressures we also expect of ourselves perfection and a continued sense of achieving. These are demands that we feel as both psychotherapists and individuals in our society (Freudenberger & Richelson, 1980). We unrealistically expect ourselves always to be at the peak of technical proficiency; to be infallible; to be emotionally available to our patients; to be clear, concise, and compassionate; and to present most of our interpretations in a meaningful fashion. These expectations are humanly impossible to meet, and if insisted upon will most likely lead to feelings of failure, despair, and cynicism; depletion of energy; and a sense of being impostors in our chosen profession. In our offices, we often work in an atmosphere of creativity and continued explorations of terrains wherein uncertainty is sometimes our main and constant companion. Therefore, how can we realistically place on ourselves the demand of being perfect? The answer, quite sensibly, is that we can not.

FAMILY, FRIENDSHIP, AND INTERPERSONAL RELATIONSHIP RISKS

It is often said that the ones who suffer most the depletion and draining effects of a psychologist's work are the spouse and the rest of the family. After spending many hours with patients, most therapists desire not to be burdened with the issues at home. How sad and unfair of us because the persons who are willing to nurture are often not given a fair hearing by us.

Cray and Cray (1977) eloquently describe the situation as follows:

> When the psychiatrist (psychotherapist) does get home to his (her) family, the very skilled listener is no longer in a mood to listen. He would like to talk for a change. He has been suppressing his talking all day. Moreover, the problems of his family seem very trite compared to the problems he has been focusing on. His sensitivity is dulled. (p. 33)

Certainly, over the course of time, this attitude on the part of the therapist may have serious negative consequences for the marital relationship. The spouse feels estranged, not invited into the life of his or her spouse, and the potential consequence might be marital discord or even divorce.

Farber (1985) and Freudenberger (1986b) both comment that "the tendency to become increasingly psychologically minded as a result of therapeutic practice also has the potential of having a detrimental effect on marital adjustment." The therapist may speak to the spouse and children in a therapeutic way that suggests that the therapist is not really listening, but rather talking in "psychologyese." Freudenberger, one of the authors, was delighted when years ago his young children would compare him to other psychologist colleagues and comment that he talked "normal," rather than "funny."

We should reflect a moment on the point that men often still perceive the woman as the nurturing object: the person who will be understanding, make allowances, always be there (no matter in what mood the husband therapist may enter the home), and continue to be "the big nurturing breast" (Freudenberger & North, 1986). But as more and more women enter the therapeutic professions, the woman's need to be mothered by the husband may raise another risk factor that appears to be gender specific to women. We do not have sufficient research on this as yet, but it would appear that the woman's need to be nurtured and emotionally supported after depleting herself all day could certainly impact on the marital relationship. This could require that the man now become the nurturer, rather than the one looking for nurturing from the woman.

Relating to our children has its own issues of risk and potential negatives. As previously pointed out, therapists may come home exhausted, depleted, and overstimulated with thinking all day. We may have a tendency to put our children off with, "Let's talk about that later," which may in effect mean never.

Kohut (1977) mentions that he has had occasion to analyze many adults, who, as children of therapists, had been negatively impacted by their parents' tendency to overanalyze and overinterpret their behavior. He states that the

> pathogenic effect of the parental behavior lay in the fact that the parents' participation in their children's life, their claim — often correctly made — that they knew more about what their children were thinking, wishing, feeling than the children themselves, tended to interfere with the consolidation of the self of these children. (pp. 146–147)

Both of us have had the same impression in working therapeutically with children of therapists. They often felt shut out by their therapist/parent and were spoken to in a manner that was replete with jargon and distancing devices.

Therapists' work also seems to make significant inroads into the socializing in their lives. Since therapists function in a one-way intimacy relationship most of their working day, they tend to find it difficult to socialize. Therapists may remain aloof and to some degree invulnerable to the spontaneity and genuine vulnerability that are part of friendship and socializing.

PRACTICAL CONSIDERATIONS

There are a host of practical considerations that must be on any list of risks of independent practice. Foremost among these is the issue of illness. Therapists can and do get sick. What then happens to their practices? Should therapists become seriously ill and be unable to work for several months, it is likely that they may have to start over at a time they are least able to withstand that stress.

Independent practitioners are *the* resource of their practice. Without their presence, there is no practice. And, if they are solo practitioners, as most therapists are, there is no one to whom they can delegate any of their responsibilities.

Serious illness will severely damage any practice. Even if patients return, they may be frightened about the physical condition of the therapist and may be reluctant to stay very long. With advancing age and the stresses inherent in independent practice, we feel that this is an issue that sorely needs airing. We also wonder how many of our colleagues have given serious thought to retiring, aging, or the possibility of becoming ill.

King (1983) speaks of aging as a critical phase in the professional life cycle of a therapist. She talks of the "depletion of skills, capacities, and abilities since psychoanalysts tend to work much longer and to retire later than people in other professions." In addition, she indicates that "the process of aging is also complicated by illnesses which exacerbate the depletion of abilities and undermine the capacity of an analyst."

Further, independent practice does not provide for sick days. If the therapist has the flu and cannot work for 4 days, those are 4 days of lost income. Similarly, there are no personal days. If the therapist has to take a day off for personal business, then he or she must cancel the appointments for that day and suffer the loss of that income as well.

Nor does independent practice provide for paid vacations. When therapists take vacations, and many are reluctant to, that is also "downtime" for the income of the practice. Many therapists consider vacations to be doubly expensive for them. To the cost of the actual vacation, air travel, hotels, meals, and so forth must be added the figure for lost income. From this vantage point, vacations can be extremely expensive, and the lack of vacations is one cause of therapists' burnout. They do not readily take the time to revitalize themselves and operate instead as machines that do not need any preventative maintenance or rest. Freudenberger, one of the authors of this article, has made it a point, against colleagues' dire predictions of loss of patients, to take a minimum of 6 weeks' vacation during the summer. This not only serves to replenish the therapist but also gives patients the opportunity to observe themselves in terms of the degree of their progress and areas that may require further exploration once they resume treatment.

There are many other practical issues facing the independent practitioner. One issue is that of the professional office. If the therapist rents office space, how does he or she negotiate with a landlord? Is a long-term lease desirable, or possible, given today's real estate climate? What happens if the landlord decides not to renew a lease? How does the therapist go about relocating? What is the impact of relocation on a practice?

What are the pitfalls if the therapist has an office in his or her home or apartment? Does this increase the therapist's isolation? Is this a violation of any zoning laws in the local community? How can he or she maintain an effective separation between the home and the home office?

Suppose a rental office is offered as a cooperative. Should the therapist buy the space? What factors and variables need to be considered? What hidden costs and problems will emerge? Can the office be shared or subletted? Or should he or she consider entering a partnership or group practice?

How should an office be decorated? Should it have a couch, plants, pictures? Should the therapist display all of his or her diplomas and membership certificates? Should the therapist eat or drink coffee or tea with a patient present? Should he or she take telephone calls during sessions? How soundproof is the office from the waiting area? Should the therapist have an answering service or will a telephone answering machine suffice? How should he or she secure confidential records and information? Should the therapist type his or her own correspondence and do the billing? What about confidentiality? Obviously, this list could go on and on, as independent practitioners are called upon to grapple with issues and decisions for which they are often poorly prepared.

In the previous section the focus was on risks and hazards that may confront therapists in their independent practice and personal life. We believe that the rewards of independent practice can more than compensate for the risks. We now turn our attention to the rewards and joys of practice, which we believe are not readily duplicable in any other work setting.

REWARDS OF INDEPENDENT PRACTICE

Tyron (1983) surveyed 300 private practitioners and found that "the satisfactions associated with clinical practice most often reported, in descending order of frequency, were professional independence, success, high income, flexible hours, relating to patients, variety, challenge of work, enjoyment of work, contacts with other professionals, serving humankind and recognition." Farber and Heifetz (1982) found that psychotherapists derive the greatest amount of career satisfaction from helping patients to change, gaining an increased understanding of human nature, and experiencing a sense of intimate involvement in their lives.

The authors believe that there are many rewards of private practice, 11 of the most important of which follow:

1. Professional independence and autonomy must rank as one of the most substantial rewards of independent practice. Therapists are free to schedule their own time, to choose which patients and which projects to pursue, and to set their own policies and ground rules within ethical guidelines. As Goldberg (1986) states, "There is a need in practice to have a variety of clients and activities. This prevents the practitioner from 'assembly-lining' his/her professional life. The contrast between different kinds of clients creates a variety of perspectives on human existence" (p. 283). The variety promotes creativity and enjoyment of one's work.

2. Independence allows therapists to be creative and pursue the dictates of their personal value system. Since they are not part of a corporate bureaucracy, they do not have to contend with office politics or strive for promotion. They do not have to be concerned with quarterly profit statements or hostile takeovers. No memos to bosses need to be written. No boring meetings need be endured. This freedom can create a climate in which therapists can do outstanding work and feel rewarded for their efforts

3. Independent practitioners do not have one boss. In a corporation, each employee usually reports to one person who is all-powerful over his or her career. That one boss can promote, recommend substantial raises for, or demote or fire the employee. Or the boss can be transferred or fired or retire, and the employee will have to contend with someone else having power over him or her. In a sense, independent practitioners have many bosses in that each patient is a separate "boss" evaluating them. But, even if one or more "boss/patients" decides to fire a therapist, the therapist will have other patients who want him or her to stay on. Furthermore, therapists can decide that they do not want to work for, or with, particular individuals, and have the freedom to transfer them.

4. Another component of professional independence is that there are many professional activities available to independent practitioners. Aside from working with patients in their offices, they can share their knowledge by writing articles or books, they can teach at a university or in adult education settings, they can consult with a variety of organizations and thus utilize their clinical skills, and they can conduct seminars and workshops and give lectures. The range of appropriate activities is limited only by the creativity, resourcefulness, and drive of the therapist. Additionally, many of these activities will help the therapist to cope with the loneliness, isolation, and burnout of a strictly office-based practice.

5. As previously indicated, the independent practitioner can earn a comfortable income. Although most therapists will never be extremely wealthy,

capable therapists can earn considerable sums of money in their practices and can have many of the comforts and luxuries of life both for themselves and for their families.

6. Being an independent practitioner allows the therapist to function at an extremely mature level. Knowing that one is making it on one's own and that he or she has the freedom and responsibility that go with the territory is exhilarating. It leads to maturity that is beneficial to the therapist and to his or her loved ones. The personal growth may also manifest itself in helping emotional growth in the spouse as well as in improving parenting skills.

7. Independent practice provides a certain status for the therapist. It tends to promote admiration and respect from members of the community.

8. Being an independent practitioner gives the therapist the opportunity to use and refine his or her skills through ongoing learning and education. There is a marvelous opportunity for learning about and revitalizing the self that is not widely available in other careers.

9. There is joy in participating in someone's growth and development. All seasoned therapists can point with pride to some of the excellent work they have done over the past number of years with their patients. It is pleasurable for therapists to know that they have had a constructive and productive impact on the lives of many patients. As therapists we are engaged in meaningful work that can and often does make a substantial difference in a person's life.

10. In connection with this is the feeling of therapists that they are a role model and mentor for some patients. The therapeutic work can assist therapists in gaining a sense of the "generativity" and "integrity" in Erikson's stages of development. Therapists have the feeling that they have been an effective and loving parent and that their professional life was led with maturity, vision, and integrity.

11. Independent practitioners can gain a unique perspective on the society and culture. Each day they have the opportunity to talk with a wide variety of people from many diverse backgrounds. It is an unusual learning laboratory and, given the diversity of patients, can offer clinicians a perspective on life, people, and culture that is poignant and personally enlightening.

In sum, independent practice has its inherent risks and rewards. It is our belief that in recent years the risks have multiplied and intensified. And, for the near-term future, the risk factors will most likely continue to impinge upon our lives as practitioners. However, forewarned is forearmed, and we believe that despite the current climate, independent practice offers a life and life-style that are not readily duplicated. The mature and creative therapist can learn to cope with the risks, maximize the rewards, and in this process have a fulfilling and productive career and life.

REFERENCES

Bermak, G.E. (1977). Do psychiatrists have special emotional problems? *American Journal of Psychoanalysis, 37,* 141–146.

Cray, C., & Cray, M. (1977). Stresses and rewards within the psychiatrist's family. The American Journal of Psychoanalysis, 37, 337–341.

Farber, B.A. (1985). The genesis, development and implications of psychological-mindedness in psychotherapists. *Professional Psychology, 22,* 170–177.

Farber, B.A., & Heifetz, L.J. (1982). The process and dimension of burnout in psychotherapists. *Professional Psychology, 13,* 293–301.

Freudenberger, H.J. (1983). Hazards of psychotherapeutic practice. *Psychotherapy in Private Practice, 1*(1), 83–89.

Freudenberger, H.J. (1984). Impaired clinicians: Coping with "burnout." In P.A. Keller & L.L. Ritt (Eds.), *Innovations in clinical practice: A source book* (Vol. 3, pp. 223–229). Sarasota, FL: Professional Resource Exchange.

Freudenberger, H.J. (1986a). The health professional in treatment: Symptoms, dynamics, and treatment issues. In C.C. Scott & J. Hawk (Eds.), *Heal thyself: The health of health care professionals.* New York: Brunner Mazel.

Freudenberger, H.J. (1986b). Chemical abuse among psychologists: Symptoms, causes and treatment issues. In R.R. Kilburg, P.E. Nathan & R.W. Thoreson (Eds.), *Professionals in distress: Issues, syndromes and solutions in psychology.* Washignton, DC: American Psychological Association.

Freudenberger, H.J., & North, G. (1986). *Women's burnout: How to spot it, how to reverse it and how to prevent it.* New York: Penguin Books.

Freudenberger, H.J., & Richelson, G. (1980). *Burnout: How to beat the high cost of success.* New York: Bantam Books.

Freudenberger, H.J., & Robbins, A. (1979). The hazards of being a psychoanalyst. *Psychoanalytic Review, 66,* 275–295.

Goldberg, C. (1986). *On being a psychotherapist: The journey of the healer.* New York: Gardner Press.

Guy, J.D. (1987). *The personal life of the psychotherapist.* New York: John Wiley and Sons.

Guy, J.D., Stark, M., & Pelstra, P. (1987). *National survey of psychotherapists' attitudes and beliefs.* Unpublished manuscript.

King, P. (1983). Identity crises: Splits or compromise—advaptive or maladaptive. In E.D. Joseph & D. Widlocher (Eds.), *The identity of the psychoanalyst.* New York: International Universities Press.

Kohut, H. (1977). *The restoration of the self.* New York: International Universities Press.

Klauber, J. (1983). The identity of the psychoanalyst. In E.D. Joseph & D. Widlocher (Eds.), *The identity of the psychoanalyst.* New York: International Universities Press.

Marmor, J. (1953). The feeling of superiority: An occupational hazard in the practice of psychotherapy. *American Journal of Psychiatry, 110,* 370–376.

Rice, D.G., Fey, W.F., & Kepecs, J.G. (1972). Therapist experience and "style" as factors in co-therapy. *Family Process, 11,* 1–12.

Tryon, G.S. (1983). Full-time private practice in the United States: Results of a national survey. *Professional Psychology Research and Practice, 14,* 685–696.

C H A P T E R
41

MENTAL HEALTH PRACTITIONERS: THE PUBLIC'S PERSPECTIVE*

Richard R. Kilburg, Ph.D.

W hen I attempted to organize this chapter, several issues immediately arose that I was forced to address before beginning to write. These issues form the foundation of the problem of public perspective/public image for all mental health practitioners.

One begins with the rather thorny difficulty of just who the public is about whom we shall speak. Our choices include the perspectives of the professions themselves, organizations and companies that purchase health insurance, third-party payers, state and federal governmental officials, governing bodies of health and human service organizations, the general population of the United States, and finally, the clients of providers and their families. The views of each of these constituencies are unique. The data available vary quite widely. They all deserve a fair hearing. However, coverage of the opinions of all of these groups is beyond the scope of this chapter. I have chosen to limit the focus of the material to the clients of practitioners, rather broadly defined to include individuals who might use mental health services.

The second issue involves the various concerns of these publics. Providers worry about market share, legal liability, professional status, funding, and various technical matters. Governments, companies, and third-party payers fret about the costs of services. Clients and their families focus on whether they get well and how much the services cost. All of these issues can be discussed legitimately under the heading of public perspectives. Here again, I have chosen to limit the chapter to the concerns of clients.

The third aspect of the problem involves what we are to believe about the perspectives of existing and potential clients. A variety of data sources are available, including research studies, public opinion polls, and anecdotal information. Do we listen to providers, clients, representatives of clients, potential clients, or families of clients? How reliable, valid, and, most importantly, useful is the information that they provide? How is the information collected? Are the data currently available useful to all practitioners or just to some? What are the limits of the available information? I hope to provide some answers to these questions.

Finally, we want to know why practitioners should care about the perspec-

*The author gratefully acknowledges the assistance of Patricia Santora, Ph.D., for her assistance in collecting the bibliographic material that supports this chapter.

tives of the public? The best and shortest answer I can think of is that practitioner survival is solely dependent on the acceptance and good wishes of clients. Providers are well-advised to ask for and listen to the opinions of the people that they serve. Clients and their families are customers in one very real and true sense. They seek and pay for services. Admittedly, there are exceptions, such as involuntarily committed or treated persons. However, these are a small minority of the clients who are served annually. Without paying customers, there is no mental health business.

Given the nature of the problem, this chapter will present a review of the data available on the opinions of real and potential clients (the general public) about mental health services, highlight a number of problems and issues raised by the data, and make several recommendations to practitioners about the steps that they can take in light of this information.

A BRIEF OVERVIEW OF THE LITERATURE

Client Satisfaction Studies

The most systematic and comprehensive source of data on clients' views about their therapists and treatment comes from studies on client satisfaction done in community mental health centers. The results of this research are based largely upon short questionnaires administered to clients during and after their treatment. Most of the reports do not specifically discuss the views of the clients about their therapists. Rather, they focus on the degree of general satisfaction with services. Since the services are usually delivered by a therapist, conclusions about them can be made responsibly.

Lebow (1982) reviewed and criticized the client satisfaction literature. Of the 30 studies covered, 27 were done solely to determine clients' satisfaction with the services in a particular facility or program. Three of the reports were part of overall efforts to evaluate an organization and its services. All of the studies were done in organized care delivery settings. The lack of information about the services of private practitioners makes it impossible to generalize the results across all types of mental health practice.

Twenty-six studies were conducted on outpatient services in community mental health centers. Three reported client satisfaction rates consistently between 91 and 100 percent. Ten reported rates between 81 and 90 percent. Eight demonstrated satisfaction between 17 and 80 percent. Four reported satisfaction for 61 to 70 percent of the clients. One study reported rates between 51 and 60 percent. Four studies were described that dealt with satisfaction with crisis intervention services. One reported satisfaction rates between 91 and 100 percent. Two reported rates between 71 and 80 percent. And one study reported satisfaction rates between 61 and 70 percent.

In general, these data lead us to conclude that the majority of clients receiving services in these studies were at least moderately pleased with their treatment. Many of the programs appeared to be doing an excellent job of meeting the demands and expectations of their clients. A smaller number reported rather mixed results, indicating that there were some problems in attaining the levels of satisfaction most desirable.

The studies revealed that variables such as age, sex, income level, marital status, and education were not significantly related to levels of satisfaction. Diagnostic, psychological, and prognostic variables were more directly related. Satisfaction levels were reported lower for clients who abused drugs or who were suicidal, psychotic, or rates as having a poor prognosis. They were also reported to be lower for clients who had little choice in the facility from which they received services, who had no choice in the therapist that treated them, or who were naive about treatment. Satisfaction was unrelated to total length of stay in treatment; it was higher when treatment terminated with the mutual agreement of therapist and client and when clients reported that treatment met their expectations.

Several factor analytic studies provide a more detailed picture of the structure of client satisfaction. Brown (1979) reported seven factors associated with satisfaction: satisfaction with therapist, outcome of treatment, clinic service, felt importance, access, confidentiality, and therapist intent. Love et al. (1979) also reported seven factors associated with satisfaction: overall care, staff responsiveness, staff behavior, center accountability, meeting of needs, medicines, and access. Studies with shorter rating scales revealed satisfaction with outcome and access (Fiester & Fort, 1978) and satisfaction with problem solving and closeness (Tessler, 1975) as components. Other authors reported a more global or unidimensional general satisfaction factor (Frank et al., 1977; Larsen et al., 1979).

These studies spring from and are consistent with the early research of Strupp et al. (1969), Hoehn-Saric et al. (1964), and Yalom et al. (1967) on the views of patients about their therapy and the preparation of clients for a therapeutic experience. These initial studies reported similar rates of satisfaction with treatment. They also provided some of the first evidence that therapists themselves could actually do something constructive to help create positive experiences with their clients.

Further illustrations of the utility of these research reports can be seen when we examine several examples of the type of work that has been done. Lorefice and Borus (1984) in one of the most recent studies examined what patients expected from treatment, what they found helpful about treatment, how they would improve treatment, what kind of therapists they preferred, and how they perceived their treatment outcome. The study found that 54.7 percent came to treatment for advice, 46 percent for ventilation, 46 percent for an understanding listener, 40.7 percent for psychodynamic insight, 39.1 percent for help in regaining control of themselves, 31.7 percent for problem clarification, 29.8 percent for psychological expertise, and 26.7 percent for medications. Less than 25 percent, the study found, came for help with a child, family member, or friend; came for help with dealing with a social, welfare, or school organization; came to talk about guilt or to see if others faced similar problems; or were unsure what they hoped for or did not feel they needed any help.

In the same study, the most helpful components of treatment were seen as problem clarification (61.9 percent), ventilation (61 percent), problem sharing (49.5 percent), self-understanding (46.7 percent), advice from the therapist (43.8 percent), and medications (24.8 percent). One-third of the clients believed that the sessions could be improved; 44.4 percent would have liked more direct advice from the therapist, and 40 percent would have wanted to know more about the opinions of the therapist. Less than 25 percent wanted medications, a change in their medications, a delving into the roots of their problems, a better listener, or a less talkative therapist.

These results highlight the importance of trying to determine what a patient wants and needs from treatment before applying particular techniques or methods. They illustrate that patients do have some idea about what will be most helpful to them. Therapists can benefit from knowing that what they do best is not always seen as useful by the people they are serving.

A second illustrative study (Edwards et al., 1978) looked at the relationship between ratings of satisfaction and treatment success by therapists and clients. They found that ratings of satisfaction climbed during and immediately after treatment but then fell slightly at a 3-month follow-up. They also reported that ratings of satisfaction were significantly related to both therapist and client ratings of treatment success. Therapist ratings of treatment success were more stringent and lower than those of patients. These authors caution that high ratings of client satisfaction do not necessarily imply treatment success.

Flynn et al. (1981) in a similar study of client improvement and satisfaction reported that 67 percent of the 22 percent of the clients who responded left the clinic when services were complete, 68 percent of the respondents stated that they improved because of the services, 54 percent terminated treatment because of improvement in their conditions, 13 percent stopped because their conditions worsened, 21 percent terminated because they could not afford the fee, 43 percent said that they would return to the clinic if they felt the need, and 84 percent would recommend the clinic to someone else. In addition, these authors pointed out that patients who were satisfied with the therapeutic relationship and had confidence in their therapists had the highest correlations with the index of therapeutic improvement. These patients also tended to stay in treatment longer. Confidence in the therapist, satisfaction with the therapeutic relationship, and longer length of treatment led to higher reported levels of client satisfaction. It is useful to note that 13 percent stated that their condition worsened as a result of treatment. This should alert practitioners to the fact that treatment is not harmless. The resulting increase in legal liabilities should focus attention on this problem.

Other interesting studies were done by Schainblatt (1980), who looked at satisfaction and outcomes in four different types of service programs; Weber and Tilley (1981), who evaluated student services at a health sciences campus; and Meyer and Zegans (1975), who evaluated the responses of adolescents to their psychotherapy. These reports are similar to those described above and those reviewed by Lebow (1982) in that they all cite fairly high levels of satisfaction with their services.

In his 1982 review, Lebow also thoroughly criticized the client satisfaction studies he summarized. His concerns included a frequent lack of reported reliability data on the instruments used in the studies; very few efforts to validate the instruments or the data collected; sampling bias in the selection of clients and their reported responses (on average only 54 percent of those receiving surveys responded); a lack of controls on data gathering procedures;

distortion in the clients' responses due to their acquiescence, their reactivity, and the social desirability of the items used in the surveys; a lack of precision in the terminology of client satisfaction; and omission of items dealing with or likely to elicit nonsatisfaction responses in the scales used.

Lebow also raised several practical problems with these reports. There tends to be a high baseline of stated satisfaction producing a lack of variability in the responses. The face validity of the instruments tends to be impaired, especially when low levels of survey response and high therapy dropout rates are considered. There is a lack of variability across aspects of treatment, suggesting the operation of a halo effect. The measures used in the studies tend not to be comparable or standardized, making generalization of results very difficult. These studies usually failed to establish baselines for satisfaction before treatment began. They also typically failed to differentiate between clients and types of treatment, rendering the impression that any treatment with any client probably yields fairly high levels of satisfaction. Other methodological variations make comparisons of the results more difficult across studies. Finally, he attacked the lack of sophistication in the methods of data analysis and reporting. These studies usually report simple, descriptive percentages on the rating scales administered. Lebow made a series of recommendations to correct these methodological weaknesses that I will not review here because of the limitations on the size of the chapter.

Public Opinion Surveys

Another source of empirical findings relevant to the core issue of how clients perceive their therapists is public opinion surveys that have been done for the past 40 years. As part of the preparation for this chapter, I called the national organizations of the four principal mental health professions, the American Psychiatric Association, the American Psychological Association, the American Nurses Association, and the National Association of Social Workers. Public affairs and professional staff members in each of these associations assured me that none of them has available results of current opinion polls about the public or client perceptions of their practitioners. The American Psychiatric Association funded an opinion study in 1977 (Clark & Martin, 1978). Only the American Psychological Association had an opinion survey in the planning stages.

Thankfully, the members of the American Psychological Association have been a little more curious about and effective in determining the views of the public about their field. Coincidentally, some of the results also speak to several of the issues central to this chapter. Not so coincidentally, I had a hand in bringing a summary of this information to the attention of the professions via a special section of the September 1986 issue of the *American Psychologist*. Three articles reviewed, summarized, and updated the available literature.

Benjamin (1986) took a brief look at the history of the public perception of the profession of psychology and some of the efforts members of that profession have undertaken to modify the public's ideas about the field. At the turn of the century, the public equated psychology with "clairvoyance, mind reading, and spiritualism" (p. 941). At the first organizational meeting of the

American Psychological Association in the home of G. Stanley Hall, the founder of the first psychology laboratory in the United States at Johns Hopkins University, Joseph Jastrow proposed that the association prepare an exhibit for the Columbian World Exhibition in Chicago in 1893. Jastrow, Hugo Munsterberg, and others arranged for and administered an exhibit that featured a testing room where individuals could have their sensory and mental abilities evaluated. This initiated an effort to understand and influence public opinion about psychology that continues today. Interestingly, the American Psychological Association, in conjunction with the National Science Foundation and a number of science museums, is planning a traveling psychology exhibition that will be seen in most of the major science museums around the country. This will coincide with the 100th anniversary of the American Psychological Association and the first exhibition at the Chicago fair.

Wood et al. (1986) reviewed the opinion surveys published in the scientific literature. Guest (1948) did the first study. This survey compared the occupation of psychologist with four other occupations — architect, chemist, economist, and engineer. Another section of the survey compared the public's understanding of psychology and psychiatry. Economists and engineers were selected more frequently than psychologists as the professionals to whom people would turn if they needed help in selecting individuals for a particular job. The respondents made little distinction between psychiatrists and psychologists. Psychologists were identified correctly as scientists. Psychology was the least preferred profession of the five mentioned when respondents were asked to name the field they would least like their children to choose. These respondents also stated overwhelmingly that psychologists would be the professionals they would be most uncomfortable with in social situations.

During the next decade, nine additional studies were reported in the *American Psychologist*. These studies presented a rich and sometimes contradictory set of perceptions about psychology and psychiatry. However, increasingly, the public seemed to be able to distinguish between the medical training of psychiatrists and the scientific and professional training of psychologists. By the late 1970s, psychiatrists were viewed by the public as "more effective in treating mental illness, which was defined as involving organic problems and antisocial behavior. Yet psychiatrists and psychologists were viewed as being equally helpful in treating emotional problems, such as inability to cope with family problems, and depression" (Wood et al. 1986, p. 948).

Kabatznick (1984) found that less than half of his respondents — scientists, business people, psychologists, and mall shoppers — thought that psychotherapists were more perceptive than other people. Over half of those interviewed thought that psychotherapists help the people they treat. Again, the respondents displayed great knowledge of the differences between the disciplines; 70 percent knew that psychologists cannot prescribe drugs.

Wood et al. (1986) performed their own telephone survey with a randomly drawn sample of the general population. They reported improvements in the public image of psychology since Guest's 1948 study. They also replicated the ability of the public to know the differences between psychology and psychiatry. Of their sample, 45.4 percent reported that psychology had had an impact on their lives; 81.3 percent were able to identify the specific effect. The majority of them mentioned the results of their own therapy and the treatment received by friends and family members as having the most impact.

Pallak and Kilburg (1986) describe the elaborate program undertaken by organized psychology to influence and change the public image of the field. I do not want to review this in detail here. What is important to realize is that the attitudes, values, and impressions of people can be modified in somewhat predictable ways. The public image of psychotherapists has seen some documented changes, at least as demonstrated in the public opinion surveys conducted by and about psychologists and other mental health professionals. Although the data are again a little suspect on methodological grounds, a somewhat coherent view emerges over the 40-year history of the research. These add to the relatively richer yield from the client satisfaction studies described earlier.

Several other more general surveys of public attitudes toward and knowledge about mental health services have also appeared in the literature. Padilla et al. (1966) conducted a sociological survey of the residents of New York City as part of a planning and evaluation study by the New York City Mental Health Board. A number of their findings stand out: 50 percent of the respondents knew someone who had been helped by mental health services. One out of every 11 persons had sought help for themselves. One-third of the sample knew someone who had been hospitalized for mental illness; 2 percent had been hospitalized for mental illness. One-sixth knew someone who was in treatment at the time of the survey; 1.5 percent were in treatment at the time of the survey.

This population knew that services were delivered by different professions but had difficulty telling the differences between them. About 50 percent could not tell the difference between psychiatrists and psychologists. Almost 50 percent did not believe that anyone else could treat mental illness besides psychiatrists. Seventy-five percent believed that psychiatrists were better at treating mental troubles than were psychologists or social workers: 67 percent stated that they thought psychiatrists were better than psychologists or social workers in treating emotional problems. The majority of respondents believed that social workers do a better job than psychiatrists or psychologists dealing with families. The respondents did not have psychotherapists as friends. Ninety percent could not name a psychiatrist, and even higher percentages could not name a psychologist or social worker. The majority did not know about the services that were available. The majority of respondents, however, did believe that mental health services were necessary.

Edgerton and Bentz (1969) reviewed several earlier surveys of public attitudes about the mentally ill and mental health services in conjunction with their own survey of the attitudes of people who lived in rural areas of North Carolina. Ninety-four percent of their respondents did not know about any services available in their communities; 98 percent felt that such services were needed in their communities. The majority believed that mental illness was the most serious health problem in the country. Eighty percent stated that they thought these problems could be treated. Ninety percent knew that psychiatrists deal with the mentally ill. Ninety percent felt that their community could benefit from the services of a mental health practitioner. Despite their otherwise enlightened views about mental illness, 69 percent believed that state hospitals were necessary to protect their communities from the mentally ill.

McWilliams and Morris (1974) surveyed the attitudes of the residents of Tucson, Ariz., in preparation for developing consultation and education services in a community mental health center. The respondents believed that drugs and alcohol (48 percent), care for the elderly (11 percent), and family problems (8 percent) were the most pressing problems in Tucson. Seventy-three percent stated that they thought people could be cured of mental problems. Psychotherapy was the service that respondents most frequently expected to find in a mental health center (14 percent). Seventy-one percent stated that they would be more likely to use the services if insurance paid for them, and 64 percent said that they probably would use the services if they needed them.

Solomon and Harris (1977) did a study to determine which of the mental health professions was most accepted by clients in their homes. They found that psychiatric nurses were the most successful in seeing their clients. Mental health therapists, mental health therapy assistants, and drug abuse counselors were also very effective in seeing their clients. Psychiatrists and social workers were most frequently turned away. Women were more successful than men, and older professionals seemed to be more accepted than younger ones.

These empirical studies of client satisfaction and public opinion suggest that the general population is aware of the problems of the mentally ill and the need for services, is increasingly sophisticated in its knowledge about such services and the professions that provide them, and is generally supportive of the mental health field. Similarly, clients are usually satisfied with the services that they receive and can be counted on to be supportive of their practitioners in most cases. The methodologies used to generate this data base raise questions about the reliability and validity of the data. However, the frequency with which the same results are reported increases confidence in the general conclusions. Let us now turn to several other sources of information that help illuminate our questions.

Opinions Of Consumers

A related source of information comes directly from consumers themselves. Several interesting articles have been written by clients. Colom (1981) emphasized the need for consumer input into the operations of community mental health centers. She pointed out that consumers have economic power, in that there would be no need for these services to exist without them. She stated forthrightly that professionals tend to respond to criticism defensively because they fear that they will be found to be inadequate professionally, that they will lose their clients, and that clients will aim their anger at them directly. Colom summarized the problems in finding and training consumers to serve on the governing boards of community mental health centers. She also emphasized the need for client education and for comprehensible and useful grievance procedures for those consumers who feel that they have been mistreated or ill served.

Allen (1974) contributed a wonderful summary of the problems and issues facing clients who use state hospitals and the community aftercare systems in California. In balanced, well-reasoned, and sensitive arguments, she made clear that there was a need for well-run state hospitals and for well-run after-care programs. She pointed out the inadequacies and the benefits of both systems from the perspective of those who have used them. She made a detailed set of recommendations for the operation of community care homes that are too lengthy to go into here but are recommended reading for any professional trying to develop such services.

Increasingly, clients have been aided by a group of professional consumer advocates, many of whom have had legal training. An article by Kopolow (1979) is illustrative of the perspective of these advocates. He directed the attention of providers to the legal rights of consumers and in particular to their right to be protected from assault and being deprived of their liberty. The abuses of power by bureaucracies and professionals in putting people in institutions against their will and performing various injurious treatments have been well documented. He urged everyone involved to aspire to higher levels of accountability in providing services, particularly when involuntary hospitalization and forced treatment must be considered. Balancing the goals of professionals to restore the lives and health of their clients with the clients' fears of loss of freedom and dignity, helplessness, and oppressive governmental policies was seen as the only way out of a difficult situation. He presented an effective and succinct bill of patients' rights as a starting place for collaboration between clients and providers on these issues.

Treatment Outcome Studies

Another tangential source of information about clients' perception of their treatment comes from studies of the outcomes of psychotherapeutic treatment. A thorough review of this topic is well beyond the scope of this chapter. However, it is very important to address the question, Do people get well as a result of their psychotherapeutic experience? Two summaries of the research in this area come to similar conclusions. Bergin (1971) concluded that there is

> modest evidence that psychotherapy "works." While most studies do not seem to yield very substantial evidence that this is so, the number that do so seems to be clearly larger than would be expected by chance; therefore, something potent or efficacious must be operating in some portion of the therapy that is routinely done, even though average effects are only moderately impressive when diverse cases, therapists, and change scores are lumped together. (p. 229)

Similarly, in what will surely be one of the classic studies in the field of outcome evaluation, Smith et al. (1980) concluded from a review of 475 controlled studies of psychotherapy that "the average person who receives psychotherapy is better off at the end of it than 80 percent of the persons who do not" (p. 87).

Documentation of the fact that in the majority of the cases psychotherapy has a positive benefit would seem to be logically related to the results reported above in the client satisfaction literature. As we have seen, most people state that they are at least moderately pleased with the services that they received. When taken together, these two streams of data appear to provide a general answer to our major question. The public's view of psychotherapy services —

and, it would seem by logical extension, of psychotherapists—is that they are useful and helpful the majority of the time. Objective evidence supports this conclusion by demonstrating that the vast majority of the problems and conditions are resolved or improved as a result of these services.

Client/Therapist Variables

One final set of empirical studies is relevant to the topic of this chapter. Over the course of the past 30 years, a series of projects has demonstrated that there are a number of specific client/therapist variables that affect the outcome of and satisfaction with psychotherapy/counseling services. Again I will not attempt a comprehensive review of this literature. Rather, the following results are presented as a way of illustrating the relevance of the studies to the central questions that I have raised here.

Garfield (1971) and Truax and Mitchell (1971) summarized the by now well-known studies involving the client-centered approach to treatment. They demonstrated that various characteristics of clients and therapists do affect therapeutic outcome. In particular they noted that "therapists or counselors who are accurately emphatic, nonpossessively warm in attitude, and genuine, are indeed effective" (p. 310).

Klerman (1969) demonstrated that clients vary in their preferences for various types of counselors. Schainblatt (1980) showed that certain social and demographic characteristics of clients such as social class and income level seem to affect how well they do in treatment. Schiff (1970) outlined various racial variables that affect the acceptance of treatment. Heilbrun (1972) indicated that the preferences of men and women differ in a number of areas in treatment. He also demonstrated that readiness for treatment improves client satisfaction with and client attendance at treatment sessions. Otto and Moos (1974) and Richmond (1984) addressed the importance of client expectations and how they affect therapy outcomes. Clients seek therapists who accept them and who are warm, genuine, empathic, nurturing, self-disclosing, attractive, trustworthy, tolerant, and expert in their work. Maskin (1974) demonstrated that the therapist's self-concept as measured by his or her degree of self-confidence and self-control can influence the amount of change in clients in the course of treatment, the amount of trust that clients have in their therapist, and clients' judgments of the therapeutic effectiveness of their therapist.

Hart and Bassett (1975) revealed cultural differences in the preferences of clients for short-term or long-term treatment. Dixon (1986) discussd the effect of families on the help-seeking behaviors of adolescents and some of the differences and issues that come with treating an adolescent population. Obitz (1975) stated that directive and nondirective approaches to treatment are preferred by different types of clients. Schmidt and Strong (1971), Kunin and Rodin (1982), and McCay et al. (1982) demonstrated that the attractiveness of therapsits increased their social influence and the approval of their clients. Birkel and Reppucci (1983) found that women preferred therapists who are more religious than those preferred by male clients, and that women with stronger social support networks were less likely to seek consultation from professionals. Berger and Morrison (1984) found that therapists thought that easy clients were those who were highly motivated for seeking help, responded openly to questions, and elaborated on their responses to questions by the therapists. Finally, Yokopenic et al. (1983) demonstrated that the likelihood of persons' seeking treatment decreases as the degree of their self-reliant attitudes increases.

Perhaps this growing area of research can be best summarized by a quote from Rogers et al. (1967) in their classic work on the therapeutic relationship.

> In those cases where the patient enters therapy with a fair degree of expressive capacity and/or motivation for self-exploration, the therapist's corresponding involvement may be enhanced. That is, the more initially expressive the patient, the richer will be the material in which the therapist can anchor his empathic efforts. The more motivated the patient for therapeutic process, the easier it will be for the therapists to become correspondingly involved in, and committed to, the relationship. The more responsive the patient, the more likely it will be that the therapist can communicate the genuiness of his concern for, and interest in, the patient as a person,. On the other hand, patients lacking these capacities for therapeutic participation will generally fail to evoke similar therapist involvement. That is, the unmotivated, defensive, and reluctant patient from a different (lower) socio-economic background may not provide the therapist sufficient opportunity to deepen the relationship, and may thus severely limit the therapist's ability to communicate and function effectively. While skillful and sensitive therapists may succeed in involving even the initially reluctant patient, and more remote or superficial therapists may dampen the motivated patient's initial enthusiasm, it seems apparent from the sample that the patient's presenting capacities and motivation contribute heavily to the establishment of a climate in which the therpiast can function effectively. (p. 308-309)

CONCLUSIONS

The empircial literature summarized above leads me to the following conclusions. First, the studies available are lacking in methodological sophistication and are relatively few in number. They tend to focus on client satisfaction with services in community mental health centers, treatment outcomes in organized care delivery settings, and public opinion surveys concerning psychology and psychiatry. The generalizations and recommendations outlined below are based on this non-too-solid foundation.

Second, and most importantly, clients seem to be satisfied with the treatment they receive the vast majority of the time. They also apear to be pleased with the effectiveness of the treatment. The research demonstrates that most people improve with treatment. The perspectives of the clients and the therapist are very different. Family members have a view of treatment that is different from that of both the therapist and the client. As clients stay in treatment longer, express more satisfaction with the relationship with their therapists, and demonstrate more confidence in their therapists, their satisfaction with treatment increases.

Third, a large number of variables have been shown to influence the therapeutic relationship, and therefore, the effectiveness of and client satisfaction with treatment. Age, sex, race, socioeconomic class, ethnicity, setting (whether urban or rural) attractiveness of the therapist and the client, therapist personality and emotional characteristics, client expectations, therapist theoretical orientation, social support networks of clients, and handling by therapists of their feelings (especially anger) about their clients are included in the list of relevant parameters. Obviously, therapists "control" only some of these variable. Understanding and tolerating the effects of the things outside of the therapist's power to control are important to becoming a good therapist.

Fourth, the general population has increased its understanding of the differences between the mental health professions. They have stated preferences in some areas—for example, to whom they will grant access to their homes. Psychiatry, psychology, and psychotherapy have all improved their status as professions in the eyes of the general public. These professionals are seen now as helpful and needed by both urban and rural communities. However, they are kept at a social distance. The public tends not to have therapists as friends or acquaintances, and they tend not to go to a therapist unless they feel a strong need to do so.

Fifth, the changing legal, social, and political climates mean that more therapists are going to be coming into contact with the law. These changes also require increased advocacy for clients and professionals alike. Professionals must adjust to the new realities, in which they share their authority with clients and their legal representatives, even as they assume a wider burden of responsibility for the effects of the treatment they provide.

Sixth, preparing clients for treatment can make a significant difference in levels of satisfaction and in treatment outcomes. Similarly, client expectations can have positive or negative effects on satisfaction and outcome. Practitioners must take these factors into account if they hope routinely to create positive therapeutic outcomes.

Seventh, although the above summary did not dwell on the negative findings, there is ample evidence to suggest that in a small minority of cases (10 to 15 percent) clients report that treatment did them more harm than good. Negative side effects identified included increased rates of family dysfunction, ingestion of drugs and alcohol, and, in the most extreme cases, death for the client. Client satisfaction cannot be take for granted despite the fact that most of the people therapists serve seem pleased with the treatment.

RECOMMENDATIONS FOR MENTAL HEALTH PROFESSIONALS

In light of the foregoing summary and conclusions, we can reasonably ask what the practical implications for psychotherapists are. What follows is a set of succinct recommendations that, I believe, flow from the available research.

1. Assume that your clients are an increasingly sophisticated group of consumers. They know something about therapy, expect to be treated well, understand something about their rights as clients, and have access to an increasingly knowledgeable group of legal advocates. Their expectations create a new climate for satisfaction and effectiveness.

2. Try to discover the expectations that clients have for you as a therapist and for the outcome of treatment. Assess whether they are ready for treat-

ment. Improve your initial intake procedures to include the above areas and to provide some preparation of the client for treatment. Extend the evaluation phase of treatment as necessary to accomplish these tasks and to know your clients as well as possible. Do not agree to see anyone who does not meet yor criteria for readiness. Know yourself as a therapist, and try not to work outside of your demonstrated limits of effectiveness and competence.

3. Use client satisfaction methodology to deal with a variety of your realistic and imagined fears. Surveys are nice if you can afford them and if you want to take the time to analyze the data. Even if you only send your terminated clients a self-addressed and stamped postcard with two or three questions, you can add to your understanding of your clients. If this seems like too much trouble, use unobtrusive measures such as attendance and cancellation rates, continuation of treatment until a mutually agreed upon termination, promptness for appointments, sacrifices made to continue in treatment, rate of early terminations, and level at which clients participate in their treatment. Knowing where you stand on these dimensions will help you deal with such things as feelings of inadequacy, patients' anger, loss of revenue, legal liabilities, and professional regulation.

4. Know your clients' rights (Kopolow, 1979). For example, allow them to participate in decisions about treatment. Protect their privacy. Advocate for them. Provide for a grievance procedure.

5. Finally, be aware that clients' satisfaction and their opinions about you as a practitioner have direct economic relevance to you. In this era of increased competition and emphasis on marketing services, keep in mind that your best advertising is still a satisfied customer. Even though you deal with a service that is stigmatized by many people, the data clearly show a trend toward increasing aceptance and utilization. Many people find their way to a therapist by asking fiends and family members. Your knowledge of the factors that influence client satisfaction and of how your own clients view your services can be an invaluable economic asset. The research clearly shows that the perceptions of clients can be influenced by a variety of factors. Your personal marketing strategy should include as much of this information as possible.

In summary, although there are methodological weaknesses in many of the empirical studies done on the opinions of the public and of clients about psychotherapy and psychotherapists, a fairly coherent view of the findings and issues can be obtained from several different sources. Clients are generally pleased with their treatment. Treatment generally produces a positive outcome. A large number of variables have been shown to influence the therapeutic relationship, and hence levels of satisfaction and effectiveness. Clients' views are increasingly important to therapists for economic reasons and in order to protect agianst litigation. The views of clients can be influenced by what the therapist does or does not do. Careful attention to this aspect of psychotherapeutic practice can have a wide variety of positive influences for both the therapist and his or her clients.

REFERENCES

Allen, P. (1974). A consumer's view of California's mental health care system. *Psychiatric Quarterly, 48*(1), 1-13.

Benjamin, L.T., Jr. (1986). Why don't they understand us? A history of psychology's public image. *American Psychologist, 41*(9), 941-946.

Berger, A., & Morrison, T.L. (1984). Clinical judgements of easy vs. difficult clients by counselor trainees. *Journal of Clinical Psychology, 40*(4), 1116-1122.

Bergin, A.E., (1971). The evaluation of therapeutic outcomes. In A.E. Bergin & S.L. Garfield (Eds.), *Handbook of psychotherapy and behavior change* (pp.217-270). New York: John Wiley and Sons.

Birkel, R.C., & Reppucci, N.D. (1983). Social networks, information-seeking, and the utilization of services. *American Journal of Community Psychology, 11*(2), 185-205.

Brown, E. (1979). The role of expectancy in ratings of consumer satisfaction with mental health services. *Unpublished doctoral dissertation.* Florida State University.

Clark, R., & Martin, G. (1978). The image of psychiatry today. *Psychiatric Opinion, 15*, 10-15.

Colom, E. (1981). Reactions of an angry consumer. *Community Mental Health Journal, 17*(1), 92-97.

Dixon, M.A. (1986). Families of adolescent clients and nonclients: Ther environments and help-seeking behaviors. *Advances in Nursing Science, 8*(2), 75-88.

Edgerton, J.W. & Bentz, W.K. (1969). Attitudes and opinions of rural people about mental illness and program services. *American Journal of Public Health, 59*(3), 470-477.

Edwards, D.P., Yarvis, R.M., Mueller, D.P., & Langsley, D.G. (1978). Does client satisfaction correlate with success? *Hospital and Community Psychiatry, 24*(3), 188-190.

Fiester, A. & Fort, D. (1978). A method of evaluating the impact of services at a community mental center. *American Journal of Community Psychology, 6*, 291-302.

Flynn, T.C., Balch, R., Kevis, S.B., & Katz, B. (1981). Predicting client improvement from and satisfaction with community mental health center services. *American Journal of Community Psychology, 9*(3), 339-346.

Frank, R., Salzman, K., & Fergus, E. (1977). Correlates of consumer satisfaction with outpatient therapy assessed by postcards. *Community Mental Health Journal, 13*37-45.

Garfield, S.L. (1971). Research on client variables in psychotherapy. In A.E. Bergin & S.L. Garfield (Eds.), *Handbook of psychotherapy and behavior change* (pp.271-298). New York: John Wiley and Sons.

Guest, L. (1948). The public's attitudes toward psychologists. *American Psychologist, 3*, 135-139.

Hart, W.T. & Bassett, L. (1975). Measuring consumer satisfaction in a mental health center. *Hospital and Community Psychiatry. 26*(8), 512-515.

Heilbrun, A.B. (1972). Effects of briefing upon client satisfaction with the initial counseling contact. *Journal of Consulting and Clinical Psychology, 38* (1), 50-56.

Hoehn-Saric, R., Frank, J., Imber, S., Nash, E., Stone, A. & Battle, C. (1964). Systematic preparation of patients for psychotherapy. I. Effects on therapy behavior and outcome. *Journal of Psychiatric Research. 2*, 267-281.

Kabatznick, R. (1984). The public's percepton of psychology: Attitudes of four selected groups. *Unpublished doctoral dissertation,* City University of New York.

Klerman, L.V. (1969). Health counseling in industrial clinics: The employee's view. *Journal of Occupational Medicine, 11*(8), 417-421.

Kopolow, L.E. (1979). Consumer demands in mental health care. *International Journal of Law and Psychiatry, 3*, 263-270.

Kunin, C.C. & Rodin, M.J. (1982). The interactive effects of counselor gender, physical attractiveness, and status on client self-disclosure. *Journal of Clinical Psycholgoy, 38*(1), 84-90.

Larsen, D., Atkisson, C., Hargreaves, W., & Nguyen, T. (1979). Assessment of client/patient satisfaction: Development of a general scale. *Evaluation and Program Planning, 1*, 42-54.

Lebow, J. (1982). Consumer satisfaction with mental health treatment. *Psychological Bulletin, 91*(2), 244-259.

Lorefice, L.S., & Borus, J.F. (1984). Consumer evaluation of a community mental health service, II: Perceptions of clinical care. *American Journal of Psychiatry, 141* (11), 1449-1452.

Love, R.E., Caid, C.D., & Davis, A. (1979). The user satisfaction surey: Consumer evaluation of an inner city community mental health center. *Evaluation and the Health Professions, 1* 42-54.

Maskin, M.B. (1974). Differential impact of student counselors' self-concept on clients' perceptions of therapeutic effectiveness. *Psychological Reports, 34,* 967-969.

McKay, J.K., Dowd, E.T., & Rollins, S.A. (1982). Clients' characteristics as mediating variables in perception of counselors' social influence. *Perceptual and Motor Skills, 54,* 522-526.

McWilliams, S.A., & Morris, L.A. (1974). Community attitudes about mental health services. *Commuity Mental Health Journal, 10*(4), 236-242.

Meyer, J.H. & Zegans, L.S. (1975) Adolescents perceive their psychotherapy. *Psychiatry, 28,* 11-22.

Obitz, F.W. (1974). Alcoholics' perceptions of selected counseling techniques. *British Journal of Addictions, 70,* 187-191.

Otto, J. & Moss, R. (1974). Patient expectations and attendance in community treatment programs. *Community Mental Health Journal, 10*(1), 9-15.

Padilla, E. Elinson, J., & Perkins, M.F. (1966). The public image of mental health professionals and acceptance of community mental health services. *American Journal of Public Health, 56*(9), 1524-1529.

Pallak, M.S., & Kilburg, R.R. (1986). Psychology, public affairs, and public policy: A strategy and review. *American Psychologist, 41*(9), 922-940.

Richman, J., & Charles, E. (1976). Patient dissatisfaction and attempted suicide. Community Mental Health Journal, 16(3), 301-305.

Richmond, J. (1984). Comparison of clients' and nonclients' expectations of counseling. *Psychological Reports, 54,* 752-754.

Rogers, C.R., Gendlin, G.T., Kiesler, D.V., & Truax, C.B. (1967). *The therapeutic relationship and its impact: A study of psychotherapy with schizophrenics.* Madison: Unviersity of Wisconsin Press.

Schainblatt, A.H. (1980). What happens to the clients? *Community Mental Health Journal, 16*(4), 331-342.

Schiff, S.K. (1970). Community accountability and mental health services. *Mental Hygiene, 54*(2), 205-214.

Smith, M.L., Glass, C.V., & Miller, T.I. (1980). *The benefits of Psychotherapy.* Baltimore: Johns Hopkins University Press.

Solomon, K., & Harris, M.R. (1977). A study of client acceptance of various professionals in psychiatric home visits. *Hospital and Community Psychiatry, 28*(9), 661-665.

Strupp, H.H., Fox, R.E. & Lesser, K. (1969). *Patients view their psychotherapy.* Baltimore: Johns Hopkins Unviersity Press.

Tessler, R. (1975). Clients' reactions to initial interviews: Determinant of relationship-centered and problem centered satisfaction. *Journal of counseling Psychology, 22,* 187-191.

Truax, C.B. & Mitchell, K.M. (1971). Research in a certain therapist interpersonal skills in relation to process and outcome. In *Handbook of psychotherapy and behavior change.* (pp.299-344). A.E. Bergin & S.L. Garfield (Eds.), New York: John Wiley and Sons.

Weber, D.J. & Tilley, D.H. (1981) Patients' evaluations of the mental health service at a health sciences campus. *Journal of the American College Health Association, 29,* 193-194.

Wood, W., Jones, M. & Benjamin, L.T. (1986). Surveying psychology's public image. *American Psychologist, 41* (9), 947-953.

Yalom, I, Houts, P., Newell, G. & Rand, K. (1967). Preparation of patients for group therapy. *Archives of General Psychiatry, 17*416-427.

Yokopenic P.A., Clark, V.A. & Anehensel, C.S. (1983). Depression, problem recognition, and professional consultation. *The Journal of Nervous and Mental Disease, 171*(1), 15-23.

S E C T I O N

B

**Patient
and
Practitioner**

CHAPTER

42

PSYCHOTHERAPY AND SUPERVISION FOR THE PRIVATE PRACTITIONER

Jerold R. Gold, Ph.D.

This chapter considers the private practitioner as a potential *consumer* of professional services rather than as a provider of services. Two particularly important services available to the practitioner—psychotherapy and supervision—will be discussed. The professional and personal needs and reasons for obtaining such services will be reviewed, as will the specific and often unique issues that assist or hinder the independent clinician in making the decision to enter therapy or supervision. The chapter will also include discussion of how private practitioners select therapists and supervisors, and of some of the finer details of the types of these experiences that are available, including potential advantages and disadvantages of each.

PSYCHOTHERAPY FOR THE PRIVATE PRACTITIONER

Reasons for Seeking Psychotherapy

The discussion that follows will focus specifically on the unique role demands placed upon the private practitioner that may influence that individual to decide to enter psychotherapy. It is not intended to lead to the conclusion that psychotherapists become consumers of psychotherapy solely, or even largely, because of their professional activities. Instead, it is an attempt to describe the reasons for seeking psychotherapy that are inherent to the maintenance of a private practice.

The psychotherapist in private practice who enters psychotherapy as a consumer (client or patient) may do so for any of the multitude of intrapsychic, interpersonal, familial, or existential reasons that the nonpsychotherapist consumer seeks out a psychotherapist. Therapists after all are people with the same vulnerabilities to anxiety, depression, loss, sadness, anger, fear of intimacy, or any of the disorders listed in the third edition of the *Diagnostic and Statistical Manual of Mental Disorders*, as any other human beings. However, often there are other factors that influence the private practitioners to seek out help, and these factors are the products of the practitioners's professional activities and the effect of those activities upon his or her psychological life.

Psychotherapy is a deeply involving, emotionally arousing, and often painful experience for patient and therapist alike. It is an experience in which the personal resources of both participants are tested, strained and often pushed to their limit. Certain schools of psychotherapy explicitly state that the therapeutic relationship is the critical, decisive factor in determining favorable or unfavorable outcome (Rogers, 1957), and almost all theoretical approaches include a strong emphasis on the importance of relational factors (Weiner, 1975). Within this emphasis, implicitly or occasionally explicitly (Rogers, 1957; Freud, 1937), is contained the notion that the therapist's level of personal development and "mental health" may be the upper limit upon growth available to the patient. Couched in such terms as "countertransference," "participant observation," "warmth, genuineness, and accurate empathy," and "personal encounter," current psychotherapeutic interest focuses intensively upon the therapist's ability to interact with his or her patients in a health-and-growth-promoting way.

Such an interaction typically is defined as one wherein the therapist keeps his or her conflicts and interpersonal difficulties to a minimum and is able to interact with patients in a strong, warm, sensitive, and empathetic manner. Such attributes generally are thought to be less available to the therapist when he or she is experiencing personal distress. These experiential and theoretical issues, with which most psychotherapists are faced during their training and then repeatedly as professional practitioners, lead many psychotherapists to construe personal psychotherapy as a necessary part of becoming and then maintaining themselves as effective practitioners. Freud (1937), in one of his last and most controversial recommendations about the practice of psychoanalysis, suggested that analysts undergo reanalysis at 5-year intervals to cope with the psychological issues generated by their analytical work and by the anxieties and conflicts of everyday life and ongoing adult development and aging.

The psychotherapist in private practice may be more vulnerable to the personal stresses imposed by the activity of psychotherapy upon its practitioners than is the institutional psychotherapist. There are several possible reasons for this heightened vulnerability. Institutional work often offers formal and informal support services to the psychotherapist, in the form of staff meetings, case conferences, supervision, seminars, and readily available companionship for coffee breaks, lunch, or normal socializing. Frequently, graduate training programs and internship or residency programs offer psychotherapists in training group experiences or group psychotherapy. It is also the case that in many institutional settings, psychotherapy is just one of the activities in which a staff member is engaged during the work day. The opportunities for collegial interchange and exchange, for socializing, and for involvement in extra-psychotherapeutic professional activities may lessen significantly the stressful impact of psychotherapy upon the therapist. Such experiences may even give that therapist important quasi-therapeutic relationships in which to work out problematic issues and to process the conflicts and emotions aroused by psychotherapeutic activity. In contrast, the private practitioner typically works in greater isolation than the institutional therapist does and the private practitioner therefore may experience more loneliness and more of a sense of total responsibility for his or her patients. The opportunities for collegial interaction, socialization, and the quasi-therapeutic effects of such interaction are less readily available. In addition, therapists in full-time independent practice often spend a much higher percentage of their time actually conducting psychotherapy than do any institutional clinicians. Such a combination of loneliness, isolation, heightened responsibility, lessened availability of professional and personal support systems, and increased temporal involvement in the provision of direct service may make the independent clinician particularly vulnerable to the demands and stresses of the work.

There are other psychosocial stresses that may impinge upon the clinician beginning a practice or moving from part- to full-time practice. Such changes in one's professional life may involve a significant change in self-image or pesonal identity, as the individual has to redefine the self in more specialized, autonomous ways. Often this change involves seeing oneself as a business person who must compete in an open marketpalce, develop new skills, and take new personal and economic risks for which previous life experiences, graduate training, and institutional work were not preparation. Such changes may eventuate in anxiety and self-doubt, which may cause significant professional and personal distress.

Many of the issues just touched upon are also raised in the extensive theoretical and clinical discussions of professional "burnout" and professionals in distress (Kilburg et al., 1986) that have entered the literature in the past 10 or so years. Obviously, psychotherapy is no more a panacea for the professional and personal problems of its practitioners than it is for the ills of the rest of humanity. Yet, it may be an ethical and moral necessity as well as a matter of personal satisfaction and comfort for the distressed therapist to seek out therapeutic assistance, as the adverse impact of the therapist's impaired functioning upon the individuals who consult him or her can be enormous. Many of the factors described above that heighten the vulnerability of the private practitioner can be prevented or ameliorated by environmental manipulation: joining professional societies, obtaining ongoing supervision or postgraduate training, establishing a social network of other practitioners. However, these efforts are often insufficient to combat the therapist's distress, and certainly cannot help significantly with the more basic affective, cognitive, or relational difficulties in the therapist with which the professional stresses are interacting. Therefore, for the therapist as for any other troubled or vulnerable person, psychotherapy becomes the intervention of choice to avert or to correct personal or professional difficulties when more limited interventions fail (and hopefully, psychotherapy will have begun prior to the failure of other efforts).

SUPERVISION FOR THE PRIVATE PRACTITIONER

Reasons for Seeking Supervision in Private Practice

The need for the practitioner to learn about the profession and to improve and redefine clinical skills does not end when he or she opens a private office. To the contrary, the added stress and responsibility of independent practice, and the absence of built-in opportunities for in-service training, review, and supervision by a department head or informal collegial guidance and discussion, may intensify the need for periodic or ongoing assistance. Many practitioners resist recognizing or acting on this need out of fear of surrendering their professional autonomy and independence. Yet it is extremely difficult to pinpoint one's blind spots without an outside perspective, and isolation from one's colleagues can often serve to make the private practitioner particularly vulnerable to getting caught in deepening vicious circles of confusion and error. Also, continuing to keep up with professional knowledge on ones' own requires a high level of self-direction and self-discipline. Such issues typically are the impetus for seeking out the assistance of a supervisor.

Venues for Supervision

Supervision in Postgraduate Education   Much of the supervision utilized by private practitioners is obtained withn the context of a postgraduate education. A wide variety of institutions including hospitals, clinics, universities, and free standing institutes, offer private practitioners the opportunity to learn and to specialize in a particular brand of psychotherapy. Such programs include, but are not limited to, postgraduate programs in psychoanalysis, family therapy, behavior therapy, cognitive therapy, gestalt therapy, transactional analysis, rational/emotive therapy, and humanistic psychotherapy. Other programs teach a more integrative or eclectic approach to psychotherapy. Most of such programs share certain common features and requirements, which include completion of a prescribed course of didactic classroom instruction, participation in extensive clinical practice, and completion of a certain, usually extensive, number of supervision hours. In such a setting, supervison typically is provided by faculty members, "approved" supervisors who are affiliated with the training program. Such supervision therefore often takes on an evaluative function as well as a purely educative role for the supervisee, as the supervisor is the representative of the program and often is asked to certify the therapist's progress and skills. Such a split role at times makes it difficult for the therapist to feel completely comfortable in presenting his or her clinical work, out of the need to impress and please the supervisor and to protect his or her own progress within the institution. Another potential source of difficulty in this type of supervision can be ideological; that is, if the supervisor or the supervisee defines the interaction as one of transmitting a particular theoretical or clinical "truth" rather than as a more individualized learning experience. While such a situation might develop in supervision outside the context of an institute setting, it is most likely to occur within this kind of setting.

Such contextual difficulties may limit the freedom of the supervisee to learn to think for himself or herself, and to work on areas of confusion or weakness that are in need of serious examination and correction. However, these difficulties are often counterbalanced or outweighed by the advantages of postgraduate education, of which there are several. They include the integration of supervision with a formalized and directed exposure to the relevant clinical and theoretical literature, and the involvement of the practitioner in a structured program, which potentially can be enriching in terms of social opportunities and chances for exchange of ideas and clinical experiences with a peer group. Such collegial contact can go a long way toward alleviating the loneliness and isolation of private practice, and can be an invaluable source of supervisory input for the therapist as well. Another advantage of the institute experience is the potential for exposure to, and supervisory experience with, some of the leaders in that specific area of psychotherapy represented by the particular program. Often, more established, innovative, and productive practitioners can be obtained as supervisors only within the context of an institute or postgraduate program.

Private Supervision   Supervision on a private, fee-for-service basis is available to the private practitioner at any time during his or her career, as long as he or she can afford it financially and temporally and there is a supervisor available. Some private practitioners use supervision as a substitute for formal postgraduate education, while others use it before, after, or along with a formal training experience.

The Private Practitioner's Resistances to Psychotherapy

As we all know too well, psychotherapy never goes completely smoothly, and each ongoing treatment relationship will be affected by the individual's ways of avoiding, denying, or otherwise resisting the significant issues aroused by the treatment. The psychotherapist patient again may bring to psychotherapy certain role-related issues and concerns that will impact uniquely and significantly on the process and outcome of therapy. Many clinicians share the same prejudices toward psychotherapy and psychological disturbance as are held by nonclinicians. They may experience their stresses, job related or not, as personal failures or as moral, ethical, or professional weakness or incompetence. Out of this outlook grows the cognitive/emotional construction of a need for psychotherapy as a stimulus for and cause of professional and personal embarrassment and shame. These attitudes are inculcated at times by the psychotherapist's own experiences in professional training programs that, subtly or openly, disparage or discourage trainees from seeking treatment, or at least do not model the positive use of psychotherapy for members of the profession.

The clinician in private practice may experience other difficulties in being a patient in psychotherapy as a result of comparisons of himself or herself with prospective therapists and with the therapist who is chosen finally. Professional and personal competition, ambitions, envy, and jealousy about personal success, competence, status, and so on are among the issues that may color the tone and progress of psychotherapy, and many clinicians will find such issues uncomfortable and will be uneasy about entering a situation in which they will be faced potentially with such ideas and emotions. Another concern typical of the psychotherapist in private practice when involved in psychotherapy is anxiety about professional autonomy. Most clinicians enter private practice after extended apprenticeships in their professions, and often the establishment of a private practice is in part an expression of and reinforcement for their sense of autonomy and personal and professional independence. Therefore, some practitioners find that asking for and receiving help leads to thinking about themselves as dependent and as unable to function professionally in an independent way.

Certainly these issues and whatever other professionally connected issues arise in the psychotherapy of independent practitioners are not unique to psychotherapists; nor do they ordinarily interfere with treatment more or less than do any other issues. Still, they remain salient features of the private practitioner/patient's experience that cannot be ignored.

Choice of a Psychotherapist

Again, the factors that influence the practitioner/patient in choosing a psychotherapist do not differ greatly from these factors that influence most patients: personal reputation of the therapist, recommendations by respected peers and colleagues, availability of the therapist, sex and age of the therapist, fee and geographic location of the therapist. In a study of how psychotherapists choose their own psychotherapist, Basile (1985) found that practicing therapists and lawyers did not differ in how they selected therapists for themselves. Both groups typically obtained names of prospective therapists from respected colleagues or friends, and most often made a final decision primarily on the basis of personal qualities such as warmth, empathy, understanding, and competence perceived in their initial contact with the therapist.

Yet other factors not included in Basile's (1985) study also seem to influence the selection of a psychotherapist by a psychotherapist to one degree or another. These include: "generation" of the therapist (most therapists choose for themselves therapists who are more experienced and at a more advanced level of professional development); theoretical orientation of the therapist; the therapist's professional status and reputation; and the therapist's potential as a future colleague, referral source, or supervisor. An interesting and as yet empirically unexplored area is the relationship between practitioners' awareness of the power of psychotherapy to elicit both positive and negative effects (Strupp, et al., 1977) and the process through which they determine who among their colleagues wold be most likely to be most effective in helping patients. Therapists probably rely on their "insiders'" fund of knowledge about the field in general as well as on the same nonobjective and secondhand sources of data as do most patients.

SUPERVISION FOR THE PRIVATE PRACTITIONER

Reasons for Seeking Supervision in Private Practice

The need for the practitioner to learn about the profession and to improve and redefine clinical skills does not end when he or she opens a private office. To the contrary, the added stress and responsibility of independent practice, and the absence of built-in opportunities for in-service training, review, and supervision by a department head or informal collegial guidance and discussion, may intensify the need for periodic or ongoing assistance. Many practitioners resist recognizing or acting on this need out of fear of surrendering their professional autonomy and independence. Yet it is extremely difficult to pinpoint one's blind spots without an outside perspective, and isolation from one's colleagues can often serve to make the private practitioner particularly vulnerable to getting caught in deepening vicious circles of confusion and error. Also, continuing to keep up with professional knowledge on ones' own requires a high level of self-direction and self-discipline. Such issues typically are the impetus for seeking out the assistance of a supervisor.

Venues for Supervision

Supervision in Postgraduate Education   Much of the supervision utilized by private practitioners is obtained withn the context of a postgraduate education. A wide variety of institutions including hospitals, clinics, universities, and free standing institutes, offer private practitioners the opportunity to learn and to specialize in a particular brand of psychotherapy. Such programs include, but are not limited to, postgraduate programs in psychoanalysis, family therapy, behavior therapy, cognitive therapy, gestalt therapy, transactional analysis, rational/emotive therapy, and humanistic psychotherapy. Other programs teach a more integrative or eclectic approach to psychotherapy. Most of such programs share certain common features and requirements, which include completion of a prescribed course of didactic classroom instruction, participation in extensive clinical practice, and completion of a certain, usually extensive, number of supervision hours. In such a setting, supervison typically is provided by faculty members, "approved" supervisors who are affiliated with the training program. Such supervision therefore often takes on an evaluative function as well as a purely educative role for the supervisee, as the supervisor is the representative of the program and often is asked to certify the therapist's progress and skills. Such a split role at times makes it difficult for the therapist to feel completely comfortable in presenting his or her clinical work, out of the need to impress and please the supervisor and to protect his or her own progress within the institution. Another potential source of difficulty in this type of supervision can be ideological; that is, if the supervisor or the supervisee defines the interaction as one of transmitting a particular theoretical or clinical "truth" rather than as a more individualized learning experience. While such a situation might develop in supervision outside the context of an institute setting, it is most likely to occur within this kind of setting.

Such contextual difficulties may limit the freedom of the supervisee to learn to think for himself or herself, and to work on areas of confusion or weakness that are in need of serious examination and correction. However, these difficulties are often counterbalanced or outweighed by the advantages of postgraduate education, of which there are several. They include the integration of supervision with a formalized and directed exposure to the relevant clinical and theoretical literature, and the involvement of the practitioner in a structured program, which potentially can be enriching in terms of social opportunities and chances for exchange of ideas and clinical experiences with a peer group. Such collegial contact can go a long way toward alleviating the loneliness and isolation of private practice, and can be an invaluable source of supervisory input for the therapist as well. Another advantage of the institute experience is the potential for exposure to, and supervisory experience with, some of the leaders in that specific area of psychotherapy represented by the particular program. Often, more established, innovative, and productive practitioners can be obtained as supervisors only within the context of an institute or postgraduate program.

Private Supervision   Supervison on a private, fee-for-service basis is available to the private practitioner at any time during his or her career, as long as he or she can afford it financially and temporally and there is a supervisor available. Some private practitioners use supervision as a substitute for formal postgraduate education, while others use it before, after, or along with a formal training experience.

There are several advantages inherent in private supervision which can be seen when it is compared with institutionally sanctioned supervision. The number of possible supervisors available to the clinician increases enormously, and is limited by personal choice rather than by institutional rules or approval. Such supervision usually is less subject to externally derived conditions of duration and scheduling, in that the contract between supervisor and supervisee can be individually tailored to meet the needs of both individuals, and does not have to satisfy any institutional requirements.

In choosing a private supervisor, the clinician has greater opportunity for exposing himself or herself to alternative theoretical and clinical modalities and approaches, and need be less concerned with the ideological and political issues that may be part of institutionally based supervision. Similarly, in a private setting the supervisor is the employee of the supervisee, and in such a situation the formal evaluative aspects of the supervisory relationship can be avoided totally, though certainly these issues may emerge in a subjective sense (see Section 3 Individual Supervision).

There are areas of weakness in the private supervisory experience. As noted above, many outstanding, experienced clinicians are available as supervisors largely or exclusively in institutional settings, or such individuals's fees for private supervision may be out of reach of many clinicians' budgets. Private supervision may avoid the political and ideological structures and entanglements of postgraduate education, but it also may miss the intellectually and socially enriching features of such a comprehensive approach, as well as the academic rigor and stimulation of the institutional environment.

Supervisory Frameworks

Supervision can be conducted within three modalities, all of which are often available within both the private and the institutional venues. These supervisory modalities are the individual supervisory experience, group supervision, and peer supervision, each of which offers practitioners unique benefits and limitations in furthering their learning.

Individual Supervision   This is the supervisory arrangement with which most clinicians will be familiar from their graduate education. In such an arrangement the practitioner and supervisor meet on a regularly scheduled, or sometimes on an as-needed, basis to review one or a few of the practitioner's cases. The advantage as to the practitioner of such an arrangement include exclusivity of the supervisor's attention and interest during the supervisory session, and the opportunity to focus in depth on whatever material is determined to be the object of study of both participants (see Technical

Orientations in Supervision, below). The ingredients for establishing a successful supervisory experience in this modality parallel the requirements for establishing successful therapeutic arrangement. The supervisor must convey a sense of respect, empathy, and warmth, and must be aware of his or her impact upon the therapist when engaged in exploration of the therapist's work or instruction of the therapist (Epstien, 1986). The therapist must over time come to trust the supervisor sufficiently to allow for an open and honest presentation of material. There must exist also a certain level of general clinical and theoretical agreement between the two participants about how to conduct clinical work, coupled with an understanding of and respect for each person's individualized and uniquely formed ideas.

The potential for the individual supervisory relationship to evoke either a master-apprentice interaction (Levenson, 1983) or a quasi-psychotherapeutic relationship (Wolstein, 1984) must be addressed by both parties as the relationship is established and as it advances. Supervision can enrich and instruct or it can limit the autonomy of the supervisee, wound his or her self-esteem, and cause the clinician to see himself or herself as second best or incapable of ever reaching the same level of competence as the supervisor. Such effects may be avoided or countered by humility and awareness of the supervisor's impact on the psychotherapist and by the supervisee's willingness to call attention to these issues as they emerge. Individual supervision works out successfully when supervisor and supervisee "match" to a necessary and sufficient degree personally and cognitively. In such situations the supervisory relationship can grow into a powerfully moving, professionally and personally important experience for both participants wherein both parties learn about their work and themselves in an enriching and vital way. Supervisory relationships that are marked by distrust, anxiety, or extreme differences in theoretical and clinical approaches will often lead to negative consequences for both participants: avoidance; "marking time" until the relationship ends (most prevalent in institutional supervision); acting out in the form of missed appointments, lateness, or concealment of clinical data; or experiences of boredom, hostility, disappointment, or depression. Such negative experience may eventuate in untoward consequences for the supervisee's patients, as well as for the supervisory dyad. As a result, some intervention in the supervisory relationship is necessary, including such possibilities as mutual exploration of the problem, consultation with a third party, or if necessary, termination of the supervisory contract.

Group Supervision   In this modality supervision is purchased from the supervisor by two or more clinicians, who attend the supervisory sessions together and who share the allotted time. Such sessions may be shared in a variety of ways; from an informal, as-needed basis to a predetermined session by session or other time-bound rotation system. In such an arrangement the supervisor theoretically shares some of his or her authority as all members are invited to participate in the discussion of the clinical material, though in practice the amount of input from group members will vary considerably as a function of the interpersonal climate of the group and of the supervisor's leadership style, interest in group input, and ability to facilitate and to promote group interaction. In advocating group supervision as the preferred modality of psychoanalytic supervision, Wolstein (1984) argues that the group arrangement facilitates the process in a number of ways. He suggests that it lessens the inclination to transform supervision into psychotherapy by diminishing the intensity of the supervisory relationship, and allows the therapist to understand his or her relationship to the patient as it is played out in parallel transferences to the other members of their group.

Wolstein's position is far from universally accepted at this time. However, the advantages he claims for group supervision have been noted by other clinicians, and there are additional advantages to this arrangement as well. Group supervision, when well conducted, allows for much interaction among members, including the supervisor, during whch differing points of view about clinical work can be debated and discussed. Such a process may allow supervision to be experienced as a collaborative, exploratory event, wherein members learn how to learn about themselves and their work in fruitful and creative ways. This ambience is likely to prevent or counter the tendencies to idealize the supervisor and to devalue one's own skills that can result from individual supervision. Certainly, such processes of idealization and devaluation can eventuate from group supervision if it is conducted by an authoritarian, directive supervisor, but the group setting may help to diffuse the impact of that variable more than an individual setting could. Another invaluable aspect of group supervision is the opportunity for the therapist to examine the effects of his or her therapeutic relationship upon relationships with other members of the group. This study of the "parallel processes" of psychotherapy and supervision may illuminate unconscious aspects of the transference–countertransference situation in the psychotherapy under discussion, and the group setting particularly is congenial to such an approach, as different facets of the therapist's relationship with the patient may be elicited and enacted with various members of the group. Group supervision obviously conveys to each participant a more pluralistic view of clinical process than often is possible in individual supervision, and the opportunities for expanding one's social and professional network are greater than they are in a one-to-one setting.

Group supervision, however, does not offer the ongoing opportunities for in-depth, continuous focus on the therapist's work, as the time must be shared or divided. Group processes and issue of competitiveness, envy and jealousy, ambitiousness, hostility, and distrust, among others, may emerge between members or between one or several members and the supervisor. Such issues must be dealt with by the group and/or the supervisor in a prompt and competent way. If the supervisor is not inclined or is unable to assist the group in dealing with such interpersonal issues, or if group members are unwilling or unable to work on such problems, the requisite atmosphere for professional and personal growth will not develop.

Peer Supervision   Peer supervison refers to the increasingly popular practice among private practitioners of establishing a regularly scheduled group for supervision that is led solely by the members themselves. The group meets at the home or office of one of its members, and cases are presented for discussion according to a prearranged schedule or on an as-needed basis. Each group member operates on an equal footing and is free to enquire about the case or to make suggestions. Organizational rules and perspectives on the nature of case material and the types of discussions will vary considerably from group to group. Some peer groups are established by colleagues who wish to have the group characterized by a particular methodological or theoretical orientation to clinical work, and members are chosen on the basis of their ideological like-mindedness as well as (or rather than) for personal compatibility. Other peer groups are formed out of a desire to study patients of a particular diagnostic grouping or in the hopes of dealing with a specific or a few pressing clinical issues, such as working with elderly patients, with men's or women's issues in therapy, and so on. Such issue-oriented peer groups may be theoretically homogeneous or heterogeneous, and at time such theory-oriented and issue-oriented groups will include, to a greater or lesser degree, a focus on relevant clinical writings as well as case material.

A third, and probably the most typical, type of peer supervision group is the group of colleagues or friends who join together out of a need for social contact, mutual support, and continued opportunities for learning. In such a group interpersonal compatibility is usually the primary factor for member selection, with theoretical or technical issues being of secondary importance.

Peer supervision is popular among its adherents for a number of reasons. It does not cost its members anything financially, and the absence of an identified supervisor/leader may allow group members an opportunity to challenge themselves and each other to question, observe, and learn from their work without having an "authority" to fall back on. Similarly, the absence of a paid supervisor, who would invariably be more senior than group members, may be liberating to the members and may allow them to present their work more openly. Finally, peer supervision, when it takes place within a congenial group setting, can be a richly invigorating social experience. Peer groups often stay together for several or even many years with the makeup of the group in a very stable state, and such ongoing groups frequently become the core source of collegial companionship and guidance, referrals, and other professional necessities for many members.

The successful peer group must be able to tolerate and to process the same interpersonal issues that were mentioned above in the discussion of group supervison, as such tensions probably are inevitable outgrowths of interactions in ongoing social groups. The absence of a supervisor makes the responsibility for such processing and resolution the equal responsibility of each member, and it is around these issues that many peer groups flounder and ultimately disband. At time the effectiveness of a peer group is limited by the very fact that its members are peers and that someone of more senior status is not present. Though it is a common enough experience for many practitioners that one's peers often are as helpful or more helpful than anyone else, there are clinical situations that can call for a particular level of expertise. Finally, one of peer supervision's most attractive features may evolve ino a potentially serious drawback. The social gratifications and rewards of peer contact for the private practitioner may be so enjoyable that the group meetings become predominantly or exclusively social events. While such regularly scheduled social meetings are vitally important for independent practitioners in combatting isolation, loneliness, and stress, they will not meet the direct professional and educational needs that led to establishment of the group. Some peer groups handle this by setting agendas and presentation schedules in advance, while others drift casually between socialization and supervision as the mood of the group dictates. Still others try to build in time for both activities on a scheduled basis. When the efforts fail to achieve a balance between social and educational needs, some peer groups give up any pretense of holding supervision sessions, while others go the opposite route and hire an outside supervisor.

Technical Orientations in Supervision

Whether supervison is obtained privately or in the context of an institution and whether it is conducted individually or in groups, the contract between supervisor and supervisee will be based on an agreement to review the clinical work of the supervisee, with the supervisor acting as teacher, guide, role model, or adviser. In practice and in principle, the supervisor–supervisee relationship will be based on certain ideas about the nature of supervision and the types of activities that are permissible and advantageous for each party within supervision. A discussion of three approaches to supervision and to the relationship between the participants in supervision will conclude this chapter. These approaches will be presented as distinct methods for the sake of clarity while it will be recognized by all that in actual practice elements of each approach will be present to some degree in most supervision experiences.

Case-Oriented Approaches to Supervision   This approach to supervision probably is the most frequently employed approach, and will be familiar to the majority of private practitioners from their earlier training experiences. The case-oriented approach is one wherein supervisor and supervisee review progress notes, audiotapes, and/or videotapes to understand and to elucidate "what happened" in a particular segment of the supervisee's clinical work. The foci of discussion are generated from the clinical data as reproduced and the supervisor's efforts are aimed at improving the therapist's understanding of the case material, enhancing the therapist's perceptions of the interpersonal transactions with the patient or patients, and helping the therapist to learn when and how to intervene within a similar clinical context in the future.

The case orientation is best understood then as a technical, "how to work" model of supervision. It can be invaluable in assisting a therapist to formulate a troublesome case in a fresh and enlightening way, or in helping a private practitioner to expand and deepen his or her ability to listen constructively and to use such an expanded appreciation of clinical material in a technically more acute and helpful way. Such an approach, however, is handicapped by its potential for turning into a master-apprentice ("I would have done this so you do it") type of relationship and by its frequent reliance on reconstructed case material or on tapes. The exclusive focus on case data, while absolutely essential, can at times exlude other invaluable sources of relevant information, which are emphasized in moderate or extreme ways in other supervisory approaches.

The Psychotherapy Approach to Supervision   This approach is at the opposite end of the spectrum from the case-oriented approach. In the psychotherapy approach, the therapist's reactions, dreams, patterns of relating, and conflicts are explored, as well as any other aspects of his or her psychology. Such exploration typically is conceptualized as "working with countertransference" or is given some other theoretical label, but the rationale in differing theoretical settings for such an approach is the same: The therapist is viewed as the agent of therapeutic change, and his or her reactions to the patient, within session or without are seen as the most important data within therapy, and as the greatest potential sources of difficulty within the clinical process. Supervision is focused largely on discussing and reviewing the therapist's experiences with, and reactions to, the patient, and the clinical material is used as a springboard for identifying and clarifying "counter-transference" phenomena. The supervisor utilizing such an approach will function in a quasi-therapeutic manner, utilizing the specific techniques and methods suggested by his or her clinical orientation, to assist the therapist in his or her quest for enhanced self-knowledge, sensitivity, and awareness.

The psychotherapy approach to supervision is beneficial particularly when issues of technique and cognitive mastery of clinical work are not foremost among the needs of the private practitioner. Such an approach requires a great deal of respect and trust between supervisor and supervisee, and the relationship can be clouded by the temptation, on the part of one or both parties, to overtly or covertly transform the interaction into a full-scale psychotherapy for the practitioner. This transformation might be valuable or in fact necessary, but it will also lead to a loss of the opportunity to learn about one's clinical work. Similarly, as Cooper and Witenberg (1985) have noted, not all clinical difficulties arise out of countertransference issues: Sometimes the therapist does not know what's going on technically and has not been able to formulate the case in a useful way. Exclusive supervisory focus on the therapist's psychology may deprive the practitioner of invaluable cognitive learning.

This approach to supervision proceeds most usefully when this orientation is known to the supervisee at the outset, and is agreed to by the supervisee. One all-too-frequent source of conflict and dissatisfaction in supervision results from a mismatch of approaches desired by supervisor and supervisee, and a supervisee who unknowingly encounters a psychotherapy approach while seeking a case-oriented approach often will be extremely distressed and disappointed.

The Process Orientation to Supervisor   This approach is eclectic and integrative in that it combines features of the case orientation and the psychotherapy orientation, while adding features unique to itself. Process-oriented supervision utilizes thorough review of case material, clinical formulation, and technical approaches, while adding the frequent study of the supervisor–supervisee relationship as an at times equal or more important source of data. The interpersonal processes that unfold in the supervision are construed as an isomorphic transformation of interpersonal processes operating within the patient–therapist relationship. That is, certain features of interaction within supervision are thought to reflect and to reproduce unwitting ways in which the therapist and patient may be interacting with each other, interactional patterns that depict particularly the character structure and interactional style of the patient in past and current significant relationships. Examination of the supervisory relationship allows both participants in it the chance to study in vivo these unwitting aspects of the patient–therapist interaction that are unnoticed by the therapist and go unreported in case notes and that may be obscured in audio or video recordings by the verbal content and more global behaviors of the dyad. These in vivo phenomena can be translated in super-vision into an expanded understanding of case material by attempts at in-tegrating the patient's verbalizations and history with his or her effect on the therapist. Alternately, process issues within the supervisory relationship may lead to the identification and exploration of a conflict or problem in the therapist's psychology or interpersonal style that is affecting the therapeutic effort.

This orientation seems to offer to the private practitioner the best features of the other two supervision orientations, as it combines intellectual, technical, and personal foci. As noted above, such an approach to supervision succeeds best when it is agreed to clearly at the outset, and this approach requires two (or more) participants who are comfortable enough to discuss openly their impact on each other. Such openness is atypical of the training experiences of many practitioners and is not easily established. Another potential dis-advantage is the eclecticism of this orientation. There are at least four possi-ble areas of study in this approach: the case material, the supervisory rela-tionship, the psychology of the therapist, and even the psychology of the supervisor. Keeping the proper balance between these components and know-ing when to shift from one component to another, or when to stay with one component, are skills perhaps as difficult to attain as the clinical skills sought after in supervision.

REFERENCES

Basile, J. (1985). *How psychotherapist choose therapists.* Unupublished doctoral disser-tation, Adelphi Uiversity, Garden City, NY.

Cooper, A. & Witenberg, E. (1985). The "bogged down" treatment: A remedy. *Con-temporary Psychoanalysis, 21,* 27–41.

Epstein, L. (1986). Collusive selective inattention to the negative impact of the super-visory interaction. *Contemporary Psychoanalysis, 22,* 389–408.

Freud, S. (1937). Analysis terminable and interminable. In J. Strachey (Ed.), *Standard edition of the complete psychological works of Sigmund Freud.* London: Hogarth, 1964.

Kilburg, E., Nathan, P., & Thoreson, L. (1986). *Professionals in distress.* Washington, D.C.: American Psychological Association.

Levenson, E. (1983). *The ambiguity of change.* New York: Basic Books.

Rogers, C.R. (1957). The necessary and sufficient conditions of therapeutic personality change. *Journal of Consulting Psychology, 21,* 95–103.

Strupp, H.H., Hadley, S.W., & Gomes-Schwartz, B. (1977). *Psychotherapy for better or worse.* New York: Jason Aronson.

Weiner, I. (1975). *Principles of psychotherapy.* New York: Wiley & Sons.

Wolstein, B. (1984). A proposal to enlarge the individual model of psychoanalytic supervision. *Contemporary Psychoanalysis, 20*131–145.

C H A P T E R
43

EFFECTS OF PRIVATE PRACTICE ON THE THERAPIST'S PERSONAL LIFE

Jerold R. Gold, Ph.D.

It is probably the case that all working persons are affected significantly by their jobs or professions beyond the specifics of their working responsibilities. The private practitioner of psychotherapy is no exception, and in fact his or her profession may be uniquely influential in the practitioner's personal and family life. In the past two decades certain writers have investigated and reported on the singular stresses and demands of practicing psychoanalysis or psychotherapy (Klauber, 1981) and of delivering health or mental health services in general (Freudenberger, 1979). However, few if any of these studies have documented the specific effects of starting and maintaining a private psychotherapy practice upon the practitioner and the practitioner's family. It is the intent of this chapter to look at those effects and to outline both the positive and negative impact of private practice on several areas of the therapist's personal and family life, including such issues as available leisure time, the therapist's self-concept, need for and availability of social and collegial interaction and support, and maintenance of useful boundaries between work and personal life. In addition, certain vulnerabilities and potential contributing factors to therapist "burnout" in private practice will be discussed.

EFFECTS OF PRIVATE PRACTICE ON PERSONAL AND LEISURE TIME

Overworking And Its Effects

Private practice rarely takes place in the conventional work week. The practitioner who has just opened his or her first office usually has done so while holding down a part-time or even a full-!time job, and therefore the hours that he or she has available to see private patients are usually drawn from hours previously available for other, nonworking purposes. Similarly, independent practitioners with established practices still may find themselves working early morning, late afternoon, evening, and weekend hours because those hours are most attractive and convenient for the large majority of patients, who have their own occupational and family responsibilities during the midday period. This need to accommodate one's workday to the needs of working patients can lead to several possible effects on the therapist's private life. At the extreme, the therapist simply will cease having much of a private life, since he or she will be working from early morning to late evening 5, 6, or possibly even 7 days a week. In other more benign situations, the therapist may work a more reasonable number of hours but find that his or her mornings, evenings, and sometimes weekends are filled with work, while the late morning and early afternoon hours are free.

Obviously, there are many combinations and permutations of hourly arrangements in private practice, but the typical and most common effects on the therapist's personal life are that the therapist has less nonworking time in which to have a personal life, and often the hours that are available do not coincide with the hours available to others. The effects of this shrinkage and alteration in time are considerable. Many private practitioners work far too long and too hard, and simply do not have enough time or energy to attend to their needs for companionship and recreation. Spontaneous get-togethers with friends or family, or such commonplace activities as a spur-of-the-moment midweek evening movie, concert, or ball game, are replaced by carefully scheduled social events that often are as frantically planned as the work week. Since most couples and families are at home together during those hours when private practice is at its peak, the therapist may find that he or she does not have enough time and energy for being a spouse, lover, or parent. It is an all-too-common complaint of spouses or children of private practitioners that the therapist member of the family spends more time with, and has more enthusiasm for, patients than family members. Such perceptions and strained interactions can lead to marital, sexual, and familial estrangement and dissatisfaction, which often have the paradoxical effect of pushing the practitioner to invest even more time and energy in work, thereby entering into a vicious circle (Wachtel, 1977) of potentially disastrous consequences.

Overwork and overscheduling may have other less dramatic but no less important consequences for the private practitioner. Simple but absolutely necessary activities such as eating, exercising, homemaking, getting one's car serviced, and the like become chores of much meaning when one is working from morning to night. As a result, poor dietary and health habits may develop, and practices such as exercising regularly may be abandoned or engaged in only sporadically. At best, this kind of erratic self-care will lead to overweight, fatigue, poor appearance, and so on; and at worst, to serious health problems. Similarly, those overworked therapists who do not have a husband, wife, or housekeeper to depend upon will find themselves tremendously hassled by and despairing of taking care of the day-to-day needs of life, again with the consequences of fatigue, tension, and possible physical problems.

There is one further consequence of overworking that should be noted. At times overworking is a symptom of some neurotic need on the therapist's part to keep every hour filled, to master some anxiety or to avoid some other personal conflict. At other times overscheduling can result from financial need or from professional zeal and enthusiasm. Regardless of its source, all work and no play can turn one's work, previously loved and appreciated, into an aversive, hated, and hateful activity.

In addition to the dire professional consequences for the therapist, such a change in his or her relationship to work can provoke psychological distress ranging from anxiety to significant depression to psychosomatic symptoms. Such distress may permeate the therapist's life away from work (what little may be left of it) and may provoke an experience akin to an existential crisis (Bugenthal, 1964) in which much of life's meaning seems to disappear.

Is private practice then an unmitigated disaster for the practitioner on the personal level? If overscheduling is anticipated and avoided by judiciously planned means, the answer is a resounding no. Private practice is lucrative in two important respects, both of which may compensate for a loss of leisure time and enrich one's available leisure. First of all, most clinicians will earn more when they work more, and such remuneration is gratifying in itself, particularly when it is used wisely in one's private life. Secondly, in private practice the clinician often will have more opportunities to do the work he or she most wants to do, with those patients he or she most wants to work with and with greater freedom from bureaucracies and institutional requirements. Some satisfaction from work will tend to generalize to one's private life, as the practitioner's sense of occupational accomplishment makes him or her a more generally satisfied individual. The caveat here is the need to build into the day time for family or social contact, exercise, proper nutrition, reading, collegial interaction, and chores. Most practitioners who combat overwork successfully do so by religiously scheduling in breaks during the day in order to compensate for the sacrifice of early and late hours. What results then is a schedule of work and leisure that is not completely conventional but that maximizes personal needs and professional time in a workable compromise.

The Calendar Of Private Practice

A particular advantage of private practice is the freedom to decide when and how long to be away from work, assuming the compulsion to overschedule is avoided. Vacations can be scheduled according to the economic and personal needs of the practitioner and the clinical needs of his or her patients, and are not subject to institutional schedules or mandated numbers of vacation days. This freedom, coupled with the economic advantages of independent practice, can lead to more vacation time used in more enjoyable and rewarding ways. Vacation time may have certain additional stresses for the private practitioner, in that his or her patients are not under the care of a team or connected to an institution, either of which might act as a substitute for a vacationing institutional therapist. Unless arrangements for adequate, responsible coverage are made (and sometimes in spite of such arrangements), the therapist's vacation may be disrupted by anxieties about, and perhaps the need to be in contact with, particularly vulnerable patients.

The private practitioner who catches a cold or the flu, or who has to decide whether to sleep off a bad night for an extra hour or two, often has a sense of obligation to his or her patients and bank account that limits the therapist's willingness to take time off compared with that of a therapist in a clinic or hospital, who has paid sick days and colleagues to handle unforeseen emergencies. On the whole, in private practice one's calendar is both more and less one's own than it is in institutional work.

ISOLATION, LONELINESS, AND THEIR EFFECTS ON THE THERAPIST

A particularly difficult resultant of private practice for the practitioner is the sense of loneliness and social isolation that grows out of spending a large part of the working day away from colleagues and friends. This problem may become more severe as one becomes more successful in private practice, in that a larger proportion of the work day will be spent providing services to others. As the therapist's caseload grows and moves toward full-time practice, the built-in opportunities for socializing and collegial interaction inherent in clinic, hospital, and university work diminish. Similarly, even those clinicians in full-time practice who are prudent (or unfortunate) enough to have open hours often are fated to spend these hours along as a result of geographic isolation or scheduling factors that make meetings with friends, colleagues, or family members impossible.

Even when the therapist is conducting psychotherapy, he or she is in a sense alone since therapy is not a social relationship and usually the therapist spends little time talking about personal concerns or interests, and in general the social gratifications available to the therapist from patient contact are minimal. As writers such as Sullivan (1953) and Fromm-Reichman (1950) have noted, psychotherapy is a very difficult and often draining occupation that one may enjoy but that will take its toll through the intense neediness, demandingness, anxiety, depression, and otgher issues that are focused upon the therapist by a succession of patients during the day.

This day-in-day-out exposure to intense emotional stimulation from patients, coupled with a relative dearth of social or collegial exchange, is one of the prime factors implicated in studies of therapist burnout (Freudenberger, 1979). Private practice and its isolation usually stand as a marked deviation from the experiences and settings in which the therapist first learned and practiced psychotherapy. Psychotherapy generally is taught in clinics, hospitals, and universities, and in these settings there are always people around with whom to interact, consult, and refresh oneself. The private practitioner, having achieved a level of competence and success in the field, finds himself or herself in a totally different setting, with few if any of the opportunities for socializing or personal renewal.

Such experiences of loneliness, isolation, and emotional depletion are frequently the primary negative characteristics mentioned by private practitioners when asked to discuss drawbacks of their work. These occupationally derived emotional consequences often have effects on the therapist's life outside of the office and contact with patients. Many private practitioners cope very successfully with these issues by building social contacts, supervision and peer supervision, recreational events, and the like into their work week on a regular basis. These efforts can go a long way toward counterbalancing and combating the depleting and depriving effects of the work. However, at times and for certain therapists, such activities may be unavailable or insufficient for a variety of reasons. In such a situation a variety of unfortunate effects on the therapist's personal life may result. Such effects will be idiosyncratic according to the character and psychological makeup of the therapist, but frequent problems include burnout and disillusionment with one's work and career; anger, depression, and irritability; countertransference problems, including inattentiveness, impaired capacity to empathize with patients, missing or coming late to work, and other similar problems. Such reactions infrequently are compartmentalized into the private practitioner's working day. Unhappiness with a career choice and path for which an individual has spent many years studying and working can cause impairments in health and interference in the ability to enjoy leisure time. Loneliness and isolation may stimulate attempts to overcompensate through overindulgence in recreation involving alcohol or drugs and may also cause the therapist to displace or transfer the responsibility for such distress onto a spouse, lover, child, or friend, leading to even greater personal distress outside of work. An overburdened, depleted therapist who has spent his or her work week attending to the needs of others may react insensitively and with irritation when faced with the emotional needs of family members and friends, as he or she may choose to construe such contacts as too demanding and too much like work.

Private practice may induce in the therapist a sense of the profession passing him or her by, in the sense that the institutional or academic transmission of new ideas or techniques is not as readily accessible as it may have been previously. In order to keep up with changes and progress in the field the practitioner will be forced to become an independent learner and to devote some work or leisure time to reading, attending lectures or conferences, or obtaining supervision or advanced training. Such a need for and interest in keeping up with advances in the field are often conflictual in that the time must come from someplace: either from a reduction in working hours, which necessitates a loss of income and other professional gratifications, or from time available for family, friends, and recreation. Whatever the source of the time, it will of course have important consequences for the therapist's personal situation.

BLURRING OF BOUNDARIES BETWEEN PROFESSIONAL AND PERSONAL LIFE

While is is certainly difficult for any professional to switch hats completely when leaving the office or business, there are factors in independent practice that contribute to lessened separation between the clinician's professional life and private life. Such blurring of boundaries is intrinsically neither positive nor negative. Its particular effect on the individual practitioner will depend upon that person's perception of a personal need for a strong separation between work and private life. Many psychotherapists experience this lessened separation as enriching, rewarding, and integrating, and are genuinely exhilarated by their ongoing intermingling of professional and private activities. Other clinicians harbor a greater need for time totally away from their profession, patients, and colleagues, and they experience work demands in their private time as intrusions to be avoided or prevented. Certain characteristics of private practice that result in this blending of personal and private worlds will be discussed in more detail below.

Taking Work Home

The busy private practitioner does much work after working hours, usually while at home. Phone calls to patients and colleagues have to be made and returned, and in order to avoid the endless round-robin of leaving and receiving messages on answering machines, phone contact often must be made from home in the early morning or late evening hours. Similarly, the practitioner must call his or her answering machine or answering service in the evening, on weekends, and on days off in order to respond to new patients or to the needs of current patients. While many therapists who work in clinics or hospitals respond to evening or weekend phone calls, most clinicians seem to perceive and to respond to the need for extended availability to a greater extent in the private setting than in an institutional setting.

In a similar vein, often it becomes necessary to complete other practice-related work at home. This work includes billing, correspondence with other professionals about patients, completing insurance and other forms for reimbursement, and other activities of this ilk. As mentioned earlier in this chapter, if the therapist is interested in pursuing advanced training or simply keeping up with current literature in the field, the chief source of the necessary time is the time spent at home. As a result, novels will go unread, family members will be left to entertain themselves in other ways, and television will go unwatched as journals are scanned, tapes are reviewed, papers are written, and case presentations are prepared. Often, the therapist's needs for education and leisure are combined as vacations and weekends away are planned around conferences in resort areas or distant cities. While there can be great personal, professional, and financial advantage to these trips, the professional requirements for attendance at workshops and lectures may strain the therapist's relations with nonclinician family members, who will be uninterested in or not welcome at these professional activities.

Socializing As An
Aspect Of Practice Building

Private practice is a business enterprise, and as such the practitioner needs a regular stream of customers (patients) in order to stay in business. The difficulties in establishing and in maintaining a thriving practice are attested to by the large and ever-growing number of books, pamphlets, and marketing programs that promise the practitioner a "gold mine" in referrals. Such materials are advertised in professional journals and through the mail, and are a reflection of the ubiquitous concern of independent practitioners about their businesses.

This concern, and the need to stay in business, assure that some percentage of the clinician's personal life will be spent in what is known as "practice building," and that at certain points he or she will evaluate relationships and leisure activities, at least in part, as to whether these experiences will be helpful in obtaining referrals.

Practice-related experiences that become part of the therapist's personal and family life may include such decisions as whether or not to join a particular church or synagogue, tennis or country club, or other social organization. In addition to assessing the fit of the organization or institution with leisure time, spiritual needs, or family needs, the practitioner may have to evaluate this organization in terms of its potential for generating referrals. Similarly, the choice of dinner and social companions, people for whom favors outside of work are priority items, and so on may be influenced, consciously or unwittingly, by one's business needs. Such an influence of professional concerns on personal decisions and on selection of friends and social activities can be the source of much distress and covert embarrassment to some therapists, who perceive a certain amount of hypocrisy and deviousness in these interactions. For others, such an intermingling of business with pleasure is experienced without conflict of dysphoria, and is actually undertaken with a sense of pleasure, excitement, and accomplishment when a social engagement works on both levels. Such differences probably reflect and are based upon important personal concerns of the therapist that will be discussed more fully in the section below on changes in self-image in private practice.

Office Needs

Establishing and maintaining a private practice require, before all else, a place to have that practice; that is, a suitable office. This seems patently obvious, yet most clinicians who are considering starting a practice are unaware often of the mundane aspects of finding, furnishing, and running an office that affect their personal lives.

The availability of attractive, appropriate, and affordable office space for the practice of psychotherapy varies considerably according to locale. In New York City, for example, as a result of construction trends and recent unfavorable court decisions, practitioners currently face enormous rents and many are threatened with eviction from offices that they have occupied for many years. In other areas there is less pressure and more choice, but in either case, finding an office can fill one's nonworking hours with worry, budgetary decisions, much pounding of the pavement, and many phone calls.

Once office space has been secured, time demands made by this office do not end. Decisions must be made about decorations, furnishings, and supplies. Some practitioners need spend little money and effort on these because they have rented furnished space that allows little modification. But, at the other end of the spectrum, many therapists completely decorate, purchase all furnishings for, and perhaps even design offices and have them constructed. To a greater or lesser degree, such things take time, which again often comes out of the clinician's nonworking hours. Spending one's time (and money) in these ways can be highly exciting, adventurous, and the source of much pride and self-esteem, if establishing one's own business and professional space is seen as adding to the self. On the other hand, these hours may become the source of resentment and other negative emotions if time spent putting together the practice is perceived as detracting from one's personal life.

Even when the office is well established and running smoothly, it may be a source of demands on private time. One must keep tissues, bathroom supplies, stationery, light bulbs, and other sundries in stock. Landlords, and sometimes cotenants or subtenants, often must be met with and dealt with during evenings and weekends, as must phone installers, plumbers, electricians, and cleaning services. These drab and mundane chores and responsibilities belong to someone else when one works in an institution, but in private practice they inevitably intrude into one's personal life.

Working At Or Near Home

The intrusion of the commonplace, as well as of occasional, more unique infringements on private life, is never more apparent than when one's practice is in one's home, or is situated very near home. With such a working arrangement, keeping one's private life private from patients and their collaterals at times can become a very difficult task.

Some psychotherapists in private practice seem to be quite comfortable encountering patients and patients' significant others when the therapist is informally (or sloppily) dressed, or is with family or friends. Similarly, certain therapists and their families tolerate and perhaps even enjoy patients coming to their homes and observing (and possibly interacting with) the therapist and family members in a way that is usually impossible in a clinic. However, many therapists find these kinds of encounters stressful, and such interactions may be particularly disturbing to spouses and children, who often impose restrictions on themselves or are asked to make themselves scarce when patients are expected. Such self-imposed or therapist-directed restrictions may be the source of marital or parent–child conflict, resentment, and mutual irritation.

Working at or near home may offer the therapist certain advantages in terms of being available for brief visits with family members during breaks in a working day or evening. Appointments can be scheduled more easily around mealtimes, children's bedtimes, and other family needs, and this interspersing of working time and personal time can combat overwork, burnout, and the sense of loneliness and isolation discussed above.

CHANGES IN THE THERAPIST'S SELF-CONCEPT AND IDENTITY THAT ARE CONSEQUENCES OF PRIVATE PRACTICE

Students of psychotherapy have noted that the psychotherapist undergoes a personal transformation of self-concept and of sense of personal identity as he or she learns the craft and gains a feeling of competence, involvement, commitment, and openness to the work. Bugenthal (1964) has likened this process to a personal journey of self-development, while writers such as Tauber (1979) describe the process as a movement toward authenticity and freedom. When a psychotherapist becomes a private practitioner, this change in work situation often is accompanied by significant and powerful changes in the therapist's self-image. Private practice is construed by many psychotherapists from a variety of disciplines as the most advanced or most desirable point upon the hierarchy of employment and professional situations. Attainment of this goal often will have highly significant and unexpected effects upon the therapist's view of himself or herself.

Changes In The Therapist's Sense Of
Autonomy and Responsibility

"Now I'm on my own," in these or related words, might be the cognitive construction of one's commencement of private work. Such a construal, as cognitive theory informs us, will have emotional sequelae that can go in several different directions, depending on the meaning to the therapist of being on one's own. This perception can lead to pride and an enhanced sense of accomplishment, self-worth, and self-satisfaction, all of which can and usually do impact upon the therapist's relationships and activities outside of work in satisfactory and additive ways. Occasionally, this sense of attainment might tip over reasonable bounds and be transformed into a swelled head full of grandiosity and snobbishness, which can be trouble for the practitioner if such attitudes are taken too seriously and are introduced into relations with others.

Other therapists will respond to independence with anxiety and fear, and will construe private practice as too separate, lonely, or difficult. Individuals with this outlook may become depressed, clinically anxious, and irritable in public and private, and may try to build in quasi-institutional supports to replace the institution they just left, in the form of supervisors, training programs, consultants, and other authorities. While such contacts obviously are important and can be highly useful resources, they also may be used to avoid the independence of private practice.

Working on one's own can be exciting because of the freedom to pursue specific interests, work in particular modalities, and have to answer only to oneself and one's patients. Autonomy also breeds responsibility, and such responsibility often elicits an alteration in the therapist's self-image: He or she now must see himself or herself as fully in charge of the treatment and of the welfare of each patient, and as capable, ready, and willing to live up to these requirements. Again, such a shift in self-perception can have very positive or untoward effects on the therapist's entire life, depending on the therapist's view of his or her capacities and the rewards or debits of such responsibilities.

Change In Professional Identity

Psychotherapy is a service provided by a plethora of professionals (and often nonprofessionals) from a variety of disciplines and backgrounds. Despite much discussion over the past 20 years or so (see Holt, 1971, for one influential collection), an autonomous profession of psychotherapy has not yet been created. Yet, when a clinician becomes a private practitioner, that person's professional identity often is redefined, as the clinician begins to think of himself or herself as a psychotherapist rather than as a psychologist, psychiatrist, social worker, or nurse. Such a shift is not easy to make, and it may be accompanied by a variety of emotional experiences, pleasant and unpleasant, that reflect each individual's internalized relations with members of his or her profession, supervisors, professors, and therapists of the same or other disciplines who made the change previously. Construing oneself as a psychotherapist in private practice may yield a sense of having "made it," a sense of joining an elite group, or a sense of having left other people in one's discipline behind, and these and other reactions may be experienced sequentially or simultaneously.

Relationships between the private practitioner and former colleagues may become strained and distant as shared professional interests (for example, credentialing of nommedical clinicians in hospital settings) are replaced for the practitioner by private practice-related issues. Similarly, new loyalties and relationships both professional and personal may be established with other practitioners who share interest in these issues, to the point that the independent therapist may experience a radical modification of his or her social boundaries, reference group, and place in the world. Such a shift obviously will impact upon one's ongoing private life in intriguing and important ways.

The Impact Of The Business Of Private Practice

It is impossible to think of any occupation or profession that is divorced from the economic realities of Western society; that is, of the vicissitudes of a competitive, capitalist marketplace. However, most clinicians do not construe themselves as businesspeople or as entrepreneurs when they make the decision to go to graduate or medical school. It is a shocking realization to many that on opening an office they also have opened a business, and must begin to think of themselves and their professional services as business activities.

Such an idea is foreign, repellent, and highly distressing to many clinicians, and the requirements of business are painful for them. Such tasks as practice building and networking, which are really efforts at advertising and promotion, setting fees, staying on top of payments, and the other business aspects of private practice, may become a source of guilt, anxiety, anger, embarrassment, and other dysphoric experiences, any or all of which may disrupt the therapist's personal life. The need to compete in a marketplace that in many areas already is highly saturated may be quite conflictual, and certain therapists react to these issues by shrinking back, avoiding the business realities, or acting out in some way. Such personal difficulties may yield a sense of incompetence, failure, and jealousy and envy of successful colleagues, experiences that don't end at the door of the office.

Other therapists enjoy and thrive upon the financial and business aspects of private practice, and take pride in and grow personally from successful efforts at marketing and running a practice. These individuals are able to integrate their role as businessperson into their larger self-schema, and find often that the new role enhances and supports their other professional and personal endeavors.

Therapists in private practice usually earn more money than do institutional therapists, at least after the practice has been established successfully. Obviously, higher income can have many immediate and long-term positive effects on one's personal life, as in our society money is the key to all sorts of otherwise unavailable possibilities. There are other, less obvious potential effects of greater income for the therapist. The opportunity for a larger income is often a critical factor contributing to overwork. As one discovers that more work yields more money and more money yields a life-style that requires more money, a vicious circle of longer and longer hours may be established. Some therapists, however, find that they are guilty or uncomfortable earning large sums, and find ways to disrupt their professional and personal lives out of guilt. Another potential effect of increased income is that increasing one's earnings may become a central motivation and prime variable against which the self and others are evaluated. If this occurs, the therapist may find himself or herself becoming cynical or careless about clinical and ethical issues, and may turn toward a snobbish, aloof orientation in relation to others whose financial status is inferior and whose attitudes differ.

CONCLUSIONS

This chapter might be thought of as a guide to the therapist who is considering starting a private practice and wondering what to expect, to look out for, and to hope for. Private practice offers many opportunities for happiness and success, but there are often serious drawbacks and disadvantages as well. If the negative side of private practice has been emphasized at points in this chapter, it has been done for precautionary reasons and not to scare anyone away from private work. All too often, these issues are ignored or denied during professional training, and come to the attention of the practitioner only when he or she is hit with them head on. It is hoped that this discussion will be useful for the reader in making informed decisions that will enhance his or her efforts in private practice.

REFERENCES

Bugenthal, J.F.T. (1964). The person who is the psychotherapist. *Journal of Consulting Psychology, 28, 272–277.*

Freudenberger, H.T. (1979). The hazards of being a psychoanalyst. *Psychoanalytic Review, 66, 224–296.*

Fromm-Reichman, F. (1950). *Principles of intensive psychotherapy.* Chicago: University of Chicago.

Holt, R.R. (1971). *New horizon for psychotherapy.* New York: International Universiities Press.

Klauber, J. (1981). *Difficulties in the analytic encounter.* New York: Jason Aronson.

Sullivan, H.S. (1953). *The interpersonal theory of psychiatry.* New York: W.W. Norton.

Tawber, E. (1979). Countertransference. In L. Epstein & A. Feiner (Eds.), *Countertransference.* New York: Jason Aronson, 1979.

Wachtel, P. (1977). *Psychoanalysis and behavior therapy.* New York: Basic Books, 1977.

44

RELAXATION TECHNIQUES FOR THE EFFECTS OF STRESS

Ninalee F. May, Ed.D.

A ny event that requires change and rapid adaptation taxes the physical and mental systems of the body and causes stress. Starting a private practice requires many changes and adaptations and can be very stressful. Not all stressful situations can or should be voided, and not all stress responses cause long-term tension. During stressful periods the entire physiology functions as if life itself were in danger. When a source of stress is clear, action is taken, the challenge is met, and the individual returns quickly to a normal functioning level. But when the cause of the stress is not defined, there is often not enough opportunity to identify the problem, take action, and recover. And when too many adjustments must be made in too brief a period of time, tension and stress develop because there is not enough time to recover. Prolonged, unabated stress eventually causes physical disorders as well as emotional discomfort. These physical problems, which include ulcers, colitis, asthma, hay fever, hyperthyroidism, and migraine headaches, occur because of the way continuing stress affects the body. They can also begin when an individual, repeatedly confronted with a situation that seems unresolvable (a "double bind"), experiences the situation as both unavoidable and overwhelming and develops a psychosomatic disorder that can incapacitate and provide a means of escape. This less than conscious choice, which initially has positive results, can be automatically repeated over time and can become a seemingly unavoidable illness as the body automatically responds to stress with a major dysfunction. Reducing stress and stress-related responses can prevent and alleviate stress-related illness. There are four steps in stress reduction: (1) self awareness, (2) specific solutions to stressful situations, (3) general relaxation, and (4) deep relaxation.

SELF-AWARENESS

Individual Stress Patterns

Each private practitioner has his or her own unique basic nature. New experiences challenge and excite some people and make others anxious. Financial insecurity, for example, is rarely pleasant, but it affects different people in different ways. The first step in stress reduction is self-awareness. If you want to reduce the stress of starting a private practice, you must first understand yourself:

How do you respond to stressful situations?

How often do you experience stress?

Are you more frequently angry (fight response) or frightened (flight response)?

What are the physical symptoms you experience from short-term stress? From long-term stress?

How do you know when you cannot handle any more stress?

What do you do to reduce your stress reactions?

What nonfunctional stress behavior do you use to respond to stress?

Do you run away into work, food, sex, alcohol, drugs, illness, or other avoidance behavior?

How do you utilize your support system to help solve your problems? To help you handle the stress?

What specific situations are especially stressful for you?

What can you find out about the underlying causes of your undefined stress?

You can become more aware of how stress affects you by analyzing, alone and with the help of friends, family, peers, and supervisors, how you usually handle stressful situations, how your body responds to stress, which situations cause you stress, and what causes your generalized stress reactions.

Frequent Causes Of Stress In Private Practice

Issues that can cause stressful situations for someone starting a private prctice fall into three categories: professional, personal, and physical. Each person will find some of the issues more stressful than others. All are discussed in detail in other chapters.

Professional Issues   Practical professional problems often occur in the areas of legal liability, fees (setting, discussing, raising, and collecting), insurance, financial records, patient records, taxes, third-party payment, office expenses, transportation and parking, scheduling, and building a practice.

Professional interactions change with the establishment of a private practice. Contact with peers must be maintained, partners are often involved, and referrals from other professionals are necessary for a successful practice. The type of practice must be appropriate for the individual therapist. Both interaction with patients and professional ethical issues can create stressful situations.

Personal Issues   A private practice causes changes in the personal life of the therapist—whether he or she is a single person, a partner in a relationship, or a member of a family. Days with no contact with peers or friends can be lonely. A variable income can be stressful. Feelings about patients and about self-image must be resolved.

Physical Issues   Private practice is not physically active. Scheduling patients whenever they prefer to come can result in no regular breaks and no exercise, poor eating habits, and late nights. Physical safety in the office and on the street can be a problem.

SPECIFIC SOLUTIONS TO STRESSFUL SITUATIONS

Stressful reactions can be treated as disasters or as opportunities for growth. Specific situations that cause stress should be approached directly. A practical solution may be possible: increased knowledge or skills to deal with the situation or a restructuring that allows either elimination of the stressful activity or accomplishment of the requirement by someone else. If the problem cannot be solved practically, reduction of the stress reaction through desensitization or therapy may be possible

Practical Solutions

Knowledge   Some situations are stressful because the therapist does not know enough about the situation, has no alternative methods for handling it, or feels so uninformed that effective action is difficult. Other chapters in this book contain useful information about most issues described above under self-awareness. Other publications; workshops; conferences; conversations with colleagues and friends; and peer, group, or individual supervision are also sources of useful knowledge.

Skills   Private practice requires skills that are unnecessary for a therapist working for a hospital or agency who is not responsible for insurance, book-keeping, obtaining patients, setting up and running an office, or keeping track of small deductible expenses. Courses in subjects like bookkeeping and public speaking can help the private practitioner develop skills he or she did not need before. Workshops and supervision groups can increase group, family, and individual therapy skills, which can help the therapist handle stressful situations more successfully and also feel more confident. Supervision and peer supervision can help resolve issues concerning transference and counter-transference.

Restructuring   Some stressful situations are not even necessary. Stress-ful states do not encourage rational approaches. Standing back and gaining perspective (which is easier with the help of peers or supervision) often results in a realization that the situation can be dealt with in another, less stressful manner. Some stressful tasks can easily be done by others such as book-keepers, cleaning services, and accountants. Some private practitioners share responsibilities, each doing what he or she does well. Other situations can and perhaps should be eliminated. A therapist who becomes a nervous wreck doing groups or an angry, resentful person working Saturdays does have the option of stopping the stressful activity.

Reducing Stressful Feelings

When no practical solution to a stressful situation can be found and the activity cannot be given to someone else or eliminated, the next step is to work on reducing the feeling state surrounding the situation. This can be done by desensitizing or by working directly on the feeling.

Desensitization   The emotional charge related to a situation or activity can be reduced. Three simple methods that can be used without outside help are described below, with specific instructions that you can follow to try each method yourself.

Affirmation and Chanting   Imagine the positive change you want in your own behavior: handling a situation calmly, feeling calm and competent, asserting yourself, or making whatever other change in yourself would eliminate the stress. Formulate one to three *positive* statements describing your goal — for example, "I am allowed to say no," "I am comfortable with patients' anger," "I am entitled to be well paid for what I do," "I am happy working on Saturdays — the results are worth it." Do not use negative suggestions such as "I am not afraid of patients' anger." Write down your affirmations and repeat them to yourself at least twice a day. The times just after waking and before sleeping can be especially effective. Don't worry if you do not believe what you are saying. Keep putting in the positive message and eventually it will become real.

An especially effective way to use affirmations is by chanting them. Reduce your statement to two to eight beats — for example, "I am / happy / with my / work," or "I / deserve / to be / well paid." As you walk, start chanting your message silently in rhythm with your steps, over and over. You will find yourself chanting and also thinking of other things. The chant will become almost unconscious, in rhythm with your walking and breathing. Your goal is to have it stay in your head the way a song sometimes does. When it is in tune with your breathing, you will find yourself repeating it over and over, beneath your other mental activity, even when you are not walking. It will become a part of you in the same way your unconscious negative messages have been a part of you, and you can begin to replace them.

Fantasy   Fantasize handling the situation the way you want to. Rehearse in your mind, over and over, the feelings you want to feel and the behavior you want to demonstrate. Block out fears and anxieties — this is just a fantasy and you can do whatever you wish. Make this picture a part of you and it can change your behavior.

Creating a Peaceful Place   Give yourself, in your imagination, a special place where you are totally calm and relaxed. It can be a place you have actually been to, seen in a movie, or heard or read about or a place you create just for yourself: on a beach, by a lake, in the woods, on a mountain, or in a special room. Even if other people are around, you must be alone and not eating or drinking or smoking anything. In your mind, create it in all its completeness — see the surroundings, the light, and the color; hear the sounds; smell the scents; taste the flavor of the air and your sweat if you are hot; feel the wind, the temperature of the air, and the ground. Write out a complete description of your special peaceful place. Focus on it until you can experience yourself as fully there.

Then, choose a minor stressful situation and fantasize it until you are fully experiencing it. Be aware of the change in your body. When you are completely involved in the stressful situation, switch back to the peaceful scene. Focus on it until you can once again be there totally; then return to the stressful scene. Go back and forth five times.

Repeat this procedure at least twice each day. The stressful scene will become boring and you will have more and more difficulty feeling upset. When you encounter the situation in real life, it will lose its power.

When this situation is desensitized, choose another. Build up from minor situations with relatively mild stress to those that are most upsetting.

Therapy   If desensitization does not work, therapy is the next step. Something about the stressful situation is familiar, causing an old response that knowledge, skill, and desensitization cannot overcome. Unless you would rather live with the stress, the time has come to uncover the cause. Remember what you tell your patients about confronting issues and take your problem into therapy.

GENERAL RELAXATION

A more relaxed life can help reduce stress. Many private practitioners need to take charge of their lives and make them better.

Taking Charge

Limits   Let yourself know what is too much for you. You have a maximum number of hours you can comfortably work in a week, in a day, and without a break. Be aware of your maximum and do not repeatedly exceed it. Establish a policy for telephone calls from patients that lets you take good care of yourself and also feel responsible, and enforce it. Decide under what conditions you are willing to be contacted at home. Define the patient population you want to work with—their functional level, life-style, use or nonuse of drugs, and so on—and stick to it. Let yourself know how much anger and criticism you can take from a patient without experiencing more than mild stress: make your limits clear to your patients, and do not work with patients who cannot keep to your limits. Set fees you feel you deserve and are comfortable with, and change them when you need to. Most therapists who go into private practice do it to have more control over their life. Take that control.

Breaks   Schedule breaks into each day, week, month, and year, and use them to be good to yourself. Five to 10 minutes between sessions can be used to stretch, get a drink, read a few pages, enter your peaceful scene (see above), listen to music, or just do nothing. Longer breaks between sessions provide time for lunch with a friend, tennis, exercise, phone calls, classes, reading, writing, or whatever else makes you feel good and provides a change from seeing patients. Sometimes reading or writing professional material or getting caught up on records can reduce stress. Everyone should have at least one entire day, preferably two, each week that is completely free of work-related issues. Vacations are essential. If finding time for yourself seems impossible, you might want to explore the possible reasons such time would be threatening.

Supervision   Every therapist deserves help, whether it be from an individual supervisor, a supervision group, or a peer group. Taking a fresh look, with help, at puzzling, difficult, or uncomfortable interactions with patients reduces stress, helps prevent burnout, and helps the patients as well.

Time With Peers Time with other therapists is important. It can give you perspective, sympathy and understanding, new ideas, a better sense of yourself as a therapist, and a chance to keep your sense of humor.

Intellectual Stimulation Studying something totally separate from your profession can provide an exciting change and add another interest to your life. Learning more about therapy can make your work more interesting and exciting. Therapists need to use their brains for more than thinking about patients, records, and the like.

Exercise Exercise reduces stress and brings both physical and emotional benefits. Stretching in the morning and between sessions relieves physical tension. Aerobics, workouts, jogging, running, walking, race walking, or biking should be scheduled on a regular basis rather than sporadically. Find time and places to play the sports you like and to learn the ones you want to try.

Clothes Wear comfortable clothes. Create a look for yourself that you like. Choose colors and textures that look good on you and make you feel good. If you enjoy the latest styles, wear them.

Office Make your office a place you want to be. Get yourself a good chair. Use colors you like that will be restful for you and for your patients. Add a refrigerator and some kind of cooking facility to help you eat well. Make your office an expression of yourself—paintings and photographs you like, plants if you want them, and some of your favorite things. You can have an office that feels personal to you and yet does not reveal more about you than you would like your patients to know.

Organization Keep your records up-to-date and your things in the kind of order that works for you. Get help if you need it.

Positive Reinforcement Remember and repeat to yourself the rewarding aspects of your private practice: the things you've done well, the changes in your patients, the positive feedback you have received. You can choose to focus on and reinforce the positive elements rather than to rerun negative tapes.

Goals Set realistic positive goals and reexamine them periodically. Know where you are heading and see the progress you are making. Remember why you chose private practice and the disadvantages of the choices you did not make.

Negative Reactions Working toward treating yourself well may cause new stress. Many therapists go into a helping profession because giving feels safer than taking and because they do not believe they deserve good things. If you find yourself resisting making positive changes in your practice, getting sick, or sabotaging your efforts, take a look at your feelings about what you deserve.

DEEP RELAXATION

Some forms of relaxation can actually cause positive changes in breath, heart rate, and blood pressure and dramatically reduce the effects of stress. For maximum effect they should be undertaken with the help of someone well trained in the method you choose. Because a positive attitude will increase your chance of success, you should choose a method you can believe in.

Self-Hypnosis

Misconceptions   Many people who are inexperienced with hypnosis have an image of weak-willed, fairly stupid "subjects" totally under the control of the hypnotist. In reality, the subjects use the suggestions given to hypnotize themselves and will do nothing against their will. The ability to use the suggestions to enter a hypnotic state requires intelligence, imagination, and concentration. A hypnotized person is not asleep and has not given up control. The hypnotic state can be described as focused attention. You hypnotize yourself many times a day: when you are reading and you do not hear someone calling you, when you are driving and thinking about something and realize you do not remember the last four traffic lights, when you are daydreaming. Learning to choose consciously to enter and leave and use this state of concentration gives you more control, not less. When your surface chatter is stilled, the messages you give yourself affect you more deeply.

Method   The suggestions you use to put yourself in a hypnotic state can come from a hypnotist, an induction tape, a book, a tape of your own voice, or, eventually, your own inner voice. Starting with the help of a hypnotist will offer you the opportunity to ask questions, deal with problems, and experience different inductions and levels of trance. Then you can use a tape of the hypnotist's voice or any of the other methods.

Relaxing the body progressively, one part after another, is a good way to begin. Then, many people imagine themselves going "down" into the hypnotic state. Others are more successful if they "float" or rise. When you are almost asleep, you probably experience yourself as either sinking into the bed or floating. If you sink, you will probably do better going down. If you float, try going up. You can select your own mode of travel. The usual image takes you down in an escalator or elevator. You can also go down the stairs, a hill, a slide, or a rabbit hole or down in a bathysphere or up in a balloon or any other image that pleases you and feels safe. You may choose to use another form of induction. Eventually you can give yourself one signal and a key phrase and hypnotize yourself quickly, unless you find you enjoy the slow induction. Adapt whatever methods you are taught or you read about to suit yourself. You are in charge. Practice going in and out of a hypnotic state for at least a week before you use it for anything specific.

Uses   You can use self-hypnosis to give yourself specific suggestions about stressful situations to relax physically stressed parts of the body or body functions, and to enter an overall state of relaxation so deep that you may be able to control pain. Suggestions must be stated in positive terms and must be formulated very carefully because the "unconscious" part of you can take them literally. For example, a man who told himself, "I will choose not to eat," found himself chewing ("chews") food and spitting it out. Suggestions for physical changes should be checked out medically. Blocking of pain should be discontinued periodically and should not be used in situations where pain is a sign of further damage. Working with a well-trained and experienced hypnotherapist in the beginning and whenever you want to make major changes is wiser and more productive than relying on a book, a tape, or untrained help.

Advantages   Self-hypnosis is easy to learn and can bring rapid results. Because it is partly verbal and results in greater control, it fits in well with the Western mind and belief system. It can be used for habit change, learning, sleep, and regression as well as for stress reduction. It is also a useful tool for a therapist to use with patients.

Meditation

Misconceptions Meditation is not contemplation, thinking about a concept, or prolonged lethargy. It involves attention. You can focus your attention on an object, a sound (a mantra), or a physiological process such as breathing. Or you can open up your attention into a state of undistracted perception of stimuli, both external and internal. Meditation, like hypnosis, involves mastery of attention.

Method In all forms of meditation, you learn to fix your attention on your chosen task for longer and longer periods of time. The surface chatter is stilled, as with self-hypnosis, but you, instead of giving yourself suggestions, work toward experiencing the part of you that comes before thought and attention. This state is called transcendental awareness or satori. A good instructor or guide is important.

The method most easily researched and most widely available in the Western world is transcendental meditation (TM). This technique involves no particular religious philosophy. Your instructor gives you your specially chosen mantra, based on your particular needs and rhythms, and you repeat it for 15 to 20 minutes one or more times daily while sitting in a comfortable position with your spine upright and your eyes closed. Many people feel they can choose their own mantra. It must be short and soft and have no associative significance.

There are two common physical positions in Eastern forms of meditation. The shavasana (corpse) pose, which involves lying on your back and making your breath the object of meditation, can be used by anyone to reduce stress. The zazen, or sitting, meditation is simple and straightforward, and you can sit in a chair if you prefer. Whichever method you choose, find a teacher. Meditation is much more effectively practiced with help, and you can reach deeper and deeper levels if you choose.

Uses Meditation can help you learn to maintain a relaxed state in stressful situations. You may also find yourself responding intensely to a situation, but returning very quickly to a relaxed state. Whichever response you learn, you can use it to avoid the consequences of prolonged stress.

You may feel you do not have the time to meditate several times a day. Committing yourself to the process and restructuring your schedule is a major step in itself and can reduce stress by giving you the feeling of taking charge of your life.

Meditation Meditation breaks the pattern of prolonged stress. Your coping capability, energy level, and overall health will improve. Meditation is the most holistic of the deep relaxation methods. It offers you a detachment that lets you see your interactions with yourself, with others, and with the environment. It brings awareness that can cause life changes. Deep meditation can open up a deeper level of reality, with an awareness of the unity of all existence that dissolves fear, including the fear of death. If you do not choose to carry your meditation to this level, you can still dramatically reduce stress.

Biofeedback

Misconceptions   Biofeedback is not a purely technical process. As in meditation, you sit quietly, working toward a state of relaxed inner awareness, developing harmony between your mind and body. You are not permanently dependent on the biofeedback machines; they are used only for the early stages of the training.

Method   Biofeedback uses biological functions that can be monitored by electronic equipment and fed back through one of the five senses, to teach you to regulate those functions. Just as a change in your emotional state changes your physical state, a physiological change can produce an emotional change. A meditative or self-hypnotic technique helps you enter a state of relaxation. You will learn to achieve deep relaxation through whatever bio-feedback channel is most effective for you. Then, in that state, you can become aware of your inner process (your fantasies, sensations, and imagery) and how it affects your physiological functioning. The same passive attention focused on breathing in meditation can be focused on any simple physiological process. The feedback from the instrumentation gradually lets you know how to control the process. The biofeedback therapist you choose must have good basic clinical skills. You must be taught the skill and be given meaningful homework exercises so you can generalize the skill you learn in the clinic with the instrumentation into your daily activity. A technician who does not help you see your inner process or give you individualized homework exercises will not be able to help you make real changes.

Uses   You can learn to recognize and change minute symptoms before they lead to more severe symptoms, and to stop a stress reaction while it is still small. You will be very aware of your personal physical manifestations of tension, and you can reverse them in the beginning stages, practicing your own preventative medicine.

Advantages   With biofeedback you can discover and control your specific physiological stress responses. Biofeedback tells you exactly how you are functioning. The physiological function you want to change is monitored; you have instant feedback on your progress. It can be used with other methods of self-exploration such as psychotherapy, behavior modification, and meditation. Successful self-healing with biofeedback involves a process of psychological development and may elicit experiences of altered states of consciousness that can bring release from old traumas, which further reduces stress and enhances life.

SUMMARY

Self-hypnosis, meditation, and biofeedback can reduce stress and offer an opportunity for intense personal growth. The awareness of self-connectedness and self-regulation coming from these states can teach you to take charge of your life.

CONCLUSION

Too much stress causes emotional discomfort and physical disorders. Private practice has many potentially stressful situations. These stressful problems offer opportunities for self-discovery and growth. For these opportunities, as well as for physical and emotional reasons, the stresses should be explored.

Therapists can become aware of how they respond to stress and of the situations that stress them. These situations can be dealt with by their learning information and skills, restructuring to eliminate the need for the situation to occur, getting someone else to handle it, desensitizing themselves, or taking the problem into personal psychotherapy. An increased state of general relaxation can be obtained by therapists' taking charge of the daily and weekly schedule, setting limits, developing pleasant activities and surroundings, and setting and assessing positive goals. Deep relaxation through self-hypnosis, meditation, and biofeedback can produce changes in the way the body responds to stress and can lead to higher states of awareness.

45

LONELINESS AND ISOLATION IN THE PRACTICE OF PSYCHOTHERAPY

Robin B. Shafran, Ph.D.

The practice of psychotherapy has been characterized as gratifying, rewarding, and enriching, as well as lonely, isolating, and leading to professional burnout. The many and varied satisfactions inherent in successful clinical work have led to the characterization of psychotherapy as the "most human" of human endeavors. At the same time, there are significant pitfalls of psychotherapeutic work, especially for therapists engaged in independent practice. These occupational hazards stem primarily from the structure of our work with patients and the reality that for the independent practitioner a typical day may consist of seeing one patient after another. For many of us, there is often little or no other interpersonal contact and little time out of the consulting room. The perhaps inevitable feelings of loneliness and isolation that arise in such a setting are the topic of this discussion.

The issue of loneliness for psychotherapists is complex, for the experience of loneliness and/or isolation in the course of ongoing psychoanalytic or psychotherapeutic work can stem from various aspects of the treatment situation. In this chapter, several of the "loneliness engendering" factors inherent in clinical work will be presented. An opening discussion of the setting and conditions for psychotherapy or psychoanalysis as an almost ideal setting for the cultivation of loneliness will be followed by some comments on the manner in which our theories and beliefs about the way we work affects our experience of loneliness during ongoing treatment. The discussion will also consider the ways in which our patients may contribute to the loneliness and isolation of the therapy situation. The impact of requirements of confidentiality and privacy and of the fundamentally dyadic nature of psychotherapy will be addressed as well. The role of collegial relationships in both contributing to and alleviating feelings of isolation and loneliness will also be considered. The chapter concludes with a discussion of a few means by which some aspects of isolation and loneliness can be managed, and other aspects at least better tolerated.

THE SETTING AND CONDITIONS OF CLINICAL WORK

Cooper (1986) characterizes the therapeutic situation as one of "extraordinary isolation." In his view, the full-time practitioner, who may spend a full day seeing only patients, suffers the "loneliness of social isolation." Similarly, Greben (1975) comments that "no person was evolved to spend eight to ten hours a day, most days a week, sitting in a room with any one other person struggling with feelings and ideas" (p. 430). Greben views the constancy and lack of stimulation of the environment of the consulting room as another source of difficulty. This is especially so for therapists practicing on their own. There is not even the opportunity to chat with a colleague for a moment or two in the hallway, reception area, or coffee room. This, then, is the breeding ground for feelings of isolation and loneliness: a consultation room inhabited by a therapist and a succession of patients, perhaps with few breaks. The day is spent focused on the "other" member of the dyad, dealing with his or her needs and wishes while one's own are put on hold.

The setting for clinical work may indeed be professionally and socially isolating, particularly for therapists working without lunch breaks, time for phone call chats with family or friends, or time for even a short walk out of the confines of the office. But is the practice of psychotherapy actually lonely? It is, in some ways, puzzling to think of spending hour after hour with individuals who speak to you in the most personal terms about intimate subjects as lonely work. One explanation is the addition of an attiude of detachment and lack of involvement, the degree to which the therapeutic relationship remains "one way," that contributes to the experience of loneliness. According to Cooper, psychoanalysis goes best if the psychoanalyst maintains an attitude which, paradoxically, includes both "therapeutic fervor and therapeutic distance" (p. 577). He speaks of the need to be totally dedicated with limited emotional involvement, and to maintain a balance between therapeutic determination and remoteness, between deep empathy and emotional detachment.

Tarachow (1963), too, speaks to this issue, commenting that the psychoanalyst "must be capable of withstanding all degrees of the necessary deprivation, tension, and task, which especially require tolerance for loneliness" (p. 11). Tarachow views the transference neurosis as vital to the success of psychoanalysis, and cautions that it "can be established only if the therapist can tolerate the isolation of not taking the patient as object." "Lonesomeness," he goes on to say, "is not to be regarded in a naive sense. A casual remark about the weather breaks the loneliness and establishes a real object relationship" (p. 12). Tarachow is speaking of enforced loneliness, necessitated by and endured for the success of the psychoanalytic work. It is essential in the conduct of this type of psychoanalytic treatment, and indeed a foregone conclusion.

While Greben acknowledges the isolation of sitting in a room all day "with a 'series of one other persons,'" he views the psychoanalytic situation differently, noting that the situation also "promises the intimacy of that most intimate of all possible relationships — the growing closeness of two people engaged in exploring the hidden, most intimate thoughts and feelings of one of them" (p. 429). Greben refers to isolation and intimacy as a two-sided coin. Speaking of the ongoing psychoanalytic relationship, he comments: "Its most healthy aspect can be the gradual dropping away of defensive postures on the part of each of the participants, allowing for them more and more to 'be themselves.' To be known as one is, at the deepest level, is a great satisfaction" (p. 429). Greben points out that he used to think of this as something only his patients should increasingly come to experience, but now believes that in a good therapeutic relationship, this satisfaction is actually available for the therapist as well. He points out that even if the therapist offers little in the way of "outside" information about himself or herself, much is revealed regarding values, strengths, and weaknesses. In this way, the analyst, too, has the opportunity of being understood. Speaking of the analyst, Greben says:

> He is, in the end, as a result of participating in any successful analysis, both more fully aware of what he is like, as his personality has been played out intimately with yet another human being, and more whole as a person, having once experienced the close interrelatedness of a longstanding working alliance. (p. 429)

And the other side of Greben's coin? What is it that is so isolating to him in the practice of psychotherapy? Simply put, therapy ends. As therapists or analysts, we are always encouraging and facilitating an ultimate separation. What is left, in the way of a residual, permanent actual relationship is often minimal. To Greben, it is this aspect of the "real" relationship that prevents the therapist's finally overcoming isolation in therapeutic practice. The analytic or therapeutic process is not one that is necessarily lonely, from this vantage point. However, it is impermanent, and so does not satisfy the ongoing, long-term need for connectedness for either patient or therapist.

Will (1979) has written eloquently about this aspect of loneliness and isolation in therapeutic practice. He characterizes the life of the therapist as "one of arrivals and departures." In his view, a therapist is a "sparring partner," not a "constant in the 'main event'" (p.571). While the therapist's feelings may be used to learn more about the field in which he or she acts, they may not be fully expressed or acted upon. This may lead to situations of aloneness, frustration, and fatigue. Therapy is, in Will's words, concerned with "problems of attachment, dependency, transferences, tantalizing and frustrating moments of approach and withdrawal, and finally, separateness" (p. 571). he elaborates:

> Repeatedly, he becomes attached to other human beings (his patients). He finds them dependent on him, struggles with his own dependencies on them, must endure their shifting transfigurations of himself. He must effect farewells. These repeated attachments and losses accent the essential loneliness of our lives (p.571).

THEORETICAL ORIENTATION AND THE EXPERIENCE OF LONELINESS

When the setting and conditions for ongoing psychoanalysis or psycho-analytically oriented psychotherapy are taken into consideration, the essential isolation of therapist or analyst from his or her colleagues seems clear. We are on our own with our patients. Some of the implications of this situation will be discussed later on in this chapter. The experience of loneliness, however, is less straightforward. Two differing aspects of therapeutic loneliness have been described thus far. The loneliness of maintaining a detached, uninvolved stance, of not being known as a person to one's patients at all, as articulated by Cooper and Tarachow, is one aspect. The loneliness and isola-tion stemming from the loss of a relationship at the point of termination, as discussed by Greben and Will, is another. These two views are significantly different and reflect essentially core differences in ideas about the therapeutic or analytic process. One cannot miss a relationship one did not really have.

It seems that these two different views raise basic issues about what con-stitutes a psychotherapeutic or psychanalytic relationship, what is appropriate, and what is actually mutative—i.e., what makes the treatment work. One view of therapeutic loneliness stems from the notion that treatment will work only to the extent that the therapist keeps himself or herself out of it. The other reflects a more interpersonal orientation. While neither prevents loneliness, each, to some extent, impacts on how it will be experienced. It seems that all therapists experience loneliness and isolation but that to some extent such ex-periences as a therapist or analyst depend on theoretical orientation.

Of interest in this regard in Gill's (1983) discussion of what he refers to as two "major cleavages" in psychoanalytic thought. The first cleavage is be-tween the interpersonal and the drive discharge paradigms. The second, having to do with the degree of participation expected of the analyst, is between those who believe that analysts should participate in a major way and those who believe that they should not. Gill emphasizes that the two do not necessarily parallel each other. These differentiations are helpful in thinking about the loneliness and isolation built into the therapeutic process, in that both the type of paradigm to which one subscribes, and the degree of participation in which one believes will influence the nature and intensity of feelings of loneliness that stem from the resultant therapeutic relationship.

One way of looking at loneliness, and the degree to which it is experienced during an ongoing therapy or psychoanalysis, has to do with the degree to which the therapist or analyst allows himself or herself to become involved and known. To some extent, this is a reflection of paradigm. Therapists who interpret Freud (1912) literally in his caution that "the doctor should be opaque to his patients, and, like a mirror, should show them nothing but what is shown to him" (p. 118) are likely to feel the most lonely and isolated throughout the therapy process. These are the working conditions set forth by Tarachow mentioned earlier in this chapter. They are conditions of a stark loneliness, which require that the analyst not permit a "real relationship" or interaction, but work solely in the "as if" or transferential realm.

Gill believes Freud's famous quote has been misinterpreted, noting the ample data that suggest that even Freud didn't work that way. He calls it a "caricature of the Freudian view to say that the analyst is a blank screen or a mirror" (p. 210). He does, however, describe the current Freudian position as that of minimal participation. Cooper (1986) also speaks to this issue, em-phasizing the need for detachment and minimal emotional involvement on the part of the therapist. However, he notes that psychoanalysis will fail if the analyst cannot find points of "empathic contact" with his or her patients, thus suggesting a softer stance that allows for some type of person to person connectedness.

Wheelis (1956) has suggested that for some analysts, problems with inti-macy may have been a determining factor in their choice of profession. He elaborates that for those individuals who may experience a conflict between tendencies toward closeness and fears evoked by that closeness, the work of analysis presents an acceptable compromise. Wishes for intimacy are met by the opportunity to hear secrets, to learn much of what is extremely personal and private about another individual. At the same time, as the analyst, one need not be involved. One can position oneself to be unseen (behind the couch) and can speak only when choosing to, with little or no self-disclosure. Cooper, too, sees the analytic situation as constructed in such a way that, as he puts it, "the analyst's safety is assured — we need not answer embarrassing questions, we need not speak when spoken to, and our quietness is hidden behind our technique" (p. 580). While such a situation may indeed be interpersonally safe, it is also interpersonally isolating and lonely.

Choice of paradigm does not entirely dictate the degree of therapist involvement, and there are adherents of psychoanalytic views who describe their engagement and participation with their patients in a way that could not be described as detached or lonely. Shafer (1979), for example, considers it a "misguided striving toward neutrality and objectivity to try absolutely to screen yourself out of the therapeutic interaction." He goes on to say that "the thing is to be as clear as possible about the kind of interaction you are establishing" (p. 355). The goal, then, is not to avoid engagement, but to know what the engagement is about. It seems that as soon as one thinks in terms of "engagement" and "interaction," the situation assumes a cast that feels decidedly less lonely.

Shafer, too, believes that analytic work calls for "significant subordination of the analysts' personality to the analytic work" (p. 355), and suggests that analysts, while doing their best work, are different than they might be in social or personal relationships. He posits the development of an analytic "second self" in which the analyst might display a greater range of empathy, acceptance, affirmative outlook, and goal directedness. Shafer comments that it "is within this forum that one expresses his or her humanity analytically. On this basis, a special kind of empathy, intimacy, strength, and love can develop in relation to the analysand" (p. 356). Again, it is just this type of closeness, which Shafer distinguished from countertransference, that can mitigate feelings of loneliness and isolation during ongoing therapeutic contact.

In discussing the degree to which one particpates in the course of psychoanalysis, Wachtel (1986) highlights the idea that it is "in the very act of participating that the analyst learns what it is most important to know about the patient" (p. 63). He does caution, however, that "just as neutrality is a myth at one end of the spectrum, so too is symmetry at the other" (p. 67). He notes that the basis of the therapy relationship is asymmetrical; one person is asking another for help, and the patterns of one life are the focus of both participants. The roles and responsibilities of patient and therapist are also different, with the patient free to say and reveal whatever he or she wishes, while the therapist must do so "judiciously" to facilitate the treatment. As Wachtel sees it it is possible and even indicated to participate and reveal oneself, in a limited way and with care, in the course of treatment. Perhaps this renders the therapeutic relationship slightly less lonely. In this framework, as therapists, we can be a bit less hidden and cut off from our patients, and, examining our participation to learn about our patients, we will be less hidden from ourselves.

Turning to the second of the two paradigms in Gill's "cleavage," the interpersonal, we see that the situation is different. Essentially differing assumptions about the way in which therapy or analysis works and about the role of the clinician lead inevitably to differing experiences in the treatment situation, including different experiences of loneliness. It is the core of the interpersonal position that the analyst is involved in the treatment and cannot be a detached, uninvolved outsider. Sullivan (1954) asserts: "There are no psychiatric data that can be observed from a detached position by a person in no way involved in the operation. All psychiatric data arise from particpation in the situation that is observed – in other words by participant observation" (p. 57). Therapists or analysts, viewed in this framework, are seen as being inherently involved; although the degree of their participation may still be circumscribed, they are indeed participants, and in their participation are not alone. Whether or not interpersonally oriented therapists feel less lonely, however, must depend on the degree and the nature of their participation and on the quality of the analytic engagement. The interpersonal paradigm offers the opportunity for a degree of relatedness and interaction that may minimize the experience of loneliness on the part of practitioners, without compromising the treatment or interfering in its outcome. This stands in contrast to classical concerns about contaminating the transference by allowing oneself to be at all known.

The concept of participant observation has remained basic to the interpersonal position and has been expanded upon in recent years. Chrzanowski (1980) views the human relationship as a "therapeutic hub." He states: "Central to my position is the assumption that the nontechnical relationship constitutes a therapeutic matrix sui generis in the analytic situation and related modes of psychotherapy" (p. 352). He elaborates that it is no longer unusual for analysts or therapists to relate to patients in a personal and spontaneous way. Chrzanowski goes one step beyond Sullivan's "participant observation," which keeps the analyst an observer, and suggests instead that the analyst's role may be more accurately described as one of "collaborative participation" (p. 349). To Chrizanowski, of more relevance to a discussion of loneliness and isolation, this adds an element of affirmation of the patient's personal worth and enlarges the field of psychoanalytic or psychotherapeutic inquiry by bringing relational aspects of the therapeutic situation into greater focus.

In Chrzanowski's recasting of the work of the treatment and the role of the therapist or analyst, it becomes clear that the day-to-day contact between therapist and patient need not be lonely. The therapist is actively engaged with the patient in the therapeutic discourse, monitoring, perhaps discussing, his or her own reactions and thoughts just as he or she monitors and discusses those of the patient. In the course of treatment, the analyst allows himself or herself to become known to the patient and better known to himself or herself, a situation which is, in its essence, neither lonely nor isolating.

Held-Weiss (1986) sees things similarly. She points out that at best, the analyst is "open and receptive to the direct and profound person-to-person contact with the patient. This creates a history together, experienced as relevant engagement, and characterized by wholeness and complexity" (p. 3). In a developing analysis, Held-Weiss describes the occurrence of greater relatedness and mutual alliance, and more personal exchange. She states: "For collaboration is not only in the sharing of responsibility for the work of the analysis, but also in the sharing of the human participation in all its fullness and complexity. After all, it is not in the use of the other as a mirror or a camera but through the human use of human beings that the definition of self-experience is achieved" (p. 3).

The interpersonal point of view clearly permits greater interaction and more opportunity for communication between analyst and patient. There is therapeutic justification for the thoughtful and considered sharing of one's reactions and impressions, which will mitigate feelings of loneliness. The choice of a theoretical framework through which to structure one's work is complex, and of course contingent upon factors other than how lonely one will feel in the course of one's work day. Clinicians who believe in the type of collaborative inquiry advocated by some interpersonalists, (e.g., Chrzanowski, Held-Weiss) may be less vulnerable to this particular pitfall of analytic work.

PATIENT CONTRIBUTIONS TO THE EXPERIENCE OF LONELINESS

Some aspects of loneliness experienced in our work as therapists may, then, be a function of the theories to which we subscribe, and the degree of participation and involvement we choose to permit ourselves. There are, however, times when feelings of loneliness and isolation arise as a result of the type of engagement and degree of involvement permitted by our patients. Feelings of loneliness are engendered, to a greater or lesser degree, by individuals with differing personalities, defensive constellations, etc., by the degree of resistance presented to the work of the therapy, by the nature of the working alliance, and by the quality of the "real," nontransferential relationship established with each individual patient.

The quality of interaction, for example, in working with someone who is schizoid and in experiencing his withdrawal and isolation and the inability to make genuine contact can feel, to the therapist, extremely lonely. Yet a different affective experience, although still one that could be considered lonely, arises in working with someone chronically depressed who is unable to make a positive connection and can drain the therapist of hopefulness and optimism. Dealing with primarily paranoid character structures may, again, in its own way, leave the therapist feeling isolated and lonely. In this situation, the therapist may have an added burden, that of sorting through the patient's projections in order to maintain a clear sense of his or her own worth and integrity. In these three examples, genuine contact and engagement are precluded by pathology, not by theories of therapeutic technique. Similarly, the gratification some therapists find in working with "good hysterics" may in part be due to the lack of loneliness, the potential for contact and lively interaction in the work.

The mix of patients seen on any particular day may also influence how people with differing presenting problems and personality constellations are experienced. Following several sessions, for example, with extremely demanding, intrusive borderline patients, an hour with a schizoid individual who makes few demands and rather focuses on his own internal processes, may be experienced by the therapist as a relief, rather than as loneliness. What feels lonely or isolating, then, is also a function of where in the day it falls, who has preceded, and who will follow.

Related to the type of pathology with which patients present themselves for treatment are the ability and motivation they have for therapeutic work. Variations in the capacity for insight will effect the ongoing treatment and the degree to which the therapist can sustain a sense of connection and intellectual liveliness in the day-to-day work. Highly resistant patients, for whom every communication is a struggle, may erect so many barriers that the therapist is frustrated, lonely, and isolated on his or her side of a seemingly impenetrable brick wall. This experience may arise in the course of ongoing work with any patient, no matter how productive, as various hurdles, presenting differing degrees of challenge and difficulty, are negotiated. In this regard, the quality of the working alliance and the ongoing real relationships become crucial, since it is these aspects of the therapeutic interaction that can sustain both participants through periods of difficulty and slow progress.

In the course of ongoing psychotherapeutic work there are, inevitably, moments when we, as therapists, are simply at a loss for what to do. Most dramatically, a situation may arise when a patient speaks of self-destructive wishes or plans and we are forced to decide what kind of intervention is required, whether to insist upon hospitalization, etc. Less dramatic and more frequent are those occasions when something not life threatening is at issue — the patient may be voicing a particular projection, or making a demand, inducing real or fantasized feelings of inadequacy and incompetence in us as therapists, and rendering us uncertain of the most helpful response. In such situations, we are left totally to our own resources, at times feeling that the course of the treatment may be at stake. Without other resources at that moment, we are on our own and may acutely feel the isolation and loneliness built into the therapy situation, two people alone in the room.

PRIVACY AS A FACTOR IN LONELINESS AND ISOLATION

This feeling, of being for the most part on one's own in one's professional life, is accentuated by the need to maintain privacy and confidentiality. Therapists become accustomed to not talking about their work, and particularly long days filled with "difficult" sessions or demanding patients become burdens that are endured privately. Guy and Liaboe (1985) describe therapeutic work as "secret and unknown to others" (p. 169). As therapists, we are the retainers of secrets, and the ongoing process of treatment is similarly secret.

Just as we as therapists live with constraints on ventilating our difficulties, we are prevented from sharing our successes. Thus, an additional manifestation of isolation and loneliness is in the inability to discuss our accomplishments in a meaningful way. This is partially due, again, to requirements of confidentiality, but goes beyond protecting our patients' rightful privacy. Much of what is gratifying, what makes therapeutic work meaningful, has to do with useful and engaging exchanges with our patients that significantly facilitate growth and enhance understanding. These interactions, lifted from their rightful context and repeated to friends, in or out of our field, may lose their momentous quality. Much of what makes therapy work simply cannot be conveyed in that way. In our inability to communicate effectively what keeps us excited about our ongoing work, we may feel its essential isolation as well.

The Loneliness of the "Expert"

There is yet another aspect of loneliness that may be present for all therapists, while exacerbated for those of us in independent practice—the loneliness of the "expert" who may grow to feel his or her life has become, in Will's (1979) words, "one of signs and symptoms" (p. 570). Essentially everything becomes data. Will elaborates that it is possible for a person to become isolated by the very esteem in which he or she is held; people tend to keep their distance. Genuine give and take, in which the therapist shares his or her own doubts or weaknesses, may become difficult.

> Very few people want to acknowledge the fact that the expert in human relationships can have grave doubts about his own life and often feel anything but expert in his dealings with people. A forbidding wall of silence can form around the expert. He may gradually disappear as a person, fading unnoticed into the mythology that replaces him (p. 571).

Freudenberger and Robbins (1979) address themselves to this issue as well, noting in addition that particularly for those therapists in independent practice, there is no respite. Professional and social lives tend to merge, and there is little time left over. Although the therapist is the expert to whom the patient turns for help, Freudenberger and Robbins not that the following scenario may develop:

> . . .in time an ironic paradox emerges. Many of the patients seem to live more fully than the therapist. . . .The therapist's controlled, objective, professional stance seems to mold all his relationships. Trained to listen in order to hear appropriately the therapist becomes trapped into the position of listening to the sounds of others. Ironically, he may be listening too intensely to be able to hear or follow his own personal drumbeat. Somewhere along this busy path of professionalism, a personal self tends to become lost. (p. 280)

Increasing feelings of social loneliness and isolation on the part of the therapist may prove to be detrimental to his or her patients. Will (15) wrote that with time, a psychoanalyst may find his world "largely peopled by patients, and he may discover (or deny) that he is in, some sense isolated and alone—perhaps lonely" (p. 29). The therapist may turn, with or without knowing it, to his patients for relief. Will elaborates that in that situation the patient, who is often quite familiar with being a confidant and parent to a parent, may meet the dependency requirements of the therapist. While the patient may experience a subsequent decrease in anxiety, he will "fail to separate from his past, having found it in his current present" (p. 29).

MANAGING AND MINIMIZING LONELINESS AND ISOLATION

In the avoidance of the type of scenario described by both Will (1971) and Freudenberger and Robbins (1979), in which the therapist's life is constricted to the point that gratifications are too related to what is available from patient contact, the cultivation of both personal and professional (collegial) relationships plays a key role. Freudenberger and Robbins emphasize the need for private time, time to cultivate one's own interests outside the psychotherapeutic sphere. The importance of satisfying personal relationships — with family or friends, individuals with whom the therapist can derive his or her own gratifications — cannot be overemphasized. As therapists, we remain outsiders in our patients' lives, observing their successes and personal satisfactions yet not completely sharing them. We need enough of our own to maintain the sense of well-being and contentment that allows us to enjoy others' success without feeling empty in contrast.

The potential danger of using patients as an antidote for isolation, as raised by Will, is of particular concern with the increasing acceptance of the interactive nature of clinical intervention. With the lessening of constraints on participation and self-revelation on the part of the analyst, there is greater risk of using one's patient contact more to meet one's own needs for contact and relationship than to further the analytic inquiry. This potential misuse of otherwise well-grounded participation on the part of the therapist or analyst adds additional weight to the importance of cultivating and maintaining social and familial contacts that provide support and gratification for the clinician.

Whether we as practicing therapists work in a manner consistent with a classical orientation and maintain a stance of detachment and limited engagement, or believe in the efficacy of greater participation and collaboration, we are still vulnerable to feelings of isolation. Regardless of theoretical orientation, we are alone with our patients, on our own and reliant on our own resources in our moment-to-moment work. Regular contact with other therapists is the most reliable antidote to such professional isolation. Relationships with other therapists, whether in groups or "institutes" or through formal supervision or individual casual contact, provide much needed intellectual stimulation and an opportunity to discuss work in progress, as well as a means of alleviating the isolation and loneliness experienced in day-to-day work with patients. Such interaction helps to remind us of the meaningfulness of the work in which we are engaged, and can provide encouragement and validation when none is forthcoming in our actual patient contact.

Regular contact and interaction with colleagues are crucial for preventing or alleviating intellectual loneliness and isolation as well. The importance of a forum in which to speak about clinical issues, and to exchange ideas about theory and technique was recognized by Freud in his invitaiton to four other analysts to join him for the 'Psychological Wednesday Society,' a weekly meeting in which the five members met to discuss Freud's work. This group was the beginning of what was to be the Vienna Psycho-Analytical Society, the first "institute" developed to share ideas and combat professional isolation (Jones, 1955). Professional societies have proliferated as the field of psychotherapy and psychoanalysis has grown, and have continued to provide opportunities for clinicians to have the kinds of exchanges unavailable to them in their day-to-day office practice.

The value of affiliating with schools or institutes has been recognized as a means of establishing and enhancing professional identity, and of providing colleagues with whom to share experiences and ideas. Shafer (1979) compared belonging to a particular school of psychoanalytic thought to sharing a "myth." He considered there to be interactive advantages in the ties to one's school, including a sense of continuity and collegiality, and a sense of confirmation from one's peers that helps to develop confidence. As he put it: "There is a sense of authenticity that comes from working within a form, a form that is a set of constraints as well as opportunities" (p. 350). This is particularly important when for so much of the day we work by ourselves, dependent on our own thoughts and reactions and sometimes uncertain about what might be most "therapeutic" at a given moment. The frame of reference provided by one's own school of thought alleviates some of the ambiguity, in its provision of a structure with which to think about what transpires in the patient–therapist interaction.

Although membership in professional societies is often sought to combat the isolation of working alone in one's office, and to provide a context for professional growth and development, intragroup relationships are not always so straightforward. Professional organizations, institutes, and schools do not necessarily provide uncomplicated affirmation and support. All too often, as Greben (1975) points out, as members of professional groups, we create an atmosphere of unrealistic expectation where "what we do and what we say we do are so different" (p. 432). Successes are presented at conferences and discussions and are written up in papers much more frequently than failures. We become reluctant to talk about our concerns, our mistakes, and our uncertainties. Consequently, what could be a setting for increasing dialogue and communicaiton among colleagues becomes a situation that only perpetuates feelings of isolation. What is needed is a situation in which information can be openly and honestly exchanged, and in which competition is minimized. Greben recommends that as analysts we strive to establish more receptive audiences among ourselves, to become more realistic about what we can and cannot do, and to increase our capacity to assess our work realistically.

Society and institute meetings and presentations, regardless of the limitations built into the setting, can provide much needed interaction and are often a primary source of "continuing professional education," in that through active membership and participation one is exposed, on an ongoing postgraduate basis, to new ideas and developments in both theory and clinical practice. As such, these meetings provide a valuable means of combating intellectual, and to some degree, social isolation. Such meetings do not necessarily aid the clinician with the day-to-day feelings of loneliness and isolation that arise from sitting alone with patients, with questions on technique or of the appropriate intervention for the particular situation, or with the feeling one's own resources are wearing thin with little replenishment. During training, this condition is typically remedied through seminars, supervision, and often training analysis. Once formal classwork, supervision, and analysis end, a satisfying solution is often found in the establishment of an ongoing peer group whose members meet on a regular basis and discuss readings and/or present cases. Leaderless peer groups are often composed of individuals of roughly equivalent background and experience, in the hope of keeping them truly leaderless and maintaining an atmosphere in which all participants feel comfortable.

Peer groups can provide a more personalized source of information than can meetings of a large society. They can be a forum for resolving specific ethical, legal, financial, and professional issues (1985). Reading groups present a structure for continued intellectual growth and encourage thoughtful consideration of the literature, either theoretical or clinical. Members choose to focus on particular issues, theories, authors, etc., for in-depth study or scan more varied topics, as the groups' interests and concerns change. The advantage over simply reading on one's own is clear. Ideas are exchanged and conversation and discussion can be lively. Additionally, with a group of colleagues counting on one's participation, one is simply more likely to read! Small groups require active participation by all members in order for the group to thrive. This necessary participation is also an excellent means of maintaining professional relationships, perhaps developing and deepending friendships, and combating feelings of isolation for the independent practitioner.

Peer supervision or consultation groups, in which practicing clinicians meet to discuss their work, are also frequently composed of six to eight individuals of roughly equivalent experience. Members either take turns presenting cases to the group, thus allowing each participant an opportunity to be "supervised," or follow the therapy process of one patient over a number of sessions. The latter, essentially a continuous case conference, permits the group to explore in depth the hour-by-hour work of psychotherapy, to examine the transferential-countertransferential interaction, the development and exploration of fantasy, or any other aspects of treatment on which the group participants wish to focus.

Peer supervision groups, especially thsoe in which members are ultimately able to speak candidly, even intimately, about their work, their feelings about their patients, and the progress or lack thereof of treatment, require care and nurturance in order to thrive. Members must take each other and the commitment to the group seriously and respect each other's needs and feelings. The group in which this author participates has gone through stages of development in which the type of discussion has clearly changed over time. Initially, much more socialization occurred, as members who knew each other professionally but not necessarily personally became better acquainted. This aspect of the group's time together, while remaining enjoyable and important, has become secondary to the primary focus of the group: to talk about the work of therapy and to learn from each other in the process. The manner in which the group approaches the data presented, in this situation an ongoing presentation of one therapy, has also undergone transition. In the initial months the participants clearly focused on the patient, her history, difficulties, symptoms, reactions, etc., or on theories of technique—i.e., when and how to make what kind of intervention. As the group coalesced, and participants became more comfortable with each other, there was more discussion of countertransference—both of the therapist and of the group—with greater freedom for the presenter and the group as a whole to discuss their reactions to the patient and the work.

Participation in a peer consultation group may be the most effective professional antidote to feelings of isolation and loneliness for the independent practitioner. Such groups can be a setting for meeting needs for support and supervision, and for staying "on one's toes" clinically. They can be used as a means of identifying and addressing sources of negative feelings, and of loss of objectivity in the patient-therapist relationship. They have a clear advantage over informal contact between colleagues, in that time and continuity lead to increased trust. As participants get to know each other better, deeper and more fruitful levels of exploration become possible.

SUMMARY AND CONCLUSIONS

In this chapter, the independent practice of psychotherapy or psychoanalysis has been considered as both interpersonally involving and isolating. For all therapists or analysts, there are moments of engagement and connection and times of loneliness. Some of what we experience, how much we participate, reveal, and interact in the course of our work day, depends on what we believe is technically and theoretically correct and appropriate. Similarly, some of the loss we feel at termination is a function of the degree of involvement we permitted ourselves.

There are, however, moments of loneliness and times of feeling extremely isolated that therapists experience regardless of theoretical persuasion. These have to do with our patients, or with moments in the treatment process when we feel frustrated or at a loss, unsure of what is happening or where to go. Furthermore, we are alone with our patients in our offices for most of the day. The isolation inherent in the situation itself is significant.

The importance of maintaining outside relationships has been highlighted as crucial in minimizing or controlling the inevitable feelings of isolation or loneliness that arise as part of the independent practitioner's working conditions. The importance of collegial relationships—in large professional settings and particularly in smaller, ongoing peer groups, which require a special commitment—has been emphasized as well. These situations serve to maintain and encourage professional development while providing much needed social contact, relaxation, and replenishment of our own resources.

Although the reality of the therapeutic setting includes moments of loneliness and isolation, even many such moments, these are not, I believe, the primary experiences we take from our day-to-day work with patients. As Shafer (1979) says: "There's so much about being an analyst that is challenging, interesting, exciting, rewarding...there are certain experiences whose marvelousness one doesn't quite encounter in any other relationship" (p. 360). Feelings of loneliness and isolation are what we tolerate in order that we may enjoy the many gratifications and satisfactions also available to the psychotherapist or psychoanalyst. As therapists, experts in human behavior and interpersonal relations, we need to put our knowledge of others to work for ourselves, and develop our own relationships as we hope our patients will, in order to counteract the isolation we encounter and maximize the gratifications and satisfaction available to us in our work.

REFERENCES

Chrzanowski, G. (1980). Collaborative inquiry, affirmation and neturality in the psychoanalytic situation. *Contemporary Psychoanalysis, 16,* 348–366.

Cooper, A.M. (1986). Some limitations on therapeutic effectiveness: The "burnout syndrome" in psychoanalysts. *Psychoanalytic Quarterly, LV,* 576–598.

Freud, S. (1912). Recommendations to physicians practicing psychoanalysis. *Standard edition, 12,* 111–120, London: Hogarth Press, 1958.

Freudenberger, H.J., Robbins, A. (1979). The hazards of being a psychoanalyst. *Psychoanalytic Review, 66,* 275–96.

Gill, M. (1983). The interpersonal paradigm and the degree of the therapist's involvement. *Contemporary Psychoanalysis, 19,* 200–237.

Greben, S.E. (1975). Some difficulties and satisfactions inherent in the practice of psychoanalysis. *International Journal of Psycho-Analysis, 56,* 427–434.

Greenberg, S.L., Lewis, G.J., & Johnson, M. (1985). Peer consultation groups for private practitioners. *Professional Psychology: Research and Practice, 16,* 437–444.

Guy, J.D., & Liaboe, G.P. (1985). Isolation in Christian psychotherapeutic practice. *Journal of Psychology and Theology, 13,* 167–171.

Held-Weiss, R. (1986). A note on spontaneity in the analyst. *Contemporary Psychoanalysis, 22,* 2–3.

Jones, E. (1955). *The life and work of Sigmund Freud,* Vol. 2. New York: Basic Books.

Shafer, R. (1979). On becoming an analyst of one persuasion or another. *Contemporary Psychoanalysis, 15,* 345–360.

Wheelis, A. (1956). The vocational hazards of psycho-analysis. *International Journal of Psycho-Analysis, 37,* 171–184.

Sullivan, H.D. (1954). *The Psychiatric Interview.* New York: W.W. Norton.

Tarachow, S. (1963). *An introduction to psychotherapy.* New York: International Universities Press.

Wachtel, P. (1986). On the limits of therapeutic neutrality. *Contemporary Psychoanalysis, 22,* 60–70.

Wheelis, A. (1956). The vocational hazards of psycho-analysis. *International Journal of Psycho-Analysis, 37,* 171–184.

Will, O.A. (1971). The patient and the psychotherapist: Comments on the unqiueness of their relationship. In B. Landis & E.S. Tauber (Eds.), *In the name of life: Essays in honor of Eric Fromm* (pp. 15–43). New York: Holt, Rinehart & Winston.

C H A P T E R
46

THE PRIVATE PRACTICE
OF GROUP PSYCHOTHERAPY:
PRACTICAL AND CLINICAL ISSUES

Robert Mendelsohn, Ph.D.

I n this chapter I will explore what I believe to be the most important issues in the private practice of group psychotherapy. While many of the issues also apply to the private practice of individual psychotherapy, group psychotherapy practice, particularly for a practitioner who also treats individuals, presents many different and complex challenges. For purposes of focus, I have attempted to gear my discussion to clinicians who are currently practicing psychoanalytically oriented psychotherapy with individuals and who are contemplating a group psychotherapy practice. Private practitioners who are already working privately with both individuals and groups will, I hope, also be able to identify with the issues raised here.[1]

The topics to be covered are beginning a group psychotherapy practice (including practical problems) and clinical problems of a group therapy practice. Included in the latter are management of resistances and transference, and countertransference issues. Conclusions and a summary will follow.

BEGINNING A GROUP
PSYCHOTHERAPY PRACTICE

New Rewards And New Challenges

For the clinician practicing individual psychoanalytic psychotherapy, the addition of a private psychotherapy group presents both new rewards and new challenges. Siegel (1972) has been most helpful in clarifying the definition of a psychotherapy group. For our purposes, the private practice psychotherapy group will be defined as a voluntary meeting on a regular basis of individuals who are preselected by the therapist for the purpose of receiving help with

---

[1] There are probably only a few clinicians who are currently engaged in a private practice devoted exclusively to psychoanalytic group psychotherapy. For example, from the vantage point of my own affiliation with the Postdoctoral Group Psychotherapy Training programs in the New York metropolitan area, I am aware of only three psychologists who limit their private practice to groups.

personal problems and who pay the therapist a fee for this service. With this definition, we can see that the private psychotherapy group differs from other social groups in that it is therapeutic and that it differs from other therapy groups in that the treatment is voluntary, the members are selected by the therapist, and a fee is paid for the service by each group member. Each aspect of this new definition points to both new rewards and new challenges.

Firstly, there are the obvious rewards of a private practice therapy group. The extensive literature on group psychotherapy (Durkin, 1964; Wolf & Schwarz, 1962; Yalom, 1970) suggests that the group is an extremely valuable treatment medium. While it is not our purpose here to evaluate group psychotherapy as a clinical technique (Toseland & Siporin, 1987), it seems clear that clinicians who feel satisfied that group therapy is effective would also see its value in their practice. Thus, one reward for a clinician practicing privately is that he or she would be adding a valuable technical approach to the practice. A clinical example follows: A number of clinical practitioners who are working increasingly with patients with borderline psychopathology have found that the combination of individual and group psychotherapy can provide an opportunity for the borderline patient to experience in vivo — i.e., in the transference — the defense of splitting. It has been suggested (Kernberg, 1975) that splitting is the major defense in borderline conditions. Thus, a borderline patient might feel that his or her therapist is "good" in the individual therapy sessions and "bad" in the group meeting (or, the reverse). A clinical practitioner who works in the combined individual therapy/group therapy approach would thereby be able to quickly and effectively work with such dynamics. A second reward of group therapy practice is that the clinician can work with many more patients in group psychotherapy than he or she can in individual practice. Thus a clinician working with two average-sized therapy groups (six to 10 members) can, in approximately 3 hours per week, have an impact on as many as 20 people, as opposed to the four individual patients the clinician would be working with if he or she were working exclusively with individuals. A third reward, as Goldman (1972) so aptly suggests, is that group practice can be helpful with a problem universal to the individual practitioner: the problem of loneliness. The loneliness that Goldman refers to is the very special loneliness that comes from the task endemic to the therapist's work: the task of focusing exclusively on the patient and the patient's needs rather than on one's own needs. With group work, an individual practitioner can temporarily shift focus — i.e., focus on the needs of the group. Further, at some periods of group life, it is helpful and effective to have group members help each other, as opposed to having all help emanating from the therapist. Of course, in the final analysis, it is the group psychotherapist who is fully responsible for, and must be continually responsive to, the needs of the group. However, what I am suggesting here is a matter of shifting emphasis, of shifting perspective, and of shifting focus. The clinician will find that an effective working group will be able, on occasion, to allow the clinician "a breather." It must be emphasized here that I am not suggesting that a clinician should exploit his or her group or patients. As I have stated above and elsewhere (Mendelsohn, 1981a, 1986a), I am suggesting that group psychotherapy offers the clinician these opportunities — as long as the clinician continues to be alert to the total clinical picture.

In a similar vein, the issue of loneliness noted above is an even more relevant one for one's patients. A well-functioning psychotherapy group can provide an excellent opportunity for the group members to work on their problems with relatedness. In many ways, a therapy group becomes a new family for the members: a family that can provide new opportunities for patients to work through problems never corrected in their own family.

There are two other rewards in group psychotherapy practice that are less frequently and openly discussed. These are the rewards of money and financial security. In our culture, both of these issues are often looked at with a somewhat jaundiced view. While it may seem somewhat paradoxical, in our capital economy, financial rewards and financial security are often not considered worthy issues for the professional to be concerned about. With a small apology to the reader, I want to say that when one fulfills professional responsibilities to one's patients, and enjoys the professional rewards that accrue in our very special work, then one ought to also be able to enjoy some financial benefit. The addition of a group psychotherapy practice can add financial benefits to the individual practitioner. Group fees are typically set at one-half the clinician's individual fee, and when this fee is multiplied by the number of group members, the amount per group session can be rewarding. My belief is that most clinicians do not practice solely for money and, further, that if a clinician is able to make a comfortable living, he or she will be less likely to act out personal conflicts regarding money, greed, envy, sharing, and exploitativeness with patients. The other financial reward mentioned above is that of financial security. An effectively functioning, therapeutically helpful psychotherapy group forms a stable core of patients in a clinician's practice. Group members are then available to help each other deal with potentially treatment destructive resistances. Yalom (1970) has suggested that group cohesiveness is a major therapeutic factor in group psychotherapy. Group cohesiveness also increases each member's commitment to the group, to the therapy, and to the therapist.

Paradoxically, introducing the possibility of group treatment to the individuals in one's practice often has an initially very disruptive effect on them and can at first even undermine the very cohesiveness in one's practice. I will say more about this below. For our purposes now, however, I want to reemphasize that the addition of a cohesive group to the clinician's practice ultimately adds to the practitioner's professional and financial security.

Training For The Private Practice Of Group Psychotherapy

As Goldman (1972) has suggested, there are few, if any, training programs that help prepare a psychotherapist for private practice. Fewer still are the training programs that prepare one for group psychotherapy work of any kind. In the New York metropolitan area, three notable programs are the Group Psychogherapy Certificate Program of the Postgraduate Center for Mental Health; the Postdoctoral Program in Group Psychotherapy of the Derner Institute, Adelphi University; and the Group Psychotherapy Program of the Washington Square Institute. The American Group Psychotherapy Association and its regional affiliates offer short, intensive workshops, courses, and continuing education programs that can be extremely helpful in increasing the beginning group practitioner's competence (as well as in sharpening the skills of the most seasoned worker). For the rest of those clinicians who wish to begin group practice, the most effective way to do so is to undertake their own course of training through private supervision, personal group psychotherapy, attendance at workshops, readings, and if they are fortunate enough to have the opportunity, peer group membership (Billow & Mendelsohn, 1987a). In contrast to the clinician practicing group psychotherapy in an institutional setting, the clinician in private group psychotherapy practice need not answer to anyone else. Yet, as one consequence of this, the clinician is also fully responsible for all decisions, each of which he or she must make alone. It would seem, therefore, that training would be useful not only in the acquisition of the clinician's knowledge and skills but also in the building of the personal confidence that the group therapist will need in order to deal effectively with the many stresses and anxieties that he or she will encounter. In this same vein, I have suggested elsewhere (Mendelsohn, 1981b; Billow & Mendelsohn, 1987a) that an increased self-awareness and the effective use of the clinician's personal reactions are very useful in a group setting. It cannot be emphasized enough that both personal group psychotherapy and peer group experiences are extremely valuable for the beginning group psychotherapist.

Practical Issues For Beginning A Private Practice Psychotherapy Group

Adjusting One's Office For The Group Siegel (1972) suggests that the optimal number of members in a therapy group is from six to 10, with a mean of seven or eight. While some writers caution against a rigid view of an ideal number of patients (Wolf & Schwartz, 1962), it is generally believed (Slavson, 1964; Yalom, 1970) that six to 10 is the best size. A beginning group psychotherapist will want to rearrange his or her office so that up to 11 people (including the therapist) will fit comfortably and each will be able to see all others present. The room should be sufficiently large that there is comfort and should have proper ventilation. Most clinicians who are adding group psychotherapy to their existing individual practice need to alter their individual consultation room by adding new furniture and fixtures. In doing so, they are revealing to all of their individual patients that a change is taking place. My choice of words here, "revealing to all of their individual patients," was planned. I would suggest that any change initiated by the clinician is always unconsciously revealed to the patient. Whether or not this change will then also be made conscious to the patient, and worked with between the patient and therapist, is a clinical decision that the therapist will need to make as it pertains to treatment goals and other considerations.

Referrals The individual practitioner who is beginning a group will most often be referring patients to the group from within his or her own practice. Initially this can be quite unsettling for both the therapist and the patients, as many patients do not wish to move from individual psychotherapy to a combined therapy of both types. Further, patient and therapist may reach a certain crucial moment when the patient wonders, "If you were not beginning a therapy group now, would you still be recommending group therapy for me at this time?" This crucial moment, if explored and understood, can provide the patient with an opportunity to alter his or her relationship with exploitiveness. That is, the patient may for perhaps the first time be able to be involved in a relationship from which both members can derive benefit. In this instance, both the patient and the therapist can derive benefit from the patient's group membership. Regarding the issue of referrals from other practitioners, the referral process for beginning group psychotherapy is somewhat less difficult than it is for beginning individual practice. With the addition of the group, the practitioner has a unique, specialized modality available, and so referrals are often more frequent. However, as a result, the group therapist is also faced with the decision whether or not to take patients for the group who are currently working in individual treatment with another therapist. Issues of competitiveness, rivalry, envy, splitting, and particularly a splitting of the transference, all must be considered before making such a decision. Typically, the stronger and more confident both the individual and group clinicians are in this circumstance, the better the prognosis for it. Finally, there are certain referral situations where a colleague will actually want to "get rid of" a patient by referring him or her for the group. A sensitive and helpful intake evaluation period will always help in clarifying this, as in all other referral situations.

Starting The Group   There is much variability in the literature with regard to the length of preparatory time needed with a patient who is beginning in a new psychotherapy group (Siegel, 1972). Whether a clinician works for two or three or 20 sessions with the patient, the most effective approach would seem to include providing the new group members with sufficient information about what might be expected to occur, assessing and managing the patient's anxieties about the group, working to uncover and understand the patient's fantasies and expectations regarding the group, and most importantly continuing to strengthen and solidify the relationship with the patient so that he or she can feel safe and supported in this new endeavor. At bottom, a paradox exists for each individual patient who did not originally request but has agreed to become a member of his or her therapist's psychotherapy group. This paradox is the following: A patient may agree (often somewhat reluctantly) to become a member of his or her therapist's group in order to get a kind of special love and approval from the therapist. Yet, to be a member of a group is, in some ways, to no longer be special. Thus, a treatment crisis can occur when an individual patient agrees to become a member of his or her therapist's group. This crisis is one of unconscious ambivalence and disappointment, and one might even liken it to the crisis that occurs between the toddler and mother at the birth of a sibling. Further, this ambivalence is often quite disruptive to the tratment. It is partly resolved, however, when the patient begins to identify with the group, so that the group itself becomes a special, loved entity. Beginning group therapists are often quite surprised at how quickly a new group will "get started" in the first session. Social anxieties and concerns, as well as the need to connect and relate to others, are extremely powerful forces in propelling the group to interact.

Selection Of Patients   The literature about group composition (Yalom, 1970; Mullan & Rosenbaum, 1962) stresses flexibility and encourages a heterogeneous group with regard to such demographic variables of age, vocation, and educational level. However, it should be noted that the social psychological literature concerned with scapegoating (Cartwright & Zander, 1962) suggests that any group member who is extremely different from other members will be more at risk. Thus, in one new psychotherapy group, all members were from 30 to 40 years old except for one considerably older man in his late 60s. This man dealt with his anxieties regarding the group experience by rigidifying old obsessive compulsive character patterns, which manifested in a rather moralizing style. This style was quite abrasive to the other group members. Soon the group coalesced, but did so in a subtle yet evident distancing from this older member. Thus, in this instance, extreme differences in age and character dynamics led to problems of scapegoating.

Fees   As I've suggested above, private group psychotherapy practice differs from individual psychotherapy practice with regard to both its rewards and its challenges. This is nowhere more obvious than with regard to fees. The most typical formula for group fees is that they be one-half the amount that the practitioner charges for an individual psychotherapy session. In metropolitan New York in the spring of 1987, this meant that a group therapist might be charging between $30 and $60 for each group session. With a group of from six to 10 members, the therapist might be earning a considerable sum for each group session. Issues of envy, competition, greed, and neediness are often stimulated under such circumstances. Further, since a therapist's fees change (usually increasing) over time and new group members are typically added over time, often from within one's practice, a group may soon become heterogeneous with regard to fees. Sibling rivalry issues are often stimulated under these conditions. A further complication arises when a therapist employs a sliding scale of fees for group and/or individual sessions. Feelings of specialness or victimization may be stimulated in individual group members, as well as in the therapist. It cannot be emphasized enough that an openness to the totality of the clinical experience is the best approach that the practitioner can apply in all such clinical situations. This openness should include an openness to the therapist's own experiences vis-à-vis sibling rivalry, competition, specialness, exploitation, and victimization.

As to the question of the missed group session, Siegel (1972) suggests that unattended group sessions be included in billing except in the most unusual of circumstances. The very structure of the group does not provide for makeup sessions, so that there can be less flexibility with fees. In every other way, however, the collection of group fees presents to the clinician many of the same complex issues as does the collection of individual fees. Resistance, transference, and countertransference issues are often prominent with regard to fees and their collection.

The Addition of Group Psychotherapy as a Change in the Clincian's Perspective   In arriving at the decision to add the modality of group psychotherapy to a private practice, the therapist is making an important change in perspective, as well as in day-to-day clinical functioning. What I mean here is that the therapist who begins to work with groups has made a shift in perspective so that group psychotherapy is now an important part of his or her work. This can be seen most clearly in the clinician's approach to the initial interview. It is here suggested that therapists who work exclusively with individuals rarely see group psychotherapy as an important treatment option in the initial interview, whereas therapists whose practice combines individual and group psychotherapy often see group treatment as a possible treatment modality. Recent work regarding the initial interview (Billow & Mendelsohn, 1982; Billow & Mendelsohn, 1987b) suggests that the clinician's own reactions are as crucial in the determination of the interview as are those of the patient. And as Bion (1959) has suggested, a change in one's perspective is often the most powerful outcome in any successful psychotherapy experience. With these issues in mind, it is suggested that psychotherapists who add the modality of group psychotherapy to their practice make a kind of therapeutic personal change that will have many implications for their future clinical functioning.

CLINICAL PROBLEMS OF A GROUP PSYCHOTHERAPY PRACTICE

In the following section, I will briefly explore what I believe to be the major clinical issues in the private practice psychotherapy group.[2] The management of resistance and crises and transference and countertransference issues will be discussed. Each of these issues is also important in the private practice of individual psychotherapy, and the contrast between individual and group work will be my major emphasis here. As an organizing principle of our purposes, it should be noted that the major difference between the private practice of group and of individual psychotherapy is that group therapy practice is never private. That is, resistance, crises, transference issues, and to a greater extent than might be realized, countertransference issues all become the public domain of the psychotherapy group. Therefore, each clinical issue concerning an individual group member must be understood with some acknowledgment that the patient is a member of a group.

The Management Of Resistance In The Private Practice Psychotherapy Group

Some practitioners (Spotnitz, 1962; Foulkes & Anthony, 1957) see the major task of group psychotherapy as the presentation and analysis of group resistances. Yalom (1970) suggests that such workers draw a parallel between the analysis of resistance that occurs in individual psychoanalytic therapy and the analysis of the resistances effected by the group. Spotnitz, Yalom, and others believe that overcoming such resistances leads to better functioning and increased self-understanding in group members. It is further suggested that as an individual group member's resistances are being worked with, other

---

[2]Many of the issues raised here are explored in more depth in the literature concerned with group psychotherapy (Yalom, 1970; Durkin, 1964; Slavson, 1943, 1956, 1964; Spotnitz, 1961; Wolf & Schwartz, 1962). My focus here concerns issues raised for the psychoanalytic psychotherapist practicing privately with individuals who has recently begun a group psychotherapy practice.

group members are a participating audience to the unfolding drama. And these members' resistances are often affected by the unfolding group process as deeply as, or at times even more deeply than, those of the individual being worked with.

In one psychotherapy group, a somewhat obsessional patient became involved in a resistance regarding lateness to the sessions. The group's therapist (who was also somewhat obsessional) began to focus on the patient's 5- to 10-minute lateness, and soon both the therapist and the patient had become involved in a "dawdler nag" kind of sturggle. This struggle is a rather common one in many relationships, and in this instance it became a reenactment of an earlier relationship for each member of the dyad. The result here was that several other group members became more introspective with regard to their own stubborn dawdling in the face of (nagging) authority. It should be emphasized here that this somewhat obsessional group therapist was not pathological and that the temporary transference–countertransference "lock" that he had become caught in is not unusual in psychoanalytic group psychotherapy (Mendelsohn, 1981; Billow & Mendelsohn, 1987a). However, the main pont is that the working through of a resistance within one group member was extremely helpful for other members of the psychotherapy group. With this in mind, the management of resistance in group psychotherapy can be seen in the larger focus of the management of group resistances. These group resistances are somewhat different from the resistances that typically appear in individual psychoanalytic psychotherapy because sibling rivalry issues are almost always manifest. Thus in the example above, several group members felt outraged that this dawdling, late group member might be able to get away with coming late to the group, while they felt constrained by the group's time schedule. The primitive appeal that infantile acting out can have on us all was operative here, as in fact these members were quite committed to the group and did not actually wish to miss any of the group time. However, these same group members did not wish to have any other group member be "special," particularly if such specialness was the result of psychopathology. In essence, then, the defiance of this late patient's resistance evoked powerful sibling rivalry and envy in other group members. These members resisted their feelings by the defenses of moralizing and righteous indignation.

Crises

Freud (1912) suggests that crises during individual psychoanalytic treatment are forms of resistance. This is equally true in group psychotherapy. Moreover, the inciting quality of the group (Freud, 1921) can intensify a treatment crisis situation.

An angry and somewhat explosively paranoid female abruptly left an otherwise stable, long-functioning group. She did so while in a rage at another group member who had, somewhat timidly, disagreed with her during one of their interactions. This woman, who liked to be called by her self-appointed nickname "Stormy," had with a series of previous outbursts bullied both the group and the group therapist. The group had begun acting toward this woman in an overly polite, timid way. The universal timidity shown to the patient was a reenactment of what had occurred in her childhood home, where her mother was frightened, polite, and distantly unrelated, while her father frequently exploded into psychoticlike rages. The group's timidity, incited by an increasing fear of the patient's violent outbursts, reinforced the patient's resistances to the exploration of her paternal identification. This ultimately led her to flee the group. Of course, at bottom this patient hated the part of her self that had identified with her bullying father. She left the group because she feared that her paternal identification was so strong that it would over-whelm her, and destory herself and the group. If the group therapist had stated that he might be willing to "leave the group" himself, the patient might have been somewhat reassured and might have been able to stay. That is, if this therapist had suggested that he would leave the group at any sign of real danger, he would have reassured the patient, as well as the group, that he was in the best position to assess danger (c.f. Saretsky, 1977, for a review of other active techniques in group psychotherapy). In any event, a treatment crisis is at bottom an expression of hopelessness by a patient. Such hopelessness in any one member is extremely frightening to all other members of a psycho-therapy group. Interpreting and working with the feelings generated by this and other crises (such as threatened termination, suicidal gestures, and fighting over fees) is the most effective approach to them. Further, if a crisis cannot be overcome and the patient terminates prematurely, the group must be encouraged to mourn the loss of this parting member. This mourning will enable group members to, in part, separate themselves from the lost member. It will also help group members to separate themselves from what the lost member represents to each. Further, the mourning will help each group member to deal with his or her partial identification ("there but for the grace of God go I"). Finally, the mourning process will help members to be reassured of the continued strength and vibrance of the group.

Transference

Menninger (1962) defines individual psychoanalytic therapy as a treatment where there is first the fostering and then the working through of a regressive transference. Further, the analysis of transference is seen as a major curative factor in all individual psychoanalytic psychotherapy (Mendelsohn, 1976). While transference analysis is also an important therapeutic factor in group psychotherapy, a number of authors (Berzon et al., 1963; Frank, 1957; Yalom; 1970) suggest that the working through of the dyadic transference between patient and group therapist may not be as important as that between patient and individual therapist, as there are many different transferences that occur within the therapy group. In fact, Yalom (1970) has suggested that the overall role of the group therapist is very different from that of the individual thera-pist. While Yalom acknowledges that in individual psychotherapy the therapist is the agent of change, he believes that in group therapy the group and group cohesiveness are the agents of change. The work of the group therapist, then, is to help the group develop into a cohesive and therapeutic unit, so that the primary therapeutic factor of group cohesiveness can operate. An opposite point of view has been suggested by Wolff and Schwartz (1962), who believe that a group therapist should employ the analysis of resistance and transfer-ence within the group setting in much the same fashion as one would conduct an individual psychoanalysis. I would suggest that while both of these points of view have merit, perhaps a more helpful way to conceptualize group work would be within a kind of midpoint on this "continuum." Thus, one may come to see that what Yalom (1970) has called "group cohesiveness" and Freud (1921) referred to as an "oceanic force" is the cohesive force that binds psychotherapy groups together. Further I would suggest that this force is an aspect of maternal transference, or "holding," that ties group members to each other and helps a group to be a therapeutic working unit. Disruptions in this transference, caused by the resistance and/or acting out of individual members, need to be continually addressed and managed in the group. This is so that the group continues to be a cohesive therapeutic organism. In this conceptualization, transference interpretation and the working through of transferences are less likely to occur with regard to this "group mother" relationship and will more typically involve sibling rivalry or father/therapist transference issues. Therefore, the main curative factor can still be seen to be the analysis of transferences, but the nature of such transferences and the techniques of transference analysis are somewhat different from those that occur in individual psychoanalytic therapy.

I have suggested above that the analysis of transference becomes even more complex when a patient is being seen in combined individual and group psychotherapy. This way of working occurs frequently in private clinical practice, as most practitioners have a somewhat limited sample of patients to draw from when constructing a therapy group. As a result, patients currently being seen in individual psychotherapy are often selected for group. Many of these patients also continue to work in individual psychotherapy after they have joined the therapy group. This combined therapy setting provides opportunities to work through many transferences, including the splitting of the therapist into "good" and "bad" parts. However, the confusing relationship that such a structure generates can be quite disruptive to the patient, particularly to the borderline patient. Massive anxiety, acting out, and fragmentation are not unusual in a borderline patient during the height of such an experience. As is true in working with borderline patients in individual psychotherapy (Kernberg, 1975; Mendelsohn, 1981b), working within the "here and now" of these splitting and transference distortions is crucial to the success of group psychotherapy with such patients (Mendelsohn, 1981a). As I have indicated above, the private psychotherapy group is not private, and so all other group members become participant observers to each unfolding relationship. The result is a paradox then. Disruptions that occur within the individual patient–therapist relationship will be felt as disruptions within the group. But the supportive "holding action" of the group will serve, at the very same time, to lessen the disruptive effects on individual members, as well as on the group as a whole. This push–pull tension within the psychotherapy group is part of what propels the group, leading to change within it.

Countertransference

I have suggested elsewhere (Mendelsohn, 1981b) that changing views of countertransference may lead us to see its understanding as just as essential in group psychotherapy as in individual psychotherapy. Because of the more public nature of the therapy group, countertransference is often noted more readily by group members. This public–private dimension seems to be a crucial factor affecting the clinician's countertransference. For example, if a group therapist "makes a mistake" in group, the mistake is a public one. If this "mistake" is not worked through within the group, the therapist must return, session after session, to an unsettling clinical situation. There is considerable controversy in group psychotherapy (Yalom, 1970) as to the value of the clinician's self-disclosure. In the clinical situation where a group therapist seems to have been in error, the group may continue to focus on the error, either primarily for the purposes of resistance and transference, or for some other reason(s) — e.g., in some attempt to "cure" the therapist. Whatever the outcome, it is important to question whether or not the clinician chooses to work with "errors." It is sadly ironic that those therapists strong enough to work therapeutically (and not masochistically) with the derivatives of their own countertransference seem to be least under its sway.

While each beginning group psychotherapist ought to have some experience as a member of his or her own psychotherapy group, I have found that an even more helpful setting for the countertransference analysis of group work is as a member of a peer supervisory group. As I have stated elsewhere (Billow & Mendelsohn, 1987a), a dual-focus peer supervisory group relates the here and now of the group experience to specific cases under the peer group's consideration. Case material is understood more clearly by an exploration of this current group experience. What is often most illuminating vis-à-vis the exploration of the group therapist's countertransferences is the parallel processes (Doerman, 1976; Ekstein & Wallerstein, 1958) that occur between supervision and psychotherapy. These processes are often reflected in the group process itself, which can parallel the emotional conflicts experienced by the group therapist and/or the group. Thus one peer supervisory group found itself under intense countertransference anxiety from aggression stimulated by an adolescent group that was being presented by one of the peer group members.[3] In parallel fashion to the adolescent group, the peer group attacked the therapist. This experience helped the therapist to recognize again his tendency to mobilize strong affects, both positive and negative.

The complex transference and countertransference issues raised in the private practice of group psychotherapy suggest that group therapists need to organize new structures to be able to work with this new clinical material. The peer supervisory group is one such structure that will hopefully become increasingly popular, as it is found to be a most helpful and effective medium for the working through of group psychotherapists' countertransferences and countertransference difficulties.

CONCLUSIONS

The psychoanalytic psychotherapy group functions in many ways like a new, and hopefully curative, family. But in a similar fashion to one's own family, therapy groups raise issues of great importance, such as sibling rivalry

---

[3] This case is presented in more detail in Billow and Mendelsohn, 1987a.

and competition, envy and greed, voyeurism and exhibitionism, oedipal and incest feelings and the defenses against such feelings, the desire for human relatedness and the fear of rejection, love and hate, and death and salvation. This complex therapeutic medium presents many complex rewards, indeed, as well as many complex challenges. Thus, it may be somewhat circular to suggest that a clinician who is contemplating beginning a psychotherapy group needs to change some aspects of himself or herself in order to function optimally as a group psychotherapist. This would seem so because the kind of therapist who would contemplate beginning a therapy group would be different in a number of dimensions (e.g., exhibitionism, activity) from the kind of therapist who would not be interested in group work. However, even if the above is so, I believe that the therapist who begins to work with groups changes in some very important ways. For example, this therapist is, for perhaps the first time, confronted directly by many of his or her patients as to how "special" they are to him or her. This can be very unnerving for a clinician who has never dealt with this issue before. It is an even more difficult issue for the clinician who has never worked through conflicts related to being able to "love" more than one person at a time. Other sibling rivalry and competition issues are also often aroused in the beginning group therapist, as are renewals of old conflicts regarding competence and exhibitionism. I would suggest that the successful resolution of much of this "stirring up" helps the psychotherapist to become stronger not only in his or her continuing group psychotherapy work but also in overall clinical functioning.

SUMMARY

In this chapter I have attempted to explore the most important issues in the private practice of group psychotherapy, and while doing so, I have attempted to contrast such issues with related issues in the practice of individual psychoanalytic psychotherapy. The most important difference between private individual and group practice is that group practice is not "private." That is, many decisions faced by the clinician in his or her work with a group member come under the "public scrutiny" of other members of the group. Beginning a private practice psychotherapy group can seem initially quite disruptive to one's individual clinical practice, as many patients, even those who had previously seemed very positively disposed toward group, now become resistant to it. Paradoxically, adding a group can be disruptive to one's individual practice initially, but as the therapy group becomes cohesive, one's practice is actually strengthened. Resistance, transference, and countertransference issues are as important in group psychotherapy as in individual psychotherapy, but each differs in both focus and emphasis. When a therapist decides to begin a private psychotherapy group within hir or her practice, that therapist has made a decision that will probably lead to changes in his or her entire clinical functioning and that will most likely include changes not only in knowledge and skill but also in perspective.

REFERENCES

Berson, B., Pious, C., & Parson, R. (1963). The therapeutic event in group psychotherapy: A study of subjective reports of group members. *Journal Individual Psychology, 19,* 204–212.

Billow, R.M., & Mendelsohn, R. (1982). Intimacy in the initial interview. In M. Fisher & G. Stricker (Eds.), *Intimacy.* New York: Plenum.

Billow, R.M., & Mendelsohn, R. (1987a). The peer supervisory group for psychoanalytic therapists. *Group 11*(1), 35–46.

Billow, R.M. & Mendelsohn, R. (1987b).On initiating the initial interview. (Unpublished Manuscript, Adelphi University, 1987).

Bion, W.R. (1959). *Experiences in groups.* New York: Basic Books.

Cartwright, D., & Zander, A. (Eds.). (1962). *Group dynamics: Research and theory.* Evanston, IL: Row, Peterson.

Doerman, M.J. (1976). Parallel processes in supervision and psychotherapy. *Bulletin of the Menninger Clinic, 40,* 3–104.

Durkin, H. (1964). *The group in depth.* New York: International Universities Press.

Eckstein, R., & Wallerstein, R.S. (1958). *The teaching and learning of psychotherapy.* New York: Basic Books.

Foulkes, S.H., & Anthony, E.J. (1957). *Group psychotherapy: The psychoanalytic approach.* Middlesex, England: Penguin Books.

Frank, J.D. (1957). Some determinants, manifestations and effects of cohesiveness in therapy groups. *International Journal of Group Psychotherapy, 7,* 53–63.

Freud, S. (1912). Recommendations to physicians practicing psychoanalysis. *Standard Edition* (Vol. 12), pp. 109–156, 1974.

Freud, S. (1921). Group psychology and the analysis of the ego. *Standard Edition* (Vol. 18), pp. 67–145, 1975.

Goldman, G.D. (972). The establishment of a private practice. In G.D. Goldman & G. Stricker, *Practical problems of a private psychotherapy practice.* Springfield, IL: Charles C. Thomas.

Kernberg, O. (1975). *Borderline conditions and pathological narcissism.* New York: Jason Aronson.

Mendelsohn, R. (1978). Critical factors in short-term psychotherapy: A summary. *Bulletin of the Menninger Clinic, 42,* 133–149.

Mendelsohn, R. (1981a). Active attention and focusing on the transference/countertransference in the psychotherapy of the borderline patient. *Psychotherapy, theory, research and practice, 18(3), 386–393.*

Mendelsohn, R. (1981b). When groups merge: Transference and countertransference issues. *International Journal of Group Psychotherapy, 31,* 139–150.

Menninger, K. (1962). *Theory of psychoanalytic technique.* New York: Free Press.

Mullan, H., & Rosenbaum, M. (1962). *Group Psychotherapy.* New York: Free Press.

Saretsky, T. (1977). *Active techniques and group psychotherapy.* New York: Jason Aronson.

Siegel, M. (1972). Special problems in group psychotherapy practice. In G.D. Goldman, & G. Stricker, *Practical problems of a private psychotherapy practice.* Springfield, IL: Charles C. Thomas.

Slavson, S.R. (1943). *An introduction to group psychotherapy.* Cambridge, MA: Harvard University Press.

Slavson, S.R. (1964). *The fields of group psychotherapy.* New York: International Universities Press.

Spotnitz, H. (1961). *The couch and the circle.* New York: Knopf.

Toseland, R.W. & Siporin, M. (1987). When to recommend group treatment. A review of the clinical and research literature. *International Journal of Group Psychotherapy 36*(4), 171–206.

Wolf, A., & Schwartz, E.K. (1962). *Psychoanalysis in groups.* New York: Grunne and Stratton.

Yalom, I.D. (1970). *The theory and practice of group psychotherapy.* New York: Basic Books.

C H A P T E R
47

THE THERAPIST'S PERSONALITY INSIDE AND OUTSIDE THE CONSULTING ROOM

Karen L. Lombardi, Ph.D.

THE NEUTRAL POSITION

The ambivalently held ideal of analytic neutrality has led therapists and analysts in training to believe that it is desirable, if not necessary to the work of psychotherapy, that they park their personalities outside the doors of their consulting rooms and enter with their feelings, values, goals, and tendencies to influence in suspension. Whether we endorse the past vogue of therapists serving as a blank screen onto which patients can freely project their thoughts and feelings or the current vogue of serving as a mirror in which patients see only their reflection, the implicit assumption is that the therapist's personality must be kept out of the consulting room so as not to interfere with the attitude of neutrality and thereby break the frame of the psychotherapeutic relationship. This chapter will examine the historical roots of the neutral position, within which I include such concepts as the blank screen, the mirror, the metaphor of the surgeon, and outermost extensions of the principle of abstinence. It is questioned whether this is a possible or a desirable positioning of the therapist in relation to the patient.

In 1912, Freud first employed the metaphor of the surgeon in his recommendations for psychoanalytic technique:

> I cannot advise my colleagues too urgently to model themselves during psychoanalytic treatment on the surgeon, who puts aside all his feelings, even his human sympathy, and concentrates his mental forces on the single aim of performing the operation as skillfully as possible. (Freud, 1912, p. 115)

Freud recommends this surgical attitude, or "emotional coldness" as he calls it in another part of the same paper, primarily to serve as desirable protection for the emotional life of the therapist. Emotional distance is recommended to guard the therapist from becoming too affected by the patient, and to guard the therapist from colluding with the patient's resistances.

Later in the same paper, Freud employs the metaphor of the mirror, which has become particularly central in recent years to Kohut (1971) and others who advocate the concept of mirroring the patient as a particular form of empathic technique. To quote Freud, "The doctor should be opaque to his patients and, like a mirror, should show them nothing but what is shown to him" (p. 118). Here, Freud is particularly cautioning against emboldened doctors bringing their own individuality directly into the relationship with their patients. An attitude of intimacy on the doctor's part, Freud believes, may help overcome initial resistances on the patient's part, but will make the resolution of the transference far more difficult.

A few years later, Freud (1915) articulated the principle of abstinence, which refers primarily to the therapist's resisting seduction by the patient's eroticized transference, and secondarily and in a more general sense to allowing the patient's needs and longings to persist so as to serve as continued motivation for the work of the analysis. Neutrality is mentioned in this passage in regard to the necessity of keeping one's countertransference in check. The principle of abstinence has come to serve both as a guidepost and as a justification for both physical and emotional distance from the patient, and even more importantly, as a prohibition against the "gratification" of any of the patient's needs or desires.

Given what is known about Freud's own personality and personal behavior in relation to his patients (as examples, that he offered a meal in his home to his now-famous patient, the Rat Man, and that he undertook the psychoanalysis of his own daughter, Anna), it is unlikely that he demanded such anonymity and detachment from himself in relation to his patients as these notions of neutrality tend to suggest. Although we would like to think that theory informs practice, it is not surprising for us to discover that we do not always do as we say, and that seems to have been as true for Freud as it is for the rest of us. However, I do believe that there are certain assumptions regarding the notion of neutrality that require reexamination and reevaluation in light of both theory and practice.

CONTROL AND DESTRUCTIVENESS

The concept of neutrality contains within it certain assumptions regarding aspects of control, influence, and destructiveness that give it particular power. Contained within Freud's discussions of neutrality, particularly as it relates to the principle of abstinence, is the paramount need for analysts to control themselves, to guard against their own impulses. The issue of control (here, primarily in a sense of self-control) is paramount. Without self-control analysts may easily be swept along by the patients' transference fantasies, particularly when of an erotic or especially deprivation-tinged sort, and may want to gratify patients, with potentially disastrous results. Neutrality is contrasted with losing control: "Our control over ourselves is not so complete that we may not suddenly one day go further than we had intended" (Freud, 1915, p. 164). As Freud conceives them, the considerations of neutrality and gratifications are absolute. One is either neutral or not neutral; one either gratifies or does not gratify. He explicitly entertains the possibility of finding a middle ground and dismisses that position as untenable. Gratification, the loss of the neutral attitude, is seen as counterproductive to analysis as it destroys the patient's "susceptibility to influence" by psychoanalysis. Interestingly, here Freud is suggesting that it is not only loss of self-control that is at issue but loss of control to the patient, who in having procured the emotional involvement of the analyst will prefer the rewards of the material over the rewards of the psychical. Alternatively, the threat to the analyst's ability to keep his or her countertransference in check threatens his or her control of the analytic situation.

Freud's concerns with such matters suggest two influences: that of the culture in which he lived and that of the theory he espoused. In order to understand Freud's emphasis on this matter we must place him in the context of his own society, or at least in the context of the society as he perceived it. Freud never lost sight of the repressive nature of his immediate world. It was a world in which, he believed, sexual tensions were so built up that they might, at virtually any moment of weakness, overcome one's socially adaptive restraint. In Freud's vision, this danger was no less compelling for the analyst than for the patient. This view of society was reflected in Freud's theory, which regarded the press of internal drive states as the primary motivating force in people. As the expression of these drives came into conflict with the demands of reality, malignant symptoms would occur as an attempt at compromise.

As a closed-system model, drive theory lends itself to regarding the anlytic relationship as one in which the action occurs exclusively *within* people, and not *between* people. The focus of attention is on the understanding of internal states within the patient that the analyst articulates through his or her intellectual understanding of the forces that operate within the patient. In the theory, there is no room for ideas, feelings, and thoughts on the part of the analyst *in relation to* the patient. The analytic ideal in this model is that of the observer and the observed, with little attention paid to the space that is shared between the two. It follows, then, that the revealing of the personality of the analyst is regarded as an imposition that will interfere with, short-circuit, or otherwise cut off the transference issues that need to be worked through.

POWER AND INFLUENCE

An ambivalent relationship to power and influence in the analytic situation is reflected in this stance. In Freud's discussion there is a paradoxical relationship to power and influence. On the one hand, there is the patient's power over the analyst, which the analyst must resist. On the other hand, there is the patient's inferiority and weakness due to illness, which the analyst must not exploit. Part of what is at issue is the fear of influence that arises from the analyst's sense of omnipotence. Part of Freud's cautions may be seen as compensatory strategies to ensure that the patient would be respected. Thompson (1938) captures this conflict by contrasting the attitude that the analyst is detached and unaffected by the patient and the therapeutic process with the attitude that the analyst, through suggestion, completely imposes his or her ideas into the patient. It is as if the myth of the detached analyst arose as a defense against a wish to influence.

Attempts to modernize the concept of neutrality to bring it in line with contemporary notions of respect for the individuality of the patient seem to me interesting but flawed. Poland (1984) contrasts the function of "neutrality" as a noun with the function of "neutrality" as a verb, and stresses the verb or action-oriented functions of neutrality as most important to preserve in analytic practice. As a noun, neutrality functions with regard to appearance, leaving us with a colorless and indifferent analyst. As a verb, however, neutrality functions with regard to power and activity, in which case the analyst would be nonaligned or nonjudgmental in relation to patients. For Poland, neutrality circumscribes the interpersonal aspect of the transference process from "eccentric intrusions" by the analyst.

Poland gives an important example of the misuse of the neutral stance by an analyst in training. This young analyst was seeing a woman who daily locked her 5-year-old son in a small room so that she could be free to attend her analytic sessions. He never questioned or commented on this woman's rather horrifying treatment of her child, as he felt that his task was not to take a position, but simply to analyze the material as it came up. Clearly, Poland views this as a distortion and a defensive use of the meaning of neutrality. It does not square, however, with his view of remaining nonaligned with regard to power and activity. Clearly, there are times when we decide to be neutral and times when we decide to align ourselves with a particular position, as most of us would have in the case of a small child's being locked in a room unattended. How, then, do we decide when to adhere to the principle of neutrality and when to abandon it? Poland does not address this question, and although he implicitly recognizes that neutrality is an ideal that is not attainable in practice, he nevertheless maintains it as an ideal.

Hoffer (1985) recognizes neutrality as an ambivalently held ideal within the field of psychotherapy and psychoanalysis. Connotations of detachment, impersonality, and indifference in the analytic attitude push up against orientations of involvement and compassion, which many of us espouse. In an attempt at integration, he asks an important question: Can one be honestly neutral and genuinely involved? Hoffer equates neutrality with empathy, by defining neutrality in an unusual way, as "the analyst's genuine appreciation of the patient's dilemmas and conflicts from the patient's pont of view" (p. 783). Hoffer's discussion of the defensive use of neutrality places the analyst's capacity for intimate relatedness at the center of the issue. The concept of neutrality, as it extends to one's relationship to conflict, to feeling, and to power, may be used in the service of isolation of affect and compartmentalization of the analytic experience (with, I believe, a concomitant denial of the dyadic nature of the experience). Hoffer's idea is that one can be both intimate and neutral if you are able to separate your *wishes for* the patient from your *needs from* the patient. This is an important idea, but it is not an idea that is primarily derived from discourse on neutrality. Hoffer's argument centers around issues of relatedness between therapist and patient in which neutrality as it was originally developed has little place. In order to make it fit, Hoffer has essentially redefined neutrality as a special form of interpersonal relatedness.

The concept of neutrality, as it was originally conceived, is an attempt to isolate the experience of the patient from participation by the analyst so as not to contaminate or influence the patient's experience. In this sense, the concept of neutrality is not consonant with a view of the psychoanalytic process as taking place within a two-person relationship. Granted, there are always aspects of individual experience that are private and unique, just as it is given that the analyst and the patient are two people who are fundamentally separate from each other. But the analytic relationship takes place within a dyad, within the shared space between the patient and the analyst. In this sense, the concept of neutrality does not fit the analytic relationship.

NEUTRALITY AND THE
RELATIONAL ORIENTATION

For those of us who espouse a theory of psychological development that stresses the primacy of relationships over the primacy of drives, the concept of neutrality has always been a troubling one. As long as 50 years ago, such more relationally oriented theorists as the Balints (1939) opposed the climate of lifelessness and sterility that the neutral position suggested. The Balints' focus was on the dyadic nature of the psychoanalytic relationship. Contrary to the commonly held view at that time that the work of the anlyst was to sit outside the transference and objectively interpret it to the patient, the Balints saw the analytic situation as the interplay between the patient's transference and the analyst's countertransference, complicated and enriched by the reactions of each to the other. The Balints' clinical attitude was consonant with the developmental point of view that they espoused, which was significantly different from Freud's. Michael Balint's (1937) conceptual contribution of primary object love posited that there is an interdependence of infant and mother from the very beginning of life that is a need in itself and not a drive derivative. According to Freudian developmental theory, primary drives are physiological (e.g., hunger, thirst, pleasure) and lead, by association and displacement, to secondary attachments to the people who satisfy those drives. In this system, object relations do not occur from the beginning of life, but are derivative phenomena. It is drives and drive satisfaction, not people and relationships, that are primary motivating and organizing forces in psychic life. This is a theory of individualism that sees life energy as concentrated on the self (what Freud calls "primary narcissism") and only gradually and secondarily, through the influence of civilizing experience, coming to be focused on or inclusive of others (what Freud calls "object cathexis"). Balint stands in opposition to this view of development when he states that object love is a primary phenomenon that is not a derivative of drive but a thing in itself. In the most reductionistic terms, in Balint's view of human development people need people, whereas in Freud's view of human development people need gratification. Clinically, Balint's position facilitates an understanding of why severely narcissistic patients do not turn away from the object world, but rather tend to be, in therapy, hypersensitive, irritable, and insatiable in relation both to the therapist and to other people in their lives.

Like Winnicott (1947) after him, Balint viewed the personality of the analyst as a special and unavoidable form of countertransference; that is, as the unique environment created by each analyst in the analytic situation, which in one way or another affects the patient. It is impossible, he maintains, for the transference of emotions in the analytic situation to be one way (that is, only from the patient to the analyst), as that would require the analyst to behave in a passive, sterile, inanimate manner. If one is animate, which one cannot help being simply by being alive, then one affects the transference situation. What goes into the creation of this unique environment? Not only whether one "gratifies" the patient or not, but whether one's voice is soft, authoritative, or soothing, whether one is parsimonious or extravagant in interpretations, whether the room is dark or well lit, whether the walls are bare or decorated, and so on.

Balint uses the analogy of the pillow to illustrate that the use to which even an inanimate object is put is affected by the analyst's personality. The pillow is a relatively standard piece of equipment in the analytic consulting room. However, there are a multitude of ways a pillow can be used. There can be one pillow for everyone, with separate tissue paper for each; there can be one pillow for each person, who must always use his or her own and no one else's; there can be two or three pillows to choose from; there can be different pillow covers for each person; and so on. Balint recounts the dream of a patient who for external reasons had to change his analyst. In his dream, the first analyst was working in a highly modern, white-tiled bathroom, whereas the second was working in an old-fashioned, dirty, smelly place.

In addition to the individual issues of the patient, which Balint does not discuss, the dream reflected that the patient drew certain conclusions about his analysts on the basis of the different ways that each of them treated the problem of the pillow. For those patients who do not use the couch, the problem of the chair is similar. In my personal experience in supervision, first in psychotherapy training and later in psychoanalytic training, I had the opportunity to be in several different consulting rooms for periods of several months at a time. In some offices the analyst's chair was opulent and the patient's chair was rather nondescript and poor; in other offices the chairs were made of the same fine material but the analyst's chair was bigger than the patient's. In other offices the two chairs were exactly alike, and in others the chairs bore no resemblance and little comparison to each other. These sorts of differences go to creating individual atmospheres that communicate something to the patient (and the supervisee) about the personality of the analyst. Balint points out that it is not that one sort of atmosphere is more desirable than another (that is, there is not one ideal way to be), but that various individual atmospheres seem to be good enough for the patient to proceed with his or her own transferences in the analysis regardless.

Balint's concept of primary object love stands in stark contrast to the Freudian idea of intrapsychic functioning as a closed-energy model. For Balint the infant and the object have a fundamental relationship with each other from the very start of life. For Freud objects are inextricably linked with the cathexis of libidinal instinctual energy, and an external object, such as a mother, is a secondary target, one that is chosen only after the primary narcissistic cathexis proves insufficiently gratifying.

Extending this contrast into the consulting room, we can see that Balint would feel that the metaphor of neutrality would fail as an attempt to symbolize either the patient's or the therapist's experience of life. Why, if both the patient and the therapist have cut their intrapsychic eye teeth in an environment in which the matter of object love was central, should either of them act as a neutral party?

FROM PERSONAL EXPERIENCE
TO SHARED EXPERIENCE

In the work of D. W. Winnicott, the relationship between the analyst and the patient is even more clearly seen to be not only primary but the very agent of change. For Winnicott, in analysis it is not just a matter of who the analyst is – the analyst's personality so to speak – but even more fundamentally it is a matter of who the analyst and the patient are together, their joint personality. In his writings we see that the maintenance of a neutral stance is viewed as essentially irrelevant since it is neither possible nor desirable, even if it were possible.

A typical example of this may be seen in one of Winnicott's (1947) earlier and most influential works, "Hate in the Countertransference." Here, he divides countertransference into three types: (1) abnormalities in countertransference feelings, which he views, as a classical analyst might, as under repression by the analyst; (2) the objective countertransference, which stresses the more modern view of the analytic setting as inherently interactional; and (3) the effect of the analyst's personality on his or her analytic work, which is similar to Balint's notion of the unique environment created by the analyst. In the third type of countertransference Winnicott is referring to the identifications and tendencies that arise from the analyst's personal experiences that contribute to making the analytic setting and the analytic work unique.

Winnicott (1962) has told us how he functions in the analytic setting.

> In doing psycho-analysis I aim at:
>> Keeping alive
>> Keeping well
>> Keeping awake
> I aim at being myself and behaving myself.

This is a reminder, it seems to me, not only of the importance of the analyst's survival of the patient's attacks of aggression, illness, and deadness within the analytic setting but also of the importance to the analyst of remaining in touch with his or her own *person*ality. This attitude is consistent with Winnicott's notion of the role of the facilitating environment in normal development. In a letter of advice (Rodman, 1987) to a mother who was troubled by difficulties in her relationship to her child, Winnicott wrote: "The only way that babies can reach anything consistent in their environment is when the parents are able to be themselves" (p. 164).

For Winnicott analysts are not, and must not try to be, alike by the virtue of their being analysts. He pointed out toward the end of his career that he himself was not the same person doing the same sort of work as he had been earlier in his career. Nor does he believe that analysts are alike on the basis of the areas in which they work best or in their adherence to the standard techniques of psychoanalysis. Just as there is no ideal way to *be* as a parent, so there is no ideal of analytic attitude or analytic technique, whether it be that of the mirror, the blank screen, the surgeon, the neutral observer, or the perfectly attuned parent/analyst who anticipates the child's/patient's needs.

A woman whose teenage daughter I was treating on a once-a-week basis was originally referred by a colleague who had treated the mother in the past. The woman herself waš seeking a referral for her brother, who lived in a distant city. "What do you call what you do?" she asked. "Psychoanalytically informed psychotherapy," I responded, "but what is it that you need?" She explained that her brother was seeing someone for psychological assistance. That person took notes and spoke little, and the brother did not know where the man was and did not feel he was being helped. "Your brother wants to feel that someone can be more involved with him?" I asked. "Yes," she said. "I think what he needs is someone more like you and Bob [her former therapist]. Can you find someone like that in his city?" Transference issues aside, there was a certain style of communication or style of being that this woman responded to, that felt comfortable and right to her, and that could not be defined by adherence to a particular theoretical orientation or technique.

The area of potential space, that area of experience that is neither inside nor outside the individual, is for Winnicott where we do most of our living and where individual growth is achieved. Productive analytic work occurs in the shared space between the patient and the analyst. Clearly, this implies that part of the analyst's personality must always be playing an active role in the therapy for the therapy to be productive. However, I think the actual implication is that the therapist's entire personality is playing an active role.

The value of the analyst's participation in the analytic situation is in the ability to be involved without interfering. Once having interfered, the analyst finds added value in the ability to use those interferences, impingements, failures of attunement, and so on to better understand both the patient and himself or herself. In the process of this participation, the reality and limitations of the analyst as a person are bound to become more visible (Khan, 1960). If the analyst is able to make use of his or her own personality in relation to the patient, the analyst–analysand dyad may share in the creation of shared experiences that expand the patient's capacities for ego-relatedness. To paraphrase Winnicott (1971), psychoanalysis and psychotherapy are playing in the potential space where the analyst's and the patient's personalities meet.

REFERENCES

Balint, M. (1937). Early developmental states of the ego: Primary object love. In M. Balint, *Primary love and psychoanalytic technique.* New York: Liveright, 1965.

Balint, M., & Balint, A. (1939). On transference and countertransference. *International Journal of Psychoanalysis, 20,* 223–230.

Freud, S. (1912). Recommendations to physicians practicing psychoanalysis. *Standard edition, 12,* 10–120, 1961.

Freud, S. (1915). Observations on transference love. *Standard edition, 12,* 157–171, 1961.

Hoffer, A. (1985). Toward a definition of psychoanalytic neutrality. *Journal of the American Psychoanalytic Association, 33,* 771–795.

Khan, M.M.R. (1960). Regression and integration in the analytic setting. In M.M.R.

Khan, *The privacy of the self.* New York: International Universities Press, 1974.

Kohut, H. (1971). *The analysis of self.* New York: International Universities Press.

Poland, W.S. (1984). On the analyst's neutrality. *Journal of the American Psychoanalytic Association, 32,* 283–299.

Rodman, F.R. (Ed.). (1987). *The spontaneous gesture: Selected letters of D.W. Winnicott.* Cambridge, Mass.: Harvard University Press.

Thompson, C. (1938). Notes on the psychoanalytic significance of the choice of analyst. *Psychiatry, 1,* 205–216.

Winnicott, D.W. (1947). Hate in the countertransference. In D.W. Winnicott, *Through paediatrics to psychoanalysis.* London: Hogarth Press, 1978.

Winnicott, D.W. (1962). The aims of psychoanalytical treatment. In D.W. Winnicott, *The maturational processes and the facilitating environment.* New York: International Universities Press, 1965.

Winnicott, D.W. (1971). Playing: A theoretical statement. In D.W. Winnicott, *Playing and reality.* Harmondsworth, England: Penguin.

C H A P T E R
48

HOW TO DEAL WITH EMOTIONAL ISSUES UPON RETIREMENT OR TERMINATION OF PRACTICE

Harold Lindner, Ph.D.

Terminating a way of life—whether by forced or voluntary retirement—must be recognized by any standards as one of the most emotionally draining decisions that a professional has to face. It is unlikely that one makes such a decision lightly. It is more likely that decisions of that magnitude are resisted until made mandatory if not in fact then in principle.

This examination of the variants involved in this process largely represents a compilation of the author's own thoughts and experiences. It also evolved from an informal survey he undertook with a dozen or so colleagues who have made the passage from practice to retirement. In deciding whom to interview in that survey, the writer elicited responses from a variety of psychologists, psychiatrists, and ancillary professional others in order to evoke a relatively wide experiential and personal range of reaction. Additionally, inherent in these choices was an effort to include people who, although coming from a history of professional practice in our discipline, independently and individually made a variety of postpractice choices along a broad continuum. All of them have carved out of their "retirement" a new direction for their lives, from absolute retirement to the other extreme of replacing their practices with new professional responsibilites. In all cases considerably different choices from their previous containments within the private practice modality were made. For the writer, the decision to terminate a psychoanalytic independent practice that spanned some 30 years of full-time commitment and the idea of "retirement" arose after a critical health problem mandated that decision (Lindner, 1985).

It appears to be universal that the immediacy of the decision to terminate a practice arouses two major emotional components: (1) anxiety and (2) depression. When the concept takes on immediacy one experiences a significant apprehension that one is contemplating leaving the real world of work, involvement, personal regard, and status and the characterological defense of being in control of one's destiny. The question almost immediately arises: Is it possible to do? For those who have experienced a life of financial, social, professional, and personal independence through the pursuits and rewards of their practices, the apprehension manifests itself in a duality. Can I do it? Can the world get along without me? The various rewards derived from practice surface to consciousness almost immediately. Even considering a termination of a practice represents a narcissistic injury that makes one blanch. In quite another context this writer published a paper some years ago that was concerned with the "shared neurosis" of therapist and patient (Lindner, 1960). In that work I examined the role of the need on the part of many therapists to be omnipotent, controlling, and, in extremity, somewhat megalomaniacal, in their insistence that patients respond to their ideas about the patients' lifestyles. To a greater or lesser degree all practitioners experience a modicum of some of these characteristics in their psychotherapeutic practices. The possibility of terminating or retiring from practice implies a necessary abdication from such character armoring. In some persons this can be catastrophic. In others it arouses a degree of anxiety that is profound. In yet others it makes for sufficient degree of apprehension that significant introspection and effort are required to ameliorate it. Even in those who have experienced a partial retirement from active practice, as in the "sabbatical," similar concerns arise: Can my patients tolerate my absence (Cooper, 1987)? Can I tolerate relinquishing my responsibility (i.e., control)? Such questions overwhelmingly bombard the person and frequently lead to a denial or a procrastination that, when ended, often becomes manifest in clinical depression. During this trying period various defensive postures occur. Reflections on the tedium, the repetition, the routine, and the obligatory schedule serve to mitigate some of these. Fantasies about the freedom from these negatives of life-styles abound: No more restrictive responsibility! Now I can be free to expand...do those things I've been unable to do...go and do whatever I choose and desire...no more detail...no more nonsense.

Following closely upon this initial reaction anxious reflections often develop. But what the hell will I do? How will I spend my time? Will I become slothful? Parasitical? Is this the end? Will it make a damned bit of difference to anyone that I'm no longer here? Will anyone care? How do I fill the void?

It is amply evident from the above that the early cognitive period is extremely difficult and demanding upon the emotional resources the practitioner can bring to bear upon the decisional activities leading to eventual resolution. Clearly, the more intact the person, the greater the ego strength available; and the more astute and comfortable with unconscious needs the person is, the more satisfactory will be the resolution and the actual making of the decision. It is too superficial to say that one has to consciously make a determined effort at decision, to be rational, and to bolster one's decision with agenda that offer positive reinforcements. These are helpful as far as they take one but only that far. Similarly, to claim sophomorically that one must engage in careful planning ignores the degree of anger (conscious and unconscious) that is inherent in this state. The power of these emotional forces is enormous. Their strength tends to exacerbate unresolved neurotic indexes that even in ordinary experience serve to debilitate one and to shrink one's horizons. One must deal very directly with these emotional facets, either through self-analysis or by consultation with colleagues, in order to achieve the emotional stability and freedom to make the final, unalterable decision to terminate the practice and retire from that period of one's life.

Once the decision has been made, the "blind spots" removed, the reality of the decisional process absorbed, action is then required and another tension state is initiated: How do I do it?

The literature is sparse on this subject, probably because therapists, like many nontherapists, have a difficult time dealing with their own internal needs, ambivalences, and defenses. They, like others, tend to repress, deny, rationalize, and displace anxieties. It appears ubiquitous that therapists — dynamic and cognitive alike — resist revealing to their patients uncertainties about their personal lives that concern critical life and health matters (Roster, 1986). They also resist informing patients about the decision to terminate a practice and to retire. They do this for a variety of reasons, not least of which is the wish to secure continuing referral sources during the interim before actually closing their doors forever. A few studies of this specific experience from the point of view of the therapist have been reported but, again, only a few. These have essentially been concerned with the perspective and experience of the therapist faced with a life-threatening crisis in his or her own life that led to either a temporary or final cessation of practice (Lindner, 1984; Abend, 1982; Burton, 1978; Dewald, 1982; Eissler, 1977; Chermin, 1976). Issues of transference, countertransference, rage, hostility, love, and hate have been surveyed in these reports. Consistently, among the various persons whom the author interviewed, very few of these emotional factors were discussed with patients by professionals who chose to retire for reasons having little or nothing to do with illness. Interestingly, however, similar emotional reactions were described to the writer by the majority of interviewees concerning the reactions elicited from the patients upon their being informed of the therapist's decision to terminate practice. Most reported a significant exacerbation of symptomology. A few reported "amazing" symptom abatements. Many reported having had to deal with (transference) neurotic behavior and ideation that they thought had been worked through previously or that had not been exhibited previously. Acting out hostile, sometimes self-destructive impulses was manifest in many. Feelings of abandonment and anxiety about loss were ubiquitous. Rageful attacks against the proposition of the therapist's sense of responsibility to the patient were rampant. Infantile, sometimes primitive behavior and thought were invoked through both dream work and familial relationships and were exhibited by some in a very primitive fashion. Suffice it to summarize, the period between the therapist's informing the patient of the date of departure and its occurrence (usually some months hence) was one of an exceedingly trying struggle between the two parties in the therapeutic dyad. Significantly, however, shortly before the actual final date a presumed resolution was almost always achieved. Parting was actualized in warm, loving, and compassionate ways by most. In those few instances where the patient could not tolerate the experience but opted to control the departure by prematurely terminating the relationship, such endings were often painful and emotionally wrenching. Sometimes the relationship regressed quite bitterly with manifest anger, resentment, and recriminations indicative of unresolved transferences. In these situations, the therapists reported frustrations in attempting to work through their own countertransferences. In situations in which resolution was achieved — by far the majority of those reported to the author — much valuable therapeutic work was done during that interim period to the advantage of the patients and to the immense satisfaction of the therapists. Of course, these experiences proved emotionally gratifying to the therapists. They helped alleviate any guilt or regret they might have been experiencing in their decision to terminate the therapeutic relationship and end their practice.

At this juncture it seems appropriate to discuss the therapists' affective states once the termination date had passed and retirement had become a reality. The experience of awakening the day after retiring with no definitive schedule, no appointments, no obligations to meet, and nobody awaiting them was somewhat disorienting but painlessly so. The sense of relief at the realization that there was no restriction to their existence was exhilarating: total freedom to be and do as they might wish. Self-indulgent feelings surfaced. This was a time for "enjoyables." One professional told me she felt as though she had "been let out of my cage" and never again would she tolerate a "defined structure." In her effort to actualize this phenomenological alteration in her existence, she symbolically took off her wristwatch, never again to wear one: She was free! Most reported a desire to "Coney Island" their lives — some by moving to a new geographical environment, others by indulging in recreational activities that previously had been denied to them because of limitations on time and resources. Invariably, all reported a desire for "change" and each defined this quite differently. For some this meant the opening of vistas previously only fantasied. For others it means new nonprofessional challenges. Still others anticipated a period of regressed, unstructured, hedonistic playtime of more libidinal character. One person claimed that he would never again use the title "Dr." Now he preferred the vernacular of a family nickname that he had previously avoided outside of the home. A few desired a narcissistic withdrawal under the guise of a marshalling of resources to prepare for a new type of social existence. Vacationing, nondemanding and nonprofessional readings, sports, recreation, entertainment, socializing, and intrigue with fiduciary matters became de rigeur. A renewal of familial and marital relationships was paramount in all reports to the interviewer — matters that previously had been given less than prominent conscious attention. In essence, there routinely commenced a shift in ideation and behavior from servicing others to servicing the self. Self-indulgence was the new order in the initial period after retirement commenced.

That period, however, was short-lived. Reality soon intruded. Those who were so joyful about not having responsibilities soon began to question their worth, no longer measured by professional responsibilities or status in the community and among peers. One interviewee reported a vignette that epitomized what most indicated their experience to be. He told of accompanying his wife to a physician's office and being asked to wait in the waiting room for her instead of to accompany her into the examining room. He was denied this privilege. Following the diagnostic examination, the wife asked for him to be present during the doctor's report of his findings and recommendations for treatment. She was told by the doctor that he did not have time to waste explaining diagnoses to family. When she reminded the doctor that her husband was a fellow physician the man shrugged it off and refused to speak to him. He was offended. He used that experience to illustrate the loss of status he felt, saying it was an awful blow to his ego. This, he said, was another of many indignities he had suffered since retirement, and he claimed that he no longer received the respect and courtesy he previously had received as a matter of course. Now, he protested, he felt castrated. He felt a narcissistic injury to his sense of worth: that he was not a contributing member of society and that he had no defined status in life. A shared phenomenon among my interviewees was the sense of existing in a hostile world, one in which society looked upon them with suspicion, as persons who are no longer contributory or valued or needed – as outsiders.

The effective state of being outsiders is also fairly common to retirees, especially when negative judgments by former peers are suspected. In fact, the most prevalent experience of all the retirees surveyed was feeling depressed at the loss of intrinsic status through belonging to the society of practitioners. Professional impotency is pervasive among this population and appears to represent the driving force behind the determination to have some form of professional renewal, either through part-time work or a consultancy. The need to become personally involved in a profession, in one form or another, rapidly became critical for all interviewees in this sampling. It seems apparent that the initial stage of rejoicing at the retirement from active professional pursuit and engaging in pleasurable alternative pursuits was not long satisfying and was soon replaced by a search for at least part-time occupational placement.

Following the time of relatively satisfying and quiescent relief from the tedium of responsibility in practice, the feeling of loss sets in and one commonly begins to worry, What will I do with myself? Some resentfully ask themselves, Am I over the hill? Those whose inner strengths are intact search for replacements. Those whose internal mechanisms are weakened flounder and suffer terrible feelings of loss. Those who are psychologically dependent hope that some paternal introject will guide and protect them and offer respite through job placement. Those whose maternal introject is debilitating will psychologically deteriorate. They tend to regress to an infantile state of depressive failure and pathos. Sometimes these people develop psychogenic and/or psychosomatic debilities that serve as protective defensive devices to ward off what is now exprienced as a hostile environment.

Clearly, the fashion in which any or all of the above is worked through and, hopefully, resolved is highly dependent upon one's character armor. If one's character state is sufficient, one will find resolutions that prove ego restorative and supportive. If one's character armor is weak, one will suffer an irresolvable need and develop pathogenic defenses and attitudes that will hinder meaningful resolution and maintain a state of unrequited despondency and despair.

The most satisfying resolution appears to reside in those whose characterological defenses are most secured in reality. Concrete thinking most adroitly directs one to simplify and substitute life choices leading to direct activity for real or imagined loss. As one interviewee commented, "Retirement should be evolutionary, not revolutionary." Introspective capacities should be used prior to and following the termination of one's practice to examine the meaning of work in one's life and the importance of relationships such as those with spouse, friends, and colleagues. One must analyze how retirement might modify or change these so that it does not necessarily mean a loss of any of them. One must develop the capacity to restructure one's life. This is precisely what successful retirement always involves and requires.

To the degree that one measures the influence of one's familiar and collegial interconnectedness (and appraises realistically one's financial and interpersonal substructure), will one be able to comfortably and without overwhelming anxiety restructure one's frame of reference and make new and egosyntonic employment decisions. One of the most satisfying aspects of this passage is being in a position of relative financial ease so that one may contemplate almost any form of restructured employment — voluntary or remunerative. Currently we exist in a social climate that tends to relieve many retirees from financial stress (through pensions, Keogh, IRA, etc.). While there is a disparity between those who were institutionally employed, and therefore able to build substantial pension safety nets, and those who were in private practice, even those in the latter category are able to subsidize their retirement period to a larger extent than were earlier generations of Americans. Furthermore, by careful accumulation of resources and lucky (if not always astute) husbanding of fiduciary manipulations, most retired professionals are free from the most damaging and restrictive anxieties of financial concern. In fact, when interviewing retirees, one gleans a universal sigh of relief and learns that, given the economic facts of life in this country today, they commence retirement with hesitation about their financial situation but soon learn that their preplanning paid off. These people enjoy relative economic stability. Often their "pensions" provide above and beyond the requirements of their new lifestyles, sans salaried or fee-for-service incomes. Obviously this state pertains only to those who have appropriately provided for this period. For those who could not, or did not, economic matters place a severe limitation on their freedom and capacity to carve out a comfortable existence without additional income, and make mandatory some form of replacement financing.

Once the matter of economic security is in place, however, retirees find the process one of opportunity. If they are not prone to depressive characterological thought processes, they soon find ways to concretize their anxieties by doing personally constructive things. These might involve avenues of professional involvement different from their previous investment in practice. If, on the other hand, they are prone to continuing depressive feelings, there is the real danger that they will find retirement a painful process and will feel that their position is precarious and that they are without power and authority and are worthless. There is the real danger that they will experience a severe loss of status and feel that they are second-class citizens. For these retirees, life can become meaningless and internalized anger has the potential to become self-directed, leading to suicidal ideation or behavior. Significantly, these retirees suffer a shifting of social position and a resulting role reversal with spouse. The frequency of and the desire for sexual relations diminish. Social and sexual impotency often occur. A psychological retreat from the world is increasingly manifest. These persons require psychotherapeutic intervention. Most interestingly, even though these people have been spending their lives in the profession of offering psychotherapeutic assistance to others, they rarely take advantage of it for themselves.

In this limited and certainly unscientific survey only two interviewees considered it necessary to seek psychotherapy. Only one person actually sought such assistance. On the surface this appears not only strange but seemingly hypocritical in view of the fact that these people spent their entire productive lifetimes in the practice of psychotherapy. More intensive examinations of this question revealed that for some there was the (ego) inhibition of appealing to a colleague for help. In yet others the lifelong pursuit of self-analysis was available and indeed proved to be ameliorative in time. All those needing assistance were struggling with issues revolving around the need to control and to maintain ego integrity. Those who had done careful and adequate preplanning and who also had a history of long-term investment in self-analysis proved the most able at resolving emotional disturbances in this critical period in their readjustments to new life-styles.

In essence, it would appear from this appraisal of the exigencies of retirement from active practice that a few factors stand out. Primarily, the prognosis is best for those who are most in touch with their intrapsychic processes and whose egos are very much intact. They seem most adequate to the task and least susceptible to emotional distresses of any significant extent. For all it is a difficult period, one with many potential psychological pitfalls. The mature (genital) ability to accept oneself comfortably without significant emotional baggage to hinder the process is probably the most important factor to be derived from this study. Those whose individuation is complete; who are not limited by unresolved needs to control their environment and environmental figures; and who can introspectively and honestly analyze their fantasies, dreams, desires, and emotional needs are of course in the best position to successfully handle new demands of a newly structured life. For those less psychologically secure, a meaningful amount of preplanning before terminating a practice and retiring is mandatory. For still others, it appears wisest to put an alternative life-style or professional activity into place before giving up what has been personally and professionally satisfying.

It also seems propitious to define as much as possible one's future environment before chancing a totally unstructured and untried new one. For some the environment of those who are peers chronologically as well as professionally is advisable. For others an entirely new or different surround would be propitious. For all becoming aware of the finiteness of life, human relations take on a more profound importance. New relationships are likely to be formed in the new experience of not being defined by identification with collegial attachments to practice or professional identity. These newly formed relationships must prove qualitatively valuable as well as quantitatively satisfactory. The retirement experience must be psychologically as well as physically bridged. The move to a totally new physical and psychological environment is fraught with pitfalls for all but the most prepared. If one is dependent upon the direct or indirect rewards derived from one's practice, whether they be financial or social/psychological, then it is essential that one carefully bridge the experience before making the total leap into the new world of the retiree or deciding that retirement is not for him or her. Finally, if "work" as a practicing therapist defines it is crucial for one's psychological stability, then to terminate the practice would place too much of a burden on him or her, one that he or she may not be able to tolerate: It shouldn't be done. But if one can project retirement from practice as an opportunity to open new horizons and vistas, he or she should go for it.

REFERENCES

Abend, S.M. (1982). Serious illness in the analyst: countertransference considerations. *Journal of American Psychoanalysis Association, 30,* 365–379.

Burton, A. (1982). Attitudes toward death of scientific authorities on death. *Psychoanalytic Review, 65,* 415–432.

Chermin, P. (1976). Illness in a therapist: Loss of omnipotence. *Archives of General Psychiatry, 33,* 1327–1328.

Cooper, A. (1987, Winter). Sabbatical year reviewed by renewed faculty. *Outlook: N.Y. Hospital, 3.*

Dewald, P. (1978). Serious illness in the analyst: Transference, countertransference, and reality responses. *Journal of the American Psychoanalytic Association,* 347–363.

Eissler, K.R. (1977). On the possible effects of aging on the practice of psychoanalysis. *Psychoanalytic Quarterly, 46,* 182–183.

Lindner, H. (1960). The shared neurosis: Hypnotist and subject. *International Journal of Clinical and Experimental Hypnosis, VIII*(1), 61–70.

Lindner, H. (1984, Winter). Therapist and patient reactions to life-threatening crises. *Psychotherapy in Private Practice, 2*(4), 73–88.

Lindner, H. (1985b). Therapist and patient reactions to life-threatening crises in the therapist's life. *International Journal of Clinical Experimental Hypnosis, XXXII*(1), 12–27.

Roster, S. (1986). The seriously ill or dying analyst and the limits of neutrality. *Psychoanalytic Psychology, 3*(4), 357–371.

C H A P T E R
49

COUNTERTRANSFERENCE: ON WHAT CONSTITUTES SHAREABLE EXPERIENCE

Karen L. Lombardi, Ph.D.

The concept of countertransference has developed from its identification by Freud (1910) as the patient's influence on the analyst's unconscious feelings — and a hindrance to the work of analysis that must be routed out and overcome — to its current status within certain theoretical orientations as a source of valuable data for understanding the patient's inner experience and for formulating more effective interventions within the ongoing therapeutic interaction. Countertransference as a useful, perhaps essential, focus of the work of psychoanalysis naturally lends itself to certain theoretical or world views and not to others, which helps account for why it remains at the center of vigorous and often vehement discussions among analysts of various persuasions.

This chapter will address one aspect of the controversy surrounding countertransference, that of countertransference as a special form of communication within the therapeutic relationship. The Kleinian and interpersonal traditions, in particular, with their various emphases on the centrality of the ongoing dyadic relationship both in normal development and in the therapeutic setting, have contributed to the notion of countertransference as communication. After a review of significant contributions to this literature, current formulations of psychic development in infancy and early childhood from data-based observations will be highlighted to afford a developmental perspective on the notion of countertransference as a special form of communication.

COUNTERTRANSFERENCE AS UNCONSCIOUS COMMUNICATION

Heimann (1950), in an early paper on countertransference, contrasts her view to the classical position, which is that countertransference is a troublesome interference with the proper analytic position of detachment, and to the position of the Hungarian school as represented by Ferenczi (1928) and the Balints (1939), who are seen by her to advocate spontaneity and "confessional" acknowledgment of countertransference feelings to the patient. Rather, her position is that the analyst's emotional response to the patient is the most important instrument of research into the patient's unconscious. As Racker will later stress, the analytic situation is seen as a relationship between two persons. What is special about this relationship is not that one person feels and the other doesn't, but that the feelings experienced in the relationship are made particular use of by the analyst: They are analyzed, sustained, and subordinated to the task of mirroring for the patient. Heimann stresses the importance of a freely roused emotional sensibility for being able to follow the affects and fantasies of the patient. The analyst's countertransference, or feelings in response to the patient, is the tool for establishing rapport or resonance with the unconscious of the patient, and is the most dynamic way in which the patient's voice reaches the analyst.

Racker (1968), like Heimann within the Kleinian tradition, regarded countertransference experiences as especially useful tools in understanding the transference problems of the patient. Racker saw countertransference as the expression of the analyst's identification with the internal objects of the patient, and as such saw transference–countertransference experiences as unconscious communications between analyst and patient. The specific characteristics of countertransference reactions (for example, the anxieties engendered, the defense mechanisms activated, the specific content evoked) help us draw conclusions about the specific character of the patient's inner psychic happenings.

Racker's pervasive attitude is interactional. He is also dialectical rather than linear in his orientation to process. Therapist and patient are seen as in the process of affecting each other through transference–countertransference experiences. The therapist does not maintain a "normal" or static attentional and affective state; rather, he or she is internally (consciously and unconsciously) reponsive to what the patient is feeling, saying, and doing. As transference is based on the patient's identifications (both projective and introjective) with the therapist, so is countertransference based on the therapist's identifications with the patient and his or her internal objects. As transference and countertransference go hand in hand in this way, neglect of the countertransference necessarily leads to incompletely understood transference.

Politically, Racker's position is antiauthoritarian without being antiintellectual or against discipline. He specifically states his opposition to the commonly to the commonly held notion that psychoanalysis is an interaction between a sick person (the patient) and a healthy person (the analyst). It is, rather, an interaction between two personalities, each of which has internal objects, anxieties, pathological defenses, identifications. One difference between them is in the analyst's objectivity toward his or her own subjectivity and countertransference, so that the analyst is in a position continually to observe and analyze the analyst–analysand interaction.

Coming from a different tradition, Tower (1956) postulates that in almost every intensive psychotherapeutic relationship there develop, in parallel with transference structures, countertransference structures. Whether large or small, they are of considerable significance for the outcome of treatment. They serve as a catalytic agent, a vehicle for the analyst's emotional understanding of the transference. Implied here is that the countertransference provides empathic linkages to the patient's inner experience that further the analyst's ability to work with the patient's transferences. Transference and countertransference are seen as intimately bound together in a living process that is the work of the ongoing analysis. Tower points out that all relationships contain transference–countertransference processes: "I doubt that there is any interpersonal relationship between any two people, and for any purpose whatever, which does not involve, in greater or lesser degree, something in the nature of this living psychological process—interaction at an unconscious and transference level (pp. 232–233).

How does this work in the analytic situation? Tower is one of the first to suggest that therapeutic encounters over the long term result in some change in each of the participants with respect to one another. Modifications in transference structures that result in major changes in the one participant probably cannot occur without at least some minor change in the countertransference structures of the other. This is a particularly interactional view of the analytic encounter, with the patient's transferences affecting the analyst's countertransferences, and the analyst subsequently adapting and adjusting his or her responses to further affect the patient's transferences.

COUNTERTRANSFERENCE AND ANXIETY CONTAGION

Cohen (1952) articulates the position of the American interpersonal school in regarding countertransference feelings as not only inevitable but welcome. Attempts to become as widely aware as possible of all one's responses to a patient, particularly those reponses that are less under conscious control and more anxiety connected, may yield valuable clues to understanding both the patient and the patient–therapist interaction. Those subjective experiences elicited in the therapist by the patient's behavior are related to early experiences with important people in the patient's life, and enable the therapist to hypothesize as to what the patient's experience has been in the past and what it is currently in the therapeutic relationship.

Cohen ties up countertransference responses with anxiety: The presence of anxiety in the therapist, when it is aroused within the patient–therapist interaction, is a signal that countertransference is present. Based on the Sullivanian (1953) notion of anxiety contagion, which has developmental roots in the ability of the primary caretaking figure to contain anxiety and to establish security in the interpersonal environment of infant and other, anxiety is seen as an altogether interpersonal (as opposed to endogenous, biological) phenomenon. Anxiety tensions are not physicochemical; they are expressed in communal existence from one person to another, with reference to a personal environment, not a physicochemical one. In infancy, the baby expresses needs, eliciting tenderness from the caretaker, which leads to integrating tendencies in an environment of interpersonal security. When, however, anxiety tensions arise in the mother and the baby hasn't a way of handling it, anxiety is induced in the baby, which leads to a snowballing of anxiety and distress between caretaker and child, and to disintegrating tendencies. In Sullivan's system, anxiety is the source of all pathology, and so would be particularly salient in the experience of transference and countertransference phenomena.

Cohen states that when the therapist catches the patient's anxiety (and this often occurs on a nonverbal, experiential, postural, or tonal level), then countertransference is present. In such cases, the patient is often applying pressure in a variety of nonverbal ways to get the therapist to be like the significant others in the patient's early life. So it is not merely a matter of transference or countertransference distortions in fantasy, but of manipulating the actual present relationship so as to elicit the same kind of behavior from the analyst. When the therapist becomes aware of the way in which he or she fits into the patient's needs, the therapist has an important source of information about the patient's patterns of interaction.

Notable in the stance of the interpersonal school, of which Cohen is an exemplary member, is the notion that there is actually something occurring between participants in the interpersonal field, so that what is represented in fantasy has some parallel, however slight, in reality. Not only is countertransference inherent in the study of the system of participant observation (Hirsch, 1986), but it is relevant to the reality of the interaction. In classical theory, patients distort through transference. In interpersonal theory, patients "read" unconscious or subtle conscious aspects of the analyst's actual self.

COUNTERTRANSFERENCE AND PROJECTIVE IDENTIFICATION

The notion of projective identification, which has been developed largely by theorists influenced by Klein or by the British object relations middle group, carries through this notion of mutual participation through unconscious influence. Originated by Melanie Klein (1946), projective identification was first discussed in relation to the defensive splitting of the schizoid position. Klein used the term to describe the development of preambivalent early object relations wherein the bad or hated parts of the self are split off and placed into the mother (and other available identificatory objects) in order to protect oneself against one's own aggressive or dangerous parts. Endangered good parts, as well, can be projected into the mother for safekeeping. Klein sees projective identification as a normal development process that allows for eventual identification with aggressive components of the personality (leading to a sense of power, potency, and strength), as well as with loving components of the personality (leading to concern, care, and empathy). The developmental task is to be able to integrate both good and bad aspects of the self, and claim them for one's own by eventually reclaiming them from the object into which they have been deposited. If projective identification is carried out excessively, good parts of the personality may be felt to be lost, with a resultingly overstrong dependence on other people as external representations of one's own good parts.

Although not explicitly stated, Klein's formulation suggests that no matter in whom it originates, projective identification seems to be an interactive process between people whereby what is projected out is identified with, and under favorable circumstances, reintegrated. The *way* it is identified with and reintegrated is dependent on a two-person field. The way in which the recipient manages the projection affects its eventual fate within the projector. This, then, can become a mutual process that is mutable.

People of varying theoretical orientations have used concepts that are nearly identical to projective identification. Johnson (1947), for example, sees parents of acting-out children as having superego lacunae. The ways in which their children act out allow the parents unconscious vicarious gratification of their own forbidden impulses, against which they are rigidly defended. Wangh (1962) uses the term "evocation of a proxy," by which he means the splitting off of libidinous and aggressive strivings and the active arousal of these strivings in another person, who then appears to the evocator as a "branch" of the self. Anna Freud (1946) uses the term "altruistic surrender" to refer to the child's unconsciously giving himself or herself over to the parent's needs. Although each of the terms has a different focus, they share the notion of unconscious communication between people in close relationship with each other who are then made to feel and act in certain ways because of unacceptable aspects of the feelings in the originator.

Bion (1959) was perhaps the first to discuss projective identification as a special form of transference–countertransference communication, and as the central dynamic of the analytic process. Bion elaborated on the concept of projective identification through his concept of the container and the contained, between which there is a dynamic relationship. In developmental terms, the infant projects a part of his or her psyche, especially uncontrollable emotions, into the good-breast container, to receive those emotions back detoxified and in a more tolerable form. The container–contained relationship can be used to represent successful or unsuccessful projective identifications. In Bion's prototypical example, the baby's death and disintegration anxieties, expressed through crying, find a loving mother who will pick up and soothe the baby. The baby calms down because the mother received the baby's anxious fear-of-death-and-disintegration projections, contained them in a confident and empathic manner, and returned them in a more tolerable form. Alternatively, the baby might find a mother who herself reacts with disintegrating anxiety and lack of understanding, who shakes the baby or withdraws from the baby, saying, "I don't understand what is wrong with this child." This baby's anxiety is at best not alleviated, and at worst escalated, so that the baby is filled with nameless dread. This also serves as a model for the psychotherapeutic process, with the therapist as the container and metabolizer of the patient's toxic parts.

Malin and Grotstein (1966) see transference and countertransference phenomena as very closely related to projective identification. They espouse a broad view of transference to include all subsequent object relations, both internal and external, that are modified by the earliest primary object relationships established in the individual's inner psychic life. All object relations are affected by transference phenomena, and all transference phenomena are affected by projective identifications. Projective identification is seen as a way of relating to objects; it may or may not be pathologically defensive. It is, therefore, a means of identification as well as a means of distortion. In psychotherapy, projective identification occurs when patients split off part of their inner psychic contents and project it into the analyst, thereby having a feeling of relatedness with the analyst. When the patient feels the projections have been received and acknowledged by the analyst, things proceed. When this does not take place the patient is left with a sense of impoverishment, futility, and doubt with regard to his or her self-worth. The analyst's ability to receive and to tolerate these projections are perhaps at the basis of the therapeutic effect in psychoanalysis.

Ogden (1979) sees projective identification as a psychological process that is simultaneously a type of defense, a mode of communication, a form of object relations, and a pathway for psychological change. As a defense, it serves to create distance from unwanted, unacceptable, and often frightening aspects of the self. As communication, it serves to induce feelings congruent with one's own unconscious feelings so as to feel understood or "at one with" the other. As an object relationship, it is a way of being with a partially separate object. As a pathway for change, it is a process wherein feelings being struggled with are psychologically processed by another person and made available for reinternalization in an altered and less toxic form.

Regarding the therapist's participation in projective identifications, Ogden refers to Winnicott's (1947) conception of the objective countertransference, which merits its own discussion. Winnicott defines the objective countertransference as the analyst's love and hate in reaction to the actual personality and behavior of the patient, based on objective observation. This Winnicott contrasts to the subjective countertransference, those countertransference feelings in the analyst that are under repression and therefore cannot be put to good use. The distinction Winnicott is making here, it seems to me, is between those feelings about the patient that the analyst is aware of and can begin to understand and manage, and those feelings about the patient that are outside of the analyst's conscious awareness and that he or she is less likely to be able to put to good use. The analyst needs to be able to acknowledge and to tolerate the experiences of love, hate, strain, and so on that the patient engenders in him or her without having to act it out in unconstructive ways. The analyst also, however, needs to be able to communicate usefully to the patient about these experiences when it is important to do so. Although Winnicott advocates the necessity of containing these experiences, sometimes for quite long periods of time, without sharing them or using them interpretively, he just as strongly advocates the necessity of communicating these experiences to the patient at some point in order for the work to truly proceed. Inherent in his work is the ability to take the point of view, often simultaneously, of both patient and analyst, without losing sight of the individuality and the needs of either. When the analyst begins to feel hate toward the patient, which the patient has had some part in engendering in the analyst, it is important both for the patient and for the analyst to be able to integrate these feelings of murderous rage without acting them out destructively and without getting rid of them through denial or projection. It is important to do so for the patient and his or her progress, so that the patient can see that the affects do not have the effect of killing off the therapist; and it is important for the therapist, as recognition of the validity of these feelings enables the therapist to tolerate hateful situations without losing his or her temper and every now and again murdering the patient.

Ogden sees the therapist's task as experiencing and processing the feelings involved in the patient's projections. The therapist then has the opportunity to observe qualities that relate to previously internalized object relations and to process this experience in such a way that the patient is not merely repeating an old relationship in the therapy. In Winnicott's language, this would represent the therapeutic use of the objective countertransference.

On the surface, Ogden is suggesting that through the analyst's receptivity to the patient's projective identifications, the analyst's understanding of the analyst-patient interaction as it reflects internalized object relations becomes enhanced. The deeper implication, however, is that in order for real change to take place, an alteration of experience within the analytic interaction must occur in both parties. Projective identification, as a subset of transference–countertransference, is a two-person experience that requires that one's projective fantasies impinge upon a real "external object" in a sequence of externalization and internalization. As mentioned above, Tower suggested that both participants, to some extent, are changed by this experience, so that they come to relate to each other differently than they did when under the sway of the original projections and identifications.

Daniel Stern's (1985) data-based observations of infants (which include his own work and a compilation of the work of others in the field of baby watching) suggest a radically different view of human nature than is presented in classical theory or ego psychology, the latter of which has come to dominate American psychoanalytic thought. Although a critical review of his work is not the subject of this paper, certain central ideas that he presents serve as a developmental framework for the notion of countertransference as a special form of communication within the interpersonal field. Briefly, Stern posits four senses of self that emerge developmentally in the context of being with another. The earliest period, which begins at least at birth, Stern calls the "emergent sense of self." During this period, neonates interact with others through head turning, sucking, looking, and so on and begin to organize themselves with reference to the external world. The second period, which predominates roughly from 2 to 6 months, concerns the development of the core self in reference to sensorimotor schemata and affective experience. There is a developing sense that self and the outside world are separate physically, emotionally, agentically, and historically. The capacity for physical intimacy develops out of the experiences of the core self. At roughly 7 to 15 months, a sense of intersubjective self predominates. Here infants begin to share their focus of attention with others, begin to attribute intentions and motivations, and sense the congruence and the incongruence of feelings between themselves and others. The capacity for empathic intimacy develops out of experiences of the intersubjective self. Last, there is the development of the verbal self, out of which arises the capacity for objectification and self-reflection. The intimacy of shared meanings arises out of experiences of the verbal self. Each of these experiences of self is not a stage, but develops in an ongoing way throughout life. And all of these experiences of self are also experiences of relatedness, both within an interpersonal context and internalized as patterns of relatedness within the self. Stern proposes that what become internalized are not objects, but object relations, that is, actions of self with reference to actions of objects. Stern calls these internalized relationships in interaction "RIGs" (flexible internal structures of abstract Representations of Interactions that have become Generalized). Briefly, he is suggesting that the earliest internalized object relations are interactional both in nature and in representation. This makes good clinical sense, because what we see in our patients are not homunculi of their parents, or even their parents' voices, but dialogic and relational patterns and conflicts that they bring to the therapy in the hopes of untangling.

Of particular relevance to the transference–countertransference process is Stern's concept of state sharing. In the realm of intersubjective relatedness, the salient shared state would be that of feeling. In the realm of verbal relatedness, the salient shared state would be that of meaning. State sharing begins with intersubjective relatedness; the sharing of affective states is its central feature. Involved is a mutual sharing of psychic states, which requires some recognition of the complementary state of separate subjectivity. What the baby discovers is that people have separate feelings, separate focuses of attention, and separate minds and that people can share the same focus of attention and the same feeling. How does the baby come to experience these shared affective states? By what Stern calls "affect attunement," which others might call "parental mirroring" or "empathic responsiveness." Affect attunement expresses the quality of feeling a shared affective state without imitating the exact behavioral expression of that inner state. It is not imitation, which would be mechanical and without its own human character; it is affective communication, being with the other person and somehow letting the other person know that. Since intersubjective relatedness begins developmentally at a preverbal stage, affect attunement is communicated nonverbally, often through cross-modal matching and matching of intensity of the experience. An example from Stern's data is a 9-month-old girl who grabs excitedly for a toy, lets out an exuberant "Aah!," and looks at her mother. In response, mother widens her eyes, lifts her shoulders, and shimmies her hands and forearms in an equally excited way. In this way, the experience of joy and discovery is acknowledged and shared; it becomes an intersubjective experience that over repeated numbers of similar experiences will become internalized in the child, and will become available in the child's repertoire of object relating.

Parental attunement to certain affective states in the child defines what constitutes shareable, knowable personal experience. Selective attunement (not unrelated to Sullivan's concept of selective inattention) implies that there will be other experiences or affective states within the realm of intersubjective experience that will be downplayed or ignored altogether. The communicative power of selective attunement reaches to almost all forms of experience: overt behaviors, attitudes, tastes, and internal states. Selective attunement, then, shapes the corresponding intrapsychic experiences of the child. All parents (and all therapists) selectively attune. One's personality dictates the pattern and the degree of selective attunement. When, however, there are areas of experience to which parents are consistently nonattuned or misattuned, the likelihood increases that there will be significant psychic experiences in the child that will become dissociated or secretly and privately guarded (akin to Winnicott's [1960] false self development or Sullivan's not-me experiences). These unshareable experiences are the very ones that are most likely to reach the analyst in the form of countertransference communications.

Recent research by Slade and Aber (1986) suggests the pervasiveness of such a state of affairs in the developmental arena. Mothers of toddlers classified on an Ainsworth-like scale as securely attached or anxiously attached were found themselves to differ in two important ways. Firstly, mothers of secure children were found to express joy in the relationship, through vivid accountings of intimate and attuned moments together, whereas mothers of anxious children placed little emphasis on intimacy, but rather stressed their children's separateness and autonomy. Secondly, mothers of secure toddlers freely acknowledged negative affect in relation to their children, and directly communicated that affect (for example, Mommy gets angry when you do that). In contrast, mothers of anxious children denied any feelings of anger toward their children and were unlikely to see their children as experiencing anger, despite reports that their children often bit and hit. These findings suggest that mothers of anxious children were less able both to acknowledge and experience intense feelings of closeness and attachment to their children, and to integrate the inevitable negative and angry feelings that arise in a close relationship. The internal affective experience of these mothers was constricted, and the degree of denial and dissociation in their relational experiences with their children is strikingly parallel to their children's insecure or anxious mode of relatedness. These children already by the age ot 2 or 3 can be seen to have shrunken possibilities for freely shareable experience.

It is the thesis of this chapter that countertransference is a vehicle for communicating experience that is not yet shareable in the more usual and direct conscious ways. Experiences and affects that through misattunements and selective attunements in early object relationships have become dissociated parts of living experience are likely to reach the analyst through countertransference communications. The analyst's task is to be attuned to these experiences, to lift them out of the realm of the dissociated and into the realm of the shareable. In serving both as an empathically attuned partner in intersubjective relatedness, and in making the transference–countertransference interaction explicit through the interpretive mode, the analyst increases the potential for shared experience. This paradigm is one of insight coupled with an alteration of relational experience within the analytic interaction. The analyst, through his or her availability for countertransference communications, offers not only interpretation but a new relationship that attempts to repair early experiences of misattunement and expands what constitutes shareability.

REFERENCES

Balint, A., & Balint, M. (1939). On transference and countertransference. *International Journal of Psychoanalysis, 20,* 223–230.

Bion, W.R. (1959). Attacks on linking. *International Journal of Psychoanalysis, 40,* 308–315.

Cohen, M.B. (1952). Countertransference and anxiety. *Psychiatry, 15,* 231–243.

Ferenczi, S. (1928). The elasticity of psychoanalytic technique. In S. Ferenczi, *Final contributions to the problems and methods of psychoanalysis.* New York: Basic Books, 1955.

Freud, A. (1946). *The ego and the mechanisms of defense.* New York: International Universities Press.

Freud, S. (1910). The future prospects for psychoanalytic therapy. *Standard Edition, 11,* 141–151, 1961.

Heimann, P. (1950). On countertransference. *International Journal of Psychoanalysis, 31,* 81–84.

Hirsch, I. (1986). Countertransference and participant-observation. Paper presented at the Manhattan Institute for Psychoanalysis, New York, December 5, 1986.

Klein, M. (1946). Notes on some schizoid mechanisms. In M. Klein, *Envy and Gratitude.* London: Hogarth Press, 1975.

Johnson, A.M. (1947). Sanctions for superego lacunae in adolescents. In K.R. Eissler (Ed.), *Searchlights on delinquency.* New York: International Universities Press, 1949.

Malin, A., & Grotstein, J.S. (1966). Projective identification in the therapeutic process. *International Journal of Psychoanalysis, 47,* 26–31.

Ogden, T.H. (1979). On projective identification. *International Journal of Psychoanalysis, 60,* 357–373.

Racker, H. (1968). *Transference and countertransference.* New York: International Universities Press.

Slade, A., & Aber, J.L. (1986). The internal experience of the parenting toddler: Toward an analysis of individual and developmental differences. Paper presented at the International Conference of Infant Studies, Los Angeles, April 10, 1986.

Stern, D. (1985). *The interpersonal world of the infant.* New York: Basic Books.

Sullivan, H.S. (1953). *The interpersonal theory of psychiatry.* New York: W.W. Norton.

Tower, L. (1956). Countertransference. *Journal of the American Psychoanalytic Association, 4,* 224–255.

Wangh, M. (1962). The "evocation of a proxy": A psychological maneuver, its use as a defense, its purposes and genesis. *Psychoanalytic Study of the Child, 17,* 451–472.

Winnicott, D.W. (1947). Hate in the countertransference. In D.W. Winnicott, *Through paediatrics to psychoanalysis.* New York: Basic Books.

Winnicott, D.W. (1960). Ego distortion in terms of true and false self. In D.W. Winnicott, *Maturational processes and the facilitating environment.* New York: Basic Books, 1975.

C H A P T E R
50

THE THERAPIST'S PREGNANCY

Estelle R. G. Rapoport, Ph.D.,
Suzanne S. Phillips, Psy.D., and
Sheri Fenster, Ph.D.

There is hardly any event that so dramatically alters the therapeutic situation as does the pregnancy of the therapist. With her pregnancy, the therapist introduces a concrete, irreversible, and evocative impingement on the treatment setting and therapeutic dyad. The pregnancy becomes an inescapable, ongoing reality attesting to the therapist's real existence as a person separate from her patient. That there are other people in the therapist's life—perhaps more important to her than the patient—also becomes unmistakable fact. The usually consistent and sheltering quality of the therapeutic situation is disrupted.

As the fact of the pregnancy becomes ever more tangible, new or formerly buried transference and countertransference material may be evoked. The "actual total personal relationship" (Stone, 1961) that subtends the transference becomes progressively accentuated. New wishes, fantasies, and anxieties are engendered by the pregnancy, for both the therapist and her patients, adding to both the burden and the promise of the therapeutic interaction at this time. Consciously and unconsciously, the pregnancy has an impact on therapist, patient, and technique. The inevitable interruption in the treatment process heralded by the pregnancy is one aspect of this impact; if the significance of the impending interruption is not explored and worked through, it may eventuate in premature termination. Predictably, patients' transference feelings of loss and displacement are underscored by the reality of the events at this time.

Other relationships of the therapist may also change. Colleagues may feel burdened if the pregnant therapist relies on them to be available to patients or to attend to other professional responsibilities. And these colleagues too may be stirred by various feelings and reactions to the pregnancy. The collaboration between therapist and supervisor may evidence the same shifts typifying other relationships. If these shifts are articulated and explored within supervision, an understanding of their impact can provide invaluable data about intrapsychic material as well as here-and-now interactions between the pregnant therapist and her patients.

Also critical for the pregnant therapist is the need to reconcile her sense of herself as both professional woman and mother. Previous identifications and relationships may be reexamined. Shifts in feeling states—such as between guilt, anger, or withdrawal on the one hand and elation and fulfillment on the other—may also accompany this time of internal consolidation and change.

THEORETICAL AND TECHNICAL CONSIDERATIONS

There are often subtle, unconscious changes that the therapist assumes in her style and technique over the course of her pregnancy. As a result of physiological and emotional factors and the presence of a time-limited, shared event in the room, the therapist may approach interactions, problems, or unconscious communications in an altered fashion. Some changes may be demanded by, and appropriate to, the modifications the pregnancy introduces into the psychotherapeutic frame; others may reflect underlying countertransference difficulties.

The Setting

The therapeutic situation provides an atmosphere and a setting, a context within which symbolic communication may develop. It offers the patient an implicit statement about the therapist's intent and function: to listen to the patient, to concern herself with the patient without requiring the patient to be concerned with her, and to protect the contact between them from impingements. This provides an environment of consistency and security that patients come to expect and upon which they rely: the appointment time; the fixed length of sessions; the fee; the analyst's person, role, and consistency of approach; her relative anonymity; and the exclusive one-to-one relationship. The reliability of these elements creates a therapeutic "holding environment" within which the process of psychotherapy may flourish.

When the therapist becomes pregnant, many of these assumptions about the therapeutic environment are altered. By introducing her pregnancy into the therapeutic setting, the therapist may emerge from the background of the setting into the forefront. Rather than screening impingements and distractions, she becomes one. Rather than seeming reliable and strong, she may appear vulnerable. Her relative anonymity is confronted: The patient glimpses the therapist as a separate and sexual person. The therapist's stability as a person, a basic aspect of the therapeutic situation, is called into question. The therapist's physical self is changing. In addition, more subtle changes are also occurring. The therapist may sit differently, the timing or character of her interventions may change, she may become more active or passive, and her responsiveness may be compromised or enhanced by shifts in mood or sensitivity.

These departures in the assumptions of the setting and role are inevitable during the therapist's pregnancy. They, in turn, demand corresponding modifications in the therapist's technique. It is the consistent recognition and understanding of such alterations, rather than the need to avoid them, that become central to the integrity of the treatment at this time.

Technical Considerations

A change in focus becomes unavoidable and necessary in order to address these phenomena adequately. From the moment of recognition of the pregnancy, and often even before, virtually all communication from the patient must be seen as potentially reflective of the meaning of the pregnancy and the breach in the setting. As the analysis becomes suffused, directly or indirectly, with the emotional reverberations of the pregnancy, the patient seeks to cope with, repair, deny, rage against, or withdraw from this breach, this new experience with the therapist. The therapist's free-floating attention must give way to an alertness to the seemingly disparate disconnected associations and implicit or explicit allusions to the pregnancy. Such a focus serves to validate reality, prevent split-off responses, confront acting out, and highlight the focus on the transference.

A special event is "anything which alters or intrudes upon the basic analytic situation" (Weiss, 1975). The therapist's pregnancy, as a special event, heightens the contrast between the therapist as a real person and as a transference figure. Therapeutic handling of the special event involves a recognition of and attentiveness to the event itself, an invitation to free associate with respect to it, an attempt to understand the genetic connections that determine the patient's particular reactions, and an acknowledgment that something special and different has in fact occurred. Central to these technical foci is the underlying assumption that a special event directly and intensively affects transference feelings. Failure to recognize the impact of the special event on the transference can result in technical errors that may jeopardize an entire treatment. Such errors can occur as both patient and therapist wish to return to the safety and regression of the analytic situation and to the gratification of the transference. In the face of the special event of the therapist's pregnancy, such wishes may be particularly powerful. Unlike the isolated special event, the pregnancy forces both therapist and patient, over a period of months, to deal with a powerful, ongoing undercurrent in the treatment. As a result, there may be a collusion between patient and therapist to act as if the therapeutic relationship remained a dyad, untouched by the real presence of the baby-to-be. Recognizing this possibly denied but critical impact on the treatment, the pregnant therapist must actively pursue—through interpretations and questions—the significance and meaning of the pregnancy and the breach in the setting for the patient. These interpretations might allude to the feelings of disruption, betrayal, shock, and anxiety that often stem from the change in the therapist.

Some changes in technique that occur as a result of the therapist's pregnancy occur more spontaneously. Overall, for example, there is an increase in the therapist's verbal activity: She tends to question, confront, clarify, acknowledge, and interpret more than usual (Fenster, 1983). This heightened verbal activity is due to (1) the increased evocation of feelings, throughts, dreams, and fantasies pertinent to the relationship and (2) the increase in acting out. The acting out especially requires more energetic questioning, confrontation, and interpretation than usual, since the continuation of these behaviors could prove destructive to the patient and/or the treatment. The therapist may need to point out elements of the patient's experience quickly, perhaps even while they are still unconscious. If acting out or intense anxiety or depression, for example, can be understood as a response to the therapist's empathic failure (by virtue of her "insensitivity" in becoming pregnant, or her preoccupation), immediate interpretation may help the patient become aware of how he or she is responding and why. It is hoped that the patient will be able to live through a potentially disruptive experience without catastrophe and with the sense that breaches are not irrevocable.

The sense of time passing and feeling of pressure as the interruption in treatment draws near also cause the therapist to intervene more actively. The time constraint imposed by the pregnancy often prompts therapeutic work akin to that done during a termination. The therapist may feel pressed to "complete" work or to review the treatment to date. There may be a return to earlier symptoms; there may be resistances to discussing the interruption or, alternatively, total preoccupation with it.

The therapist's increased level of intervention is overdetermined, being a response to the upsurge of new material, the patient's acting out, and the press of time. An active response is not only warranted but crucial to the integrity of the therapeutic work at this time. This more active stance occurs within the framework of the ongoing psychotherapy. There must be a constant effort to explore with patients the meaning and relation to the past and present of their responses to the pregnancy. In this way, even while changes do occur, the analytic attitude of the therapist remains constant.

The Real Relationship And Self-Disclosure

The therapist's pregnancy forcefully confronts the patient with the real aspect of the therapist's life and person. While much about the therapist or her office may have already suggested her tastes, values, and points of view, the pregnancy provides direct information about her outside the consulting room. The patient's awareness of the therapist as a real person, then, goes on alongside of his or her ongoing transference relation to her. The real relationship is a legitimate and necessary aspect of the therapeutic situation that, during the therapist's pregnancy, ought not be minimized. Acknowledging and addressing the patient's reactions to the "real" therapist, particularly at this time, can strengthen the therapeutic alliance and facilitate the acceptance of transference interpretations when necessary (Greenson & Wexler, 1969).

Because the therapist's pregnancy enters so directly into the treatment as an unavoidable aspect of the therapist herself, it provides fertile ground for a consideration of the real relationship. Indeed, there is an internal push to be more self-disclosing on the part of the therapist as well as external pressure from patients for information. Such pressure toward self-disclosure at this time serves a critical function in the real relationship. It is an acknowledgment that the pregnancy is an event that is shared by patient and therapist. It expresses a recognition that the patient is part of the process of the pregnancy and may realistically need to have certain information about the therapist's experience. . It is an expression of the therapist's own pleasure in her pregnancy and the experience of having a baby—an important role-modeling function for many patients who grapple with ambivalence regarding children. In the sharing of this most basic human experience, the genuine connection between therapist and patient can be a bond enhancing patients' ability to tolerate the new tension in the analytic work.

Such nonanalytic interventions as limited self-disclosure reflect an altered or new interactional process that results from the pregnancy. Now, more often than before, patients begin to voice fantasies or ask questions of the therapist. The fact of the pregnancy in the room seems to offer them a sense of license or an avenue for questions not previously open. The therapist appears more human, more real, and patients may thus seem more curious, more interested.

In her interaction with her patients the pregnant therapist must address and acknowledge these elements of their ongoing real relationship, while being vigilant for the unconscious material and the implicit or explicit derivatives of the transference. Such responsiveness preserves the therapeutic process while validating the nontransferential, real feelings prompted by the pregnancy. For some patients it allows a respectful inclusion, a mutuality that enhances ego growth.

A therapist's response to the issue of self-disclosure is obviously determined by the clinical needs of the individual patient as well as her own personality. A full cognizance of these factors should serve as her guide. When in doubt, a stance of active questioning and exploration of fantasies before the therapist reveals personal information is recommended. This position may be altered somewhat with adolescent and child patients, who require a more immediately interactive and personally disclosing approach.

Most importantly, it must be recognized that the real relationship between patient and therapist does not require continued self-revelation for its development. It is more the fact of the pregnancy, the therapist's continuing recognition and acknowledgment of its impact on herself and her patients (both real and transferential), that fosters the genuine connection between them.

The therapist's pregnancy is an intrusion by the analyst herself into the good-enough therapeutic setting, the unarticulated constants that make up the analytic space. A sensitive exploration of the meaning of the disruption in the "holding" dyadic nature of the therapeutic setting is essential. Maintenance of the usual therapeutic stance will reassure the patient that the therapist can sustain or restore the holding aspects of the setting despite this temporary, but ongoing, impingement on the relationship. It offers both therapist and patient an unusual, evocative, and reparative moment within the treatment, a chance to meet each other more simply and directly.

Therapeutic technique that allows for an honest assessment of reality and unreality, especially regarding the therapist herself, is critical to the ongoing working alliance, to the patient's receptivity to interpretation, and to his or her ultimate integration of the reality of the analyst as a person.

TRANSFERENCE

Central to understanding the impact of the pregnancy are issues of transference. Transference may be considered a person's patterns of thought, feeling, and behavior that reflect early object attachments and conflicts and that are reactivated in the relationship with the therapist. Transference issues during the therapist's pregnancy potentially enhance the progress of the treatment by heightening each patient's dynamics, as well as eliciting formerly repressed or suppressed material engendered by the in-vivo experience with the therapist.

For the pregnant therapist to understand and utilize the patient's response to her pregnancy it is important for her to consider the timing and nature of the patient's response as well as the differences that can be expected as a function of a patient's sex and diagnosis.

Recognition Response

Patients use their own styles and reflect their own dynamics in recognizing and acknowledging a pregnancy. Some directly ask the therapist about the pregnancy; some allude to it through dream material or other derivatives like content themes of abandonment, children, weight gain, secrets in the room, or something being unusual or queer. Others respond to the pregnancy by acting out with missed appointments, rage outbursts, sexual promiscuity, telephone calls to the therapist, silent sessions, or premature termination.

Many therapists allow patients to recognize the pregnancy in their own way and in their own time rather than informing them about it. This position, which involves waiting for a patient to ask directly about the pregnancy or show derivatives of some unconscious recognition of the pregnancy, can provide a wealth of information about the patient that can be utilized within the treatment situation.

Initial Reactions And Responses

On learning or deducing the therapist's pregnancy, patients often respond most strikingly with either initial pleasure or shock. Generally, even when congratulatory feelings are the first reaction, they are quickly followed by anger and a fear of abandonment. The patient's expression of pleasure and happiness for the therapist may last for only one session; in the next session there may be a beginning expression of both rage and fear. Patients' expressions of fear of abandonment may take the form of a concern that the therapist will be emotionally unable to attend to them, or will literally stop seeing them. Some patients become unwilling to work; others terminate as a way of protecting themselves from the therapist's abandonment.

Concurrent with such fears are anger, hostility, even outrage at the therapist for becoming pregnant, for causing an inevitable disruption in the therapeutic relationship, and for feelings of dependency on her. Escalating both the patient's discomfort and aggression is often the cultural and self-imposed restriction that it is not acceptable to be angry with someone who is pregnant.

Some patients react with solicitousness, tenderness, and helpfulness. Although such responses may actually defend against negative feelings, they are often a function of genuine connection and caring induced by this real-life event. Other initial reactions to the therapist's pregnancy include flight into health, idealization or devaluation of the therapist, intense feelings of humiliation or betrayal, and acting out in the form of missed sessions, cancellations, terminations, pregnancies, and abortions.

Common Themes And Issues

There is a degree of consistency in the themes and issues that emerge in treatment when the therapist is pregnant. Underscored by the patient's own dynamics is an increased focus on sexual themes; identity themes; themes regarding siblings; and issues of trust, abandonment, and secrets being withheld. There is often some reflection on the movement from a dyadic relationship with the therapist to a triadic one with the therapist, the patient, and the baby. This brings to consciousness issues regarding the triangle of mother, father, and baby. Often the pregnancy elicits new material and themes while simultaneously focusing and crystalizing old ones.

Sex Differences In Recognizing The Pregnancy

A significant factor in the consideration of both a patient's recognition and response to the pregnancy of the therapist is the patient's sex. Female patients, especially those who are mothers or want children, respond earlier and more directly to the therapist's pregnancy than do male patients. Male patients tend to wait and, rather than inquire directly, often respond in the form of dreams or derivative themes related to the pregnancy.

This differential response may be a function of cognitive, developmental, and emotional factors. The therapist may seem different in some intangible way to both male and female patients, but female patients have a frame for identifying this difference as pregnancy. From a developmental perspective, the male patient's failure to recognize and directly confront the pregnancy may be a function of his early need to separate from his mother and move outside the orbit of female identification. Another facet in the male patient's nonrecognition may be his denial of the therapist's evident sexuality and obvious sexual involvement with another man. Whereas such dynamics operate in any treatment situation with a male patient and a female therapist, they may reach heightened proportions when the therapist becomes pregnant.

Sex Differences In Responding To The Pregnancy

Beyond the initial recognition phase, male and female patients tend to respond differently over the course of the therapist's pregnancy as well. Male patients most often react to the therapist's pregnancy with some degree of denial, isolation of affect, and suppression of thoughts and feelings. They seem generally less willing than female patients to entertain transference issues related to the pregnancy. Men often insist that the pregnancy does not affect them. They avoid the emotional impact of the event and focus instead on the concrete details, such as upcoming schedule changes or the interruption in treatment. Evidence of unexpressed and unanalyzed feelings is found in increased acting out by male patients in the form of missed sessions, forgetting things in the office, and abrupt terminations. The dreams and theme derivatives in conjunction with this acting out suggest feelings of rage, envy, deprivation, and exclusion.

Female patients most often react to the therapist's pregnancy with identification, competition, and envy. For some there is the need to view the therapist as a role model whose behavior implies that marriage is acceptable; that childbearing is safe; and that the combination of career, marriage, and children is possible. For other patients, notably mothers, the therapist's pregnancy provides them with a ground of commonality. As such, it increases intimacy and reduces fears and inhibitions in responding to the therapist. Some patients act on the wish to proffer advice and mother the therapist, often a significant alteration in the transference. A negative outcome of the identification with the therapist is an increased incidence of unrealistic pregnancy wishes and some actual unexpected pregnancies. Such acting out through identification may involve a wish to compete with the therapist, or an attempt to ward off loss of the therapist by becoming like her.

Other reactions of female patients to the pregnant therapist include envy and jealousy. Envy is generally expressed in the feeling that the therapist has "everything"—a profession, a man, and now a baby—while the patient has nothing. There are feelings of resentment, emptiness, and despair. Jealousy expressed to the pregnant therapist is often directed at the fantasied relationship the therapist has with her husband and baby. There is a sense of being replaced in importance by the real baby and of having to grow up. There is jealousy that this baby will have the idealized mother the patient longs to have.

Diagnostic Differences In Patient Recognition And Response

How patients deal with the pregnancy is greatly affected by their diagnosis or level of ego strength. This is particularly true of borderline patients, who as a group are strikingly similar and visible in their reactions to the pregnant therapist. Patients falling within the borderline range of pathology often voice their conviction earlier than others that the therapist is pregnant. Notably less disturbed patients (i.e., neurotic range) and very disturbved patients (i.e., psychotic range) generally do not recognize the pregnancy as readily.

For the borderline patient, who is often described as having only a partial ability to differentiate between self and object, changes in the therapist may be immediately felt and registered within the self system. Conflicts surrounding separation/individuation may lead borderline patients to be exquisitely attuned to situations that may precipitate feelings of abandonment and aloneness. The pregnancy of the therapist certainly poses such a threat. In response, borderline patients evidence more acting out, crises, clinging rage, emotional withdrawal, and abandonment fears than other patients. Needing an idealized object with which to merge, they respond to any alteration in the treatment setting with feelings of deprivation, betrayal, and rage.

Negative Influences Of The Therapist's Pregnancy

A patient's inability or refusal to react overtly to the therapist's pregnancy is difficult to address. Many overtly nonresponsive patients "know" but feel it too intrusive to ask the therapist about the pregnancy. Their reluctance to intrude may unconsciously be an attempt to maintain the therapeutic frame, which has already been intruded upon by the therapist. Patients must deal with the reality of the therapist as a person with an outside, separate life and a sexual relationship, and may need to avoid the resentment, hostility, humiliation, and fear that they may be feeling. This avoidance serves to protect the therapeutic relationship from disruption.

Sometimes a therapist's pregnancy makes treatment impossible, and a patient terminates. For some, the pregnancy is used as a resistance to treatment, which would have ended for other reasons had the pregnancy not emerged. For others, there is an understanding of the dynamics involved in the wish to terminate, but an inability to get past them; and in some cases, neither patient nor therapist parts with a clear understanding of why the treatment has ended.

Positive Influences Of The Therapist's Pregnancy

The therapist's pregnancy underlines and advances transference issues. It places the therapist — and the patient in response to her — at center stage. Conflicts and feelings both negative and positive are heightened and more directly expressed. The pregnancy makes resistance more difficult because it is a reality event that becomes more and more difficult to ignore. While often complex and at times intimidating for both therapist and patient, the recognition and analytic understanding of the patient's response are an invaluable avenue to therapeutic gains. They call upon the resources of the working alliance between patient and therapist. The result is that the patient and therapist share an event beyond the usual frame of treatment. Their willingness to make it their mutual history is the basis for therapeutic empathy, repair, and growth.

COUNTERTRANSFERENCE

It is crucial for the therapist to examine and understand her countertransference as it emerges and is experienced over the course of the pregnancy. Countertransference may be defined in terms of two factors: therapist responses (behaviors, impulses, images, and defense mechanisms, etc.) that stem from her own conscious and unconscious issues and therapist responses made in reaction to the patient and the treatment situation.

Personal Issues

As soon as she is aware of being pregnant, a woman is confronted with a number of issues involving her self-image, integration of roles, identification as mother, awareness and exposure of sexuality, and reassessment and redefinition of male–female relationships. She must face the question of who she is and whether she can maintain a sense of self while making an investment in another who will be an integral part of herself. She must come to grips with her changing body image and her new physical and emotional vulnerability. She must redefine old roles and integrate new ones without a sense of panic or narcissistic loss. She must integrate her fantasy of the maternal ideal with the reality of her experience with her own mother and resolve some issues of dependence and independence. She must confront her sexuality and shift from the dyadic relationship with a man to a triadic unit that includes a baby.

Professional Issues

Such issues are significantly compounded for the pregnant therapist. Whereas her image of herself professionally may be characterized by a relatively anonymous, neutral stance, the obvious nature of the pregnancy makes this impossible. She must negotiate a new image of herself, one that allows for disclosure and can accommodate a human, changing, less idealized sense of self. There is anxiety associated not only with the integration of this new image but also with the anticipation of patients' responses to it.

In terms of her sexuality, for example, the therapist must deal not only with her own conflicts and history but also with the expectation of patient responses to her disclosed sexuality. Similarly, she must not only identify and integrate a mothering role that is often historically and culturally different from that of her own mother but also deal with the resulting fears and needs in tandem with patients' real and transferential demands. Whereas the wish to be the idealized mother exists at times for all therapists, for the pregnant therapist, the pull may be intensified. In her personal life, she must blend family and career roles. As therapist, she must be able to differentiate her personal and professional "mothering." Her need to be the idealized, "all available" mother to all, makes her vulnerable to those patients (usually narcissistic or borderline) who need an idealized parent and respond to any alteration with feelings of deprivation and rage.

Countertransference Implications
Across The Trimesters

The physical realities and emotional responses associated with the trimesters of pregnancy have particular relevance to the pregnant therapist's countertransference responses. The first trimester dates from conception to the quickening, or perception of fetal movement, usually in the beginning of the fourth month. Characteristically, it is a time of strong mixed emotions — excitement and joy in the anticipation of a child coupled with anxiety and fear. Such fears are often exacerbated by general physical fatigue, nausea, and discomfort, as well as by the inability of the outside world to visually validate the pregnancy. It is a time of self-absorption and concern for self and baby. The countertransference anxieties at this time involve the feeling of not being objective and of carrying a secret, the fear that in some way the pregnancy will harm or otherwise negatively affect the patient and her or his treatment, and the fear that anger will be directed at the therapist and negatively affect her and her baby. The impact of this anxiety, and the attempt to deal with it, add to the self-absorption and distraction experienced by the pregnant therapist in the first timester.

The second trimester, usually the calmest, dates from the beginning of the fourth month to the end of the sixth month. During this time most women experience "the quickening," which both confirms the pregnancy and relieves some of the fear of losing the child. The visibility of the pregnancy at this stage also underscores its reality as it allows for validation and support by the outside world.

The countertransference position at this time reveals less anxiety, increased empathy, selective disclosure, and awareness of and interest in patients' responses to the pregnancy. Because of the therapist's lowered anxiety at this time, it often becomes possible for her to use the feelings engendered in her to further understand patient reactions.

The third and final trimester dates from the end of the sixth month to the beginning of labor and delivery of the child. It is a time marked by an increase in self-absorption and concern with issues of life, death, separation, and attachment. The task of the therapist is compounded by the need to face these issues not only in her personal life but also with her patients and in her relationship with them. In reality, there is often an urge comparable to "nesting behavior" to prepare and be ready for the baby. It manifests itself in the urge to effect closure with patients, to make arrangements for leave-taking, to simplify patient records, and to prepare for someone else's possibly having to take over.

For some therapists such responding may be propelled by a fear of death during or following delivery, a feeling of impending physical jeopardy. For others, the fear is less tangible. It is more a conscious awareness and fear of never being the same again.

Another issue the therapist faces at this time is separation. One of the realities of the third trimester is that the treatment has become time limited — both therapist and patient live with the awareness that interruption and separation are inevitable. The countertransference anxiety experienced is not only the fear of losing patients in the practical sense but the awareness of emotional loss often associated with separating from patients. This is experienced at times as a loss of one's sense of self, a loss of one's identity as therapist, which has heretofore been validated by the presence of patients.

During the third trimester, the baby becomes an imminent reality and a primary preoccupation. The therapist longs for the time to be alone and fantasize about the baby and her mothering role. There is often a need and a desire to separate these fantasies from work with patients. Possibly as a reaction to the therapist's preoccupation there is often a resurgence of patients' interest in and concern about the reality of the baby in the third trimester. Often patients' anxieties about the therapist going into early labor or suddenly not appearing for their sessions take the form of comments, questions, and nurturing gestures toward the therapist. The urge at times to dismiss such comments or to move quickly away from them can reflect the therapist's need to protect involvement with the baby from involvement with her patients.

Ultimately, the pregnant therapist leaves her patients to have and be with her baby. The events surrounding this departure in their plan and in their final reality have an unforgettable impact on the therapist and her patients. Their meaning to the therapist and her understanding of this facilitate her use of countertransference as a vehicle for expanding treatment.

SUPERVISING THE PREGNANT THERAPIST

It often happens that a therapist is in training, or chooses to be in supervision, when she becomes pregnant. Probably little in the therapist's learning or experience has prepared her for the often intense, varied, and unexpected reactions engendered by her pregnancy. There is both rationale and a particular need for seeking the support, feedback, and advice of colleagues and supervisors at this time.

However, this helping process can be fraught with the same complex relational patterns that characterize the process of therapy during the therapist's pregnancy. The issue of the pregnancy, and the often special needs of the pregnant therapist, can be evocative stimuli to which supervisors, as people, may find themselves unwittingly reacting. The therapist's new role, the impingement of the pregnancy on the therapeutic and supervisory relationships, the therapist's vulnerability, the many unknowns — all these can cause the supervisory process, like the treatment process, to take on new dimensions.

Many therapists find that supervisors, to their dismay, tend to focus supervision away from rather than toward the issue of the pregnancy. Thus, indirect references or increased acting out on the part of the patient are not viewed in supervision as linked to the therapist's pregnancy. Sometimes supervisors will actively steer the therapist away from the issue of the pregnancy, seeing it as a neurotic or narcissistic tendency to focus on oneself rather than on the patient. A patient's lack of reaction, for example, would then not be pursued, questioned, or interpreted.

Alternatively, supervisors may stress the impact of the pregnancy so strongly that almost all reactions are viewed within this framework. This can engender a sense of panic and guilt in the therapist who cannot escape the havoc she has wreaked on the treatment.

A useful way to examine such pitfalls in the supervisory process at this time is to consider the supervisory process itself as a tool (on a par with transference, countertransference, dreams, free association, and resistance) that may offer up essential, and often preconsciously known, information about a parallel process that may be occurring between patient and therapist. Thus, the supervisory process itself offers another dimension for analysis and understanding of the therapeutic process. Supervision is more than simply a didactic or consultative experience; there are emotional reactions on both sides that warrant intelligent examination and exploration, particularly at this time.

Fenster (1983) found striking similarities between pregnant therapists' interactions with their patients and with their supervisors. Many of the therapists interviewed described a sense of feeling less open, more distant, and newly uncomfortable in supervision during their pregnancies. These therapists perceived their supervisors as having difficulty with their pregnancies, particularly within the realm of the supervisor's possible jealousy or envy. Upon questioning, it evolved that the therapists were reacting in a similar way to the envy displayed by their patients and their supervisors, with distance and discomfort. Had the supervisors been more willing to discuss the possibility of their own jealousy, this willingness might have been communicated to the therapists, who might have been more comfortable confronting their patients' envy in the treatment situation.

Other dynamics that were reflected within the supervisory process and that occurred in the treatment situation include the following: the supervisor's feelings about the therapist's termination of supervision; the therapist's increased vulnerability to criticism or disapproval in supervision; the therapist's preoccupation, which manifests itself in supervision; the supervisor's increased protectiveness or criticalness at this time; a new sense of closeness that evolves in supervision as a result of the pregnancy, advice giving, and personal sharing and anecdotes; new feelings of attachment and dependency toward the supervisor; the supervisor's maternal transference to the therapist. All of these dynamics can be experienced by supervisors, therapists, and patients. A recognition of them provides the supervisory dyad an unusual opportunity to explore and understand often unverbalizable feelings and fantasies.

Guidelines For Supervision

When the therapist learns she is pregnant, the supervisor and therapist should spend a block of time considering each patient's dynamics and history in light of the issue of the pregnancy. This should take place, if at all possible, before the pregnancy becomes known. Discussions should include a review of the patient's major areas of conflict; his or her usual defensive styles; his or her style for dealing with separation, displacement, anger, and abandonment; and expectations for how the patient might go about handling the fact of the pregnancy.

In particular, transference issues and the real relationship between patient and therapist should become more focused and central to the work during the pregnancy. It is recommended that these issues be addressed systematically and regularly in supervision. It is particularly relevant that supervisors become aware of their own feelings and reactions to the therapist, her pregnancy, and her baby-to-be. They must observe how these may be enacted in the supervisory sessions and utilize these data when possible as a potential point of reference for understanding the therapist's and the patient's dynamics.

Both positive and negative reactions and interactions hold useful and often untouched information within them. Supervisors' exploration of their own feelings will ensure a facilitation of the supervisory process rather than an acting out or mutual denial of underlying issues.

MANAGEMENT OF PRACTICAL ISSUES

Side by side with the necessity for a dynamic understanding of the impact of the pregnancy is the need to make many decisions concerning the management of the practice. It is crucial to realize that the therapist's vision of herself will fluctuate during her pregnancy; hence, she will feel differently about her decisions at different times. The hallmark feeling is conflict — conflict between proving herself a reliable professional and proving herself a good mother. The therapist may initially deny her increased physical and emotional vulnerability, and the consequent limitations in her capacity for work, in order to continue to be the "reliable" therapist. She must be realistic and make allowances for her special needs without feeling that this makes her an inadequate therapist.

Recognition

When and how to tell patients about one's pregnancy is usually the first concern. This decision is tied to when the therapist plans to stop working, how long the maternity leave is, and if she is in fact going to return to work after the baby is born. It is often more useful to wait either for the patient to openly address the pregnancy or until derivatives or behavior make it apparent that the issue has been attended to, albeit unconsciously. If such derivatives are not forthcoming at least 3 months prior to the anticipated interruption, it is incumbent upon the therapist to address the pregnancy so that there is an adequate time frame for therapeutic exploration. It is never appropriate to let the patient go on indefinitely without bringing the pregnancy into discussion.

The advantages to waiting for patients to display signs of recognition are, first, that waiting gives the patients some degree of control over their psychological readiness to deal with the pregnancy. Second, the therapist gains an understanding of how a person may continue to react during the pregnancy. Patients who act out awareness, for instance by coming late or missing sessions, may continue to act out during the course of the pregnancy. Patients may also display their awareness of the pregnancy through dreams and increased discussion of matters related to children, mothers, pregnancy, and weight gain. Faced with this material or behavior, the therapist must work to bring the pregnancy into the conscious arena. Such questions as "Do you think there is any particular reason that you are dreaming more frequently of your mother at this time?" or "Do you think missing sessions a lot lately has to do with something happening in the therapy?" or "I wonder if your desire to have children right now is related to something about me?" may be useful in eliciting patients' awareness.

Waiting till patients notice the pregnancy can, of course, reach an extreme where the patient never spontaneously verbalizes awareness or derivatives of awareness. This is not uncommon. It is therefore necessary to set cutoff dates by which time all one's patients have to know. In this way, a patient's denial of and reaction to the therapist's pregnancy and the impending interruption of treatment may be worked with more actively. As stated earlier, the patients should have at least 3 months prior to the interrupiton of treatment to grapple with the issue of the pregnancy openly.

New Referrals

It is essential, from the outset, for the therapist to tell prospective patients of the pregnancy and the eventual interruption in treatment. If patient and therapist feel this is a workable arrangement, treatment can begin. Some therapists may choose not to take any referrals at this time, particularly those planning to take a maternity leave of over 3 months.

Not telling new patients about the pregnancy, either before treatment is started or as soon as the therapist herself knows, is very disruptive for these patients. It seems as if, not having had the opportunity for an alliance with the therapist before the pregnancy, new patients feel particularly betrayed and overlooked. Transferrentially, they seem to have no frame for expanding the perception of the therapist; rather, their initial experience of the therapist is of deprivation and imminent disruption.

The therapist may want to consider carefully whom she does take on as a new patient. Excessively hostile or suicidal, extremely dependent, or borderline patients may be inappropriate to take on at this point and are best referred to colleagues. The therapist's increased emotional and physical vulnerability may make these patients' demands or crises difficult to manage.

The Period Of Interruption

When should the therapist stop working? At first, she may believe that she can work virtually until labor begins. It has been our experience that it is preferable and necessary to plan an interruption date with patients. This allows the therapist some conflict-free time to care for herself and prepare for the baby. For all concerned, a preset date to interrupt the treatment prior to one's due date will usually relieve the anxious fear that the "water may break" or labor begin during a therapy session. Most importantly, it provides closure and control for all, underlining the reality of the pregnancy and birth. By providing a frame, a preset date engenders work regarding the interruption or termination. It allows for a focus on separation, abandonment, dependency issues, and the like. To fail to set a date is to collude in the denial that the therapist is pregnant and to encourage the misbelief that there will be no interruption and no baby.

The decision about the length of maternity leave is a personal one. Some therapists feel that they want to go back immediately, and some feel that they never want to go back. This issue is made more difficult because tentative decisions need to be made early in pregnancy, when the therapist has no idea, especially in the first pregnancy, how she may feel after giving birth. Many therapists underestimate the time they need for maternity leave (Fenster et al., 1986). They do not anticipate the intensity of attachment to their babies in the first 3 months postpartum and their own consequent reluctance to return to work. Concern for oneself, one's baby, and one's patients must be juggled at this time. A 3-month maternity leave is a reasonable time period for all concerned. Shorter spans seem stressful for the therapist, and much longer leaves seem difficult for the patient.

Both therapist and patient need to understand clearly the plans for the interruption and return to treatment. It is important that patients know the approximate date of the therapist's planned return to work, barring any complications. Although logistics may vary, one possibility is for patients to be told to expect a letter or call 1 month prior to the therapist's return. The letter can contain an appointment date for an initial return appointment, at which time a regular schedule can be set up. If the initial appointment time is impossible, patients can be urged to call to reschedule. We have found this method to be very effective and clear, with the letter serving as a transitional connection to the therapist for the patient.

Contact During The Interruption

The issue of contact with patients during one's absence can be handled in a variety of ways. Patients are often unsure that the therapist will survive the birth, return to work, and stay. It is useful to offer some information to the patient regarding one's well-being. This can be a birth announcement, a note telling of the birth, or a phone call.

Contact with patients regarding a crisis or serious problem is another matter. Many therapists feel excessively guilty about having little contact with patients about their problems during maternity leave. Having willingly brought about this break in treatment, the therapist may offer contact as an effort at reparation.

There will inevitably be some crises during the therapist's leave, and the therapist needs to have a procedure for handling such requests for contact. Some therapists see their patients for emergency sessions. Some take emergency calls and refer the patients to a colleague if the crisis warrants further attention. Some take no calls and give patients the name of a colleague to call in the interim. Whatever arrangements are made, the therapist should clearly think through her personal and professional motivations.

Gifts

A sensitive situation often develops concerning gifts. Many patients will bring gifts prior to the interruption or send gifts during the hiatus or on resumption of treatment. How should this be handled? Most therapists accept these gifts from their patients, but not without a certain degree of conflict about the appropriateness and discussion with patients regarding the meaning of gifts. It is often felt, however, that because the baby has been such a major part of the interactional system for so many months, it seems unfair and confusing to patients to have their gesture of goodwill refused. Although one may not usually accept gifts, this particular circumstance seems to call for different behavior. The acceptance of such gifts may be considered reparative in nature, in that patients have no choice but to become part of this external event in the therapist's life. To do other than accept seems double binding. The exploration of the meaning of these gifts may occur later in the treatment in the context of the continuing discussion of the patient's reaction to the interruption of the treatment and his or her concerns about changes in the therapist now that she has a child or more children for whom to care.

Colleagues

An important issue is the reaction of colleagues to the therapist's pregnancy and the effect it can have on the therapist. One reaction we noted quite consistently was an intolerance for the therapist's increased vulnerability and encouragement for her to work far beyond what is realistically manageable for her during the time of her pregnancy. The pregnant therapist is particularly vulnerable to this type of pressure. If she herself is uncomfortable with her heightened emotionality and increased personal needs, she may blame herself for what she sees as self-indulgence. She may deny her needs and may even take on more work to prove her capability. If the therapist has counterphobically overworked to the extent that she has diminished her effectiveness, she may feel guilty or depressed when she perceives her failure. It conflicts with an image of herself as having unlimited capacity.

Colleagues may take an unpredictable stance in relation to the pregnant analyst and her work. Their responses may include oversolicitous concern, a demand for overcompensation at times of weakness or need for help, jealousy, envy, identification with and anxiety about the burden the therapist is taking on, fear of neglect of themselves, and hostility. We found that in a psycho-analytic training institute there was very little support for the pregnant thera-pist's needs for flexibility. It is vital for the therapist to hold on to her sense of self and her needs in the face of such varied and often strong reactions.

THE IMPACT OF MOTHERHOOD
ON THE THERAPIST

Every woman changes dramatically after giving birth. Motherhood in-volves a reorganization of a woman's self-concept in many areas: her relation-ship to her own mother, her husband, her child, and society. There is a con-tinual stress on the therapist, an unresolvable conflict that began with her pregnancy—that of being a "good" mother and simultaneously being a "good" therapist. This becomes the backdrop of her life.

Stages In The Return To Work

The attempt to integrate the roles of mother and therapist can be concep-tualized in two stages (Fenster et al., 1986). The first stage, termed "anticipated loss," is characterized by a fear of loss in both spheres of career and mother-hood. The second stage, termed "dual role integration," is characterized by the ongoing struggle to balance both roles comfortably.

In the stage of anticipated loss, the idea of returning to work with patients brings anxieties and excitement. The anxieties are part of the fear of loss in both areas. As part-time mother, the therapist fears losing connectedness with her baby, fears the baby's preference for other mothering figures, feels a sense of loss at missing out on her baby's special moments, and fears that her choice will inevitably damage her child's emotional growth and development. As part-time therapist, she fears a loss of connection and effectiveness with her pa-tients, anticipates a loss of patients' commitment to treatment, and fears that her lack of total commitment will irrevocably damage her patients. Despite the intensity of these fears, it is the actual return and beginning of work with patients that allow the therapist to relax and start integrating her dual roles.

In the dual role integration stage, the therapist repeatedly grapples with the quandary of separation from her baby and reconnection with her patients. To do this, she must be able to move in and out of merger with her infant into a working alliance with her patients.

There seem to be immediate changes in the emotional involvement with work for one who has had a baby. Most therapists develop a greater emotional distance from their patients, which they feel enables them to do better work. Many therapists perceive themselves as having been overinvolved with their patients prior to their motherhood, treating patients as surrogate children. With motherhood they become more comfortable with defining emotional boundaries as well as setting limits regarding appointment schedules, avail-ability for phone calls, payment deadlines, and abusive behavior.

As she builds up a continuing sense of her own capacity to shift roles suc-cessfully, the therapist/mother finds that she is comfortable bringing the increased emotional openness developed with her child into the treatment process. She is better able to maintain an empathic stance and to tolerate chaos and frustration without feeling excessively frustrated herself. She can fine-tune her concentration level, and she can use her experiences as a mother as a frame for understanding her patients' needs. As a parent she also broadens her experiential frame. She is in a much better position to understand the at times overwhelming intensity of emotions engendered by parenthood.

Winnicott (1963) makes the point that in handling the dependency needs of our patients and in protecting a fragile ego from being overwhelmed "there is nothing we do that is unrelated to child care or infant care. In this part of our work we can in fact learn what to do from being parents." Therapists confirm that the quality of their work changes at this time. There is an increase in empathic responses to parents, families, and children and an increased respect for the complexity of feelings and issues between parent and child and between parents. There is a new level of emotional understanding for the memories and fantasies of childhood reported by patients because of the therapist's more intense involvement in the ongoing unfolding of these experiences. Becoming a mother and raising children bring to a therapist an empathy, a sensitivity, an openness, a richness of emotional experience, and practical wisdom that can only increase her effectiveness with her patients. It is difficult to imagine any other life situation that could produce such a plethora of change and learning.

REFERENCES

Fenster, S. (1983). Intrusion in the analytic space: The pregnancy of the psychoanalytic therapist. *Dissertation Abstracts International.* (University Microfilms No. 83–17,555.)

Fenster, S., Phillips, S., & Rapoport, E. (1986). *The therapist's pregnancy: Intrusion in the analytic space.* Hillsdale, New Jersey: The Analytic Press.

Greenson, R., & Wexler, M. (1969). The non-transference relationship in the psychoanalytic situation. *International Journal of Psycho-Analysis, 50,* 27–39.

Stone, L. (1961). *The psychoanalytic situation.* New York: International Universities Press.

Weiss, S. (1975). The effects on the transference of "special events" occurring during psychoanalysis. *International Journal of Psycho-Analysis, 56,* 69–75.

Winnicott, D.W. (1963). Dependence in infant-care, in child-care, and in the psychoanalytic setting. *International Journal of Psycho-Analysis, 44,* 339–344.

C H A P T E R
51

A MINORITY EXPERIENCE OF PRIVATE PRACTICE

James F. Lassiter, Ph.D.

It is difficult to begin a discussion about the experience of being a minority private practitioner without first considering the components that make up life for any private practitioner. As well, it seems impossible to discuss only the experience of functioning in a private practice without addressing the experience of being a minority in the field of psychology as a whole. The advantages of the work appear obvious: income, mobility, access to learning and emotional as well as intellectual growth/stimulation, and the opportunity to help identify and remediate the social problems that produce psychological ones—often from the inside. It is in the spirit of the last that this paper is offered. The stresses involved, in the author's opinion, need to be highlighted, and as such this chapter will touch on several to raise consciousness (something that has been of a concern as we have moved away from the 1960s) and hopefully to cause others to help look for solutions.

It is this author's notion that satisfaction and security; the ability to work, love, and play; and integration of acceptable images of self and other into a respectable internal ego representation are the core components of several of the more popularly practiced personality theories of the day. They suggest formulas for what comprises the emotionally "healthy" individual and imply certain "shoulds" necessary to achieve this development. They also serve as signals (i.e., when one or more is missing) for amelioration. No one develops perfectly, achieving optimum levels of these components, and everybody must overcome some deficits and appreciate the differences inherent in the specifics of individual experiences during maturation. With this in mind, a brief description of one view of the minority experience of the independent practice of psychology follows. This is not a definitive statement, and I make no claim to speak for every practicing minority therapist in the country. Also, it is a given that healthy professional development depends on the above-listed hallmarks for personal growth. In the case of minority private practitioners, the same racism/cultural bias that threatened successful personal development (including amelioration—even when the signs were clear) can be seen in parallel for their professional development as well (Wispe et al., 1969). This leaves room for others (colleagues and laypersons) to ponder the age-old question, especially when considering issues of quality and ability: Can "deficit" and "difference" really be two separate things or is one a euphemism for the other?

For any professional working in the private sector, some things are mandatory for satisfaction, security, integration of an acceptable self-image for working, loving, playing, etc. From my experience and informal interviews with 10 other minority private practitioners in the area, a consensus was reached concerning the importance of adequate training, a palatable work environment, and supportive collegial (as well as personal) relationships. Certainly, coming to grips with internal issues also received a primary ranking. Achieving this intrapsychic success, however, is still related to working through personal history and remediation in the present, which always seems to involve the way people attain and coordinate the other three major portions of their life.

These needs are of special significance for the private practitioner because possible institutional support structures probably are not readily available owing to the solitary nature of the work. Most minority psychologists interviewed expressed feeling on the fringe of their professional communities, socially and politically (Norcross & Brochaska, 1983). Considering the paucity of minorities in private practice and the built-in isolation of the work, one is left with a group of individuals that, at one time or another, feel alienated and dissatisfied with their choice of vocation. The work becomes a very lonely business when you are a rare bird looking for others of your genus. All minority psychologists in private practice are not unhappy, but one must recognize that the risk factors are enhanced and the effort necessary to make a successful practice is beyond that of our colleagues who are readily accepted and find their communities more accessible. The attraction to enter the field is lessened, and this occurs at a time when there is a substantial upward shift in the minority population across the country (Wyatt & Parham, 1985).

Between 1970 and 1980, the nonwhite population for the country approached 25 percent; by 1990, this figure will probably have been surpassed. During that same time period, the number of minority PhDs went from 2 percent (Wispe et al., 1969) to 3 percent (Norcross & Prochaska, 1983). This last figure, the authors report, is an accurate reflection of overall minority membership in the American Psychological Association (APA). Both PhD figures represent only those legitimately licensed to practice independently throughout the nation. This point is underscored because the few studies that have addressed the issue, particularly the older ones, were prone to inflate the numbers of minority psychologists by including all persons who majored in the discipline at any level, possibly to emphasize the size of the group being disenfranchised. This obfuscates the very real absence of licensed minority PhDs and the investigation of the continued causes of the problem. Dr. George Goldman, a noted psychoanalyst of the New York metropolitan area, remarks the obvious when describing the advantages and disadvantages of going into private practice: "You will meet few blacks, fewer poor people, and only a modicum of the middle class" (Goldman & Stricker, 1981, p. 8).

There are some discernible reasons for this obvious lack. It is suspected that they lie in the differences in the very areas considered most significant for the making of a satisfied, secure, happy private practitioner: work environment, training, and support.

TRAINING

Over the past decade, the influx of Asians, Hispanics, and Caribbean blacks has increased. They, along with our minority American populations, cluster in the coastal regions and major urban centers. These are the same centers that purport to be the bastions of psychological research, theory, and general development of the field. Our major universities and institutes are located there, yet we have not been able to recruit efficiently, monitor the complexion of the courses offered, or address adequately—programwise—the minority elements that make up substantial proportions of these populations that increasingly are part of the patient groups we are asked to treat (Wyatt & Parham, 1985). It has been the author's experience that given any group of two or more academicians involved in the graduate training of clinical psychology students at least one of whom represents a minority, the conversation turns to the very small number of minority students that apply and are accepted into programs. This is not a problem unique to psychology, as Jones and Jordon (1984) attest to the same problem for social work training programs and in the mental health field overall (Dean et al., 1976). On the surface, this appears to be a major concern. There is, to the author's knowledge, only a minimal effort to interest, excite, and maintain this enthusiasm for the field for our students on an undergraduate level (Bayton et al., 1970). This was an issue suggested to the APA a number of years ago by the Black Student Psychological Association (Simpkins & Raphael, 1970) as an avenue toward meeting the deficit of minority applicants. It also appears, and I suspect gets communicated, that our major programs are not geared to address the issues that would attract and be efficacious for minority students (Jones, 1985) and that the number of culturally sensitive courses in no way would satisfy these students or prepare them for working with their own ethnic groups, let alone others (Wyatt & Parham, 1985).

Part of the problem, which almost begs the question, is, how do we ensure larger numbers of minorities in the field? This has to do with the make-up of the faculties (Russo et al., 1981). Few qualified minority students appear interested in teaching; those in private practice (from intgerviews) find teaching less than cost-effective, and the narrowness of the curricula does little to encourage their desire to participate (Dean, 1977). Of course, one may answer that students in these programs show little interest in the more culturally sensitive courses that these would-be professors might offer. Nonetheless, the irrelevance of the curricula for the minority student ensures that fewer will enroll in the programs, leading to a smaller professor pool to be drawn on later— as well as to a group of professionals who missed the same training in their own graduate student careers (Fooks, 1973). One might also argue that, given the increase in minority patient populations, it could be considered a loss to all graduate students in psychology that culturally related courses are not sufficiently available (Wyatt & Parham, 1985). One might continue the argument by making the case, therefore, that these courses ought to be a mandatory and integral part of the core courses in any graduate psychology program (Jones & Block, 1984). Recognizing these issues and their limited training, clinicians who attempt to practice privately or otherwise must on their own go about completing their education by filling the holes left by programs that are difficult, rigorous, lengthy, expensive, and especially for them, questionably relevant. For many, feeling so much on their own during and after formal graduate training lessens the likelihood that they will find the notion of private practice as a "life's work" attractive.

For many, ethical issues arise concerning the learning and practicing of theoretical approaches of a psychology steeped in white, western European traditions. Not all cultures conform to these notions, yet only a few scholars have come forward to make the theories applicable to nonwhite experiences (Evans, 1985). One young man recently confronted this author with the question, "For a minority American, is subscribing to standard psychoanalytic theory a sophisticated form of identification with the aggressor?" Certainly it didn't feel like that, but the question gives one a big pause for thought. The years of experience needed to learn how to tailor these theoretical frames so that different cultures might still benefit from the tremendous amount of important research and effort put into them are not easily communicated in a few short hours' conversation, aside from their deserving more than that.

These are some of the things that are missing for our young clinicians-in-training, and I might add, part of the frustration that helps keep new minority professionals from running the private practice obstacle course along (Mataragnon, 1979). There are many issues that are rarely, if ever, addressed for these students. Courses on psychological testing of the minority inner city child area excellent example. With standard materials, these children often look abnormal—"so then must I be" is what gets communicated to minority students training to use the materials, since they are often a product of that same experience. To add further insult, they are evaluated by the same genre of tool for their intellectual appropriateness for college and graduate training. How does one prepare for understanding the spiritualism that resides heavily in many black and Hispanic homes, and the part it plays in personality structure? The whole psychology of upward mobility, trying to move into the mainstream of American life for minorities, has had little attention, especially from groups that realize that it is not just a class issue, but a perceptual one as well (i.e., for some reason—color, sound, facial features—you clearly stand out from everybody else and historically it has been a sin: from Step-and-Fetch-it to the Yellow Peril). Our students must be prepared for dealing with that part of the therapeutic process when it inevitably turns to this material, even as they are part of and identify with the struggle. It becomes clinically a problem to try and work with clients who transferentially tap areas in one that no one addressed at school (and as a result in analysis) because it was considered not part of the curriculum—e.g., inbred racial hatred. Being confronted with one's own confusion and inner skepticism because one has grown up in a society that presents blacks with a negative self-image, not knowing if a patient's negative transference is his or her own or one's own projected, and never having been able to deal with it appropriately in training in a psychology program, seems ludicrous, but it exists. Apparently, according to the numbers, few minority students are willing to undergo the personal stresses to survive the training, and fewer still believe they can make a difference privately practicing what they have been taught (Calnek, 1970).

It would be remiss of me not to mention one of the biggest obstacles to minority graduate training in this field and thus to the numbers of minority psychologists eventually entering the private practice marketplace: funding. As a member of the faculty of one of the most prestigious institutes in the country (and probably abroad), I feel confident in stating that most minority students can compete academically with their nonminority counterparts. They cannot, however, do the same financially. Many are the first in their family to enter graduate training — there is no history of psychology traditions or economic sources to draw upon. It is foreign territory to begin with, and since they are faced with various states of penury for several years along with all the above-listed liabilities of psychology programs for minority students, it is no wonder that a host of other competitive professions look much more inviting. Thomas and Sillen (1972) offered a challenge to the profession in their book *Racism and Psychiatry* some 15 years ago: namely, to redirect training, employment, and practice toward equity to ensure an "open market." This has not happened.

THE WORK ENVIRONMENT

Of vital importance to the private practitioner is accessibility to patients and referral sources. Especially when starting out, the private practitioner is dependent on colleagues and other agencies that respect his or her work and believe that he or she is qualified to handle cases. What is often part of this referral process, however, is a type of "case conferencing/assessment" (it is as easily done by an individual as a group) to try and match patients with a therapist they might work best with. When two or three such possibilities are arrived at, the list of potential therapists is given to the patient for follow-up. This procedure is not unusual and is done in clinics and agencies every day, as well as by individual colleagues on a private basis. For the most part, it seems to work extremely well, until one considers the minority clinician in the pool of possible therapists. Now the attributes of clinical awareness, years of experience, style, and type of oreintation become qualified by that practitioner's ethnicity. The notion of whom a patient will feel most comfortable working with becomes colored by racial considerations. In part, this may be necessary because of the present state of our graduate training and the climate of the nation: Patients of a particular ethnic background may in fact fare better with a like therapist. It is, however, limiting (privately, even a restraint of trade), and when referrals are made solely on this basis, therapeutically unsound.

I suggest that it may even be done on an unconscious level. As therapists, we make decisions about patients all the time, based initially on how they appear. Part of any good mental status examination will include a section bout this. Often we make decisions about patients referencing intellectual capacity, income, ability for insight, regularity with which they might attend sessions, and projected success of the therapy — on the basis of how they look. This is dependent on our experience with others who look like that, and the general matrix of stereotypes we have experienced from our own biased developmental histories, which includes the neighborhoods we have lived in and the biases we were taught by parents and grandparents, etc. Something similar probably occurs when therapists are considered for referrals, and particularly when a minority therapist is included as a possible referral. Questions are raised such as, Will this patient be able to relate to someone nonwhite? Or, will the non-white therapist be able to identify adequately and thus be sufficiently empathic? When referrals are made to minority therapists, are class differences ever considered, or are we still seen as all the same because we "look alike" (Wolkon et al., 1973; Griffith, 1986)? I have been at conferences where a practitioner's qualifications were held in question because it was known that his entrance to graduate training was in part due to an affirmative action campaign, suggesting that he was probably moved along in that program because of its need for "window dressing."

When a referral is made privately, another question often arises: Will the patient get there? For most, it is a concern about the patient following through. When the minority private practitioner is referred to it may mean, will the white patient travel to this neighborhood? Minorities are concerned about where one can live in peace and quiet with unintrusive neighbors. It is no different for the minority therapist in private practice: Where will office space be available? When one's office is part of one's home, residential restrictions determine professional availability. Wispe et al. (1969) made the dismal observation that being a black psychologist (I believe any minority psychologist) may give one greater mobility and more access to the "American dream" than other blacks have, but it does not remove one from the experience of being a minority. Many of us testify to the veracity of this notion almost 20 years later.

If office space is restricted, does this suggest that one's income is restricted as well? Some of my white colleagues have commented that the reason I keep a full practice is because of the shortage of blacks in the field, which ignores any relevance of clinical acumen. It does suggest two things: (1) that the speaker has a one-track mind regarding the way patients are referred and (2) that more blacks have become attractive patients as they have moved above the poverty level. As such, what the statement overlooks is that many potential minority patients have the same reservations about minority therapists as do their white colleagues. The system works so well that many still believe that they themselves are second-rate and second-class and so are minority therapists, their training, and the quality of their treatment. We are all not as fortunate as the late Godfrey Cambridge, who in the film *Watermelon Man* portrayed a bigoted insurance salesman who woke up black one morning and after many trials and tribulations of trying to "get white" again decided to accept his new status, only to find he had an incredible market available to him and he was doing better than he ever did when he was white.

A minority private practitioner reports consistently getting better referrals from an advertisement in the local telephone directory than from colleagues. She believes this is because there is no way to make a clear ethnic distinction from her name and credentials. She has a varied ethnic practice, and her patients seem to stay for average lengths of time and have the same success and failure rates as those referred by other sources, perhaps even better. One must ask if referral sources are more concerned about the therapist's ethnic background (à la the perfect match for the patient) than patients are (Harrison & Butts, 1970). Could this get communicated to the patient on some level when the referral process is begun—even if it is indirect, nonverbal, or consciously unintended (e.g., inherent in the referrer's developmental makeup, so much so that it is second nature)? While this is an excellent topic for research, Thomas and Sillen (1972) note: "The subject of referral is always a touchy one for private practitioners and it is hardly surprising that the professional literature has bypassed it" (p. 151). Fifteen years later, a computer search revealed no significant change.

Before further discussion about minority therapists and patients, a final note needs to be made about restriction of office space. Although some minority therapists have become established after many years of hard work, and some are fortunate enough to be in neighborhoods that recently have been regentrified, many experience the problems of segregation. Consider the plain economics of the situation. Even in urban centers, where it is more difficult to segregate openly, if minority therapists are screened out of the poor for referrals of better-paying clients because they "won't relate" (which really is a euphemism for the "old boy" type of systematic exclusionary tradition), then these private practitioners will have a restricted income. A restricted income most certainly restricts one's place of residence and, in the case of a private practice, where one can afford to rent. Therefore, minority therapists are either nonexistent or few and far between on the "shrink rows" of the Park Avenues of the metropolises of this country.

Patients all enter treatment with sets of ideas, agendas, desires, and expectations that more often than not are modified in the course of treatment. More often than not, issues arise that they did not anticipate would ever need to be dealt with. What if one of these issues is their need for a course in race relations while they are really very comfortable with their present position? Many see bigotry as a personal choice (Harrison & Butts, 1970). Should bigotry be shielded under a liberal laissez-faire attitude, or must one understand it clinically as another form of delusional thought disorder? As it stands, this poses an interesting theoretical/ethical debate for the profession; for the minority psychologist, it becomes a real life issue that calls into question not only the therapist's political/professional beliefs but also his or her personal history, mores, and dignity as a human being (Jackson, 1973).

A Hispanic colleague confided about her shame, anger, and confusion at having the telephone hung up on her repeatedly, she believed, because she has a clearly discernible accent. "Freud had one," she said, "but it didn't sound like el barrio." The author has had the experience of patients tripping on the steps to his office on their initial visit because, they said, "You do not sound the way you look." What eventually is uncovered from this behavior is their surprise at finding a black analyst. The ordinarily expected difficulties of working through negative transferences are confounded when they are racially based (Garonex, 1971). Standard techniques quickly take on parameters. As one example, something other than the usual interpretation is called for when dealing with patients' fantasied longing for the traditional symbiotic "you and I are one" phase when the therapist doesn't look like someone the patient could be part of. Patients, being aware of this on several levels of consciousness, develop a resistance to the expression of the wish and, by preventing that expression, hinder the development of it and hence its working through. The potential for leaving a major piece of the analysis untouched is tremendous.

To deny countertransference motives is just as difficult when the therapist and the patient are aware of the tensions both live under and the therapist most definitely holds opinions about this (Fooks, 1973). Some white patients question the therapist's altruism and desire to help. The author has been confronted by the possibility that he now had an excellent opportunity to "get even" for all the ills suffered at the hands of white folk. At other times, the patient's alliance was cemented because of a belief that being black was tantamount to being downtrodden and therefore was the basis of the therapist's empathy. Of course, the patient could get better, but the therapist would always be black. Patients' reactions run the gamut from total denial of the therapist's differences to being devastated by them (Gardner, 1971). One patient collapsed in tears as she told the author that as a child, her mother often threatened her with being abandoned to a black family, "and look where I've ended up," she said. Another, rather brilliant, verbose patient in analysis suddenly became tongue-tied, developing a very disruptive stammer. After some investigation, a fear of offending the analyst was revealed becaue of "glib" associations kept to herself because all had some reference to "black" in them. This had apparently started when the phrase "black humor" had come to mind, and it quickly generalized to any such use of the word in adjective form. One patient very proudly exclaimed/proclaimed several months into her first analysis that because I was so unusual to her and she had no real experience with black folk in her life, I was the perfect blank screen for her to project onto (she had obviously been reading).

Minority patients also have racial issues; they may assume an intimate knowledge of the therapist's politics and home life or question the therapist's ability to work as effectively as a white psychologist. As described earlier, often the anger, racial self-hatred, and identification with the aggressor of a minority patient, when projected onto the minority therapist, can be confused with that therapist's own difficulties and one truly becomes embroiled in the proverbial "forest" as one of the "trees" (Turner, 1981). The job of the minority therapist now is to avoid the very attractive pitfalls of commiseration while helping that patient to make an honest, real assessment of the situation. This does not happen with all patients, and most of the minority psychologists interviewed have learned to handle adeptly these situations for themselves and their patients' benefit. However, there is a potential for correcting bizarre perceptions of reality when racial material is handled properly and not treated as taboo or avoided as a possible source of countertransference resistance or, at the very least, an empathic breach. It is the author's experience that treatment is enhanced and progresses in a rich and fulfilling manner if the issues are confronted openly and the fears concerning differences/separateness are addressed.

For the private practitioner, it becomes an added concern because of the need to resolve these difficulties in a manner that allows one to continue to build a practice. Without appropriate training, and there is a paucity of culturally sensitive senior supervisors to work with, it adds to the burden of functioning in isolation. One may feel the conflict and/or the temptation to compromise personal integrity for the sake of economics or to do just the opposite by taking a rigid, hostile, militant stance, thereby all but ensuring the collapse of a fledgling career. Again, choosing patients is intimately tied to the question of where referrals emanate from and what those sources consider to be the type of patient you work best with. Having patients referred solely on the basis of ethnicity can prevent proper growth of professional skill and economic stability. An excellent example is offered by a black colleague who noted that he was being referred an inordinate number of young black males by a white colleague in an agency setting because it was that person's belief that these children needed an experience with a mature, accepting black male (vis-à-vis the developmental model of the "best family" as an "intact nuclear one"). This therapist's relative lack of training in child therapy did not seem to be a concern for either. Both professionals seem at fault by operating under the misconception that ethnicity alone suggests expertise. When asked why he continued to accept these children, the black therapist replied that he doubted if they would receive treatment at all otherwise, and at least he was motivated to learn and care for them even though he felt his practice flooded by this large number of lower-fee patients. One questions the soundness of both these responses—the one for its narrowness of theoretical perspective and the other for the ethics of working with patients without a demonstrated expertise. These issues are magnified by the numbers games that agencies and private practitioners alike must contend with (i.e., more children than therapists and more available hours than scheduled hours), but still one has to question the benefit gained overall. The referrer learns nothing new by maintaining a traditional philosophy; the therapist is pressured to handle a population he or she is uncomfortable with and, by filling in the time in this manner, makes himself or herself unavailable for more appropriate patients; and the patients lose the opportunity for the best possible therapeutic experience. Hopefully, this is the exception and not the rule, but it does illustrate the type of ills that can be generated when this restricted criterion is foremost in the referral process. It also again highlights the need for preparation oriented toward culturally relevant issues for private practitioners prior to and during professional vocational development. With experience and a more established practice, this may become less of a concern as one is able to choose more of the patients one wishes to work with.

Regardless of the number of years of training or specialty of practice, one seems expected to do casework with minority clients and to keep a sliding scale of fees. The assumption appears to be that minority practitioners will take lower fees more regularly than their white counterparts (Thomas & Sillen, 1972). Clients often seem surprised to learn that a minority therapist's rates are competitive. Some minority patients expect to be given a reduced fee, become indignant at not receiving one (regardless of their ability to pay), and frequently will not return after a few sessions, citing the expense as the major reason. If the patient is of the therapist's ethnic group, it appears as if others believe that the therapist is obligated to provide treatment. In a clinic setting, in which the demands of cost-effective management dictate policy, this is probably more easily handled than in a private setting. Many minority private practitioners admit to holding several hours aside for the purpose of seeing lower-fee patients rather than alienate an existing referral source.

SELF-PERCEPTION AND
THE NEED FOR SUPPORT

While many minority therapists hold hours because they have a commitment to servicing the less financially fortunate minority patient, another major purpose of this practice is related to survival guilt (Whitten, 1987). The former reason may keep us tied more closely to the community, but the latter reason interferes with ongoing professional growth because mandatorily keeping a foot in both worlds can have a regressive and binding effect. For many the question is: Do we have a right to a better life-style when others, some of whom may even be close relations, are suffering in poverty? It can leave one in a perpetual mode of reparation for the failures of the nation and our disenfranchised brothers/sisters. This speaks of a still bigger issue for the minority psychologist and private practitioner: one's professional and personal self-images, which are inextricably tied together.

The efficacy of the self is involved on both these levels. Of the psychologists interviewed, each one handled the issue differently, but the concern revolved about whether or not they believed their work to have value to those they treated and to be respected by their colleagues. All were concerned as well with helping to change the consciousness/conscientiousness regarding ethnic bias of those they come in contact with. All were focused on understanding and developing innovations in treatment approaches that would help address the nature of the problems of cultural specificity for their patients. Most acknowledged the need to look outside the mainstream of the independent practice of psychology for support and acceptance. In trying to "fit in," especially in places where one may not be wanted, one runs the risk of perpetuating the problem — i.e., one becomes so accustomed to experiencing racial bias that, even when it is not there, the potential to act as if it were is great.

With perseverance and some luck it is hoped the lot of the minority private practitioner will change. As it stands, however, it appears that the future of these professionals is pretty much in their own hands. The frustration develops when intervention that is early enough to improve the conditions is blocked by the rigid wall of tradition, especially for issues of training and referral sources. As the nation seems to be in the process of philosophically swinging to the right on many fronts, it is questionable whether a joint national effort by all psychologists in private practice (or otherwise) to effect these needed changes can be expected. James Jones (1985), past director of the Minority Fellowship Program of the APA, points out that "we should note that for each of the past four years, the Reagan administration budget for clinical training support has been $0. The Minority Fellowship Program as well as many university training slots filled by ethnic minority students are directly threatened by this policy position" (p. 453).

All of the above contribute to the minority practitioner's self-image and influence his or her choice of avenues for support. Home, religion, family, and other environmental roots are used to fill the gaps when the usual professional channels are blocked. Those of us who are practicing recognize the many obstacles and are succeeding, and so it must be concluded that the obstacles are not insurmountable. It must be said that of those I interviewed (and they share this notion), no minority private practitioner has had to leave a practice because of a paucity of patients. Bilingual practitioners are especially in demand, and in general most minority psychologists find employment when others cannot, differential income notwithstanding (Russo et al., 1981). There is room and the need is great on all levels of clinical practice. Our job now seems to be to meet that need. The row may be difficult for us to hoe, but our 40 acres are fertile acres and our mules are strong and dedicated.

There are certainly many other areas that have not been touched on here. Again, I emphasize that the purpose of the chapter has been to underscore some major difficulties, recognizing that another chapter could be devoted to enumerating the several positive aspects of the experience. I have highlighted what I felt to be things well known to only a few of us and seldom written about for the majority to know. The scope of this chapter necessarily limits the discussion, but hopefully it will spark others to enter the field, to make a difference in the private sector, and to enlighten those that need to be enlightened the most, those who have more resources and better access to the process of becoming an independent practitioner in psychology.

REFERENCES

Bayton, J., Roberts, S.O., & Williams, R.K. (1970). Minority groups and careers in psychology. *American Psychologist, 25*(6), pp. 504–510.

Calnek, M. (1970). Racial factors in the countertransference: The black therapist and the black client. *American Journal of Orthopsychiatry, 40*(1), pp. 39–46.

Dean, W.E. (1977). Training minorities in psychology. *Journal of Non-White Concerns in Personnel and Guidance, 5*(3), pp. 119–125.

Dean, W.E., Parker, B.A., & Williams, B.C. (1976). Training mental health professionals for the black community. *Journal of Black Psychology, 3*(1), pp. 14–19.

Evans, D.A. (1985). Psychotherapy and black patients: Problems of training, trainees, and trainers. *Psychotherapy: Theory, Research, Practice and Training, 22*(2S), pp. 457–468.

Fooks, G.M. (1973). Dilemmas of black therapists. *Journal of Non-white Concerns in Personnel and Guidance, 1*(4), pp. 181–191.

Gardner, L.H. (1971). The therapeutic relationship under varying conditions of race. *Psychotherapy: Theory, Research and Practice, 8*(1), pp. 78–87.

Griffith, E.E. (1986). Blacks and American psychiatry. *Hospital and Community Psychiatry, 37*(1), p. 5.

Goldman, G.D., & Stricker, G. (1981). White psychiatrists' racism in referral practices to black psychiatrists. *Journal of the National Medical Association, 62,* pp. 278–282.

Jackson, A.M. (1973). Psychotherapy: Factors associated with the race of the therapist. *Psychotherapy: Theory, Research and Practice, 10*(3), pp. 273–277.

Jones, J.M. (1985). The sociopolitical context of clinical training in psychology: The ethnic minority case. *Psychotherapy: Theory, Research, Practice and Training, 22*(2S), pp. 453–456.

Jones, J.M., & Block, C.B. (1984). Black cultural perspectives. *Clinical Psychologist, 37*(2), pp. 58–62.

Jones, J.M., & Jordan, A.R. (1984). Part-time education for minorities: A black and white issue. *Journal of Continuing Social Work Education, 3*(1), pp. 53–57.

Korchin, S.J. (1980). Clinical psychology and minority problems. *American Psychologist 35*(3), pp. 262–269.

Mataragnon, R.H. (1979). The case for an indigenous psychology. *Philippine Journal of Psychology, 12*(1), pp. 3–8.

Norcross, J.C., & Prochaska, J.O. (1983). Psychotherapists in independent practice: Some findings and issues. *Professional Psychology: Research and Practice, 14*(6), pp. 869–881.

Prochaska, J.E. & Norcross, J.C. (1983). Contemporary psychotherapists: A national survey of characteristics, practices, orientations and attitudes. *Psychotherapy: Theory, Research and Practice, 29*(2), pp. 161–173.

Russo, N.F., Stapp, J., Olmedo, E.L., & Fulcher, R. (1981). Women and minorities in psychology. *American Psychologist, 36*(11), pp. 1315–1363.

Simpkins, G., & Raphael, P. (1970). Goals of the Black Students Psychological Association. *American Psychologist, 25*(5), XXII–XXVI.

Thomas, A., & Sillen, S. (1972). *Racism and Psychiatry.* New York: Brunner Mazel.

Turner, S., & Armstrong, S. (1981). Psychotherapy: What the therapists say. *Psychotherapy: Theory, Research and Practice, 18*(3), pp. 375–378.

Whitten, L. (1987). Survival guilt. Presented as a panel presentation to The One Hundred Black Men of Nassau/Suffolk, Inc., The Plight of the Black Male.

Wispe, L., Awkard, J., Hoffman, M., Ash, P., Hicks, L.M., & Porter, J. (1969). The Negro psychologist in America. *American Psychologist, 24*(2), pp. 142–150.

Wolkon, G.H., Moriwaki, S., & Williams, K.J. (1973). Race and social class as factors in the orientation toward psychotherapy. *Journal of Counselling Psychology, 20*(4), pp. 312–316.

Wyatt, G.E., & Perham, W.D. (1985). The inclusion of culturally sensitive course materials in graduate school and training programs. *Psychotherapy: Theory, Research, Practice and Training, 22*(2S), pp. 461–468.

52

THE EMOTIONAL IMPACT
OF A HOME OFFICE

Robert H. Keisner, Ph.D.

A t a conference recently I was presenting a paper that included a discussion of my work with a very difficult patient. After my description of a particularly stormy phase of treatment with the patient, someone in the audience asked what I thought precipitated the phase. I thought for a moment, then replied that this patient was probably reacting to a recent change in my office location. I had just moved my practice from a professional building to my home. It was my understanding that any major change would have created intense anxiety for this patient, but that he had to see me in my home office aroused considerable envy, rage, and terror in him and had an enormous emotional impact on both of us. As a result of the way he treated me, I felt a range of awful emotions—from uselessness, hatred, ineffectiveness, detachment and despair to relief and satisfaction that we both survived the ordeal. Even though these emotionally tumultuous experiences may have been precipitated by other circumstances, it is my sense they were a result of my practicing in a home office.

Actually, the private practice of psychoanalysis began when Freud opened an office in his home. There in the space of his consulting room he created the psychoanalytic situation. He expressed his own characterological needs and enacted his countertransference with his patients (Kurz, 1986). Since then many psychotherapists have chosen to establish their private practice in rooms located in their own homes. Although mental health practitioners tell numerous stories and express various feelings about working in the space of their homes, there is no formal literature that examines the reasons for such a choice and the emotional impact that having a home office has for patients or practitioners. This chapter will focus on the emotional consequences of working at home, especially the impact on one's professional conduct and experience with patients. Consideration will be given to conscious and unconscious reasons and reactions to practicing in a home office with special emphasis on the patient's transference as a vehicle to understanding the practitioner's feelings.

A CASE OF SELECTIVE INATTENTION

Whenever there is little or no formal discussion of a facet of practice, or for that matter any professional or personal activity, Sullivan's (1956) principle of selective inattention becomes relevant. Selective inattention occurs "when the significant is not attended to" (p. 43). Generally, Sullivan saw this process of overlooking something important and relevant as self-system motivated, designed to facilitate security through success in dealing with others.

I would like to suggest that one reason for practitioner inattention to the causes and effects of working in a home office is the incongruency between the unnoticed benefits to the practitioner and the "dedicated physician" role (Searles, 1979a). Whenever there are nonobvious benefits to the practitioner, besides the undeniable factors like collecting fees for their services or "doing good work," there is likely to be a lack of self-awareness regarding the nature and origin of these benefits. I hope to make it clear that therapists have much to gain, consciously and unconsciously, by working at home and that they use selective inattention to avoid knowing about some of the benefits and emotions associated with using a home office.

Let me go further. First, the history of transference–countertransference in the psychoanalytic tradition has been to identify and understand transference prior to countertransference. It is true that we have come a long way from this perspective, but we may still be oriented toward considering the emotions of our patients as primary and our own motives and feelings as secondary. According to the traditional intent of psychotherapy, we are not there to be influenced or impacted. Our patients are the ones we are there to change, improve, or cure. Second, the place we practice is literally and figuratively "under our own noses." We are inclined to focus our attention on our patient's feelings, cognitions, or behavior—depending on our orientation. Perceptually, therefore, practitioners do not usually look very curiously at their own rooms or homes with the hope of gaining relevant insight from such observations. Another possible explanation for not attending to the impact of working at home is that negative emotions are sometimes (if not often) associated with working at home. Feelings such as guilt, anger, and anxiety are real emotional consequences of our work, but the fact that they may be partly elicited by working at home is something we may not wish to know. Being in our own home is supposed to be relaxing. We hope to feel "at home" there and not to feel tension, guilt, anger, or any other negative emotion. Finally, if our theoretical orientation is psychodynamic, it becomes part of our professional life to focus on individual variables such as defenses, conflicts, diagnoses, and development—all aspects of the patient, not the setting. Whether we are behavioral, cognitive or humanistic, we focus respectively on altering, modifying or expanding the clients' actions, thoughts or personal awareness. Settings are usually considered by practitioners to be superficial, impermanent issues, generally unimportant in the tratment process, much as classical psychoanalysts consider culture to be a secondary determinant of unconscious processes. This is not the case for therapists from all psychological orientations. Barker's (1965) work on ecological psychology has identified settings as the best predictors of human behavior. According to him, "behavior settings," such as classrooms and churches, have social properties and facilitate the satisfaction of a variety of motives. This view is consistent with the plethora of observations made by Goffman (1961) regarding institutional effects on personalities and communication patterns. As Stricker and Keisner (1985) have pointed out, since practitioners lose their enthusiasm for research when they make the transition from student to professional, the large majority are probably unaware of empirical evidence that focuses on the role that setting, institutional, or situational variables play in psychotherapy.

CONSCIOUS MOTIVES

What are some of the motives and emotional consequences involved in practicing psychotherapy at home? First, practitioners who work at home benefit from the convenience of an office located "at their doorstep." They don't have to travel to work, which enables them to escape frustrations that many others have to put up with, including the discomforts of bad weather, traffic, air and noise pollution, and high social density. This becomes especially salient when there is inclement weather or when a patient reports considerable difficulty in getting to the office because of naturally occurring events beyond the patient's control (e.g., road construction, train delays, etc.). At such times, therapists working in home offices are reminded of how comparatively easy they have it, and how much relative control they actually have. Second, there is the economic benefit from tax deductions for the use of space in one's home for a professional office. This is probably the most conscious reason therapists have for using their homes as a place to work. There is also the availability of need-satisfying people and places at one's "fingertip": families for interpersonal contact, kitchens for snacks, couches or beds for resting, and so on. When a therapist is "between" patients or when cancellations occur, he or she can easily take advantage of these comforts or pleasures. Finally, there is a more amorphous but no less significant feeling of ease associated with working in one's home. In his paper "House, Home and Identity in Contemporary American Culture," Hummon (1987) has described how people report "feeling at home" at home, doing what they like, being themselves, and generally being more relaxed and comfortable in the space of their own homes. Practitioners, like anyone else, undoubtedly prefer places where they feel more comfortable and secure.

Working at home also establishes and maintains a dialectical relationship between a practitioner's patients on the one hand and his or her family members on the other. With the exception of practitioners who live alone, a practitioner who works at home is in very close proximity to the other places (rooms) in the home, and is reminded (usually as a result of direct sensory impingements, including noises and cooking smells) that he or she is "with" a patient and not "with" his or her family. This can arouse guilt about abandoning one's spouse and children or anger toward the patient for taking one away from the family. This can create resentment toward a patient who may be seen as responsible for these guilty or angry feelings. In addition, going from home to office and back involves almost no time or place separation. Only a few seconds and steps are required to make the trip, and while this is extremely convenient, there are occasions when difficulties may develop. For instance, moving from one room (e.g., the kitchen) to another (the office) in a mater of seconds requires a rapid transition from a personal to a professioal relationship. Just as we need a few moments to make the transition from one patient to another, we also need some time to adjust ourselves to the often highly demanding work of psychotherapy. A number of possible scenarios come to mind. We may be enjoying a meal with our family, playing with one of our children, having an argument with our spouse, or being confronted with an adolescent's problems only to be required to suddenly shift our attention to a depressed, angry, or frightened patient. With little chance to recover our balance because there is no separation in time and space, we may be called upon to be instantly sensitive to a demanding, rejecting, or sadistic patient. Even under conditions of maximum attention and energy this is a most difficult task. Another disconcerting situation may occur when patients either come very early to a session or linger well beyond their session time, causing a therapist to make necessary adjustments in his or her personal activity. Certainly these acts are meaningful expressions of a patient's wishes, feelings, defenses, and/or character style, but they are more likely to create negative emotional reactions for therapists working at home than for those working in an office or waiting room located in a more "neutral" professional building. These "invasions" of privacy are, of course, not completely without a context. After all we do "invite" patients into our home, although we implicitly or explicitly communicate to them our expectation that they refrain from entering other rooms or areas in our home and that they recognize that our time with them is limited to 45- or 50-minute sessions. However, since patients have been "invited" and often do develop intense feelings toward their therapist, it is not surprising that they may experience a strong and irrational attachment to their therapist's home. For example, they may feel safe spending long periods of time in their therapist's waiting room before or after a session precisely because the waiting room is in their therapist's home and represents a safe haven or sanctuary. It might be said that such experiences can serve as growth opportunities for patients who need to develop a stable sense of separateness between themselves and others.

UNCONSCIOUS MOTIVES

I would like to discuss some unconscious reasons that motivate therapists to have an office in their home. They can stay "close to home" and minimize or even avoid travel away from home. This may allow them to successfully defend against separation anxiety. More specifically, working in one's home may even reflect back upon certain stages of the separation/individuation process (Mahler et al., 1975). As Kurz (1986) pointed out, Freud most likely gratified certain symbiotic needs by placing certain antiques, pictures, and furniture in his consulting room. The same may be said of having the opportunity to "go to work" without leaving the security of one's nest. In addition to the gratification of symbiotic needs, a home office involves a process of frequent coming and going during the course of a single workday. This resembles the rapprochement subphase of separation/individuation, perhaps representing for some therapists an acting out of contradictory needs to separate and re-attach in their movements away from the "personal" part of the home (kitchen, living room, etc.) to the "professional" part of the home, and then back to the "personal" areas, and so on. Since it has been pointed out that mothers spend more time at home than fathers and generally identify more with home (Hummon, 1987), it may be said that a practitioner who works in a home office is staying closer to home and mother.

Narcissistic needs, both pathological and normal, may also be in the picture. It is possible that therapists use a home office in order to "show" their patients the level of social rank and class membership they have attained. Hummon (1987) has pointed out that individuals and groups will often display their homes, the content of their homes (such as sculptures, large potted plants), and their communities as public messages to others that they belong to a certain social group and have "made it" in our society. Therapists, like most people, are undoubtedly aware of this manner of nonverbal communication and in all likelihood assume their patients are also cognizant of this relationship between home appearance, style, size, location, and personal status. On a pathological level, this could be an indication that a therapist has the need to have patients admire his or her accomplishments. If so, there would no doubt be other indications of such needs, such as offering interpretations or advice in order to be admired.

"Everyday" narcissism may also be at stake for some practitioners. In a paper extending Freud's 1901 article "The Psychopathology of Everyday Life," Burstein and Bertenthal (1987) have proposed that analysis of pathological narcissism can be extended to secondary or everyday narcissistic disturbances that occur in individuals with a "firmly consolidated self." Using a Kohutian analysis, they identified restaurants as settings where one's grandiosity can be gratified by waiters who anticipate a diner's every wish, or where narcissistic injuries and rage are common reactions to frustrated grandiosity and omnipotence resulting from a lack of attention. Having an office in one's home may be considered an attempt to have patients, family members, and the comforts of home (especially the kitchen) all within close proximity. Given these possibilities, there is a range of narcissistic needs that therapists may be seeking to satisfy, from "normal" self-stabilizing needs to the confirmation of a grandiose fantasy of being in total command of one's world (as in "my home is my castle"). Furthermore, "territoriality" research with humans suggests that when people are in their own place they are more dominant and powerful. This research, which compared task performance of residents and visitors of dormitory rooms, lends support to the notion that individuals who are in their own home setting are more dominant and powerful than those who are not (Martindale, 1971). A home office is obviously far more neutral territory but is a place where the practitioner has certain advantages. This needs to be kept in mind and recognized as a realistic obstacle to the expression of normal dominance and power on the part of patients who visit therapists in a home office.

Another set of needs that can be gratified and expressed through one's home office have to do with identity and individualism. Cooper (1976) has pointed out that dwellings express the self as a unique individual, although there is literature that suggests an important distinction between female identity expression (which is connected to the interior decoration) and male identity expression (which is connected to the more public exterior space). Complicating this distinction, however, is the observation that women have greater role involvement with the home, are more emotionally satisfied from their homes, and generally use their homes more than men do for self-expression and self-definition (Hummon, 1987). Thus, while male therapists may be expressing themselves through the publicly visible areas such as lawns and driveways, there may be a general (but unspoken) consensus that female therapists are disclosing more of their "emotional" selves through their homes than male therapists are. Thus, when there is a male therapist working in the home, his patients may assume that his home is at least partly an expression of his wife's identity, values, and tastes. And they may be making a correct assumption.

Finally, choosing to have an office in one's home is somewhat like deciding to create a private space within which one can be segregated from one's family members. It is like "having your own room." Perhaps this is a strong but unacknowledged reason for working at home. Having a place that is "all yours," to which you can go to get away from other family members, to which you are the only family member with access, that you are the only one with knowledge about, and that is mysterious to other family members can be an attempt to recreate a childhood space or to finally establish one's own room as an adult. This, incidentally, is a question that can be developed into a testable hypothesis for empirical verification.

CONSEQUENCES FOR THE PRACTITIONER

Having considered these unconscious motives for working at home, I would like to look at the indirect consequences that any and all of these factors may have on the practitioner. As motives that our outside of the practitioner's awareness they are more likely to have an inadvertent influence on patients. The first set of motives for working at home, which may have an emotional impact on the practitioner after filtering through the patient's experience, are the separation/individuation ones — symbiosis and rapprochement. As temporary motivating forces they are probably less significant than they would be if they were permanent. But, practitioners who remain stuck in any one of these phases — that is, with unresolved conflicts — are likely to create iatrogenic consequences for their patients and undoubtedly will engage in therapeutic misalliances. Although there is a potential for a variety of such misalliances, one such hypothetical case should be enough to illustrate how this can impact on a practitioner. For instance, if a practitioner is working at home because of symbiotic needs, he or she may experience patients (especially demanding ones) as threatening his or her attachments to family members. Emotions such as anger, anxiety, and guilt are likely possibilities in such circumstances, depending on the therapist's neurotic style. A therapist who resents patients for separating him or her from family members may create a vicious circle of countertransference rejection causing patients to be more demanding or withdrawing, with the patients in turn causing the therapist to experience even greater resentment or possibly manic relief when the session is over or the treatment ends. The central issue here is that the unconscious needs of the therapist that contribute to his or her establishing a home office may very well come "home" to haunt the practitioner in the sense that patients are likely to react to these needs and fulfill the therapist's prophecy. If the practitioner resents a patient for getting "in the way," then the patient will probably act or be perceived to act in consistency with the therapist's expectations.

Similar circles may be set in motion by narcissistic or identity-related factors. Seeking admiration from our patients through such a subtle medium as the size, style, and location of our home stands to gratify only the therapist. In general, such events will enhance gratification for therapists instead of facilitating maturation for patients. We all agree that practitioners' satisfaction should come from genuine service to others who are in need rather than from gratification of their own previously unmet desires.

Before closing this discussion, I would like to look at this issue from a different perspective. Searles (1979a) has hypothesized that "innate among man's powerful striving toward his fellowman...is an essentially therapeutic striving...the more ill a patient is, the more does his successful treatment require that he become and be implicitly acknowledged as having become, a therapist to his officially designated therapist" (p. 381). Therefore, when a therapist chooses to work at home for neurotic reasons, he or she must be conscious of the possibility that the patient can serve as his or her therapist. According to Searles, only if patients actually help the therapist to become more mature can they succeed in freeing themselves from the guilt regarding failure to benefit or repair early objects. While it may be considered a mere justification for self-gratification, it does seem that if working at home is symbiotically, narcissistically, or otherrwise neurotically motivated, patients are not necessarily sacrificed so long as the therapeutic task is accomplished.

We could find out what practitioners feel when working at home by asking patients what their impressions are. However, they may not know, they may give socially desirable answers, or they may be unable to formulate their ideas. Another way to approach patients as a source of data is to look for derivatives in the associations they have and thus unobtrusively gather data on their impressions of the practitioner's experience of working in his or her own home.

I would like to accomplish this by turning to a model of transference-countertransference that has recently been developed in the writings of Merton Gill (1983), Irwin Hoffman (1983), and others. This paradigm conceptualizes transference as the patient's selectively attending to certain aspects of the therapist's conduct and experience and engaging the therapist in an interpersonal process inadvertently designed to elicit responses that will confirm the patient's impressions of the therapist's character. Another member of this "school," Sandler, said that "in the transference...the patient attempts to prod the analyst into behaving in a particular way and unconsciously scans and adopts to his perception of the analyst's reaction" (1976, p. 44). He referred to the countertransference as "role responsiveness" to the patient's prodding. Furthermore, Benedek (1953) saw the patient as "boring his way into the unconscious mind of the therapist and emerging with...preconscious awareness of the therapist's personality and even his problems" (p. 203). If we operate, as Hoffman (1983) has suggested, with skepticism about what therapists know of themselves then we may be prepared to recognize the patient as an astute observer of the therapist's own resisted motives and experience. The patient's prejudice, therefore, can be used as a source of information about the therapist's unformulated emotions. This is not to say that the patient knows better or more, but that there are times when his or her perspective (transference) can serve as a window into the therapist's enacted but unacknowledged experience. As a result, we may find that certain transference-countertransference transactions are characterized by the patient knowing and expressing what the practitioner is feeling and not knowing. Working in a home office setting, as previously discussed, may well be an example of just such a situation. Let me present a few clinical vignettes to illustrate my understanding of these circumstances.

TWO CASE ILLUSTRATIONS

A 40-year-old female patient reported the following dream after about a year of treatment. During this period, our sessions took place in my home office, which was located on one side of my home. The dream reflected some unacknowledged feelings I had about working in my home office that the patient had apparently detected. She dreamt that she walked into my house at 2:00 P.M. and tried to call her office to tell a man she worked with to have somebody bring her car to my office. In the dream I had a different setup. There was a separate garage with a pay phone where she could make her call. She got here early and went to the phone, but I was speaking to someone so she hung up. She then met two or three young boys, one with dark or black hair and long eyelashes and another who looked just like me. There was also a little girl who came running through, and I told her to be careful and slow down.

The emotional impact of my working at home with this patient was, I believe, inadvertently revealed by her perception of certain aspects of our relationships. Her associations revealed that she saw herself as having to make the effort and arrangements for our meetings, that she saw herself as deferring to me, and that she was an intruder. She also saw me as a father of many children, one of whom was attractive and another of whom (the little girl) I was carefully supervising. This dream described a central aspect of my countertransference and represented a degree of correspondence between the way she experienced me and the impression I wanted to make. Understanding her dream this way gave me insight into the gratification that I was receiving from knowing that she saw me as the authority figure deserving of her effort and deference and also that she idealized me as a good, productive, and supportive father. Not only did this fit with her characterological need to sense what men wanted and satisfy them as if she were following an internal command, but it also alerted me to how important it was for me that she confirm my self-perception as an important person worthy of her deference and idealization. Although an absence of baseline data prevents me from concluding that the home office setting was a contributing factor, it seems plausible that she "knew" I liked the fact that she "came to me" in my "castle" and further that since we met in my home I wanted her to see me as a "good father in his home." This latter issue represented a blend of what she actually needed and my need to show her that I was the one who could satisfy that need. The home setting surely did not create these complementary needs but did bring them out into the open for therapeutic inquiry.

I had been seeing the second patient, a 37-year-old man, in a professional building office for about 5 years when he started attending sessions in my home office. Shortly after making the switch, he became noticeably enraged and especially frightened. So strong was his fear that I would harm him that for 7 months he sat on the end of a couch very close to the waiting room door. Only after this crisis ended and he felt safe enough to sit in a chair closer to me (which, he realized was where my patients usually sat), did he make it clear that the home location of my office contributed to his reaction. He reported feeling like an unwanted intruder who was looked upon as a burden by me and my family, a position he often experienced in his own family. In addition, the home setting aroused strong feelings of inadequacy and failure since he made comparisons between his unhappy and frustrating life and what he believed to be my trouble-free, well-organized, and happy life. While these feelings made therapy into an unusually difficult ordeal for him, they also clarified an important idiosyncratic dynamic. Because he felt lacking in moral and ethical qualities and saw himself as without compassion, he constantly attacked my morality, ethics, and capacity for compassion. It was, for me as well as him, a draining and distressing period of time. As the therapist, I experienced feelings of anxiety, guilt, hatred, relief that it was over, and then genuine satisfaction that we both survived the process. There is little doubt that his character and the home office setting had interacted to create the events as I described them. There is also no question but that all therapists subject some of their patients to intense emotional reactions when they invite them into their home office consulting room. Practitioners must be cognizant that what is done for their own convenience or unconscious motives, or both, is likely to have an impact on the therapeutic experience of their patients and consequently themselves. Then again, so long as the therapist respects the patient's views and doesn't "blame" the patient by considering the effects to be entirely a result of the patient's transference, the therapist remains in a position to use whatever develops as a means to better understand any mutual reactions that occur.

CONCLUSIONS AND SUGGESTIONS

The impact of a home office setting on the participants depends on a number of complex issues. Why a practitioner chooses to establish a consulting room in a home setting and how the patient experiences the practitioner's motives and conduct are significant determinants of how the process unfolds. A practitioner's unconscious motives, be they related to separation, identity, narcissism, or dominance, are likely to influence patients in unique but observable ways. Two clinical examples have been presented to illustrate how a home office setting can affect the therapeutic process and the emotional experience for both participants.

It was my intent to alert practitioners to the importance of situational determinants of psychotherapeutic outcomes. The home office setting represents one such determinant. An example of how situational variables interact with characterological and dynamic factors may be found in a recent article by Grey and Fiscalini (1987) on parallel process in psychoanalytic supervision. They concluded that there are "similar features in the authority structure of supervision and analysis...that they both are dyads with one person participating as the socially defined superordinate expert and the other as a client requiring help.... The clients are expected to provide personal information whereas the experts are not required to be especially self-disclosing" (p. 138). My point here is that a home office setting implies an institutional norm for both participants that further intensifies the already unequal authority structure. And, as Grey and Fiscalini (1987) point out, such structures contain pressures toward concealment of motives and enactment of defensive maneuvers. Notwithstanding the unique personal contributions of therapist and patient, a home office practice takes place in the practitioner's "castle" or territory and the patient is at best granted a limited visa. Practitioners always have the home court advantage and are in a unique position to turn the advantage into benefit for the visitor.

Beyond being alert to these issues and how they interact in different interpersonal fields, at this time only a general suggestion appears to be appropriate. Each practitioner will express countertransference through such factors as the location and privacy of the psychotherapy office. But whatever home variables are established must be considered relevant. After all, we expect our patients to accept the determinism of their decisions—why not ask the same of ourselves?

REFERENCES

Barker, R.G. &1965). Explorations in ecological psychology. *American Psychologist, 20,* 1–13.

Benedek, J. (1953). Dynamics of the countertransference. *Bulletin of the Menninger Clinic, 17,* Burstein, A., & Bertenthal, M. (1986). A note on everyday psychopathology and narcissism. *Psychoanalytic Psychology, 3, 269–276.*

Cooper, C. (1976). The house as a symbol of self. In H.M. Proshansky, W.H. Ittleson, & L.G. Rivlin (Eds.), *Environmental psychology,* pp. 435–448. New York: Nolt, Rinehart and Winston.

Gill, M.M. (1983). The distinction between the interpersonal paradigm and the degree of the therapists' involvement. *Contemporary Psychoanalysis, 19, 200–237.*

Goffman, E. (1961). Asylums. Garden City, N.Y.: Doubleday.

Grey, A., & Fiscalini, J. (1987). Paralleled process as transference countertransference interaction. *Psychoanalytic Psychology, 4,* 131–144.

Hoffman, I. (1983). The patient as interpreter of the analysts' experience. *Contemporary Psychoanalysis 3,* 389–422.

Hummon, D. (1987). *House, home and identity in contemporary American culture.* Unpublished manuscript.

Kurz, S. (1986). The analyst's space. *Psychoanalytic Review, 73,* 41–55.

Mahler, M., Pine, F., & Bergman, A. (1975). The psychological birth of the human infant. New York: Basic Books.

Martindale, D.A. (1971). Territorial dominance behavior in dyadic verbal interactions. *Proceedings of the 79th Annual Convention of the American Psychological Association, 6,* 305–306.

Sandler, J. (1976). Countertransference and role responsiveness. *International Review of Psychoanalysis, 3,* 43–47.

Searles, H. (1979a). The "dedicated physician" in the field of psychotherapy and psychoanalysis. In H. Searles, *Countertransference and selected papers, pp. 71–88.* New York: International Universities Press.

Searles, H. (1979b). The patient as therapist to his analyst. In H. Searles, *Countertransference and selected papers,* pp. 380–459. New York: International Universities Press.

Stricker, G., & Keisner, R. (1985). The relationship between research and practice. In G. Stricker & R. Keisner (Eds.), *From research to clinical practice.* New York: Plenum Press.

Sullivan, H.S. (1956). Clinical studies in psychiatry. New York: Norton.

C H A P T E R
53

WOMEN THERAPISTS: SPECIAL ISSUES IN PROFESSIONAL AND PERSONAL LIVES

Anna C. Lee, Ph.D.

As a discipline, psychotherapy—its multiple forms, impact on patients, outcome, and factors contributing to overall effectiveness—has been investigated extensively in recent years. Less studied, however, has been its effect on the practitioners of psychotherapy. Of late some authors who have undertaken such exploration have come to view it as complex at the very least and incredible at the extreme. Indeed, Malcolm (1982) has described it as the "impossible profession," echoing Freud's comment years ago that the therapeutic situation was one that gave little satisfaction to either of its participants. Its immense benefits notwithstanding, objections raised by patients about the process are known to any psychotherapist who has withstood hours of listening to and grappling with resistance, transferential love and hatred, and so forth. Until recently, moreover, therapists have maintained or even colluded in a silent stoicism about the toll exacted from them for conducting the psychotherapeutic enterprise—that is, for listening intently without many quick or easy gains obvious or forthcoming. At last, more recognition has been given to the needs of the therapists themselves as they continue the task of conducting psychotherapy. In one of the finest essays written on the subject, Arthur Burton (1975) underscores the need to examine therapist satisfaction with these wry but cogent remarks:

> There is almost a silent conspiracy in the refusal to look at the treatment needs of the psychotherapist. This of course derives from general medicine where healing had a quasi-religious function extending back at least to Aesculapius and Hippocrates and where no personal reward for the healer could be countenanced. For this reason, even the economic aspects of medicine today come as a great or small shock to patients who expect their doctors to be directly modeled after St. Francis. Observations of psychoanalytic psychotherapists reveal that they are indeed quite human, perhaps even on the sensual side, and need constant personal reward and reinforcement to maintain steerage. (p.115)

For female psychotherapists the situation may be even worse than it is for their male colleagues. Externally, this seems directly related to and exacerbated by the demands of this particular culture, one where the expectations exist both overtly and covertly for women to maintain primary responsibility for hearth and home. Hence, undertaking a profession or career has traditionally been considered of secondary importance to a woman's being a wife and mother. The situation seems no different for female psychotherapists. For the most part, those who choose to engage in the psychotherapeutic enterprise in addition to maintaining traditional feminine roles do so by juggling multiple roles simultaneously. For women who devote their time exclusively to their careers, the hazards center on dealing with the effects of not subscribing to roles deemed socially appropriate. They thus are confronted with the burden of guilt and even ostracism for eschewing societal approval and its multifaceted sanctions. I state the foregoing with caution, knowing full well the potential protest such a statement might draw from feminist quarters. It seems especially important here to address the various problems and conflicts faced by many female psychotherapists, mostly due to the special difficulties, internal and external, faced by many career-minded women in the American culture, regardless of the nature of the career or job, the gains of the feminist movement notwithstanding. The purpose of the present chapter, hence, is to examine the particular dilemmas faced by female psychotherapists both within the context of the psychotherapeutic situation and within their personal lives.

The present chapter will focus on the various factors impinging on the female therapist and the particular problems she encounters in working with patients, both female and male. It is the premise here that while special issues have always existed for women psychotherapists during the conduct of psychotherapy, little attention has been paid in the psychotherapy literature to the impact of conducting psychotherapy on the personal lives of the women psychotherapists. Hence this chapter will focus on specific countertransferential difficulties that are pertinent to female gender role issues rather than on the gamut of countertransferential issues that are likely to impinge on therapists. The most recent impetus for the interest in the study of female therapists has been the increasing number of patients requesting and obtaining female therapists. Such has been spurred in large part by the impact of feminism, thereby stimulating the wish and even insistence of many women that they work with a female psychotherapist or psychoanalyst.

This chapter will proceed by presenting an introductory discussion of the variables pertinent to the practice of psychotherapy itself. These include the changing pattern of referrals (from fewer to more women requesting a female therapist), differential resistance, transference and countertransferential reactions for female versus male patient–therapist dyads, managing issues of sexual seduction and abuse, and issues of personal safety. Subsumed in this section will be specific concerns of female therapists in dealing with particular patient populations (i.e., lesbian patients) who maintain sex role orientations and attitudes diametrically opposed to those of the therapist. The importance and contributions of feminism will be discussed in terms of its effects on the short- and long-term goals for treatment, whether or not a feminist perspective changes the criteria for internal changes. Given space restrictions, I have chosen to confine most of my remarks on treatment to the interaction between female therapists and female patients, with the understanding that many similar issues arise as well in the therapy of male patients. Following the discussion of the technical aspects of treatment as they affect female psychotherapists, the focus will turn to the personal "occupational hazards" for the therapists themselves. This section will examine more closely the costs as well as the benefits of the work for female practitioners, the very real concerns they face daily in maintaining a steady course in their work. The potential for burnout, depletion, depression, and even suicide as one goes about trying to meet the demands of the "impossible profession" will be discussed. Of particular interest here will be the role conflicts and strains that women assume when they opt for a career in addition to more traditional gender roles. The stresses placed on the female practitioner who must "juggle" all demands and maintain a delicate balance will be considered. For the single therapist, there is the very real possibility of working in greater isolation than her married or coupled counterpart, with a dearth of resources from which to draw the emotional sustenance so necessary to the vitality of the psychotherapist. Finally, for the lesbian therapist working in a community wherein her sexual orientation and life-style are less than fully accepted or condoned, the question arises about ways to negotiate her private life with the role as a therapist and member of her community. The final section of the chapter will address possible solutions or alternatives to the dilemma raised in the preceding sections. Of concern will be the particular stresses women psychotherapists face in both their professional and personal lives. Ways for female psychotherapists to seek different solutions to "burnout" and depletion will be examined, through which it is hoped women practitioners will be able to develop more satisfying, creative ways to integrate the polarities of work and home which confront them more urgently than their male colleagues. This by no means presupposes that undertaking a career as a psychotherapist would pose difficulty for all women. It merely highlights the reality of a type of life particularly prone to the "occupational hazard" of turmoil and depletion should its stresses go unrecognized and unalleviated.

TECHNICAL CONSIDERATIONS

A study of changes in the practice of psychotherapy for women practitioners should, first of all, take into account the changing pattern of referrals during the past two decades. Since the inception of the feminist movement in the 1960s, increasing numbers of women have sought psychotherapy with women psychotherapists and analysts (Turkel, 1976; Person, 1983). These authors attribute the trend to various motivations on the part of the female patients. These include the search for a female role model or figure of identification who may condone more readily the patient's career and achievement orientation and the active avoidance of male psychotherapists or analysts (whatever their competence or sympathy to feminism) arising from a fear that a male therapist will seek to control them or to undermine their hard-fought-for sense of autonomy and independence. Other reasons include the belief that it is too easy and tempting to fool a male therapist and thereby avoid problem areas, the wish to avoid an erotic transference or countertransference, and the explicit desire to have a strong competent women with whom to make a positive identification (Person, 1983). This shift dramatically highlights, moreover, the greater choice of patients now open to female psychotherapists, which hardly existed before. No longer are they restricted to those rejected by male therapists for one reason or another. Turkel (1976) comments on this trend of referral to female therapists:

> Male therapists are reluctant to make referrals which may somehow offend their patients, for example, it might hint at latent homosexuality. Thus, for many years, my referrals consisted primarily of adolescent girls (they need a good mother), homosexual males (they might feel homosexual panic with a male therapist), lesbians (they are too hostile to men), and those patients for whom I was a reanalyst (as long as they are changing analysts, they might as well try a woman).

While it seems obvious that a more favorable climate exists today for female therapists and analysts as far as sheer number of patients now seeking their services, various treatment issues have arisen as well. The challenge posed by the task of absorbing and grappling with varied transference reactions takes on a special cast when women therapists find themselves perforce the repository of a host of positive and negative therapeutic reactions. In her excellent review of the importance of therapist gender on the outcome of treatment, Mogul (1982) notes the differential, more critical effect of therapist gender in those psychotherapies that are less intensive than traditional psychoanalysis. Though the outcome of the latter is less affected by therapist gender than by therapist training, experience, and so forth, this seems less true for shorter-term therapies:

> The course of therapy is more commonly affected, with differences in the nature of the alliance, the development of different transference feelings and content, and possible differences in overt difficulty and conflict. With some patients, in shorter forms of psychotherapy, or with therapists who are less experienced and skilled, such factors can be powerful enough to substantially affect outcome. (p. 9)

Female therapists have reported a number of consistent trends in transference and countertransference reactions that have arisen in work with both male and female patients. In addition to the stereotypical reactions to the woman therapist as the earth mother who heals all wounds, there is the envy of the all-powerful mother and frustrated rage toward her for nurturance seemingly withheld. The development of dependency, hostile or otherwise, accelerates a maternal transference and is exacerbated by passivity typically experienced with maternal images. The combination of appropriate external cues — female therapist plus traditional role — seems to speed up the occurrence of the maternal transference. Person (1983) draws some conclusions about the female–female therapist–patient dyad more specific to the therapist's gender:

> In sum, the female therapist is sought not just as a role model. More important, she is sought as a stand-in for the mother. In this role, it is her permission to compete and to achieve that is required. In short-term therapies, such permission may lead to a transference "cure." In long-term therapy, an intense rejecting mother transference is frequent. Current cultural attitudes may sometimes engender idealizing transference attitudes in female analysts that encourage and, thereby, short-circuit the working through of underlying conflicts. (p. 202).

Other typical reactions include heightened Oedipal dynamics in the form of competition with the woman therapist in the area of femininity, devaluation and depreciation of the patient's self and of the therapist, and the equation of assertion with hostility and phallic aggressiveness. Women are seen as rivals for men, not to be trusted, and are unconsciously or consciously felt to be second-rate. The deep conviction of the unworthiness of female gender often leads particularly competitive women to view themselves and their mothers (and therapists by way of transference) as incomplete creatures who cannot function without the "sponsorship" of a man (Eisenbud, 1986). Symonds (1976) notes that socialization of aggression in females has effected a significant impact on the psyche of women, suggesting that a lifetime spent in the repression of hostility presents a dilemma for both women patients and therapists. Since women have not been allowed to fight for themselves in this openly competitive society, having to deal directly and aggressively, as they are called upon to do in demanding careers, may challenge women to learn lessons in the workplace that men have known all along. Women are, in essence, facing issues as adults that men have confronted since early childhood. These effects of socialization are apropos for women therapists as well. As they take their place in the professional world they may also feel less equipped than their male colleagues to deal with the competition of building a practice. For instance, men are more open about seeking avenues for developing their practices and professional roles. Female therapists may be more passive and perhaps even masochistic in developing their professional roles and networks. In this respect, Bernay (1983) enjoins women practitioners to overcome their passivity and masochism in the interest of developing their practices and participating more fully in their professional roles.

Though the issue of sexual acting out with patients in terms of seduction and abuse is relevant for women therapists as it is for men. It must be noted that women therapists are less noted for actual instances of sexual behavior with patients. Person (1983) notes here that the relative subordination of the patient to the authority of the therapist is not congruent with the predominant types of female sexual fantasies. Yet female therapists do have sexual fantasies about male patients that, because of cultural prohibitions, are less likely to be considered or openly acknowledged than are those of male therapists about female patients. Nonetheless, grappling with her sexual attraction to the patient may pose some countertransference burden for the therapist who has not fully resolved it in her own mind.

Countertransference reactions and pitfalls also run the gamut from over-identification with patients to unconscious rejection, envy of the patient's dependent way of life, competition with the patient in the areas of youth and appearance, elitism, and excessive proselytizing about the need for women patients to choose careers (Turkel, 1976). While many women therapists fall squarely on the side of emancipation of women and greater freedom of choice and self-definition, they too can be subject to reactions of avoidance and disdain for the gender-related conflicts of their women patients. In her survey of female therapists presently involved in personal psychotherapy, Coche (1984) highlights the dilemma faced by several respondents when confronted with patients whose ongoing conflicts resembled too closely unresolved issues in their own lives, especially in the areas of femininity, role conflicts, conflictual interpersonal relationships, and "leading a balanced life."

Many countertransferential reactions occur even as most women therapists are cognizant of the pernicious effects of long-term socialization of women and at times may cause them to endorse such dynamics as masochism, helpless dependency, deference to male authority, and shared fears of female destructiveness, all at the patient's expense. Bernardez-Bonesatti (1978) warns, for example, that women therapists are as likely as male therapists to disapprove strongly the anger or competitiveness of their female patients, especially if the target of the patient's hostility is a male. Concurring with this observation, Lerner (1984) also comments on the oedipal dynamics aroused here:

> Not only is a protectiveness for males aroused, but the female therapist who unconsciously fears that her own unrestrained anger may be hurtful to men is threatened by her identification with a female patient whom she perceives as "destructive" and "castrating." I have also been impressed by the need for female therapists to avoid identifying with women who are angry with men, even if they perceive themselves as having a legitimate cause (p. 279).

While countertransferential reactions abound for female therapists working with female patients, perhaps the most taxing, difficult, and "stickiest" involve situations where the maternal transference creates inordinate demands on the therapist to provide a neutral "holding environment" for patients in the midst of intense pulls for symbiosis and fusion. Balsam (1974) aptly describes the dilemma of the female therapist who, though sympathetic with female goals for herself and her patients, must nonetheless maintain therapeutic distance:

> The maintenance and nurture of symbiotic tendencies is, I think, natural in women, patients and therapists alike. The talents of empathy, creative projective identification, the enjoyment and expression of feeling in interaction, are examples of the strengths brought to exploratory work by symbiotic functioning in either male or female therapists. . . . Many female patients use their proclivity for symbiosis defensively. They yearn to luxuriate in this state of affairs, symbolically still in utero, and they do everything they can to ignite an answering quality in the female therapist that they, of course, intuitively know is likely to be a part of her womanhood, too. The infantile mother-daughter bonds, with their implications of homosexuality and boundariless interrelatedness, can combine to produce intense attachment but little therapeutic movement. The tolerance of aggression in the progressing relationship is part of this therapeutic tie. Many women subtly or less subtly turn aggression against themselves, and the female therapist is no exception. Under attack from another woman, self-doubt often emerges. This tendency may represent guilt in the women therapist for maintaining her own separateness. . . . In other words, pregenital maternal dynamics may be triggered in either patient or therapist or both, especially because they are both women. (pp. 312–313).

Secondly, the tendency for the transference to become erotized gives rise to intense homosexual yearnings that may challenge the therapist to the extreme. The therapist's own sexual orientation and comfort with homosexual dynamics are of importance here in providing the context by which she will react to the regressive pulls of the patient's longings for sexual involvement in whatever form. In a related vein, Gartrell (1984) cites issues that typically arise in the treatment of lesbian patients to include therapists' understanding of the etiology of heterosexuality and homophobia; the advantages and disadvantages of "coming out of the closet," with its attendant effect on self-definition and self-esteem; and the realities of the sociopolitical context of heterosexuality on individuals who have opted for a homosexual orientation.

These issues can pose potentially problematic areas for the woman therapist since, like her patients, she is conditioned from early on to be more sensitively attuned to the interpersonal surroundings than males are. Gilligan (1982) notes, for example, that masculinity is defined through separateness while femininity is defined through attachment. Hence, the male gender identity is more easily threatened by intimacy while femininity is threatened by separation. As such, different relational styles exist for women (and women therapists) and for men, posing potentially more conflict for more nurturant individuals to turn away from or reject the press of someone's need, and attendant guilt over maintaining separateness from their patients exists more for women therapists than for their male counterparts. One must consider that these reactions are likely to arise as much out of social conditioning as out of intrapsychic pressures, as these differences have existed early on between men and women in their formative years. Underscored here is also a need for a comprehensive developmental study of the socialization process of the female as it is similar to or different from that of the male (Hare-Mustin, 1978; Welnar et al., 1979).

PERSONAL LIVES OF THERAPISTS

We turn our attention now to the ramifications of conducting psycho-therapy on its practitioners. Despite its many positives, chief among these the rewards of involvement in the emotional growth of another individual, the cost of devoting one's professional life and energy to it is high. Various studies have cited the higher degree of psychopathology and suicide within the profession when compared with other professions, with the trend even more marked for female practitioners (Racusin et al., 1981). Troubled family dynamics also characterize the families of origin of a number of therapists, as Racusin and colleagues have suggested. These include the therapists' enmeshment in the conflictual marital relationships of their parents, provision of parenting in the form of responsibility for family functions or nurturing, and care for at least one family member with a physical or behavioral difficulty involving presumed psychogenic factors. Physical disorders included cardiovascular disease and diabetes, while psychological factors included neuroses, character disorders, and child abuse.

Thus, it should come as no surprise that many therapists enter the helping profession in order to perpetuate the roles they may have assumed in their families of origin, especially within a setting of controlled intimacy. Unfortunately, this role exacts a toll for those clinicians who exhaust their supplies of nurturance, resulting in a feeling of giving without receiving like recompense in return. Burnout and stress in therapists have reached alarming proportions and women therapists have more than their fair share, as Freudenberg and Robbins (1979) note in their article on the "hazards" of the profession:

Feelings of depression, loneliness, futility, cynicism, loss of vitality, authenticity, anger, frustration, psychosomatic symptoms, chronic fatigue, sleeplessness, and poor interpersonal relationships are characteristic of the impaired therapist. Over a period of time the feelings do not necessarily dissipate. Quite the contrary, for some they may increase.

In addition to the stress of grappling with the strains of ongoing emotional arousal, the therapist is expected to maintain objectivity and neutrality without suffering excessive detachment, callousness, or depletion. Along with this curious admixture of demands the female therapist is expected to cope with and manage another entire set of demands related to her gender role. As if to remind women of the price they must pay for being "superwoman," symptoms of fatigue and depletion may occur. Chief among these are themes related to feelings of inadequacy in female therapists' ability to merge the polarities of assertion and nurturance, feelings of being hypocritical and an imposter, constant role strains, and the lack of clear role models and mentors to guide and support their efforts in combining professional and personal lives. We shall examine each accordingly.

As professionals and career women, female therapists are indeed called upon to martial their energies in the area of assertion or instrumentality— that is, to accomplish goals and objectives in the larger world. At the same time, women respond compellingly, by way of biology and social conditioning, to the press for nurturance of others, most typically their children and mates. These two polarities reflect, moreover, the ends of a continuum referred to by various writers as the instrumental–expressive dimension and require the individual who seeks to have both sets of qualities to confront potential areas for conflict and confusion. Not achieved without some measure of internal conflict, the synthesis of instrumentality and expressiveness is nothing less than creative integration of typically defined masculine and feminine attributes existing in all of us. Their integration has also been defined as psychological androgyny, a state whereby stereotypical notions of gender and sex role compartmentalization are surpassed by a synthesis of the best of both gender identities.

In their study of these very aspects in male and female therapists, Jones and Zoppel (1982) found women therapists to be superior in the expressive aspects of therapy. Speculating about this trend, Gibbs (22) opts for the presence of androgyny in therapists, such that both male and female therapists will possess balanced proportions of instrumentality and expressiveness and integrate them for the sake of the work of therapy. She points out, however, that the pressure toward instrumentality involves some role conflict for women since it also means pressure to move out of the stereotypically feminine role into a masculine one that might be perceived negatively, either as deviance, rejection of femininity, or envy of male instrumentality.

One by-product of moving out of the feminine gender role has been what is described by Clance and Imes (1978) as the "imposter phenomenon" in high-achieving women. Elaborating on this phenomenon for women therapists, Gibbs (1984) notes that the fear of being shown up for the fraud that one is may be due, first of all, to ambiguity about one's effectiveness.

Spontaneous remission rate lies between 43–53% with 20% of patients improving in therapy who otherwise would not have improved.

Secondly, the therapist has little way of determining an individual success rate in comparison to the overall success rate for the profession. Thirdly, even when one manages to feel successful as a therapist it is extremely difficult to pinpoint which of many interventions, interpretations, and aspects of the therapy situation led to the patient's improvement. . . . Cultural attitudes about therapy may affect the therapist's confidence. Expectations from patients range from the hope of the magic cure, which the therapist knows is impossible to fill, to complete distrust and lack of understanding (pp. 23–24).

Our patients' expectations of our competence also work in tandem with our own. In a panel discussion about the analyst's emotional life during work. Tolpin (1974) suggested that the child's view of the "higher, wiser father" as contrasting with his or her view of the mother who cares for bodily and psychological needs persists into adulthood, raising expectations in both patient and analyst for the latter to provide the magical cure. There exists also the ubiquitous tendency of analyzable patients to idealize the needed functions of the analyst-mother-father-teacher-model unique to the analytic situation. Little wonder that the psychic burden on the analyst looms large and contributes to the stress experienced in the work. Other stresses underscored include the impact of life stresses and other intercurrent events, such as the illness or pregnancy of the analyst, which exert undeniably significant impact on the analyst's countertransference.

The conflict imposed on women therapists by role strains has been discussed at great length, though more in popular and feminist writing than in therapy/therapist literature. Though much attention has been paid to the issue of egalitarianism or parity within the marriage, especially in dual-career couples, the experience of most women in such relationships during the past 20 years, since the inception of the feminist movement, has been one of emancipation in some quarters and slow-changing division of labor in other quarters. Child care and domestic superivsion of the home still remain, for example, more clearly the responsibility and turf of the woman than of the man. While fathers are evidencing more involvement in their parenting roles, as a product of both individual and societal change in attitude about fathering, the daily oepration of the home is relegated to the woman. Hence, her assumption of a profession or career has the cumulative effect of adding on another set of responsibilities to the existing one of nurturing her family. She is usually not relieved of that primary burden simply because she has opted for a career or profession. Though written at least 10 years ago, the observations of Johnson and Johnson (1976) note unquestionably that the burden of family development concomitant with high aspirations in women with careers posed obvious dilemmas for the woman rather than for her spouse. Many of the high-achieving women they surveyed reported feelings of deviance in assuming roles other than the traditional gender role, often assuming another role or roles that posed constant, competitive demands and concerns. One result was a persistent sense of diminishment and guilt about the fact that, under the pressure of many disparate roles and obligations, they were inadequate in fulfilling any one particularly well. The disproportionality of male-female interdependency in marital pairs can be partly explained by the role served by the nurturing female figure of childhood. It is the loss of such a mother that stimulates the gender differentiation between the sexes.

> The unconscious and obligatory nature of the primary dependency needs satisfied by women seems strongly related to the profound anxiety connected with the threat of loss of gender identity in both males and females. This intrapsychic reaction is reinforced by ubiquitous social and cultural standards which hold women accountable for fulfilling these primary demands. On the other hand, men ordinarily deny such dependency needs, partly since the awareness tends to stimulate feelings of abject helplessness. Helplessness in men may also be connected to a phobic disidentification with mother, with the consequence that consciousness of succorant and nurturant needs leads to anxiety about loss of male gender identification. (Johnson & Johnson, 1976, p. 33)

A more personal account of the realities of contending with a career as a therapist simultaneously with being a wife and mother can be found in Davis (1984). In analyzing the complexities of manging her own role proliferation, the author clearly proposes four criteria that facilitate the ease of merging them. These are (1) the woman's ability to merge her need to be assertive and nurturing, (2) the acceptance of the priority of the husband-wife relationship, (3) consideration of the age and stage of the family, and (4) the man's acceptance of his paternalistic role and domestic assistance outside of the immediate family network. She observes that women with tripartite identity have needs for nurturance and support, especially given the emotional drain that our work is on our lives. Our needs for communication, comfort, and loving support can be met more by our spouses than anyone else to allow us to reenter our professional relationships feeling replenished. When our own needs for empathy are met at home we are better protected against inadvertently reaching toward our patients to satisfy our personal longings for intimacy and contact.

Though somewhat less complicated for the single therapist in practice, the problem of isolation and loneliness comes into sharper focus for her. To be sure, her life is less filled with role proliferation than is that of the married therapist with children. On the other hand, however, she is likely to have to confront managing the burden of maintaining home and practice without the benefit of consistent physical or emotional support. As Lerman (1984) has observed, it is frequently the case that single unpaired therapists, busy in their juggling of work and life demands, have little time to provide much emotional support to one another. For those with marriage as an eventual life goal, the prospect of finding a suitable partner diminishes with the passage of time. Time is already a commodity in short supply to those with busy work demands. The search is also complicated by the awareness that accrues by way of training. One judges potential partners, for instance, through the lens of therapeutic knowledge, and is more sensitized to immaturities, personality flaws, and hidden motivations that may or may not exist. There is also the undeniable difficulty of finding a male partner who can and will tolerate a competent woman rather than a seemingly "weaker" one. Even for those who choose not to marry, the eventual toll of living a life where much of the giving is directed toward others rather than toward oneself can be depletion and disillusion. Though not a large risk, there is also a potential hazard of personal safety if one chooses to practice in the home, where the possibility of having patients intrude unpredictably always exists. The latter alternative also complicates one's life by the physical lack of separation of work and living space, creating possible complications for both therapist and patient.

The lesbian therapist must ever keep in mind the issue of her sexual orientation in her professional and personal lives. Whether or not she chooses to deal openly with her sexual orientation can render more complex the entire treatment process, especially since the issue of homophobia is likely to pervade many aspects of the therapeutic relationship. Gartrell (1984) emphasizes the therapist's need to deal with revealing her own sexual orientation and any existing homophobia since it will undoubtedly surface in some fashion to affect the therapeutic work. Additionally, given its relatively small population, the therapist's participation in any lesbian community will most likely render her more exposed to the scrutiny and possible criticism of its members.

Lastly, female therapists in general are likely to be affected by the dearth of female mentors and role models to advise and guide their efforts in the practice of therapy and in weaving it into the fabric of their lives as women. Until the recent developments in feminism and the influx of women into the mainstream of professions and careers, women have had mostly traditional role models in their mothers and grandmothers. Even those mothers who worked were most closely identified with or regarded as primary their roles as wives and mothers. Working outside the home was in all likelihood a necessity rather than an alternative embraced for the woman's enhancement. The presence of professional role models who helped to steer fledgling women therapists in their careers was unlikely. The number of women analysts and therapists, though not disproportionately small when compared with that of their male colleagues, has been nonetheless far too few for the number of women now entering the field. The few women who have achieved professionally are often too burdened or invested in maintaining their hard-won status to interest themselves in serving as models for younger women colleagues. As Goldstein (1963) has pointed out, men in psychology take for granted their same-sex mentors and facilitative effect; women cannot do this, however, and must exert heroic and somewhat isolated efforts to achieve their goals. Until more women enter the field and devote themselves to the process of mentoring others, many will continue to experience the isolating and lonely effects of the paucity of professional role models.

CONCLUDING REMARKS

This chapter has attempted to address the more prevalent themes and concerns of female therapists in both their professional and personal lives and complicating factors that impede the harmonious integration of the two. Among the issues of discussion, those related to transference and countertransference are the most challenging. In the personal sphere, dealing with role conflicts, feeling like an "imposter" and feeling the associated inadequacy, and struggling without the benefit of a mentor are some of the more pertinent issues. Perhaps new directions need to be taken, both theoretically and practically, to improve the quality of life of female therapists in particular.

In the first place, there exists a compelling need for a revised theory of female development, a hope advocated by Freud as he witnessed the proliferation of female analysts working with female patients. Though this trend has not taken hold aggressively in either analytic therorizing or research diretions, some headway can be noted in the writings of Chasseguet-Smirgel (1970) and Gilligan (1982). Simply put, these authors are foremost proponents of the ways in which feminine sexual identity is formed in relation to significant object relations rather than to the fulfillment of drives or their derivatives. Rather than the phallocentric model of development, much criticized in feminist thinking and writing today, the model of female identity development proceeds along different, more complex paths precisely because of its emphasis on the relational context. While many differences exist between the sexes in the socialization process, they should not preclude a finer examination and analysis of the various ways in which present theories of development subtly or insidiously relegate the differences to biological, sociological, or psychological differences that defy alteration or change. At this point, acknowledging the insidious, subtle effects of sexism as it affects all areas of psychological development and its effects on psychotherapy seems an important first step toward fuller examination and eventual change. As Clamar (1980) notes, women therapists must remain flexible and open to all possible life styles and options for their patients, no matter their sex or sexual orientation. Such an attitude will assist in fighting the gender role stereotypes that have pervaded the traditional theories of feminine personality development. In other words, women therapists should maintain the standards expected of all good therapists: to assist their patients to grow in the fullest and most authentic way possible.

As for practical concerns of women psychotherapists, it has already been noted that many of these relate to the profound changes brought about by the impressive increase in the number of women moving into the professional world. Whether or not women therapists eschew their traditional feminine role of nurturing their families, the conflicts seem inevitable in view of the recency of these changes, thereby rendering still fresh for the present generation the effects of a traditionally feminine background. In this context women therapists need to reconsider the impact of their own rearing, especially if it was traditional in nature, and the demands it now makes on their roles as professional women. This would hold especially true for women attempting to fulfill dual or even tripartite roles. Recognition of the demands of each may make more manageable the task of setting clear priorities in fulfilling each role successfully. Women therapists are herein cautioned about the high cost of being "superwomen" whose field and professional roles are known for their demanding emotional nature and intensity. It is often difficult to bridge the gap to share the burden of the intensity with another in an effort to enlist emotional support, even when that person is a supportive significant other. For the single or unpaired woman therapist, the task of finding consistent emotional support is even more difficult and requires more effort. Perhaps, as Lerman (1984) has suggested, such a therapist would need to take special care of her physical and emotional well-being, though this need not always be through other people. Possible avenues for women therapists to provide more nourishment and replenishment for themeslves are peer supervision, support groups, and professional networks wherein the demands of professional and personal lives can be aired and addressed. Directing one's energy to interests completely separate from psychology and psychotherapy, as well as giving oneself private time, may provide added relief from the pressures and possible exhaustion of the work. For many women who nurture others, giving oneself some time seems indeed a luxury. Sharing one's ideas with supervisees or working with women's groups may also provide avenues for mentoring of younger colleagues, thereby providing for them needed role models, which were more scarce after the first generation of feminist thrust for wider career choices for women. In so doing women therapists may also provide for the continuity of theory building in female development and in enlarging more emphatically the scope, challenge, and benefits of a career as a woman therapist.

REFERENCES

Aaron, R. (1974). The analyst's emotional life during work. Scientific proceedings panel reports. *Journal of the American Psychoanalytic Association, 22*(4), 160–169.

Balsam, R.M. (1974). Women therapists and women patients. In *Becoming a Psychotherapist. R.M. Balsam & A. Balsom (Eds.), Chicago: University of Chicago Press.*

Bernardez-Bonesatti, T. (1978). Women and anger: Conflicts with aggression in contemporary women. *Journal of the Medical Women's Association, 33*(5), 215–219.

Bernay, T. (1983). Making a practice: Overcoming passivity and masochism. *Psychotherapy in Private Practice, 1*(1), 25–29.

Brodsky, A. & Holroyd, J. (1981). Report of the task force on sex-bias and sex-role stereotyping in psychotherapeutic practice. In *Women and Mental Health.* E. Howell & M. Bayes (Eds.), New York: Basic Books.

Burton, A. (1975). Therapist satisfaction. *American Journal of Psychoanalysis, 35,* 115–122.

Chasseguet-Smirgel, J. (1970). Feminine guilt and the Oedipus complex. In *Female sexuality: New psychoanalytic views.* J. Chasseguet-Smirgel (Ed.), Ann Arbor: University of Michigan Press.

Clamar, A. (1980). The "empty couch" syndrome. *American Journal of Psychoanalysis 40,* 313–317.

Clance, P.R., & Imes, S. (1978). The imposter phenomenon in high achieving women: Dynamics and therapeutic intervention. *Psychotherapy: Theory, Research and Practice, 15,* 241–247.

Coche, J. (1984). Psychotherapy with women therapists. In *Psychotherapy with psychotherapists.* F.W. Kaslow (Ed.), New York: Haworth Press.

Davis, B. (1984). Wife, mother, therapist…Which comes first? *Psychotherapy in Private Practice, 2*(4), 17–24.

Eisenbud, R.J. (1986). Women feminist patients and a feminist woman analyst. In *The psychology of today's woman.* T. Bernay & D.W. Cantor (Eds.), Hillsdale, NJ: The Analytic Press.

Freudenberger, H.J. (1983). The hazards of psychotherapeutic practice. *Psychotherapy in Private Practice, 1,* 83–89.

Freudenberger, H.J., & Robbins, A. (1979). The hazards of being a psychoanalyst. *The Psychoanalytic Review, 66*(2), 275–296.

Gartrell, N. (1984). Issues in the psychotherapy of lesbians. In *The gender gap in psychotherapy.* P.P. Rieker & E. Carmen (Eds.), New York: Plenum Press.

Gibbs, M.S. The therapist as imposter (1984). In C.M. Brody (Ed.), *Women therapists working with women: New theory and process of feminist therapy.* New York: Springer Publishing Company.

Gilligan, C. (1982). *In a different voice.* Cambridge: Harvard University Press.

Goldstein, E. (1963). Effect of same and cross-sex models on the subsequent academic productivity of scholars. *American Psychologist, 34,* 407–410.

Hare-Mustin, R.J. (1978). A feminist approach to family therapy. *Family Processes, 17,* 181-194.

Jones, E., & Zoppel, C. (1982). Client and therapist gender in psychotherapy. *Journal of Consulting and Clinical Psychology, 50,* 257-272.

Johnson, F.A., & Johnson, C.L. (1976). Role strain in high-commitment career women. *Journal of the American Academy of Psychoanalysis, 4*(1), 13-36.

Lerman, H. (1984). The solo heterosexual woman in practice. *Psychotherapy in Private Practice, 2*(4), 3-8.

Lerner, H.E. (1984). Special issues for women in psychotherapy. In *The gender gap in psychotherapy.* P.P. Rieker & E. Carmen (Eds.), New York: Plenum Press.

Malcolm, J. (1982). *Psychoanalysis: The impossible profession.* New York: Random House.

Mogul, K.M. (1982). Overview: The sex of the therapist. *American Journal of Psychiatry, 139*(1), 1-11.

Person, E.S. (1983). Women in therapy: Therapist gender as a variable. *International Review of Psychoanalysis, 10,* 193-204.

Racusin, G.R., Abramowitz, S.I., & Winter, W.D. (1981). Becoming a therapist: Family dynamics and career choice. *Professional Psychology, 12*(2), 271-279.

Symonds, A. (1976). Neurotic dependency in successful women. *Journal of the American Academy of Psychoanalysis, 4*(1), 95-103.

Turkel, A.R. (1976). The imapct of feminism on the practice of a woman analyst. *American Journal of Psychoanalysis, 36,* 119-126.

Welnar, A., Marten, S., Wochnick, E., Davis, M., Fishman, R., & Clayton, P. (1979). Psychiatric disorders among professional women. *Archives of General Psychiatry, 36,* 169-173.

Part
Four

Legal
and
Ethical
Issues

Charles Patrick Ewing, J.D., Ph.D.
Editor

C H A P T E R
54

PROFESSIONAL ETHICS AND THE PSYCHOLOGISTS' CODE OF ETHICS:
An Introduction and Overview for the Private Practitioner

Leonard J. Haas, Ph.D.

T his chapter presents a basic discussion of professional ethics theory, current ethical concerns in the area of mental health practice, and related legal issues relevant to the private practitioner. While space prevents a full treatment of each of these issues, I hope that by identifying the major standards of ethical practice and examining some of the ethical dilemmas facing today's practitioners, I will encourage readers to search for additional information and generate new ideas for ethical practice.

The chapter uses as its foundation the *Ethical Principles of Psychologists* (American Psychological Association, 1981). Although each of the mental health professions has developed a code of ethics specifically related to its goals and population, the APA code is viewed as a foundational work because it is the one most followed by psychologically trained professionals, and because it addresses essential issues that *every* mental health professional must face. As I point out elsewhere (Haas & Malouf, 1989), there are enormous similarities between the various codes of ethics; the reader is encouraged to compare the various codes if interested.

The chapter presents summaries of the guidelines to be found in the *Ethical Principles*. After each major section, problematic situations are presented to illustrate particular standards (or the violation of those standards). These examples are for the most part rather clear-cut ethical violations, although I leave it to the reader to determine what, if any, actions on the part of the practitioner would have prevented or remedied the problem. Almost all of the examples are from "real life", of course suitably disguised to prevent identification of particular individuals. The incidents have been provided by graduate students in my professional ethics courses, participants n professional ethics workshops I have offered to practitioners, members of groups to whom I have presented papers at professional meetings, and by respondents to surveys my colleagues and I have conducted (e.g. Haas, Malouf, & Mayerson, 1988).

The examples are followed by brief indications of legal principles related to the ethical standards discussed in each section. It should be emphasized at this point that the legal aspects of practice are evolving at least as rapidly as the ethical dimensions, and the conscientious practitioner is well-advised to obtain current legal information. In part, the legal portions of this chapter are not presented in depth because legislatures, courts and licensing boards in each state differ in the nature and degree of regulation they impose on psychologists and other practitioners.

Following each of the sections focused on legal principles is a discussion entitled "Current Controversies." In these I have tried to pick out issues that seem to present current difficulties to many practitioners, and ones that can often be resolved *before* they turn into ethical problems. The reader is encouraged to consider his or her response to the issues, and perhaps to use the controversy as the focus for a discussion with colleagues. The consultative approach is one that helps to put a large number of apparently insoluble ethical dilemmas into perspective rather quickly. Even in areas where standards are rather straightforward, honest and open discussions with colleagues can help enormously in clarifying ways to practice ethically that also are practical and clinically effective.

ETHICAL THEORY

Overview of Ethical Theory

This section provides an introduction to ethical theory and moral philosophy. It is obviously not a substitute for a detailed analysis of the issues and concepts of moral philosophy, the study of which has occupied countless scholars over centuries; it is, rather, an attempt to provide the psychologist with the rudimentary concepts that are likely to be useful in further analysis of problems in professional ethics, and to give a general overview of the domain in which professional ethics lies.

One of the major facets of the philosophy of ethics about which the chapter does *not* go into detail is its history. A good introductory text on ethics such as that by Frankena by (1970) will provide sufficient information to allow the psychologist some grasp of the general currents of moral philosphy, but a very brief overview of historical trends may prove useful here.

Briefly, major themes in ethical philosophizing initially involved the development of schemes for moral justification of action. Many of these schemes are still used as the foundations of modern ethical frameworks. Twentieth-century ethical theory focused on the analysis of linguistic elements in moral reasoning, largely consisting of the attempt to demonstrate that many moral dilemmas were actually just linguistic mistakes or confusion. Most recently (e.g., within the past 20 years), "applied ethics" has become popular. This branch of moral philosophy attempts to apply ethical principles to real-world problems. Professional ethics as a subspecialty of ethics can be considered within the applied tradition. Surprising as it may seem to the professional, until fairly recently philosophers of ethics had little interest in the kind of decision-making problems typically emphasized in practice. Professional ethics, as we conceptualize it for the purposes of applied decision making, is a branch of ethical theory best located within normative applied ethics. A discussion of this follows.

What Is Ethics?

One useful method for distinguishing ethics from other major standards for determining whether an action is right, good, or proper is to contrast it with those frameworks. Law (especially criminal law) and etiquette can be thought of as domains similar to ethics, since each focuses on aspects of proper or good behavior and each specifies penalties for deviation.

Although each set of standards is in some respects the consensus of the society or culture that promotes it, moral frameworks are (or should be) developed largely thorugh rational processes; legal standards, on the other hand, are primarily developed through political processes, while norms of etiquette are developed for the most part by historical precedent.

Ethical standards, in theory at least, focus on behavior and on motivations that aim at the highest ideals of human behavior. Criminal law, in contrast, focuses primarily on behavior that may harm other members of society, and etiquette focuses on behavior that establishes one's standing within a subgroup.

Actions that violate moral or ethical standards can result in censure, guilt, or social criticism. Illegal behavior, on the other hand, results in actual punishment, at least in theory; impolite behavior results in social ostracism, or perhaps mild social criticism.

In the view of many moral philosophers, ethics is distinguished by three main features: (1) it is based on *principles*; (2) the principles are *universalizable*; and (3) proper behavior may be deduced from the principles by *reasoning*. Thus, ethics proper should involve adherence to a consistent set of principles assumed to be relevant for all actors in similar situations, which result (deductively) in obligations to take particular actions.

Two relevant facts follow from this. First, professional ethics in psychology is not pure ethics, but rather a combination of ethics, law, and etiquette; and second, no existing ethical theory (especially no theory of professional ethics) meets the standard set forth above. Thus, we are dealing with an ever evolving topic.

Types of Ethical Theory

Moral philosophy can be subdivided into three major areas: descriptive ethics, meta-ethics, and normative ethics. The emphasis of most ethics issues in psychology will be in the third area.

Descriptive ethics is most closely related to anthropology, and is at present not a prominent subfield within the discipline. Its emphasis is empirical. What types of behavior are considered right and wrong, and by whom? Meta-ethics is most closely related to what was described as moral philosophy above. Its focus is conceptual: Why is a particular action considered ethical? What do we mean by the term "ethical"? Normative ethics focuses on prescriptions for action in particular circumstances and attempts to resolve dilemmas: What is the ethical course of action in *this* situation?

Ethical Justification

Meta-ethics can also be considered the study of justifications for calling particular actions ethical or unethical. At the risk of vastly oversimplifying, the theories of meta-ethics can be characterized as adopting one of two basic positions: (1) the justification for considering an action ethical rests on the nature of the act itself, or (2) the justification for considering an action ethical rests on the consequences produced by the act. The first position is known as deontological justification or deontology and the second as teleological justification or teleology.

Deontology Immanuel Kant is often cited as the paradigmatic deontolgist. Deontological theory is well characterzied by Kant's famous epigram, "Let justice be done though the heavens fall" (Kant, 1949). The appeal of deontological approaches is that they are internally consistent; once a characteristic of an act has been identified, the determination of its ethical value unequivocally follows. Criticisms of deontology are of two major types: (1) if more than one characteristic is considered to mark an act as ethical and two contrary courses of action each has one of those characteristics, an unresolvable dilemma results, and (2) deontology seems to make it too easy for an intuitively immoral action (e.g., one that demonstrably harms someone) to be justified as ethical.

Classical examples of these problems are as follows:

1. A youth considers stealing medicine needed to save his severely ill but impoverished mother; since it is unethical to steal, he decides against it and allows the mother to die.

2. A hospital administrator in Nazi Germany is asked by the Gestapo whether the hospital has any Jewish patients. Since it is unethical to lie, he tells the truth.

Examples that stem more directly from psychological practices include:

1. A psychologist is asked to evaluate the "parental fitness" of a father suspected of child abuse and pedophilia. When the father asks if the testing is voluntary (which it is), the psychologist answers truthfully. The man thereupon refuses further testing.

2. A subject in a social psychological experiment provides test results that indicate thought disorder. Since it is ethical to be honest, the psychologist informs her of the results.

Teleology Utilitarianism (Bentham, 1823; Mill, 1863) is the best-known teleological approach. A well-known epigram that well characterizes the approach is Mill's "the greatest good for the greatest number." Western culture and American society, in particular, are strongly utilitarian. The appeal of the approach is that acts are judged by their outcomes. The major criticisms of the approach are of two types: (1) the ends can too easily justify the means, and (2) the calculation of benefits (or of costs) can be subjective and can change depending on who does the calculating.

A classic example used to criticize teleological approaches is that of the dropping of the atomic bomb on Hiroshima. Its use was justified by the argument that ending the war quickly would ultimately save a great many more lives, both American and Japanese, than would be lost in the bombing.

Examples more closely related to psychology that illustrate means-ends problems are:

1. In order to "shake up the defenses" of a patient whom he considers resistant, the psychologist tells the patient that his wife is having an affair with a close friend as a result of the patient's persistent alcohol abuse. To the best

of the psychologist's knowledge, this is a lie.

2. The psychologist receives a call from an unidentified male who asks for treatment for his incestuous behavior, but indicates that he will refuse to enter treatment if the psychologist abides by the state's mandatory child sexual abuse reporting statute. After discussing the case with the caller, the psychologist agrees not to abide by the law if the man will agree to a minimum of six months of therapy.

Mixed Teleological-Deontological Systems   In practice, most individuals use some admixture of teleological and deontological frameworks. Since there are good arguments for (and against) each theory of ethical justification, it is useful to understand the difference between them, and to describe the major criticisms of each. A useful outline of a mixed system specifically applied to problems of professional ethics may be found in Beauchamp, Walters, and Childress (1978). They advocate a combination of the principles of *justice, autonomy,* and *non-malificence.* Detailed discussion of the benefits of this approach is beyond the scope of the present chapter, but the issues are better considered in the work by Haas & Malouf (1989) as well as by Beauchamp et al.

Ethical Rules

Regardless of the justification system used, any moral framework does eventually arrive at a set of prescriptions or proscriptions. Though these may vary in specificity, they generally fall into one of two types of moral rules. The two sorts of ethical rules or obligations are known as mandatory and aspirational (Gerts, 1981).

Mandatory Ethical Obligations

Mandatory obligations establish the "floor" or minimal criteria for ethical behavior. They can typically be identified by their proscriptive elements; that is they indicate what behavior is to be avoided. The *Ethical Principles of Psychologists* (APA, 1981), contains a number of mandatory obligations or mandatory principles, such as: testimonials from clients are unethical, sexual intimacies with clients are unethical, and fee-splitting is unethical. Three features of mandatory or "thou shalt not" rules are useful to point out: (1) Upholding them is minimally ethical, and no particular praise is due the psychologist who does uphold them. (2) Violating the mandatory obligations does involve censure or liability of punishment. (3) Confusing mandatory ethics with aspirational ethics (e.g., aspiring to the minimal level of ethical behavior) results in a very low standard of professional conduct.

Aspirational Ethical Obligations

In contrast to mandatory obligations, aspirational ethics constitutes the "ceiling" of ethical conduct. Aspirational ethics denotes the ideals to which the ethical person aspires. The *Ethical Principles of Psychologists* contains a number of aspirational obligations as well as mandatory obligations. For example, "in providing services psychologists maintain the highest standards of their profession"; psychologists work to actively and objectively inform the public to help them make choices in their best interest; and psychologists make efforts to avoid relationships that could impair their professional judgment. There are three important features of aspirational, or "thou shalt" obligations: (1) It is difficult clearly to establish violations of aspirational obligations, although not impossible: thus, it is rare for censure to be applied to a psychologist who "violates" them. (2) Psychologists who are especially skillful at achieving aspirational objectives (although they are never completely achieved) are frequently commended. (3) Confusing aspirational with mandatory obligations — that is, assuming the minimal requirements for ethically appropriate conduct involve achieving the highest ideals of the profession — can lead to paralysis and pervasive feelings of inadequacy.

Current Controversies in Professional Ethics

In this section, I briefly note several issues that are of current concern in professional ethics, although there are no universally accepted resolutions to them.

Professional Versus Ordinary Morality   The question at hand in this controversy is whether or not professionals are bound by a different set of moral obligations than are ordinary citizens. An example that might highlight this conflict is the psychologist who decides that a chronically depressed patient is "bringing him down" and notifies the patient that the psychologist's services are no longer available. Note that this puts at issue the private individual's freedom of choice versus the professional's obligation not to abandon his or her client.

Another example involves the psychologist who is routinely late to appointments with clients. Her response to clients who express concern about this is that "everybody makes mistakes." At issue in this case is the qustion of whether a psychologist is "allowed" to make the kind of mistakes that the private individual can make or whether the professional has additional obligations to persons who are clients.

Moral Reasoning Versus Moral Behavior   Recent research in the area of moral development has questioned the relationship of moral action to moral reasoning (Blasi, 1980). The issue is of central concern to those who teach professional ethics since the underlying assumption of such courses is that instruction in moral reasoning will lead to more ethical behavior. Beyond this, however, the issue should be of concern to practitioners since the link between what one does and how one justifies it immediately calls up the question of ethical justification (cf. deontology and teleology).

Cases that illustrate such problems are as follows:

1. A psychologist agrees to provide organizational consultation to a paramilitary white-supremacy organization. When it is pointed out that his presence in the organization may legitimize it, he replies that he will attempt to reform the group from within. This type of case can illustrate the line between sophisticated moral reasoning and self-serving rationalization. A question that may be usefully discussed is whether the psychologist's reasoning or his actions are morally questionable.

2. A psychologist who is a devout member of a religious sect routinely informs church authorities about the nature of clients' problems if the clients belong to the group. The clients are not informed of this practice; the psychologist justifies the practice by claiming that it is in the clients' best spiritual interests. Although this example does cut across the reasoning versus behavior controversy into the professional versus ordinary morality controversy, it does highlight the issue of whether a psychologist may justify behavior that would be considered professionally unethical by appeal to a "higher code."

3. A psychologist falsifies research data when testifying about the funding for a new child-abuse-prevention center. The psychologist justifies this behavior by claiming that the benefits of building such a center outweigh the problems potentially emerging if the data falsification is discovered. This case also highlights the difference between moral justification and rationalization.

4. A psychologist faithfully upholds each of the proscriptions in the *Ethical Principles of Psychologists*. When asked how she manages to do this, she replies, "I'm so afraid of being caught and having my license revoked that I monitor myself scrupulously." This case highlights the issue of moral reasoning as a justification for moral behavior and raises the question of whether there are "better" or "worse" reasons for behaving ethically.

Cost-Benefit Analysis   One of the most popular tools for resolving (utilitarian) ethical dilemmas is cost-benefit analysis. There are three questions that center on cost-benefit analysis: (1) Who calculates the cost and who calculates the benefits? (2) Over what period of time are the costs and benefits calculated? (3) Do the costs and benefits fall on different target groups and is this distribution equitable?

Religion, Ethics, Science, and the Identification of Proper Conduct   This controversy actually consists of two related questions: the relationship of scientific to nonscientific methods of establishing proper conduct, and within the realm of ethics, the role of religious versus nonreligious frameworks for establishing proper action. The first centers on the issues of whether science or scientifically based professional activity is value-laden or value-free. This controversy will no doubt be familiar to most readers in its form of criticisms of therapist-directed behavior change or the values underlying psychological diagnosis.

The second controversy involves the role of religious values and centers on the place of religiously motivated standards or religiously derived standards in ethical theory. Although there is some disagreement about this point, most religiously derived frameworks are considered subcategories of deontological ethics. That is, it is the nature of the behavior (e.g., commanded by God) that determines whether or not it is ethical.

ETHICAL PRINCIPLES APPLICABLE
TO ALL PSYCHOLOGISTS

Regardless of the specific roles in which they function, psychologists are bound to a set of general ethical obligations codified in the *Ethical Principles of Psychologists* that together constitute the highest ideals of the profession as a whole. This section notes each of those general ethical obligations and describes them in broad terms. Each is applicable to the specialized functions described in later sections.

Reduced to one principle, the highest ideal of the profession of psychology is the promotion of human welfare. In the pursuit of this ideal, psychologists take on themselves the general obligations to be responsible, competent, honest, respectful of colleagues, cooperative with duly constituted committees of their professional association, and aware of community, moral, and legal standards.

The obligation of psychologists to be responsible implies accountablity and autonomy. That is, as psychologists, they are considered to be free to choose and to accept responsibility for their choices and the consequences of those choices. In particular, when psychologists are functioning in an institutional context, they are accountable for the use to which their services and products are put. Given the primary priniciple noted above, this further implies that psychologists accept the responsibility to attempt to correct practices that diminish human welfare. That is, they do not condone illegal, discriminatory, deceptive, or injurious practices.

Since psychology claims for itself the status of an independent profession not subject to the supervision of any other profession, psychologists themselves bear the burden of maintaining and monitoring their own competence. Psychologists only provide services or operate as psychologists within the boundaries of that competence. Within such domains, psychologists recognize the need for continuing education and maintain awareness of developments in their fields. Maintaining competence also implies obligations to recognize when one is *not* capable of delivering effective service and taking steps to become more effective, whether this involves seeking personal assistance, developing greater awareness of differences among people, or changing customary procedures.

Psychologists, as members of a scientific discipline, also take on themselves the obligation to be accurate and honest in making public statements. This honesty includes the presentation of personal qualifications and characteristics; the obligation to correct others who misrepresent one's services, qualifications, and so forth; and the avoidance of situations or manipulations that might compromise the fair and accurate presentation of information.

Psychologists have an obligation to be respectful of colleagues. In part, this implies that they do not act in ways that make professional activities for other psychologists more difficult. Consideration of colleagues does not, however, include condoning their inappropriate behavior; the psychologist has an obligation to bring ethical violations to the attention of colleagues if it seems appropriate, or to bring more serious cases to the attention of appropriate ethics committees. With regard to non-psychologist colleagues, psychologists respect the prerogratives and special training of associated professions.

Finally, psychologists incur an obligation to be aware of prevailing community standards and an obligation to conform to those standards if violating them would compromise their own or their colleagues' ability to function professionally. In part, this obligation refers to the standards imposed on psychologists by the various legislative bodies that have jurisdiction over their activities; in part, it refers to general community standards. With regard to either set of standards, if they are discriminatory or injurious, psychologists are obliged not to conform to them and not to condone them.

Examples that illustrate clearcut violations of ethical principles.

1. A psychologist's research assistant coerces research participants to submit to a harmful aversive stimulus. The psychologist excuses herself from responsibility, since the research assistant made this decision on his own. (Problem of denying responsibility)

2. A psychologist trained in psychodynamic psychotherapy is a guest on a radio call-in talk show and a caller describes continual problems with headaches. The psychologist assures him that the headaches are in no way physically based but rather are related to suppressed hostility. (Incompetent service)

3. A psychologist prescribes psychedelic drugs for his patients in group psychotherapy. (Violating law; incompetent service)

4. A psychologist treating a depressed housewife suggests forcefully that she adjust herself to her role and "count her blessings." (Imposing values on client)

5. A psychologist in solo independent practice describes himself in advertisements as "The Personal Growth Institute, Dr. _____, Director," and includes in his advertisements, "testimonials from satisfied customers." (Misleading or fraudulent advertising)

6. Dr. X has turned to the bottle for comfort since his office was vandalized and burned. When it is suggested that he has a drinking problem, he refuses to acknowledge this. (Offering services when incapacitated)

Related Legal Principles

It may be useful to differentiate between legal notions of responsibility and psychological concepts of responsibility. Legal concepts of responsibility imply causation and bear on issues of liability and negligence. Some court cases, especially those having to do with wrongful death and alienation of affection, turn on the notion of legal responsibility for the consequences of one's actions.

The obligation to be competent raises the legal question of usual, customary, and reasonable professional practices. Malpractice law and concepts of professional liability typically involve issues of what is nationally seen as the standard duty to clients or consumers ("feasance") and what is seen as the ordinary and minimally competent fulfillment of this duty in a particular branch of psychology.

The obligation of honesty is related to legal principles of contract law. The psychologist should become familiar with the notions of fraud, false advertising, and breach of contract.

The general obligation to promote human welfare touches on the legal issue of civil rights. Although it may be far afield from many professional ethics issues, the practitioner should have some understanding of the protection granted to him/her, clients, employees, colleagues, through the Civil Rights Act, the Bill of Rights, equal opportunity guidelines, or related statutes.

Current Controversies

1. In moral philosophy, it is sometimes suggested that when more than one actor is involved, "responsibility multiplies, rather than divides." This concept raises many questions in relation to joint activities with other professionals or other psychologists. Psychologists must balance their ethical duties with the need to maintain harmonious working relationships.

2. The concept of competence is elusive. Competence to practice may be considered competence in a given area of knowledge—or, more generally, competence to produce a particular result. As the psychotherapy "marketplace" becomes increasingly competitive, how can psychologists "market" themselves while remaining ethically appropriate?

3. The obligation to attempt to correct ethical or moral violations that one encounters may have repercussions for one's personal well-being. How much personal risk should psychologists take in attempting to "police themselves"?

ETHICAL ISSUES IN SPECIAL CLINICAL FUNCTIONS

This section is intended to highlight ethical issues particular to clinical functions not easily subsumed under the usual individual service paradigm. This paradigm (which in many ways is implicit in many of the ethical principles), is that the consumer of psychological services is (1) an individual adult (2) competent to negotiate a contract to (3) meet personal needs for (4) treatment that is well established and known to be effective, to be (5) provided to that individual. This section focuses on variations from each of the elements of that paradigm.

1. Consumers who are not individuals, but are groups or families.
2. Consumers who are not competent to give informed consent for services (e.g. minors, psychotic or retarded individuals).
3. Consumers who are third parties rather than the target client.
4. Treatments that are not well established.

Multiperson Services: Group and Family Therapies

Ethical Issues.   Two primary issues—distinct from the general obligations to provide ethical clinical services—are important in considering the group and family therapies. These are, first, the special problems with protecting confidentiality and preserving privileged communication in multiperson settings and, second, the fact that these are specialty services that require advanced training to ensure the competence of the provider.

When more than one nontherapist is present for treatment, psychologists must take special care to protect confidentiality since the other nontherapists are not bound by a code of professional ethics. The participants in treatment must be informed of this limitation. In addition, the therapist must be aware that in many states there is no legal privilege existing when more than one person is present, and must take steps to inform the clients of this.

In addition, since group and family treatments are specialized services, therapists must be competent in delivering them. With regard to family therapy, where the issue of coercion may arise (Margolin, 1982), the psychologist has an obligation to inform family members of their right to choose participation in treatment. If family therapists are of the school that requires all family members to be present before treatment can be provided, they should inform the family of this and note that not all therapists enforce this rule.

Examples of Unethical Decisions

1. A child-clinical psychologist with no training in family therapy has been working with a seven-year-old boy. The client begins to talk about arguments that the parents have in his presence, and the psychologist decides to invite the family into the sessions. (Problem of competence)

2. A member of a therapy group discusses the content of previous sessions with her friend. The friend is a co-worker of another member of the group. The group therapist has not discussed issues of confidentiality with the group members. (Problem of protecting confidentiality)

3. A family therapist firmly adheres to the principle that unless all members of the family are present, no family session will be held. A family is referred for concerns about their withdrawn 11-year-old son; the family includes a 16-year-old daughter reluctant to attend, and the therapist does not inform her of her freedom to leave the session. (Problem of denying voluntary participation)

4. A psychologist is subpoena'd to testify about a parent's fitness to retain custody after he has been seeing the couple in marital treatment. The psychologist agrees to testify, even though no discussion of this possibility had taken place with either partner. (Problem of failure to obtain informed consent)

Related Legal Principles   The psychologist should become familiar with emerging case law regarding group therapy. These precedents involve the difficulty in ensuring that members of therapy groups (who are not professionals) are subject to the same obligations to protect confidentiality as is the therapist. In addition, privileged communication is likely inapplicable in group settings. Privileged communication statutes for the state in which the psychologist practices should be reviewed. For family therapists, the above will be useful, as will a review of child-custody statutes.

Current Controversies

1. The question of court testimony about parental-fitness or child-custody decisions when family or marital therapy has been conducted presents many ethical dilemmas. Psychologists should carefully consider how to proceed when requested to testify and should explain their policies clearly to clients at the beginning of therapy.

2. Psychologists who lead groups should consider how best to protect the confidentiality of group members. Haas & Malouf (1989) suggest some options in this regard, particularly involving "contracts" among members.

Consumers with Diminished Competence to Consent

Ethical Principles.   Despite the obligation to provide informed consent, not all persons who consume psychological services are capable of doing so. Specifically, minors, involuntarily committed patients, prisoners, and psychotic and retarded individuals all have diminished capacity. In such cases, psychologists work to uphold the best interests of the client and to avoid violating or diminishing the individual's rights. In cases where competence to consent may make the protection of confidentiality an issue, psychologists should negotiate suitable arrangements with a legal guardian or representative of the individual. However, attempts should be made to clarify the nature of treatment arrangements with clients regardless of whether or not they have the capacity to provide truly informed consent.

Examples of Ethical Problems in Procedure.

1. A 16-year-old girl requests therapy from a private practitioner to discuss aspects of her sexuality. Her parents are very strict in these matters and she does not want them informed. She does not ask and the psychologist does not describe his practices regarding confidentiality. The parents call to inquire about the progress of treatment and the psychologist informs them fully. (Failure to consider how to protect confidentiality)

2. A psychotic patient who has not responded to various conventional treatments, including medications, is a candidate for an aversive conditioning paradigm designed by the ward psychologist. The treatment involves administration of painful shocks, and the psychologist decides to administer the shocks without discussion with the patient, since the patient is incompetent. (Failure to obtain even substituted consent)

3. The warden of the prison in which a psychologist works requests the names of any prisoners who have discussed their involvement in a recent riot. The psychologist provides these names. (Loyalty to employing agency versus loyalty to clients; question of who is the client.)

Related Legal Principles   The psychologist should become familiar with the notion of substituted consent and with relevant case law in the area of informed consent and its management.

The psychologist should also become familiar with legal considerations that may compromise the rights of persons receiving services at the request of third parties. This is an issue of particular concern in schools and in federally supported institutions. Two federal statutes are of relevance here. One is PL 94-142, the Education for All Handicapped Children Act (1975), which guarantees the rights of parents to approve or withhold approval for services proposed for their children. The second, PL 93-380, is the Family Education Rights and Privacy Act (or Buckley Amendment) of 1974, which guarantees parents access to their children's records.

Psychologists working with patients who may have been involuntarily committed should review the federal court cases concerned with patients' rights to both participate in and refuse psychological treatment. In addition, state law regarding emancipated minor status is relevant to the issue of children's ability to provide informed consent. Recent court cases at the federal level have focused on (and generally upheld) the rights of minors to consent to treatment, and psychologists who work with minors should review these findings. Haas & Malouf (1989) and Cohen & Mariano (1982) are useful resources in this area.

Current Controversies

1. Providing too detailed a statement of informed consent can actually reduce prospective patients' motivation for treatment. Psychologists must carefully consider how to balance the arousal of hope with the provision of accurate information.

2. Not only failure to provide informed consent but also providing too detailed a promise of benefit may expose the psychologist to risk. The nature of the information provided, and the form — written or verbal — needs to be carefully considered.

Services Provided at the Request of Third Parties

Ethical Principles The fact that psychologists frequently provide organizational consultation, community interventions, court-ordered psychological services, school psychology services, and other such third-party-requested services makes a focus on the special ethical considerations in these situations important. The general ethical obligations enumerated previously all hold in these circumstances. In addition, the following ethical principles are relevant.

Informed consent of the directly affected individuals is often difficult to obtain in third-party-requested services; nonetheless, psychologists work to provide as much opportunity for it as possible.

If the nature of the service is such that individuals involved in it may not have the opportunity to provide informed consent (organizational development efforts and prevention programs are particularly of relevance here), psychologists have an obligation to protect the interests of such individuals.

Conflicts of interest between the demands of the organization, payor, or third party and the needs of the particular person with whom the psychologist is interacting may arise; in such cases, the psychologist works to inform all "stakeholders" (Mirvis & Seashore, 1979) of the situation and to work toward a resolution.

In organizational and community work, the psychologist has an obligation to be aware of individual differences in client groups.

If the initiators of community or organizational intervention request assessment results, psychologists take responsibility for the consequences of the assessments or diagnoses that are delivered.

If in the course of community or organization work psychologists become aware of practices that diminish the rights of members, they attempt to rectify the situation.

Psychologists also have an obligation to clarify the nature of their services to organizational members who may come in contact with them.

Psychologists are also obliged to ensure that the organizations that employ them will not misuse the results of their work or exploit them or their work.

When providing training to community or organization members, psychologists have an obligation to avoid misleading them into believing that they possess competence in psychological service delivery that they do not possess.

Examples that Illustrate Poor Ethical or Legal Decision Making in Relation to Third Parties.

1. A psychologist is developing a community intervention to prevent drug abuse. It involves interviewing junior high school students about their parents' use of illegal substances. The plan is for paraprofessionals to visit the homes of high-risk parents and discuss alternative stress-reduction methods.

2. An organizational psychologist discovers that several middle-management employees are "burned out." When she proposes to develop a support group for these managers, upper-level executives decide that it would be more cost-effective to replace them, and on the basis of her findings, fires them.

3. An organizational consultant discovers that one of the consultees with whom he is working is severely suicidal. He begins weekly treatment sessions with the person.

4. A community psychologist feels that many of the lower-class black parents with whom she is working in a poverty-reduction program discipline their children too harshly. She refers several of them for investigation of child abuse.

5. An organizational psychologist is hired to conduct stress-reduction workshops in an organization. He discovers routine sexual harassment in the course of his efforts but decides not to do anything about it for fear of being fired.

6. An organizational psychologist is hired to improve the mangement skills of supervisors in a manufacturing plant. Many of them begin to confide in him about marital problems and alcohol abuse. Because a portion of his job involves screening for employees with greater managerial potential, he reports those with more problems as having less potential. He does not inform them of these reports.

7. A psychologist has developed a peer support group for preventing drug abuse among airline employees. A drug-abuse scandal hits the airline, and the psychologist is asked to provide the names of group members to management. She does so.

8. A psychologist has trained several paraprofessional community groups in stress-management techniques for poverty-level mothers. She finds that group members are promoting their services to other community groups (e.g., drug abusers) with the claim that they are "relaxation experts." She does nothing to halt this practice.

9. A school psychologist is assigned a group of high school teachers who have discipline problems in their classrooms. Her job is to help them learn new classroom-management techniques. The psychologist discovers that the teachers have been told that if they refuse to attend the group, they will be reassigned to less-desirable schools. She does nothing about this.

Related Legal Principles   The psychologist who works in organizational consulting or in school contexts should become familiar with case law and statutory law regarding civil rights and informed consent. Here too the work by Cohen & Mariano (1982) on legal issues may be helpful.

Current Controversies

1. Third parties may expect (and may have legal rights to expect) access to data regarding services. Psychologists on the other hand have an obligation to protect confidentiality and should be clear with all parties about such obligations. This raises questions about balancing customary practice in non-professional contexts with ethical obligations.

2. Licensure and credentialing for organizational and community psychologists is hotly debated, since the type of service (and the level of regulation needed to protect consumers) may be quite different from traditional clinical work.

3. Employers increasingly demand that psychologists perform services outside their areas of competence; ethical practitioners face the dilemma of protecting their jobs versus upholding their professional standards.

Innovative Treatments and Services

Ethical Principles   As noted previously, psychologists have a general obligation to provide competent service. In specialty areas where established standards exist, psychologists who wish to deliver such services have an obligation to obtain training or supervision in the new specialty. However, many forms of psychological service involve new or innovative techniques for which clear standards of competence have not as yet been established. Three forms of innovative services are discussed in this section: novel forms of clinical treatment, "media psychology," and computerized testing.

With regard to novel clinical techniques, psychologists should become aware of them as a part of their general obligation to be competent providers of services and use them as needed. Insofar as possible, psychologists attempt to allow the prospective client to give informed consent.

Media psychology, in which psychologists provide personal advice or general opinions about particular problems via electronic or print media, is emerging as a specialty service. Psychologists are obliged to be aware of possible negative impacts on the audience and to exercise careful professional judgment. Psychologists also have a duty to avoid exploiting the needs of callers or writers seeking advice, and must take care not to overstep the boundaries of their competence. Some useful guidelines are presented by Haas & Malouf (1989).

In the area of computerized testing, psychologists are obligated to maintain high standards. The psychologist should become familiar with the emerging standards of practice in computerized services and obtain the American Psychological Association guidelines for the provision of automated testing services (APA, 1986).

Examples That Illustrate Ethical Violations.

1. A group therapist has developed a technique entitled "deprivaton breakthrough," which requires that group members restrain the person who is "it" until he or she becomes emotionally aroused. The technique has not been used elsewhere, and patients report that it is terrifying.

2. A psychologist who has read about "neurolinguistic programming" in a recent journal article begins to employ it with her patients.

3. A psychologist who has had one course in sex therapy during graduate school decides to continue treatment with a female client who has sexual concerns even though the presenting problem was smoking cessation, which is his specialty.

4. A psychologist who is the host of a call-in radio show complies with instructions to limit the time he spends with the "less interesting cases" presented by callers.

5. A psychologist on a radio talk show receives a call from a woman whom he thinks is in treatment with an incompetent therapist. He advises her (on the air) to quit the therapist and read some self-help books.

6. A psychologist develops her own scoring system for the Bender-Gestalt test and markets it as a "repressor screening protocol." Purchasers receive printed paragraphs describing the personality characteristics of the test takers. No validation has been undertaken on the descriptors.

Related Legal Principles   The psychologist should become familiar with case law regarding novel treatments. Examples include state law regulating the use of sexual surrogates (almost always illegal, as a form of pandering) and court cases that establish precedents for providers' liability for damages in the case of untried services. In addition, the psychologist may want to refer such cases as *Hammer v. Rosen* and *Abraham v. Zaslow,* which establish the notion that certain actions (in this case, striking a patient) are in and of themselves evidence of malpractice regardless of professional justifications.

In addition, legal standards for informed consent should be reviewed here.

Current Controversies.

1. Some critics have questioned whether "media psychology" should be conducted at all; does it cause too many problems for the profession? Or is it a way to reach previously underserved populations?

2. Psychologists have been on the forefront of computerized testing, but currently risk loss of control over testing procedures. At issue is the best way to provide testing services without allowing unqualified individuals to offer such services.

3. What constitutes a specialty in psychology? Are the existing specialties clearly distinct from one another? The American Psychological Association has decided to declare a moratorium on recognizing new specialties, although other credentialing bodies (and quasi-credentialing bodies) continue to certify specialists. The practitioner must decide whether, and how, to specialize in areas where additional credentials are offered, and must decide how to best promote the public's understanding of what various "specialists" can do.

REFERENCES

American Psychological Association (1981). *Ethical principles of psychologists.* Washington, D.C.: Author.

American Psychological Association (1986). *Guidelines for computer based tests and interpretations.* Washington, D.C.: Author.

Beauchamp, T.L., & Childress, J.F.(1979).*Principles of biomedical ethics.* New York: Oxford University Press.

Bentham, J. (1863/1948). *An introduction to the principles of morals and legislation.* New York: Hafar Publishing.

Blasi, A. (1980) Moral reasoning and moral action: A critical review. *Psychological Bulletin. 31,* 1–21.

Bloch, S., & Chodoff, P. (1981). *Psychiatric ethics.* New York: Oxford University Press. This edited volume covers a wide variety of topics in its 18 chapters. Of particular relevance to the present discussion are chapters focused on ethics in suicide and involuntary hospitalization. Other chapters that may be of interest focus on drug treatment and psychosurgery.

Cohen, R.J., & Mariano, W.E. (1982). *Legal guidebook in mental health.* New York: Free Press.

Faden, R., Beauchamp, T., & King, N. (1986). *A history and theory of informed consent.* New York: Oxford University Press. This volume covers both legal and ethical theory of informed consent and reviews cases from both research and practice.

Frankena, W.K. (1973). *Ethics.* Englewood Cliffs, NJ: Prentice-Hall.

Haas, L.J., & Malouf, J.L. (1989). *Keeping up the good work: A practitioner's guide to mental health ethics.* Sarasota, FL: Professonal Resource Exchange.

Haas, L.J., Malouf, J.L., & Mayerson, N.H. (1986). Ethical dilemmas in psychological practice: Results of a national survey. *Professional Psychology: Resaerch and Practice, 17,* 316–321.

Kant, I. (1949). *Critique of practical reason and other writings in moral philosophy.* Chicago: University of Chicago Press.

Lowman, R.L. (1985). *Casebook on ethics and standards for the practice of psychology in organizations.* Society for Industrial and Organizational Psychology. Recent compilation of cases that illustrate ethical issues for organizational psychologists and consultants.

Mill, J.S. (1863). *Utilitarianism.*

Monahan, J. (Ed.) 1980). Who is the client? The ethics of psychosocial intervention in the criminal justice system. Washington, DC: American Psychological Association. This edited volume is a product of the APA task force on psychologists in the correctional system; it provides a series of useful papers focused on the roles, difficulties, and ethical obligations of psychologists in such correctional settings as courts, prisons, police agencies, and the juvenile justice system. Included is a set of recommendations from the task force, and an interesting survey regarding ethical dilemmas (mostly focused on confidentiality) that occur to psychologists practicing in such settings.

Public Law 93-380 (1974). *The family educational rights and privacy act* (The Buckley Amendment). United States Code.

Public Law 94-142 (1975). *The education for all handicapped children act.* United States Code.

C H A P T E R
55

THE PROFESSIONAL LIABILITY OF BEHAVIORAL SCIENTISTS: AN OVERVIEW*

Ronald Jay Cohen, Ph.D.

A record amount of malpractice litigation against phsycians during the last decade has sensitized practitioners in all health-related professions to the need for an adequate understanding of the legal framework in which they function. Practitioners in the field of behavioral science, including psychologists, psychiatrists, social workers, psychiatric nurses, occupational therapists, and others have taken cognizance of a foreboding constellation of societal factors that may make them more vulnerable than ever before to the receipt of a summons and complaint alleging malpractice (Bernstein, 1978; Cohen, 1979; Cohen & Mariano, 1982; Stone, 1977; Green & Cox, 1978). Thorough knowledge of a professional specialty is a necessary but no longer sufficient condition for the successful practice of that specialty; a knowledge of the law is essential.

NEGLIGENCE, MALPRACTICE, AND PROFESSIONAL LIABILITY

Stated generally, all adults have a legal duty to conduct themselves in a fashion that at least measures up to the way that any ordinary and reasonable person would behave under the same or similar circumstances. If a person's unintentional behavior falls short of this "ordinary and reasonable person" standard, the behavior is described as "negligent." Negligence is formally defined as "conduct which falls below the standard established by law for the protection of others against unreasonable risk of harm."[1,2] In litigation, the burden of proof is on the plaintiff; the plaintiff must prove by the preponderance of the evidence that the defendant was indeed negligent.[3] The elements of proof required to prove the tort of negligence are (1) duty on the part of the defendant, (2) breach of that duty, (3) causation, and (4) damages.

Members of professions, like the citizenry in general, are also legally bound to behave in ways consistent with the proverbial "ordinary and reasonable person." However, persons acting in their professional capacity are additionally

---

* Reprinted from Cohen, R.J. (1983). *Behavioral Sciences and the Law, 1*(1), 9–22.

held to a higher standard, that of any ordinary and reasonable person in their profession acting under the same or similar circumstances. If the professional's behavior unintentionally falls below this higher standard, the term "malpractice" applies; malpractice refers to negligence in the execution of professional duties. If the professional is a lawyer, one speaks of legal malpractice; a physician, medical malpractice; a psychologist, psychological malpractice; and so forth. The elements required to prove malpractice are the same as those described above for negligence. The place of malpractice within the general schema of the law is illustrated in Figure 1.

An understanding of what malpractice is, is best complemented by a knowledge of what it is not. It is not malpractice if the professional fails to bring an extraordinary amount of skill, knowledge, or expertise to bear on the problem; the professional, as stated by Chief Justice Tindal in the 1832 case of *Lamphier* v. *Phipus,* is not charged by law to be brilliant: "Every person who enters into a learned profession undertakes to bring to it the exercise of a reasonable degree of care and skill; he does not undertake, if he is an attorney, that at all events you shall gain your case, nor does a surgeon undertake that he will perform a cure, nor does he undertake to use the highest possible skill." Jurow and Mariano (1972) have emphasized that professionals are not guarantors of good results:

Table 55-1. Some Intentional and Unintentional Torts

Intentional	Unintentional (Negligence)
Torts to person — Battery — Assault — False imprisonment	Negligence based on duty of due care — Breach of duty of due care (malpractice) including special affirmative duties to prevent harm — Duty to prevent suicide — Duty to prevent assault to third parties
Torts to property — Trespass to land — Trespass to chattels — Conversion of chattels	Other — Negligent misrepresentation — Negligent causing of emotional distress — Negligent invasion of privacy
Other — Intentional or fraudulent misrepresentation (deceit) — Intentional causing of emotional distress — Intentional invasion of privacy — Malicious prosecution — Abuse of the process of law	

> Professionals, including psychologists, physicians, attorneys, engineers, accountants and others, do not guarantee to accomplish a particular result or cure. But once he undertakes treatment of a patient, the psychologist, in the same way as the physician and surgeon, is obligated to conduct his examination and treatment in a skillful, competent and professional manner. The psychologist holds himself out as possessing the skill and knowledge commonly possessed by members in good standing of the psychology profession, and is consequently liable for harm or injury for failure to meet current professional standards. (pp. 224–225)

Technically, it is not malpractice if the act or omission in question was intentional on the part of the professional. As we have noted, malpractice is to the professional what negligence is to the layperson and both imply that the negative effect or outcome was unintentional. Still, the wide range of actions or omissions that professionals could potentially be held liable for is referred to as "malpractice" in common parlance. An illustrative listing of some intentional as well as unintentional torts appears in Table 1.

A psychiatrist, for example, who is instrumental in committing an involuntary patient to a mental institution and who then administers medication to the patient against the patient's will might be sued for "malpractice" on grounds such as assault, battery, false imprisonment, and malicious prosecution. For protection against such claims, insurance companies offer *professional liability* insurance—colloquially but inaccurately referred to as *malpractice* insurance—the former term being all-inclusive with respect to intentional and unintentional acts and omissions.

The Duty Of The Professional

When the elements of proof for malpractice are reviewed it can be seen that it is the plaintiff's burden to prove that the defendant owed a duty of due care. This element is usually, but not always, a straightforward matter of establishing that a professional–client or doctor–patient relationship arose. In *O'Neill* v. *Montefiore Hospital,*[4] for example, a question before the court was whether or not a doctor–patient relationship arose as the result of a telephone conversation. The now-deceased Mr. O'Neill had presented himself with his wife (the plaintiff) at the Montefiore Hospital emergency room complaining of chest pain and asking to see a Hospital Insurance Plan (HIP) doctor. He was told by the nurse that the hospital had no connection with HIP but that she would try to get him an HIP doctor. The nurse telephoned an HIP doctor, and Mr. O'Neill was overhead to say during the course of the conversation, "Well I could be dead by 8 o'clock." What happened next appears in the court record:

> When the deceased concluded the telephone conversation, he informed the nurse that Dr. Craig had told him to go home and come back when HIP was open. Mrs. O'Neill, however, asked the nurse to have a doctor examine her husband since it was an emergency. Disregarding the request, the nurse told her that their family doctor would see Mr. O'Neill at 8 o'clock, to which he again replied, "I could be dead by 8 o'clock."

When examination or treatment at the hospital was refused, the plaintiff and the deceased left and returned home on foot, pausing occasionally to permit him to catch his breath. After they arrived at their apartment, and as the plaintiff was helping her husband to disrobe, he fell to the floor and died before any medical attention could be obtained.

The appellate court in *O'Neill* held that "the jury could have concluded that Dr. Craig undertook to diagnose the ailments of the deceased and could have decided whether he abandoned the patient, inadequately or improperly advised him, or, conversely, made a proper diagnosis fully appropriate under the circumstances, or offered an examination which was rejected." The court therefore reversed the lower court's dismissal of Mrs. O'Neill's complaint and ordered a new trial. Although *O'Neill* is presented here primarily for illustrative purposes, the possibility of a comparable situation arising with respect to the duty of a mental health professional is ever present. That, for example, is the duty of the clinician contacted by telephone by a suicidal or homicidal person wishing to undertake therapy but uncertain about what he or she will do in the next hour or so?

Another question of duty arose in *Rainer* v. *Grossman*,[5] wherein it was alleged that the opinion of a medical school professor expressed at a professional conference made the professor liable for malpractice. The *Rainer* court did not find this to be the case:

> As a teacher of doctors, defendant used as a teaching vehicle cases presentd to him by his pupils. It is conceded that his opinion became part of the total information upon which one of those pupils, Dr. Rainer, drew in giving advice to his patient.
>
> Presumably every professor or instructor in a professional school hopes, expects or foresees that his students will absorb and apply in their own careers at least some of the information he imparts. Does he thereby assume a duty of care and potential liability to those persons who may ultimately become the clinets or patients of those students? We think not.

Another exceptional situation with respect to the professional's duty involves the duty not to the client but to some third party. Physicians as well as other health professionals are required by law to report to the appropriate authorities the diagnosis of certain contagious diseases, ccases of child abuse, and related diagnoses deemed to be in the interest of public health and safety. Additionally, physicians have a duty to warn a patient or responsible family members of the dangers to the family of a contagious disease (*Hoffman* v. *Blackmon*).[6] An extension of this duty to warn endangered third parties to the field of behavioral science appears in the decision by the Supreme Court of California in *Tarasoff* v. *Regents of University of California.*[7] Tatiana Tarasoff died at the hands of Proenjit Poddar.[8] Mr. Poddar had been in therapy with a psychologist employed at the University of California, Berkeley, Counseling Center and had indicated to his therapist his intention to murder an unnamed but readily identifiable person (Tatiana). As a result of the civil suit brought by the parents of the deceased, the Supreme Court of California ruled that psychotherapists have a duty to warn endangered third parties of their peril; in the oft-cited words of the court, "The protective privilege ends where the public peril begins."

Professionals who supervise the psychotherapeutic or psychodiagnostic work of others may themselves be "endangered third parties" with respect to legal jeopardy if substandard supervision leads to a negative result. According to the legal doctrine of *respondeat superior* ("let the master respond"), "masters" (employers, supervisors, corporate entities) can incur vicarious liability for the acts of their "servants." Cohen and Mariano (1982) elaborate:

> Psychologists, psychiatrists, and other mental health professionals who supervise the work of training psychotherapists must be responsive[9] to the needs of the needs of the supervisee and of the patient if they are to avoid liability under the doctrine of *respondeat superior.* In too many training institutions today, psychotherapy supervision is et up on a *pro forma* once-a-week or once-a-month basis. It would seem to the present authors that this standard, upon which the profession has expressed approval by its silence, is too low. If some harm or injury befalls the patient of the student psychotherapist because the supervisor improperly failed to take into account the specific and unique needs of the patient and the supervisee, then it would seem that the doctrine of *respondeat superior* would be applicable. (p. 351)

In addition to exposure to legal jeopardy for improper supervision, mental health professionals must exercise due care in their referrals to fellow practitioners lest they be liable for the malpractice of another; the referral is an act of professional judgment and as such is capable of incurring liability.[10] Professionals who serve on peer review committees are exposed to the possibility of a malpractice lawsuit when a claim is made that they failed to exercise their responsibilities with due care.[11] In his survey of malpractice claims against psychologists, Wright (1981) noted that an "area of substantial exposure to claims of malpractice is service in the governance of psychological organizations and structures, particularly as an ethics committee member, a member of a licensing board, and so on" (p. 1,492).

Breach Of Duty

The yardstick used by the court to determine if a legal duty was in fact breached is referred to as the *standard of care.* The court will under most circumstances look to the standards of the profession and examine how the ordinary and prudent practitioner of the profession would have acted under the same or similar circumstances in order to define the applicable standards. Exceptions to this general rule occur when the applicable standard is defined by statute and when the court deems the profession's standard to be too low (as in *Tarasoff*[12] and in *Helling* v. *Carey*).[13] "Ordinarily, a doctor's failure to possess or exercise the requisite learning or skill can be established only by the testimony of experts" (*Lawless* v. *Calaway*).[14] An exception to this rule is the instance where the court invokes the doctrine of *res ipsa loquitur* ("the act speaks for itself"), which holds that the mere fact that injury occurred under a particular set of circumstances bespeaks negligence. This doctrine was invoked in *Rodriguez* v. *State,*[15] a case involving injury of a 5-year-old, profoundly retarded resident of a state mental hospital. Another instance that obviates the need for expert testimony is where, in the opinion of the court, a jury is qualified to determine if malpractice occurred. This *doctrine of common knowledge* was invoked by the court in *Steinke* v. *Bell,*[16] a case in which a dentist extracted the wrong tooth: "We think laymen, looking at this case in the light of their common knowledge and experience, can say that a dentist engaged to remove a lower left second molar is not acting with the care and skill normal to the average member of the profession if, in so doing, he extracts or causes to come out an upper right laterial incisor." In *res ipsa loquitur* cases, the plaintiff is only required to prove injury and not a particular standard of care or a specific act or omission. In cases in which the doctrine of common knowledge is invoked, the plaintiff has already proved damage and an act or omission by the defendant and the effect of the invocation of the doctrine is to let the jury decide what the applicable standard is.

Defining the applicable standard of care in the mental health profession tends not to be as straightforward a task as it is with respect to other professions. Stated succinctly, the problem is that if you ask two psychotherapists — even two psychotherapists who subscribe to the same school of psychotherapy — about their opinion on a particular course of treatment, you are likely to get two (or more) different opinions. In treating phobias, for example, one behavior therapist might have a predilection for systematic desensitization while another might believe that implosion is the treatment of choice. Needless to say the variance of opinion increases exponentially if expert psychotherapists from other schools of therapy are consulted. The law prefers no one form of treatment over another, and it will usually measure a practitioner's professional behavior by the standards of his or her own school of treatment,[17] provided that that form of treatment is supported by at least a "respectable minority" of the members of the profession. Harris (1973) has noted that such minorities are legion in the field of psychotherapy and that the courts have in some cases "shifted the burden to the doctor to justify the use of unorthodox methods" (p. 419).

Persons who hold themselves out to the public as specialists in some professional area will be held to a higher standard of care — that of the specialist — than the presumably less-trained nonspecialist. This is so even if the professional in question has falsely represented herself or himself as a specialist.[18] Nonprofessional psychotherapists cannot, technically speaking, be sued for malpractice as that cause of action is reserved for licensed members of a recognized profession:

> Those persons who are either licensed or members of professions sanctioned by the state must follow the standards of care of their professions or they may be subject to either liability for negligence, or loss of license, or criminal penalties. Those people who practice outside the law are either quacks or non-professionals not yet under the state's statutory umbrella. Since no standards are established for their reputed professions, someone injured by their "care" will have to rely on tort theories other than malpractice. (Harris, 1973, pp. 408–409)

Although the quack[19] cannot technically be sued for malpractice, he or she will be held to the same standard of care that the properly credentialed professional being (mis)represented would be held to.[20] Sometimes the court, on tghe basis of the fact situation before it, will elect not to hold the defendant to the standard of a mental health professional despite the fact that the defendant's work closely resembled or was in many respects indistinguishable from the work of a psychiatrist, psychologist, social worker, or other licensed mental health professional.[21]

Causation And Damages

Causation in the legal sense is a relatively complicated concept that encompasses factors such as the foreseeability of the outcome and the effects of intervening variables. Damage is defined as "loss, injury, or deterioration, caused by the negligence, design, or accident of one person to another, in respect of the latter's person or property" (Black, 1968, p. 446). In its plural form, damages additionally refers to monetary compensation for a loss. *Compensatory* damages are awarded by a court to compensate a successful plaintiff for her or his loss. *Punitive* damages are awarded by a court to the plaintiff to punish a defendant for the recklessness, wantonness, or heinousness of his or her actions or omissions. As Rothblatt and Leroy (1973) note, proving the elements of causation and damage in a malpractice proceeding involving a mental health professional is no easy task.

> Besides proving that the psychiatrist has breached the requisite standard of care in some specific detail, the plaintiff must also demonstrate causation and damage. Because the natural pathological development and prognosis of mental disease is not well known, it is frequently difficult to state to a reasonable degree of medical certainty whether the application or omission of a particular procedure at a specified time caused mental injury to the patient. Thus it is often difficult for the plaintiff to prove the element of causation. The task is simplified, however, if the alleged negligence in some manner caused or encouraged the patient to sustain or inflict tangible physical injuries upon himself or others. Indeed, this characteristic is typical of almost every successful suit. In this situation, proof of the injuries in addition to proof that ordinary and prudent therapeutic techniques would have prevented the damage may sustain the burden of proof.
>
> The plaintiff who complains of exclusively mental injuries may also have a difficult time proving the element of damages. Not only are his allegations intangible and difficult to demonstrate to the judge and jury, but they also tend to be somewhat speculative because of the state of knowledge about mental illness. Even where improper procedures have been used to institutionalize a person in need of mental care, the courts may absolve physicians from liability by finding that the patient was not injured by receiving the treatment he needed. (p. 264)

The courts have increasingly become more liberal with respect to their recognition of — and compensation for — emotional distress as an injury. Illustrative of the types of actions that have succeeded in this area are the following: In *Chavez* v. *Southern Pacific Transportation*[22] the claim of "severe traumatic neurosis" was made after a Hispanic railroad worker injured his back, an injury that healed after 9 months but left him depressed. It was alleged that the depression was intensified as a result of his Mexican-American "machismo" tradition. Mr. Chavez was awarded $1,300,000 and the verdict was not appealed. In *Vanoni* v. *Western Airlines*[23] it was held that "shock to the nerves and nervous system" constituted physical harm. The shock in this case was fright as a consequence of the negligent operation of an airliner. In *Cauverian* v. *DeMetz*[24] it was alleged that the negligent infliction of emotional distress caused the victim to become mentally unbalanced. In *Samms* v. *Eccles*[25] damages were awarded to the plaintiff as a consequence of the emotional distress she suffered when the defendant exposed himself and propositioned her.

WHAT CAN YOU BE SUED FOR?

As a mental health professional, regardless whether you are primarily involved in psychotherapy, psychological assessment, consulting, research, or some related professional endeavor, you are exposed to the potential of professional liability. A cause of action is the basis of a lawsuit, and the causes of action that have been cited in suits against behavioral scientists have been quite varied. In general, any intentional or unintentional action or failure to act that impinges on the patient's rights is actionable.[26] Thus, for example, you may be sued on grounds such as assault, battery, wrongful death, sexual or marital harm, abuse of psychotherapeutic process, breach of confidentiality, breach of contract, breach of right to informed consent, false imprisonment, defamation, the list goes on. Detailed description of these and related causes of actions appear in Cohen (1979), Cohen & Mariano (1982), Danzon (1983), Horan & Milligan (1983), Slovenko (1983), and Wettstein (1983).

Psychiatrists, as physicians, will of course be more prone than their colleagues in the field of mental health to be sued for allegedly improper conduct with respect to the prescription and administration of medication, the administration of electroshock therapy, and hospitalization. Wright (1981, p. 1487) has observed that for psychologists "the greatest (malpractice) risks are incurred in those areas of psychological practice designated as *evaluation*." Indeed, the import of a psychological evaluation can have momentous consequences for the person being evaluated. The evaluation may result in the denial of employment, denial of promotion or transfer, denial of child custody, denial of probation, and the diagnosis of, or failure to diagnose, suicidal or homicidal potential.[27] In contrast to the situation in psychotherapy, where the professional and the client have ample time to establish a good working relationship, the assessment situation is more often than not brief, to the point, and almost adversarial in nature from the perspective of the (frequently unwilling) examinee.

AVOIDING LEGAL JEOPARDY

If one day you are served with a summons and complaint alleging professional misconduct or substandard service, (1) expect to read a laundry list of horrible things about youself since lawyers will frequently cite every possible cause of action they can scare up, hoping to prevail on at least one, (2) do not panic and do not call the patient to reconciliate, berate, or apologize and beg for mercy—do not call the patient, (3) notify your malpractice insurance broker or carrier immediately,[28] and (4) discuss the case only with your attorney, and no one else except under the advice of your attorney. If your attorney has been appointed by your malpractice insurance carrier, question him or her as to prior experience in this area and satisfy yourself that this is the right person to defend your personal savings and professional reputation. If your codefendant in the suit is your employer (e.g., a private hospital; the state, etc.) I would strongly advise that you retain your own counsel and politely reject your employer's offer of joint legal representation by one attorney; the rationale here is that you will be better off if you have someone in the courtroom representing your interests exclusively. Never assume that your family attorney or lawyer friend is capable of representing you in the action by virtue of the fact that he or she is admitted to the bar; retain a specialist in the area. One psychologist for whom I acted as a consultant had made the grave error of allowing a lifelong attorney friend to represent him. Suffice to say that the results of that error in judgment were rather disastrous in terms of the psychologist's personal health and economic well-being.

Most malpractice actions are settled out of court at the claim stage; it is simply more economical to do it that way as opposed to the potentially long and expensive litigation route. Out-of-court settlements do not impute blame but instead merely indicate that the suit is being dropped for some unspecified reason in return for an agreed-upon dollar amount. If your insurance carrier wants to settle but you insist on "going the distance," be prepared to do so at your own cost and expense. If, for whatever reason, the case does go to trial, thorough preparation is essential. Organize all of your notes and reports so that you can crisply recite what was done on what date, your interpretations if any, your plans if any, and so forth. Thoroughly review the professional literature pertinent to the issue and have your attorney brief you on how best to comport yourself in pretrial discovery proceedings and in court.[29] In court, communicate effectively and avoid what I have elsewhere referred to as "WWT" errors:

> Many mental health professionals, to their detriment, make what might be termed "What's-wrong-with-that?" (WWT) errors in their court testimony. When a supposedly revealing statement about a patient's pathology compels the majority of the jury to ask themselves, "What's wrong with that?" a WWT error has been made. For example, suppose "Mr. Citizen," the patient, is forcibly taken from his home by the police, handcuffed, and packed into a police car in full view of his friends and neighbors. And suppose "Dr. Smith," a psychiatrist, testifies that the patient was verbally abusive and hostile to the therapist on admission. Jury members are likely to ask themselves. "What's wrong with that? Who wouldn't be verbally abusive and hostile under such conditions?" This is especially true if Mr. Citizen appears to be composed and "normal" in the courtroom. Smith may compound his WWT error by going on to say something like, "Further, Mr. Citizen denied that he was mentally ill." Again, jury members—who are more likely to identify with a patient than a psychiatrist—are likely to ask themselves, "What's wrong with that? I would deny it under the same circumstances." To weaken his testimony still further, Smith might testify that the patient's denial of mental illness demonstrated lack of insight, which was evidence of mental illness. Although all of Smith's statements might make sense to experienced mental health professionals, they will probably not make much sense to the lay people in the jury. WWT errors can be avoided with some forethought, factual documentation, and practice in presenting professional opinion to lay audiences. (Cohen, 1979, pp. 280–281)

If you are dissatisfied with the final disposition of the matter you can, on the advice of your attorney, appeal. Regardless of the disposition of the case one option you may want to discuss with your attorney is that of instituting a countersuit. The countersuit will be most effective when the initial suit was instituted on patently frivolous grounds and the plaintiff's lawyer might be held liable for abuse of process of law, malicious prosecution, or barratry. The countersuit is least effective — even something that will get you into a lot more trouble — when it is employed in reflex action fashion as a retaliatory measure.

Claims Prevention Strategies

An oral surgeon who was sued for malpractice after a patient swallowed one of his tools reflected, "No man sued for malpractice ever wins completely. . . . You can't know what it's like to go through such an ordeal — until you do it. One day you're a respected, confident professional man. The next day your ability is being debated in court, with all your friends and patients looking on — and wondering" (Balliet, 1974, p. 73). Indeed, given the amount of apprehension, loss of time, and loss of income most malpractice actions entail, it is meaningless to talk about winning or losing and more constructive to speak of how losses can best be cut. What follows are some claims prevention strategies designed to keep the process server away.

Perhaps the primary triggering factor in most malpractice litigation against private practitioners — regardless of the cause of actions listed in the complaint — is a fee dispute; to allow a client to run up a large bill is to invite litigation when you try to collect. Personally, I have tried to make it a policy for therapy patients to pay on a per session basis. Such a policy is not only a good claims prevention strategy but it also cuts down on bookkeeping time and time spent preparing and mailing out bills and notices. I make it a policy to collect fees for psychological assessment and for certain types of consulting in advance, if possible. Exactly how the individual practitioner handles fee collection will depend on the nature of the practice, personality factors of the practitioner, and related factors. The point here is that *some* policy that prevents the running up of large bills is a necessity.

If your work is primarily in the area of psychological evaluation, be conversant with the validity of the tests and methods you use and take care to employ the appropriate test or measure for the particular situation and the particular examinee. You should also have a well-defined and systematic method of interpreting test findings and be able to support your conclusions in court. If the results of the testing are to be transmitted to any third party, the examiner should be aware of this prior to the testing and should, if necessary, give his or her informed consent for such transmittal of results. Test records, protocols, reports, and related documents must be stored in a manner that makes them reasonably secure from persons not privileged to read this confidential material.

Like the psychological assessor, the psychotherapist must also take reasonable precautions to safeguard from unauthorized eyes privileged information such as therapy notes, records, and reports. Assure your individual patients of confidentiality and get assurances from your therapy group members regarding the confidentiality of the communications there. If you do marital and family therapy[30] or consulting to business,[31] you should be familiar with the legal issues of privacy and confidentiality as they apply in those settings. If you use an automated test-scoring service in your clinical practice you had best have a sound understanding of the test and its scoring and interpretation lest you look rather foolish in court. If you treat persons who may at some point become dangerous to themselves or others, it is important for you to have a contingency plan to put into action if the need arises. You are not obligated to accept into treatment all prospective patients who show up at your door. However, once you do accept a patient, you are legally obliged not to abandon her or him; continue the treatment until the patient leaves for whatever reason or you mutually agree that therapy should be undertaken by another therapist or terminated. All policies with respect to matters such as missed sessions due to sickness, vacation, and so forth should be clearly set forth at the onset and informed consent to treatment, to the extent that such consent is feasible,[32] should be obtained. If, in your treatment you employ methods involving touching or physically cathartic behavior, you are probably much more likely to be sued for injury arising out of therapy per se than the therapist who relies exclusively on verbal behavior.

Concluding this brief, noncomprehensive list of claims avoidance strategies, I should point out that in supervising the professional work of others it is best you structure the number of hours given to the unique needs of the supervisee and the client as opposed to some pro forma schedule. Remember that if you are in a partnership you can potentially be held liable for the tortious behavior of your partner. Permises liability can be avoided by keeping your work space neat and in reasonably good repair. Know the limits of your competence and do not practice beyond those limits. If your ability to work effectively should at some point be compromised, take some time off to obtain personal help; this is the most cost-effective way of handling such a situation in the long run. In general, keep in mind that you owe your patients, clients, research subjects, corporate consultees — anyone whom you deal with professionally — a duty to act skillfully and carefully. Finally, keep abreast of the law as it impacts on professional practice in the behavioral sciences through regular perusal of pertinent literature. As was noted at the outset, sound professional practice is a necessary but insufficient condition for avoiding allegations of malpractice; a knowledge of the law is essential.

REFERENCES

Balliet, G. (1974). Thirteen ways to protect yourself against malpractice suits. *Resident and Staff Physician, 20*(4), 70–75.

Bernstein, B.E. (1978). Malpractice: An ogre on the horizon. *Social Work, 23,* 106–112.

Black, H.C. (1968). *Black's law dictionary* (rev. 4th ed.). St. Paul: West Publishing.

Carey, J.P. (1981). Business ethics, employee privacy and the management of insurance information. *Review of Business, 3,* 21–24.

Cohen, R.J. (1979). *Malpractice: A guide for mental health professionals.* New York: The Free Press.

Cohen, R.J. (1977). Socially reinforced obsessing: A reply. *Journal of Consulting and Clinical Psychology, 45,* 1166–1171.

Cohen, R.J., & DeBetz, B. (1977). Responsive supervision of the psychiatric resident and clinical psychology intern. *American Journal of Psychoanalysis, 37,* 51–64.

Cohen, R.J., & Mariano, W.E. (1982). *Legal guidebook in mental health.* New York: The Free Press.

Cohen, R.J. (1988). *A student's guide to psychological testing: Laboratory exercises in assessment.* Mountain View, CA: Mayfield Publishing.

Cohen, R.J., Montague, P., Nathanson, L.S., & Swerdlik, M.E. (1988). *Psychological testing and assessment.* New York: St. Martin's Press, *in press.*

Cohen, R.J., & Smith, F.J. (1976). Socially reinforced obsessing: Etiology of a disorder in a Christian Scientist. *Journal of Consulting and Clinical Psychology, 44,* 142–144.

Danzon, P.M. (1983). An economic analysis of the medical malpractice system. *Behavioral Sciences and the law, 1*(1),

Green, R.K., & Cox, G. (1978). Social work and malpractice: A converging course. *Social Work, 23,* 100–105.

Harris, M. (11973). Tort liability of the psychotherapist. *University of San Francisco Law Review, 8,* 405–436.

Horan, D.J., & Milligan, R.J. (1983). Recent developments in psychiatric malpractice. *Behavioral Sciences and the Law, 1*(1),

Jurow, G.L., & Mariano, W.E. (1972). Law and private practice. In G.D. Goldman & G. Sticker, *Practical problems of a private psychotherapy practice.* Springfield, IL: Charles C. Thomas.

Margolin, G. (1982). Ethical and legal considerations in marital and family therapy. *American Psychologist, 37,* 788–801.

McLemore, C.W. (1982). *The scandal of psychotherapy: A guide to resolving the tensions between faith and counseling.* Wheaton, IL: Tyndale.

Prosser, W.L. (1971). *Law of torts.* (4th ed.) St. Paul, MN: West Publishing.

Rothblatt, H.B., & Leroy, D.H. (1973). Avoiding psychiatric malpractice. *California Western Law Review, 9,* 260–272.

Slovenko, R. (&1983). The hazards of writing or disclosing information in psychiatry. *Behavioral Sciences and the Law, 1*(1), 109–127.

Stone, A.A. (1977). Recent mental health litigation: A critical perspective. *American Journal of Psychiatry, 134,* 273–279.

Wettstein, R.M. (1983). Tardive dyskinesia dna malpractice. *Behavioral Sciences and the Law, 1*(1),

Wright, R.H. (1981). Psychologists and professional liability (malpractice) insurance: A retrospective view. *American Psychologist, 36,* 1485–1493.

FOOTNOTES

[1]Restatement 2d, Torts § 282 (1965).

[2]Our presentation of the concept of negligence and of related terminology is necessarily brief and simplified. The interested reader is referred to Prosser (1971) for a detailed and thorough discussion of these legal concepts.

[3]This is true except for the relatively rare instance where in a case is decided on the basis of a doctrine, that the negligent act need not be proved; it is sufficient to demonstrate that but for the negligent act, the plaintiff could not have been injured.

[4]O'Neill v. Montefiore Hospital, 11 App. Div. 2d 1332, 203, N.Y.S.2d 436 (1960).

[5]Rainer v. Grossman, 31 Cal.Appl.3d 539, 107 Cal.Rptr. 469 (1973).

[6]Hofman v. Blackmon, 241 So.2d 752 (Fla. App. 1970).

[7]Tarasoff v. Regents of University of California, 131 Cal.Rptr. 14, 551 P.2d 334 (1976).

[9]People v. Poddar, 10 Cal.3d. 750, 111 Cal.Rptr. 910, 518 P.2d 342 (1974).

[9]See, for example, "Responsive Supervision of the Psychiatric Resident and Clinical Psychology Intern" (Cohen and DeBetz, 1977).

[10]Cestone v. Harkavy, 243 App. Div. 732, 277 N.Y.S.2d 438 (1935).

[11]Corleto v. Shore Memorial Hospital, 138 N.J.Super. 302, 350 A.2d 534 (1975).

[12]Both the American Psychological Association and the American Psychiatric Association filed an *amicus curiae* brief in *Tarasoff* (citation is in note 7) arguing that the duty to warn was not required by professional standards and in fact would be counter to the psychotherapeutic process.

[13]Helling v. Carey, 83 Wash.2d 514, 519 P.2d 981 (1974).

[14]Lawless v. Callaway, 147 P.2d 604.

[15]Rodriguez v. State, 355 N.Y.S.2d 912.

[16]Steinke v. Bell, 107 A.2d 825 (1954).

[17]Nelson v. Dahl, 174 Minn. 574, 219 N.W.941 (1928).

[18]In Simpson v. Davis (219 Kan. 584, 549 P.2d 950) for example, a dentist who performed endodontic work was held to the standard of an endodontist.

[19]According to Black (1968, p. 1403) a quack is a "pretender to medical skill which he does not possess; one who practices as a physician or surgeon without adequate preparation or due qualification." We might substitute "psychotherapeutic" for "medical' and "licensed mental health professional" for "physician or surgeon" in this definition but we are still left with a disturbing question; to what standard should the burgeoning number of formally unlicensed psychotherapists be held?

[20]Whipple v. Grandchamp, 261 Mass. 40, 158 N.E.270, 57 A.L.R. 974.

[21]See for example the discussion of *Bogust v. Iverson* (110 Wisc.2d. 129, 102 N.W.2d 228) and Previn v. Tenacre, Inc. (70 F.2d 389) in Cohen and Mariano (1982).

[22]Chavez v. Southern Pacific Transportation, Los Angeles Superior Court No. C-134638, October 2, 1979.

[23]Vanoni v. Western Airlines, 247 Cal.App.2d 793.

[24]Cauverien v. DeMetz, 188, N.Y.S.2d 627.

[25]Samms v. Eccles, 11 Utah 2d 289, 358 P.2d 344.

[26]This is not to imply that professionals will be held liable for honest errors in professional judgment that result in negative outcome. The courts have long recognized that behavioral science is not an exact science (e.g., St. George v. State, 283 App. Div. 245, 127 N.Y.S.2d 147) and that prediction of violence and other behavior cannot be made with precision (e.g., Taig v. State, 19 App. Div. 2d 182, 241 N.Y.S.2d 495). The court in Taig held, "If a liability were imposed on the physician or the State each time the prediction of future course of mental disease was wrong, few releases would ever be made and the hope of recovery and rehabilitation of a vast number of patients would be impeded and frustrated." This is one of the medical and public risks which must be taken on balance, even though it may sometimes result in injury to the patient or others.

[27]For an elaboration of these and related issues, consult Cohen et al. (1988, pp. 35–45 and pp. 602–614) and Cohen (1988, pp. 6–7 and pp. 186–190).

[28]Notwithstanding the fact that many clinicians have argued against the "tyranny of the shoulds," you *should* carry malpractice insurance.

[29]Fifteen guidelines with respect to handling pretrial dispositions as well as other suggestions regarding courtroom behavior appear in Cohen (1979, pp. 276–281).

[30]A review of some of these issues appears in Margolin (1982).

[31]An analysis of some of the issues here is provided by Carey (1981).

[32]For a real-life illustration of the problems in obtaining informed consent prior to beginning therapy consult Cohen (1977). The article is a rejoinder to the many comments generated by an earlier case study (Cohen and Smith, 1976) in which a Christian Scientist relinquished her obsessive symptomatology only after she stopped believing in Christian Science. Further discussion of the issues raised by this study appear in Cohen (1979, pp. 76–83) and in McLemore (1982).

C H A P T E R
56

THE IMPACT OF LITIGATION ON PSYCHOTHERAPY PRACTICE: LITIGATION FEARS AND LITIGAPHOBIA

Stanley L. Brodsky, Ph.D., and
and Joseph E. Schumacher

A peculiar thing is happening in psychotherapists' offices and meetings all over the United States. Where once upon a time psychotherapists engaged in excited, intense discussions about what works in psychotherapy, a large part of such discussions now concerns self-protection from litigious clients and unscrupulous attorneys. And these animated discussions about being sued are hardly unique to psychotherapists. They are heard also among educators, nurses, corporate executives, dentists, and realtors, to select just a few categories from a burgeoning list. Indeed, in some fields the concern about litigation has profoundly influenced the nature of fundamental practices. Stockbrokers, for example, now frequently tape-record meetings with clients who wish to proceed with risky investments against the brokers' advice. University tenure meetings often split their debating time between a discussion of the merits of candidates and the probability that rejected candidates will sue.

When fears about litigation worm their way into the minds of psychotherapists, something even more problematic may happen: The effectiveness of the psychotherapy may be reduced or altogether sabotaged. After all, in psychotherapy the relationship between professional and client is more personal and more central to the objective of the tratment than it is in most other professions. If the therapist sees the client as possible litigant, the potential exists for a compromise of the trust, acceptance, and regard so essential in the practice of psychotherapy.

This chapter addresses the impact of litigation on the practice of psychotherapy. Four major areas will be explored. First, we ask: Is there truly an increase in litigation against mental health professionals involved in direct service delivery? We answer that question affirmatively, but go on to conclude that the extent is decidedly less than commonly perceived and that it is specific to certain areas of service delivery.

The second question we ask is: How did the perception of lawsuits as raindrops falling continuously on all our heads develop? We answer by looking at the ripple effect from the *Tarasoff* decision. This court case produced what is a lasting skinned-knee sensitivity to lawsuits among psychotherapists.

The third question raised is: How are psychotherapists responding to this perception? The answer is that most therapists are concerned, and that in about 5 percent of all psychotherapists this concern gets out of hand. The excessive and irrational fear of litigation is discussed under the label "litigaphobia."

The final question is: What can be done about both the garden-variety, mild fears of litigation and the full-blown litigaphobias? A series of possible answers are put forth. These solutions range from mastery of legal/psychological concerns to specific suggestions relating to the duty to warn. With this outline completed, we may now move to the topic proper: Is there truly an increase in lawsuits against psychotherapists?

LAWSUITS AGAINST PSYCHOTHERAPISTS: A 10-YEAR PERSPECTIVE

Until the late 1970s, malpractice suits against psychotherapists were relatively rare. Hogan (1979b) observed that with the upsurge in litigation in general, there has been a concomitant rise in suits against therapists. Articles in law reviews have described such a trend as well. Psychotherapists and psychiatric hospitals have offered anecdotal evidence that their patients are more willing to sue than ever before. Furrow (1980), for example, maintained that in light of changing consumer expectations, society has become increasingly dissatisfied with products and services, individuals are more aware of the limitations of psychotherapy, and they are willing to use litigation as a means to solve their disputes. Furrow went on to predict that psychotherapy clients will employ more varied forms of litigation in the future.

A comprehensive examination of all reported malpractice suits against therapists brought to trial through 1977 was published by Hogan (1979a). It is the only thorough, archival research on lawsuits against psychotherapeutic practices. Three hundred cases involving psychotherapeutic malpractice in treatment, diagnosis, care, or combinations of the three were collected and analyzed. This study provided empirical evidence for uncovering the trends and etiology of psychotherapeutic malpractice litigation.

Hogan reported that the total number of malpractice suits involving psychotherapists rose substantially in recent years. One-third of all known decisions occurred within the 10-year period from 1960 to 1969, and another third occurred through 1977. Overall, plaintiffs won roughly 30 percent of all of these suits, but the 1970s found decisions in favor of plaintiffs rising to nearly 40 percent. A geographic concentration of suits was also reported. New York State was the venue for 40 percent of these suits against psychotherapists. California followed with 8.7 percent, Texas was next with 3.7 percent, and no other state had more than 3 percent. In fact, 11 states had no suits against psychotherapists.

Nearly two-thirds of all complaints occurred as a result of practices in mental hospitals. Suits against private practitioners accounted for 6.9 percent of all cases and for 8.1 percent of cases in the 1970s. The plaintiff had the best chance of winning if the suit involved the government or the state as defendant.

In the Hogan study, most suits alleged negligence in the diagnosis, treatment, or care of clients. The most common charges were of physical and sexual abuse, inappropriate commitment and release actions, improper prediction of dangerousness, and inadequate physical supervision resulting in accidental injuries. Plaintiffs' chances of winning were good in suits involving physical assault and sexual abuse. Less successful were allegations of inappropriate release of confidential information, failure to recognize a suicide, improper failure to release, and failure to warn third parties.

A jury was the trier of facts in only one out of five cases. Juries were found to be more favorable to the plaintiffs than were judges. Judges decided in favor of the plaintiffs only 26 percent of the time, while juries did so 43.5 percent of the time.

Hogan (1978a) concluded that "suits against psychotherapists, hospitals, and others responsible for the diagnosis, treatment, and care of the mentally ill were increasing exponentially" (p. 25). He emphasized, however, that the technical difficulty in effectively establishing a case against a psychotherapist makes liability suits a chance proposition. Proof of allegations was reportedly a monumental task, except in the most serious cases, such as those involving negligent custodial care, physical assault, and sexual abuse. It was predicted that plaintiffs would continue to have difficulty winning psychotherapeutic malpractice cases.

In a review of claims against psychologists covered by professional liability insurance, Wright (1981) analyzed claims for a 54-month period prior to July of 1980. The aggregate premium paid by psychologists enrolled in this plan exceeded $5 million, and the total projected loss was judged to be approximately $435,642. Sixty percent of the total claims were settled for less than $5,000. The average claim valued approximately $3,571. One particular suit alleging negligence resulting in wrongful death resulted in a $250,000 settlement. This single case consisted of over half of the total projected losses for the period under investigation.

The percentage of claims per thousand insured psychologists did not increase during the time period assessed. Wright (1981) concluded that "the frequently heard comment of a wave of malpractice actions reflecting an increasingly litigious public, or concern about increasing sexual involvement of psychologists with their patients, is not readily substantiated" (p. 1,489).

Galanter (1983) attempted to assess the more general contention that courtrooms are being overwhelmed by an unprecedented flood of litigation attributable to the excessive litigiousness of the general populationg. His findings revealed that only a small portion of all injuries result in legal disputes. Of those that do, the vast majority are dropped, settled, or routinely processed without extensive adjudication. Galanter reported that comparisons of current with past litigation rates showed a recent rise but that present levels are not without precedent.

Galanter stated that the "litigation explosion" is fictional, and he attributed this myth to changes in patterns of governmental activity, organization of legal work, and relation of the media to the law and to the increased education and knowledge about the availability of the courtroom to handle disputes.

Our own parallel conclusion is that the so-called malpractice crisis in psychotherapy has been exaggerated. The probability is low that a typical practitioner will become involved in malpractice litigation in any one year. Plaintiffs are generally awarded insubstantial amounts of money, even where allegations involve obvious disregard of responsible practice. That there has been an explosion of professional litigation has also been challenged by Rust (1986), who observes that even experts disagree about its existence.

IMPACT OF MALPRACTICE LITIGATION ON MENTAL HEALTH PROFESSIONALS

Our reading of the existing data supports the notion that malpractice litigation against psychotherapists is not increasing at the geometric rate feared by experts. Psychotherapists, however, continue to fear the threat of malpractice litigation and often react in maladaptive ways. The impact of the *Tarasoff* doctrine has reverberated through the practices of all psychotherapists. Its effects have been extensively studied. Fear of litigation encompasses areas of professional practice far beyond *Tarasoff.* We will discuss these fears and their substantial effects on psychotherapists' lives and practices.

Duty To Warn

Tarasoff v. *Regents of University of California* (1976)[1] has had a seminal impact on the regulation and practice of psychotherapy. In 1974, "the California Supreme Court ruled that psychotherapists owe an affirmative duty of reasonable care to third parties whose persons are threatened by patients under the psychotherapists' treatment" (Wise, 1978, p. 165). In 1976, the ruling in "Tarasoff II" held that the decision to break confidentiality was no longer within the full discretion of the therapist. "The California court made clear that the obligation to protect a patient's confidences must yield when a therapist determines (or should determine) that a patient presents a serious danger of violence to another person" (Wise, 1978, p. 166).

An empirical survey by Wise (1978) was conducted approximately 1 year after the implementation of the second *Tarasoff* ruling to assess its impact on psychotherapists. Questionnaires were completed by 1,272 psychotherapists, most of whom indicated that the *Tarasoff* decision had influenced their practices. Some psychotherapists reported concentrating more carefully on minor threats made by their patients and directing therapy sessions more toward the subject of dangerousness than they had previously. Others avoided probing into sensitive issues that might elicit threats of physical harm. The majority of the respondents felt increased anxiety when the subject of dangerousness was discussed during therapy. Over half reported an increased fear of legal liability directly related to the newly recognized duty to warn.

It has been argued that the success and trust of psychotherapy itself is compromised by lack of total confidentiality. Stone (1976) echoed the views of many psychotherapists when he asserted that imposing a duty to warn poten-

---

[1]Tarasoff v. Regents of California, 17 Cal.3d 425, 131 Cal. Rptr. 14, 1976.

tial victims is counterproductive. Such a duty, he explained, is incompatible with an effective therapeutic relationship and will deter both patients and therapists from dealing with potentially threatening material. Kermani and Drob (1987) reported that *Tarasoff* has elicited three common objections from by psychotherapists: "that mental health professionals cannot reliably predict violence, that successful psychotherapy is predicated on the trust engendered by strict confidentiality, and that a duty to warn actually increases acts of violence by placing a chilling effect upon potentially violent patients' disclosures in treatment" (p. 284).

The impact of *Tarasoff*-related issues has spread into broader contexts. George (1985) wrote that "cacophonous wails of unlimited liability and doomsday forecasts concerning confidentiality and the therapeutic relationship again are reverberating throughout California" (p. 291). This response was initiated by *Hedlund* v. *Superior Court* (1983).[2] *Hedlund* involved a psychologist and a psychology assistant who failed to warn an adult woman of threats made against her by the defendants' patient. She ultimately was shot by the patient. Her minor son allegedly suffered emotional injuries as a result of witnessing the attack upon his mother, and he successfully brought suit against the psychologists.

Since then, *Hedlund* has been misread by mental health practitioners and caused fears of persecution that have been referred to by George as "Hedlund paranoia"! George emphasized that *Hedlund* did not imply that the psychologist has a duty to warn or protect the offspring of potential victims threatened by their patients. The ultimate issue remains whether practitioners exhibit the degree of skill, knowledge and treatment required by members of their professional organizations.

The *Tarasoff* cases have influenced the practice of psychotherapy after a decade of controversial interpretation. Kermani and Drob (1987) identified the emergency of two general trends. At one extreme, courts have narrowly interpreted the duty to warn as applying only when a therapist is aware of a serious threat directed at a specific individual. At the other extreme, courts have broadened the decision to include warnings about clients who do not make threats and whose potential victims are unknown to both the therapist and client himself or herself. The latitude allowed by the courts has perpetuated the fear of being sued by creating the illusion of a "no win situation" for therapists trying to decide how to respond to threatening or potentially threatening clients.

Since 1976, the *Tarasoff* ruling has been followed by a number of cases that extend the duty to warn beyond its original context. Recent cases, however, have limited the liability of psychotherapists to specific situations in which threat of harm to identifiable victims is present. In *Currie* v. *United States,*[3] a federal district court in North Carolina strictly limited the duty to warn by employing a good faith test for determining liability (Miller, 1986). This court found that psychotherapists were not liable for simple errors made in good faith and with reasonable professional judgment.

The *Tarasoff* brouhaha has changed the understanding of psychotherapeutic practice. At the least, practitioners have shown a heightened awareness of issues of legal liability. At most, a serious and pathological impediment has appeared in psychotherapeutic practice in the form of litigaphobia.

---

[2]Hedlund v. Superior Court (1983), Cal. 3d 695, 194 Cal. Rptr. 805, 1983.

Litigaphobia

Fear of litigation extends far beyond *Tarasoff* and duty to warn issues. Patients' rights, suicides, institutional negligence, improper diagnoses, and breach of contracts are areas of mental health practice perceived as vulnerable to litigation. Many practitioners have taken significant actions to avoid litigation and in the process have sometimes emotionally overresponded to the fear of being sued.

Brodsky (1986a) coined the term "litigaphobia" to describe the excessive and irrational fear of litigation among health professionals. Breslin et al. (1986) developed a psychometric instrument to measure and understand the phenomenon of litigaphobia. The responses of 123 physicians and clinical psychologists were factor analyzed, yielding two main underlying factors: (1) fear of lawsuits and (2) felt vulnerability to lawsuits. It was concluded that the excessive and irrational fear of litigation could now be studied with a reliable scale. We contend that concern about litigation may be part of a widespread adaptation to a real and present threat. However, in its extreme form, the fear becomes litigaphobic and meets the criteria for a simple phobia.

According to the *Diagnostic and Statistical Manual of Mental Disorders, Third Edition* — Revised (American Psychiatric Association, 1987), the essential feature of a simple phobia is a persistent fear of a circumscribed stimulus. Exposure to the stimulus object or situation typically provokes an immediate anxiety response. Anticipatory anxiety occurs when the individual is confronted with the necessity of entering into the simple phobic situation. Generally the individual recognizes that his or her fear is excessive or unreasonable. Attempts to avoid the phobic stimulus may have significant effects on social or professional adaptive functioning.

The litigaphobic responds to the devastating fear of being sued for malpractice in the same way the acrophobic responds to the devastating fear of falling from a tall skyscraper. The phobic practitioner suffers significant distress when confronted with a phobic stimulus like a threatening client or a court subpoena. Drastic and often irrational measures are taken to avoid perceived consequences such as overwhelming embarrassment and career and financial loss. The apprehension about confronting anything resembling a litigious experience is disproportional to the actual dangerousness of the feared experience. This often leads to maladaptive responses.

The *actual* experience of being sued can be devastating. Charles et al. (1984) examined the impact of malpractice suits on 140 Cook County physicians. This study reported that 57 percent of these physicians felt that they had suffered as a result and that 19 percent reported experiencing a "loss of nerve" in some clinical situations. Approximately three-fourths of the sample reported some symptoms associated with major depression, anger and tension, or onset of physical illness during the litigation. The investigators concluded, "A malpractice suit was considered a serious and often devastating event in the personal and professional lives of the responding physicians" (p. 565). Our present concern is with individuals who are not being sued, who have never been sued, who probably never will be sued, but who are intensely afraid of being sued.

Our best estimate is that 5 percent of mental health practitioners suffer

---

[3]Currie v. United States, No. C-85-0269-D (M.D.N.C. Oct. 3, 1986).

from litigaphobic symptoms. Excessive worry and preoccupation about one's own vulnerability typically arise after one becomes aware of a well-publicized local malpractice suit. One of the authors (JES) experienced overwhelming frustration and anger when a jury held a colleague responsible for prediction of the future behavior of a released inpatient. This colleague was sued successfully in part because "forcing" the reluctant patient to take the MMPI would allegedly have yielded information enabling a more accurate prediction.

> Instantly, I began planning ways to avoid being sued. Avoiding "risky" clients, specializing, and overinsuring were thoughts racing through my mind. Conversations with colleagues revealed even more drastic reactions. They spoke of excessive anxiety and preoccupation with becoming sued, manipulating records, frequent consultation with attorneys regarding potentially liable practices, and consideration of changing careers.

Why do psychotherapists react in these ways? What can be done? In order to answer these questions, we move to the theoretical bases of litigaphobia and then to recommendations for managing the perceived threat of litigation.

A THEORETICAL PROPOSITION

As humans we naturally seek to explain the meaning of events in our world. The discovery of patterns allows us to make predictions and gain some adaptive control over life. We often seek out consensual and statistical information for validation of our ideas and decisions. Stanovich (1986), however, asserts that characteristics in many people make it difficult for them to understand and accept the nature of statistical information and probability.

The concept of litigaphobia can be understood by analyzing how we process information gained from statistical base rates and phenomenological experiences. We propose that the fear of litigation is elicited and maintained through exposure to isolated but salient life experiences. The representativeness of these experiences is overgeneralized and overweighted during information processing. Professionals who suffer from litigaphobic symptoms tend to rely on anecdotal evidence and refuse to allow other sources of information to challenge set beliefs. Single-trial learning and the "man who" phenomenon will help us understand litigaphobia from an information-processing perspective.

The effect of the single trial on learning and changing attitudes has been studied. Borgida and Nisbett (1977), for example, found that beliefs and attitudes are formed by significant isolated life events. Kahneman and Tversky (1973) describe examples of belief formation that overly weigh individual case evidence and insufficiently weigh statistical base rates and sample size information. We believe that the excessive and irrational fear of litigation can be directly or vicariously conditioned through single-trial exposures. Sensational media coverage, testimonials, and intraprofessional gossip are potential single-trial stimuli in this case.

The tendency for people's judgments to be dominated by a single, salient event, while discarding more accurate and reliable statistical evidence, is known as the "man who" phenomenon. Stanovich (1986) states that well-established trends are disregarded because someone knows a man who went against the trend. If a particular isolated experience validates a belief or myth held by an individual, then overgeneralization to similar experiences occurs. Irrational beliefs become strengthened by anecdotal evidence resistant to contradictory hard data. Litigaphobic professionals are reluctant to allow factual evidence to challenge their fearful beliefs.

Fellow colleagues who fear being sued consistently refer to isolated cases of colleagues who have been sued and have suffered drastic and traumatic consequences. Emotions from anger to depression are commonly exhibited. These colleagues become preoccupied with isolated lawsuits and show maladaptive methods of coping and avoiding being sued. Feelings of unfairness arise when professionals believe they may be held responsible for the prediction and control of clients' behavior.

Rotter's notion of locus of control and Seligman's concept of learned helplessness are helpful in understanding litigaphobia as a dehabilitating phenomenon. The acceptance of "fate" or control by external forces has been studied by Rotter (1966). The degree to which one accepts external forces as being controlling varies with the extent to which we have had the experience of our actions making a difference. Rotter contends that "internal" personality types perceive that consequences are contingent on their own behavior and/or their own personal attributes. "Externals" perceive that consequences occur independently of their actions and are controlled by unpredictable external forces. While Rotter viewed locus of control as a trait, we have come to see it in this context as a transient state. A hazard of the fear of litigation is that a state of externality is created. The practitioner feels that he or she is out of control, vulnerable, and often helpless.

In learned helplessness both animals and humans exhibited fear and helplessness when they had no effect on a traumatic event or on minimizing its impact. The inability to control the consequences of behavior is the basis of learned helplessness. Anger and frustration, then apathy and inaction, are the consequences of helplessness (Seligman, 1975). In litigaphobia, helplessness arises from a perception of the law as an unfair and uncontrollable entity.

The fear of being sued may be perpetuated by those practitioners who feel controlled by external circumstances. The fear of litigation can arise after they read a newspaper article about a sensational malpractice case, pay an increased insurance fee, or talk about a colleague who has been threatened with legal action. Practitioners frequently feel helpless to avoid both suits and the consequences of being sued. Excessive and irrational beliefs, intense negative emotions, and avoidance behaviors can arise in the face of these threatening perceptions.

Further empirical experimentation is necessary to validate these theoretical assumptions. Brodsky (1986b) suggests taking the following steps in order to understand the meaning of litigaphobia: (1) gather survey data to assess the extent and nature of fear of litigation among practicing professionals (special attention should be given to those who meet published criteria for phobic reactions), (2) document the effects of litigation on professionals, (3) trace the developmental patterns of the fear of litigation, and (4) conceptualize and test intervention models.

COPING WITH FEAR OF LITIGATION

The excessive and irrational fear of litigation appears in several areas of psychotherapeutic practice. We turn to methods of coping with fears of litigation. While our concern has been with excessive fears, a range of quite rational and appropriate fears exist as well. Our recommendations are intended to address fear of litigation in general.

Mastery vs. Avoidance And Anxiety

One constructive approach to the fear of litigation is to develop a personal and professional mastery of the threat. We have noted that many mental health professionals perceive the threat of lawsuits as being external to themselves, and as a consequence a sense of helplessness is their primary reaction. Some professionals therefore actively avoid all clients and situations that may lead to litigation. This act of avoidance becomes increasingly difficult as the scope of mental health lawsuits expands. An equally frustrating alternative pattern is for professionals to continue with their work while experiencing considerable distress. A sense of mastery can substitute positive actions for avoidance. Our suggestions for mastery of the fear of litigation include these steps.

1. Acquisition of an appreciation of the legal process related to mental health practice. This step encompasses reading, attendance at workshops, and a general cognitive mastery of the issues.
2. Skill development related to courtroom appearance. For many professionals, a key part of the threat is the belief that aggressive attorneys will humiliate them on the witness stand. Practitioners without such courtroom experience are advised to seek out practical, experiential training in coping with such situations.
3. Routine peer consultation or supervision in the most difficult, litigation-prone cases. While this step is always good advice, it has special relevance for ensuring that the practitioner does not feel alone, and indeed is not alone, in making case management decisions.

Disclosure Of Client Information

One of the most touchy and litigation-focused decisions is how and when to respond to information about potentially violent clients. Kermani and Drob (1987) recommend a three-tiered hierarchical conception of disclosures. The first tier consists of disclosures based upon the therapists' subjective clinical judgment and not the clients' words or actions. Release of minimal suspicions is neither appropriate nor justified, and the clinician might be liable for damages that follow the misues of such information.

The second tier consists of disclosures prompted by clients' threats that are not serious or specific enough to meet the strict interpretation of the *Tarasoff* doctrine. Such disclosures are based on the verbal report of the client and can be documented and justified as such. Release of this type of information is more dependent on the judgment of the therapist and is less vulnerable to liability than the first tier.

The third tier consists of disclosures that are serious and specific enough to meet the *Tarasoff* criteria. The practitioner is not only justified in making but required to make the disclosure in this case and may be liable to potential victims for failing to do so.

This system leaves ambiguous cases to the discretion of the practitioner while clearly mandating disclosures in obvious situations. Such discretion is both clinically sensible and legally appropriate. Conscientious documentation of verbal threats and overt behaviors is recommended to justify and support appropriate disclosures. Practitioners can gauge their duty to warn by these standards.

Documentation

Several attempts at coping with fear of litigation through record keeping have been observed. We have in mind leaving out potentially liable information or adding information to records in an attempt to create a favorable evidentiary document in case of a lawsuit. Keeping two sets of records, one public and the other private, is a common practice among those who fear having their words interpreted. These are dangerous and unethical practices. Remember, private records can be subpoenaed. Deliberate omissions or defensive additions to records are justly suspect. Destruction of potentially liable records sometimes also occurs. Such record shredding appears in court as proof positive the clinician has something to hide.

Our message is unequivocal. Record manipulation in response to fear of litigation is always inappropriate and is a sign of professional inadequacy. Clinicians should routinely be prepared to justify their statements and conclusions. Proper record keeping begins with common sense and ends with honesty.

Fees

One of the surprisingly frequent allegations of professional misconduct is in the area of fee collection. The typical fee-related lawsuit occurs when a practitioner allows substantial unpaid fees to accumulate, terminates the client, and attempts to collect the outstanding bill. Unsuccessful efforts at collecting the fee personally often result in the practitioner's turning the account to a collection agency or initiating a civil suit. A not unusual response of the client is a malpractice complaint!

The accumulation of fees may foster indulgence, unrealistic dependency, and angry retaliatory reactions on the part of clients. Some clients deprecate the worth of the practitioner and the services. "Complaints of professional malfeasance are rarely seen in a context in which fees are straightforwardly structured or are dealt with as important data in the professional relationship" (Wright, 1981, p. 1,492). Responsible private practitioners do not neglect delinquent balances.

Evaluations And Confidentiality

Legal complaints about the evaluation process do not generally allege inappropriate evaluation methods or procedures. Instead they relate to violations of confidentiality or invasions of privacy. Complaints in this area typically reflect a distress over the findings and their implications. Some clients resent labeling and wish diagnoses and conclusions to be stricken from all records.

Wright (1981) recommends a full and complete disclosure to the patient of the purpose of the evaluation and of the findings and recommendations prior to release of that information. He particularly discourages what he calls the "technician mentality," in which the practitioner caters to the paying third party and ignores the rights and feelings of the client. Other related evaluation hazards include unknowing misinterpretation of results, failure to consider a critical piece of information, and inability to substantiate conclusions.

Sexual Involvement With Clients

Psychotherapy typically involves intense and close interpersonal relationships. Therapists need to be familiar with the nature of the therapeutic relationship and to be trained to cope with issues of transference and countertransference. Sexual involvement with a client is considered taboo by all governing professional organizations. Allegation of sexual abuse of patients are fairly frequent and are one of the most successful bases for clients' suing therapists. Holroyd and Brodsky (1977) found that 5.5 percent of male psychologists and 0.6 percent of female psychologists admitted to having had sexual intercourse with their clients. Such unprofessional activity is an invitation to malpractice litigation.

Consultation

An attorney friend who defends doctors in malpractice suits tells of physicians who call him daily to check out their legal risk with particular clients and procedures. Such excessive consultation with an attorney is absurd and unnecessary. This is not to say that practitioners should not know the laws specific to their practice; they should. Consultation is most effectively offered by peers and supervisors who specialize in the particular problem or type of client with whom you are dealing. It is more common today than it was previously for practitioners to hire consultants and join discussion groups to improve their practices and to cope with difficult cases and the stresses of the profession.

LITIGATION AS A CURSE, LITIGATION AS A GIFT: A CONCLUDING PERSPECTIVE

To many mental health professionals, litigation is a curse, an unwanted, intrusive evil visited upon the practices of good-minded, good-willed professionals by greedy lawyers and ungrateful clients. Professionals who see it this way feel hurt at the accusations, upset at the loss of time and income that results, and distressed that they should have to deal with such unpleasantness. Our view is that it is indeed an annoyance to many mental health professionals. Outrageously large and seemingly inappropriate jury awards are indeed sometimes made in malpractice suits. The practice of psychotherapy surely is complicated by the potential for litigation.

Although we agree that these aspects of litigation are troublesome, we also see litigation against psychotherapists as a gift to the profession and to the public. The gift is that litigation is a vehicle for making public many actions that are private and problematic. If it were not for litigation against psychotherapists who sexually engage their clients during sessions, our professions would have been far slower to actively condemn this practice. Litigation has done more than lead to condemnations; it has served to rid us of unethical people who should never have been harming the lives of their clients behind the privacy of closed psychotherapeutic doors. Getting our hands washed of these unthinking, self-centered therapists has been a gift from lawsuits against therapists.

A second gift has been the mild anxiety many psychotherapists have felt about litigation concerns. A number of good practices, such as keeping accurate, complete records, used to be weaker, background issues. Now they have become strong, foreground issues. Practices have changed since the fear of litigation blossomed. We grant that some people are following good practices for extrinsic reasons, such as protecting themselves in the case of lawsuits. However, if these practitioners were not and still are not motivated by intrinsic reasons, then let the societal mechanisms of potential legal actions push them into doing what they should have been doing anyway.

In this chapter we have explored the role of litigation and the fear of litigation in psychotherapeutic practice. We do not suggest it has been the best thing in the world for psychotherapists; that is simply not so. However, we conclude that neither has it been the worst thing in the world. Psychotherapists who overreact unnecessarily make these new concerns into catastrophies.

Litigation is a potential event for almost all Americans. As psychotherapists we need to let go of the prima donna belief that we should be exempt and take simple, sensible actions to ensure what we do is reasonably, rationally, and professionally what we should be doing. Only then can litigation fear fade to the background issue it truly is.

REFERENCES

American Psychiatric Association. (1987). *Diagnostic and statistical manual of mental disorders* (Third Edition, Revised). Washington, DC: Author.

Borgia, E., & Nisbett, R.D. (1977). The differential impact of abstract vs. concrete information of decisions. *Journal of Applied Social Psychology, 7,* 258–271.

Breslin, F.A., Taylor, K.R., & Brodsky, S.L. (1986). Development of a litigaphobia scale: Measurement of excessive fear of litigation. *Psychological Reports, 58,* 547–550.

Brodsky, S.L. (1986a). Litigaphobia: When fear of litigation becomes irrational. In a symposium, *Litigaphobia: The escessive and irrational fear of litigation.* Annual convention of the American Psychological Association. Washington, DC, August, 1986.

Brodsky, S.L. (rev. 1986b). Fear of litigation in mental health professionals. Presented to the Sixth Annual Conference of State Mental Health Forensic Directories, San

Francisco, and to the Annual Convention of the American Psychological Association, Washington, DC, 1985.

Charles, S.C., Wilbert, J.R., & Kennedy, E.C. (1984). Physicians' self-reports of reactions to malpractice litigation. *American Journal of Psychitary, 141,* 563–565.

Furrow, B.R. (1980). *Malpractice in psychotherapy.* Lexington, MA: Lexington Books.

Galanter, M. (1983). Reading the landscape of disputes: What we know and don't know (and think we know) about our allegedly contentious and litigious society. *UCLA Law Review, 42,* 4–71.

George, J.C. (1985). Hedlund paranoia. *Journal of Clinical Psychology, 41,* 291–294.

Hogan, D.B. (1979). *The regulation of psychotherapists: A review of malpractice suits in the United States,* vol. III, Cambridge, MA: Ballinger.

Holroyd, J.C., & Brodsky, A.M. (1977). Psychologists' attitudes regarding erotic and nonerotic physical contacts with patients. *American Psychologist, 33,* 5–7.

Kahneman, D., & Tversky, A. (1973). On the psychology of prediction. *Psychological Review, 80,* 237–251.

Kermani, E.J., & Drob, S.L. (1987). Tarasoff decision: A decade later dilemma still faces psychotherapists. *American Journal of Psychotherapy, XLI,* 271–285.

Miller, R.D. (1986). Currie v. United States: Tarasoff comes south. *Mental and Physical Law Reporter, 10,* 577.

Rotter, J.B. (1966). Generalized expectancies for internal versus external controls of reinforcement. *Psychological Monographs, 80* (1, Whole No. 609).

Rust, M. (1986). Experts differ on lawsuit explosion. *American Medical News, 28,* 1–3.

Seligman, M.E.P. (1975). *Helplessness: On depression, development and death.* San Francisco: W.H., Freeman.

Stanovich, K.E. (1986). *How to think straight about psychology.* Glenview, IL: Scott, Foresman, and Company.

Stone, A.A. (1967). The Tarasoff decisions: Suing psychotherapists to safeguard society. *Harvard Law Review, 90,* 358–378.

Wise, T.P. (1978). Where the public peril begins: A survey of psychotherapists to determine the effect of Tarasoff. *Stanford Law Review, 31,* 165–190.

Wright, R.H. (1981). Psychologists and professional liability (malpractice) insurance: A retrospective review. *American Psychologist, 36,* 1485-1493.

C H A P T E R
57

CONFIDENTIALITY IN PSYCHOTHERAPY

David J. Miller, Ph.D.

E thical considerations continue to pose complex, often contradictory mandates for mental health professionals. Issues such as informed consent, civil commitment, sexual relations between client and therapist, and the confidentiality of information discussed in the context of therapy continue to be subjects of much professional debate.

Issues related to the confidentiality of information obtained in the context of therapy permeate our professional lives. Such issues arise every time a client enters treatment; whenever homicide, suicide, or child abuse is involved; and every time a call is received from a family member or insurance company requesting information. It is not surprising that confidentiality was a consideration even in the early days of psychotherapeutic intervention. Freud, for example, struggled with the issue when documenting case histories:

> If the distortions [of relevant material] are slight, they fail in their object of protecting the patient from indiscreet curiosity, while if they go beyond this they require too great a sacrifice. . . . It is far easier to divulge the patient's most intimate secrets than the most innocent and trivial facts about him, for, whereas the former would not throw any light on his identity, the latter by which he is generally recognized would make it obvious to everyone. (Freud, 1963)

The following review will explore issues related to confidentiality in psychotherapy, including the relevance of moral philosophy to clinical decision making about confidentiality, the interface between legal and ethical considerations, current research, and applied considerations for the individual practitioner. Most of the information in this chapter is for the individual private practitioner and does not specifically address the concerns of professionals working in institutional settings (e.g., maintenance of records in large decentralized computer data bases). Because few persons would maintain that "gossip" or "story telling" at parties or informal nonprofessional gatherings is justifiable (although it happens more than professionals would care to admit), this discussion of confidentiality is limited situations that arise within the professional psychotherapeutic context.

For the purposes of this paper, confidentiality consists of the *ethical* obligation that protects clients from unauthorized disclosures of information that are given in the confidence that they will not be divulged to others. Privileged communication, on the other hand, involved *legal* considerations and enables a patient to bar a court from compelling the therapist to disclose information about him or her.

PHILOSOPHICAL ISSUES

Historically, the professional's duty to keep information confidential has never been an absolute principle. When Hippocrates urged medical secrecy, he and his followers were in a minority. Nonethtless, according to the Hippocratic oath the physician pledges, "Whatsoever I see or hear in the course of my profession in my intercourse with men, if it be what should not be published abroad, I will never divulge, holding such things to be holy secrets." However, as with most ethical codes, the oath helps little in deciding when and to whom physicians should reveal information because the proscription gives no specific criteria for determining "what should" be spoken. In fact, during the Roman Empire and Middle Ages, physicians freely disclosed information about patients. During the 16th century, however, the role of the physician more closely approximated that of the priest as the concept of confessional secrecy spread throughout the Catholic countries (Slovenko, 1973). Since then, the necessity for "secrecy" of information revealed in a therapeutic setting has been the predominant attitude of the medical/psychotherapeutic community.

Ethical theories provide a set of principles to be used for the assessment of what is morally "right" or "wrong" with regard to human action. Psychotherapists (through their own internalized set of moral beliefs) as well as professional organizations (through their ethical guidelines) use ethical theories to justify the adoption of particular positions. Such ethical theories are usually classified as teleologic or deontologic.

From a teleological perspective, no class of actions (e.g., the taking of human lives) is viewed, in and of itself, as morally right or wrong. It is the *consequences* (direct or indirect) resulting from an action that determine whether a given action is morally correct. The teleological ethical theory that has received the most prominence in biomedical ethics is known as "utilitarianism." A deontological position, on the other hand, mandates that morally correct behavior is not exclusively (and in the extreme case, not at all) a function of the consequences of an action. Therefore, a class of behaviors would be viewed as morally right or wrong *independently* of the consequences of those behaviors. After professionals clarify their own moral positions on ethical issues such as confidentiality, a second decision must be entertained: whether to tell the patient of the therapist's position.

Applied Philosophical Positions

If one maintains that confidentiality should not be broken under *any* circumstance, justification may come through a deontological stance that posits that the confidentiality of the communications in the psychotherapeutic setting is sacrosanct and the interpersonal relationship that psychotherapy fosters must not be broken. Philosopher Benjamin Freedman (1978) defends the principle of psychotherapeutic confidentiality by viewing it as a corollary to the preeminent moral position of *primum non nocere*. He claims the following:

> Society ought to, and does grant freedom to those with fanatical adherence to an ideal. We recognize that not all of us have the same moral tasks, that some values are especially dear to some of us. When the value is attached to a profession of great worth to society, the recognition is yet more clear. By our desire that physicians [and psychotherapists] be zealots for health, we must allow its corolarries.

Thus, his assumption is that psychotherapy is an endeavor of "great worth" to society and that society must allow psychotherapists, as "zealots," the privilege of totally confidential communications. There are those who support the same position through a utilitarian view that maintains that the therapeutic relationship must be preserved even in specific situations that may indicate breaking the confidential relationship (e.g., potential suicide). The potentially negative consequences of breaking confidentiality (e.g., individuals in society come to fear psychotherapeutic disclosures to commitment officers or police) are such that under no circumstance must confidentiality be broken. Also, arguments regarding the necessity of confidentiality in psychotherapy are often made from a position that is ultimately utilitarian in nature (i.,e., that confidentiality in psychotherapy promotes other "desirable goals" such as participation in psychotherapy).

Nonetheless, many clinicians justify breaking confidential communications under certain circumstances. For example, a deontological position might maintain that certain actions (e.g., suicide) are morally wrong, that individuals attempting such behaviors are not capable of rational decision making, and that as responsible free-willed agents, practitioners must take steps to prevent harmful actions regardless of possible negative ramifications to the therapeutic relationship. Alternatively, a utilitarian might postulate that for the preservation of an "ordered society," certain behaviors (e.g., potential homicide) fall outside the realm of acceptability. Therefore, professionals must take steps, for the good of all, to reduce the likelihood of negative occurrences.

Sharing With The Client

After the clinician has determined his or her own moral stance regarding potential limitations to confidentiality, a decision must be made regarding whether or not to share this decision with the patient and/or under what circumstances. The question for many clinicians, based upon either teleological or deontological principles, is whether to tell the client, in advance, of the limitations to absolute confidentiality. For example, Siegal (1976) states that "those who work with me in a clinical situation know my position in advance, and know that I will *never* betray a confidence." There are also those who support therapeutic confidentiality and maintain that clients should be directly informed of the legal and ethical limitations, but believe that there are specific limitations to the mandate of absolute confidentiality. For example, Everstine et al. (1980) state:

> When in doubt, provide your client with information; this is the "informed" aspect of informed consent and implies that almost any kind of

information concerning the nature of therapy and the therapeutic experience, provided to the client in advance, can be beneficial.

Educating the client about the limitations fo confidentiality prior to the initiation of therapy is seen as critical. As these authors state, the duty to warn "implies an obligation to warn a client that such a duty exists; it is only fair to let your client know, in advance, that certain statements are inadmissible to therapy. This means that once uttered, such a statement will cause at least temporary interruption in the therapeutic process." Nonetheless, it is implied that the therapeutic relationship can continue despite the limitations delineated and may indeed benefit from addressing the issues. However, Robert Langs (1982) believes that in some instances exceptions to confidentiality should not be openly discussed or focused upon. For example, in a clinic setting where exceptions to confidentiality are "apparent" to the patient, "the therapist should accept these realizations implicitly, without direct confirmation to the patient, because direct revelation of the existence of these alterations in the frame tend to be highly disruptive to the patient and the therapeutic experience" (p. 476). When supervision of a case is necessitated, "it is best...not to directly reveal this deviation to the patient" (p. 478).

It is clear that clinicians and philosophers utilize a variety of ethical theories to support their particular positions regarding confidentiality. Given the current state of disarray in philosophical discussions regarding confidentiality, it appears that individuals can justify (or perhaps rationalize) many apparently discrpant moral positions. While ethical guidelines often note exceptions to the general principle supporting confidential communications (e.g., imminent dangerousness), individual practitioners disagree about the moral correctness of any disclosures. Given this less than desirable state of affairs, one must ask whether there exists any empirical evidence that can clarify the situation or support any of these positions.

CURRENT RESEARCH

Psychotherapists' Knowledge
Of Legal/Ethical Issues

Practitioners in the mental health professions have been criticized for possessing less than adequate knowledge of their legal and ethical obligations (Keith-Spiegel, 1977). Unfortunately, empirical evidence indicates that these appraisals may be accurate. For example, Tancredi and Clark (1972) found that admissions personnel in a mental health center were basically ignorant of patients' rights, including those rights that would be decisive in whether patients would remain incarcerated or be let free. Jagim et al. (1978) surveyed mental health professionals in North Dakota and found support for the importance of confidentiality in the therapeutic relationship. However, the results showed a wide variation in the respondents' knowledge regarding privileged communication, suggesting that the legal implications of privilege statutes are blurred in the minds of many mental health practitioners. Finally, Swoboda et al. (1978) reported that a significant proportion of psychologists, psychiatrists, and social workers were unaware of laws related to privileged communication and the required reporting of child abuse.

Psychotherapists' Attitudes About Confidentiality

Jagim et al. (1978) found that mental health professionals (e.g., psychologists, psychiatrists, and social workers) agreed that confidentiality was an integral aspect of the therapeutic relationship. Confidentiality was seen as essential in maintaining a functioning therapeutic relationship by 98 percent of the professionals. Additionally, 98 percent felt a professional obligation to keep information about a client confidential. However, Jagim et al. also found that a majority of their respondents would "break" confidentiality under certain circumstances (e.g., danger to third parties and/or statutory requirements to disclose information). Swoboda et al. (1978) found that 87 percent of mental health practitioners who were aware of the reporting requirement still refused to comply in a hypothetical case.

While much attention has been given to external pressures (e.g., legal statutes) that threaten confidentiality, Faustman (1982) found that 60.8 percent of professional psychologists have not maintained a position of absolute confidentiality by virtue of their use of collection agencies to receive compensation for their services. Only 48.9 percent of those psychologists using collection agencies had informed their clients regarding the limitations to confidentiality.

Studies Of Patients/Clients

It has been maintained that the reason for confidentiality in social research and psychotherapeutic practice is the "social injury" that might occur if the information discussed were not confidential.

Studies conducted in the 1960s indicated that some outpatients were not concerned about the issue of confidentiality. More recently, however, studies have documented that individuals considering psychotherapeutic contact are indeed aware of and concerned about the issue of confidentiality. For example, Lindenthal and Thomas (1982) questioned 76 psychiatric patients who had been in psychotherapy for at least 3 months. Twenty-two percent of the sample stated that fear of disclosure had held them back from seeking psychotherapy initially. They also found that, compared with a sample of psychiatrists, patients significantly overestimated the likelihood that psychiatrists would break confidentiality in particular situations. Similarly, 29 percent of a group of psychiatric outpatients had asked their psychiatrists about confidentiality when they began therapy, and 54 percent reported that it was an area of concern (Shuman & Weinger, 1982). Ethical obligations were given by 96 percent of the sample as the reason that the privacy of their communications would be maintained.

Limited research has been conducted on clients' attitudes about "release of information" forms. Rosen (1977) reported that patients refused to authorize disclosures of personally identifiable mental health data to state officials if they were specifically informed that refusal would not jeopardize the availability or quality of treatment. In a subsequent study, all patients (n = 1,620) at a community mental health center who were simply asked to release information to state agencies agreed to do so. However, the clients may have perceived that they had little choice in the matter. Of those who were given an explicit option of refusing disclosure, 65 percent declined to authorize release. The author concludes that mental health clients sign release forms either in habitual obedience or in the belief that signing is a prerequisite for receiving care.

Appelbaum et al. (1984) examined 58 psychiartic outpatients and reported that the subjects

> were quite receptive to their therapists disclosing information when it might aid them (e.g., to a consulting therapist), or at least when it would be unlikely to cause them harm (e.g., to mental health professionals not involved in the case). When breaches might lead to difficulties, however, as with family members and courts, and especially with employers, patients were much more likely to be upset by such behavior. (p. 114)

Also, the majority of outpatients were confident that their therapists would protect their privacy. However, when compared with a group of 30 inpatients who were studied earlier (Schmidt et al., 1983), outpatients were much more aware of their rights and options if breaches should occur (e.g., legal recourse). Additionally, Schmidt at al. found that 95 percent of their sample of inpatient psychiatric patients were upset at the thought of information in their charts being automatically released to third parties; 80 percent of the patients said an assurance of confidentiality improved their relationship with staff; 67 percent said they would be angry or upset if information were released without their permission; and 17 percent said that, in the event that information was released without their permission, they would leave treatment.

In a recent study, 532 subjects from three populations (high school, college, and former outpatients) were given open-ended questions assessing knowledge and attitudes regarding confidentiality (Miller & Thelen, 1986). The study suggests that the general population, independently of previous therapeutic involvement, may have a similar conception of issues germane to the confidential relationship. Beliefs relating to therapeutic communications appear to be established by young adulthood and are similar to those held by older adults. The majority (69 percent) of respondents believed that everything discussed in the context of psychotherapy is considered confidential by psychologists. Additionally, most subjects (76 percent) maintained that there are no exceptions to confidentiality. Only 11 percent of the total population maintained that confidentiality *should* be broken when danger to self or others is a consideration, while 13 percent believed that psychologists feel danger to self or others overrides the mandate requiring confidentiality. For that small percentage of respondents who did *not* believe that all information was considered confidential by psychologists, there existed a fairly even split between the stated rationales. Specifically, there were those who thought that it was in the best interest of the client that certain information not be confidential (e.g., danger to self); those who felt that psychologists had an obligation to others for viewing certain information as nonconfidential (e.g., potential homicide); and finally, those who thought that anonymous information was not viewed as confidential by psychologists. All subjects responded to a hypothetical situation as if they were clients (for those who had been clients this was only a matter of reflection). The majority (56 percent) of that subgroup of subjects who did not believe that all was considered confidential by the psychologist felt that issues related to the client (e.g., so the client can be helped) were sufficient reasons for disclosure of certain information. Nearly all (96 percent) of the subjects desired to be apprised of information pertaining to confidentiality. Of note, the greatest single percentage (47 percent) desired to be told of the exceptions to confidentiality *before* the first session, while the second largest group desired discussions at various points throughout the therapeutic process. Finally, while subjects desired to be told of the limitations to confidentiality, the majority (54 percent) felt that they would experience a "negative" reaction from such information (e.g., discontinue therapy or not speak of topics that are not confidential). The vast majority (73 percent) of respondents believed that psychologists are ethically ogligated to uphold confidentiality because the mandate is critical for the development of the therapeutic relationship.

Overall, the research with clinical populations is sparse and limited in scope. However, it does offer some information about clients' reactions to possible breaches of confidentiality. First, the research to date suggests that most clients assume that information conveyed in therapy is confidential and, if informed of potential limitations, may have negative reactions. Second, clients may comply with a request to release confidential information only because they assume that they have no option to refuse. When clients are informed that they may refuse, many do so. Third, several recent studies suggest that clients are upset or inhibited at the prospect that certain material would not be confidential. Nonetheless, when philosophers and clinicians look to empirical evidence they will find, at most, general trends without specific direction. After examining discrepant philosophical positions, vague professional ethical guidelines, and limited empirical evidence, one may have a tendency to look to the courts for guidance—if for no other reason than to facilitate a perceived reduction in ambiguity.

LEGAL CONSIDERATIONS

Rooted in ecclesiastical courts, which held that the "truth will be discovered" by ordeal or combat, the Anglo-Saxon system justified the legal demand for access to all information on the basis that, if this were not the case, justice would not be served. In one of the first English legal rulings, the court decreed that the "king had a right to know" any information possessed by his subjects. Working within this framework, an Anglo-Saxon law in 1776 forced a physician, Dr. Hawkins, to testify against the Duchess of Kinston in a suit involving bigamy (Slovenko, 1973). Within the U.S. legal system, Wigmore (1961) quotes from the Massachusetts Constitution of 1788 regarding privileged communications between patient and physician:

> This inconvenience which he may suffer, in consequence of his testi-
> mony, by way of enmity, or disgrace, or ridicule or by other disfavoring
> action by fellow members in the community is also a contribution which
> he makes in payment of his duties to society in its function of executing
> justice. (p. 818)

Hence, a general principle of law is that the courts have a right to every person's testimony. There are, however, some justifiable exceptions. Wigmore's
authoritative view on the subject lists four criteria for the establishment of
a privilege: (1) the communications must originate in a confidence that they
will not be disclosed; (2) the communications must be essential to the full and
satisfactory maintenance of the relationship; (3) the relationship must be one
that, in the opinion of the community, ought to be fostered; and (4) the injury that would "inure" to the relationship by the disclosure of the communication must be greater than the benefit thus gained by the correct disposal
of litigation.

The concept of privileged communications is based on the theory that
public release of certain information restricts the open and necessary communication between professionals and their clients. Presumably, the value of
full disclosure between the two parties outweighs the potential benefit to
justice that would occur if testimony were required in court. Thus, the legal
impact of privileged communications is, in essence, a restriction on the otherwise required disclosure of information inside the courtroom. Nevertheless,
although statutes exist that "guarantee" privileged communications, the required "duty" to testify is the most prominent attitude of the legal profession
today regarding the "confidentiality" of information given between psychotherapist and client. In fact, Ralph Slovenko (1973) recommends that therapists
also be clergy in order to guarantee complete confidentiality.

Finally, statutory mandates regarding the required reporting of child abuse
or recent court decisions requiring the warning of endangered third parties
(e.g., *Tarasoff*) interact with the "confidentiality" of the therapeutic relationship. As we saw earlier, clinicians give mixed messages about what they believe
and what they would do in any given situation (Jagim et al., 1978; Swoboda
et al., 1978). Additionally, there exists great variation between states on specific
mandates regarding the reporting of child abuse, potential homicide, or potential suicide. It is critical that therapists be aware of what their obligation is
in a given jurisdiction.

DISCUSSION

The judgment of whether to maintain confidentiality is both complex and
confusing. Patricia Keith-Spiegal (1977) echoed the futility of attempting to
set specific standards of professional behavior when she stated the following:

> The APA ethics committee cannot, unfortunately, offer any rules of
> thumb to assist psychologists with this difficult decision because each case
> has its own unique features. What we can say, however, based on our ex-
> perience, is that deliberate disclosure should be made only after the ut-
> most consideration, and psychologists must be able to defend such action.
> (p. 292)

Even if we recognize that our ethical codes specify exceptions to confidentiality, radical differences exist regarding the pragmatics of whether we should openly discuss the issue with clients. If the issue of confidentiality is not discussed, clients may act on incorrect assumptions about the therapist's position on this matter. At present, if the issue is discussed, the effects remain relatively unknown. It may be that only after we determine the specific effects of limiting confidentiality can potential societal gain be weighed against the cost to the therapeutic effort.

As a result of litigation in the courts, there has been increased attention to the issues of confidentiality and privileged communications by the legal profession. Unfortunately, the ramifications of court decisions or statutory law and the ethical responsibilities of therapists may be at odds. One reason for this potential conflict is that ethical and legal statements have differing conceptual bases and pragmatic implications (Schwitzgebel & Schwitzgebel, 1980). As noted earlier, most ethical codes consist of statements that are "guidelines" for minimal standards of conduct within a profession. Frequently, ethical proposals speak of "rights," "duties," "intentions," responsibilities," etc., all of which are based on a subjective, moral sense of current attitudes or behavior. Thus, they rarely provide specific guidance to either practitioners or clients. However, Associate U.S. Supreme Court Justice Oliver Wendell Holmes advised that if an individual wishes to understand the law, he or she must examine it as does an immoral man who cares only for material consequences and not about the "vaguer sanctions of conscience" (Holmes, 1921). If psychotherapists are to maintain the therapeutic "privilege," it will be because of "amoral," not "immoral," research that documents the negative effects of limited confidentiality.

Widiger and Rorer (1984) provide an excellent illumination of the fact that "the torment [of ethical decisions] is greater than has been acknowledged, because it is not possible to have a single set of ethical principles that is consistent with currently extant therapeutic [or philosophic] orientations" (p. 513). They go on to suggest the following:

> [If] some relativism is unavoidable, then a possible solution would be to require each therapist to formulate and to leave on file with a designated ethics committee a set of principles that would be made available to each prospective client. Each therapist's action would be judged according to his or her set of ethical principles. (p. 513)

Until there is greater clarification (both empirical and philosophical) of these issues, one possible solution is for each mental health professional to submit a set of ethical principles to a designated committed and let the *committee* decide whether or not one's positions are acceptable for membership in a given organization. Individual organizations would then have to determine whether therapists must disclose ethical positions with patients.

Ethical issues such as these are affectively laden and theoretically complex, have vaguely formulated questions, and as of yet, show little in the form of conventional, "scientific" answers. Hence, it is of no surprise that precious little systematic attention has been given to the issue of confidentiality. While acknowledging inherent difficulties, mental health professionals must continue efforts to increase the clarity and breadth of knowledge in this area. The topic has affected and will continue to affect how clinicians conduct their day to day functions, as well as what messages they send to society about their professional obligations regarding the ethical aspects of psychotherapy.

REFERENCES

Appelbaum, P.S., Kapen, G., Walters, B., Lidz, D., & Roth, L.H. (1984). Confidentiality: An empirical test of the utilitarian perspective. *Bulletin of the Academy of Psychiatry and the Law, 12,* 109–116.

Everstine, L., Everstine, D., Heyman, G., True, R., Frey, D., Johnson, H., & Seiden, R. (1980). Privacy and confidencitality in psychotherapy. *American Psychologist, 35,* 828–840, 1980.

Faustman, W.O. (1982). Legal and ethical issues in debt collection strategies of professional psychologists. *Professional Psychology, 13,* 208–214.

Freedman, B. (1978). A meta-analysis for professional morality. *Ethics, 89,* 1–19.

Freud, S. (1963). *Three case histories.* New York: Collier.

Holmes, O.W. (1921). *Collected legal papers.* New York: Harcourt Brace Jovanovich.

Jagim, R.D., Wittman, W.D., & Noll, J.O. (1978). Mental health professionals' attitudes toward confidentiality, privilege, and third party disclosure. *Professional Psychology, 9,* 458–466.

Keith-Spiegel, P. (1977). Violations of ethical principles due to ignorance or poor professional judgement versus willful disregard. *Professional Psychology, 8,* 288–296.

Langs, R. (1982). *Psychotherapy: A basic text.* New York: Jason Aronson.

Lindenthal, J.J., & Thomas, C.S. (1982). Psychiatrists, the public and confidentiality. *Journal of Nervous and Mental Disease, 170,* 319–323.

Miller, D.J., & Thelen, M.J. (1986). Confidentiality in psychotherapy: Knowledge and beliefs about confidentiality. *Professional Psychology: Research and Practice, 17,* 15–19.

Rosen, C.E. (1977). Why clients relinquish their rights to privacy under sign-away pressures. *Professional Psychology, 8,* 17–24.

Schmidt, D., Appelbaum, P.S., Roth, L.H., & Lidz, C. (1983). Confidentiality in psychiatry: A study of the patient's view. *Hospital and Community Psychiatry, 34,* 353–355.

Rosen, C.E. (1977). Why clients relinquish their rights to privacy under sign-away pressures. *Professional Psychology, 8,* 17–24.

Schmidt, D., Appelbaum, P.S., Roth, L.H., & Lidz, C. (1983). Confidentiality in psychiatry: A study of the patient's view. *Hospital and Community Psychiatry, 34,* 353–355.

Schwitzgebel, R.L., & Schwitzgebel, R.K. (1980). *Law and psychological practice.* New York: Wiley.

Shuman, D.W., & Weinger, M.F. (1982). The privilege study: An empirical examination of the psychotherapist-patient privilege. *North Carolina Law Review, 60,* 893–942.

Siegel, M. (1976). Confidentiality. *The Clinical Psychologist, 30*(1), 23.

Siovenko, R. (1973). *Psychiatry and the law.* Boston: Little, Brown.

Swoboda, J.S., Elwork, A., Sales, B.D., & Levine, D. (1978). Knowledge of and compliance with privileged communication and child-abuse-reporting laws. *Professional Psychology, 9,* 448–457.

Tancredi, L., & Clark, D.C. (1972), Psychiatry and the legal rights of patients. *American Journal of Psychiatry, 129,* 104–106.

Widiger, T.A., & Rorer, L.G. (1984). The responsible psychotherapist. *The American Psychologist, 39,* 503–515.

Wigmore, J.H. (1961). *Evidence in trials at common law* (Vol. 8, McNaughton Revision). Boston: Little, Brown.

C H A P T E R
58

THERAPIST-PATIENT SEXUAL CONTACT: CLINICAL, LEGAL, AND ETHICAL IMPLICATIONS

Kenneth S. Pope, Ph.D.

The phenomenon of therapist–patient sexual contact affects every private practitioner in one way or another. It is the major basis of complaints against clinicians before state licensing boards, courts, and professional ethics committees (Pope, 1989). As the extent of this practice and its consequential damages becomes known, the public attitude toward mental health professionals becomes more cynical, and people needing help are less willing to trust practitioners.

As the mental health professions have failed to take effective action to clean their own houses in this regard, the courts and other external regulatory bodies have intruded more and more into the professional lives of clinicians. Because of the abuses of some practitioners, all clinicians have become subject to a growing complexity of legislation, case laws, regulations, standards, guidelines, and criteria for professional liability insurance coverage. Currently, professional liability policies for the major mental health professions either exclude or severely limit coverage in the area of sexual relations with patients. This change in coverage was necessary to prevent even more drastic increases in premiums, which were needed to pay off the settlements and court awards — some for several million dollars — related to therapist–patient sexual intimacy claims.

Furthermore, the research suggests that virtually any clinician is likely to encounter patients who have been sexually intimate with a former therapist (Pope & Bouhoutsos, 1986). In order to meet the highest legal and ethical standards of care, practitioners must therefore be able to identify and to assess adequately the clinical sequelae of this prior involvement, and to provide — either firsthand or through referral — a comprehensive treatment approach.

In summary, therapist–patient sexual intimacy is a phenomenon with consequences and implications for all private practitioners. We can no longer avoid or minimize the topic. It is important for every clinician to become knowledgeable in this area.

Table 58-1.
Percentages of Professionals Reporting
Sexual Involvement with Patients

Publi-cation	Profession	Reference	Location	Return Rate (%)	Male (%)	Female (%)
1968	Psychologists	(Forer, 1980)	L.A. County	70	13.7	0
1973	Psychiatrists	(Kardiner et al., 1973)	L.A. County	46	10.0	N/A
1976	Psychiatrists	(Perry, 1976)	CA & NY	33	N/A	0
1977	Psychologists	(Holroyd & Brodsky, 1977)	National	70	12.1	2.6
1979	Psychologists	(Pope et al., 1979)	National	48	12.0	3.0
1986	Psychiatrists	(Gartrell et el., 1986)	National	26	7.1	3.1
1986	Psychologists	(Pope et al., 1986)	National	59	9.4	2.5
1987	Psychologists	(Pope et al., 1987)	National	46	3.6	0.5

Source: Adapted from Pope and Bouhoutsos (1986) with permission.

THERAPISTS WHO SEXUALLY ABUSE PATIENTS

While malpractice, licensing, and ethics complaints concerning therapist–patient sexual intimacy have shown dramatic increases in recent years, such complaints probably underrepresent the problem. The research tends to suggest that such formal complaints account for only about 4 percent of the instances in which therapist–patient sexual intimacy occurs.

Anonymous self-report surveys have attempted to provide better estimates of the prevalence of sexual involvement with patients. Table 1 summarizes the findings of these studies for psychiatrists and psychologists.

First, male therapists become sexually intimate with their patients at significantly higher rates than female therapists. Second, the recidivism rate is high: about 80 percent of such therapists repeat the involvement with more than one patient (Holroyd & Brodsky, 1977; Pope & Bouhoutsos, 1986). Third, in a substantial number of cases, therapists become sexually intimate with minor clients, some as young as 3 (Bajt & Pope, 1989). Fourth, nonsexual dual relationships, while unethical and harmful per se, foster sexual dual relationships. A study of 4,200 clinicians found that 78 percent of those who reported engaging in nonsexual dual relationships later engaged in sexual dual relationships (Borys, 1988; see also Ethics Committee, 1988). Fifth, therapists who become sexually intimate with their patients share significant similarities with both those who engage in incest with children and those who rape (Pope, 1989a). Sixth, individuals who, as students, engaged in sexual intimacies with their professors are later, as therapists, significantly more likely to engage in sexual intimacies with their patients (Pope, Levenson, & Schover, 1979).

THE FUNDAMENTAL PROHIBITION

The most important statement this chapter can make to any private practitioner is to avoid any and all sexual intimacies with patients. No matter what the patient says or does or thinks or wants or hopes. No matter what the situation is. No matter what.

This fundamental prohibition against sexual intimacies with patients can be traced back at least as far as the Hippocratic oath. It is now clearly and explicitly stated in the formal ethics codes of every major mental health profession.

The courts have affirmed the authority of state licensing boards to revoke the license of a clinician who engages in sex with a patient. As mentioned earlier, therapist–patient sex is becoming or has become the major focus of malpractice suits against clinicians, and thus is firmly established as part of case law. Moreover, at least 15 states have passed legislation making therapist–patient sex illegal, so that expert testimony is no longer needed to establish the fact that such behavior violates the standard of care (Pope, 1986b).

Legal actions taken against therapists who engage in sex with their patients may be not only civil (malpractice) and administrative in nature but also criminal. Masters and Johnson urged that any health care professional engaging in sexual intercourse with a patient be charged with rape (Masters & Johnson, 1976). A number of states have enacted legislation making therapist–patient sexual intimacy a felony.

These ethical and legal prohibitions have been established in light of the often devastating consequences of therapist–patient sex for the patient. Taken en masses, the research studies establish beyond doubt the harmful nature of this phenomenon (Pope & Bouhoutsos, 1986; Ethics Committee, 1988).

Clinicians who wish to be most careful in protecting their patients from harm and in minimizing legal liability should avoid attempting to use termination as a justification for later sexual intimacies with a patient (Pope & Bouhoutsos, 1986; Gabbard & Pope, 1989). Research, theory, or expert testimony justifying posttermination sexual liaisons with patients is difficult to locate. Indications that such behavior violates the standards of care, on the other hand, are prevalent. The authors of the landmark national study of therapist–patient sexual intimacies among psychiatrists review the issue and conclude:

> Neither transference nor the real inequality in the power relationship ends with the termination of the therapy. . . . [P]ragmatic efforts to define a posttermination waiting period, after which sexual relations might be permissible, disregard both the continued inequality of the roles of the therapist and former patient and the timelessness of unconscious processes, including transference. (Herman et al., 1987, p. 168)

Such statements are consistent with a multiyear study of state psychology ethics committees and state psychology licensing boards that found that "psychologists asserting that a sexual relationship had occurred only after the termination of the therapeutic relationship were more likely to be found in violation than those not making that claim" (Sell et al., 1986, p. 504). It is important to note that the cap on coverage concerning therapist–patient sexual intimacies in the professional liability policy provided to members of the American Psychological Association specifies sex with former as well as current clients.

AWARENESS OF RISK

Beyond the commitment simply to observe the fundamental prohibition at all times and under all circumstances, perhaps the most important first step clinicians can take to avoid placing themselves at risk for sexual involvement with patients is to acknowledge, accept, and take into account their own sexual attraction to patients. A national study of this phenomenon indicated that an overwhelming majority (87 percent) of psychologists experienced sexual attraction to at least one patient; that over half found that this attraction made them feel guilty, anxious, or uncomfortable; and that only 9 percent reported that their training or supervision in this area was adequate (Pope et al., 1986). About one in five treated this attraction as an absolute taboo, not mentioning it to anyone else in any context. To the extent that individual therapists treat their own attraction to patients with neglect or even denial, they place themselves at increased risk to act out or otherwise express indirectly—perhaps harmfully—this phenomenon.

The second step clinicians can take to reduce risk is to be knowledgeable about the diverse ways in which therapists become sexually involved with their patients. If they feel themselves to be slipping into one of these roles, they can take immediate and vigorous action to ensure that they deal safely with the slippage. The following chart—taken from *Sexual intimacies between Therapists and Patients* (Pope & Bouhoutsos, 1986) and used with permission—summarizes the 10 most common scenarios of therapist–patient sexual intimacy.

The third step clinicians can take to reduce risk is to conduct a periodic self-evaluation in terms of specific risk factors. The following dozen items were presented by Pope and Bouhoutsos (1986). Examining this list from time to time—especially during periods of great stress or "burnout"—can help ensure that we handle appropriately any risk factors associated with therapist–patient sexual intimacy.

1. Becoming preoccupied with personal problems and devoting large portions of therapy sessions to discussing these problems with a patient

2. Playing "know it all" with a patient: providing authoritative answers to all the patient's questions and becoming angry when challenged or caught in error

3. Telling the patient to engage in certain kinds of sexual behaviors, so that you can derive vicarious enjoyment and feel a sense of control over someone else's sexuality

4. Instructing a patient to refrain from sexual relations or to discontinue certain relationships on the basis of your jealousy

5. Dressing or talking in a seductive manner

6. Telling a patient to dress or talk in a seductive manner

7. Meeting your patient for drinks, dinner, or a "date"

8. Scheduling your patient's session (at night, as the last patient of the day, and so on) on the basis of your sexual attraction rather than on the basis of the patient's clinical needs

9. Discussing sexual issues and material with the patient on the basis of your sexual interests rather than on the basis of the patient's clinical needs

10. Finding yourself sexually attracted to or aroused by the patient without examining this response in light of the treatment dynamics and the appropriate handling of this response

11. Isolating the patient (for example, not referring to a physician for screening medical problems, to a psychologist for psychological and neuropsychological testing, to a colleague for adjunctive treatment or a "second opinion") so that you become the patient's only lifeline and so that any improper activity between you and the patient will more likely go undetected by others

12. Isolating yourself (not seeking out customary consultation, supervision, support, and so on from colleagues regarding your work with a particular patient

Scenario	Criterion
1. Role trading	Therapist becomes the "patient" and the wants and needs of the therapist become the focus
2. Sex therapy	Therapist fraudulently presents therapist-patient sexual intimacy as a valid treatment for sexual and other kinds of difficulties.
3. As if...	Therapist treats positive transference as if it were not the result of the therapeutic situation
4. Svengali	Therapist creates and exploits an exaggerated dependence on the part of the patient
5. Drugs	Therapist uses cocaine, alcohol, or other drugs as part of the seduction
6. Rape	Therapist uses physical force, threats, and/or intimidation
7. True love	Therapist uses rationalizations that attempt to discount the clinical/professional nature of the relationship with its attendant responsibilities
8. It just got out of hand	Therapist fails to treat the emotional closeness that develops in therapy with sufficient attention, care, and respect
9. Time out	Therapist fails to acknowledge and take account of the fact that the therapeutic relationship does not cease to exist between scheduled sessions or outside the therapist's office
10. Hold me	Therapist exploits patient's desire for nonerotic physical contact and possible confusion between erotic and nonerotic contact

Fourth and finally, clinicians who feel that they are at considerable risk for engaging in sexual intimacies with a patient would do well to seek professional help. Personal therapy may help them to explore, understand, and handle safely unresolved issues and impulses that—if acted out—would harm a patient. Specific techniques are currently being developed for therapists who identify themselves as being at risk but who have not yet sexually abused a patient (Pope, 1987) and for those who have already perpetrated sexual acts (Schoener, 1986; Pope, 1989a & c).

RECOGNIZING THERAPIST–PATIENT SEX SYNDROME

As stated earlier, in light of the statistical likelihood that any private practitioner will encounter patients who have been sexually intimate with a former therapist, it is important for practitioners to be able to identify and assess adequately the destructive sequelae of such involvements. Negligence in the assessment and treatment of this specialized area is no more excusable—ethically, legally, or otherwise— than it would be in such other specialized areas as the sequelae of rape, incest, or child battering.

The sequelae of therapist–patient sexual involvement may form a distinct clinical syndrome for the patient, with possible acute, chronic, and delayed aspects. Therapist–patient sex syndrome (Pope, 1985, 1986a, 1988) includes 10 major aspects.

First, the patient tends to experience a persistent *ambivalence*. This phenomenon is similar to aspects of child abuse in which the abused child may—virtually simultaneously—seek to both cling to and flee from the abusing parent. This ambivalence is an understandably agonizing experience for the patient. It is frequently a demoralizing force in the subsequent therapy: Just when the patient (after perhaps months or years of work) begins to achieve a sense of autonomy, perspective, and distance from the prior, abusing therapist, he or she suddenly returns (psychologically if not literally) to the prior therapist. This process may be repeated numerous times. It may make the patient—and in some cases the therapist also—feel as if all intervening therapeutic work has been lost.

The ambivalence also constitutes an often insurmountable obstacle to the patient's careful consideration and pursuit of formal complaints against the prior therapist. Unfortunately, by the time the ambivalence has been sufficiently worked through, the statutes of limitations may have run in the various arenas. Even if formal complaints are still possible, the patient must contend with the question, "Why did you wait so long in filing this complaint?"

Second, the patient may experience a sense of *emptiness and isolation,* in which there is a lack of feeling related—in a fulfilling way—either to oneself or to the external world. The emptiness is often described as a hollowness that only the prior therapist could fill up. It is as if there is no self without the boundary-blurring connection with the therapist. The sense of isolation is similar to that experienced by many survivors of rape, incest, and child or spouse battering. Whatever the patient may or may not understand on a cognitive level, the feeling is that this catastrophic event is unique, a singular horror with one sole victim. The patient feels that he or she is absolutely alone in the universe.

Third, the patient frequently experiences *sexual confusion.* The patient may have originally sought therapy for a sexual problem, or the abusing therapist may have defined — in however farfetched a manner — the presenting problem as a sexual one, or at least one requiring a sexual treatment. In any event, the smokescreen of jargon, confused concepts, denial, and distortions that the therapist must use to justify to the patient the sexual contact often leaves the patient extremely confused about his or her own sexual nature, desires, and activities.

Fourth, the patient tends to experience a profound and persistent sense of *guilt.* Again, therapist–patient sex syndrome shows its similarities in this regard to rape trauma syndrome, reaction to incest, and the sequelae of child or spouse battering. In the same way that a rape survivor — regardless of the circumstances of the rape — may experience a deep guilt (e.g., "If I only would have dressed differently," "If I only would've taken a different route home," or "Why didn't I try to fight him more?"), the patient who has been sexually intimate with a therapist will tend to blame himself or herself despite the fact that it is always and without exception the therapist's responsibility to avoid sexual contact with a patient. Even when the patient intellectually understands transference, appreciates the fact that patients may say and do a wide variety of things in the course of therapy, and acknowledges that he or she knows that therapists are prohibited by law from engaging in such destructive acts, there is still the feeling that the patient is the cause of the problem.

Unfortunately, this understandable but irrational sense of guilt is sometimes aggravated by insensitive subsequent therapists, attorneys, or "friends" who tell the individual that the therapist–patient sexual intimacy (or the rape, or the incest, or the battering) was the fault of the victim. The principle that must be understood by patients and therapists alike is that no behavior on the part of the patient (e.g., seductive clothing, a direct proposition) justifies a therapist's sexual involvement with that patient just as no seductive or provocative behavior on the part of a child justifies incest, no activity of any kind on the part of an adult justifies rape, and no so-called misbehavior on the part of a child or spouse justifies child or spouse battering.

The guilt may also make the patient treat the subject as "taboo," even if the prior therapist–patient sexual involvement is dominating his or her life. The patient may be ashamed of the involvement — just as many rape, incest, and battering survivors are ashamed of their victimization. In all such areas, the clinician must be knowledgeable, careful, and conscientious in conducting a comprehensive evaluation while remaining respectful of and sensitive to the patient's feelings.

Fifth, the patient tends to experience an *impaired ability to trust.* This reaction is understandable. The patient has put his or her trust in the hands of a professional clinician, and has likely developed the customary feelings of dependence and transference. When the therapist violates this deep and vulnerable trust, the very ability to trust is injured. Consequently, individuals who have been sexually intimate with therapists may avoid any future contact with therapists. In any event, the issue of trust is likely to be a focus of any subsequent therapy.

Sixth, there is frequently an *inversion of tasks or roles.* In the sexualized therapy, the patient often becomes the "therapist" of the nominal therapist, just as in many families fostering child sexual abuse, the children become the "parents" of their nominal parents, attempting to take care of them not only sexually but in other ways as well. In some cases this inversion becomes the focus of the sexualized therapy, as in the role-trading scenario mentioned earlier in this chapter.

Seventh, there may be intense *emotional liability.* The inability to maintain a moderated emotional tone may be as much a source of demoralization during the subsequent therapy as the ambivalence mentioned previously.

Eighth, the patient may during the course of the subsequent therapy become aware of *suppressed rage.* This reaction is likewise similar to the blocked rage felt by many survivors of incest, rape, and battering.

Therapists who become sexually involved with their patients generally dissuade their patients from expressing any anger toward them. The therapist tends to assume a virtually omnipotent, omniscient, and infallible stance, and thus is beyond criticism, let alone anger. In some cases the therapist may use threats or actual physical force to intimidate the patient from expressing anger. In other cases the therapist may use psychological manipulations, such as, "Here I am doing all this good for you—virtually saving your life—and you have the gall to get angry at me!," "I'm well educated and very intelligent and you know very little, so don't you dare question my words or behavior!," or "If you want to cause me any trouble at all, then I'll throw you out of here and never see you again."

The sexually exploitive therapist who is aware of legal liability may also threaten to kill the patient (or a relative of the patient) should he or she report the sexual contact to any third party, or may convince the patient that no one will believe him or her (i.e., it will be a "crazy" patient's word against the word of a prestigious therapist). Thus the patient may have to contend with a variety of barriers to the awareness, understanding, and expression of the suppressed rage.

Ninth, there tends to be an *increased suicidal risk.* This vulnerability to self-destructiveness may be related to the suppressed rage.

Tenth, the patient tends to experience *cognitive dysfunction,* especially in the areas of attention and concentration, often involving intrusive thoughts, unbidden images, nightmares, and flashbacks. The unwanted cognitions often have an "as if it were happening now" quality. In this aspect, therapist–patient sex syndrome bears similarities to post-traumatic stress disorder.

Conducting an assessment to identify and assess therapist–patient sex syndrome is an initial responsibility of a clinician working with a patient who has been sexually involved with a previous therapist. If the involvement with the prior therapist and destructive sequelae are identified, specialized treatment should be implemented. Approaches to treatment of patients who have been sexually involved with a prior therapist have recently been evolving (Pope, 1985, 1986a; Pope & Bouhoutsos, 1986; Sonne, 1987).

CONCLUSION

This chapter has attempted to summarize for the independent practitioner some essential information about therapist–patient sexual intimacy, a phenomenon with implications for all therapists. Practitioners need to understand and be alert to the factors that may put them at increased risk for engaging in sex with a patient, and need to accept and handle carefully any sexual attraction they may feel toward patients. Practitioners are likely to encounter patients who have been sexually involved with a prior therapist, and must meet the ethical and legal standards of care by assessing the consequent damage and developing an adequate treatment plan. Most important, practitioners must observe without exception the fundamental prohibition against sexual intimacies with patients.

REFERENCES

Bajt, T.R., & Pope, K.S. (1989). Therapist-patient sexual intimacy involving children and adolescents. *American Psychologist, 44,* 455.

Borys, D.S. (1988). *Dual relationships between therapist and client: A national survey of clinicians' attitudes and practices.* Unpublished doctoral dissertation, University of California, Los Angeles.

Ethics Committee of the American Psychological Association. (1988). Trends in ethics cases, common pitfalls, and published resources. *American Psychologist, 43,* 564–572.

Forer, B. (1980). The therapeutic relationship: 1968. Paper presented at the annual convention of the California State Psychological Association, Pasadena, CA.

Gabbard, G.O., & Pope, K.S. (1989). Sexual intimacies with patients after termination: Legal, ethical, and clinical aspects. In G.O. Gabbard (Ed.), *Sexual exploitation in professional relationships.* Washington, D.C.: American Psychiatric Press.

Gartrell, N., Herman, J., Olarte, S., Feldstein, M., & Localio, R. (1986). Psychiatrist–patient sexual contact: Results of a national survey. I: Prevalence. *American Journal of Psychiatry, 143,* 1126–1131.

Holroyd, J.C., & Brodsky, A.N. (1977). Psychologists' attitudes and practices regarding erotic and nonerotic physical contact with patients. *American Psychologist, 32,* 843–840.

Herman, J.L., Gartrell, N., Olarte, S., Feldstein, M., & Localio, R. (1987). Psychiatrist–patient sexual contact: Results of a national survey. II: Psychiatrists' attitudes. *American Journal of Psychiatry, 144,* 164–169.

Kardiner, S., Fuller, M., & Mensch, I. (1973). A survey of physicians' attitudes and practices regarding erotic and nonerotic contact with patients. *American Journal of Psychiatry, 130,* 1088–1081.

Masters, W.H., & Johnson, V.E. (1976). Principles of the new sex therapy. *American Journal of Psychiatry, 133,* 548–554.

Perry, J.A. (1976). Physicians' erotic and nonerotic involvement with patients. *American Journal of Psychiatry, 133,* 838–840.

Pope, K.S. (1985). Diagnosis and treatment of therapist–patient sex syndrome. Paper presented to the annual convention of the American Psychological Association, Los Angeles, August, 1985.

Pope, K.S. (1986a). Therapist–patient sex syndrome: Research findings. Paper presented to the annual convention of the American Psychiatric Association, Washington, D.C., May, 1986.

Pope, K.S. (1986b). Research and laws regarding therapist–patient sexual involvement: Implications for therapists. *American Journal of Psychotherapy, 40,* 564–571.

Pope, K.S. (1987). Preventing therapist–patient sexual intimacy: Therapy for a therapist at risk. *Professional Psychology: Research and Practice, 18,* 624–628.

Pope, K.S. (1988). How clients are harmed by sexual contact with mental health professionals: The syndrome and its prevalence. *Journal of Counseling and Development, 67,* 222–226.

Pope, K.S. (1989a). Identifying and rehabilitating abusive therapists. Paper presented at the annual meeting of the American Psychiatric Association, San Francisco.

Pope, K.S. (1989b). Malpractice suits, licensing disciplinary actions, and ethics cases: Frequencies, causes, and costs. *Independent Practitioner, 9,* 22–26.

Pope, K.S. (1989c). Rehabilitation of therapists who have been sexually intimate with a patient. In G.O. Gabbard (Ed.), *Sexual exploitation in professional relationships.* Washington, D.C.: American Psychiatric Press.

Pope, K.S., & Bouhoutsos, J.C. (1986). *Sexual intimacies between therapists and patients.* Praeger: New York.

Pope, K.S., Keith-Spiegel, P.C., & Tabachnick, B. (1986). Sexual attraction to clients: The human therapist and the (sometimes) inhuman training system. *American Psychologist, 41,* 147–158.

Pope, K.S., Levenson, H., & Schover, L.R. (1979). Sexual intimacy in psychology training: Results and implications of a national survey. *American Psychologist, 34,* 682–689.

Pope, K.S., Tabachnick, B.T., & Keith-Spiegel, P. (1987). Ethics of practice: The beliefs and behaviors of psychologists as therapists. *American Psychologist, 42,* 993–1006.

Schoener, G.R. (1986, September). Assessment and development of rehabilitation plans for the counselor or therapist who has sexually exploited clients. Paper presented to the Sixth National Conference of the National Clearinghouse on Licensure, Enforcement, and Regulation, Denver.

Sell, J.M., Gottlieb, M.C., & Schoenfeld, L. (1986). Ethical considerations of social/romantic relationships with present and former clients. *Professional Psychology: Research and Practice, 17,* 504–508.

Sonne, J.L. (1987). Proscribed sex: Counseling the patient subjected to sexual intimacy by a therapist. *Medical Aspects of Human Sexuality, 16,* 18–23.

C H A P T E R
59

THE POTENTIALLY VIOLENT PATIENT: CLINICAL, ETHICAL, AND LEGAL CONSIDERATIONS

James C. Beck, M.D., Ph.D.

P otentially violent patients raise unique and complex problems for psychiatrists. When psychiatrists fear that violence may occur, their responsibilities may extend not only to the patient but also to potential victims, or even to society at large. The clinical difficulty inherent in managing such patients has been compounded for many psychiatrists by the fear of suit. Typically, psychiatrists are uncertain of what their legal duties are and unaware of how to reconcile potentially conflicting clinical responsibilities and legal duties.

The thesis of this chapter is that legal duties and clinical responsibilities seldom conflict, and that psychiatrists' fears are exaggerated. Knowledge of the law coupled with good clinical judgment should permit the psychiatrist to make decisions that are not only ethically and clinically sound but legally defensible as well.

The plan of this chapter is as follows: First, there is a review of the relevant law. Psychiatrists must understand what the courts have said before they can understand how it relates to clinical practice. Next there is a review of clinical assessment of potential violence and of clinical decision making when the psychiatrist fears violence. Finally, there is a discussion of risk management: how one can protect oneself in the event that a patient should kill or seriously injure another person.

THE CLINICIAN'S DUTY TO PROTECT

Legal Duty Before Tarasoff

At the outset, it is important to distinguish ethical duties from legal ones. If I see a person crossing a busy street apparently about to be hit by a car, I have an ethical duty to shout. If I see someone drowning, I have an ethical duty to try to help. However, I have no legal duty to either potential victim. One person owes a legal duty to another only if there is a special relationship between the two.

The physician–patient relationship is a special relationship, and physicians have long owed legal duties to their patients. However, before *Tarasoff,* this special relationship implied that physicians had only a limited duty to control their patients: to control hospitalized patients and to use due care in deciding on their release. After *Tarasoff,* the legal duty and the therapist's potential liability expanded considerably.

The Tarasoff *Case*

In 1974, the California Supreme Court issued its landmark decision in *Tarasoff* v. *Board of Regents of the University of California.*[1] The court held that the psychotherapist–patient relationship is a special relationship, and that the therapist of an ambulatory patient may have a duty to protect a person whom the patient threatens to harm. The decision dismayed psychotherapists because it greatly expanded their potential liability for the violent actions of their patients.

The facts.   In 1968, a psychologist in a California university health clinic treated a graduate student from India, Prosanjit Poddar, in outpatient psychotherapy. Mr. Poddar had become depressed after another student, Tatiana Tarasoff, had rejected his advances. Mr. Poddar told his therapist that he was thinking about killing Ms. Tarasoff, and the therapist learned from a friend of Mr. Poddar's that he had purchased a gun. Convinced that Mr. Poddar posed a threat to Ms. Tarasoff, the therapist consulted his supervising psychiatrist. They tried, unsuccessfully, to have Mr. Poddar committed. Shortly thereafter, the patient terminated therapy and moved into an apartment with Ms. Tarasoff's brother. Two months later, Mr. Poddar went to Ms. Tarasoff's home and tried to talk with her. When she refused, he first shot her with a pellet gun, and then fatally stabbed her with a butcher knife.

Poddar was convicted of second degree murder and served time in a California prison. He then returned to India. In response to a letter from Alan Stone, M.D., past president of the American Psychiatric Association, Mr. Poddar wrote saying he was happily married.

Ms. Tarasoff's survivors sued, charging the professionals involved with negligence in failing to confine the patient, and in failing to warn Ms. Tarasoff of her peril. A lower court held that the defendants had statutory immunity on the question of failure to confine, and no legal obligation to warn the potential victim. The survivors appealed.

The Opinions.   Following a number of interim court actions, the California Supreme Court held that, on the facts alleged in the case, the psychotherapist had a duty to warn.

> When a doctor or a psychotherapist, in the exercise of his professional skill and knowledge, determines or should determine, that a warning is essential to avert danger arising from the medical or psychological condition of his patient, he incurs a legal obligation to give that warning. (p. 914)

This opinion provoked such an outcry by psychotherapists of all disciplines that the court agreed to rehear the case, and in 1976 the court issued a second opinion.[2] Following the second opinion, the case was settled for an undisclosed amount.

The second opinion agreed with the first, but it contained language that was significantly different. The court said:

> When a therapist determines or pursuant to the standard of his pro-
> fession should determine, that his patient presents a serious danger of
> violence to another, he incurs an obligation to use reasonable care to pro-
> tect the intended victim against such danger. The discharge of this duty
> may require the therapist to take one or more of various steps depending
> upon the nature of the case. Thus it may call for him to warn the intended
> victim or others likely to apprise the intended victim of danger, to notify
> the police, or take whatever steps are reasonably necessary under the cir-
> cumstances. (p. 346)

The first opinion was widely publicized in psychiatric newsletters, so that almost all psychiatrists understood that they had a duty to warn. Relatively few psychiatrists understand that they have a broader duty to protect that requires them to use their professional judgment when they are concerned about potential violence. Some psychiatrists believe they can fulfill their legal duty by giving a warning whenever a patient threatens, but that course of action has its own pitfalls. Most psychiatrists believe they have an ethical duty, independent of the law, to prevent violence (Givelber et al., 1985). The *Tarasoff* court said, however, this ethical duty is also a legal duty.

Recent Court Decisions

The *Tarasoff* decision is legally binding only in California, but courts in more than 20 other jurisdictions have now considered the *Tarasoff* doctrine. The courts have repeatedly been asked to consider whether the *Tarasoff* duty applies when a psychotherapist is treating an outpatient, and whether it, as well as the duty to use due care, applies when a hospitalized patient is released.

Although a few courts have declined to find a *Tarasoff* duty in a particular case, most often courts hold that there is a *Tarasoff* duty, and no court has rejected the *Tarasoff* duty as a valid principle. A few courts have extended the duty to unarmed third parties and to property. Today, *Tarasoff* has become a national standard for psychiatric practice. Every prudent psychiatrist should practice as if *Tarasoff* were the law in his or her jurisdiction, regardless of whether any court has yet said that it is.

In determining whether there is a duty to protect, judges typically focus on two factors: (1) whether the violence was foreseeable and (2) whether the element of control was sufficiently present. Prosser, in a classic legal text, explains foreseeability as follows:

> The test as regards foreseeability is not the balance of probability,
> but the existence, in the situation in hand, of some real likelihood of some
> damage and the likelihood is of such appreciable weight and moment as
> to induce, or which reasonably should induce, action to avoid it on the
> part of a person of reasonably prudent mind. (Prosser et al., 1982, p. 148)

The question of foreseeability has been relatively easy for courts to answer affirmatively when a patient threatens a named victim. When the patient is a threat to a class of persons or to society at large, the question of foreseeability is more difficult. On the question of control, courts have not been consistent. Some courts find that the outpatient therapeutic relationship involves sufficient control to entail a duty; others do not.

Although the wide acceptance of the duty to protect and its expansion to unnamed victims have substantially increased potential liability for therapists, actual liability is rarely found. A recent review found a total of 36 published cases since 1974 that involved the duty to protect (Beck, 1987). Three psychiatrists have been found liable: two state hospital psychiatrists and one in the Veterans Administration. In two of those three cases, the court found that the defendant had also violated the duty to use reasonable care. Except for the absence of due care, there appears to be no clear fact pattern or legal theory distinguishing cases in which courts find *Tarasoff* liability from those in which they do not.

Thirty of these 36 cases involved state hospital psychiatrists, V.A. psychiatrists, or public mental health outpatient facilities and staff. Only six involved psychiatrists in private practice. Five of these six cases were decided in favor of the psychiatrist, and the sixth is currently undecided. Thus, no psychiatrist in private practice has been found to be negligent in a published case involving the duty to protect.

Published cases are those in which the trial court verdict is appealed. Possibly there are many other unpublished cases, in which psychiatrists who have been found liable chose not to appeal, but there is little evidence to suggest this. A recent informal poll of state mental health attorneys revealed no active *Tarasoff* suits involving the state's psychiatrists in 20 states (Beck, 1987). The finding was consistent with two other small surveys of psychiatrists who practice privately (Beck, 1981, 1985), which also failed to find any *Tarasoff* suits.

Case Examples

In *McIntosh* v. *Milano*,[3] a state appeals court held that the *Tarasoff* doctrine applied in New Jersey. Later, a jury found no negligence. The patient, a 16-year-old with a drug problem, who was being treated in outpatient psychotherapy, murdered the plaintiff's daughter with whom he had apparently had a prior sexual relationship. The psychiatrist testified that the patient told him that he had fired a BB gun at a car in which he thought the victim was riding. The psychiatrist also testified that the patient had never expressed any feelings of violence toward the victim, or made any threats to hurt or kill her. Although the psychiatrist failed to predict correctly in the presence of actual danger to the victim, the jury found no negligence.

This case illustrates that the existence of a legal duty does not imply that psychiatrists will always be found liable for violating it whenever someone is injured. After *Tarasoff*, psychiatrists feared that they would be held to a legal standard that was impossible to meet: a standard of accurate prediction of violence. *McIntosh* undercuts therapists' fears that they will be found liable for failing to predict accurately.

In *Heltsley* v. *Votteler*,[4] the plaintiff sued a psychiatrist whose patient struck her with a car. The assailant/patient had separated from her husband, and the plaintiff/victim was dating him. The victim knew that the patient had hit her husband with an iron pipe. Furthermore, the patient had threatened her directly the night before she ran her down. The plaintiff testified that she ignored the patient's threats against her but would have taken them seriously if the psychiatrist had told her to. There was no allegation that the psychiatrist had failed to use due care. The Nebraska court said, "We do not believe the *Tarasoff* rule should be stretched to support a finding of a cause of action against the therapist in these circumstances" (p. 762). This case illustrates that courts usually look realistically at the facts before asserting that a duty exists. Here, since the court found no duty, there is not even the possibility of a finding of negligence for breaching it.

Jablonski v. *U.S.*[5] extends therapists' liability to patients who commit violence without prior threats. Philip Jablonski murdered his live-in girlfriend, Melinda Kimball, and Kimball's daughter sued for wrongful death. Several weeks prior to the murder, Mr. Jablonski had attempted to rape Melinda Kimball's mother. She complained to the police. They referred Jablonski to the V.A. Hospital, and they warned a V.A. psychiatrist of his possible violence. The V.A. psychiatrist failed to pass on this message. Another V.A. psychiatrist, after eliciting the fact that Jablonski had served 5 years for raping his wife, diagnosed an antisocial personality and suggested hospitalization. Jablonski refused to be hospitalized or to release his prior medical records. However, he accepted outpatient treatment and kept several appointments, accompanied by Ms. Kimball. She told several different psychiatrists she was afraid of Mr. Jablonski, and each of them advised her to leave him. She did leave Mr. Jablonski, but when she returned to the apartment to pick up some diapers, he murdered her.

The Calfornia trial court found the defendant's psychiatrists liable for failing to record and communicate the warning from the police, failing to secure the patient's prior records, and failing to properly warn the victim, stating that "the warnings from both doctors, if given, were totally unspecific and inadequate under the circumstances" (p. 396). On appeal, the California Supreme Court affirmed, noting that although this victim was not named, violence against her was clearly foreseeable because of the patient's history of violence toward his wife.

In *Jablonski* the defendants foresaw the potential for violence. However, there was evidence that the defendants' professional behavior fell below the usual standard of care. As a result, the court found the defendants negligent.

The lesson for clinicians who wish to avoid liability is clear: A psychiatrist who identifies a patient as potentially violent should make sure to meet or exceed the usual standard of care. Should violence occur and a suit follow, the argument that professional behavior met or exceeded a usual standard of care will be stronger than the argument that professional behavior is essential to a successful defense.

One unique case, *Cole* v. *Taylor*,[6] involved a patient who murdered his wife and then sued his former psychiatrist claiming that the psychiatrist was negligent in failing to prevent him from murdering her. The Iowa Supreme Court held that *Tarasoff* created a duty to protect the victim, not the patient, and that it would be "wrong as a matter of public policy to allow recovery" for a wrongful action (p. 159).

In an unpublished case that is quite instructive, a psychiatrist who gave a *Tarasoff* warning was found liable for breach of confidentiality. In *Hopewell*

v. *Adibempe*,[7] the plaintiff told her psychiatrist that she would "blow up and hurt somebody very seriously" if the harassment on her job did not stop. Without the patient's consent, the psychiatrist wrote a letter to her supervisor quoting the remark, but noting that this information "was not to be taken as an estimate of the probability that the threat will actually be carried out." The letter carried a stamped endorsement stating, "The information disclosed was confidential and is protected by state law. State regulations prohibit you from making any further disclosures of this information without the prior consent of the person in respect to whom it pertains."

Apparently, the psychiatrist's concern about the duty to warn led him to an act without clinical justification. He sent the letter, not because he thought there was any actual likelihood of violence, but because he feared a *Tarasoff* suit.

This case illustrates what can happen when psychiatrists make decisions that are contrary to their clinical judgment and based on their fear of suit. This is a recipe for trouble.

In summary, potential liability for patient violence has expanded substantially, but few psychiatrists have actually been found liable. Statistically, the chances of being found liable for breach of a *Tarasoff* duty are almost vanishingly small. However, there are practical steps one can take to minimize the possibility of a suit resulting from a patient's violent action. One fundamental principle applies: *The psychiatrist who makes decisions based on a careful exercise of clinical judgment has the best protection against being sued.*

CLINICAL IMPLICATIONS
OF THE DUTY TO PROTECT

It is mathematically impossible to predict rare events with near 100 percent accuracy (Beck, 1985, p. 83). Serious patient violence is rare. Therefore, psychiatrists cannot predict this violence accurately. Although study after study shows this to be true, many psychiatrists, myself included, believe they can tell when there is a serious possibility of violence. While this belief may be correct, the psychiatrist is wrong who imagines that his or her ability to predict violence is a sufficient shield against error. It is in part a matter of luck if our predictions are right or wrong. Therefore, due care is our shield.

Assessment Of Violence

Certain variables are associated with potential violence. The clinician should ask the questions that will elicit information about those variables. These variables are being male, having a past history of violence, moving frequently, being unemployed, living in or growing up in a violent subculture, abusing drugs or alcohol, having low intelligence, coming from a violent family, having weapons available, and having victims available.

The most important clinical variable that predicts violence is motive. It is important to ask, "Are you angry at anyone?" and "Are you thinking about hurting anyone?" If the answer to either question is yes, it is important to follow up with questions about what specific thoughts the patient is having: who, when, where, and how long these thoughts have been occurring; if the patient is worried about being able to control the impulses; and if the patient has acted on them or come close to acting on them.

It is important to ask about past history of fighting, hurting others, and being in trouble with the law. Twenty percent of juveniles in some studies have had legal trouble, so this is not a rare event. Positive answers should be followed up.

Is there evidence of weak controls? Psychotic illness, paranoid suspiciousness, organic brain syndrome such as frontal release syndrome, or more commonly drug or alcohol use? Is there any history of impulsive behavior? If there are threats, does the person have the means to carry them out?

As with self-destructive thoughts, specific intent stated in the active voice is more serious than generalized remarks in the passive voice. It is important to distinguish in order of increasing concern, "I wish he was dead," "I'd like to kill that son of a bitch," and "I may stick a knife in that bastard if he keeps on bothering my wife." Always, it is important to follow up positive responses until one is satisfied that one has learned as much as one needs to know about the person's state of mind. Longer-term, one should decide on diagnostic measures including medical and neurologic exam, and EEG and neuropsychological investigation.

Strategies For Dealing With Potential Violence

The clinician who has done an adequate job of assessing violence will usually have a reasonably clear sense of whether a patient is one of the great majority for whom serious violence is not a concern or one of that small group for whom it is. In the former case, there is no problem. In the latter case, the question is what to do next.

Once the psychiatrist has concluded that violence is a possibility, the choice of action is limited, broadly speaking, to one of three: (1) deal with the problem with the patient, within the therapy; (2) discuss the problem with some third person, such as the victim or the police; or (3) hospitalize the patient, voluntarily if possible, involuntarily if not, assuming the patient meets legal standards for commitment.

A psychiatrist who believes his or her patient may be violent has an obligation to the patient as well as to the potential victim to try to prevent the violence. Patients' proposed violent actions are seldom entirely ego-syntonic or conflict free. The first responsibility of the psychiatrist is to treat the proposed violence as a therapeutic issue. This means *discuss it with the patient*.

When a warning appears indicated, psychiatrists fear that the proposed breach of the patient's confidentiality may damage the therapeutic alliance. In a series of cases in which psychiatrists did warn, the therapeutic alliance was rarely damaged when the psychiatrist discussed the warning with the patient first (Beck, 1981). However, when the psychiatrist discussed the patient with a third party without first discussing it with the patient, the case often ended badly. Discuss your concerns with the patient.

The therapist who takes the threat seriously and discusses a proposed course of action with the patient demonstrates the ability to remain concerned in the face of imminent danger. In most cases, this strengthens the alliance. Consider what it would mean if the psychiatrist stood passively by and failed to act to contain the threat. The responsibility to prevent a patient from harming others is at least as great as the responsibility to prevent a patient from harming himself or herself.

There is a legal duty, but it is secondary to the ethical and clinical duty. The clinical duty requires the psychiatrist to explore the situation with the patient and take whatever action may seem most appropriate. Note that, contrary to some writing on this subject, there is no inherent conflict between the duty to the patient and the duty to third parties. There is an overarching ethical duty to prevent violence, a duty that runs to both the patient and to third parties.

The decision about what course to follow is based on an estimate of imminence of violence. If the psychiatrist thinks the patient is unlikely to act before the next scheduled appointment, then the psychiatrist can afford to deal with this purely as a therapeutic issue — i.e., without involving any third party. Further discussion with the patient and/or more or different medication are possible options.

If there appears to be danger of imminent violence — i.e., if it appears that the patient may hurt someone today or tomorrow — then hospitalization is the intervention of choice. Issues involving discharge of hospitalized patients are discussed below.

In the intermediate case, which is the most uncertain, the psychiatrist should consider involving some third party. Warning the potential victim is often indicated. In this situation, I usually warn by telephone, and I almost always telephone with the patient present, so that the patient knows firsthand what I have said. This serves several functions. First, it ensures that the psychiatrist talks about the patient in a way that will stand scrutiny. If one is frightened about potential violence, it is easy to talk about the patient in language that is less than measured. If the patient is present, this acts as a useful brake on the tendency to rush into immoderate remarks. Second, it diminishes the likelihood that the patient will develop psychotic or paranoid fantasies about what the psychiatrist may have said behind his or her back.

Psychopharmacology

Recent clinical experience suggests that lithium is useful not only for manic depressive disorder but also for persons who have chronic difficulty modulating their affect (Schatzberg & Cole, 1986). Persons who are potentially assaultive and who give a history of chronic difficulty controlling their feelings may benefit from lithium carbonate 300 mg qd or bid. Tegretol has been useful in the control of aggressive behavior in persons with organic brain syndrome or psychotic disorders (Yudofsky et al., 1987). Propranalol has also been effective with some recurrently violent patients (Yudofsky et al., 1987). Neurologists who have much more experience with tegretol than psychiatrists have thought that psychiatrists' concerns about white cell suppression are exaggerated, and that properly monitored, tegretol is an effective, safe drug.

Hospitalized Patients

Control of violence is a routine aspect of hospital treatment and will not be discussed here. Prior to releasing any patient for whom potential violence is an issue, the psychiatrist should evaluate that potential and write a careful note. If the patient wants to be discharged and the psychiatrist agrees that discharge is clinically indicated, the note should document this. If the psychiatrist thinks there may be potential for violence but does not think the patient meets standards for involuntary hospitalization, it is essential that the psychiatrist write a careful note explaining this (see below, under Risk Management).

Consider, for example, an acutely psychotic, chronic schizophrenic patient who drinks heavily and has been assaultive. He reconstitutes in the hospital after treatment that includes medication. The patient is no longer psychotic, and wishes to leave. The psychiatrist knows that there is a risk of violence if the patient stops taking his medication, and that he has taken his medication inconsistently in the past. Nevertheless, the patient is not currently committable. It is essential that the psychiatrist refer the patient for appropriate outpatient treatment, and that the psychiatrist make some effort to ensure that the patient connects with outpatient treatment. It is not sufficient to tell the patient to go, and then do nothing if the patient fails to appear.

It is difficult to know what to do if the patient does not show up, but at the least some discussion with the outpatient facility about how to proceed, and possibly some discussion with either the patient, if possible, or a responsible family member, if there is one, is indicated. The psychiatrist must make a reasonable effort, so that if there is violence, it does not appear that the violence is the result of psychiatric neglect. Courts look for evidence that the psychiatrist has made a good faith effort to protect; they do not require success in every case. But, if there is violence and there is not good evidence that the psychiatrist made some effort to ensure that the discharged patient received follow-up treatment, a court may find that the psychiatrist was negligent.

One difficult scenario occurs when the patient wants to be discharged, the psychiatrist thinks the patient is committable and petitions for commitment, and the court finds that the patient is not commitable and discharges the patient. In this situation, the psychiatrist should make certain that his or her concerns are on the record, and should, as always write a careful note documenting not only observations of the patient but also the psychiatric thinking that underlies the choice of action. Again, the psychiatrist should also discuss his or her concerns with the patient, and try to reach some agreement on how to proceed. Agreement may not be possible, and the psychiatrist may decide to breach the patient's confidentiality in opposition to the patient's wishes. If so, it is better to make the telephone call with the patient present for the same reasons as apply above. It is also essential to make an appropriate referral for outpatient treatment and to discuss your concerns about the patient with the outpatient treatment agent, if this is not yourself. If the patient refuses treatment, document the refusal.

Case Examples From Private Practice Cases

Case 1.   An outpatient in his forties, seen in a private office, was abusing his children, and the psychiatrist told him it was necessary to discuss this with his wife. The psychiatrist discussed the child abuse with her in the patient's presence. The psychiatrist commented, "It was enormously helpful to psychotherapy. It got the wife to take him more seriously. She took seriously the things he was pleading for. Before he would yell at her and ask for answers, and she would be silent. That changed." On 6-month follow-up there had been no further violence. Comment: In this case violence had already occurred, and the action taken appeared to prevent further violence. The breach occurred with the patients knowledge and consent. The *Tarasoff* intervention appeared to have a beneficial effect.

Case 2.   In consultation, a psychiatrist was asked by a therapist how to treat a schizophrenic who was threatening his mother. The psychiatrist advised warning the intended victim. The therapist discussed the warning with the patient first, and then warned the mother by telephone and letter. No violence occurred. Comment: The warning was discussed with the patient and no violence occurred. If the patient's internal controls are poor, the addition of external controls can tip the balance so that acting out is controlled. Knowledge that there is a responsible third party who will take appropriate action if violence occurs appears to be a deterrent to violence in these patients.

Two cases demonstrate psychotherapeutic relationships that were damaged as a result of the *Tarasoff* intervention.

Case 3.   A man whose marriage was dissolving was seen in office psychotherapy. He reported that he had threatened his wife and told his psychiatrist, "I can't be responsible for what I might do." The psychiatrist decided that a warning was necessary, but he could not recall whether he had discussed it with the patient prior to breaching confidentiality. He discussed the threat with the wife, her attorney, and the probate court. The patient terminated, complaining that the psychiatrist was on the wife's side. The wife installed a security system in her home. There was no violence.

Case 4.   A man who used heroin and cocaine was evaluated in a private psychiatric hospital. He reported that he had confronted and threatened his divorced wife and her boyfriend. In the admissions conference, the patient said, "I'll kill him." The psychiatrist informed the patient that a warning was necessary. Later the psychiatrist reported the threat to the ex-wife, and she reported it to her boyfriend. The patient signed out against medical advice. The psychiatrist knew nothing further about the case. Comment: These two cases illustrate the chiling effect of *Tarasoff* envisioned by Stone (1984). Stone suggested that patients who had engaged in criminal behavior would be reluctant to enter into or remain in psychotherapy if their confidentiality was threatened.

Case 5.   A schizophrenic woman seen in a private office threatened to kill her husband. The psychiatrist notified the husband and had repeated discussions with him, but never told the patient he was doing this. The patient eventually stopped taking her medicine, made a serious suicide attempt, and was committed to the state hospital. Comment: The breach of confidentiality was not discussed with the patient, and the outcome was poor.

Case 6.   This patient was a borderline woman who was a private outpatient. She reported that she had assaulted her children. The psychiatrist discussed with the patient the legal requirement that he report the assault to the authorities. After two sessions, she agreed that the report was necessary, and she understood that it might be helpful to her and the children. Some time later, the patient terminated, partly for financial reasons and partly because she was unhappy about the report of child abuse. After the appropriate investigation, her children were allowed to remain with her. Eventually they assaulted her with a deadly weapon. Comment: After the *Tarasoff* intervention, the patient was not again violent toward her children, as far as is known. There is evidence that the intervention interfered significantly with the therapeutic alliance, and ultimately there was further violence in this case.

These are difficult cases. They do not always end well. Following the suggested practices should help to minimize the risk of serious violence. But the worst occasionally happens, and if it does, the psychiatrist who has practiced so as to minimize risk will sleep easier.

RISK MANAGEMENT

When a doctor is negligent, this negligence is called malpractice. To win a malpractice case, a plaintiff must convince a jury that four conditions have been met: First, that someone has been damaged; second, that the damage was directly caused by something the defendant did that he or she shouldn't have, or didn't do but should have done; third, that the defendant had a duty to the injured person; and fourth, that the defendant was derelict in his or her duty. In malpractice cases, dereliction of duty is shown if it can be shown that the defendant failed to use due care. The definition of due care is what the average practitioner would have done in the same or similar circumstances.

In general, there is no malpractice if it can be shown that the defendant used due care—i.e., practiced according to a usual or average standard of care. Even if someone is badly hurt or killed, the law says that the injured party cannot recover from the doctor if the doctor has met this standard. Thus careful exercise of professional judgment is the best protection against being sued. And, as we have seen, this holds true for *Tarasoff* suits just as it does for other malpractice actions.

Cynical malpractice lawyers say that doctors' notes are more important than their clinical practices. They exaggerate, but the point is essentially correct. If suit comes, the defense must rely on the notes written at the time. After-the-fact explanations, written or oral, are of little use.

Violence rarely happens out of the blue. Psychiatrists usually suspect it may happen. When a psychiatrist has such a suspicion, it is essential that he or she write careful, detailed notes. This means full and complete documentation of what the patient has said, what you have observed, what you thought about, and what you concluded. Verbatim notes taken during an interview are the best evidence to support a conclusion. A note that says only, "Patient was paranoid" or "patient not violent," is a conclusory note in which evidence is lacking. Contrast the first with a note that quotes the patient, "I have to keep my guns because the communists are after me." Or, in the second case, contrast, "Patient denies ever having hurt anyone, and denies any thoughts currently of hurting anyone else." A note should always include the psychiatrist's conclusion about the likelihood of violence, citing clinical data; the proposed course of action; and the reasons why this course is likely to be effective or at least better than any other choice.

When violence occurs, courts look for evidence that professionals made thoughtful decisions. Psychiatrists are not trained to explain why they did something and why they did not do something else. Courts understand that the choices are often difficult, but they look for evidence that the decision making was thoughtful.

When in doubt, obtain a consultation. Two heads are often better than one. Questions of assessment and of appropriate action are often clarified through the process of review and discussion with another person. Again, this is evidence that demonstrates that the psychiatrist made decisions carefully and thoughtfully. Either the consultant should write a note, or the psychiatrist should write a note summarizing the consultant's opinion.

When there is an immediate concern, get an immediate consultation. Consultation may be informal, and can occur over the telephone. If the consultant can see the patient, so much the better, but if not, it is better to have an immediate consultation if an immediate decision is called for than to have nothing until later, when it may be too late.

Attorneys' advice is different from the advice of a forensic psychiatrist. For example, attorneys sometimes advise warning by registered letter. A lawyer is not a doctor, and clinical judgment should take precedence over legal judgment. If a registered letter makes clinical sense, then send it, but do not be afraid to argue clinical considerations with an attorney.

Recent litigation in several states, supported by the American Psychiatric Society or the District Branch, states that a psychiatrist is protected from liability except in the situation where a patient threatens a named victim and the psychiatrist fails to warn or take other responsible action. This narrowing of potential liability is welcome. However, not withstanding, if the psychiatrist has reason to fear violence and fails to exercise reasonable professional judgment, there is still a likelihood of successful suit. Court decisions generally reflect common sense, and judges will often find a legal basis for holding professionals to a standard of professional behavior.

Note that the usual advice in avoiding malpractice suits does not apply in the *Tarasoff* situation. Experts say that doctors can minimize the risk of suits by establishing a good personal relationship with their patients, but in *Tarasoff* cases there is rarely a relationship with the victim. For that reason, the strategies for risk management described above are essential.

This chapter has at every point urged upon the psychiatrist a course of action that is clinically and ethically sound, whether there are any concerns about possible legal consequences or not. The unlikely eventuality of a *Tarasoff* suit should not distract the clinician from the tasks at hand.

REFERENCES

Beck, J.C. (1981). When the patient threatens violence: An empirical study of clinical practice after *Tarasoff. Bulletin American Academy of Psychiatry and Law, 10,* 189–201.

Beck, J.C. (1985). Violent patients and the *Tarasoff* duty in private psychiatric practice. *Journal of Psychiatry & Law, 13,* 361–376.

Beck, J.C. (1987). The Psychotherapist's duty to protect third parties from harm. *Mental and Physical Disability Law Reporter, 11,* 141–148.

Givelber, D., Bowers, W., & Blitch, C.L. (1985). In Beck (Ed.), *The potentially violent patient and the* Tarasoff *decision in psychiatric practice.* Washington, DC: American Psychiatric Press.

Prosser, W.L., Wade, J.W., & Schwartz, V. (1982). *Torts: Cases and materials,* 7th ed. Mineola, NY: Foundation Press.

Schatzberg, A.F., & Cole, J.O. (1986). *Manual of clinical psychopharmacology.* Washington, DC: American Psychiatric Press.

Stone, A.A. (1984). *Law, psychiatry and morality.* Washington, DC: American Psychiatric Press.

Yudofsky, S.C., Silver, J.M., & Schneider, S.E. (1987). Pharmacologic treatment of aggression. Psychiatric Annals, 17, 397–407.

FOOTNOTES

[1]Tarasoff v. Regents of Univ. of Cal., 529 P.2d 553, 118 Cal. Rptr. 129 (1974).
[2]Tarasoff v. Regents of Univ. of Cal., 551 P.2d 334, 131 Cal. Rptr. 13 (1976).
[3]McIntosh v. Milano, 403 A.2d 500, 168 N.J. Super. 466 (1979).
[4]Heltsley v. Votteler, 327 N.W.2d 759, 213 (Neb. 1982).
[5]Jablonski v. U.S., 712 F.2d 391 (9th Cir. 1983).
[6]Cole v. Taylor, 616 F.Supp.157 (D. IOowa 1985).
[7]Hopewell v. Adibempe, No. Gd78-82756, Civil Division, Court of Common Pleas of Allegheny County, Pennsylvania, June 1, 1981.

C H A P T E R

60

CLINICAL AND LEGAL ISSUES RELATED TO PSYCHOLOGICAL/PHYSICAL CRISIS INTERVENTION

Michael Thackrey, Ph.D.

Aggression against the mental-health clinician is simply a fact of professional life. Far from being a phenomenon limited to the public-sector emergency, inpatient, or forensic facility, such violence is known in almost every applied setting and with nearly every patient population (Lion & Reid, 1983; Roth, 1987; Thackrey, 1987; Turner, 1983). Although incidence is difficult to estimate with precision, and the percentage of patients who actually threaten or enact violence against the therapist may be quite low, the more patients one sees, the greater are one's chances of eventually being the object of an assault. Such an eventuality has been characterized (Whitman, Armao, & Dent, 1976) as an "inevitable phenomenon that may occur at some time to every therapist" (p. 428). Therefore, it behooves each mental-health professional to understand the fundamental clinical and legal principles relevant to psychological/physical crisis intervention.

CLINICAL ISSUES

Phenomenology And Judgment

Although some general statements might be offered concerning the relative likelihood of assaultive behavior posed by different categories of patients and of the relative efficacy of various approaches to intervention, such generalizations are so riddled with exceptions and contingencies as to render them of little practical utility. The well-known "base rate problem" makes unbiased statistical prediction of any rare event (such as assault) mathematically impossible (Megargee, 1981); also, even rather minor differences among patients, clinicians, and circumstances may lead to major differences in the way situations are perceived by patients and clinicians, and thereby to profound differences between even relatively similar situations in terms of the proper course that must be pursued for effective crisis management and resolution. Therefore, instead of employing diagnostic and prescriptive criteria that purport to identify the violent patient and to specify proper management, the clinician must instead utilize an approach to assessment and intervention that is based on clinical phenomenology and judgment. Although such an approach is fallible, there is no practical alternative.

For purposes of predicting and managing assaultive behavior, the clinician always has immediately available two sources of data: (1) the patient's present behavior in context, and (2) the clinician's internal reactions to the patient. The patient's present behavior refers to both verbal and nonverbal events, which may be quite subtle yet telling (the more volatile the situation, the more salient are the nonverbal aspects of behavior and communication); the context of the behavior (subsuming both circumjacence and previous history) is crucial to its meaning. Some patients characteristically threaten yet do not act; others may never threaten without genuine intention; still others may attack without apparent warning or provocation. Furthermore, differences in even minute aspects of the patient's behavior or in the context within which the behavior is embedded may signify that the patient will act out behavior that contrasts with previous history. Often the most important indicator of imminent outburst is some deviation from the patient's typical behavior. Prior to assault, the talkative patient may become quiet or the quiet patient talkative, and so on.

The clinician's internal reactions ("hunches," "gut reactions") to the patient may represent effects of nonverbal, qualitative, and often elusive yet important aspects of patient behaviors. The clinician may actually perceive and react to such molecular behaviors of the patient without recognizing these reactions or their source. The clinician should become sensitized to these internal affective reactions and responses. Rather than ignoring or avoiding (especially unpleasant) feelings, the clinician should cultivate and utilize them as a source of valid data. The clinician should also recognize that the patient reads and reacts to subtleties of the clinician's behavior that reflect the clinician's thoughts and feelings. At times, the clinician's nonverbal communications will be louder and clearer than words. The clinician must become perceptive to and utilize effectively the two forms of phenomenological data that will be available in any encounter: the patient's immediate behavior in context and the clinician's internal reactions to the patient. Judgment is the mechanism whereby such forms of information are integrated meaningfully, and whereby the clinician decides what to make of a situation and what to do about it. Judgment is the fundamental basis for sound mental-health practice in general, and for effective psychological/physical crisis intervention in particular.

Crisis Adaptation

The patient's adaptive mechanisms function so as to maintain overall physical and psychological equilibrium. However, in a crisis situation, the capacity of the patient's (and clinician's!) coping mechanisms may be exceeded, resulting in erratic or impulsive behavior. Although there are no pathognomic signs of impending violence, precipitous assault is quite rare, if indeed it exists at all (of course, warning signs may be subtle). Typically, the crisis process entails (1) a prodrome, (2) an identified "incident," and (3) a reintegration/restabilization period. The clinician can optimize crisis outcome through early identification and intervention (depending on clinician sensitivity and judgment), and by adopting the therapeutic stance of collaborating with the client in working through the various stages of crisis adaptation. The clinician must participate in rather than attempt to short-circuit this process.

Aggressive behavior results from the patient's experience of fear or anger. Both affects are meaningful and potentially understandable reactions (defensive and offensive, respectively) to the patient's (perhaps accurate, perhaps inaccurate) perception of threat. While most clinicians seem to assume that aggressive patient behavior is indicative of anger, most aggressive behavior in the clinical setting may instead be a reflection of fear. A fearful patient must be approached differently than an angry patient, yet this crucial distinction is frequently overlooked. All people direct their behavior according to the channels or alternatives that they perceive. Even a gentle person may fight when feeling cornered without alternatives. In working through the crisis process with any patient, the clinician must take great care not to inadvertently structure a situation so that the patient's only perceived option to meet essential needs is through dysfunctional means. An acceptable alternative must be allowed to any inappropriate behavior.

The Assessment/Intervention Matrix

Just as the aggressive patient typically experiences either fear or anger, the clinician's actions can be conceptualized as either yielding or firm. These possibilities form the matrix shown in Table 1; its four cells may help the clinician to conceptualize four prototypical approaches to working with the aggressive patient. Here, assessment entails differentiating the fearful patient from the angry; intervention requires choosing between the yielding and the firm approach. Of course, sound clinical judgment is central to both assessment and intervention.

In response to the fearful aggressive patient, the clinician may attempt to reduce the degree of threat that the patient perceives, verbally (e.g., "It's safe here now") or nonverbally (e.g., allowing plenty of interpersonal distance). Alternatively, the clinician may attempt to help the patient feel able to cope

Table 60-1. The Assessment/Intervention Matrix

| | | *Clinician's response* | |
		Yielding	*Firm*
	Fear	Reduce perceived threat	Increase perceived coping capacity
Patient's experience			
	Anger	Appease	Set limit

with the perceived threat (e.g., "I am on your side, and I will help"). Just as one fearful patient may respond better to yielding threat reduction, another may respond better to firm support and enhancement of perceived coping capacity. Similarly, in response to the angry patient, the clinician may employ a yielding strategy in order to appease the patient and so defuse aggressive potential (e.g., "I am sorry that I hurt your feelings"), or alternatively may respond firmly and inhibit aggressive expression through limit setting.

Good judgment is required for the clinician to choose between the yielding and the firm approach to the angry patient, and the practical test of the chosen approach lies in the resulting behavior of the patient. One angry patient may only attempt further to "push around" the yielding clinician, yet another angry patient may be "pushed over the edge" into violence by the firm clinician. Although appeasement is not synonymous with inappropriately pacifying a bully (it is indeed possible to defuse anger through appeasement without sacrificing the essential interests of both patient and clinician), many clinicians seem loath to react gently in the face of anger. It seems likely that the most common precipitant of unnecessary patient violence is clinician counterhostility.

Limit Setting

The ultimate goal in external limit setting is for the patient to develop internal controls; however, limit setting may be instrumental in the course of the patient's development of autonomous self-regulation. Limit setting can be a positive therapeutic technique inasmuch as it allows the patient to understand which behaviors are prescribed and which are proscribed. It also gives the patient realistic expectations regarding the behavior of others, thus allowing the patient to gain approval rather than disapproval. Moreover, limit setting may prevent the patient from doing something humiliating or harmful, and it can convey clinician concern and competence. Some degree of patient resistance to limit setting is a positive sign — generalized, docile acceptance of the clinician's will is dysfunctional. And, of course, whenever any of the patient's intention is blocked, an acceptable alternative must be allowed.

Limit setting should be presented to the patient as a statement of fact, never as a request, as a bribe, as advice, as punishment, or as a challenge or threat. Reality-based, natural consequences of behavior are a more productive focus than are consequences contrived and maintained by the clinician. Fairness and consistency in limit setting are absolutely essential. Expected and prohibited behaviors must be described concretely in terms of actions that can be performed immediately. The clinician must know the actual enforceable limit, and must never describe either positive or negative consequences that he or she is unable or unwilling to deliver. On the whole, limit setting is often utilized too late rather than too early by well-meaning but inexperienced clinicians; timely implementation can prevent undue deterioration of the patient and the therapeutic milieu. Once the need for a behavioral limit has been established, the clinician may briefly explain the limit and its rationale but must avoid being drawn into superfluous discussion or argument.

There are two major methods of limit setting: direct and indirect. The former involves presenting the patient with one specific directive, and the latter involves presenting the patient with choices among acceptable alternatives.

Direct technique   Essentially, the direct technique of limit setting consists of stating clearly and specifically the required or prohibited behavior. (Although the clinician may additionally describe consequences of violating the limit, such a statement is not a defining aspect of this method.) Whenever possible, a directive should be expressed in a positive format ("do this," which describes acceptable behavior), rather than in the negative ("do not do that," which does not describe acceptable behavior). The direct method is often preferable for the confused or emotionally overwhelmed patient.

Indirect technique   Essentially, the indirect method of limit setting consists of keeping the patient in a state of choosing among acceptable behaviors, thus dividing the patient's will to resist. Although it may be easy for the patient to oppose a single directive, attention cannot be focused simultaneously on two or more alternatives and so resistance to any particular one is diminished. The clinician subtly maintains control by limiting the choices while giving the patient the opportunity to choose among them ("you can sit down and we can talk about how you are feeling, or you can leave"). Should the patient refuse to make any choice, the clinician can then make a time-bound conditional choice on behalf of the patient ("if you do not choose to sit down in 10 seconds, I will take that to mean that you choose to leave and I will have the security guards escort you out"). Even when the situation develops in this way, any resistance demonstrated is typically far less than had the patient not been given a choice.

The clinician must exercise sound judgment in deciding which limit-setting technique to employ. Some patients will be angered by and vigorously resist directives; others will be confused or disorganized by choices. At an appropriate time after such an intervention, the meaning of the limit setting within the context of the therapeutic relationship must be addressed with the patient. Ultimately, clinician actions with the patient's best interests at heart are likely to be understood and appreciated.

Physical Intervention

Not every episode of potential or actual aggressive behavior can be resolved without physical intervention (e.g., an individual who is so afraid or angry that sustained, meaningful interaction is not possible and with whom an attempt at nonphysical intervention might be dangerous to patient and clinician alike), and even in those episodes in which nonphysical intervention might have been possible, less than optimal clinical technique may fail to prevent (or may even precipitate) a physical attack. Just as cardiopulmonary resuscitation (CPR) training is preparation for an emergency situation that may occur only infrequently, brief training may be adequate for the relatively rare event of overt physical aggression and be of critical therapeutic benefit. While an in-depth presentation of proper clinical techniques for humane, safe, and effective physical management of the aggressive patient is beyond the scope of this discussion and is available elsewhere (Thackrey, 1987), a few comments are in order here.

Physical intervention principles are a conceptual subset of psychological intervention principles. Applied physical techniques are effective only insofar as they utilize psychological as well as mechanical/kinesiological principles. Aggressive behavior is a psychologically meaningful event for both the patient and the clinician. Just as sound clinical judgment is required to determine the best psychological intervention, sound judgment is also required of the clinician in implementing the proper physical intervention. There is no single physical response for every possible situation; instead, the clinician must apply principles to the situation at hand. Effective physical intervention is possible because the clinician is mentally prepared, anticipates the actions and reactions of the patient, and optimizes mechanical/kinesiological factors (e.g., leverage, torque).

Applied physical intervention techniques must facilitate therapeutic psychological intervention while protecting both clinician and patient. They are treatment procedures, and must meet a number of essential criteria. First, they must be effective. Second, they must be safe for clinician and patient alike. Third, they must be absolutely nonabusive, inflicting neither injury nor pain, and preserving the humanity and dignity of the patient. Fourth, they must require a minimum of clinician training for motor-skill acquisition and retention. As are principles and techniques of therapeutic psychological intervention, physical intervention technology is evolving continuously. Innovations in physical technique should be evaluated by the practitioner according to the four essential criteria presented above.

Although some persons have expressed the concern that inclusion of physical management techniques in the context of training clinicians to prevent and manage patient aggression might lead to overutilization of these methods, such a concern may be allayed by substantial research evidence (Thackrey, 1987) demonstrating that appropriate training actually decreases the incidence of assaults and the utilization of restraint, seclusion, and so on. High-quality training that presents physical management methods within their proper clinical and legal context can serve as one means of helping to preserve the patient's rights, consistent with the values traditionally associated with professional mental-health services.

LEGAL ISSUES

The clinician may be understandably uncertain about legal rights and responsibilities in crises requiring physical intervention. Ultimately, reasonableness in light of specific circumstances forms the legal basis for appropriate practice in such situations.

The rights and responsibilities of both the patient and clinician are defined by legal standards from three sources: (1) statutes generated by federal, state, or local legislature; (2) regulations generated by administrative agencies empowered by the legislatures; and (3) case law consisting of precedents set by judicial decisions in similar cases. Failure of the patient or clinician to meet relevant legal standards can constitute crime or tort. A crime is an action that is legally prohibited; a tort is a wrongful act resulting in injury to another person (or that person's property) for which that person is entitled to compensation, even though that act might not be illegal. The law may prescribe punishment for crime (imprisonment, fine, etc.), and financial or other liability may ensue from tort. Negligence, which can be crime or tort, is failure to exercise sufficient care in the protection of other persons or their property. Malpractice is negligence in a professional matter.

In general terms, the patient has a right to protection from harm by the clinician and others, and a right to appropriate treatment by the least restrictive methods available. Similarly, the clinician has a right to protection from harm by the patient, and a right to exercise sound professional judgment in providing appropriate treatment in emergency situations.

Patient's Right To Protection

By virtue of the patient–clinician relationship, the patient has a right to be protected from harm resulting from the actions of the clinician, from the actions of other patients, and even from the patient's own actions. The clinician must exercise reasonable care in order not to harm the patient, must protect the patient from other patients, and even must protect the patient from self-harm. Failure to protect the patient may result in criminal or tort liability for the clinician.

Assault is an attempt or threat to do violence against another person, regardless of whether the attempt or threat is actually carried out. Battery is an actual, unlawful attack upon another person. Even touching the person's clothing or an object held by the person can constitute battery. Abuse is maltreatment of a patient, and can be crime or tort consisting of an act of omission or of an act of commission. There are many varieties of abuse. Physical abuse may consist of bodily mistreatment such as striking, rough handling, and inflicting injury or pain; psychological abuse may consist of verbal or nonverbal actions, such as demeaning or humiliating words or demeanor, exploitation, coercion, or threat. Other abuse may consist of neglect, or failure of the clinician to take therapeutic action, to protect the patient, and to report abuse by another clinician.

Appropriate Treatment

The appropriateness and adequacy of treatment rendered to the patient are defined by the standard of care which is the general level of expertise and skill that other competent professionals deliver. From a practical standpoint, the concept of "standard of care" means that the patient is entitled to services that utilize the best of currently known, commonly available information and technology. Failure of the clinician to provide services consistent with the standard of care places the clinician in legal jeopardy. However, an unfavorable treatment outcome per se does not necessarily imply professional liability so long as the treatment rendered meets the standard of care.

The concept of the "least restrictive alternative" for adequate treatment has proved difficult to define and to apply to actual clinical situations. Rather than representing a simple unidimensional continuum from the least restrictive to the most restrictive treatment methods, "relative restrictiveness" is actually a multidimensional construct. Whether a given treatment method is relatively more or less restrictive than some alternative may be a function of each method's behavioral intrusiveness, physical instrusiveness, effectiveness, reversibility, safety, painfulness, effect on the patient's dignity and responsibility, treatment setting, voluntariness, and so forth. There is no consensus among legal experts as to the relative restrictiveness of such procedures as medication, seclusion, and mechanical restraint. Although perhaps counterintuitive, some experts argue that medication may be more restrictive than even mechanical restraint because medication is invasive; others argue that seclusion may be more restrictive than restraint because seclusion restricts access to other persons; and so on. In the applied situation, while the clinician must be mindful of the requirements for implementing the least restrictive treatment, the decision as to actual method of intervention cannot be made on a priori grounds but must be made with respect to the individual patient and the particulars of the situation and possible treatment approaches.

Clinician's Right To Protection

The clinician has a right to be free from unreasonable behavior by the patient and to take appropriate action for self-protection. However, a major difference between the clinician's private response to aggressive behavior in a nonclinical situation and the behavior required of the clinician in the professional setting is that, in the latter case, the clinician's self-protective actions will be also judged by quality-of-care criteria. Care and treatment of the patient will always remain a consideration, even when the clinician is justifiably protecting the self. The clinician has a right and responsibility to use reasonable force in the therapeutic course of physical intervention involving self-protection and patient control; failure to use sufficient, reasonable force to prevent a patient from harming another patient or from harming the patient's self may render the clinician legally liable. Of course, even in response to extreme patient provocation, the use of excessive force is intolerable whether in the course of self-protection or otherwise. The amount of force that is considered appropriate is a matter of judgment, dependent on the context of the specific persons and situation involved.

Patients are required to conduct themselves appropriately within the limits of their capacity to do so. A patient can incur criminal or tort liability for assault or battery. In years past, the judicial tendency may have been to consider the patient as not responsible for aggressive conduct in the clinical setting; however, contemporary legal thinking seems to hold that unless the patient's capacity to do so is substantially compromised by major mental disability, the patient is legally required to conform to standards of behavior expected of other members of society, and the clinician technically has the right to sue a patient for damage resulting from willful aggression, and even to file criminal charges. Civil or criminal proceedings may be therapeutic in some cases in that the patient is given a clear message as to the inappropriateness of assaultive or destructive behavior.

Discharge from professional care is also an option to be considered for some aggressive patients. Treatment occasionally produces deterioration in functioning, and when this deterioration takes the form of aggressive acting out, discharge should be considered. At times, such a discharge may make the patient more amenable to subsequent treatment by another clinician or in another setting. Decisions concerning such actions as lawsuits, criminal charges, therapeutic discharge, and so forth should be made in terms of the patient's clinical picture and needs rather than the clinician's emotional reactions to the assault.

Clinician's Exercise Of Judgment

In situations requiring emergency action, the clinician has substantial authority and responsibility to take necessary steps (such as physical intervention, medication, seclusion, and restraint) to protect the patient, the self, and others (Roth, 1987; Tardiff, 1984). Behavior that is destructive to the patient, to others, or to the therapeutic environment legally warrants immediate intervention even without the consent of the patient. Similarly, preventive intervention when such destructive behavior appears to be imminent but has not actually occurred (even in the absence of a specific threat or act) may be considered appropriate legally. In an emergency, the clinician is given a great deal of legal flexibility to exercise judgment in determining the necessity of and particular methods for immediate intervention. The clinician's judgment in such emergency situations is typically presumed to be valid; the clinician is typically held liable only if the intervention performed is such a substantial departure from the usual standard of care that it calls into question whether judgment was in fact exercised (Roth, 1987; Tardiff, 1984). As a legal protection and (more important) as a clinical validation, the clinician is well advised to consult with colleagues whenever possible in important matters requiring judgment, and to document the consultation appropriately.

Documentation

In addition to the actual clinical procedures implemented, the clinician is also required to document the procedures appropriately. Inadequate record keeping can in itself be considered a substandard practice. Because not all emergency situations can be reasonably anticipated, and the ultimate cannot always be foreseen, special attention to careful documentation is essential. The clinical record must be complete, factual, and scrupulously honest. The clinician must not misstate or omit facts that indicate that the clinician may have committed an error in procedure or judgment—the documentation of such errors attests to the honesty and integrity of the record, and may protect the clinician from untrue allegations that could be even worse than any actual shortcomings.

The clinician, however, should avoid speculation in the clinical record. To be included are a description of facts that caused the clinician to consider the situation an emergency, a rationale for the choice of intervention method (including explicit discussion of less restrictive alternatives considered and reasons for rejecting each), specific criteria for the implementation of less-intensive intervention (e.g., release from restraint), the steps taken to prevent another, similar incident, the exact time and duration of intervention (e.g., manual or mechanical restraint, seclusion), a description of care given during intervention, the time of notification of other appropriate professionals (e.g., a physician) and other appropriate follow-up actions (e.g., incident review), and a description of property damaged or of injuries suffered by the patient and the clinician. If trauma is visible, color photographs should be taken.

SUMMARY

Both the patient and the clinician have rights and responsibilities in the therapeutic setting. The patient has the right to be free from harm and to be treated appropriately by the least restrictive methods; the clinician has the right to self-protection and to intervene in an emergency. Both the patient and the clinician may be criminally or civilly liable for their actions. Judgment is central to the evaluation of the actions of both patients and clinicians.

The clinician must know the general principles that relate to the legal aspects of professional mental-health practice. Ultimately, however, the clinician's decisions about the patient's treatment should be made on clinical grounds. Actions that make the most clinical sense will typically be best for both patient and clinician.

REFERENCES

Lion, J.R., & Reid, W.H. (Eds.). (1983). *Assaults within psychiatric facilities.* New York: Grune & Stratton.

Megargee, E.I. (1987). Methodological problems in the prediction of violence. In J.R. Hays, T.K. Roberts, & K.S. Solway (Eds.), *Violence and the violent individual.* New York: Spectrum.

Roth, L.H. (Ed.). (1987). *Clinical treatment of the violent person.* New York: Guilford Press.

Tardiff, K. (Ed.). (1984). *The psychiatric uses of seclusion and restraint.* Washington, DC: American Psychiatric Press.

Thackrey, M. (1987). *Therapeutics for aggression: Psychological/physical crisis intervention.* New York: Human Sciences Press.

Turner, J.T. (Ed.). (1983). *Violence in the medical care setting: A survival guide.* Rockville, MD: Aspen.

Whitman, R.M., Armao, B.B., & Dent, O.B. (1976). Assault on the therapist. *American Journal of Psychiatry, 133,* 426–429.

C H A P T E R
61

LEGAL ISSUES IN
TERMINATING TREATMENT

Charles Patrick Ewing, J.D., Ph.D.

Once you, the psychotherapist, agree to treat a patient and begin treating that patient, you have established a relationship that is governed by both law and professional ethics. Although the patient is entirely free to terminate that relationship at any time thereafter, for any reason or for no reason at all, you are not. You have an ethical and elgal duty to avoid abandoning the patient (Barker, 1982; Gutheil & Appelbaum, 1982; Ewing, 1985; Smith, 1986).

This chapter deals with that duty and related legal issues in terminating treatment. Specifically, this chapter examines legal and ethical issues related to (1) terminating treatment for therapeutic reasons, (2) terminating treatment for nontherapeutic reasons, (3) dealing with patients who terminate unilaterally, (4) being available to patients in emergencies, (5) arranging coverage for patients while you are unavailable, and (6) referring patients to other mental health practitioners.

TERMINATION FOR THERAPEUTIC REASONS

There are numerous situations in which it is therapeutically advisable to terminate psychotherapy. Among the most common are those where therapy has accomplished its purposes, where therapy has not accomplished its purposes but is not progressing sufficiently to justify continuing it, and where another type of therapy or another therapist seems indicated.

In these situations, psychotherapists have an ethical if not a legal duty to terminate (Barker, 1982) and may do so without fear of liability as long as the patient is given reasonable notice of the therapist's intent to terminate and the termination is handled in an appropriately therapeutic fashion (Ewing, 1985; Smith, 1986). To continue treating a patient with no reasonable expectation for improvement or where it is clear that the patient needs another therapist and/or therapeutic modality is clearly unethical and could result in legal liability for malpractice, fraud, or both.

Legal and ethical problems are unlikely to result from therapeutically indicated terminations as long as the terminations are handled properly (Ewing, 1985; Smith, 1986). Ideally, the decision to terminate psychotherapy should be made jointly by patient and therapist. Not infrequently, however, patients seek to avoid terminating treatment even though termination is therapeutically indicated (Ewing, 1978). Their motives are understandable: Terminating any relationship is painful and people generally try to avoid pain. Under these circumstances, however, the therapist's ethical and legal duty is to proceed with termination in a therapeutic fashion.

Even where termination is appropriate if not required, however, the therapist must give the patient reasonable notice of plans to terminate treatment and make a good faith, therapeutically proper effort to smooth termination for the patient. A therapist who simply breaks off the therapeutic relationship with a patient without adequate notice or without making a reasonable effort to work through the patient's termination concerns not only has behaved unethically but also has set himself or herself up for a potential lawsuit for abandonment (Barker, 1982; Gutheil & Appelbaum, 1983; Ewing, 1985; Smith, 1986).

Although the law has never provided a certain or even universal definition of abandonment (Ewing, 1985), the principle behind the concept is clear and simple. Health care providers (including mental health professionals) have a relationship with those they serve that is built upon trust — the patient's trust that once the provider has assumed the patient's care, the provider will be reasonably available to provide care to the patient until care is no longer needed or desired. If the provider violates that trust and, as a result, a patient is harmed, the provider may be found guilty of abandonment and held liable for money damages (Smith, 1986).

TERMINATION FOR
NONTHERAPEUTIC REASONS

A lawsuit charging a psychotherapist with abandonment is most likely to result not from a therapeutically indicated termination but rather from a termination that has no therapeutic basis. There are numerous nontherapeutic reasons for terminating psychotherapy, but perhaps the most common are lack of patient cooperation in treatment and failure to pay for professional services rendered (Ewing, 1985; Smith, 1096).

Where a patient refuses to cooperate in treatment, termination may in fact be therapeutically indicated. However, there is often a fine line between normal resistance and refusal to cooperate. Therapists have an obligation to help the patient work through resistance to treatment, but that obligation goes only so far. Once it is clear that the patient will not cooperate in treatment, it is both ethically and legally proper to terminate treatment (Ewing, 1985).

Even then, to avoid any question of abandonment, the therapist must provide the patient with reasonable notice and make a good faith effort to see that termination is carried out in a therapeutically proper fahsion. Therapists who terminate with patients under these circumstances are also well advised to document in writing the reason(s) for termination, the amount of notice given the patient, and the efforts made by the therapist to ensure a smooth termination (Ewing, 1985). Not infrequently, the most resistant patients also turn out to be the most litigious (Smith, 1986). So, in any event, it is always wise to err on the side of caution when terminating with these patients.

The more difficult nontherapeutic termination is one precipitated by the patient's failure to pay the therapist's fee. Many mental health professionals donate some portion of their time to professional work that is not economically remunerative. Some private practitioners routinely provide free treatment to one or more patients. But, for the most part, mental health professionals expect to be paid for the services they render.

Patients who fail to pay for their treatment not only threaten the economic interests of the therapist but also raise difficult transference and countertransference issues. Once the patient and psychotherapist assume the roles of debtor and creditor, there is bound to be an adverse effect on the therapeutic relationship. Thus, in some cases, there are good reasons both economic and therapeutic for considering terminating the treatment of a nonpaying patient.

Perhaps the foremost consideration in such cases is the patient's current status. If the patient is in no crisis at the moment and no crisis seems imminent, the therapist may terminate treatment without fear of liability as long as the therapist gives the patient reasonable notice, offers the patient assistance in finding another psychotherapist, and makes the patient's records available to the new psychotherapist if the patient so requests. Where a patient is in crisis, however — especially one in which the patient is at risk for injury to self or others — termination is contraindicated, both therapeutically and legally (Ewing, 1985; Smith, 1986). Terminating with a patient in crisis under any circumstances, but particularly for the sole reason of nonpayment, places a psychotherapist at grave risk for legal liability. As Gutheil and Appelbaum (1983) note perceptively, "Courts are likely to look least favorably upon therapists who have stopped seeing patients for failure to pay their bills than [upon] those who have terminated patients for any other cause" (p. 155).

PATIENTS WHO TERMINATE UNILATERALLY

Not infrequently, a therapeutic relationship is terminated unilaterally by the patient (Ewing, 1978); Smith, 1986). In some instances, the patient informs the psychotherapist that he or she is ceasing treatment, but many times the patient simply fails to keep an appointment and is never heard from again. Although patients have an absolute right to terminate treatment unilaterally, their exercising that right does not necessarily relieve the psychotherapist of his or her duty of care. Ironically, even where a patient terminates treatment unilaterally, the psychotherapist may still be at risk for abandonment unless he or she takes certain steps (Ewing, 1985; Smith, 1986).

Where a patient notifies the therapist that he or she is terminating treatment, the therapist should at a minimum attempt to ascertain the reason for termination and also should record it. If in the therapist's judgment the patient still needs treatment, the therapist should indicate that to the patient and, if appropriate, offer to resume treatment at the patient's request and/or refer the patient to another therapist. If the patient is in crisis, the therapist should recommend against termination and make a reasonable effort to convince the patient to continue treatment with the therapist or with another mental health professional. If the patient in need of treatment persists in his or her desire to terminate, the therapist should make clear to the patient verbally and in writing that termination is against professional advice. And, of course, the therapist should indicate the same in the patient's record.

The more difficult unilateral termination case is that in which the patient simply ceases treatment without notice or explanation — e.g., the patient who misses an appointment and then never again calls or writes. The legal duty of the therapist under these circumstances is unclear, but to avoid any question of abandonment and resulting liability in the event of harm to the patient, the therapist should make a good faith effort to contact the patient, determine the patient's reason(s) for terminating, and take appropriate therapeutic steps to deal with the termination — e.g., discussing the patient's need for continued treatment, referring the patient to another therapist or agency, and offering to resume treatment if and when the patient desires (Ewing, 1985). Naturally, the therapist should also make a written record of these efforts and their results. Where the termination is against professional advice, it is advisable to indicate that in a letter (sent by registered or certified mail) to the patient, with a copy to the patient's record (Smith, 1986).

If in the course of following up on a unilateral termination without notice, the therapist discovers that the patient is at risk for injury to self or others, the therapist may be held to a higher duty of care (Barker, 1982). Under these circumstances, if the patient will not resume treatment with the therapist or another mental health professional, it may be necessary to take appropriate action to keep the patient from hurting himself or herself or others. Naturally, such action will vary depending upon the situation, but therapists should not assume that their duty to the patient (or to those who might be harmed by the patient) has ended simply because the patient has dropped out of treatment.

BEING AVAILABLE TO PATIENTS
IN EMERGENCIES

Mental health professionals should be aware that they may be held liable for abandonment even where neither they nor their patients have terminated treatment. Liability for abandonment may result where therapists simply fail, even briefly, to make themselves available to a patient already in treatment. Such liability is most likely to arise from a situation in which there is an emergency, the patient (or the patient's family) is unable to reach the therapist, and as a result the patient or someone else is harmed (Ewing, 1985; Smith, 1986).

This form of abandonment can easily be avoided by simply making oneself reasonably accessible to patients at all times (arranging coverage for those times when one cannot be available to one's patients is discussed below). Modern technology makes this kind of accessibility relatively painless. One alternative — the cheapest in economic terms — is simply to make one's home telephone number available to patients. Therapists who are frequently on the go and/or those who do not wish to take unscreened calls from patients at home can rely upon a telephone answering service. Those who wish to maintain constant availability can combine a telephone answering service with a portable electronic paging device.

Clearly no one — not even the law — expects a psychotherapist to be available to patients every minute of every day. Reasonable availability is all that is required (Ewing, 1985; Smith, 1986). Thus, making one's home telephone number available (Smith, 1986) and/or maintaining a live answering service will generally suffice to prevent liability for abandonment. One pitfall worth noting in this regard, however, relates to modern technology. Telephone answering machines now make it possible to have one's phone answsered in one's absence and for the caller to receive and leave a recorded message. But unless such machines are used to provide callers with a number where the therapist can be reached in an emergency, or unless these machines are checked constantly for messages, they have little value for the patient in an emergency, and a therapist's reliance upon them may help establish rather than prevent legal liability for abandonment.

ARRANGING COVERAGE WHILE
YOU ARE UNAVAILABLE

Obviously, no psychotherapist can be available to patients every day, 365 days a year. Therapists suffer illnesses, take vacations, leave town for conferences, and have other commitments that occasionally take them away from their practices.

To avoid potential liability for abandonment, therapists who plan to be unavailable to patients at certain times should arrange coverage by another clinician and, wherever possible, should give patients advance notice of such coverage (Gutheil & Appelbaum, 1983; Ewing, 1985; Smith, 1986). Where advance notice is impractical, the therapist must make it possible for a patient to reach the covering clinician should an emergency arise. In such instances, a telephone answering service or at least a telephone answering machine should be available to explain to patients who call who the covering clinician is and how he or she may be reached. An alternative is to have one clinician cover all absences and to tell all patients at the start of treatment to contact that clinician in the event of an emergency in which they cannot reach you.

Arranging for coverage of one's practice while one is away is essential but is not by itself sufficient to relieve the therapist of potential legal liability. The therapist must take care in selecting a covering clinician. The therapist will not be held liable for the negligence of the covering clinician but may be held liable for his or her own negligence in selecting the covering clinician (Gutheil & Appelbaum, 1983; Ewing, 1985; Smith, 1986). At a minimum, therapists should select only qualified and reputable clinicians to cover for them while they are unavailable (Smith, 1986). If a therapist knows or should have known that his or her covering clinician is not qualified or has a reputation for failing to provide proper care to patients, and one of the therapist's patients is harmed as a result of the covering clinician's negligence, the therapist may well be held legally responsible for that harm (Gutheil & Appelbaum, 1983).

Additionally, thereapists need to make sure that their covering clinicians are equipped to provide adequate care to their patients. First of all, this means providing the covering clinician with sufficient information or access to information about patients who may seek care from him or her while the therapist is unavailable. Additionally and probably more importantly, the therapist should be sure that the covering clinician will in fact be available to cover while the therapist is away.

Simon (1987) tells a story that, though perhaps apocryphal, makes the point. Dr. B agreed to cover the psychotherapy practice of Dr. A for the month of August, a traditional vacation period for many mental health professionals. Once August rolled around, Dr. B discovered that the other psychotherapists in the area, including his own, had arranged to have Dr. A cover their practices for the same month. As a result of his agreement with Dr. A, Dr. B ended up covering for his own psychotherapist.

The point, of course, is that therapists need to make sure that those they select to cover for them will, in fact, provide coverage. Where possible, therapists may find it helpful to secure two or more colleagues to cover for them when they are unavailable for long periods of time. A system of multiple covering clinicians provides greater assurance that any emergency will be handled by a clinician selected by the therapist, and thereby decreases the likelihood of liability for abandonment.

REFERRING PATIENTS TO OTHER PRACTITIONERS

As noted earlier in this chapter, there are instances in which it is therapeutically appropriate to refer a current patient to another therapist. In such circumstances, if the transfer is handled properly by the therapist, he or she should have no worry of liability for abandonment. The same is true even where the referral is made for nontherapeutic—e.g., economic—reasons.

The legal issue that may arise as a result of such referrals is likely to be not abandonment (unless the transfer is not handled therapeutically or with reasonable notice) but rather negligence. Just as in the case of coverage, a therapist is not liable for the negligence of another therapist to whom he or she refers a patient. But the referring therapist may be held liable for negligence in selecting the other therapist to whom the patient is referred (Appelbaum & Gutheil, 1983; Ewing, 1985). And the answer here, as in the discussion of coverage, is simple: Refer patients only to qualified therapists whose work you know and trust.

REFERENCES

Barker, R.L. (1982). *The business of psychotherapy: Private practice administration for therapists, counselors and social workers.* New York: Columbia University Press.

Ewing, C.P. (1978). *Crisis intervention as psychotherapy.* New York: Oxford University Press.

Ewing, C.P. (1985). Mental health clinicians and the law: An overview of current law governing professional practice. In C.P. Ewing (Ed.), *Psychology, psychiatry and the law: A clinical and forensic handbook* (pp. 527–560). Sarasota, FL: Professional Resource Exchange, Inc.

Gutheil, T.G., & Appelbaum, P.S. (1982). *Clinical handbook of psychiatry and the law.* New York: McGraw-Hill.

Simon, R.I. (1987). *Clinical psychiatry and the law.* Washington, DC: American Psychiatric Association.

Smith, J.T. (1986). *Medical malpractice: Psychiatric care.* Colorado Springs, CO: Shepard's/McGraw-Hill.

C H A P T E R

62

THE COMPUTERIZED CLINICIAN: ETHICAL, LEGAL, AND PROFESSIONAL ISSUES IN AUTOMATING PSYCHOLOGICAL SERVICES

David E. Hartman, Ph.D.

During the past decade, computers have become mental health professionals. Software packages have been developed to handle a full range of clinical duties, from mundane activities having no direct effect upon psychological treatment and decision making (e.g., data collection and billing) to "expert system" software that substitutes for or bypasses the judgment of the expert clinician (e.g., "report writers" and psychotherapy programs). Controversy increases as a function of how completely the computer is asked to assume the duties of the clinician in that very few clinicians would object to automated patient accounting procedures, while software psychotherapy remains highly controversial.

A remarkable variety of practical and fanciful computer applications are currently available for professional and lay purchase. Versions of traditional psychological tests like the MMPI coexist on the software shelves with programs that purport to manipulate a child's behavior, coax a partner into a sexual relationship via a computerized analysis of his or her personality, or hire the person most likely to fit in with the emotional styles of other employees. These computerized clinicians are a new but rapidly expanding mental health industry. As early as 1984, when most clinical software was processed by mainframe computer services, more than 300,000 computerized test reports were being generated each year (Johnson, 1984). There is every reason to suppose that the use of psychological software has increased since then, paralleling the rapid assimilation of the personal computer into society at large.

Psychologists view the computerization of their services on a continuum ranging from enthusiasm to anger. On the one hand, supporters of automated methods predict that computerized methods will become so universally adopted that "practitioners who fail to understand the impact of computer technology will soon be surpassed by [their] more enlightened colleagues" (Pressman, 1984), p. vii). On the other hand, American Psychological Associa-

---

The author gratefully thanks Deborah J. Hartman, J.D., for her assistance with portions of this manuscript.

tion treasurer Ray Fowler has stated that "any clinician who *can* be replaced by a computer *should* be," and Joseph Weizenbaum (who programmed the Rogerian therapy simulation, "ELIZA") has termed the prospect of computerized psychotherapy a "monstrous obscenity" (Weizenbaum, 1976, p. 226).

The divergence of opinions about automated methods reflects the complex issues involved in computerizing clinical psychology. Since the technology exists and the genie cannot be put back in the bottle, the most appropriate response for psychology as a profession is to become computer literate, regardless of preexisting prejudice. This new literacy is necessary to address the scientific, professional, and social questions generated by new technology. Thus, psychology must concern itself not only with the construction of the program but also with larger issues about the marketing of the software, appropriate use by the purchaser, the interaction of programs with ethical and legal standards, and perhaps most importantly, determination of the degree of professional equivalence between clinician and computer.

Most reviews of psychological software have concentrated on the scientific aspects of computer program use: the psychometric properties of particular software packages and their equivalence to existing noncomputerized methods. Only a short review of these concerns will be summarized here, since the issues are covered in ample depth elsewhere (e.g., Hartman, 1986; Matarazzo, 1985; Wilson et al., 1985). The remainder of the chapter will address the "nonscientific" but equally important issues—the ethical and legal ramifications of automating the profession.

SCIENTIFIC ISSUES

Proponents of automated clinical methods frequently cite Paul Meehl's (1956) advocacy of scientific "actuarial" methods over imprecise human clinical methods. In fact, computers are superb processors of actuarial formulas. They are far faster, more accurate, and more reliable than their human counterparts at processing repetitive and probabilistic details. Computers can process complex formulas quickly and perform calculations beyond the time constraints or patience of the average clinician. They have no preconceived biases or expectations (Kleinmuntz, 1984) and do not become bored or sulky when required to interview every single patient using the exact same questions in the exact same order. Barring a system malfunction or power outage, computers are always ready for work without complaint, salary, coffee break, or holiday.

Not all psychologists accept the scientific validity and utility of automated methods. Opponents counter that Meehl's advocacy of actuarial methods should not apply to "inadequate" and "aggressively marketed" psychological software (Lanyon, 1984, p. 689). Critics of present-day automated methods point out that little actual validation research is available for automated clinical methods (Matarazzo, 1985). The need for validation research is crucial because of the many patient and hardware/software variables that make for nonequivalence between computer and clinician. Patient variables include familiarity with the computer, age, and cultural background (Hartman, 1986; Mooreland, 1985). Hardware and software are very different in their presentation from noncomputerized psychological services. The materials are different — e.g., CRTs and "mice" or keyboards instead of paper and paper test or interpersonal clinical interview. Variations between and within computer systems may also greatly affect norms. The "expandable" character of most personal computers permits many very basic characteristics of information presentation to vary, including levels of processing speed, degree of graphic resolution (pixels), monitor size, presentation in color or monochrome, to name just a few. Even without the complications produced by patient reactions, the rapid cycle of technological change in personal computing works against the basic necessity for standardized materials and presentation in psychological software.

PROFESSIONAL ISSUES

Equivalence Of The Computer To The Clinician

In the rush to technologize psychology, the distinction between the services of clinicians and computers can become blurred or lost. Marketing that touts the equivalence of automated methods to human activities further clouds the distinction. Nonetheless, recent reviews have emphasized a possibly irreducible difference between computerized and human clinical activities. Tallent (1987) notes the distinction between "testing," an activity amenable to computerization, and "assessment," which is a multivalued, problem-solving activity that depends upon active information searching by the human clinician. Matarazzo (1985) also emphasizes the contextual nature of the computer evaluation, claiming that "even if today's computerized interpretations...were valid...the same results can and do...take on differential meaning based on the unique characteristics and related context of each and every individual being assessed" (p. 248). The courts recognize this unique contribution of the human clinician and view trained psychologists as "experts" able to testify about human behavior. The same cannot be said of the automated simulation of a psychologist's services (Matarazzo, 1985).

The proposal of equivalence between human clinician and computer is most controversial in the case of psychotherapy programs. The idea of computerized psychotherapy has captured the imagination of scientist and artist alike. Sagan (1975) predicts the advent of "psychotherapeutic terminals...like arrays of large telephone booths" where large numbers of patients can be treated "for a few dollars a session" (p. 10). Further in the future, Poul Anderson's novel *Gateway* imagines a character who undergoes computerized "psychoanalysis." While the patient lies on the couch, his defenses are probed by a televised construct of Sigmund Freud himself. The digital "Sigmund" puffs a cigar reflectively and employs powerful artificial intelligence programming to analyze his patient's speech and arousal level (using sensors inside the couch) before delivering a psychological interpretation.

Present-day applications of software psychotherapy are far more prosaic and limited in their capabilities. Much of the available software falls in the "self-help" category, available to the public through computer outlets or local bookstores. Some programs specialize in focused treatment and coach the user through specific cognitive or behavioral strategies of symptom reduction. Programs that treat depression, stress, impotence, and other dysfunctions are in this category. Other software purports to serve more general counseling functions. For example, a program called "Psyche," selling for $49.95, is viewed by its creator as "a modern software simulation of a. . .counselor who will hold a delightfully real keyboard conversation with you on more than 50 topics." The program is said to "stay with your feelings like a real therapist" but presumably unlike a real therapist, "has unlimited time and patience and never judges you or hands out advice" (Balis, cited in Pothier, 1984).

While psychotherapy softrware attempts to inspire and encourage its patient/users toward improved psychosocial function, it simultaneously inspires a wave of professional controversy. The issue is that there is no legal or ethical standard of care required by such software. The computer, functioning as an unlicensed therapist, does not have a diploma ensuring basic competence in the field, has not taken an internship or a state licensing examination, and perhaps even more importantly, has no malpractice insurance in the event of harmful outcome. Such maltreatment can be easily imagined: e.g., a "depression management program" that does not measure the degree and severity of depression in the user and thus refer him or her to a human clinician in the event of serious suicidal symptoms. Similarly, the manufacturer of a biofeedback program that encourages the use of relaxation techniques to reduce headaches may someday be named in a suit by a patient whose brain tumor became inoperable while he or she learned to temporarily ameliorate symptoms using the program.

The ethics of developing unsupervised, automated psychotherapy for the lay public is not specifically addressed by the ethical codes of the American Psychological Association. However, analogous principles relevant to automated test interpretation clearly prohibit the providing of computer interpretations directly to the patient.

Research vs. Restriction

The development of psychological software highlights what may be an inherent conflict between business and science. Software developers whose companies spend money to develop and market a product are usually loathe to "give away" the programming and decision rules that constitute that product. This restriction, reasonable from a business perspective, frustrates the equally reasonable aims of psychometric researchers, who would ordinarily require such detailed information to conduct validity studies. The present "compromise" has been for interested companies to conduct research "in-house." However, having the developer (who has a substantial economic investment in the product) also perform all the validation studies may damage the real or perceived impartiality of the research. The developer may selectively sponsor certain studies but withhold materials from others. One prominent researcher who independently attempted to compare the output of several psychological testing programs was unable to procure evaluation services from selected companies (Kleinmuntz, 1986).

ETHICAL ISSUES

Marketing

Advertised Claims   The dichotomy between "the needs of the professional psychologist to uphold the ethics of the profession" and the psychological entrepreneur whose primary motivation is profit (Kleinmuntz, 1982, p. 237) is exemplified by the problems of psychological software marketing. While many software purveyors produce responsible product ads, there are several types of marketing methods that could be construed as violating the American Psychological Association's *Ethical Principles of Psychologists (EPP)* (APA, 1981) and the newly published *Guidelines for Users of Computer-Based Tests and Interpretations (GCBTI)*, 1986).

Exaggerated claims for the clinical software product are an obvious concern. A widely advertised assessment program called "Mind Prober" asks readers if they have "Read any good minds lately?" and suggests that the program can produce "a scientifically accurate personality profile of anyone. . .the things most people are afraid to tell you. . . . Their strengths, weaknesses, sexual interests and more" (*Psychology Today,* Sept. 1984). This is disputed by *Infoworld,* whose review of Mind Prober notes that the manual provides no validity data about the program.

Mind Prober is a good example of another marketing concern — the promulgation of suggestive ads that would be inappropriate for a licensed human mental health provider. The Orwellian character of "Read any good minds lately?" is perhaps surpassed by another ad for the same program, a Machiavellian enticement suggesting the program will "help you get into her head, the rest is up to you" and ambiguously adding that after you meet the "perfect woman," Mind Prober will teach you how to "insert yourself into her psyche" (cited in Eyde and Kowal, 1985). *Infoworld* also disputes this claim, noting that the clinical-sounding and somewhat brutal descriptives generated by trhe program should not be used to evaluate a significant other "unless you are prepared for a short relationship" (cited in Eyde & Kowal, 1985).

If Mind Prober's statements advertised the 'abilities' of a human psychologist, they would immediately provoke ethical censure. The advertisements would violate *EPP* Principle 4b, which prohibits public statements claiming unusual, unique, or unjustified abilities, and also Principle 4g, which prohibits sensational, exaggerated, or superficial public statements.

As many state licensing laws are written, programs like Mind Prober have only to a avoid mentioning any variant of the word "psychology" to escape the ethical and legal requirements of the American Psychological Association. It is likely, however, that such marketing claims damage the credibility of the psychological profession, regardless of wording. Moreover, such programs are in a legal limbo as to their equivalence to the profession of psychology; it is unclear whether they must adhere to any standards, ethical or legal, required by psychologists performing similar services. The ambiguous status of psychological software may be a by-product of licensing laws that regulate the *title* but not the *practice* of psychology. Such lenient laws could allow harmful software simulations of psychological services to be marketed. The stronger licensing statutes of the medical profession are probably the reason why analogous diagnostic and therapeutic "software physicians" have not become available to the public.

Violating the relationship with the clinician   Another common ethical violation of clinical software advertising is to propose product use in a manner that subverts the proper relationship between clinician, software, and patient. The American Psychological Association clearly intends that clinical software should be utilized in the context of assessment or treatment managed by the clinician (*GCBTI*, Principle 9). Potential violators of this relationship include companies that tout their product as capable of equalizing the skills between good and poor clinicians. Since poor clinicians presumably do not know enough to perform their skills adequately, they must rely on the computer's expertise, a violation of *EPP* Principle 2b, which requires psychologists to perform their duties "on the basis of careful preparation," and Principle 8f, which prohibits psychologists from encouraging "inappropriately trained or otherwise unqualified" persons to use assessment techniques.

Trivial Pursuits   A related subversion of the relationship between clinician and software is promoted by advertisers who promote software for its profit-generating capability rather than for the welfare of the consumer, a violation of the Preamble to Principle 8 of the *EPP.* One such promoter advocates the use of its software in "high volume profit centers" where "hundreds of reports" are "processed" each day. This type of use removes the clinician from the process of testing. Mass testing militates against appropriate supervision of test performance by responsible clinicians and forces the data from the test to stand in place of a true clinical assessment. Thus, it may violate *GCBTI* Principle 6, which emphasizes the importance of monitoring test behavior, and Principle 9, which explicitly requires the test output to be used only in conjunction with (and not in place of) the professional's judgment. Unsupervised mass testing, in addition to generating reports with questionable validity, also implicitly condones a "mechanical" nonselective approach to testing that debases the use of testing procedures and by implication, the practice of psychology.

Marketing to Undertrained and Untrained Users   There is considerable concern among psychologists that computer software will target professional and lay buyers untrained in psychometric theory or artificial intelligence limitations, but whose professional status, income, or marketability could be enhanced by adding automated procedures to their repretoire. This prospect could occur both inside and outside of the health professions. Physical and psychiatric medicine welcome the possibility of automated psychological methods. Medical journals like the *Lancet,* for example, have termed computerized psychological testing "immensely economical" because "long run marginal costs are negligible" ("Psychological Assessment," 1983, p. 1024). Similarly, the *American Journal of Psychiatry* suggests that computerized diagnostics produce "none of the possible embarrassment, expense or inconvenience of using a consultant" ("Computers and Diagnosis," 1980, p. 62).

Other service professions that may fall into this group include law, nursing, social work, and nonaffiliated counselors. Businesses and industries may respond positively to the claims of psychological software marketing. Even many marginally trained psychologists are not exempt from the lure of automated methods. Because automated psychological procedures may not require the end user to have any idea what the computer is doing, or why, the end user may not even be required to read the manual, much less to learn about validity or the appropriate use of the automated procedure. Companies that market to clinicians whose licenses do not require understanding of test construction or computer principles may be more likely to have their materials misused, with subsequent ethical and legal consequences. If harm occurs to the patient as a result of software use by untrained individuals, it is likely that *both* the clinician *and* the manufacturer (who should have foreseen this inappropriate use) would be legally liable (see under Legal Issues below).

If psychologists market to untrained or undertrained personnel, they violate *EPP* Principle 8f, which prohibits just such activities, and the *GCBTI* Principle 9, which states that computer-generated interpretive reports should be used "only in conjunction with professional judgment."

Other Ethical Concerns

Plagiarism   Despite the apparent purpose of automated "report-writers" that generate a grammatical "psychological" report from input data, clinicians who hand in such a report or even copy the output into their own evaluation without attribution are guilty of plagiarism (Keith-Spiegel & Koocher, 1985). Including the content of computerized evaluations directly into clinical reports also violates *EPP* Principle 8e, which considers the offering of assessment techniques to be a "professional-to-professional" service.

LEGAL ISSUES

Copyright Violations

Psychological software may also cause problems in the domain of copyright law. Copyright violations are especially likely to occur when paper and pencil tests are adapted to computer use. Programmers may be required to employ tables, data, formulas, etc., from the original copyrighted test manual to produce automated scoring output. This issue has not been tested by the courts as of this writing, although it seems almost inevitable that litigation in this area will be initiated.

Liability

Mental health software is quite controversial from a legal point of view, with both attorneys and psychologists expecting the next decade to bring a wave of legal action from patients who claim harmful effects from psychological software. Some of the potential for harm may stem from incorrect programming—a likely possibility, since the removal of "all errors from a computer program...is a difficult if not an impossible task" (Brannigan & Dayhoff, 1981). However, even a program that has been scrupulously "debugged" may cause significant harm to an unsuspecting client. Some possibilities can be easily imagined:

1. A patient is misdiagnosed as psychotic or dangerous by a software diagnostic program and is inappropriately hospitalized.

2. A depressed patient attempts to alleviate her serious depression with a self-help program and subsequently attempts suicide, causing serious self-injury.

3. A parent is denied custody of a child in a divorce settlement on the basis of a computer-generated personality test profile.

4. A patient follows a software treatment regimen for impotence and delays additional treatment until he is hospitalized for diabetes and is discovered to have penile neuropathy.

At issue is the legal responsibility (liability) for damage caused by defective or harmful software. The two types of tort liability relevant to psychological software use are (1) *negligence* (malpractice), which applies to the performance of services and (2) *strict liability,* which addresses injuries caused by defective materials.

For negligence to be proved in the use of automated psychological methods, they must be considered "services" much like any other provided by the clinical psychologist. All services are judged according to a court-determined "reasonable standard of care" common to the particular profession. A psychologist can be held liable for the consequences of using harmful automated procedures because they are considered as harmful services for which he or she always holds final responsibility. A patient who wishes to prove negligence in the courts has to show that the psychologist in his or her use of psychological software violated the "reasonable standard of care" by providing a harmful service, automated or not.

Current standards suggest that psychologists would certainly be considered negligent if they employed harmful software, since the reasonable standard of care in the psychological community clearly prohibits slavish reliance upon software in the provision of those services. Even if the particular software package is inaccurate or defective, the psychologist would still be negligent, since he or she is reasonably expected to intelligently select correct instruments and techniques in the provision of clinical services. If the software is not defective but its use is inappropriate (e.g., examples 1 and 3 above), the psychologist's liability is also clear; psychologists are supposed to know the psychometric properties and appropriate uses of their clinical software.

From the viewpoint of the plaintiff there may be circumstances where negligence (software as service) does not provide redress. First, a patient who has been harmed by defective software may not recover damages if it has been determined that the clinician *has* exercised a reasonable standard of care, especially if the practitioner could not have reasonably prevented the error. Second, viewing psychological software as a service could make the assignment of liability quite difficult in cases when the patient buys the program directly from the retail vendor. "Because of the multi-stage process of perfecting a computer program, the plaintiff would have difficulty finding the proper defendant" (Brannigan & Dayhoff, 1981, p. 129). Finally, increased use of software by psychologists could actually *decrease* the clinician's liability if software is viewed as a service. This paradoxical result could occur if use of psychological software becomes so popular and widespread that reliance upon it *becomes* the "reasonable standard of care" for the profession. It is not so difficult to imagine a future where there is "mandated" use of certain software to determine diagnosis, placement, or treatment. Computer use would become the de facto reasonable standard of care in this scenario, reducing the clinician's liability. Indeed, a psychologist, like a physician who failed to utilize state-of-the-art technology, could be held liable for failing to employ computerized methods (Miller et al., 1985).

Because of such possibilities, Brannigan & Dayhoff (1981, 1986) argue that software be considered a *product* rather than a *service,* and so be subject to *strict liability.* The authors claim that under strict liability laws, there is no need to make a complex determination about reasonable standard of care; instead, there must be a claim of product defect that has caused harm.

Another advantage for the plaintiff if software is viewed as a "good" rather than a service is the possibility of redress even if the clinician is *not* negligent. It would also appear to be especially applicable to mental health software sold directly to lay purchasers who bypass a clinical service provider but then become harmed in the course of self-treatment (e.g., examples 2 and 4 above). The manufacturer (who does not provide a service) could be held liable for the production of a defective or harmful "product."

Not all legal authorities consider it advantageous for software to fall under the domain of "strict liability." Miller et al. (1985) point out that if clinical software "product" manufacturers are to be proved liable, their program's defects must "render the product 'unreasonably dangerous.'" In the case of software, it is unclear whether an unreasonably dangerous product is a product of bad design or defective manufacture; therefore, "proof of the existence of a defect can be very difficult" (Miller et al., 1985, p. 532). In addition, the products most clearly applicable to strict liability are those programs upon which a clinician must rely completely—e.g., blood test lab results or programs that monitor the continuous output of an EKG. When this criterion is used, it is unlikely that psychological programs administered by a clinician would be considered products subject to strict liability.

In summary, it appears that there is some ambiguity as to the legal status of clinical software. Differential liability may accrue depending upon whether psychological software is viewed as a product or a service. It is certain, however, that the plaintiff will attempt to establish liability in whatever way is likely to fit the context of the case and provide redress. Attorneys are not limited to proposing one type of liability or the other; any and all combinations may be employed. Both the psychologist who administers the program and the manufacturer/designer could be held liable: the psychologist for improper service and the manufacturer for marketing a product whose defective use was "foreseeable" (Miller et al., 1985).

Privacy vs. Piracy

Computer storage of medical records is clearly becoming the norm for hospitals, partially because in this age of strict health care financial management, every single procedure, equipment use, and medicine must be recorded for later billing. In addition, requirements for rapid transmission of patient data to health care specialists, government accounting requirements, and "heavy increases in volume of paperwork" all suggest that computerized information transmission systems "will inevitably become ubiquitous in hospitals" (Hiller & Beyda, 1981, p. 465).

The problem of maintaining confidentiality is a difficult issue in the face of these competing requirements. Further complications arise when computerized records eliminate the single access point through which information flow could be controlled. While noncomputerized hospitals could funnel all information requests through a medical records department, centralized data base storage of patient medical and psychological records eliminates this single access point along with its gatekeeping function. Centralized computers allow (and encourage) the hospital to have multiple terminals each with easy access to patient records. Remote telephone access via a modem permits potentially unrestricted availability of records to anyone with knowledge of the system, access to a personal computer, and a telephone. The result could be theft of information, violation of privacy, and a potentially serious legal problem (Brannigan & Dayhoff, 1986).

Contrary to patients' expectation, the privacy of their hospital psychological records is only partially protected by the Constitution of the United States, state statutes, common law, and "the fiduciary nature" of the psychologist–patient relationship, which binds the psychologist to act only in the patient's best interest (Miller et al., 1985; Hiller & Beyda, 1981). In addition, the federal Privacy Act of 1974 provides some guidelines for maintaining private patient records; however, it suffers from numerous shortcomings, not the least of which is that it "does not apply to state or local governments or to private agencies" (Hiller & Beyda, 1981, p. 472). There are no laws regulating the confidentiality of records in settings other than licensed hospitals or clinics. Thus, "visiting nurse associations, drug addiction treatment centers, [and] alcoholism centers have only "professional and ethical codes" to regulate the privacy of patient records (Hiller & Beyda, 1981, p. 473). However, despite the incomplete or ambiguous protection of current privacy laws, "if the disclosure of confidential health information violates the patient's rights of privacy, monetary damages can be awarded to the patient for any emotional distress, humiliation, embarrassment, loss of wages or profits, or any other advantageous economic relationships that are affected adversely" (Miller et al., 1985, p. 533).

Because of these legal and ethical consequences, psychologists who employ computers for patient record storage, whether in hospitals or group practices, should make every effort to ensure the confidentiality of computerized patient records. Accessibility to the individual clinician's software and patient data can be protected with passwords to lock out unauthorized users. Single floppy disks can be locked away when not in use, as can removable mass storage like Bernoulli media. Nonremovable hard disk systems can also have password protection. For added security, patient data can be "encrypted": Software packages are readily available to render stored data unreadable without a special descrambling code.

When systems are designed for remote entry and dial-up of information, special "dial-back" modems can be installed that check a user's password and then, instead of logging the user on directly, dial back to the site of the correct owner of the password. For added security and to monitor system use, all access to the machine by terminal or modem should be recorded by the computer, including the user's name, time of use, and information about what was accessed, whether anything was copied, and whether data were altered.

Restricting modem access and limiting information disbursement to within hospital may eliminate the dangers from remote access but do nothing to prevent in-hospital personnel not involved in patient care from scanning records. Limited local area networks instead of completely centralized mainframe storage may likewise contribute to confidentiality; however, no externally imposed method can be truly effective without intensive education of clinical personnel about the patient's right to privacy in the computer age.

CONCLUSIONS

Psychological Software: A Scientific Issue?

The types of concerns presented in this chapter suggest that the scientific validation of psychological software must be considered just one issue in the automation of psychological services. In fact, scientific validation may prove to be a more easily solvable problem than the questions of ethics, legal responsibility, and professional equivalence raised by clinical psychology software.

Given this perspective, it appears to be in the best interest of both professionals and patients to emphasize the *differences* rather than the *similarities* between the psychologist and software that simulates psychological services. Psychologists are licensed health professionals who provide (and are legally responsible for) clinical services. No computer program has that legal status. Psychological service is also fundamentally different from any computer simulation because psychologists independently direct an active search for personal, interpersonal, historical, and other contextual informationn for the purpose of providing the best care possible for the patient. Psychologists can assay these data directly from the physical world and are not limited to the fixed modalities of software input and programming code. Computer simulations lack both the ability to integrate such a wide realm of accumulated data and the moral responsibility to integrate these variables over the shifting, ambiguous, and context-bound standard of providing the "best possible care."

Some computer problems, like the protection of computerized data bases, can be corrected with present-day methods. However, these are not applications where computers substitute for clinical decision making. The ethical, legal, and professional difficulties inherent in simulating psychological services are not correctable with present-day technology. Viewed as a purely technological problem, it is possible to imagine the substitution of psychological service with present-day software. Viewed in the larger context of current ethical standards, legal liability and overall professional capabilities, it seems obvious that software simulations are not very similar to psychologists after all. Automated psychological services are not artificial intelligence but only artificial psychology.

REFERENCES

American Psychological Association. (1981). Ethical principles of psychologists. *American Psychologist, 36,* 633–638.

American Psychological Association. (1986). *Guidelines for computer-based tests and interpretations.* Washington, DC: Committee on Professional Standards (COPS) and Committee on Psychological Tests and Assessment (CPTA).

Brannigan, V.M., & Dayhoff, R.E. (1981). Liability for personal injuries caused by defective medical computer programs. *American Journal of Law and Medicine, 2,* 123–144.

Brannigan, V.M., & Dayhoff, R.E. (1986). Medical informatics. The revolution in law, technology, and medicine. *Journal of Legal Medicine, 7,* 1–53.

Computers and diagnosis. (1980, January). *American Journal of Psychiatry, 137,* 61–62.

Eyde, L.D., & Kowal, D.M. (1985). Psychological decision support software for the public: Pros, cons, and guidelines. *Computers in Human Behavior, 1,* 321–336.

Hartman, D. (1986). Artificial intelligence or artificial psychologist? Conceptual issues in clinical microcomputer use. *Professional Psychology: Research and Practice, 17,* 528–534.

Hiller, M.D., & Beyda, V. (1981). Computers, medical records and the right to privacy. *Journal of Health Politics, Policy and Law, 6,* 463–487.

Johnson, J.H. (1984). An overview of computerized testing. In M.D. Schwartz (Ed.), *Using computers in clinical practice.* New York: Haworth, 131–133.

Keith-Spiegel, P. & Koocher, G.R. (1985). *Ethics in psychology.* New York: Random House.

Kleinmuntz, B. (1982). *Personality and psychological assessment.* New York: St. Martins Press.

Kleinmuntz, B. (1984). The scientific study of clinical judgment in psychology and medicine. *Clinical Psychology Review, 4,* 111–126.

Kleinmuntz, B. (1986). Retrospective and prospective views of automated assessment. Paper presented at the 1986 Annual Meeting of the Illinois Psychological Association, Chicago.

Lanyon, R.I. (1984). Personality assessment. *Annual Review of Psychology, 35,* 667–701.

Matarazzo, J.D. (1985). Clinical psychological test interpretations by computer: Hardware outpaces software. *Computers in Human Behavior, 1,* 235–255.

Meehl, P.E. (1956). Wanted—A good cookbook. *American Psychologist, 11,* 263–272.

Miller, R.A., Schaffner, K.F., & Meisel, A. (1985). Ethical and legal issues related to the use of computer programs in clinical medicine. *Annals of Internal Medicine, 102,* 529–536.

Mooreland, K.L. (1985). Computer-assisted psychological assessment in 1986: A practical guide. *Computers in Human Behavior, 1,* 221–234.

Pothier, D. (1984, July 22, section 3). Depressed? Heal thyself bit by byte. *Chicago Tribune,* pp. 1, 8.

Pressman, R.M. (1984). *Microcomputers and the private practitioner.* Homewood, IL: Dow-Jones-Irwin.

Psychological assessment by computer. (1983, May 7). *Lancet, 1,* 1023–1024.

Sagan, C. (1975, January). In praise of robots. *Natural History, 89,* 8–20.

Tallent, N. (1987). Computer-generated psychological reports: A look at the modern psychometric machine. *Journal of Personality Assessment, 51,* 95–108.

Weizenbaum, J. (1976). *Computer power and human reason.* San Francisco: W.H. Freeman.

Wilson, F.R., Genco, K.T., & Yager, G.G. (1985). Assessing the equivalence of paper-and-pencil vs computerized tests: Demonstration of a promising methodology. *Computers and Human Behavior, 1,* 265–276.

C H A P T E R
63

PROBLEMS ENCOUNTERED IN THE PREPARATION AND PRESENTATION OF EXPERT TESTIMONY

David L. Shapiro, Ph.D.

Several recent volumes on forensic psychology and psychiatry, as well as several recent collections, have dealt with the basic parameters of expert testimony in a series of different substantive areas (Blau, 1984; Shapiro, 1983; Ewing, 1985; Everstine & Everstine, 1986). All of these works address many of the basic issues in expert testimony.

This chapter, rather than reviewing or summarizing any of these materials, will focus on specific problems encountered in the preparation and presentation of expert testimony. Many of these problems result from limitations on the role of the expert witness imposed by recent litigation, and others are issues suggested by such litigation but not yet actually "put to the test." Other topics to be covered are a variety of ethical issues posed by various areas of psychological evaluation and expert testimony.

PSYCHODYNAMIC MECHANISMS AND CRIMINAL RESPONSIBILITY

Psychoanalytic theory and methods of treatment have contributed in a major way to our understanding of human behavior and, especially, of maladaptive manifestations of such behavior. The basic assumption, however, of psychic determinism can pose many problems if the expert witness utilizing this framework does not "check" the validity of the assumptions derived through a psychoanalytic process against the objective reality of the circumstances of the offense charged. That is, even if a particular offense "makes sense" when viewed from a psychodynamic point of view, this cannot automatically be translated into an absence of criminal responsibility under the law, unless the examiner pays close attention to secondary sources of data such as police reports, witness statements, videotape confessions, etc., to see whether the psychodynamic assumptions do indeed comport with the reality of what actually occurred.

Perhaps one of the foremost proponents of a theory of unconscious determinism and its direct equation into an absence of criminal responsibility is Abrahamsen (1974), whose volume *The Murdering Mind* is exceedingly thought provoking. Abrahamsen, however, makes little attempt in his analysis to integrate objective sources of data into his understanding of the motivations of the defendant being examined, and tends to equate unconscious determinants of behavior with legal insanity.

The following example will illustrate the phenomenon described above, that while some seemingly bizarre and senseless behavior of a defendant at the time of a homicide could be explained from a psychodynamic perspective, careful analysis of witness statements, police reports, videotaped interviews, and actual interviews with family and friends cast serious doubt on the validity of the psychoanalytic formulations in explaining the defendant's behavior and in reaching an opinion on criminal responsibility.

Example One

The defendant, Mr. G, was the owner of an apartment building, and had had a long-standing rent dispute with one of the women who lived in the building regarding her rent and occupancy in the building.

One day, he chased the woman into her apartment with a shotgun, shot her in the back, and then shot at her mother who was asleep on the couch, grazing the mother. He then went into a rear bedroom and mortally wounded a sister of the first victim, went back to the first woman who was still alive, dragged her outside, poured a flammable liquid on her, and set her afire. While she was on fire, he shot another blast into her, then shot out the windows of the apartment, and waited for the police to arrive.

The two decedents were the granddaughters of a woman who had previously lived in the same apartment, in one of the two buildings that Mr. G. owned. Following the death of the grandmother, Mr. G had attempted to have the two sisters move out of the grandmother's apartment, insisting that they were not the tenants, that their grandmother had been, and that he, as landlord, had a perfect right to put them out. Mr. G had made repeated references to the fact that these women were drug dealers and prostitutes and that he did not regard them as suitable tenants for his building.

A prior psychological evaluation performed on Mr. G by a psychoanalytically trained psychologist had included a clinical interview, a Wechsler Adult Intelligence Scale, a Bender Gestalt, the Human Figure Drawings, and the Rorschach, as well as a review of a transcript of the videotaped confession, the newspaper account of the offense, and various letters that Mr. G had written to various tenants of his buidling.

This psychological evaluation resulted in a diagnosis of Mr. G as a narcissistic personality disorder and stated that the defendant "viewed himself as one who had been deprived of love and nurturance." The defendant, according to this report, also "revealed a grandiose sense of his self-importance, as well as feelings of chronic uncertainty and dissatisfaction with himself." He was also described as very constricted in his emotional life and having several depressive equivalents. This evaluation described the patient as having a stormy and abusive relationship with his father, a military attaché who physically abused the patient. It was further noted that the patient, who was overindulged by his mother, had grown up in Haiti, the illegitimate son of a union between his natural father and his father's maid.

The psychological test data, according to this evaluation, revealed feelings of uncertainty and a low sense of self-esteem, which was in marked contrast to the need to be a "real man," which was "synonymous with the military man that his father was." The psychological evaluation described Mr. G as having "a basic weakness in his impulse control and frustration tolerance." The psychological test data further substantiated the difficulties in controlling aggression. The psychologist performing the evaluation described the sense of tenuous control that Mr. G had in modulating aggressive feelings. The report also noted that the patient "becomes overwhelmed in the face of emotionally-charged stimuli and at times reality testing is compromised."

The patient described, in this initial evaluation, the fact that when he saw one of the sisters leave the apartment on the day of the offense, he became "a beast," got his gun, entered the apartment, "and I shot her and after that I just went into the apartment and went for everything that moved." He described his state as one of "blind fury," and stated that it was as if he were "blind and deaf." He insisted "I had no reason to do these things, I was a beast."

The psychologist indicated, regarding the issue of criminal responsibility, that Mr. G suffered from a narcissistic personality disorder, and "it appears highly likely that he experienced a transient psychotic episode (third edition of the *Diagnostic and Statistical Manual of Mental Disorders* [DSM-III] Brief Reactive Psychosis)." The psychologist noted that, according to the DSM-III, narcissistic personalities may be particularly vulnerable to the development of such transient psychotic states. The patient had described to the psychologist a series of repeated humiliations at the hands of the decedents who, on many occasions, had thrown him out of the apartment, had laughed at him, had called the police to arrest him, and threatened to "blow his brains out." In the face of the repeated humiliations, according to this evaluation, "Mr. G decompensated and suffered a transient psychotic episode, losing the ability to test reality, and his identification with the aggressive military man father became complete for the hours preceding the murder." He became the powerful one, developing a mission to free his property of the "invaders," which in point of fact was a word he had used to describe these very tenants. The psychological evaluation noted that the manner in which the crime was committed lent support to the patient's loss of reality testing and identification with the military man, especially his dragging the decedent into the front yard after shooting her and setting her afire in full view of neighbors and passers-by on the street. The psychologist opined that Mr. G experienced himself, in that psychotic episode, as being in military action, heaping atrocities on the enemy in order to "build up self-esteem and demoralize those who are still alive, those who will see the humiliation." The description that the patient gave of going into the apartment and "shooting everything that moved" was the description of a soldier in battle, according to the psychologist.

As noted above, this psychological evaluation, which made "perfect sense" from a psychodynamic point of view, failed to incorporate any possible sources of external verification. It will be recalled that this evaluation was based on one interview plus a series of psychological tests. No witnesses to the offense were interviewed, the videotape of the patient's confession was not viewed, no family or friends were interviewed, and no records were reviewed.

If all of the inferences from all of the test data and the clinical interview of Mr. G were accurate, whether or not he was actually experiencing a brief reactive psychosis at the time of the offense could be determined only by interviewing people who had observed his behavior immediately before, during, and after the offense. There are, according to the DSM III, objective criteria for the diagnosis of such a brief reactive psychosis, and if indeed the patient were experiencing such an episode, some, if not all, of the symptoms would be apparent to the witnesses to the offense.

As noted in my earlier volume, *Psychological Evaluation and Expert Testimony* (Shapiro, 1983), one must make every effort possible to obtain as complete a chronology as one can of the patient's behavior prior to, during, immediately after, and subsequent to the time of the offense, up to the very time that one examines the patient in order to determine consistencies and differences in the patient's behavior.

The evaluation that was later performed included not only three psychological evaluations, including extensive history taking, but a review of the videotapes of the confession and interviews with a number of witnesses, including his ex-wife, his two daughters, his girlfriend, the mother of the decedent, a friend of his who had attempted to restrain him at the time that he set the body of one of the decedents on fire, and an interview with a woman who lived in the apartment building who had spoken with the defendant approximately 15 minutes prior to the shooting. In addition, there were interviews with police officers who had been present at the time of the arrest in order to ascertain the defendant's behavior and demeanor immediately following the offense. In short, a series of interviews were conducted with people who saw him just prior to, during, immediately after, and a few hours subsequent to the offense. If indeed the patient had been suffering from a transient psychosis, some of the symptoms should have been evident to these individuals. The psychologist in the initial examination had not talked to any of these witnesses. Review of the history preceding the offense did indeed reveal several incidents in which the patient had been arrested following his demanding of rent money from the woman in the apartment. He did indeed describe these incidents as profound humiliations, and indeed the second psychological evaluation was totally consistent with the initial one, viewing Mr. G as an exceedingly narcissistic individual who regarded himself as "the king" in his neighborhood, and who felt that the residents of the neighborhood revered him and that such incidents of his being arrested and publicly humiliated were profoundly traumatic events.

An interview with Ms. R, a resident in Mr. G's apartment building, revealed that approximately 15 minutes prior to the shooting, she had asked Mr. G to fix a venetian blind in her apartment that had come off its bracket. He did so, and according to Ms. R, he was coherent, rational, and pleasant, showing no evidence of incoherence of speech, delusions, hallucinations, or any disorganization of behavior.

An interview was also conducted with Mr. J, a young man who had known Mr. G for several years and tried to restrain him at the time of the offense. This interview revealed no evidence of bizarre behavior at the time of the offense. Mr. J stated that a child ran up to him and told him that Ms. B, one of the victims, needed him. Mr. J ran around the corner and saw Mr. G in the dooway of Ms. B's apartment. She was lying on the floor, holding her leg, and Mr. G pointed the shotgun at Mr. J and said, "Bob, this doesn't concern you, get out of here." Mr. J backed down to the front gate. He then described Mr. G's dragging Ms. B down the front steps and throwing her in the front yard, where he poured a flammable liquid on her and lit her. Mr. J begged Mr. G to put the gun down as the defendant, Mr. G, was walking around the burning body. Mr. G then found more shells in his pocket, reloaded the shotgun, and fired once more into her body and twice into the windows of the apartment.

While the behavior is certainly extremely violent, when Mr. J was questioned whether or not the patient manifested any indications of psychotic behavior such as loosening of associations, incoherence, delusions, or hallucinations, Mr. J responded in the negative.

Several police officers were interviewed, all of whom noted nothing unusual in Mr. G's presentation. When Mr. G was read his Miranda rights, he stated, "I understand my rights and don't want to say anything."

The importance of this particular series of interviews sets the offense within some time frame. An interview had been conducted with witnesses who had observed Mr. G 15 minutes prior to the offense, at the time of the offense, and immediately after the offense. None of these witnesses, either spontaneously or in response to specific questions, noted the presence of any of the symptoms suggestive of a brief reactive psychosis.

The next piece of data that was important to evaluate was the videotaped confession that was taken approximately 3 hours after the offense. Here again, the patient described himself as a beast, recounted the sense of humiliation that he had encountered at the hands of the women in the apartment, and said that he became irrational and went into the apartment and "shot everything that I saw alive." There was also some evidence that he was planning to shoot the victim, for when he saw her exit the apartment a few minutes prior to the offense, he took his gun and, addressing his gun, stated, "Mister, when she comes back in I'm going to turn you loose."

Given the absence of any prior evidence of psychotic behavior, it would be highly unlikely that 3 hours after a brief psychotic reaction, had it indeed occurred, an individual would have insight to speak about his being irrational or having a beast or monster take over his character. His statement that he was shooting at everything that moved was inaccurate since the children, in fact in the same bed with her, were unharmed. This suggests that despite his apparently agitated state, he was capable of distinguishing the children from the other people in the apartment. Furthermore, when approached by Mr. J, Mr. G showed a capacity to inhibit his rage, stating that this did not concern Mr. J and that he should back away or he would shoot him too. Again, this casts some doubt on Mr. G's statement that he had gone "completely wild." A review of prior police reports, which again the first psychologist had failed to make, revealed that in an earlier arrest for simple assault Mr. G had expressed some outrage at the fact that he had been arrested, stating that in his own country "we take such matters into our own hands." Finally, interviews with the patient's ex-wife and daughters revealed the fact that, while had had never done anything previously as violent as the current offense, his interactions with them consisted of repeated beatings and extreme humiliation, especially of his daughters.

Finally, the idea of the patient's identifying with an aggressive military man and being in the midst of combat was explored, with the rather striking fact being revealed that his father, according to both the patient and a subsequent interview with the father, was a "passive bureaucrat" who had not ever seen battle. The father, in fact, never even spoke to his son about military exploits, and the defendant himself read romantic books rather than novels about war. In point of fact, the patient may well have identified with his father, but what he identified with was his father's brutal and sadistic means of punishment, not with his being a military man.

What is critical here, of course, is the difference between a traditional clinical and a forensic evaluation, with special emphasis on the way that a very elegant psychoanalytic hypothesis may be totally inconsistent with the objective facts revealed by a careful review of witness statements and other external sources of data.

QUALIFICATIONS OF EXPERT OPINIONS

Although the model suggested above of a comprehensive forensic evaluation — including not only clinical data but also the integration of a wide variety of external sources of verification — should be followed if at all possible, on some occasions such material is simply not available, witnesses refuse to be interviewed, or various rules of discovery inherent in the adversary process interfere with the availability of, or access to, many of these data sources. As a practical matter, it protects the expert from the typical onslaught of cross-examination in which opposing counsel will inevitably confront the expert with all of the things that he or she "didn't do but should have done."

In rendering the opinion in the evaluation, the expert should make reference to the specific data sources that it would be important to have available for a final opinion and that again were not made available. Again, this presents to the trier of fact the statement that the witness knows the relevant dimensions and is qualifying his or her opinion specifically because of the absence of those elements.

Example Two

A psychologist had been retained by a defense attorney to perform a criminal responsibility evaluation on a defendant charged with an armed rape. The defendant was a young man who had had an extensive history of psychiatric hospitalization and was in outpatient treatment at the time of the offense. There was verification from his family that the patient had been acting in a rather bizarre manner for several days prior to the crime but no verification from the arresting officers that the defendant in any way behaved in an irrational manner at the time of arrest, which took place about an hour after the offense. The victim of the sexual assault, an adolescent girl, was quoted in the police report as stating that after the assault had occurred the defendant was "talking out of his head."

This, of course, was a critically important piece of data, for it might have meant that the patient was acting in a bizarre and psychotic manner at the time that the offense occurred. On the other hand, the phrase "talking out of one's head" is often "street parlance" and has little or no reference to psychosis. It may merely mean that the individual in question was talking rapidly, was drunk, was high on drugs, or was talking about some unrealistic way of making money.

What was critical, of course, was to be able to interview the complaining witness in this case to find out exactly what she meant by "talking out of his head." The problem became one of discovery, with the government refusing to allow an expert retained by the defense to interview one of their witnesses. In a series of pretrial hearings initiated by defense counsel, it was explained to the court that an opinion on criminal responsibility could not be rendered without the defense's expert interviewing the complaining witness. The government continued to object adamantly to this, and the judge eventually, as a compromise, suggested that the defense-retained psychologist provide a list of questions that the U.S. Attorney would then ask the complaining witness, that the session be tape-recorded, and that a transcript of this recording then be provided to the doctor. Hopefully, the doctor would then be able to render an opinion on criminal responsibility.

Something was "lost in the translation," and the psychologist retained by the defense did not, in good conscience, have enough material to render such an opinion. For this reason, the conclusion of the report was qualified in the following manner:

> There is evidence that on or about the date of the alleged offense, the patient was suffering from a Schizophrenic Disorder, characterized by auditory hallucinations and delusional thinking. These phenomena were verified by family and friends. Whether or not the patient was actually under the influence of these delusions and hallucinations at the time of the alleged offense cannot be answered in any conclusive manner because the only witness to the offense, namely the complainant herself, was not made available for interview. Therefore, while the patient was manifesting signs of a psychotic disorder at that point in time, it is unclear whether or not that disorder substantially contributed to his behavior at the time of the offense.

In summary, then, it becomes important for the examiner not only to provide the details of a comprehensive forensic psychological evaluation but also to qualify an opinion when critical data are lacking.

ETHICAL ISSUES IN FORENSIC EVALUATION

Ethical principles affect forensic practice in many ways. This has been addressed in many excellent publications, most notable of which is the work by Monahan (1980) entitled *Who Is the Client?*, published by the American Psychological Association. One can see the impact of virtually every one of the ethical principles in the daily conduct of psychological evaluations and expert testimony. For instance, forensic practitioners must be constantly alert to the potential for misuse of their data within the legal system and for that reason must be exceedingly careful in the way that data are presented, being frank about the limitations of the data and what questions can and cannot be answered with the data. It is an unfortunate truth that many attorneys in attempting to represent their clients vigorously will ask psychologists to present data in a distorted way or to present only "half of the picture" in order to assist in their advocacy. Such efforts must be firmly resisted.

With the qualification as an expert witness, there is a constant temptation in forensic work to go beyond the limits of one's competence and to render opinions in areas in which either the psychologist has no particular training or the state of knowledge is so meager that opinions should not be rendered. There is also a strong temptation and pressure on the part of expert witnesses to present data as "classic examples" of particular syndromes, which in turn result in a particular legal conclusion. Again, the psychologist must remain scrupulously close to the data, present only material that is solidly documented, and present only conclusions that can be firmly supported by the data.

The ethical principle prohibiting "a partial disclosure of relevant facts" likely to mislead or deceive is particularly relevant to the cautions noted above. The presentation of qualifications, a necessary part of expert testimony, can easily give rise to a violation of Principle 2, Section B, Subsection 1, of the APA Code of Ethics, which states: "Presenting a false, fraudulent, misleading, deceptive, or unfair statement." In a sense, the very process of qualifying an expert witness invites these deceptive or unfair statements, especially when one is involved in a "battle of the experts." Again, of course, one must not attempt to overemphasize one's qualifications in such a manner. One should certainly not present affiliation with any organization "in a manner that falsely implies sponsorship or certification by that organization." A number of psychologists who are applying for Board Certification, for instance, have referred to themselves as "Board Eligible," and utilize this designation in their correspondence and in their qualifications as expert witnesses. This is clearly unethical, since there is no such status with a certification board as "Board Eligible."

The issue of confidentiality in forensic examinations is often misunderstood. In general, if a psychologist is performing a court-ordered evaluation, then the confidentiality of the proceedings is not a factor and the privilege is generally waived. This is, in fact, noted in Principle 5 of the APA Code of Ethics, which states, "Where appropriate, psychologists inform their clients of the legal limits of confidentiality." While this most likely refers to situations in which a psychotherapy client threatens to do bodily harm to an identifiable third party, it has equal relevance to the forensic evaluation and testimony. That is, many patients participating in a forensic evaluation are not aware of the fact that whey they say to a psychologist is not privileged in a court-ordered evaluation and that it will become part of the report to the court on such issues as competency or criminal responsibility. This must be made clear to patients in advance of their participation in an evaluation. The exact nature of this informed consent to evaluation will vary with a number of factors, and these will be discussed in a subsequent section that deals more specifically with the issue of informed consent. However, at this point, from the point of view of professional ethics, it is important that patients participating in pretrial court-ordered evaluations be aware of the fact that the material they share with the psychologist is not confidential.

Although the dual relationship is prohibited by the APA Code of Ethics (Principle 6, Subsection A: "Psychologists make every effort to avoid dual relationships"), this concept has been poorly understood within the forensic domain. In my previous volume, *Psychological Evaluation and Expert Testimony* (Shapiro, 1983), I have discussed, in a section entitled "Therapist or Examiner" in Chapter 6, the practical reasons for avoiding such a role conflict. From the point of view of professional ethics, there is also an important point to be made: One cannot be an effective therapist, in terms of helping the patient deal with his or her difficulties, if one has also been involved in a comprehensive forensic evaluation of that individual. That is, if one has done a comprehensive assessment, interviewed many witnesses, reviewed many reports, assessed the possibilities of malingering or secondary gain, then one, in a sense, "knows too much" to be of assistance to the patient and to maintain the "free-floating attention" necessary to truly help that patient unravel personal difficulties. On the other hand, the therapist should make every effort to avoid becoming involved in any litigation as an expert witness. Therapists frequently feel that since they know the patient so well they can answer relevant legal questions, but, of course, given the comprehensive model noted above, it is virtually impossible to address these issues because psychotherapy is not directed toward such issues as obtaining external verification of the patients perceptions and assessing malingering. If a therapist does become involved in litigation, he or she must scrupulously avoid rendering any opinions relevant to the legal matters at hand and simply describe what the course of the psychotherapy was and how the patient may have changed. That is, the treating therapist is essentially testifying as a lay witness, not as an expert witness. This is a crucial distinction that many attorneys fail to recognize. Attorneys customarily refer a patient to a physician for examination and treatment if deemed necessary. Indeed, when the examination is solely for the purpose of diagnosis in order to render appropriate treatment, the mixing of roles is permissible. Forensic psychologists and psychiatrists need to inform attorneys, however, that a diagnosis made as part of a treatment program is *not* the same as an expert opinion rendered in a legal proceeding and that a treating therapist should never be called as an expert witness.

Within legal contexts, a particular problem frequently arises when an opposing counsel will demand, as part of discovery, the raw psychological test data obtained by a psychologist. While this is not directly addressed by the ethical code, the code does speak repeatedly of psychologists' needing to avoid the misuse of assessment results, and states, "Psychologists make every effort to maintain the security of tests and other assessment techniques within the limits of legal mandates. They strive to assure the appropriate use of assessment techniques by others" (Principle 8 Preamble). This issue is addressed more directly by the APA *Standards for Providers of Psychological Services.*

In Principle 2.3.5, these standards state, "Raw psychological data (e.g., test protocols, therapy or interview notes, or questionnaire returns) in which a user is identified, shall be released only with the written consent of the user or legal representative and released only to a person recognized by the psychologist as competent to use the data." In short, if a psychologist receives a request from opposing counsel for raw psychological test data, the psychologist should inform the attorney that he or she cannot provide such material directly to him or her, but that if the attorney will provide the psychologist with the name of another duly licensed and qualified psychologist whom the recipient of the subpoena recognizes as competent to interpret the data, then the raw data can be sent directly to the other professional but not to the attorney.

THE DUTY TO WARN IN
EXAMINATION SITUATIONS

The "duty to warn," or as it has emerged in subsequent cases, the "duty to protect" identifiable third parties against harm threatened by one's patient, has in virtually all of the recent litigation applied to treatment situations. There is little information or case law dealing with whether an individual performing an evaluation, who becomes aware of a patient's violent tendencies, incurs the same duty to protect.

Malpractice litigation, of course, does recognize the heading of "negligent diagnosis" that results in harm to the individual patient, and there are several malpractice cases against mental health practitioners based on this very principle. Several cases in which there has been violence done to third parties who were not identifiable have had recovery based on the fact that a negligent diagnosis had been made and had the correct diagnosis been made the patient would not have been in the position to have acted out his or her violent impulses. That is, the assumption is that, had the correct diagnosis been made, the violence would have been recognized, and the patient would probably have been hospitalized and therefore have been incapable of carrying out his or her violent activities.

It would appear, therefore, that the "handwriting on the wall" indicates that the duty to protect does indeed involve the examination as well as the treatment situation, and that one's role as a forensic examiner comes under the definition of the "special relationship" that is continually referred to in the litigation dealing with the duty to protect.

LEGAL CONSTRAINTS ON
PSYCHOLOGICAL EVALUATIONS

A striking example of the misuse of forensic evaluation emerged in the case of Estelle v. Smith (Cert. granted 48 USLW 3602, March 17, 1980). In this murder case, the American Psychiatric Association filed an *amicus curiae* brief before the U.S. Supreme Court in which it declared that psychiatrists' predictions of future dangerousness are unreliable and should not be taken into consideration when sentencing a defendant to capital punishment. The individual in question was indicted for murder after participating in a robbery in which a victim was fatally shot by the man's accomplice.

A competency evaluation was conducted by a court-appointed psychiatrist who concluded that the patient was competent to stand trial. Competency was uncontested, and the defendant was found guilty of murder in the first phase of a bifurcated trial. In the penalty proceedings, the second phase of the bifurcated trial, the critical question dealt with whether the defendant would commit further violent acts and thus pose a continuing threat to society. Without prior notification to the defendant, the government called as its only witness the psychiatrist who had performed the competency evaluation. On the basis of the competency evaluation, the doctor concluded that the patient was an antisocial personality, according to the diagnostic and statistical manual, and that by definition he would be certain to commit further acts of violence and would therefore pose a threat to society. On the basis of the psychiatric testimony, the jury returned a verdict mandating the death penalty. A district court set aside this sentence because the state failed to give prior notice of the psychiatric testimony. The Fifth Circuit Court confirmed that defendants could not be compelled under the Fifth Amendment to talk to a psychiatrist when their statements could later be used against them at the sentencing stage of a trial for a capital crime. In its *amicus curiae* brief to the U.S. Supreme Court, the American Psychiatric Association supported the earlier opinion of the circuit court, arguing that psychiatric assessments of the probability of future dangerousness are unreliable, especially in the absence of a prior history of violent activities, and that such a prior history must serve as a base rate for prediction. The brief contended that if psychiatric testimony is ruled admissible, the defendant must be guaranteed an opportunity to challenge and rebut such testimony. There is also a clear implication that the defendant, or patient, must be given fully informed consent, knowing precisely how the data in the examination are to be used.

Several courts have gone so far as to state that the forensic examiner must give the patient a full Miranda warning prior to the commencement of a forensic examination, indicating that the material obtained in the examination "can and will be used against him in a court of law." In the opinion of this author, this, while seen as an appropriate legal safeguard, is far too extreme for a clinical setting and could well influence the nature of the data obtained in the course of such an evaluation. Rather than needing to give a full Miranda warning, one should merely inform the patient of the fact that the material obtained in the examination is not confidential and of the exact manner in which it will be used.

The general reasoning behind the *Estelle* v. *Smith* opinion had led many attorneys to question even the use of an expert witness retained by the government to assess an issue of criminal responsibility. Much of the impetus for this line of attack stems from the case of United States v. Byers (740 F. 2d 1104, D.C. Circuit, July 24, 1984). Byers was an individual who was charged in the District of Columbia with murdering his girlfriend with a sawed-off shotgun. Psychological and psychiatric evaluation resulted in an opinion to the court that Mr. Byers had suffered an acute psychotic episode at the time of the offense and should therefore not be held legally responsible for the shooting. The specific delusional system concerned the decedent's having cast spells on him through the use of "roots" as well as her having the power to control his mind through her menstrual cycles.

The U.S. Attorney's Office sought and obtained a second opinion from another psychiatric facility. The second opinion found not only that the patient showed no evidence of mental illness but that in the discussion about "roots" he was malingering. The critical aspect of the government's case was that when Mr. Byers was interviewed at the second facility and asked why he had shot his girlfriend, he replied that he did not know (i.e., he did not mention roots, menstrual cycles, or mind control). When asked about the roots, Mr. Byers indicated that he and his wife had talked about that possibility while he was a patient at the first facility. The doctors at the second facility concluded from this that Mr. Byers and his wife had "concocted" the roots delusion after the offense was committed, that it had nothing to do with the motivation for the shooting, and that in fact telling it to the doctors at the first facility was a deliberate attempt to feign mental illness. However, the opinion about the patient's malingering was not contained in the letter sent by the second set of doctors to the court. Rather, it was "sprung" on the defense at the time of trial, which clearly gave the defense no opportunity to rebut this line of reasoning.

Mr. Byers was convicted largely on the strength of the government's presentation of the theory that he was malingering. The prosecutor, in his closing argument, described the defense's position as having come "crashing down," and the trial judge described the government's evidence as "devastating to the defense."

The case was appealed, largely on reasoning analogous to that in the case of *Estelle* v. *Smith* in which, as noted, the defendant was not informed that his statements could be used against him in a capital sentencing phase of the trial. Mr. Byers, it was argued, had his statements taken out of context and interpreted as malingering. The court was not informed of this in advance of the trial, and the opinion was not rendered until the defense's case was being rebutted.

The U.S. Court of Appeals rejected this argument, but in a strongly worded dissent, Judge David Bazelon agreed with the appeal and cited violations of both the Fifth and Sixth Amendments when a defendant is ordered to submit to a "government compelled psychiatric examination." Judge Bazelon spoke of the fact that the Springfield staff had "transmogrified" Mr. Byers' comments and, in effect, used his own words to testify against him. Judge Bazelon noted that while such violations occur rarely, there is the potential for widespread abuse of examinations conducted by "government doctors." He suggested, as possible safeguards, either having the defense attorney present at the examination or having a video or audio recording made of the examination. There would then be an opportunity at a pretrial evidentiary hearing for the "government doctor" to present his or her opinion and be questioned on its congruence or lack of congruence with the material contained on the tape or in the attorney's notes. *Amicus curiae* briefs were submitted to the court by both the American Psychological Association and the American Psychiatric Association. The brief of the American Psychological Association was basically supportive of Judge Bazelon's position that there was a potential for widespread abuse and that there must be procedures to prevent violations of Fifth and Sixth Amendment rights.

In its brief, the American Psychological Association maintained that a defendant's communications during a court-compelled clinical interview on the issue of insanity were incriminatory, even though admissions made during such an interview could not technically be used against him or her in an evidentiary sense. If the evidence gained from a clinical interview established that the accused could appreciate the wrongfulness of the act or control his or her conduct, it would negate the defense of insanity, and was therefore probative of criminal intent because there was not mental disorder to interfere with or diminish the intent and therefore indirectly incriminate the accused. If the defendant admitted the crime, testimony negating insanity increased the probability of conviction. In order to prevent the admission of such indirectly incriminating evidence and also to provide some data base for cross-examining the "government witness," there should be, according to the American Psychological Association brief, a complete and definitive record of precisely what occurred at the interview—that is, a video or audio recording. This would prevent the government expert from selecting out of context certain statements and giving them certain interpretations. Psychologists serving as government experts should fully inform the defendant of the purpose and nature of the evaluation, the limits of confidentiality, and the possibility of self-incrimination. Furthermore, the government, according to this brief, should be obligated to demonstrate that the clinical interview is necessary before the court grants it.

While the thrust of this brief is to limit what was certainly some inappropriate conduct on the part of witnesses, such as those from the second psychiatric hospital who testified for the government, one may wonder, in the interests of justice, whether or not the defense expert should be subject to the same constraints, producing a video or audio recording, such that statements would not be taken out of context.

The American Psychological Association brief further argued that following much of the research that Rosenthal has done, people controlling the situation can unwittingly evoke the data they expect. Therefore, since the staff at the second hospital knew that the U.S. Attorney's Office was displeased with the first evaluation, they implicitly felt the need to reach a different conclusion, one that supported the government.

In its brief, the American Psychological Association further proposed that, rather than a government expert's being allowed to evaluate the patient at all, the prosecution, in order to challenge defense testimony, should rely only on cross-examination of the defense experts and use its own experts to testify only on hypothetical material that might rebut the defense position, rather than allowing the "government psychiatrist" any access to the defendant whatsoever.

The brief filed by the American Psychiatric Association was quite different from that filed by the American Psychological Association. It held that there was essentially no constitutional need for the presence of counsel or for the provision of other safeguards in "government sanity examinations."

The American Psychiatric Association laid emphasis on the fact that the principles of medical ethics that dictate the limits of confidentiality should be closely and carefully explained to the defendant. In fact, as we have noted above, the American Psychological Association Code of Ethics also advocates the same point. The American Psychiatric brief stated that if such limits are explained to the defendant, the elaborate procedural safeguards advocated by the American Psychological Association are unnecessary. Specifically, this brief recommended that the examiner should explain that he or she is not the defendant's doctor and that the examination is not being conducted for therapeutic purposes, and should reveal who it was that requested that the examination be performed. The defendant should further be told that if the examiner finds no evidence supportive of exculpability, he or she may be called as a prosecution witness. The examiner was also urged to refrain from examining a defendant for competency or criminal responsibility until that defendant has had an opportunity to consult with counsel about his or her participation in the examination.

Both briefs, as well as Judge Bazelon's lengthy dissent, eloquently dealt with a variety of complex legal issues. However, they all overlooked some rather important clinical considerations—though the position advocated by the American Psychiatric Association, stressing that the safeguards are contained within the Code of Ethics, appears to be moving in the appropriate direction. Initially, the actions of the "government doctors" in the *Byers* case are a poor example on which to base legal precedent. It is clear that because of their interpretation of an ambiguous statement as clear evidence of malingering, their ignoring of many other clinical details that suggested a bona fide mental disorder, and their failure to fully inform the court of their opinion or the basis for that opinion, they had basically lost their objectivity and were becoming advocates for the government rather than for their own opinion.

In addition, the expert witness must remain objective in order to maintain his or her credibility. Complete examinations must be performed in order to render accurate opinions, whether or not those opinions comport with the position of the side by whom the expert was retained. Therefore, when one is truly functioning as a forensic expert, the term "government doctor," or for that matter "defense doctor," is a misnomer and is totally irrelevant. One's opinion should be open and objective in court. One is an advocate only for one's own opinion, not for the defense and not for the prosecution. Therefore, since there is no "government doctor" who will automatically be a prosecution witness, the concern over possible violations of Fifth and Sixth Amendment rights becomes moot. That is, the well-trained forensic expert presents an opinion based on the available data, is impartial, is not tainted by association with one side or the other, and is therefore not violating any of the defendant's constitutional rights.

DISCLOSURE OF NONSUPPORTIVE EXPERT TESTIMONY

As has been noted in several of the preceding sections, the issue of informed consent to forensic evaluation is exceedingly important. However, recent court decisions point to the fact that the nature of the informed consent, and the specific information given to the defendant regarding the individuals to whom the results of the evaluation will be made available, vary from state to state and from one federal circuit to another. It therefore behooves the expert to be highly aware of which decisions and which assumptions are applicable in the jurisdiction in which he or she is practicing in order to word properly the statement regarding informed consent.

As noted above, if the evaluation is being performed for the court, then the statement is relatively clear — namely, that the results of the evaluation are not confidential, that a report will be sent to the court, and that the court will make the report available to both the defense and the government. The situation becomes more problematic, however, when the expert is retained either by the defense or by the government, because, as noted above, different laws governing disclosure of opinions apply depending on the jurisdiction in which the individual is practicing.

On occasion, an expert who has been retained by defense counsel to perform an examination of competency or criminal responsibility may render an opinion that is not helpful to the defense. That is, the defense may be interested, for example, in pursuing an insanity defense and retain an expert to perform an evaluation. That expert then, upon completing an objective and impartial examination, may find that he or she cannot support such a defense; the expert may reach the conclusion that under the law the patient is criminally responsible or, in an even more extreme example, may find that the defendant is malingering. Under such circumstances, can the results of that examination be made available to the government — i.e., the prosecution — and can the original expert retained by the defense then be called as a government witness, in a sense compelling him or her to testify for the opposing side and to be cross-examined by counsel who initially retained him or her?

As is the situation with so many cases, the findings of the various courts on this issue are highly inconsistent; some courts maintain that such crossover is forbidden and others that it is permissible. As we shall see in a review of some of the more salient and recent cases, after much of the excessive legalistic verbiage has been penetrated, there are two basic issues that determine the way in which the court makes its decision: (1) whether or not the opinion of the expert retained by the defense is covered by attorney–client privilege — that is, whether the opinion is regarded as part of the "work product" and (2) whether or not the raising of an insanity defense by a defendant effectively constitutes a waiver of the attorney–client privilege, in a concept analogous to that found in civil litigation. (In civil litigation, if a patient places his or her mental or emotional state into litigation, it constitutes an implicit waiver of privilege.)

As regards the argument against the government's use of a defendant's psychological expert: The most well-known case in federal courts denying the government the right to call the defendant's expert is United States v. Alvarez (519 F 2nd 1036, 3rd Circuit, 1975). In the *Alvarez* case, the defendant was convicted of kidnapping and conspiracy to kidnap. During the insanity phase of this bifurcated trial, the government called a psychiatrist whose testimony was strongly objected to by the defense. The defendant's attorney had retained a well-qualified forensic psychiatrist to conduct a psychiatric examination. That psychiatrist concluded that the defendant was sane at the time of the alleged offense. The government then subpoenaed that doctor, and he was permitted to testify about statements made to him by the defendant. Defense counsel strenuously objected to the doctor's testimony, claiming violations of the defendant's privilege against self-incrimination, the physician–patient privilege, and the attorney–client privilege.

The court quickly dispensed with the defendant's Fifth Amendment objection, declaring that "because the disclosures made to the doctor were entirely voluntary, the privilege against self-incrimination was irrelevant." The court also found that the physician–patient privilege was not implicated because the doctor's consultation was for purposes of litigation, not for diagnosis or for treatment. However, regarding the issue of whether a defense attorney in a case involving a potential defense of insanity must run the risk that a psychiatric expert, whom the defense attorney hired to advise him or her with respect to the defendant's mental condition, may be forced to be an involuntary government witness, the court declared, "Such a rule would have the inevitable effect of depriving the defendant of the effective assistance of counsel in such cases. Disclosures made to the attorney cannot be used to furnish proof in the government's case. Disclosures made to the attorney's expert should be equally unavailable at least until he is placed on the witness stand." In essence, the court found that the defendant's communications to an examining psychiatrist or psychologist are protected by the attorney–client privilege: "If the defendant does not call the expert to the stand, the same privilege applies with respect to communications from the defendant as applies to such communications to the attorney himself." The court's decision in *Alvarez* was largely an elaboration by analogy to a previous case in the Second Circuit, United States v. Kovel (296 Fed. 2nd 918, 2nd Circuit, 1961).

In a similar manner, a recent state court decision in the State of Maryland followed a similar principle. The Maryland Court of Appeals reversed a defendant's conviction for second degree murder, finding that the attorney–client privilege was violated when, over objection, a psychiatrist who was retained by defense counsel to examine his client was permitted to testify at the insistence of the prosecution (State v. Pratt, 398 A. 2d 421, Maryland Court of Appeals, 1979). The Maryland court stated, "It is now almost universally accepted in this country that the scope of the attorney/client privilege, at least in criminal cases, embraces those agents whose services are required by the attorney in order that he may properly prepare his client's case." The court further stated, "We have no hesitancy in concluding that in criminal cases, communications made by a defendant to an expert, in order to equip him with the necessary information to provide the defendant's attorney with tools to aid him in giving his client proper legal advice, are within the scope of attorney/client privilege."

As regards the argument in favor of permitting the government to call defense experts: This argument has primarily been based on the concept of waiver of the attorney–client privilege by the defendant. As noted before, the raising of an insanity defense, in the reasoning of these decisions, effectively waives the attorney–client privilege. This is a concept largely borrowed from civil litigation involving personal injury claims for emotional distress. In such cases, for example, if the patient is in psychotherapy and wishes to claim, as part of the damages in some form of accident, emotional distress for which he or she is being treated in psychotherapy, the mere raising of the lawsuit constitutes a waiver of the privilege between the treating doctor and the patient. That is, once the patient's emotional condition is placed into litigation, the records of that therapist are no longer regarded as privileged, and the opposing side is entitled to examination of those portions of the records related to the ongoing litigation.

This waiver doctrine was articulated in the case of Edney v. Smith (425 Fed. Supplement 1038, Southern District of New York, 1976, affirmed without opinion 556 F. 2nd, 556 2nd Circuit, 1977). In *Edney,* the defendant was found guilty in a New York State court of kidnapping and murder. During the trial, the government called as its witness a psychiatrist who had examined the defendant at the request of the defendant's attorney. The psychiatrist testified that in his opinion the defendant knew what he was doing at the time of the alleged offense. The defendant appealed, claiming that the government had violated his constitutional rights by calling the psychiatrist. The New York Court of Appeals upheld the defendant's conviction, hodling that where a defense of insanity is asserted and the defendant offers evidence tending to show his or her insanity, a complete waiver of the physician–patient and attorney–client privilege is effected, and the prosecution may call a psychiatric expert who examined the defendant at the defense counsel's request. In the appeal, the defendant claimed that his Sixth Amendment guarantee to effective assistance of counsel had been violated. In ruling on the defendant's writ, the court declared that, while a majority of other courts had followed the *Alvarez* ruling extending the attorney–client privilege to communications to expert witnesses in litigation, the privilege was qualified, not absolute, and its infringement could be justified by the defendant's actual or implied waiver, further stating that the raising of the insanity defense constituted the implied waiver.

The court ventured the opinion that whether such a waiver existed in any specific case depended on considerations of fairness, viewed in light of the concept that the trier of fact should have adequate access to as much psychiatric evidence as possible when the defendant puts his or her sanity at issue. More recently, in a case from the State of Missouri (State v. Carter, 51 USLW 2221, 1982), a defendant charged with murder raised the defense of insanity. Two psychiatrists were hired by the defense to examine the defendant. One concluded that the defendant did suffer from a mental disease or defect excluding criminal responsibility, while the other concluded that the defendant did not. The prosecution moved that the defense be compelled to release the latter report, and the trial court granted the request. The defense appealed the eventual conviction on the grounds that the compelled disclosure violated the attorney–client privilege and undermined effective assistance of defense counsel.

The Missouri Supreme Court denied the appeal, ruling that not only must the defense surrender an adverse report, but the witness may also be called by the prosecution. This in essence is the exact opposite of the reasoning followed by the Maryland court in the *Pratt* decision. The court ruled that such reports were not covered by attorney–client privilege and, further, even if they were so covered, the privilege had been waived by utilizing the insanity defense at trial. In analyzing the reasoning followed in *State* v. *Carter,* some issues raised are: (1) Would jurors weigh the testimony of such a witness more, knowing that the witness had originally been retained by the defense? and (2) Would the defendant be as candid with an expert who might later be a witness against him or her?

In several of the cases, many issues regarding Fifth Amendment rights against self-incrimination have been dismissed on appeal because disclosures made by the defendants to experts were regarded as completely voluntary. In a similar manner, the issue of the violation of the doctor–patient privilege has largely been dismissed because the defendant was being examined solely for litigation. The issue clearly revolves around the matter of attorney–client privilege. In essence, the court can find either way, depending on its characterization of the pertinent issues. If the court focuses on the matter of whether or not the expert witness was an agent of the defense attorney, it is likely that the government would not be allowed to call the defendant's expert. In short, that expert would be covered under attorney–client privilege. On the other hand, if the court could be persuaded that the crucial issue was not the fact of the privilege, but rather whether the privilege was waived by the raising of an insanity defense, the government might be allowed to call the expert employed by defense counsel. The government might argue, on the grounds of providing the jury with all available information as to insanity, that the court should find that the defendant waived his or her attorney–client privilege by introducing the defense of insanity (i.e., placing his or her mental state into litigation).

How then is the expert witness to deal with this dilemma? While no formal statement obviously can be made, several recommendations are in order. First, the rather venerable concept of the expert being a true *amicus curiae,* or friend of the court, is highly relevant. That is, if an insanity defense is to be raised, both attorneys should, in open court, agree on an expert who would then be appointed by the court. In such a proceeding, the report would be made to the court, rather than to one side or the other, and would therefore be made available to all concerned. An extension of this doctrine, in fact, is now being used in several states in which a panel of experts, agreed to by both defense and government, is appointed by the court with, once again, the reports being made available to all parties concerned. This truly preserves the concept of the impartiality of the experts since there is no pressure, implicit or explicit, to "help out" the attorney who has retained them.

The second suggestion is to be followed where such an impartial panel, or friend-of-the-court model, is not practical. In such a case, the experts should, informally, inform both sides that their reports are impartial and objective, that there is no "ax to grind," and that the expert is willing to provide reports to both sides and to discuss findings with both sides in a mutual discovery procedure. This discovery procedure could be conducted either on an informal basis or in a more formal setting of an evidentiary hearing, but this would all be done prior to the actual trial.

In my opinion, if either of these models is followed, there would be far less of the legal hairsplitting that has seemed to go on in the conflict between the two approaches that I outlined earlier: trying to decide whether the more important issue was the attorney–client privilege or whether that privilege had been waived by the raising of an insanity defense.

The emphasis, of course, in all of the decisions just reviewed is the disposition of a report prepared by an expert retained by the defense and whether or not the government is able to gain access to it.

It is important to understand that any findings made by an expert retained by the government *must* be turned over to the defense under the provisions of a federal case called *Brady* (373 U.S.L.W. 63 [1963]). What is not made clear in the *Brady* decision, however, is the extent to which, and in how much detail, that government opinion must be disclosed; for, as seen in the *Byers* case discussed earlier, while the opinion of the second psychiatric hospital, the one retained by the government, indicated that Mr. Byers was not suffering from any mental disorder, it did not mention in its report the fact that it felt that Mr. Byers was malingering. This material was brought up only at the time of trial.

In summary, then, if an expert is retained by the government, he or she essentially need not be concerned about the disposition of the evaluation since federal law dictates that the evaluation must be turned over to the defense regardless of what the finding is.

Despite this fact, the expert should proceed with the informed consent, letting the patient know that the report is being prepared at the request of the government, that the examination will be impartial and objective, and that if the results of the evaluation are supportive of an insanity defense, then the witness may well be called by the defendant's own counsel; while, if the results of the evaluation support a finding that the patient is responsible for his or her action, then the examiner may be called as a prosecution witness.

If the expert is retained by the court or is working for a facility that operates under court order, then the examiner merely needs to inform the defendant of the fact that the examination is not confidential and that a report will be prepared for the court and will be made available to both defense counsel and to the government.

If the examiner is retained by the defense and is conducting his or her evaluation in one of the states or federal jurisdictions bounded by the *Alvarez* logic—namely, the protection of the work product by attorney–client privilege—the defendant should be told that the examination is being conducted at the request of his or her defense counsel and that a report will be prepared for that attorney. If the attorney chooses to pursue an insanity defense based on the expert's recommendation, then and only then will the material be made available to the government. If no such opinion is reached and no such testimony requested, it should be explained to the patient that the material will not go beyond his or her attorney.

Finally, if the examiner is practicing in a jurisdiction covered by the logic in the *Edney* case of the *Carter* case, the defendant should be told that he or she is being examined at the request of defense counsel, that the results of the examination are not confidential, and that whatever the results of the evaluation, the defense attorney must provide a copy of the evaluation for the government. In the event that the examiner reaches a conclusion that does not support the insanity defense, that examiner could conceivably be called as a witness for the prosecution.

SUMMARY

This chapter has outlined some of the issues that forensic practitioners run into in their daily practice. Some of these issues are related to matters of professional ethics, conduct of the examinations, and the differences between traditional/clinical and forensic examinations. Other issues dealt with are changes in practice that have been dictated by recent court decisions.

REFERENCES

Abrahamsen, D. (1974). *The murdering mind.* New York: McGraw-Hill.

Blau, T.H. (1984). *The psychologist as expert witness.* New york: John Wiley.

Everstine, L., & Everstine, J.S. (Eds.) (1986). *Psychotherapy and the law.* New York: Grune & Stratton.

Ewing, C. (Ed.) (1985). *Psychology, psychiatry and the law.* Sarasota, Fla: Professional Resource Exchange.

Monahan, J. (1980). *Who is the client?* Washington, D.C.: American Psychological Association.

Shapiro, D. (1983). *Psychological evaluation and expert testimony: A practical guide to forensic work.* New York: Van Nostrand Reinhold.

C H A P T E R
64

ETHICAL ISSUES IN
FORENSIC ASSESSMENTS

J. Roy Gillis, M.A., and
Richard Rogers, Ph.D.

The psychologist in private practice, within the course of his or her career, is likely to be involved in cases that originate in the civil courts or the criminal justice system. Most often, these cases will involve either child custody disputes or psychotherapy with mentally disturbed offenders, and less frequently they will involve court-referred assessments of offenders. Within these settings, the practice of forensic psychology (defined by Howard [1981] as "the branch of applied psychology concerned with the collection, examination and presentation of evidence for judicial purposes") will normally be guided by the ethical principles and standards set out by the American Psychological Association (APA, 1981) in the "Ethical Principles of Psychologists." However, because of competing alliances between the referral source (frequently either an attorney or the court) and the client encountered in forensic practice, some of the ethical principles developed by the APA will require a critical review prior to their adoption.

This chapter will highlight several major problems encountered by psychologists when working with forensic clients. The primary objective is to provide a resource base for the psychologist negotiating the often "murky waters" of forensic psychological practice. Since most forensic assessments occur at a pretrial stage, issues of particular concern at this stage will be emphasized. Specific topics include agency, informed consent, confidentiality, duty to warn, and limits of expertise. A review of these topics should enable the psychologist involved in a forensic assessment to clarify his or her role vis-à-vis the legal system and to provide an increased awareness and sensitivity to the issues discussed.

AGENCY

The scope of agency as noted by Rogers (1987) is more broadly defined than as the strict contractual or financial arrangement under which the assessment was initiated. Rather, agency impinges on all aspects of the assessment process, periodically requiring the psychologist to address the question of who the client is (see Monahan [1980] for an excellent discussion). Historically, psychologists have been accustomed to the view that their goal is to "further the best interests of the client," and this ideal has been reinforced in our ethical code (APA, 1981). Adherence to a client's "best interests" in most nonforensic settings — with the exception of work with children where the parents are often the clients — is relatively uncomplicated. In contrast, the purpose of most forensic assessments is to address specific psycholegal issues rather than the needs of the client. Thus, with forensic cases, the psychologist could alternatively be described as working to further the "best interests of society" through enabling justice to be served.

Though the "Ethical Principles of Psychologists" recognizes the need to work for the best interests of society, it provides no guidelines to resolve situations where the best interests of the client and society are at odds. Thus, there is a possibility that psychologists may become confused about whose interests are being served. For example, in criminal cases (e.g., competency to stand trial, insanity, and sentencing evaluations), a psychologist may see himself or herself as the agent of the defendant, the defense attorney, the prosecuting attorney, or the court itself. Civil cases have the potential for being more complicated. For example, in child custody cases, psychologists may perceive themselves as working for one or all of the children, either parent, either attorney, the legal guardian, or the court. It becomes apparent that the number of possible allegiances can generate substantial conflicts. Thus, agency should be the first issue to be settled before a psychologist agrees to participate in a forensic assessment.

A psychologist should be aware, however, of the potential biases that can occur as the result of an overidentification based on agency. Rogers (1987) has pointed out some ethical concerns that can emerge from a consideration of agency, namely: Are psychologists unduly influenced by agency? Do psychologists engage in either self-deception or conscious misrepresentation regarding whom they see as the client? Does agency necessarily compromise objectivity? If the psychologist can answer the above questions in the negative, it is probable that subsequent ethical dilemmas involving confidentiality or impartiality can be avoided.

INFORMED CONSENT

Informed consent has a broader scope than merely the client's implicit or explicit agreement to participate in the assessment. Truly informed consent requires that the client not only understand what type of assessment or procedure he or she is consenting to but also understand the implications and the likely outcome of the decision. Legal scholars have proposed that valid consent usually requires three basic components. According to Grisso (1986), these general requirements are (1) that the individual has the capacity to choose, (2) that the individual understands what he or she is consenting to, as well as the alternatives, and (3) that the consent was voluntary. Unfortunately, research has found that in practice informed consent is rarely obtained (Lidz et al., 1984).

Before any assessment procedures are conducted, it is essential that the informed consent of the client be obtained. Curran et al. (1986) have suggested that the *minimum* information a client must have to give informed consent for a forensic assessment is (1) the name and background of the examiner, (2) the circumstances of the evaluation, (3) the relationship of the client's problems to the evaluation, (4) the knowledge that the examination is for legal purposes and is not for psychological treatment, and (5) the awareness of the client that he or she may decline to participate in the assessment process. A client should also be cautioned about the limits of confidentiality and about any specific legal obligations, such as the duty to report child abuse or to warn of dangerous behavior. Ideally, this consent should be obtained in a written form with a signature, witness, and date, so that it would be possible to introduce it as documentary evidence in a subsequent legal proceeding.

In cases where the client is grossly impaired, the psychologist must determine whether the client is, in fact, competent to give informed consent. Considerable progress has been made in developing standardized measures to assess informed consent to a forensic assessment, as well as to the other forms of competency (Grisso, 1986). Obtaining informed consent must be an essential element of psychological practice and should never be dispensed with or assumed. When the psychologist obtains truly informed consent before initiating the assessment, many of the ethical concerns to be discussed in the following sections can be avoided or successfully resolved.

CONFIDENTIALITY

The commonly held belief of both psychologists and their clients is that any information communicated to a psychologist will remain confidential and will not be divulged to any person or agency without the client's consent. In fact, confidentiality is not absolute in any setting in which a psychologist may work. For instance, statutes exist in all states that require the reporting of suspected or actual child abuse. Additionally, many states have established by statute or case law, a "duty to warn" of dangerous behavior under certain conditions (Cavanaugh & Rogers, 1984). The APA (1981) has also recognized limits to confidentiality, providing for disclosure where there is "a clear danger to the person or to others" and advises informing clients of the legal limits of confidentiality.

Ethical conflicts emerge when the client is under the expectation that the information he or she has related to the psychologist will be held in confidence. This assumption is often unintentionally supported by psychologists who may appear "helpful" or "well-intentioned" toward the client without specifying their actual role. Thus, any contacts with a client should detail the limits of comfidentiality, specifying what information is required to be reported and the extent of that reporting.

It must be remembered that the psychologist who conducts a forensic evaluation on a client may very well be requested to appear in court to testify regarding that report. In most states, communications between a psychologist and a client do not have the legal status of a privileged communication, as communications between lawyer and client do. Furthermore, the psychologist must recognize that, in addition to reports, files, tapes, notes, or transcripts can also be called into court as evidence. Thus, the psychologist must be thorough and precise in documenting his or her assessment.

Promises not to reveal sensitive information cannot always be honored and therefore should be avoided. This practice is meant to protect both the psychologist and the client. A psychologist who has information regarding child abuse or dangerous behavior that was obtained with the assurance that it would be held in confidence, is in a dilemma between legally mandated reporting and professional ethics. While psychologists can maintain control over the content of the reports they prepare, they are not usually in a position to ensure that information is not revealed during a court trial or to another agency. Therefore, it is preferable to have the client refuse to reveal information than to have sensitive material disclosed that the client believed was to be held in confidence.

Concerns about safeguarding confidentiality extend also to family and friends of the client. Informed consent in writing must be obtained from the client before any individual, including family members, or any agency is contacted for information about that client. In addition, the psychologist has a responsibility to protect the confidentiality of the client when speaking to family or friends by not divulging information concerning the client's background, criminal history, or clinical status. A release to obtain information does not in any way imply reciprocity. Thus, a psychologist must not share knowledge about the client with another person or agency, even if he or she was given permission to contact that person or agency.,

The psychologist must never divulge information unless the written permission of the client has been obtained or the material has been subpoenaed. Furthermore, the discussion of a particular assessment conducted, even without the use of the client's name, would violate confidentiality if sufficient details were revealed to allow for the identification of that person. It is vital to the interests of both the client and the profession that confidentiality be maintained for all assessments. A psychologist should remain aware of the advedrsarial nature of forensic assessments and should adequately caution all clients, we well as respect their privacy.

DUTY TO WARN

No recent judicial decision has caused as much concern among mental health professionals as the decision handed down in California in the 1974 case of *Tarasoff* v. *Regents of the University of California.*[1] Briefly summarized, the case involved a wrongful death suit brought by the parents of Tatiana Tarasoff, a woman killed by Prosenjit Poddar. Mr. Poddar, a student at the University of California, had developed a romantic fixation upon Ms. Tarasoff, also a student at the same university, and became extremely upset when she did not respond to his interest. Mr. Poddar had initially seen a psychiatrist at the university student counseling center and was subsequently referred to a psychologist at the center. During psychotherapy with his psychologist, he stated his intention to kill a woman readily identifiable as Tatiana

---

[1]*In re* Tarasoff v. Regents of the University of California, 118 Cal Rptr. 129, 529 P.2d 553 (1974) *reargued,* 17 Cal. 3d 425, 551 P.2d 334 (1976).

Tarasoff. The psychologist, fearing that Mr. Poddar would act on his threat, and after consultation with colleagues, called the campus police to have Mr. Poddar detained. A letter was also sent to the campus police informing them of Mr. Poddar's intentions toward Ms. Tarasoff. Mr. Poddar was brought in for questioning by the campus police, but was released soon after when he gave assurances that he would not harm Ms. Tarasoff.

Subsequently, however, he arranged to share accommodations with Ms. Tarasoff's brother. Ms. Tarasoff was on vacation while these events transpired. On her return, she was killed by Mr. Poddar. A wrongful death suit was brought by Ms. Tarasoff's parents charging that the psychologist, the psychiatrist, the campus police, and the university were negligent in their duty to warn Ms. Tarasoff of the danger posed to her by Mr. Poddar.

In 1976, a California court handed down the initial ruling, excerpted below, establishing the "duty to warn" doctrine:

> Once a therapist does in fact determine, or under applicable professional standards reasonably should have determined, that a patient poses a serious danger of violence to others, he bears a duty to exercise reasonable care to protect the foreseeable victim of that danger. While the discharge of this duty of due care will necessarily vary with facts of each case, in each instance the adequacy of the therapist's conduct must be measured against the traditional negligence standard of the rendition of reasonable care under the circumstances.

Subsequently, the duty to warn has been upheld in other jurisdictions and has become a generally accepted legal doctrine (Cavanaugh & Rogers, 1984). Some states have extended the boundary of the ruling and have imposed a duty to warn even if the intended victim is unknown or impossible to identify (Cavanaugh & Rogers, 1984). Simply put, the duty to warn doctrine assumes that mental health professionals, because of their specialized training in human behavior, possess certain skills in assessing the likelihood that an individual will carry out a violent act. The doctrine requires mental health professionals to take appropriate action to warn an intended victim and to safeguard the community if they determine that a client is dangerous (Cavanaugh & Rogers, 1984).

Objections to this doctrine have centered on the fact that because the research indicates that the prediction of dangerousness is so inaccurate, mental health professionals are being asked to perform an impossible task (Appelbaum, 1985). However, all the doctrine requires is that the assessment of dangerousness be undertaken according to the prevailing standards of the profession. Another mmisconception pertaining to this doctrine is that once a warning is given to the individual at risk, the legal and moral obligations are satisfied (Cavanaugh & Rogers, 1984). Rather, the duty to warn doctrine involves a more complex and flexible response and could be more accurately characterized as a "duty to protect" (Appelbaum, 1985).

Appelbaum (1985) has proposed a three-stage model for fulfilling the duty to warn. The first stage of the model is the collection of relevant data and the determination of dangerousness. Following assessment, the psychologist must select a course of action that will protect potential victims. The final stage of the model involves implementation and follow-up. The psychologist must ensure that the recommended course of action has been effectively implemented and must continually monitor the progress of the client.

Appelbaum has suggested that discussing the threat made by the client and informing the client of the obligations in such situations may be effective at resolving the conflict. If clinical intervention is unsuccessful or impossible or if the threat is very immediate, a more intrusive intervention such as contacting the intended victim or the authorities may be appropriate. Considered in these terms, the duty to warn, rather than being an unfair burden imposed upon professionals, becomes an extension of the duty to protect society required of all citizens. (Appelbaum, 1985).

LIMITS OF EXPERTISE

The "Ethical Principles of Psychologists" (APA, 1981) stipulate that psychologists must not undertake work in areas where they have not been appropriately trained. Therefore, psychologists who have had no formal training or supervised experience working with children should not function as child psychologists. Similarly, psychologists in forensic contexts must not overextend the limits of their training by rendering services in areas where they have not been specifically trained. Further, the licensed psychologist testifying in court concerning an assessment performed on a client must adhere to the standards for test usage, administration, and interpretation elucidated by the American Psychological Association in the *Standards for Providers of Psychological Services* (APA, 1977). The use of psychological measures that have high standards of reliability and validity for reports to the court is essential. Serious, and often irrevocable, decisions are made as a result of the information conveyed in a psychologist's report.

The greatest potential for abuse in forensic assessments, however, is in the domain of "expert opinions." One particularly problematic issue is the prediction of dangerous behavior (Monahan, 1981). Forensic psychologists are often asked to give a global assessment of a client's "dangerousness." However, it has been argued that a psychologist should not render expert opinions on matters that are outside the expertise of the profession (Monahan, 1980). Some authorities have held that predictions of dangerousness are within the expertise of the profession and can be made ethically under well-defined restrictions (Blau, 1984). Other authorities have argued that predictions of dangerousness are made with a degree of accuracy that is little better than chance and fall outside the areas of psychological expertise (Monahan, 1980; Webster et al., 1985). Whether or not predictions of dangerousness are outside the expertise of psychologists may be controversial, but it is already clear that there is a strong bias among mental health professionals toward overprediction of dangerousness (Webster et al., 1985).

Concerns have also been raised about the expertise of psychologists to testify on such diverse issues as competency to stand trial, insanity, custody issues, and personal injury cases (Blau, 1984; Shapiro, 1984). Nevertheless, the point of view of some authors is that if these psycholegal judgments are going to be made anyway, it is best that they be made with explicit opinions offered by mental health professionals (Megargee, 1980). Mental health professionals, as the argument is presented, at least have sufficient familiarity with the clinical issues involved to offer such opinions.

PROFESSIONAL ISSUES

Fee Arrangements

It is considered unethical for psychologists to render services under any kind of a contingency fee arrangement (i.e., where payment of the fee is linked to the judicial outcome (Curran et al., 1986). The reasoning behind this prohibition is clear. A psychologist accepting a contingency fee may be consciously or unconsciously influenced by the monetary incentive to favor one position over another.

Opinion Shopping Or The "Hired Gun"

Psychologists must avoid giving the impression to lawyers or the public that their opinions are for sale (Curran et al., 1986). Thus, any practice, such as misleading advertising, that would suggest that the psychologist can guarantee an outcome or has unique skills is unethical. Such practices may also contravene state regulations governing the licensure of psychologists. Additionally, it has been suggested that regularly appearing as an expert witness for either the prosecution or the defense may create a strong perception of bias (Curran et al., 1986).

Preparation Of Reports
Based On Third-Party Information

It is optimal that a psychologist interview a client rather than rely solely on third-party information, previous reports, or testing conducted by others. This recommendation is consistent with principles of test interpretation and reporting advocated by the APA (1977) in the *Standards for Providers of Psychological Services.*

Avoiding Direct Involvement In Punishment

The involvement of psychologists in such areas as competency-to-be-executed evaluations and inmate tribunal hearings is a very controversial area. Issues such as capital punishment raise very strong feelings that make an objective discussion difficult. In any event, it should be remembered that the codes of many mental health professionals prohibit them from directly participating in any form of punishment (Curran et al., 1986).

A PRACTICAL EXAMPLE

The following hypothetical case vignette is presented to highlight some of the issues considered in this chapter.

John, a young married male with two children, has been charged with committing an aggravated sexual assault and has pleaded guilty to this charge. Although he has no previous criminal record, the prosecution has indicated its intention to ask the judge to sentence John to the maximum penalty allowed for this crime. The judge has requested that you conduct the evaluation on John because you previously saw him for therapy. The judge has asked you to comment upon his personality, family life, dangerousness, and suitability for treatment. You agree to evaluate John and warn him that any information he might give you will not be confidential. The results of your assessment suggest that John would benefit from behavioral treatment available in the community. In addition, you determine that he would pose a high risk for reoffending should he not receive treatment. John has also confided in you that he values his family life above all else and that his wife has threatened to leave him should he go to prison. John has made it clear to you that he would accept treatment on an outpatient basis, but would refuse treatment if separated from his family and sent to prison.

This vignette brings into focus the complex issues of agency, confidentiality, impartiality, and limits of expertise faced by psychologists conducting forensic assessments. Many questions come to mind when one is considering a case like this, but the overriding concern is whether or not the psychologist should have participated in the assessment considering his or her previous therapeutic involvement with the client. Certainly, it would have been preferable for the psychologist to have informed the judge that the previous therapeutic relationship with the client would compromise his or her objectivity and prior confidential relationship. The psychologist could then ask to be excused from performing the assessment. However, in this instance, the psychologist agreed to conduct the assessment, which raises a multitide of concerns.

How will previous contacts with the client influence the psychologist's report to the court? Is the psychologist acting as an agent of the court, as an agent of the client, or as an agent of both the court and the client? Does the psychologist have the requisite expertise to give an opinion on the issue of treatment for sexual offenders? Should the psychologist recommend treatment in the community, thereby allowing the offender to maintain his family relationships and obtain treatment? Does the psychologist inform the court of the defendant's ambivalence about accepting treatment and his attempts to manipulate the recommendations? Given the defendant's ambivalence, does the release of this offender represent an unacceptably high risk to the community? Do the possible benefits accruing to the offender outweigh the risks assumed by the community? Moreover, would your answers to the above questions have changed if you had been retained by the defense attorney or the prosecution rather than appointed by the court?

Answers to the above questions may vary as a function of attitudes toward sexual offenders, awareness of available treatment options, appreciation of ethical principles, and attitudes toward the penal system, to name but a few of the potential vairables involved. What is important to recognize, nevertheless, is the existence of unavoidable conflicts in the case vignette described. By failing to resolve the issues of agency and confidentiality before proceeding with the assessment, the psychologist in the vignette may be forced to choose between duties to the court and responsibilities to his or her client. As a general guideline, psychologists should be clear about whose interests are being served by their written recommendations and what subsequent risks or benefits will accrue to others. Another consideration in this vignette is the psychologist's own attitudes concerning sexual offenders and the potential bias that they may introduce. Should a psychologist have strong negative reactions to an offender or a class of offenders that would compromise his or her objectivity, then the psychologist should decline to work with that client and provide an appropriate referral to another professional.

SUMMARY

This chapter has raised some important ethical concerns for psychologists in forensic practice. Working with both the mental health and legal systems presents some unique ethical challenges because the two systems operate according to different principles. The legal system operates under an adversarial system that assumes that the "truth" will be arrived at through a critical examination of opposing sides of the issue at hand. The mental health system, in contrast, is much more collegial and beneficent in nature and assumes that diagnostic or treatment "truth" will be arrived at through a careful consideration of all potential sources of information. Because of the differing philosophies of fact finding, the guiding principle that a psychologist "work in the best interests" of his or her client is not always adequate for forensic cases.

It was stressed that the psychologist must make explicit his or her perceived agency and obtain informed consent prior to initiating the assessment. The psychologist has the additional responsibility to make certain that the client understands the exact nature of the assessment, the implications of any findings, the likely outcomes resulting from the assessment, and any limits to confidentiality. When agency and informed consent have been established from the onset, the likelihood that unsolvable ethical problems will emerge later is greatly reduced. Although ethical conflicts in forensic assessments may never be totally resolved, an awareness and a sensitivity to the issues involved can prevent major barriers to ethical professional practice.

REFERENCES

American Psychological Association. (1977). *Standards for providers of psychological services.* Washington, DC: Author.

American Psychological Association. (1981). Ethical principles of psychologists. *American Psychologist, 36,* 633–638.

Appelbaum, P.S. (1985). Tarasoff and the clinician: Problems in fulfilling the duty to protect. *American Journal of Psychiatry, 142*(4), 425–429.

Blau, T.H. (1984). *The psychologist as expert witness.* New York: John Wiley & Sons.

Cavanaugh, J.L., & Rogers, R. (Eds.). (1984). Duty to warn third parties. *Behavioral Sciences and the Law, 3*(2).

Curran, W.J., Hyg, S.M., & Polack, S. (1986). Ethical perspectives: Formal codes and standards. In W.J. Curran, A.L. McGarry, & S. Shah (Eds.), *Forensic psychiatry and psychology: Perspectives and standards for interdisciplinary practice.* Philadelphia, PA: F.A. Davis Co.

Grisso, T. (1986). *Evaluating competencies: Forensic assessments and instruments.* New York: Plenum Press.

Haward, L.R.C. (1981). *Forensic psychology.* London: Batsford Academic and Educational Ltd.

Lidz, C.W., Meisel, A., Zerubavel, E., Carter, M., Sestak, R.M., & Roth, L.H. (1984). *Informed consent: A study in decisionmaking in psychiatry.* New York: The Guilford Press.

Megargee, E.I. (1980). The prediction of dangerous behavior. In G. Cooke (Ed.), *The role of the forensic psychologist.* Springfield, IL: Charles C. Thomas.

Monahan, J. (Ed.). (1980). *Who is the client? The ethics of psychological intervention in the criminal justice system.* Washington, DC: American Psychological Association.

Monahan, J. (1981). *Predicting violent behavior: An assessment of clinical techniques.* Beverly Hills, CA: Sage Publications.

Rogers, R. (1987). Ethical dilemmas in forensic evaluations. *Behavioral Sciences and the Law, 5,* 149–160.

Shapiro, D.L. (1984). *Psychological evaluation and expert testimony: A practical guide to forensic work.* New York: Van Nostrand Reinhold.

Webster, C.D., Ben-Aron, M.H., & Hucker, S.J. (1985). *Dangerousness: Probability and prediction, psychiatry and public policy.* New York: Cambridge University Press.

Part
Five

Philosophical, Theoretical and Technical Issues

Richard Robertiello, M.D.
Editor

C H A P T E R
65

TYPICAL MISTAKES OF THE BEGINNING THERAPIST

Carl Goldberg, Ph.D.

This chapter and the next, I must point out at the onset, could be reasonably written in two basic and distinctively different ways. Of course, in the reality of psychotherapeutic practice, these perspectives become conjoined. To properly emphasize what I believe is most essential to therapeutic work in the space allowed, however, I must make a choice.

With the first perspective, the operational skills of the psychotherapist as a professional would be examined. Like Buckley and his associates (1979) or Tourney and his associates (1966), I could consider specific therapist "mistakes" in terms of errors of commission (e.g., overidentification with clients, inappropriate or poorly timed interpretations, unnecessary advice, controlling behavior) and errors in omission (e.g., insufficient empathic response, failure to ask appropriate questions, failure to interpret, inability to set clear and appropriate limits).

With the second perspective, therapist "errors" would be viewed from a consideration of the ongoing personal growth of the practitioner as an emergent person. This examination would consider the mistake of practitioners (beginners or veterans) as based upon the difficulties and resistances they are experiencing in their own psychological growth, rather than as due to lack of technological information and psychological knowledge of proper therapeutic procedure.

I have chosen the latter approach in keeping with my own view of psychotherapy. Consequently, the therapist "mistakes" I will be discussing are not so much errors as they are misdirected therapist responses and stance emanating from unfinished aspects of the practitioner's own growth as a person as well as a practitioner. Psychotherapy is too complex and interactive in terms of variables beyond the control of the therapist, to say nothing of its propensity for untestable subjective judgments as to proper procedure, to regard its practices as capable of scientific precision, as "error" or "mistake" would imply.

The point I am attempting to make should become obvious when we realize that the vast volume of material examining clinical practice focuses almost exclusively on understanding the client. In contrast, there are few works that address both the personal and professional effect of the therapeutic endeavor on the practitioner. I find it ironic that, in discussing the most human of sciences, authors have largely ignored an extremely significant component of this process—the practitioner. It would appear that those who write on the subjects of psychoanalysis and psychotherapy have made the assumption that once practitioners acquire clinical skills, they should be able to maintain them over a lifetime. Those who make this assumption poorly serve their readers. We can no longer disregard the process of disillusionment that has seriously afflicted a considerable number, if not all, practitioners at some point in a full-time career. Clearly, serious work dissatisfactions will reduce clinical effectiveness. But no less significantly, they will concomitantly jeopardize the clinician's physical and emotional well-being.

If you follow me to this point, you may realize that the primary common mistake of the psychotherapy practitioner, the first, much too common error, is made prior to becoming a practitioner. This mistake is the selection of a profession. This pronouncement baldly stated may seem extreme and unfair. When we examine it more carefully, we find it a more complex and less obvious indictment than it initially seemed to be.

The major theme of this chapter and the next is that since the person and the practice of the psychotherapist are inexorably related, wise and effective practice requires deep personal satisfaction in one's personal life and in one's work. This becomes more apparent over time as we immerse ourselves in our work. The stresses from the serious responsibilities of practicing psychotherapy usually militate against a career that is sedate and harmonious. It is not that there are not those in our ranks who practice psychotherapy the way others sell cars, process customer complaints, or practice constitutional law. They may be quite friendly, readily informative, and responsible to the ethical standards of the profession; but they clearly see their work as a rather circumscribed job and find effective means for avoiding more complications and difficulties than are necessary to make their practice a convenient, profitable, and time-limited endeavor. Work concerns are left at the office at the end of the day. They are rarely bothered by telephone calls at night from clients who threaten suicide or present other difficulties that cannot be safely contained within the regular therapeutic session. They are able to practice in a 9 to 5 framework. Such practitioners generally refer the less affluent, more demanding and difficult prospective clients to other practitioners, or request that these people contact public agency clinics.

THE IMPOSSIBLE PROFESSION

This chapter and the next are not written for the practitioners described above, who would have absolutely no use for them. They are written for those who realize the extraordinary difficulties that seem to be inherent in the practice of psychotherapy. Many of these issues have not been addressed adequately in training or supervision, and cannot simply be relegated to being concerns that will be worked out by additional personal psychotherapy. A meaningful career decision to practice psychotherapy requires knowledge of the hazards of practice, and these cannot be reduced to the misunderstanding and mishandling of transference and countertransference, despite what most textbooks on psychotherapy claim. Freud himself seemed to hold a pessimistic view regarding the avoidance of pitfalls in practice. If, however, the practice of psychotherapy is not the impossible profession Freud (1937) regarded it as, it is still an extremely demanding one for those of us who are not willing to relegate our commitment to a comfortable and convenient business. There are factors inherent in the work we do, as well as qualities of those who experience a calling to the profession, that transcend a conscious, vocational choice.

In short, there are factors that create pitfalls for the practitioner's calling. Wheelis maintains that the vocation of psychotherapy misleads those who wish to pursue it as a career. According to Wheelis (1957), psychotherapy is experienced quite differently by the practitioner than by the outsider. Psychotherapy has certain qualities that cannot properly be communicated in words and that can be found out only by experiencing it. Therefore neophyte practitioners can realize only by gradual steps what is required of them and the effect it will have on their inner resources and vulnerabilities. The Jungian analyst Goresbeck (1975) states the case for the danger even more caustically than does Wheelis. He points out that in other risky occupations, such as fire fighting, recruits and apprentices are warned of the inherent dangers of the work. But no such warning is given to neophyte psychotherapists. This is unfortunate because a considerable period of their life may have elapsed before practitioners learn whether or not they are in the right profession. Such a long time, says Wheelis (1957), that in fact "he may no longer be a young man, but at the midpoint of life and deeply committed. Indeed, he may never realize his mistake, for there are powerful forces opposed to such awareness." If this picture is accurate, and I believe it is, then it would appear that psychotherapists have not devoted adequate time and attention to understanding the stress inherent in their work.

PROMISE AND REALITY OF PRACTICE

The stress of practice has to do with what the practitioner and others expect are the results of psychological examination and treatment. (I will discuss these expectations later in this chapter.) Also involved are the quintessential skills that the practitioner must possess at the outset to effectively fulfill these expectations but that can be developed only over many years, I cannot extensively examine the qualifications essential to practicing psychotherapy here. The interested reader is referred to chapter seven of my recent book, *On Being a Psychotherapist* (Goldberg, 1986). I will indicate here, however, that the practice of psychotherapy is not for everyone. It takes a special kind of person to be a psychotherapist. We should realize that although a person may be intelligent, insightful, interested in other people, and concerned about their well-being, these qualities alone are not sufficient for being a practitioner. Being a competent psychotherapist also involves the willingness to touch upon personal problem areas of the person of the practitioner, as clinical work absorbs the practitioner's entire being, often very deeply. Consequently, people who practice psychotherapy have to examine very thoroughly their motives, interests, and expectations for practice. Practitioners have to ask themselves why they are choosing this profession rather than some other. Practitioners need to examine not only what they expect to get from it but also what they need to give in order to be successful and satisfied.

Many of us who choose to become psychotherapists do so with the hopeful prospect that we can experience, and be the ascendant agent in intimate relationships, without some of the risks for hurt and disappointment that we experienced in our earlier attempts at love and friendship, particularly within the practitioner down emotionally. People who are quite insightful, psychologically knowledgeable, and interested in studying people in depth, but whose emotional vulnerabilities are overly compromised by working with those in suffering, may do better in some capacity other than psychotherapist. They may have contributions to make in teaching, research, consulting, writing, or even practicing counseling in nonclinical settings, such as in the educational, vocational, or industrial areas of psychology. People who have thoroughly examined their motives and expectations for being a psychotherapy practitioner need to decisively commit themselves to a willingness to touch the deeper recesses of themselves in their work. Practitioners cannot allow themselves to become inordinately fearful of the people they work with or of their own internal processes evoked by these therapeutic encounters.

What then should be the basis for becoming a psychotherapist if intelligence, psychological insight, and desire to help people are not sufficient?

THE PRACTITIONER'S FAMILY OF ORIGIN

The choice of career as a psychotherapist is shaped by the role provided for the psychotherapist-to-be in the family of origin (Goldberg, 1986). Responding to the calling of being a psychotherapist suggests that the role of being responsive to the emotional substratum of human experience is central to the identity of the practitioner. As such, the practitioner's identity is continually being defined by clients. The ways clients respond to the practitioner's family role, in regard to how the practitioner employs it in therapeutic relationships, will affect the ongoing tempering of the practitioner's identity. Therapists whose identity is ill defined and still tentative and whose self-esteem is contingent upon the momentary satisfactions and disappointments of clients' responses will experience an identity crisis when their family role is frustrated.

Many of us who choose to become psychotherapists do so with the hopeful prospect that we can experience, and be the ascendant agent in, intimate relationships without some of the risks for hurt and disappointment that we experienced in our earlier attempts at love and friendship, particularly within our own families. This conscious intention, wedded to a somewhat less witting need to help and understand ourselves through others' plight and suffering, may create a tenacious gravitation toward the healing professions in ways we have little understood when we entered the field.

How does this translate into practice? It is difficult to face, hour after hour, day after day, certain aspects of oneself that one has tried to distance oneself from and to deny. Yet, when we scrupulously examine the therapeutic situation without rationalization and altruistic bias, we are faced with the startling realization that psychotherapy practitioners may well be touching some of their own deepest vulnerabilities each day of their practice. A well-known, seasoned practitioner makes a clear statement of this position when he writes, "I am no longer willing to accept anyone as my patient to whose pain I do not feel vulnerable" (Kopp, 1976, p. 23).

From this vantage we might regard practitioners as trapped masochists, while at the same time realizing the source of their continuing concerns and apprehensions. Nonetheless, it is probably more valid to view the practice of psychotherapy as practitioners' courageous endeavors to come to terms with their own demons — the denied and disintegrative aspects of the self — than to understand it as a masochistic enterprise. This in no way suggests that the practice of psychotherapy is essentially a self-serving profession for the practitioner. As psychotherapists we realize, at least ideally, that by using a deeply subjective understanding of ourselves we have the most potent human instrument available for understanding and responding to the hurt and suffering of our fellow beings. This belief, I assume, is not contested. What is contested, however, is the required state of vulnerability of the psyches of practitioners in order that they be maximally responsive to those with whom they work.

Now let us look at the misdirected motives that prevent neophyte practitioners from being maximally responsive to their new vocation.

IDENTIFICATION DENIAL

The motives that draw a person to the process of psychotherapy influence the roles practitioners take with clients. For some misdirected practitioners — a small number, hopefully — practicing psychotherapy is a means of denying their own conflictual issues. There are practitioners, according to Groesbeck and Taylor (1977), who have had serious illnesses of one sort or another in their lives but have never fully acknowledged that they were actually ill. In short, they have denied for themselves need to be a patient, and have not assimilated the archetype of the wounded healer (Goldberg, 1986). Nevertheless, they are fascinated by the patient role for others. Because of their own "identification denial" they cannot get very close emotionally to their clients.

Since we are so similar to the clients we select to work with, as the research of Henry and his associates (1973) clearly indicated, it may not be clear why we have so much difficulty at certain times in understanding and helping these clients. I will try to explain this in terms of identification denial. There is a natural tendency for us to identify with people with whom we are significantly emotionally involved. However, we may also overidentify — we may be more concerned with what the clients are doing destructively in their lives than are the clients themselves. When the therapist becomes more concerned than the client about the client's suffering, the client is prevented from adequately examining conflictual concerns. In such situations, therapists attempt to protect the clients and do the work for them. Or, on the other hand, therapists may become threatened by a sense (usually not conscious) that they share with clients certain traits and attitudes that they find unacceptable in themselves. In short, there are threatening personal concerns of practitioners that are touched on in encounters with clients who are struggling with similar issues.

When either client or therapist or both deny their commonality with one another, magical rather than realistic expectations and demands are potentiated. The unwitting need of practitioners to gain distance from their own unacceptable attributes, which they encounter without conscious awareness in the client, makes therapeutic alliance unattainable. Ostensibly, these practitioners work arduously to develop a relationship with these threatening clients. Covertly, they resist this relationship. These incompatible aims inevitably foster conflict (Goldberg, 1983).

THE "AS IF" PRACTITIONER

There is another class of misdirected people — those who become psychotherapists from their intense identification with their own therapist. They have experienced considerable conflict in their own lives. They have found personal psychotherapy so helpful that they may even regard it figuratively, if not actually, as having saved their lives. With gratitude for their own survival, they are willing to devote the rest of their lives to saving others. This is a commendable motive. However, some of these fervently dedicated practitioners have never resolved in their personal psychotherapy a pervasive denial of their shameful feelings of unworthiness. They see themselves through the eyes of their own therapist. In this light, they are appalled by their desperation, dependency, and deep oral craving. To deny this painful picture of themselves they become "as if" people. They desperately try to convince themselves they "are" their therapist. This is to say, they are their therapist's strengths, wisdom, and interpersonal skill. In short, they are able to partially disown their wretched feelings by projective identification with their own therapist.

To maintain this "as if" salvation, they find practical ways to become psychotherapists themselves. Many of them, because they come upon this solution later in life (generally midlife) feel they have little time left to gratify the "solution" they have found. They find the quickest route to practice, with or without sufficient training and supervision. The unconscious rationale they give themselves is, if other people come to them and regard them as helpful, or at least as impressive, then maybe they are not really wretched after all. Under these circumstances they may deny their own dissatisfactions and conflictual issues. But what is harmful for both them and their clients is their desperate need for their clients' admiration. Their denial of wretched feelings is abetted by intellectual strivings. For them, psychotherapy is the pinnacle of intellectual and psychological knowledge. The psychotherapist knows things that other people do not. The "emotional truth" with which the practitioner is conversant is not confined to cognitive knowledge. For the "as if" practitioner, these intellectual rationalizations prevent full recognition and effective resolution of psychic suffering.

We also need to look at an insidious aspect of using personal therapy as a training component. I will touch on this only briefly. Many people who have come from other fields of endeavor have used their experience as a patient in psychotherapy as the sole criterion and justification for being a practitioner. They conduct themselves as practitioners with little or no training. I believe that this begs the question of what a practitioner is. I think being a practitioner requires experiences that cannot be derived simply from being a patient. I believe that personal psychotherapy should be only one of the components of psychotherapeutic training. A well-trained therapist has a balance of experience and training in all areas of psychological education. It would be injudicious to consider only one or two of these areas as sufficient for competence, or to assume that an abundance of training in some areas can compensate for a deficiency of training in others. All of these areas of training blend with the necessary intellectual and emotional equipment into a dynamic and mature gestalt.

Once the question of proper qualification has been addressed, the next issue concerns the practical and existential preoccupations of the neophyte practitioner.

THE CONCERNS OF THE BEGINNER

In attempting to understand the foundations of therapeutic practice, neophyte practitioners search for the ingredients of success, such as developing a sound therapeutic model, and methods of making a good livelihood. They question whether they have sufficient professional qualifications and proper personal attributes for being a competent and successful practitioner. They also question whether they are able to practice independently or still require supervision, consultation, and additional training. Deciding that further training is necessary, beginners inquire where to get this training. They ask themselves which doubts, mistakes, and other concerns should be shared with colleagues and supervisors and which should not. For practitioners who decide that they are competent with their present skills, questions about getting sufficient referrals and competing with more seasoned practitioners come to mind. There are also latent concerns about being sufficiently loved, admired, and appreciated by clients that cannot be easily put aside.

These concerns rest on a certain uneasiness between therapist and client, which is predicated upon a number of unrealistic and questionable societal attitudes and expectations of practitioners. I will examine some of these.

THE DANGER OF SUPERIORITY

Let us be frank with one another! Beginning therapists do not generally regard themselves as ordinary people; they believe they are special in a number of ways. They assume they are more intelligent, more compassionate, and more perceptive than most people. They feel that they are more willing than most people to express their perceptiveness about others in caring and concerned ways. This is their conscious reason for entering the field. For some practitioners this constellation of beliefs may be more exaggerated than for other practitioners and result in what the British analyst Ernest Jones referred to as "the God complex." In discussing Jones's classic paper "The God Complex," Judd Marmor (1953) suggests that many who are drawn toward the professions of healing have disavowed their own sense of impotence through an identification with the Supreme Being. People with this type of character structure demonstrate intense scopophilia and curiosity about the private lives of others, together with a strong need to be recognized and admired for superior skills in helping others.

This air of superiority creates serious dangers for practitioners. If they are not ordinary people, then they cannot allow themselves the same excuses and rationalizations that ordinary people use to defend themselves from their own fears. Consequently, many beginning therapists appear to believe that they are not entitled to use the same methods of dealing with anxiety that other people use. By regarding themselves as being more than ordinary, practitioners force themselves to assume responsibility for living life more exceptionally than the ordinary person. In fairness to practitioners, we should recognize that this attitude is not simply a product of defensive grandiosity. As I point out elsewhere (Goldberg, 1986), it is a part of a mutually induced relationship with the public.

The public expects a certain kind of life-style from psychotherapists. They are on duty constantly in how they conduct their lives and comport themselves. Only people in the public eye (politicians, ministers, ministers' children, entertainers, atheletes) have this kind of exposure pressure. Two of the areas in which this issue has considerable bearing are availability and money.

Psychotherapists are unlike certain other professionals such as attorneys and physicians whose "avarice" has now been firmly "accepted" by the public. Like the minister, the practitioner is viewed as having a spiritual calling and, as such, is supposed to be caring and available at all times, without consideration of fee or personal convenience. This causes many problems for the beginning practitioner who feels guilty about business practices. One young practitioner was referred a client by a former client who was a business partner of the man he was referring. The new client, after a couple of months of excuses for not paying the bill, gave the therapist a large check that was subsequently returned by the bank because of insufficient funds. The practitioner found out, to his dismay, that the client had left town. Nevertheless, he was reluctant to check on the whereabouts of the deadbeat client by contacting his business associate. The practitioner felt checkmated by concerns about confidentiality and by embarrassment about his lack of business acumen.

Many beginning psychotherapists would like to practice in a kind of ivory tower, where the financial concerns are taken care of by someone else. In most instances, however, the business and financial concerns of practice cannot be separated from the psychotherapeutic issues.

Weinberg (1984) indicates two typical causes that together contribute to clients' not paying bills. The first is overidentification with the client. Practitioners who overidentify find it difficult to make firm demands on people who are suffering or undergoing personal difficulties. These practitioners experience themselves as an ally, someone with unlimited empathy, patience, and understanding. They find it hard to admit that they are doing psychotherapy for a living.

The second cause is an even more unconscious and disabling attitude toward practice. These independent practitioners harbor a pervasive sense of inadequacy and a lack of credence in the psychotherapeutic method. Weinberg points out that in conveying that "money isn't important," therapists are actually indicating that they don't deserve to be paid. It is essential, Weinberg indicates, that neophyte practitioners acknowledge to themselves, as well as to clients, that they do this *for a living*. This can serve as an antidote to clients who don't like to part with their money or who wish for a "pure" relationship with the therapist.

Now let us look more specifically at the common errors beginning practitioners get involved in.

COMMON DILEMMAS FOR
BEGINNING PRACTITIONERS

The most common and resistant mistakes of beginning therapists are those involved with handling threats to their emergent identity as persons who empathically care about and demonstrably help clients resolve psychological dilemmas and become self-actualized people. Consequently, the clinical situations that portend the greatest arena for stress, conflict, and inappropriate therapist activity are situations in which the clients come in acute suffering and despair. If we as therapists feel competent about our skills (or are insensitive to our limitations), working with these clients feels challenging. However, if we are not able to offer palliatives and quick solutions or if we question the impact of what we do, we frequently feel helpless to assuage clients' suffering. For beginning practitioners, open-ended listening leads to feelings of ignorance, confusion, and impotence in the face of the complexity of the material. These practitioners may feel the need to do something active in order to reassure themselves and the client that they have the wisdom and capacity to help. Even those of us who feel that we are effective practitioners may have to wait a long while to be able to ascertain that we have helped a particular client. There is something about being with someone in pain and not being able to do something actively at that distressing moment to alleviate the pain that is excruciating to the practitioner.

Compounding this stress, neophyte practitioners are confronted by the dilemma of trying to realize the impact of clients' feelings while at the same time trying to avoid being adversely affected by them. These feelings are referred to in psychotherapy literature as "countertransference." The use of this term frequently has a pejorative implication, suggesting that practitioners, in reacting intensely to what occurs in sessions, are somehow at fault in allowing clinical work to have a deep effect upon them. Beginning practitioners, however, come to realize that it is necessary to remain vulnerable in order to be most available and responsive to clients' communications. Nevertheless, beginning therapists are threatened by their countertransference, and it takes some time for them to become comfortable and effective in properly utilizing it. Inappropriate therapist activity often results from dealing with this conflict. For example, it is generally deleterious to therapeutic outcome for the practitioner to make an active intervention before properly understanding what the client requires. The anxious beginning practitioner often does this to the detriment of a conversant alliance with whom the client *is* rather than whom the practitioner *assumes* the client to be.

NORMAL STRESS OF PRACTICE

Countertransference is only part of the story. An important point posited by Spensley and Blacker (1976) is that the typical stress in therapeutic work is not necessarily predicated upon the practitioner's existing vulnerabilities. It may be inherent in the nature of the psychotherapeutic process itself. There is a "normal" stress that is not reducible to the countertransferential stress induced by the practitioner's unresolved conflicts and psychic vulnerability.

The very process of working intimately with human suffering presents the practitioner with real and painful psychic discomfort. In few other situations in life is there a continual direct onslaught of emotionally jarring communication like that experienced in the therapeutic relationship. Because psychotherapy is frequently an emotionally evocative encounter, strong affect — including hurt and anger — is more often demonstrated in the practitioner's consulting room than in most other professional offices. Effective therapeutic work, from a psychoanalytic point of view, cannot be done unless the client transfers the resentments and hurts, including overwhelming rage experienced toward parental and other significant figures in the client's life, to the practitioner. The unconscious strategy of the client in this process is often to reverse the feelings of anger, helplessness, and fright felt in the presence of a hurtful authority figure in the past by inducing the therapist to feel as frightened and helpless as the client did in the past. Confronting this unconscious strategy is essential to reconstructive work. In a real sense, then, there are professional dictates to encourage the reception and retention of emotions provoked by the affective interchange. This leaves the practitioner continually with a residue of powerful and, often noxious, affect.

In short, there are numerous typical situations that place considerable emotional stress on the practitioner. Spensley and Blacker (1976) give a number of examples, such as when a well-liked client, previously very positive toward the therapist, explodes with intense rage. And there is the termination of a therapeutic relationship with a person the practitioner has worked with intimately for a number of years. Here again, inappropriate therapist activity frequently results if the practitioner is not aware of his or her responses.

Of course, some types of stressful situations are more consistently recognized than others. Handling a client who is suicidal is a situation that would raise considerable anxiety for anyone. Also, there is the danger that a highly disturbed client might take physical action against the practitioner. Almost every practitioner encounters, at least once in a career, an agitated client who actually carries a weapon, threatens an assault, or expresses strong hostility toward the practitioner. If the therapist is not wary, or is unlucky, one such incident may be sufficient to end a career, if not a life. Despite this ominous possibility, there is very little discussion in the professional literature about the causes of these dangers and how to recognize them beforehand.

Practitioners with considerable expertise with violent patients, such as John Lion, caution practitioners to properly monitor countertransferential reactions to agitated patients (Madden et al., 1976). Practitioners who work in urban hospitals, which are magnets for highly disturbed people, face seriously agitated and violent patients regularly. This is particularly true of practitioners who work in crisis services and emergency rooms. Many of the victims of attacks by agitated patients are younger practitioners, who inevitably treat the most difficult clients.

Madden et al. (1976) report a study of practitioners who were assaulted by patients. They found that more than half of the assaulted practitioners had acted in a provocative manner toward the assaulted client prior to the attack. They indicate that many of these incidents can be related to the inexperience of the practitioner, who was too insistent that a client deal squarely with upsetting material.

Even when no actual attack occurs, the fear and threat of not being able to manage agitated clients occupies the thoughts of many young therapists. The first psychotherapy patient I was assigned as a clinical intern in a large city hospital when I was in my 20s was a rather beautiful, sensual-looking black woman. She had been recently discharged from the inpatient unit of the hospital. I read in her clinic folder that her husband was a paranoid Black Muslim who had been recently released from prison for armed robbery. He and the patient were separated. In the folder was a statement reputedly made by the husband that he would shoot anyone he found his wife with. The woman had come to the clinic for a prescription for medication. As a psychologist I could not, of course, prescribe medication. I was told by my supervisor to convince her that she needed psychotherapy on a weekly basis in the clinic. As she and I climbed three flights of steps of the 100-year-old clinic building to a small room on the fourth floor, I wondered what I was going to tell her. At the same time, I had a fantasy of her husband charging up the stairs after us demanding to know what I was doing with his wife. As an inexperienced practitioner with my first psychotherapy case, I wasn't sure myself. In short, I have tried to demonstrate that there is normal stress inherent in the process of psychotherapy that is over and beyond the issues of countertransference and therapist psychopathology.

Underlying the normal stress of practice are unrealistic assumptions and attitudes of practitioners and clients alike about psychological inquiry (which I referred to earlier in this chapter). Let us look at two of those important dilemmas.

PSYCHOTHERAPY AS AN INEXACT SCIENCE

For many practitioners, if not most, the inexactness of practice is a constant stress factor. Emotions are, of course, a highly uncertain dimension of experience. We have no reliable, scientifically agreed upon methods for assessing the validity of our inferences about the intricate interplay of emotions at work. This assessment of validity is not just a matter of idle curiosity. The well-being of our clients, if not their very lives, may rest upon our ability to sense their experience and respond appropriately. Psychotherapy is such a complex process that the clinician is never certain about the effect that saying something, or saying nothing, will have upon a client. This can be contrasted with other service professions, such as medicine, where physicians clearly recognize in most cases the effect of interventions; in short, they have a distinct sense of saving lives.

As I have discussed elsewhere (Goldberg, 1986), there are different types of personalities drawn to practice psychotherapy. Those whose intellectual and scientific attitudes require certainty about what they are doing are rarely satisfied with their own skills. Insofar as their emotional character militates against their taking clinical risks, they are plagued by the unpredictability of their clients' behavior and the therapeutic methods available to guide their understanding. These practitioners, whose scientific orientation is highly operative in their work, prefer errors of omission to errors of commission. The preference for a particular type of psychological risk generally is built into the instructional philosophy of training programs in psychotherapy. Young psychoanalysts, for example, are taught that the best therapeutic attitude for an inexperienced therapist is to say as little as possible. My psychoanalytic supervisor during my internship as a clinical psychologist required me to keep verbatim notes of what both the client and I said during the sessions. This compilation required so much attention that I had little or no time to think about what to say to the patient. I quickly realized that the main function of the compulsive note taking was to avoid errors of commission. I was uncomfortable being so inactive, and I started using a tape recorder during sessions. My rather conservative supervisor was not entirely satisfied with that strategy.

In contrast to practitioners who fear errors of commission, there are therapists who more closely identify with their clients' suffering than with a scientific framework for their work and find themselves thwarted by not being able to be helpful enough. Finding their theoretical formulations limited, as I did, they may become more active in trying to reach their clients and gain their cooperation than their training orientation generally has recommended. Therefore, they are more likely to commit errors of commission than are their more cautious and scientifically oriented colleagues.

I will cite a recent example of this. I supervised an inexperienced practitioner who worked in a low-cost mental health clinic. Because he was being paid only $12 per session, he saw about 15 clients a day, generaly seven or eight in a row, without a break. Most of the clients were severely impaired people who had been diagnosed as suffering from psychotic and borderline conditions. Many had had several psychiatric hospitalizations, and some had made suicidal attempts in the past. In supervision the young practitioner indicated that the mother of a child he was treating had been recently hospitalized in a nonpsychiatric hospital after a suicide attempt. The family of the woman wanted her to be at home and not sent to a psychiatric hospital. They told the practitioner that they would be willing to see him weekly if he would work with them as a family. The practitioner, although inexperienced with family therapy and having never before worked with a client who had made a recent suicide attempt, nevertheless said he was eager to do anything to help the woman. He confidently indicated to me that family therapy could get her over her difficulties. He said he didn't believe that inpatient treatment helped patients. I asked him if he had spoken with the hospitalized woman about treatment plans. He said that he had. The woman, he reported, was quite agitated and felt hopeless and trapped in her domestic and occupational situations. She expressed considerable anger that the emergency personnel of the hospital had resuscitated her. She promised to try to take her own life again.

She also demanded to be taken out of the hospital. At the same time, she agreed to see the practitioner with her family in return for being allowed to leave the hospital.

I was concerned that the practitioner wasn't taking the woman seriously, nor was he recognizing and accepting his own therapeutic limitations. I pointed out that it was one thing to be unrealistic about what he could do therapeutically to help a person who had sufficient ego strength to deal with his or her frustrations if therapy wasn't helpful. It was quite another matter to be unrealistic with a person who had made a suicide attempt and promised to do it again. He became quite defensive and plaintively indicated that if he recognized and accepted his present clinical limitations, then he could not continue to practice psychotherapy because all his clients were psychodynamically similar to this woman. Apparently, therefore, he needed to deny his limitations by a reaction formation in which he unrealistically assumed that, with the blessing of providence, he could help anyone, under any circumstances. His optimism would have been commendable if it had been amalgamated with common sense and compassion for himself and for his clients; but he set an impossible task for himself by assuming that he was not allowed to recognize and accept his own limitations as a practitioner and the inexact nature of the profession in which he practiced.

In short, many beginning practitioners work in a climate of uncertainty and intense emotional transaction. To the extent that their clients are not agitated they may feel safe and intellectually challenged by the transactional undertainty. On the other hand, it may be a very different experience for the practitioner whose clients are highly agitated and who can find no effective means of reaching them.

The second dilemma I alluded to is concerned with the illusion of responsibility. It is related to the inexact science of psychotherapy.

RESPONSIBILITY AND ILLUSION

The psychotherapist is a professional who is asked to help people, many of whom have failed to find resolution with numerous other helpers. We are given a very heavy responsibility for other people's lives. In assuming this clinical task, we actually have very little power. Rarely, unless we work in a custodial institution, do we have real control over our clients' lives. The power we do have generally derives from transferential and magical attributes given to us by our clients. At best, we have some influence through reasoning and persuasion, but this rests upon an often fragile alliance. Moreover, unlike practitioners from other professions — for example, the police officer — we don't have a codified standard of procedure and clear limitations for dealing with dire situations. Nor do we have a clear idea whether we will be supported for our actions, or reacted to, by our colleagues. This situation stands in sharp contrast to that of the law officer or the attorney, whose codes do not speak in broad vagaries as do the professional codes of the mental health disciplines.

These considerations make quite clear again the fallacy of acting as if psychotherapy were a scientific and regulated profession. It isn't, and we as practitioners are thrown back on our own resources to handle critical situations as best we can. The need to share these concerns with our colleagues is heightened in clinical situations, in which formal procedures are vague and open to free interpretation. Beginning practitioners have great difficulty in sharing their concerns; too often, they regard asking for assistance as a sign of their incompetence. Inappropriate therapist activity frequently occurs when practitioners foolishly believe they must handle every clinical difficulty alone.

We do not handle crises every day of our practice, of course, unless we specialize in this work. Nevertheless, our typical unmotivated client — the client who succeeds in threatening our image as a concerned and competent practitioner — raises in subtler form issues similar to those raised by the client in crisis.

I will touch on one more important inappropriate response of the beginning therapist.

A RECOGNITION THAT THE CLIENT'S "ABERRANCE" IS AN ATTEMPT TO MAKE MEANING OF EXISTENCE

Much of the problem in training young psychotherapists is that they are oriented to look for (and to believe in) only what is wrong with the client; that is to say, to find what is hidden, denied, or pathological. This continual searching for the pathological is very stressful for practitioners. Therapists need to balance the search for the pathological with looking for what is right, healthy, and hopeful in the lives of those with whom they work. Consequently, practitioners must free themselves from concentrating on the "patient" aspects of the client; otherwise, the healthier aspects of the client's personality will be "frozen." Practitioners must respond to the client's emotional needs, not simply render these needs intelligible by interpretation. If psychotherapy is a process within a relationship, the relationship must be nurtured so that the enabling processes can be activated.

REFERENCES

Buckley, P., Karasu, T.B., & Charles, E. (1979). Common mistakes in psychotherapy. *American Journal of Psychiatry, 136,* 1578–1580.

Freud, S. (1937). Analysis terminable and interminable. *Standard edition of the complete works of Sigmund Freud.* London: Hogarth Press, 1955.

Goldberg, C. (1983). The function of the therapist's affect in therapeutic conflict. *Group, 7,* 3–18.

Goldberg, C. (1986). *On being a psychotherapist — The journey of the healer.* New York: Gardner Press.

Groesbeck, C.J. (1975). The archetypal image of the wounded healer. *Journal of Analytic Psychology, 20,* 122–145.

Groesbeck, C.J., & Taylor, B. (1977). The psychiatrist as wounded physician. *American Journal of Psychoanalysis, 37,* 131–139.

Henry, W.E., Sims, J.F., & Spray, S.L. (1973). *Public and private lives of psychotherapists.* San Francisco: Jossey-Bass.

Kopp, S.B. (1976). *If you meet the Buddha on the road, kill him!* New York: Bantam.

Madden, D.J., Lion, J.R., & Penna, M.W. (1976). Assaults on psychiatrists by patients. *American Journal of Psychiatry, 133,* 422–425.

Marmor, J. (1953). The feeling of superiority: An occupational hazard in the practice of psychotherapy. *American Journal of Psychiatry, 110,* 370–376.

Spensley, J., & Blacker, K.H. (1976). Feelings of the psychotherapist. *American Journal of Ortho-Psychiatry, 46,* 542–545.

Tourney, G., Bloom, V., Lowinger, P.L., Schrorer, C., Auld, C.F., & Grissell, F. (1966). A study of psychotherapeutic process variables in psychoneurotic and schizophrenic patients. *American Journal of Psychotherapy, 20,* 112–124.

Weinberg, G. (1984). *The heart of psychotherapy.* New York: St. Martin's Press.

Wheelis, A. (1957). The vocational hazards of psycho-analysis. *International of Psycho-Analysis, 37,* 171–184.

C H A P T E R
66

TYPICAL MISTAKES OF THE
SEASONED THERAPIST

Carl Goldberg, Ph.D.

Therapists have a tendency to be reactors rather than initiators in life. A considerable part of the stress some seasoned practitioners experience has to do with finding themselves snowed into an empty existence because they have lost sight of what they want of life, other than being there for their clients. Some practitioners actually feel shameful about attending to their own needs.

My thesis in this chapter is that practitioners often deny in themselves the very issues they are concerned with in their clients. Certainly, this is an issue for neophyte practitioners during their initial years of practice. However, young practitioners are more likely than seasoned therapists to be in their own therapy or in close supervision. A competent training therapist or supervisor will quickly spot this issue and help the neophyte effectively examine it. On the other hand, senior practitioners who still suffer from a need to be available to those with whom they work, at a cost to their well-being, are less likely to be in treatment and may be ashamed to seek supervision for such an issue.

Marmor (1953) indicates that the greatest strain for practitioners occurs in mid-life when they measure themselves in terms of wealth, prestige, and power, on which great emphasis is placed in American culture. The public assumes that the skills and knowledge of the trade will forge the way practitioners vivify life outside of the office as well as how they conduct themselves at work. Unfortunately, as Freudenberger and Robbins (1979) indicate, while psychotherapists are experts about problems in living, they are not necessarily proficient in living their own lives.

THE DANGERS OF
VICARIOUS EXPERIENCES

Practitioners may unconsciously attempt to accomplish through influencing clients' lives what they have not directly been able to attain for themselves through the years. Through mechanisms of voyeurism, manipulation, and projective identification, practitioners may act out their own impulses.

Therapists in many ways can be viewed as people whose lives center on learning from and identifying with their clients in terms of their excitement and fantasies about the clients' lives, rather than on actively participating in their own lives. There is a danger of "starvation of reality" inherent in being a practitioner. Therapeutic practice needs to be balanced by active involvement in the real world of the therapist. A sense of well-being requires a balance of psychic energies — those directed toward both reflective behavior and initiative behavior. To the contrary, unfortunately, practitioners too often tend to be inordinately reflective. Many have learned early in life that it is safer to observe than to be observed. Consequently, their major source of pleasure throughout the years has been from vicarious identification with their clients. There is a cost to this identification. The price is competition with and envy of those through whom we live vicariously. Practitioners may get themselves caught up in a vicious bind of needing clients to succeed in order to satisfy their own need to offer succor, while at the same time needing clients to fail in order not to foster their competitive and envious sentiments. On the other hand, to the extent that practitioners are actively involved in their own social world, the force of this vicious circle is lessened. The practitioner generally takes an active participant role in therapy from experiencing an energetic, refurbishing, and gratifying life outside the consulting room.

Ralph Greenson (1966) has pointed to the importance of a safe haven for practitioners. This is a place where they can be less than perfect — a place to be a husband or wife, a mother or father, a son or daughter or friend — and not be a special person with omniscient and omnipotent qualities. The need for a safe haven at home, close friendship, interesting activities, and involvements outside their practice seems vital when we recognize that the times of greatest stress for practitioners are generally those when they must face the everyday onslaught of emotional issues of clients without feeling that their own emotional needs are being met. For practitioners whose marriage or caring relationships are depressing, attraction to clients, as well as loosening of defenses against looking toward them for emotional sustenance, may follow. No one but a masochist would endure endless therapeutic practice without having his or her own needs met.

In short, for many veteran practitioners, one of the most serious "mistakes" is that their practice has consumed their whole being. I can give numerous examples that illustrate well that for many practitioners clients become home, family, mission, and destiny. It was said of Harry Stack Sullivan, for example, that his clients were his closest companions. At various times, apparently, several of them boarded with him in his large townhouse. Research of Henry et al. (1971) verified that for most mental health practitioners their relationship with clients is more emotionally intense and satisfying than their involvement with their own spouses and children. In my view, therapists need to balance the labors of their practices with satisfactions, gratifications, and interests in other aspects of life and human existence. To the extent that this does not transpire, they will become fused with their clients. If they cannot appropriately be there for their clients, they will begin to use clients to meet their own needs and satisfactions.

What I mean by this is that therapists who can't share professional concerns with family, friends, or colleagues will feel increasingly insulated, and, as a result, clients will become more important for them than other people. Inevitably the concerns of practice are experienced by both therapist and client. It is reasonable to infer that practitioners will feel closer to those clients with whom they share the most personal thoughts and feelings. It may be to those clients that practitioners unwittingly or even intentionally turn during prolonged and painful periods of estrangement.

PERSONAL INVOLVEMENTS WITH CLIENTS

In an emotional setting with people who have become significant to them over time, therapists may be drawn and attracted to clients sexually, intellectually, or emotionally. If they don't realize this, or can't make clear to themselves the appropriate function and purpose of their being together, serious problems may develop.

Of course, I should indicate that it is certainly not unusual, nor is it untoward, for an attraction to arise toward some patients practitioners work closely with — patients they care about and who they feel care about them. This may not be particularly difficult to examine therapeutically if the client's feelings are "eroticizing" rather than "erotic." What I mean by this is that, for example, the client who says, "I think I love you," or "I fantasize about being physically close to you," implicitly recognizes the transferential quality of the romantic feelings toward the practitioner. In sharp contrast, the client who says, "I love you — let's have an affair," probably doesn't and poses a far more difficult situation for the practitioner.

The problem arises when the practitioner, because of advancing age and the accompanying loss of vitality and fear of diminished interest and attractiveness to others, feels the need to act on a client's feelings, particularly when they are erotic rather than eroticized. The problem is dynamically compounded, as Harold Searles has shown in many of his brilliant clinical papers, by clients rather apperceptively picking up on the therapist's loneliness, sexual frustration, and so forth, and attempting to provide what the therapist needs. Searles tells us that the client's unconscious motive is to help the therapist integrate and become whole in order to be able to provide the emotional resources required for the client's own integration. Analogously, it is like children's trying to save their mother from danger because they unconsciously realize that they will starve to death if the mother perishes.   In short, if the spouse or significant others in practitioners' lives are not available, and they feel neglected, they may manipulate clients into taking the role of caretaker. What is missing existentially in practitioners' lives that may be generating their assuming innapropriate roles toward clients?

LONELINESS AND BOREDOM IN PRACTICE

When the practitioner loses curiosity and enthusiasm for therapeutic work so that the details of people's lives are no longer of excitement or interest, the practitioner will become bored. This is particularly true of analysts and other practitioners who work only with individual clients and without much interaction transpiring between client and therapist. When practitioners see client after client, day after day, in this way, their professional lives become rather lonely. In essence, they may feel hopeless and cynical. When they do not see the potential for realization about themselves by learning from clients, boredom sets in. This often comes from a depression in which the whole of life has become restricted, painful, and ungratifying.

A feeling of boredom in practice is generally symptomatic of a more pervasive ennui in one's life. People who are drawn toward practicing psychotherapy are generally people who are highly stimulated by and responsive to the inner life; a state of boredom in the seasoned practitioner stands in sharp contrast to the practitioner's usual stance. If the onset has been sudden, it may be due to acute hurt and disappointment in life and with sense of self. However, if it is chronic, it may have to do with practitioners' having gradually lost touch with the goals, purposes, and directions with which they began their career. But in almost all instances the feeling of boredom signals the abandonment of the examined inner life. It evinces the externalization of satisfactions. It represents the requirement that other people provide practitioners with sources of contentment that formerly they hoped could be found within themselves.

What are the expectations about the psychological inquiry that may have failed the seasoned practitioner?

THE QUEST FOR REASON

In our discussion of the frustrations and disillusionment inherent in the practice of psychotherapy, we should not lose sight of the fact that one of the cardinal principles of psychotherapy is a working relationship in which therapist and client can reason together. There is, therefore, a kind of certainty that practitioners, particularly if they are psychoanalytically oriented, struggle to find. The basic professional commitment of the practice of psychotherapy for most practitioners is to the assumption that each person they work with is capable of a self-understanding that will lead to self-modification and a sense of purpose in life. In short, for the seasoned practitioner, the disillusionment of practice often stems from the ultimate failure of talk and reason. Many of us, as practitioners, have gone into the field because we have been led to believe from significant figures in our backgrounds and from the ways we ourselves have tried to handle our conflicts that all problems can be resolved if only we face up to them and talk them out in a reasonable way to someone else. As psychotherapists, we find, I think, that often this is not enough.

The problem with this emphasis on rationality, Wheelis (1957) soberly indicates, is that the most common illusion of clients and psychotherapists alike is the belief that insight actually helps. Consequently, the most common disappointment in psychotherapy for the veteran practitioner after seasons of reasoning with clients is the fully developed realization that insight frequently does *not* lead to change. Wheelis states the dilemma rather poetically: "Analysts are purveyors of insight; patients are applicants for magic." What makes this situation inherently antagonistic, according to Wheelis, is that the analyst by disposition and training is the least likely of all people to rely upon methods of reaching clients that eschew self-examination. At the same time, the seasoned practitioner over the years becomes "the object for the most intense and continuous demand for magic performance."

To do their job competently, practitioners soon learn that the theoretical formulations they have been taught in training cannot be depended upon for accurate predictability and insight, as they can in other sciences. Wheelis indicates that the analyst is "forced to realize that insight is not for his patient the edged tool that it is for him." Although practitioners are expected to uphold the highest standards of scientific objectivity, they observe that it is actually how effectively they utilize their personality that enables them to emotionally reach and gain the therapeutic cooperation of clients. In short, the success of therapeutic work actually rests upon the interpersonal skills of the practitioner.

On the other hand, practitioners who cannot or will not transcend talk and reason, refusing to realize the need for their own and their clients' courage in the immediate encounter in which they take part, come to believe that what is being experienced in the here and now is not real. What is more real for them is the transferential implication of the present moment. The practitioner, so believing, is now engaged in reductionism. Psychological reductionism has the unfortunate consequence of fostering intellectualism rather than a vibrant therapeutic relationship. It implies that our behavior at the moment has nothing to do with the immediacy of the experience—the actual feelings we are experiencing toward one another—only with how this moment stimulates associations to another time, another place, another face. The special world of the psychotherapist replaces everyday words and meanings with a psychodynamic language that is regarded as more truthful (Henry et al., 1973).

Wheelis (1956) points out that the failure of insight to bind analyst and client together leaves few courses open to the analyst. He states, "The least painful is a retreat into dogma. . . . Such a development marks the end of the analyst as a creative scientist. He has become a true believer."

It is unfortunate that in holding up Sigmund Freud as a practitioner to emulate, many of us focus exclusively on his intellectual gifts and not on certain of his highly admirable character qualities, such as personal courage. Ernest Jones (1957) in his biography of Freud tells us that when Freud learned that there had been some trepidation about whether to inform him that he was suffering from a malignancy, he responded with profoundly felt resentment. He angrily demanded to know what right anyone had to keep this knowledge from him. He brushed aside the possibility that kindness and care, rather than patronizing arrogance, were the motives that kept his family and friends from telling him about his physical condition. He told his concerned friends that no truth was so painful that fear to face it was not more painful.

THE THERAPEUTIC SEARCH FOR TRUTH

Psychotherapy represents an authentic search for the meaning of one's existence. Some systems of therapy, certainly psychoanalytic therapies, purport to seek the real motives of behavior, as if there were a solitary reality and a single truth. When therapy is unsuccessful, practitioners may feel that in some way they have been involved in a fallacious endeavor. They may question their own limitations and truthfulness. Consequently, it is important for practitioners to recognize that although psychotherapy searches for truths, these truths are actually "functional truths."

Functional meaning has to do with the practical considerations of how people come together and deal with their human existence. It has to do with the specific kinds of meaning that they give to their existence. Psychotherapy is a very important place for examining functional truth. However, if the search in psychotherapy is for objective truth, the work is illusionary, and ultimately disappointing. Nietzsche, in his caution, said it well. He indicated that all truth needed to be confronted with the question, "Can it be lived?" In a word, can the beliefs that we as practitioners hold be meaningfully lives by both our clients and ourselves?

Part of this functional truth is to recognize that inappropriate therapist activity has to do with the inherent struggle in psychotherapy between therapist and client.

THE STRUGGLE IN PSYCHOTHERAPY

There is always a struggle in psychotherapy about how each shall make himself or herself known to the other. The underlying conflict existent in every therapeutic encounter is how therapist and client will address their personal concerns with each other. Awareness of this prevents the therapist from managing the life of the client and moving the client to therapeutically logical conclusions that may be in contradiction with the existential needs of the client's existence. The practitioner's therapeutic system represents value orientations as to how the practitioner requires the client to address his or her human condition. Unless the practitioner is comfortable in exercising considerable power in the client's behalf and unless this influence is openly explored with the client, their work together will be replete with implicit, if not manifest, struggles of will and moral persuasion. Psychotherapists' power resides not in the validity of their explanations but in the audacity of their being willing — with clients' conviction, or at least desperate need — to reduce all matters of importance to psychological terms, which therapists know better than do clients. Under these conditions, the client is not obliged to validate the therapist's explanation in terms of his or her own experience. Therapists who do not examine their own power ploys in their work operate from theoretical models that try to induce the client to play the game by the rule of the therapist's psychological system rather than to accept and work where the client is. In this enterprise, the only power left to the client as long as he or she remains in the therapeutic system — conceptual or real — is the utilization of subversive power. Each of us as a practitioner has experienced our clients' subversive power — the various indirect strategies clients employ to negate our misdirected efforts to help them or protect ourselves.

Therapeutic struggles, of course, should not be encouraged, but neither should they be discouraged or avoided. They need to be viewed as both inevitable and important consequences of significant human interaction. Most theories of psychotherapy tend to disregard therapeutic conflict (Friedman, 1975). These positions tend to attribute the struggle either to the client's distortions or to those of the therapist (or, in a few theories, to the nature of their coming together). But generally, therapeutic conflict has been regarded as that which gets in the way of allowing the practitioner to get on with the business of proper psychotherapeutic procedure (Goldberg, 1977).

The problem of the practitioner's "getting on with the business of proper psychotherapeutic procedure" is that trying to help frequently antagonizes difficult clients. Their experience with "helping" and "nurturing" has been anxious and adversive. The client experiences aloneness as unbearable. What the client actually wants the therapist to do is just to be there and do nothing. The therapist frequently gets caught up in therapeutic conflict because the practitioner doesn't really want to be there because it is boring or painful, but since he or she must be there, the practitioner insists on trying to help. What lies behind this struggle between therapist and client?

A major theme in Western thought is that happiness is the goal of living. A corollary to this thesis is that to harbor self-doubts and to engage in extensive self-examination prevents happiness. Not surprisingly then, most people erect defenses to deny unpleasantness, dissatisfaction, and fear. These defenses collide jarringly with the contrasting belief system of the psychotherapist. The practitioner proclaims, from the Socratic stance, that life is meant to be examined because the unexamined life is not worth living. Moreover, it is enduring meaning, not momentary pleasure, that is the goal of life, according to the psychotherapist. Psychotherapists come from a markedly circumscribed sector of the social world, representing a high congruence of ethnic experience and religious, political, and philosophical values (Henry et al., 1971). They share an orientation toward resolution of problems by means of rational discussion and compromise, working within and accomodating to the established social order (Goldbert and Kane, 1974a; Goldberg and Kane, 1947b). It is small wonder then that the middle-class mental health professional's attitudes best prepare the practitioner to provide ameliorative modalities that are insight oreinted and to direct them toward clients who have a conscious philosophical stance toward life, who are capable of abstract and symbolic reasoning, and who have sufficiently conflict-free areas of psychological functioning to permit them to withstand day-to-day frustrations, tensions, and problems, so that they can struggle with the meaning of their existence and develop a viable sense of identity (Goldberg & Kane, 1974b). Even experienced practitioners may have a great deal of difficulty reaching clients who do not share these same personal and work values.

As a result of ungratifying efforts with difficult clients, practitioners may place themselves in a position that Haveliwala et al. (1979) have referred to as "whitemail." These are clients who, through attractive physical characteristics or personality or rapid improvement in therapy, readily reward us for out time spent with them. For such clients there are countless ways the practitioner unwittingly may pay back the client, such as providing special appointments, remaining overtime, and not broaching embarrassing issues. The problem presents itself when we catch ourselves doing these extras and we try to stop doing them; as a result, the client becomes enraged at our unwillingness to continually play Santa Claus. Some of these clients may stop at nothing in order to resurrect the holiday spirit, not even at self-destructive threats and attempts.

We must face the serious nature of our work. Unless we select clients who wish only cosmetic touches and we choose to indulge them at a perfunctory level, we must accept the inevitable. Sooner or later we will have a client attempt suicide, become psychotically decompensated, or regard our sincerest efforts as incompetent practice. How far will we go in trying to reach these clients? Bared to its core, the crucial issue that is involved in the hazards and mistakes of practice may be examined by answering the following questions: How far should we go in trying to help others? What are the limits of our obligations? How far are we personally willing and able to go beyond these obligations? How we address these questions has much to do with the misappropriated efforts we experience in our work.

DISILLUSIONMENT IN THE SEASONED PRACTITIONER

I have contended in this chapter that practitioners' ability to avoid inappropriate responses and stances has to do with how skillfully their personality and temperament are forged to struggle with inherent antagonism between client and therapist. When clients choose certain ways of handling their anxieties that run counter to therapists' belief systems, anxiety and threats to personal security systems become activated in both participants. To the extent that the idealized imago of the practitioner is threatened, considerable stress may result in controlling and defensive behavior. Disillusionment about the possibility of a meaningful human encounter may also ensue.

Those who are called to the profession of healing generally have an intense interest in learning about themselves. They find a career that will allow them continuous means for examining their own lives while being concerned with the lives of others. Practitioners who feel that they know themselves sufficiently after personal therapy, many seasons of supervision, and many more of clinical practice will find their work as practitioners dull and mechanical.

To the extent that seasoned practitioners no longer consciously experience the struggle with their own humanity in the encounter with clients, they tend to regard the therapeutic relationship as a function. The therapeutic relationship under these conditions becomes an abstraction, appropriate for description and convenient for observation, but at the same time unavailable as a meaningful human encounter in which client and practitioner share concerns in regard to their being in the world.

Disillusionment about meaningfully being involved with those one sees hour after hour, day after day, year after year, breeds loneliness and separateness. The loneliness of practice, when it is not a passionate and inquiring one involved with productive and creative inner dialogue, breeds arrogance and feelings of superiority. Yet, at the same time, practitioners are generally people who have a deep concern for others and a desire to be close but who require a special structure in which to exercise closeness. Within the therapeutic enterprise, there are manifold illusory powers that come to the therapist by virtue of clients' transference distortions and magical hopes. For clients, the therapist becomes the most significant and powerful figure in their lives—the embodiment of every person they have ever known, cared for, feared, or hoped to encounter. To those who are uncomfortable with real power, the illusory power bestowed by clients is ideal. They can choose to nurture their sentiments as genuine when they are ego syntonic or, on the other hand, to interpret and disarm them when threatened by the client's wish to act upon these sentiments in ways uncomfortable to the therapist.

I have tried to show heretofore in this chapter that seasoned practitioners frequently experience the deleterious effects of practice to the extent that they are not sufficiently aware of, or feel that they are not entitled to address, their own emergent needs. Inappropriate therapist activity among veteran practitioners generally is due to the fact that their sensitive empathy and insight are directed toward their clients' needs too exclusively. The character of practitioners, because it gives their life purpose and direction, has been forged from a need to care for others and, at the same time, from a feeling of shame for addressing their own immediate and long-term needs. The very significant rates of "burnout," deep depression, broken relationships, and suicide among psychotherapists attest to the ambivalence many have about their own well-being.

There are, in contrast, some inappropriate therapist activities that result from insufficient sensitivity to the clients' needs. I will address one particularly serious error of omission here.

INAPPROPRIATE THERAPIST FEARS OF COMPASSION

Strict adherence to the specific theoretical principles and their implications for technique and treatment methodology is necessary for scientific validation of theory. On the other hand, although practitioners may be inclined to wish for scientific validation of their clinical work, they are first and foremost an agent of the client and therefore clinically responsible to the client. Practitioners are responsible for abetting the client, even if this requires deviating from the cardinal tenets of the theoretical position with which they identify. It is inhuman and improper to withhold an intervention that will help the client because it does not accord with a theoretical position.

I still vividly remember when I was a candidate in a psychotherapy institute some 15 years ago, sitting and watching a seasoned practitioner conduct psychotherapy with a very fragile, suicidal young woman, while my classmates and I watched from behind a one-way mirror. The patient became inordinately upset during one of the sessions. She was in tears, screaming that the therapist was like everyone else who claimed to want to help her but was actually indifferent to her. She jumped up, promising never to return to therapy because life wasn't worth holding on to. My classmates and I, concerned about the upset woman, called for the therapist to go after her. I don't know if he heard us. I don't know if it would have mattered. He sat there and didn't move. In our postsession discussion with him, he justified his actions on the basis of his theoretical position. His theory said that if he went after the woman, he would be manipulated time and again. The patient never returned.

Many therapists have the notion that they can be most helpful to clients by not gratifying any of the clients' needs except self-understanding. This attitude fosters a rather barren atmosphere in which to relate. It is also a misunderstanding of Freud's dictum about the therapist getting too involved. There are times when it is clinically necessary for the client to feel the therapist's compassion. The practitioner must not be afraid to show compassion and concern. Sidney Jourard (1964) indicates this ethic in his eloquent statement about the I–thou relationship in psychotherapy: "No patient can be expected to drop all his defenses and reveal himself except in the presence of someone who he believes *is for him,* and not for a theory, dogma, or technique" (p. 65).

In curious contradiction, the preponderance of the training for mental health practitioners that I have found available over the past several years has been concerned with psychotherapeutic technique. This is particularly true of workshops held at professional psychotherapy conferences conducted by seasoned practitioners. These workshops emphasize the theoretical and methodological considerations in how to practice therapy: consideration that are designed to help the practitioner work with certain types of difficult, borderline, and narcissistic client populations; techniques that Gestalt practitioners, for example, claim have have more impact than analytic techniques; techniques that psychodynamic practitioners believe to be better thought through than those of transactional analysis or psychodramatic methodologies (Goldberg, 1977).

I believe a curbing of the operational orientation to psychotherapeutic practice is seriously needed. I have emphasized fear of compassion because some practitioners after many seasons still undergo considerable distress in struggling with whether or not to underscore their own values in their therapeutic encounters. Sigmund Freud stated his belief that practitioners' style and technique must be in keeping with the type of person they are, not based upon a ritualized technique for all. Freud (1919) indicated this rather clearly:

> The technical rules which I bring forward here have been evolved out of my own experience in the course of many years, after I had renounced other methods which had cost me dearly. . . . I must, however, expressly state that this technique has proven to be the only method suited to my individuality; I do not venture to deny that a physician quite differently constituted might feel impelled to adopt a different attitude to his patients and to the task before him.

Considering the misdirected therapist activity heretofore discussed, how can seasoned practitioners avoid the ruts of boredom and alientation, or at least climb out upon finding themselves in the dark hours of isolation and despair? I cannot, of course, adequately address this vital question in a few pages. I have examined this in detail elsewhere (Goldberg, 1986). Briefly, however, the following considerations should be of help.

THE PRACTITIONER'S
LIFE PLAN AND GOALS

Just as many practitioners explicitly suggest to their clients that they develop life plans and goals, so too this existential project is valuable for practitioners in assessing the course of their career. Practitioners should examine what they devote their time to in practice. In this examination, at least, the following three questions should be asked: (1) Is the practitioner specializing too exclusively in certain types of clients, which limits the practitioner's effectiveness with other kinds of clients? (2) Have the limitations the practitioner has imposed on himself or herself resulted in feelings of staleness and boredom? and (3) How can the practitioner broaden (or, in some cases, narrow) the directions he or she wishes to take in life?

To provide a broad enough perspective for the practitioner's planning and examination, it may be helpful to formulate a 5- or 10-year plan. The following considerations should be included in the practitioner's life plan.

First, it is important in the growth of all practitioners that no matter how conservative their practice is, or even how successful, they take on one or a few clients who are different from, or even more difficult than, the type of client they usually work with. It may be useful to experiment with, even if only to a limited extent, some therapeutic approaches other than the ones they customarily employ. Like travelers who learn more about their own culture through the eyes of the foreigner, practitioners can learn more about their own practice by these occasional journeys into previously unexplored areas of clinical work.

In short, there is a need in practice to have a variety of clients and activities. This prevents practitioners from assemblylining their professional life. The contrast between different kinds of clients creates a variety of perspectives on human existence. A perspective on human existence becomes artless and slanted whenever practitioners assume the position of having finally figured out human existence. Contrasts among the clients they see should constructively challenge these beliefs. Practitioners who believe that they are capable of formulating their work into a universal scheme of human nature will have clients who suffer from unknown aspects of their complexity as human beings even after many years of treatment. Human existence requires a continual response from each of us. It rejects all final answers. In return, we will reject human existence only if we attempt to impose final answers upon our human condition.

Second, just as seasoned practitioners need to accept new types of clients for their own growth, so should they reject those who do not promise growth and instead would perpetuate stagnation. Maintaining the growing edge in practice, Burton (1969) maintains, requires a careful selection of those with whom we work. "After more than 25 years in the practice of psychotherapy, I have come to the place where I accept only those clients for a therapeutic relationship where there is not only some promise that I can help them, but who offer something to me for my own growth."

Third, it is important that neither practitioners' financial nor their therapeutic satisfactions depend upon one or a few clients. The practitioner should never keep a client for personal satisfactions, whether they be financial, intellectual, or emotional.

Fourth, because of the built-in frustrations and limitations of dealing with very disturbed clients, it helps practitioners to balance their energies by applying their talents to other areas of psychological work. Seasoned practitioners who work only with difficult borderline and schizophrenic clients may receive little positive regard from these clients. By sharing their experience, knowledge, and concerns with students and supervisees, or simply in devoting professional time to those areas of interest and skill that they do not normally use in private practice, practitioners may receive satisfactions not obtainable in their daily clinical practice.

Fifth, practitioners who work exclusively with individual clients may profit from devoting some of their practice to group or family work. Among other values, it may serve as an invaluable tool for understanding their own counter-transferences.

A final issue that I would like to briefly address concerns the question of whether there is life after practice.

LIFE AFTER PRACTICE

The practitioner's knowledge, skills, and experience can be effectively utilized for ventures other than psychotherapy. Psychotherapy need not be a terminal career! Notwithstanding, many practitioners hold on to the saddle to the very end. There is nothing else they want to do or believe they can do well enough to pursue as a second career. There are others who retire to fish, take the boat out, play tennis or golf, visit the grandchildren, or travel around the globe. Many of them feel that after so many years spent as a psychotherapist it is too late to learn new skills and pursue another field of endeavor.

Still other practitioners feel that they would like to pursue another field, but to do so would be tantamount to admitting to themselves and to others that they have failed in their careers as healers. In order to protect their integrity, they look upon their psychotherapeutic practice as necessarily final. Yet, many of us tell our clients that their psychotherapeutic experience should open a world of possibilities for them. This should be valid for ourselves as well. To pursue an allied, or even a distant field after years as a psychotherapist is hardly a statement of failure. It is no more a failure than to terminate a marriage, not because it wasn't once enriching for both but because one or both have matured over the years and have moved in different directions, requiring different kinds of experience for increasing their capacity for intimacy and self-development. There are some people who are "born" therapists. By this I mean that their programmed needs are continuously, throughout life, satisfied by working as therapists. There are many other practitioners, however, whose maturation is different. After a number of years or practice, they have achieved for themselves the most that they can reasonably expect to derive from practice. They experience the need to move in different directions to relate to and be in the world with others. I have written about life after practice in the belief that turning to other fields is not necessarily a sign of failure and because I hold that the seasoned practitioner has much to offer society in undertaking new and expanded ventures.

In summary, the growing concerns practitioners relate to the origins of our interest in self-examination and understanding of others. To the extent that practitioners work arduously to understand self and clients, and to the extent that they are not dutifully recognized or rewarded for their skills and compassion, they may begin seriously to reconsider a career as a healer.

There are, of course, many different ways practitioners may react to their growing concerns. They may rationalize their practice and relegate it to being a business, concerning themselves rather exclusively with financial considerations. This may be reinforced by the feeling that, because practitioners have spent more years than most other professionals in training, they are now owed a good income. Or practitioners may join or initiate new theories, schools of thought, and psychological movements that offer new meaning to the work. In this regard, I am leary of those practitioners who spend considerable time on television talk shows or promotional tours for their books or for their radical new psychotherapy institutes. At best, these practitioners have little available time for careful work with clients. Moreover, many of them may be more concerned with selling their clients a technique and a life-style than with helping the clients come to terms with where they are "at." Just as the best teachers go unsung, so perhaps do the best psychotherapists. They don't write books, give lectures, or even teach. They are known only to the clients.

On the other hand, bored practitioners may gradually shift their time, energy, and interest to new pursuits or fields of interest peripheral to clinical work or simply devote more time to teaching, research, or supervision than they formerly did. Or, more unfortunately, they may become increasingly iatrogenic for their clients. That is to say, they may deleteriously affect their clients because they are not aware of their own needs and how they use their clients to meet these needs. If they continue in this way, they will sooner or later experience a burnout. Some of us forget too quickly that the source of our ability to touch others lies in our being human. We heal others by courageously heeding our own suffering.

Therapy is the most human of the arts and sciences. A responsive vulnerability is the basis of practitioners' sensitivity, compassion, and receptivity to others' suffering. But, as such, it is by necessity a double-edged instrument. It is potentially their most sensitive tool for responsively attending human suffering, while at the same time, it is a wound that may become exacerbated by excessive, painful stress and self-doubt.

I recommend that practitioners may best maximize the advantages of their highly attuned responsiveness by treating self and clients with liberal amounts of compassion and common sense. Whatever practitioners do, it must make sense to them and to those with whom they work. Clients, whatever their specific symptoms, all undoubtedly suffer from lives that were bereft of sufficient common sense and compassion. If practitioners do no more than offer clients both sincere compassion and common sense, they can do no harm; indeed, practitioners will more likely serve as a meaningful human bridge to the world they share. Competent practitioners well know this in terms of their clients. The common sense and compassion of which I speak are, therefore, in the treatment of oneself. One needs to take seriously one's own humanity and must sensibly be cognizant of what is and is not possible to accomplish as a practitioner, without unreasonable risk to health and well-being. One needs to use common sense to provide in one's practice and in one's personal life those satisfactions, securities, and provisions of well-being necessary to apply oneself meaningfully and energetically to this important and difficult human task.

In a word, this chapter has attempted to help practitioners deal with the strain of being an idealized person during those times when they experience themselves as merely human—all too human. For no matter how intelligent, well trained, experienced, caring, and well-meaning we are as professionals, we are at the same time host to the same fears, ambitions, and temptations as those we treat. We can be no more than that and no less if we are to treat meaningfully those who petition us with their suffering. Burton (1975) points out that psychotherapy is a business, but it takes a more or less vulnerable person to do it well. This is to say, the practitioner must remain vulnerable and, at the same time, professional and skillful. We must be openly human, which means being less than the ideal for which we strive, without regarding our limitations as weaknesses or our efforts as failures. To view our limitations as weakness is to regard ourselves as superordinary beings who should be the fulfillment of our ego ideal at all times. Our vulnerabilities are the bridges to our clients. If we carry out this complex task without pretense or apology, we cannot fail.

REFERENCES

Burton, A. (1969). To see and encounter critical people. *Voices, 5,* 26–28.

Burton, A. (1975). Therapy satisfaction. *American Journal of Psychoanalysis, 35,* 115–122.

Freud, S. (1919). *Lines of advance to psychoanalytic therapy.* Standard edition of the complete works of Sigmund Freud. London: Hogarth Press, 1955.

Freudenberger, H.J., & Robbins, A. (1979). The hazards of being a psychoanalyst. *Psychoanalytic Review, 66,* 275–296.

Friedman, L. (1975). The struggle in psychotherapy: Its influences on some theories. *Psychoanalytic Review, 62,* 453–462.

Goldberg, C. (1977a). *On being a psychotherapist: The journey of the healer.* New York: Gardner Press.

Goldberg, C. (1977b). *Therapeutic partnership: Ethical concerns in psychotherapy.* New York: Springer.

Goldberg, C., & Kane, J. (1974a). A missing component in mental health services for the urban poor: Services-in-kind to others. In D.A. Evans & W.L. Claiborn (Eds.), *Mental health issues and the urban poor.* (pp. 91–110). New York: Pergamon.

Goldberg, C., & Kane, J. (1974b). Services-in-kind: A form of compensation for mental health services. *Hospital and Community Psychiatry, 25* 161–164.

Greenson, R.R. (&1966). That "impossible profession." *Journal of the American Psychonalytic Association, 14,* 9–24.

Haveliwala, Y.A., Scheflin, A.E., & Ashcroft, N. (1979). *Common sense in therapy.* New York: Brunner/Mazel.

Henry, W.E., Sims, H.J., & Spray, S.L. (1971). *The fifth profession: Becoming a psychotherapist.* San Francisco: Jossey-Bass.

Henry, W.E., Sims, J.H., & Spray, S.L. (1973). *Public and private lives of psychotherapists.* San Francisco: Jossey-Bass.

Jones, E. (1957). *The life and work of Sigmund Freud.* New York: Basic Books.

Jourard, A. (1959). I–thou relationship versus manipulation in counseling and psychotherapy. *Journal of Individual Psychology, 5,* 174–179.

Marmor, J. (1953). The feeling of superiority: An occupational hazard in the practice of psychotherapy. *American Journal of Psychiatry, 110,* 370–376.

Wheelis, A. (1957). The vocational hazards of psycho-analysis. *International Journal of Psycho-Analysis, 37,* 171–184.

C H A P T E R
67

BOREDOM AND BURNOUT—
HOW TO AVOID THEM

Lucy B. Smith, C.S.W.

Very early one morning, soon after I began in private practice, as I was walking to my office I saw a man come out of an apartment building and walk in my direction. It was a clear, sparkling day; he sniffed the air approvingly, straightened his tie, and walked briskly to his car. As he unlocked the door, I noticed a familiar, oversized sign on top of the car advertising a driving school. He was a driving instructor and was on his way to work, just as I was. A cheerful thought crossed my mind: "Hey, I could do that. I could teach people how to drive!" Later that day, on my way to a supervision session, a woman approached me on the subway platform and asked a complicated question about subway directions. After giving her the answer, I realized that that was the first time that day I *really knew* what I was talking about! I mentioned these two instances to my supervisor, who asked me if I had been feeling "burned out" lately. At first, I did not understand her question. I thought burnout was something that happened only to old-timers, seasoned therapists who, after years and years of private practice, "burned out," like used-up candles. But these two incidents revealed an incipient burnout syndrome in me, and I had been practicing for less than two years. What was happening to me, and why? What could I do to check it?

Usually, when we think of burnout in the psychotherapeutic community, what comes to mind are the aggravating conditions faced by social workers and other therapists in agency settings. Clinical conditions, such as the vast number of cases and the magnitude of the task, irksome, endless administrative chores, and pressures, can combine to demoralize an entire staff. Overworked, overwhelmed workers in agencies and clinics often burn out, and some leave the field altogether. But burnout also occurs in therapists in other, less desperate settings. In private practice, where the conditions seem serene compared with agency settings, therapists are still vulnerable to syndromes of boredom and burnout. Here, the causes of burnout are apt to be internal stresses as well as external ones. Personal qualities, needs, and motivations, as well as professional attitudes, can dramatically increase or decrease the susceptibility to burnout.

The term "burnout" describes an occupational stress syndrome frequently seen among people working in the human services (Maslach, 1976). Symptoms of burnout include the loss of motivation and effectiveness in connection with work; reduced energy, interest, and satisfaction in work; and even a dread of work. The metaphor is a vivid one. In addition to spent candles, burnout evokes the image of an overloaded electrical system. Fuses, unable to withstand the power input, melt and burn out, and the current is interrupted. What burns out in human-service professionals, according to Christina Maslach (1982), one of the earliest writers on the subject, is the capacity to involve oneself in the painful emotions of others. Maslach sees emotional fatigue as the crux of the burnout syndrome.

Maslach's perspective is particularly relevant to burnout among older, seasoned professionals. Years of intense emotional involvement may have taken their toll; changes in the therapist's personal life may result in a loss of inspiration; or burnout may be the end point in a long process with complex, personal origins. A large percentage of professional burnout, however, takes place early in careers. Ironically, as Freudenberger (1977) points out, burnout often occurs in young professionals who bring the most dedication, sensitivity, and commitment to the field. In this discussion, I will focus, for the most part, on the causes of emotional fatigue in therapists who are in the early stages of their careers.

Stress, for therapists, derives from social interaction (Maslach, 1982). As therapists, we listen to patients and we try to help them with our words, through a therapeutic relationship. Research by Farber and Heifetz (1982) indicates that professional gratification, for psychotherapists, is related to the ability to develop a helpful, therapeutic relationship. When we see and hear that our verbal responses have had a soothing, reassuring, or otherwise helpful effect on patients, we feel effective as therapists. The research shows that as long as we therapists feel this effectiveness, as long as our efforts seem to "pay off," the difficult and stressful nature of our work is acceptable (Farber & Heifetz, 1982). For beginning therapists, there is an especially strong correlation between a sense of success, or effectiveness, and resistance to emotional fatigue. When burnout develops in a beginning therapist, its roots usually can be found in painful feelings of ineffectiveness.

In studies of professional burnout in private practice, three predisposing factors emerge: conditions of the profession; inner qualities and personal characteristics of the therapist; and attitudes toward work. As we examine these factors as they pertain to the private practitioner, their correlation to a diminished sense of effectiveness in the therapist is apparent. Symptoms of burnout develop as a defense against feeling ineffective.

CONDITIONS OF THE PROFESSION

Arnold Cooper (1986), in a discussion of burnout and psychoanalysis, outlines several conditions inherent in the profession that, he believes, predispose the practitioner to burnout. All psychotherapists, Cooper emphasizes, work in a setting of emotional intensity. The degree of empathy, emotional awareness, and tolerance for ambiguity that is required can be exhausting. In her study of burnout, Maslach (1982) described how a therapist's adjustment to this degree of emotional intensity—an adjustment that is made to avoid emotional exhaustion—can actually lead to burnout. In an effort to put emotional distance between themselves and distressed people whose needs may be overwhelming, therapists develop detachment. The right balance of detachment and concern enhances effectiveness, and can prevent emotional exhaustion, but what frequently happens, according to Maslach, is that detachment, serving as a defense against emotional involvement, gradually increases to the point where the therapist has developed a hardened, dehumanized stance toward patients. At this point, genuine empathic responses to patients are blocked, and, as a result, the therapeutic relationship breaks down.

Such a breakdown can occur on a smaller scale, intermittently in treatment. For example, when I am feeling tired during a session, I tend to detach more. I become silent and less responsive, and there is a temporary break in the relationship. While everyone agrees that a degree of detachment is necessary for effectiveness, therapists cannot reduce significantly the emotional intensity in the therapeutic setting without running the risk of losing their most valuable tool, the personal connection.

Another "hazardous" condition of private practice, according to Cooper (1986), is the extraordinary degree of social isolation in which we work. Psychotherapists in full-time private practice are often lonely. Unlike other professionals in human services, therapists in private practice seldom have social contacts other than patients during the course of a normal working day. Between sessions, moreover, therapists usually spend their time reading or writing, both solitary activities. On longer breaks, therapists may go alone to movies. Most of our free time arises during the middle of the morning or afternoon, when friends or spouses are busy. This social isolation is less felt by therapists who work in clinics, who are part of a staff and may meet with colleagues during breaks, meetings, and so on. But for the therapist in private practice, the combination of emotional intensity and extreme social isolation can have a debilitating effect. Some therapists try to counter this by attending or holding classes or workshops or by supervision. Participating in a peer or therapy group whose memebership is made up of other therapists can greatly relieve the effects of isolation.

In addition to social isolation, Cooper (1986) notes, psychotherapists are isolated from a base of scientific data concerning the results or effectiveness of the profession. There are few statistics or precise records of treatment. Psychotherapists must rely on their own experience and on broad accounts by others, both to set goals and to assess progress in treatment. Although recently there has been a trend toward efforts to standardize diagnostic criteria and treatment techniques — and efforts in this direction will increase because of the exigencies of a third-party payment system — the scientific nature of data about the results of psychotherapy will always be compromised because of the uniqueness of every patient. Psychoanalytic or psychotherapeutic treatment is not the same as, for example, medical treatment of a bacteriological infection, where the specific bacteria can be isolated and treated. Psychotherapy, with the exception of certain behaviorist techniques, involves the entire personality of the patient, including his or her life history.

What research we do have on treatment effectiveness underscores the therapeutic importance of the relationship between the patient and the therapist. Not only is every patient different, but the personality of the individual therapist is also a significant variable. There may be more than one effective treatment model, for example, when the "right" therapist is working with the "right" patient, whereas a preferred treatment may be ineffective if patient and therapist are mismatched. A consequence is that we can never be sure about our long-term effectiveness, even with our own patients. Though significant efforts are being made to remedy the lack of data and research in our field, it is likely that the practice of psychotherapy will always be part science, part art. This may be an acceptable condition to most therapists, even a desirable one, but it has its "down side": we do not fully understand our own profession—its limitations, its possibilities, its boundaries. We are continually reviewing our profession.

Finally, Cooper (1986) points out, we are isolated from our patients in a formal way that other helping professionals are not. It is ironic, he notes, that as involved as we may be with a patient for months, or even years, once treatment ends we are cut off from knowing this person. Unlike medical doctors, we do not, for the most part, acquire new friends through our patients. When a relationship with a patient develops into a lasting friendship, it is considered exceptional. In spite of the intimacy, closeness, and trust that the therapeutic relationship affords, it is not quite the same as a "normal" friendship. There is a certain remove, a certain distance dictated by the structure and special nature of our relationship with patients.

Uncountered, these isolating conditions can, with the passage of time, lead to a sense of ineffectiveness and to burnout. Boredom, a weariness toward work, sets in as a defense against long-felt frustrations. This weariness is not considered pathological; it is reactive, a symptom created by the vexing nature of the profession.

PERSONAL CHARACTERISTICS

There are personal qualities, however, that can inhibit the practitioner's ability to counter the tensions and uncertainties created by the conditions of the profession. Personal characteristics and needs can predispose a therapist to feeling ineffective. By far the most common personal characteristic connected with the syndrome of burnout is compulsivity. Burnout is pathological (and almost inevitable) when there is a compulsive element in the psychotherapist's relation to work.

Like other helping professionals, therapists often are attracted to psychotherapy as a profession because of a great need to help or rescue others. The sense of mission and omnipotent wishes around rescuing others may have a compulsive quality. They may mask a need for expiation, for making reparations (Edelwich, 1980). The therapist whose unconscious motivation is to make reparations works harder and harder, keeping longer and longer hours. But underneath all the "dedication" and "commitment" is the compulsion to expiate a neurotic guilt. When the need to be an all-powerful rescuer is thwarted—as it surely will be—the "guilty" therapist feels helpless and frustrated. To escape these intolerable feelings, the therapist may begin to feel bored. He or she may lose concentration or interest, and may feel relieved when a patient cancels a session; the therapist's mind may begin to wander during sessions. These are "soft signs," or precursors, of a burnout syndrome.

Some patients have a special ability to tap into our neurotic guilt. For example, patients who continue to be deeply depressed after weeks or months in treatment can have a demoralizing effect on a therapist with a rescue fantasy. Frustrated at not being able to relieve the depression, the therapist may lose perspective on the treatment, which, overall, may be going very well.

In addition to inner guilt, omnipotent wishes around rescuing others may conceal inner sources of self-doubt. Therapists with a compulsion to rescue others make exaggerated demands on their own performance. As Cooper (1986) indicates, when they fail, they are prone to vicious self-recriminations. They never give themselves credit for doing the best they can; instead, they experience an agony of self-doubt. To defend against these painful feelings, the therapist develops a burnout syndrome. Self-doubt generated a compulsivity in relation to my practice in those first few years. At that point in my career, my need to help people was far greater than my ability to be effective with patients. If these feelings are not analyzed in supervision or in personal therapy, a sense of dread in connection with work may develop. Eventually, burnout takes the form of negative attitudes toward patients and a generalized negativity toward the profession itself. Patients begin to seem all the same, or all sessions the same. Impatience with and resentment and hostility toward patients increase, and a burned-out, nihilistic, angry stance develops with regard to the profession.

Christina Maslach (1982) examines other "selfish" reasons that people enter helping professions. One, which applies particularly to psychotherapists, is the need for close personal relationships. Thereapists who have difficulty in establishing close relationships may use their patients to satisfy their own needs for intimacy. In the patient–therapist relationship, the therapist is in the "safe," passive, less-vulnerable position. Relationships with patients are intimate and intense, since they focus on deeply personal issues, but it is the patient who initiates the relationship and the patient's issues are the focus of treatment. The therapist can attempt to fulfill a personal need for closeness without personally taking the risks involved in an intimate relationship. An inner deadness remains in the therapist, however, as personal needs for intimacy may be partly, but never fully, met by our patients.

Another personal need that therapists often try to satisfy through therapeutic relationships is the need for control over their own personality problems. Many therapists are drawn into the profession by way of their own therapy, to work out—or avoid working out—their own pathology. Focusing on other people's problems can be an attempt to relieve the tension around one's own issues. The tension of the therapist's own neurosis or characterological issues, however, is then revived in the debilitating countertransferences that develop toward patients in the course of treatment.

But, as Maslach (1982) says, therapists who attempt to meet personal needs for expiation or self-esteem through their work can still provide a high quality of care to patients. Nevertheless, there are dangers. One danger is that personal motivations *can* interfere with the quality of care, particularly when therapists are unaware of their underlying motivations. Unconscious, compulsive motivations become the source of emotional burnout, because patients do not provide all the intimacy or identity or approval that the therapist needs or wants. Frustration around one's own needs being thwarted is eventually expressed in hostility toward patients, who respond accordingly—by getting worse. The therapist's effectiveness and self-esteem are reduced, leaving the therapist ripe for burnout.

Unfortunately, many therapists respond to the initial stages of burnout in a way that aggravates the syndrome. By increasing steadily the number of patients seen and dramatically extending working hours, therapists work even harder in an attempt to get affirmation or other personal needs met. This is done compulsively, without reflection or a sense of option, and usually results in a chronic sense of being overburdened.

This is the time to be alert for burnout symptoms. As a therapist, one has to assess how much one can do in a week for optimum effectiveness, enjoyment, and creativity. If one continually exceeds that limit, there is apt to be a compulsive component to one's work. The overburdened therapist should ask himself or herself: Why am I overworking? Am I being competitive with other therapists? Am I being greedy? Does my work have an expiative function? Am I making reparations? We may not be successful in ridding ourselves altogether of compulsivity; many of us are, or become, unreconstructed workaholics. But if we can analyze and understand the compulsive component of our work, we can avoid or analyze countertransferences that inevitably develop when personal needs are not met. Our countertransferrences can wreak havoc on treatment for our patients and leave us feeling ineffective and demoralized.

WORK ATTITUDES

Attitudes that may predispose a therapist to the syndrome of burnout are often closely related to personal characteristics. Every contributor to the literature on burnout stresses the importance of expectations, role definitions, and realistic goals in therapy. Unrealistic self-expectations, an exaggerated sense of responsibility, and too much therapeutic zeal are attitudes that lead to excessive energy output. Overcommitment and overdedication to a job end in exhaustion and disappointment. Burnout develops as a defense against exaggerated personal expectations that have been frustrated. The therapist's loss of energy and interest serves as a defense against an underlying disappointment and anger.

The appropriate therapeutic stance, according to most writers, is a contradictory one. It includes therapeutic fervor and therapeutic distance. Therapists must be involved, dedicated, and optimistic, but they also must realize that they cannot, ultimately, be responsible for rescuing patients from pain, nor can they be solely responsible for positive change in their patients' lives. All therapists should be dedicated and concerned, and in extreme situations, where there is a threat of suicide, homicide, or spouse or child abuse, must assume complete responsibility and intervene immediately. At these times, there is a genuine rescue operation. But in the normal private-practice treatment setting, there should not be an ongoing sense of emergency (Friedman, 1985).

A certain therapeutic distance provides the therapist with space to reflect, improvise, and work creatively with patients. When there is a balance between optimism and concern, on the one hand, and distance, on the other, there is an atmosphere conducive to spontaneous thought and inventiveness. The therapist is open to a wider range of ideas and can take risks. He or she can explore an issue with a patient that does not conform neatly to psychoanalytic theories. It is the exploration of these issues that so often provides a patient with a realization of the idiosyncratic aspects of himself or herself, and a heightened experience of individuality. Excessive therapeutic zeal, with its emphasis on theory, its unrelenting search for the pathological, its sense of urgency, and its goal focus, does not permit this kind of "diversion."

By emphasizing therapeutic distance, Cooper and other writers do not imply a support of "abstinence" on the part of the therapist, or a reduction of involvement with patients. Involvement with patients is not what causes burnout; excessive performance demands and overcommitment to unrealistic expectations are the attitudes that lead to therapeutic burnout.

Therapists least susceptible to the syndromes of boredom and burnout may be those who maintain dialogues with themselves as well as with patients. A great deal has been written about therapists being drawn to the field in an effort to control their own pathology. While the dangers of this are real, and some of them have been underscored in this chapter, there can be an advantage to having a "selfish" motivation. Therapists who are still engaged in their own "soul searches" may, through the analytic process with patients, continue to make discoveries about their own lives. For example, a patient may say something about his or her childhood that changes the therapist's perspective on the therapist's own childhood. Or a patient may touch on something else in life with which the therapist identifies strongly. These experiences stimulate positive feelings toward our patients and the profession.

In order to experience profound identifications with patients, however, the therapist must have an "other" life, outside the profession. As committed to and excited by our work as we may be, we cannot live through our patients. Our patients terminate with us; they leave us and move on, living their lives. As much as our work deals with the "stuff of life," it cannot *be* our life. We must have other interests and involvements and relationships that provide us with experiences and feelings to associate to, process, and understand as we listen to our patients and try to help them understand their lives.

For the practitioner in private practice, in addition to having a full personal life, it is helpful to have another professional dimension to supplement work with patients. Workshops, seminars, and study groups are excellent sources of contact and stimulation. In my own experience, individual and group supervision provided a supportive milieu in which to analyze countertransferences and personal attitudes that would have caused burnout early in my practice. Over the years, a therapist's own "soul search" can be continued through personal analysis, individual supervision, group supervision with a leader, and peer group supervision. Not only do these experiences provide stimulation and contact with and support from other professionals, but they also serve to monitor our internal conflicts and stresses and countertransferences.

REFERENCES

Cooper, A. (1986). Some limitations on therapeutic effectiveness: The "burnout syndrome" in psychoanalysis. *Psychoanalytic Quarterly, 55*(4), 576–598.

Edelwich, J. (1980). *Burnout: Stages of disillusionment in the helping professions.* New York: Human Sciences Press.

Farber, B., & Heifetz, L. (1982). The process and dimensions of burnout in psychotherapists. *Professional Psychology, 13,* 293–301.

Freudenberger, H. (1977). Speaking from experience—burnout: the organizational menace. *Training Development Journal, 31,* 26–27.

Friedman, R. (1985). Making family therapy easier for the therapist: Burnout prevention. *Family Process, 24*(4), 549–553.

Maslach, C. (1976). Burned out. *Human Behavior, 5,* 17–22.

Maslach, C. (1982). *Burnout: The cost of caring.* Englewood Cliffs, NJ: Prentice-Hall.

C H A P T E R
68

THE MANAGEMENT OF CRISES IN PSYCHOTHERAPY

William C. Normand, M.D.,
Edwin S. Robbins, M.D., and
Lillian Robbins, Ph.D.

In this chapter, we discuss some general principles and specific guidelines regarding the prevention and management of crises and emergencies in the private practice of psychotherapy. We consider psychodynamic issues, but the emphasis is on clinical and administrative aspects that may lead to tension and anxiety in the therapist regarding therapeutic outcome and necessary pragmatic decisions in areas in which many therapists have had little experience.

DEFINITIONS OF CRISIS AND EMERGENCY

Although the terms "crisis" and "emergency" may be used interchangeably, in the context of psychotherapy it is useful to distinguish between the two (Chrzanowski, 1977). In psychodynamic theory, "crisis" refers to a turning point, a period in which new demands on the ego cannot be met successfully by the usual coping mechanisms. At such times, powerful emotions, such as anxiety and guilt, are intense, and cannot continue for long. The possible outcomes of a crisis can be formulated in general terms as:

- Return to the previous state;
- Growth process, with an increase of ego strength;
- Destructive process (i.e., suicide, homicide, assault) or the emergence of new psychopathology.

To complicate matters, crises may resolve into some combination of the above. Erikson (1959) referred to the universal developmental phases of life as "developmental crises," and to individual traumatic events as "accidental crises." Caplan (1964) provides examples of the latter, such as "the death of a loved person; loss or change of a job, a threat to bodily integrity by illness, accident, or surgical operation; or change of role due to developmental or sociocultural transitions, such as going to college, getting married, and becoming a parent." In psychotherapy, acting out and transference and countertransference distortions are additional common sources of crises.

The term "emergency" refers to danger that demands immediate intervention. An unresolved crisis can be considered a nascent emergency. There is an extensive literature dealing with crisis theory, crisis intervention, psychiatric emergencies, and brief psychotherapeutic interventions in emergencies, but we found only two articles written specifically about crises that arise in the course of ongoing psychotherapy (Chrzanowski, 1977; Birk & Birk, 1984).

DEALING WITH CRISES

Formulating The Problem

An effective response to a crisis depends in part on the characteristics of the crisis and in part on the therapist's comprehensive understanding of the patient, including both manifest clinical circumstances and psychodynamic formulation. Perry, Cooper, and Michels (1987) describe the elements that make up a workable formulation:

> 1) A summary. . .that describes the patient's current problems and places them in the context of the patient's current life situation and developmental history; 2) a description of nondynamic factors that may have contributed to the psychiatric disorder; 3) a psychodynamic explanation of the central conflicts, describing their role in the current situation and their genetic origins in the developmental history; and 4) a prediction of how these conflicts are likely to affect treatment and the therapeutic relationship.

Among nondynamic factors they include such issues as genetic predisposition, mental retardation, overwhelming trauma, and drugs or any physical illness affecting the brain. In assessing current life problems, we would add that the therapist should be on the lookout for changes in biological (including physical illness), psychological, and social circumstances of the patient's life.

Chrzanowski (1977) defined several common categories of crisis:

• The emergence of an acute psychosis, which may or may not require hospitalization.
• Self-destructive acting out often associated with alcohol or drug abuse, promiscuity, or delinquency.
• Major illnesses or serious accidents involving the patient or people close to him or her.
• Family disturbances, including separation and divorce.
• Economic crisis.
• Severe transference distortions (i.e., psychotic transference).
• Serious countertransference distortions.
• The paradoxical upsurge of disturbed and disturbing emotion and behavior when the patient is threatened by success in the therapy, including the prospect of termination, as cause of crisis.
• The response of a significant other who perceives the patient's improvement as a threat.

Whether such circumstances lead to an emergency depends on the interactions among the severity of the stress, the strength of the patient's ego and support network, and the therapist's skill. Some patients with relatively weak egos (schizophrenics; chronically depressed, narcissistic, and borderline personalities; substance abusers; and some adolescents) are especially prone to developing crises that become emergencies. In treating vulnerable people, the therapist should be vigilant for personality and behavioral changes that indicate increasing tension or problems in adjusting to routines of daily living. When problems are anticipated, especially early in the course of treatment, the therapist is well advised to meet with the family and lay the groundwork for working together if the need arises.

The Management Of Crises

True emergencies are rare in the practice of psychotherapy, but crises are not, since transference and countertransference distortions, as well as stressful life events, are common. How can the therapist prevent crises from becoming emergencies? Of course, no absolute rules are possible. The aim is to strengthen the ego relative to existing inner and outer pressures. This can be done by reducing demands, increasing the person's ability to cope and, when possible, by a combination of the two. Birk and Birk (1984) state, "The challenge is to find ways of managing the crisis that protect the patient from undue risk, yet do not infantilize him, encourage dependency, or otherwise set back the goals of his ongoing psychotherapy."

There are many ways to reduce pressure on the ego. Modifying the therapeutic process to provide more support, to focus upon reality, and to assist the patient in developing coping mechanisms are useful techniques. It is critical, however, to be certain that the crisis indicates a serious threat that requires significant changes in the therapeutic approach, rather than a vicissitude of the therapy (such as fear of improvement or of termination) best dealt with by interpretation.

External pressures may be reduced by what is commonly called manipulation (Bibring, 1954). The term is pejorative, though what is done is therapeutic. We prefer to call it exerting therapeutic influence, that is, encouraging the patient to carry out or to avoid certain activities, according to the therapist's understanding of the meaning of such activity for the patient; for example, advising the patient to go ahead or to postpone asking his or her boss for a raise. In selected cases, hypnosis (Zeig, 1980) and behavior modification (Wolpe, 1973) are useful techniques in teaching people how to cope with stress. Role playing can help a patient develop the skills and techniques necessary for mastery of the problem. When utilizing role playing consider having the patient sequentially take the part of both the adversary and himself or herself. Quite often, an excellent understanding of the other person's thinking develops when the patient has to present another's alternative viewpoint. The therapist can be of great assistance during role playing by offering suggestions for change while acting as one of the protagonists.

In psychoanalytic therapy, crises may be attenuated by modifying the parameters of treatment in the direction of providing more support. Some examples are increasing the number of sessions, changing from couch to chair, scheduling or permitting telephone calls during certain hours, involving family members, and using medication. Kliman (1978) illustrates the flexibility of a therapist in her book on crisis intervention. Today, of course, many family therapists would not consider dealing with a crisis if all family members were not available and actively involved in the therapeutic process.

In the following two illustrations, the therapist used therapeutic influence to help patients resolve crises.

> A couple, who lived at opposite ends of the country, met at a resort and had a torrid time, which they continued for the next year by spending romantic weekends together each month. They maintained contact by telephone in the intervening time. In the course of the year, they decided to marry. Since he had more job opportunities, they agreed that he would quit his job and move to her city. A date was not fixed, so he decided to surpirse her. When he arrived, she told him that she did not wish to hurt him and so had not been able to bring herself to tell him that she had become seriously interested in another man. When he learned that she no longer wanted him to move in with her, he became severely distressed and sought therapeutic assistance.
>
> Both were seen jointly for several sessions and individually for a month. Their feelings were explored, and each was helped to feel that a decision to separate was in his or her best interest. At the end of a month, the man felt no further need for treatment. A year later, he called to say that he had had an excellent year, had been promoted to a senior executive position, and was relocating. She remained in treatment, came to understand more of the developmental factors that had led her to fear closeness and commitment to men, and married the second man.

The next case illustrates how role playing and rational exploration of alternatives may help a person arrive at a decision, even though the resolution of the crisis is, in many ways, equivalent to accepting the "least worst" of several available options.

> An intelligent woman, who had been married for 20 years to an alcoholic husband, initiated steps to resume working when he successfully conquered his drinking and began to perform well in his job. She became absorbed in her career and was recognized as being very competent, and was unable to pay as much attention to him and the household as in the past. He became overtly competitive with her, resumed drinking, and again performed poorly at work. His therapist, who had an ongoing relationship with the woman, had a series of conferences in which a variety of scenarios were explored through role playing and discussion. She sadly concluded that, if she wished to remain married to the man, she would have to capitulate to his emotional blackmail and resume her previous role as dependent housewife. His goal achieved, he again became abstinent and his work performance improved.

Use Of Medication

Psychotropic medication is increasingly being used as an adjunct in psychotherapy, psychoanalytic as well as supportive (Normand & Bluestone, 1986). It may be the critical factor in preventing destructive acting out of unbearable anxiety, rage, or guilt, or psychotic decompensation. Lack of sleep, per se, can exacerbate the crisis and may be ameliorated by the judicious short-term use of hypnotics and tranquilizers. However, medication should not be introduced without careful consideration of the risks, such as addiction and side effects.

EMERGENCIES

Problems Reported By Practitioners

An informal survey among psychiatrists, psychologists, and social workers in the department of psychiatry at Bellevue Hospital Center in New York showed that few have ever experienced an emergency in their private practice, but that many have had episodes of discomfort that are still remembered. Nearly all reported dealing at one time or another with aberrant behavior, ranging from having a patient directing traffic outside the office to being asked to see a woman who was stopped by other women in the playground from throwing her child off the slide. One respondent described a case in detail, writing, "The only case I considered an emergency turned out to be Munchausen's syndrome or malingering. . . . I see a wide variety of patients, many referred from psychiatric hospitals or with a history of psychosis. I have never felt such an emergency as in this feigned illness. . . . I was so concerned that I actually *took a cab* with her to the Bellevue ER (I have never done this before or after with any patient)."

Stress for the therapist proved to be a major component of the reports. Examples included a patient who had a psychotic episode in the doctor's office, a patient who had an epilaptic seizure while on the couch, and an intoxicated woman who accused the doctor of having an affair with her. Other serious concerns were illustrated by a mother who threatened to throw her child out of the window and a man who said he wished to kill his boss.

Another colleague requested that a former patient be hospitalized during a manic episode because she stood outside his office handing Mickey Mouse balloons to his current patients, telling them he was a Mickey Mouse psychiatrist.

Occasionally, a therapist had been threatened during a session by a physically strong adolescent or young adult. Only one reported being struck by a thrown object.

Suicide, Homicide, and Criminal Behavior

Evaluating the threat of suicide may be extremely difficult. The therapist must be alert to changes in a patient's behavior that indicate increasing distress. Schneidman (1985) suggests that the most common stimulus to suicide is unendurable psychological pain, and the common stressor is frustrated psychological needs. He argues that the common purpose of suicide is to seek a solution, and end the pain through cessation of consciousness. Emotionally, people who attempt suicide feel helpless and hopeless and perceive their options as constricted. Klerman (1986) has edited a book focusing upon suicide and depression among adolescents and young adults that describes current thinking about risk factors and interventions. Robins (1985) notes that alcoholism and the depressed phase of affective disorder are the two psychiatric diagnoses predominantly associated with completed suicide (about 70 percent of suicides that are studied). Schizophrenics account for 5 percent and hysteria for 1 percent of successful suicides. While the numbers may be small, the risk in acting-out borderline patients must be considered, as must the threats of young people with character disorders who have strong feelings of rage and depression and whose suicidal gesture may lead to death if intervention is not timely.

Men are three times more likely than women to succeed in killing themselves, while women make suicidal attempts more frequently. This is a function of men's choice of more violent methods, such as guns and jumping from heights, in contrast to pills or cutting wrists, more often selected by women. The risk for both sexes increases with age. Younger women have a higher incidence of making attempts than older women, but a lower success rate.

Many therapists are reluctant to discuss the possibility of suicide openly with a patient, fearing that this could prove to be embarrassing or might encourage the act. It is almost always good practice to ask. Openness may help the expression of tabooed feelings, and enable the therapist to offer alternatives that the patient had been unable to consider. Such discussions may also help in assessing the seriousness of the patient's intent. Though there are no hard and fast rules defining seriousness, some guidelines exist. Depression, especially in the recovery stages of major mood disorder, when the patient is regaining energy, can be a critical time. Alcoholics who feel despair are also in a high-risk group, as are some people who feel unbearably lonely, or have serious physical illness, financial problems, command hallucinations, or a past history of suicide attempts. For a fuller discussion of assessment and intervention, see Robbins and Stern (1976) and Rothman (1976).

Homicide And Other Serious Crimes

Laws regarding the necessity of reporting crimes vary from state to state. Many crimes do not have to be reported, nor is it required, in New York City, to inform the police that you know the identity of a person for whom the police have a warrant. Therapists who treat people who are involved in criminal activity should be certain of their state's laws, lest they be considered violators. It may be difficult to find exact rulings about some situations. New York requires reporting anyone who is suspected of child abuse to the state's Division of Family and Children's Services. Yet it is unclear whether New York requires routine reporting of pedophilia or to whom it should be reported. When we have been puzzled about the appropriateness of specific actions, we have found it best to contact our malpractice attorney, as well as therapists experienced with forensic matters.

Therapists are in an extremely difficult position when they suspect that a patient intends to murder someone. The California Appellate Court ruling in *Tarasoff* v. *Regents of University of California* mandates that police and the potential victim be notified. Since this decision, Appelbaum (1984) has reviewed the literature and concluded that there has been a trend from negligence toward liability, which places psychotherapists at greater risk. He notes that courts are becoming stricter in their rulings and tend to hold psychotherapists responsible for any violence committed by their patients. Many therapists, as well as therapeutic facilities, therefore dislike having to treat potentially violent patients.

Responsibility for reporting homicides that occured in the past appears to remain within the bounds of confidentiality, but people who have recently committed a felony may need to be reported to the police or the therapist might be considered an accessory to the crime. Patients who wish to discuss these matters must be told that the rules of confidentiality do not apply, and that the therapist is legally obligated to report violent crimes to the police. It is essential that informed consent be given before the patient continues. This may lead the patient to become silent, to terminate the therapeutic relationship, or to threaten the therapist if any action is taken, but the law permits no easy alternative.

The following case illustrates the role of informed consent in a recently committed homicide.

> An alcoholic man sought consultation for impending delirium tremens. In the course of the workup, he stated he had a confession to make regarding a homicide. He was told that anything he said might have to be reported to the police, if the crime was a recent one. He said that he wished to continue, and described a recent murder he committed, giving exact details regarding the location of the body and its appearance. When he concluded, the police were notified and located the body. They came to the office and arrested the patient, who was hospitalized in a prison psychiatric service.

The following case illustrates the treatment of a young schizophrenic who threatened to murder his uncle.

> The patient, who was recently discharged from a state hospital, grew worse in spite of increasing doses of psychotropic medication. When he confided in the psychiatrist that he was finding it increasingly difficult to resist command hallucinations telling him to murder his mother's brother, the psychiatrist told the patient he would have to call his mother. He contacted the mother, rather than the uncle, because he felt she could have the patient hospitalized without alarming her brother. Had she been unwilling to have her son hospitalized, it would have been advisable to contact the uncle directly.

When therapists fail to listen attentively to the patient, they may unwittingly facilitate a homicidal act.

> A delusional young man stated that his father was a communist, which happened to be true. The patient felt it was his mission to kill his father. When he was transferred to a state facility, the facts were clearly written so that the hospital staff would recognize the seriousness of the situation, and long-term hospitalization was recommended. The state hospital staff did not correctly assess the strength of the patient's homicidal urge. Within days of discharge, he murdered his father.

There is limited latitude in dealing with potentially homicidal people. The expressions "drop dead," "I wish you were dead," or "I'm going to kill you" are familiar to all of us. When patients express these fantasies, it is necessary to judge how much is hyperbole and how much is potentially lethal. The therapist who endeavors to continue therapy must be reasonably sure that the patient is unlikely to enact the fantasies. Risks may be greater in psychotic patients who have command hallucinations or are severely paranoid. These must be distinguished from the many who have homicidal fantasies in response to feeling wronged. Depending upon the therapist's assessment, which should take into account the status of the therapeutic process, decisions must be made about continuing treatment, notifying others, or recommending hospitalization.

Clinical Assessment

Many of the factors to be considered in the evaluation of emergencies are discussed by Robbins and Stern (1974).

Appendix I contains a list from Bronx-Lebanon Hospital in New York City of factors the therapist should consider in assessing the probability that suicide and homicide will be carried out.

Organic Psychiatric Syndromes

Emergency disorders frequently have an organic basis. The therapist should be mindful that organic pathology may be a causative factor in any form of disturbed behavior, particularly when the psychosocial circumstances are not commensurate with the clinical picture.

Psychiatrists are often asked to help with cases in which a previously stable person has become acutely psychotic. Frequently the family is puzzled about the behavioral changes and tries to explain or deny them. The patient may be dimly aware that something is amiss and may fluctuate between seemingly rational behavior and bizarre or unusual acts. Patients with acute symptoms may come to the psychiatrist's office or be taken to an emergency room where the private practitioner is called upon as a consultant. The precipitant is likely to be an organic process.

Endocrine Diseases

Many endocrine illnesses are associated with organic brain syndromes or exacerbation of underlying psychosis. Among those seen most frequently in our practice are hypoglycemia, usually secondary to an insulin overdose, or gastric resection, and thyroid disorders. Pituitary and adrenal disorders have been less common.

In an office setting, the therapist may be faced by a patient who appears extremely anxious. The patient described below was referred for treatment of his anxiety and hysterical visual changes by an ophthalmologist who could not account for periods of diplopia and blurred vision.

> The patient was a 38-year-old married man who was deeply distressed because of "blackouts" that occurred without relationships to stress. He described falling off a ladder and finding himself on the floor, and said that he was fearful of continuing his job as a bus driver. There was no history of soiling or tongue biting, which would have indicated seizures. Past medical history revealed a subtotal gastrectomy six months earlier

for bleeding ulcer. His surgeon said he healed well and had no complications. His internist also said there were no medical problems and referred him to the ophthalmologist. Blood drawn at the termination of the psychiatric interview showed marked hypoglycemia. Once this was treated, his subsequent course was uneventful.

In a review of psychotic hyperthyroid patients admitted to Bellevue, the majority had been seen by internists who failed to recognize that hyperthyroidism was the "steam" behind the agitated psychosis. The diagnosis was suspected because of the noisy, unmanageable quality of the patients, coupled with symptoms of hyperthyroidism, such as rapid pulse and fine tremor. Ophthalmological changes were infrequent. Treatment of both psychosis and hyperthyroidism is required for good management.

Other Causes Of Organic Mental Disorders

Illnesses may be primary, such as meningitis, subarachnoid hemorrhage, or impending cerebrovascular accidents, or secondary to other conditions, such as pulmonary anoxia following heart attacks. If the patient with an acute brain syndrome is seen in the practitioner's office, referral to a hospital for detailed workup and probable admission is indicated.

Meningitis rarely presents as a behavioral disorder but at times, acute behavioral changes are the first sign that something is wrong. Frequently, a low-grade fever, explained by dehydration, is the only physical concomitant. Only later do the typical meningeal symptoms appear, when it may be too late to save the patient's life.

Subarachnoid hemorrhage may be insidious in onset — presenting as a behavioral disturbance associated with an organic brain syndrome, rather than as a major catastrophe. In these cases, the altered behavior of the patient may lead to a psychiatric consultation rather than the more appropriate neurological one.

Impending stroke may have prodromal behavioral symptoms of confusion, difficulty in calculation, visual changes or feelings of depersonalization, as well as transient blackouts.

Substance Abuse   Alcohol and other drug abuse are virtually epidemic in our society. Because of embarrassment, patients may conceal their addiction from their internist. The condition may be suspected by a psychotherapist because of behavioral changes such as slurring of speech, bruises on the face from falling, or memory deficits. It is helpful if the therapist is familiar with the patient's nondrug state and can identify the personality changes that may be brought about by intoxication. With alcohol, the breath may be a telltale sign. Some therapists are too uncertain of their observations to be confident of their conclusion. A question may be sufficient to confirm the diagnosis. For example, a secretary drank before coming to work; when questioned, she said that her mouth wash was flavored with whiskey.

For patients recently hospitalized or who have just entered psychotherapy, the precipitant of a delirious reaction may be withdrawal from a drug. People who take Xanax, Valium, or other benzodiazepines or barbiturates may be reluctant to tell their therapist or admitting physician, or may be too sick medically to be concerned about this at the time of admission. As withdrawal begins, a medical emergency can develop.

Occult Medical Illness   A certain number of people will be seen in practice who develop severe depression without having prior behavioral indicators or appropriate recent life experience. While most of these people will have a functional basis for their illness, the role of an occult physical illness, such as a neoplasm, should be considered in the differential diagnosis. Whenever possible, people should be encouraged to have a thorough physical examination if they have not had one within the past year.

Laboratory Tests   Many adults are careless about having routine physical examinations. Psychiatrists rarely perform routine examinations, but we have found that blood tests (CBC and SMA 6 and 12) performed annually may have useful psychiatric spinoffs. Recently, a patient with increasing signs of depression that did not respond well to treatment was found to be severely anemic.

Medication Interactions   The possibility of drug interactions always exists. We make it a general rule to ask patients the names of every medication they take when treatment is initiated and to tell us whenever a new medication is prescribed. From time to time, it then becomes possible to link the appearance of symptoms with medicines, such as depression with contraceptive pills or impotence with hypertensive medication. Parenthetically, it should be noted that many internists prescribe psychotropic medications, even when they know the patient is in psychotherapy. Patients are also told to tell any physician whom they consult what their psychotropic medications are — and never to take a psychotropic medication prescribed by an internist without prior discussion with a knowledgeable psychiatrist.

Functional Psychosis

The tratment of an acute psychosis is an emergency, which may require medication, immediate hospitalization, or, in rare instances, supervision at home while waiting for the medication to take effect. In treating people who have had an acute psychosis in the past, it is critical for the therapist to be alert for the early signs of recurrence and, if possible, to train the patient to monitor his or her symptoms so that quick intervention is possible. Many patients can be drug-free, or on low doses, and increase medication when symptoms appear. Among the common indicators are the onset of paranoid ideation, early signs of hypomania (feeling too good, becoming more energetic), and changes in sleep pattern or other aspects of physiological functioning. One of our patients knows that she is becoming depressed as soon as she finds it impossible to make a decision about which meat to purchase when she goes shopping.

In dealing with acutely psychotic patients, good clinical judgment is required to determine whether hospitalization is indicated or if the patient can be treated at home. In addition to a supportive network, the doctor–patient relationship is a determining factor. When a positive therapeutic alliance exists, it may be possible to keep the patient at home, rather than insist upon hospitalization, provided that suicide or homicide is not a concern. When an acutely psychotic patient is seen in consultation, hospitalization is often the only alternative.

SPECIAL PROBLEMS
RELATED TO EMERGENCIES

The Previously Unknown Patient

It is obviously easier to exercise good judgment and obtain cooperation when the patient knows and trusts the therapist.

When an unfamiliar person who expresses suicidal preoccupation is seen in consultation, it is most prudent to insist upon hospitalization, especially if there is no supporting network. The therapist is more likely to prevail if he or she practices in a clinic or hospital setting, where other staff members may be called upon, than in a private office, where physical confrontation could become a possibility if the patient refuses to accept the therapist's recommendation or threatens to walk out. The therapist must be a judge at all times of his or her control of the situation and of the likelihood that the patient can be trusted to follow recommendations.

It is quite difficult for a therapist to be certain what to do when a person is seen in consultation, does not provide the names of any significant others, is judged to require hospitalization, and refuses to accept the recommendation. If the therapist insists upon calling the police, an altercation may result in a lawsuit. The patient may sue if he or she is not admitted to a hospital or feels that hospitalization was forced. It the therapist does not act immediately, but contacts the police later, there can also be multiple unpleasant outcomes, especially if the person feels that the appearance of the police officers led to embarrassment.

In the following tragic case, the patient was seen late at night, in an isolated private office, as a favor to a colleague.

> A tall, physically strong student came to the office alone. He was agitated, paranoid, but denied hallucinations, although he acknowledged that he was homesick and found it difficult to make friends with anyone in his dorm. He expressed suicidal ideation, but said that he had no intention of trying. The judgment was made that he was a poor risk, but he refused hospitalization and indicated that he would leave the office and not return home if the police were called. Because it would have been humiliating to have the police called to his dormitory, the therapist decided to try to create a therapeutic alliance by asking him to call if he felt more agitated as the night progressed. The student was given a sedative to help him sleep and an appointment to be seen first thing in the morning. He committed suicide several hours after the consultation.

THE THERAPIST'S FEELINGS:
REALISTIC AND COUNTERTRANSFERENTIAL

Emergencies constitute a severe stress for therapists, as well as for patients and families, since they inevitably evoke feelings of distress in the therapist, both reality based and countertransferential. Either may interfere with judgment and the ability to act. When it is questionable if the therapist can distinguish between reality-based feelings and those stemming from countertransference, we recommend consultation with colleagues before taking action. During treatment, all therapists must monitor their reactions, paying particular attention to anxiety about the consequences of an error in diagnosis; the implications of failing to act or overreacting; and the risk of danger to the patient, others, the therapist, or the therapist's family. Loss of face, feelings of abandonment or powerlessness, and the legal consequences of therapeutic action or failure to act all must be considered, as well as conscious and unconscious emotions such as disgust, fear, envy, or admiration.

Therapists have been warned through the years to consider several behaviors as indications of countertransference — including free-floating anxiety, drowsiness, competitiveness, wandering attention, depression, and the desire to share experiences that ordinarily would not be discussed with the patient.

We are aware of an instance in which a therapist, who had esthetic interests similar to those of his patient, a professional artist, became increasingly competitive with her, to the detriment of therapy. He converted sessions into discussions in which he attempted to demonstrate that he was more knowledgeable than she and became irritable when he failed. She became increasingly anxious. He was unable to recognize that a problem existed until she attempted suicide as a means of escaping from the therapeutic quagmire.

Threats

Patients may threaten the therapist in the course of treatment or return some time afterward in a paranoid state to air their grievances. In dealing with an angry patient, it is better to try to remain clam and to rely on logic and trust the patient's positive feelings and social controls than to express fear. People who continue in treatment will usually have some positive feelings, even if they have a negative transference. The therapist must try to establish verbal contact and make some effort to dissuade the patient. There are no rules about the correct thing to say. Often it is a case of intuitive judgment, based on the therapist–patient relationship. Sometimes a variation of a behavioral technique described by Fensterheim and Baer (1975), asking directly if the patient is trying to terrorize, can be a useful introduction to an exploration of feelings and behavior. Once the patient can begin to talk, his or her feelings may subside, permitting therapy to progress. If the therapist becomes so frightened that it is impossible to continue treatment, the reasons for termination should be discussed, and an effort made to find a new therapist.

Angry former patients who enter the office in order to injure or kill the therapist obviously pose a more serious problem since they have been nursing a grudge for some time. No guidelines exist for dealing with this situation either, other than remaining calm and trying to open a dialogue. The angry former patient may feel relieved to be able to express his or her angry feelings, rather than feel compelled to act them out. When the patient begins to talk, continue talking until the patient appears to be more settled. At this point, it may be possible to negotiate a peaceful resolution. Few therapists will have panic buttons in their office, which they can push to obtain help.

One instance in which the director of a mental hygiene clinic showed great courage was based upon her knowledge of the patient and belief that he could control himself.

The patient was a schizophrenic man known to behave impulsively. The director of the clinic, who was familiar with the case, and a colleague were discussing a research project when a therapist was heard to scream and run down the hall. Practically at the same time, a shot was heard. The two psychiatrists ran to the office where the patient was still sitting and asked him for the gun. He gave it to them and permitted himself to be hospitalized. His therapist had panicked when he saw the weapon and had run from the room.

Threats To Family Members

Threats to family members are more likely when the therapist practices at home or in the same apartment building where the family resides. The admonition not to socialize with patients can have special reference for paranoid, threatening patients. Some therapists do not hang family photographs in their office so as to reduce the possibility of identification.

When a threat is made, the therapist should endeavor to judge its seriousness. One of our paranoid schizophrenic patients, who generally was very friendly, spoke of fantasies of harming the therapist's wife, whom he had met by chance on several occasions. The judgment was made that he was having transferential problems that would respond to interpretation and would not act out after he discussed his feelings toward the therapist. Fortunately, this was correct.

Homicidal Attempts Against The Therapist Or Family

Such attempts are rare, but we all know of cases from reading the tabloids. In one instance, a disgruntled patient called her therapist, who refused to talk with her. She then ambushed his wife and murdered her. Although we do not know the details, this case illustrates the general principle that it is preferable to be available to talk with such a patient, rather than to try to avoid the matter. In this view, some of her anger might have been understood and defused, rather than intensified by rejection.

Telephone Calls

Threatening Calls   Telephone calls from violent or angry patients usually are intended to frighten or annoy the therapist. Calls may be anonymous, which can be of great concern when the therapist works in a hospital or clinic setting, and may not have any idea who is calling. If the therapist happens to answer the phone, it is best to listen and not become involved in responding to accusations or to show fear about the threat. If the person can be identified, he or she should be addressed by name and told that the police will be notified. If the threats persist, it is necessary to work with the police and develop a strategy of self-protection. A court order of protection may be necessary. When told that one will be sought, threateners sometimes desist. A colleague reported that a patient who had been threatening him for six months apologized after a court order was invoked, saying he did not realize how uncomfortable he made the therapist.

When confronted by a threatening patient, the therapist should inform another person, giving full details so that the patient can be located if he or she actually attempts physical harm. In addition, a file should be maintained for all relevant information. A person close to the therapist should be aware of the file's existence.

Annoying Calls   The answering machine has proved to be a boon for people dedicated to annoying others. They usually know when the therapist is unavailable and time calls for those periods. The tapes should be saved since evidence may be needed if the harassment escalates.

The telephone company should be notified about annoyance calls. In New York City, little will be done initially other than to advise you about the correct statements to make and ways in which the telephone can be manipulated to make it sound as if an official is listening. The company will not take any action unless ordered by a court. Local telephone calls are not traced, but long-distance calls are recorded on telephone bills. The telephone company does not release bills to the victim of the annoyance call unless charges are pressed, but will verify that a long-distance call was made from a specific number. When this is done, the company can be requested to retain a copy of the bill for several years—just in case charges will be filed. Most often, annoying calls terminate after a period of high intensity.

Precautions To Take In The Office

One of the risks the private practitioner faces is the isolation of treating people in an office setting, in which only the therapist and patient may be present. Some recommendations that increase the therapist's security are:

- Do not display any heavy objects that can readily be lifted and thrown.
- Locate your chair and the patient's chair or couch in such a way that your egress from the office cannot easily be blocked.
- Install a second telephone outside the office so that an emergency call to the police or a relative could be placed.
- Place a smoke detector in the waiting room so that you can be alerted to a fire.
- When possible, have two doors to your office. (This makes it possible for patients to enter and leave without having contact with each other.)
- Have papers for emergency hospitalization available.
- Anticipate methods that the patient could choose to attempt suicide and try to prevent them; that is, do not leave poison in a kitchen or medication in a bathroom or have windows from which a patient could jump.

RESOURCES HELPFUL IN EMERGENCIES

Community

Therapists should be aware of their community's resources. Those who practice in a hospital or clinic setting have learned how to deal with the police, prepare papers for hospitalization, and feel comfortable in consulting with relatives or other key people in the patient's life. Those who work only in private practice may need to refresh their knowledge about the many agencies that are available to provide assistance in moments of emergency. These include the police and fire departments, voluntary ambulance service, child welfare and social welfare agencies, county and state professional societies, and specific self-help groups such as Alcoholics Anonymous, Narcotics Anonymous, Gamblers Anonymous, and phobia groups. There may be coalitions of self-help agencies such as New York City's Self-Help Clearing House, Inc. Each therapist should consider developing a network of other therapists whose judgment can be trusted, and discuss cases on a regular basis or in times of stress. A resource that few therapists may think of, but that can be helpful in a crisis, is the malpractice attorney, who can be reached through the insurance carrier.

Police

The police officer who encounters mentally ill people in the course of his or her work often intervenes on the street or responds to calls to evaluate, and possibly remove, people from their dwellings. About 20 percent of the people admitted to Bellevue are brought by the police.

The training level and human relations skills of officers vary widely. A study of those who took people to Bellevue Hospital (Stern & Robbins, no date) showed that the officers were sincere in their desire to help, were not always well informed about departmental regulations regarding their role, and desired more training because of the sensitive and potentially dangerous nature of their work. Police officers, in our experience, have almost always been cooperative with professionals, but are fearful of lawsuits or of being accused of racial insensitivity. They are more likely to remove an acutely disturbed person from a residence if given papers for emergency hospitalization than if asked by family or neighbors to go to the residence and evaluate the disturbed person themselves. If the patient is verbal, educated, and able to present a cogent case, the officer is unlikely to insist on forcible removal to a hospital.

The therapist who desires to have a person hospitalized should be certain of the laws governing hospitalization and, if possible, have the necessary papers ready before the police arrive. In the rare instance in which we have had to request police assistance in our office, response has been immediate.

The following cases illustrate two ways in which the police have been very helpful.

> A young man with diagnoses of bipolar illness and hysterical psychosis had a long history of fantasizing that he would murder strangers on the street. He spoke of carrying a gun. He left the city for several months and had no contact with any therapist. He called at 10 o'clock one night to reestablish contact, stating he was in Grand Central Station with a gun and finally was ready to murder people as they walked in the lobby. There was no way to ascertain if this was fantasy or reality. He was thanked for calling, given an appointment to come to the office the next day, and asked to remain in the station until the psychiatrist arrived to talk with him. After the telephone conversation was terminated, the police

were called and asked to help deal with the patient. The psychiatrist went to the station to locate the patient and establish contact. When this was done, the police joined them. The patient did not have a weapon, but was sufficiently disturbed that hospitalization was indicated.

The second illustration is that of a young woman with a history of self-immolation.

She had come to the office in an agitated state shortly before her session was to begin. She lingered in the bathroom instead of coming to the office to begin her session. Suspecting that something was amiss, the psychiatrist went to investigate and insisted that she open the door. When he entered, he saw she had a can of kerosene and threatened to ignite herself. They fought, and she was subdued. The police were called, and took her to the hospital.

Family And Networks

In current psychotherapeutic practice, there is great variability in the type and amount of contact that therapists seek with patients' relatives. Some are extreme in their avoidance of families; the despair of parents of a suicidal child who were refused communication with the therapist is movingly described by Wechsler (1972). Some make it a practice to have communication, often on a regular basis, with key relatives. Family-oriented therapists believe they can help most effectively by involving significant others in the treatment program. It is good practice to have telephone numbers of people to contact, if necessary. These can be obtained at the time of the initial interview, by having the patient complete a brief questionnaire.

While many patients respond positively to a family's nurturance and willingness to become involved, some become paranoid and angry, often threatening the relative physically or stating they will break off future contact with the therapist. In these circumstances, it is foolish for the therapist to persist. The therapist can accept the refusal without approving of it, and bring it up again later, when the patient may be more receptive.

SUMMARY

Crisis, as a turning point, is common in psychotherapy. Emergency, as danger requiring immediate action, fortunately is rare. Therapists can help patients deal with crisis by applying their clinical, psychodynamic knowledge in a flexible way to provide additional support.

When an emergency does arise, the therapist should be able to assess rapidly and accurately what clinical and administrative matters require attention, and have the courage to act appropriately. He or she should be familiar with community resources, and know how to arrange for hospitalization.

A significant proportion of emergencies have an organic basis, and the therapist should be skilled in recognizing the behavioral manifestations of physical disorder. Medical consultation is often the essential core of successful management.

A good relationship with the family can be of inestimable value in helping the therapist cope with emergencies, both in carrying out treatment decisions and in diminishing the strain on patient, family, and therapist.

Appendix I

Bronx-Lebanon Hospital Center
New York, N.Y.

A. *Dangerousness*

1. *Suicide risk assessment*

2a. *Current thoughts*

- Intense wish to kill oneself with plan
- Wish to kill oneself but no plan
- Command hallucination with suicidal intent
- Ambivalent wish to end life
- Passive suicidal ideas or feelings
- No suicidal wishes or ideas

2b. *Recent behavior*
(within few weeks)

- Serious suicide attempt, e.g., gunshot, jumping, hanging
- Development of specific suicide plan
- Suicide attempt with little chance of discovery
- Minor attempt with good chance of discovery
- Behavior indicating little interest in or hope or plan for future
- No evidence of suicidal behavior

2c. *Past history*

- History of one or more suicide attempts
- Anniversary of important significant events
- Family history of death by suicidal behavior

2d. *Risk factors*

- Patient is single, living alone
- Young adult or geriatric patient
- Major psychiatric disorder
- Serious medical illness or disability
- Substance abuse

2. *Homicidal potential*

1a. *Current thoughts*

- Intense wish to kill someone
- Command hallucination
- Ambivalent wish to kill someone
- Nonspecific feeling of anger, rage
- No thoughts of homicide

1b. *Recent behavior*

(within few weeks)
- Trying to strangle, stab, shoot
- Physical abuse causing harm
- Slapping, pushing, punching
- Unpredictable, impulsive behavior causing destruction of objects
- No behavioral disturbance

1c. *Past history*

- Commission of violent acts in past in different unrelated situations
- Arrest or assault in the same repetitive situation
- Carrying of weapons (gun, knife, etc.)
- Criminal record, chronic problem with authority
- No past history of violent, antisocial, or disruptive behavior

1d. *Other risk factors*

- Young male
- Little education, lower socioeconomic background
- Psychotic patient with delusions
- Substance abuse
- Character disorder (antisocial, borderline)
- Delirium

B. *Support system*

- Has no home, family, friends, or institutional involvement
- Has home but has nobody who can observe the patient
- Has family but not motivated and interested in patient
- Has willing fmaily members but patient has tenuous connection with them
- Has strong, willing, competent support system

C. *Ability to cooperate with treatment*

- Patient refuses to cooperate
- Patient is unable to cooperate

- Patient demonstrates limited participation
- Patient actively seeks treatment and is able to make plan

D. *Substance abuse*

- Drug intoxication or withdrawal
- Long-term continued substance abuse
- Intermittent substance abuse
- Recreational drug use
- No history of drug use

Appendix II

Bellevue Hospital Center, Department of Psychiatry
Unit Admitting Note   Rev. 9 25 87
Mental Status Examination

Appearance:

aloof ____	distractible ____	lethargic ____	psychomotor
anxious ____	elated ____	neat ____	retardation ____
dejected ____	hyperactive ____	peculiar dress ____	restless ____
depressed ____	hyperalert ____	postural	slovenly ____
		problems ____	tense ____
Other _____			vigilant ____

Attitude:

cold ____	deprecatory of	evasive ____	self-
condescending ____	others ____	frank ____	deprecatory ____
cooperative ____	disdainful ____	hostile ____	sensitive ____
demanding ____	disinterested ____	overidealizing	superior ____
	egocentric ____	others ____	suspicious ____
			vain ____
Other _____			

Behavior:

aggressive ____	cheerful ____	guarded ____	manipulative ____
angry ____	critical ____	helpless ____	negativistic ____
argumentative ____	dependent ____	hostile ____	passive ____
arrogant ____	dramatic ____	indecisive ____	seeking
assertive ____	exploitative ____	ingratiating ____	reassurance ____
assaultive ____	exhibitionistic ____	irritable ____	subdued ____
belligerent ____	friendly ____	irascible ____	obsequious ____
bizarre ____	grossly	limited	secretive ____
	disorganized ____	empathy ____	verbally abusive ____

Other _____

Affect:

aloof ____	blunted ____	inappropriate ____	temper ____
apathetic ____	cold ____	irritable ____	outbursts ____
appropriate ____	flat ____	labile ____	

Other _____

Mood:

Anxious ____	elevated ____	depressed ____	within normal limits ____

Other _____

Supplemental information regarding mood:

Is *anxious mood* associated with:

compulsions ____   obsessions ____   panic attacks ____   phobias ____

Is *depressed mood* associated with:

agitation ____	decreased enjoyment ____	guilt ____
early-morning awakening ____	feeling worse in the morning ____	loss of interest or enjoyment in sex ____
decreased effectiveness at: school__ home__ work__	feeling inadequate ____	pessimism ____
	feeling slowed down ____	tearfulness ____

Is *elevated mood* associated with:

decreased need for sleep ____   hypersexuality ____ distractibility ____   poor judgment ____

excessive involvement with pleasure ____

increased: creativity____ energy____ feelings of omnipotence____ optimism____
physical activity____ talkativeness____ inappropriate joking____ laughing____
or punning____

Speech and thought progression:

Rate: average ____   decreased ____   increased ____   mute ____   pressure ____

Other _____

Progression:

blocking ____	concentration	indecisive ____	perseverative ____
circumstantial ____	loss ____	irrelevant ____	poverty of
clang ____	digressive ____	loosening of	content ____
concrete ____	echolalic ____	associations ____	stereotypy ____
condensed ____	flight of ideas ____	neologistic ____	tangenital ____
	incoherent ____	overelaborate ____	vague ____
			verbigeration ____
Other _____			word salad ____
None of the above ____			

Thought content:

autistic: yes ____   no ____

Delusions or feelings of:

being controlled____	hypersensitivty ____	jealousy ____	religious nature ____
blamelessness ____	inability to express	knowledge ____	self reproach ____
body image	warmth ____	limited pleasure in	special identity ____
disorder ____	ideas of	life ____	somatic ____
disorganization____	reference ____	losing control ____	stubbornness ____
dying ____	inadequacy ____	magical thinking____	suspiciousness ____
entitlement ____	indifference ____	nihilism ____	thought:
forgetfulness ____	indecisiveness ____	objectivity ____	broadcasting ____
going crazy ____	ineffectiveness ____	paranoia ____	insertion ____
grandiosity ____	inflated worth ____	persecution ____	withdrawal ____
guilt ____	insistence upon	poverty ____	unreality ____
helplessness ____	having own way ____	power ____	worthlessness ____

Other _____
None of the Above ____

Hallucinations:

Auditory ____   Olfactory ____   Tactile ____   Taste ____   Visual ____

Depersonalization: Yes ____   No ____

Fears or phobias: Yes ____   No ____
If Yes, are they: social ____   spatial ____   animal ____   Other _____

Illusions: Yes ____   No ____   Intellectualization: Yes ____   No ____

Obsessions, compulsions, and recurrent thoughts   Yes ____   No ____
ego dystonic ____   ego syntonic ____   both ____

Overdetermined ideas, preoccupations, and trends: Yes ____   No ____

Level of consciousness: clear ____   clouded ____   comatose ____
    Memory impairment: Yes ____   No ____   If Yes is there:
        impairment of: immediate recall ____   recent recall ____   past recall ____
        confabulation ____
    Orientation: person ____   place ____   time ____
    Calculations: Normal ____   Impaired ____
        aphasia ____   agnosia ____   difficulty in naming parts of the body ____
    Level of Information: average ____   average ____   average ____
    Intelligence: superior ____   bright ____   average ____   dull normal ____
                    borderline ____   retarded ____

Judgment and insight:
judgment: adequate ____   impaired ____insight: adequate ____   impaired ____

Disturbance of organs of special sense:
Auditory   Touch   Visual
    deafness ____   anesthesia ____   blindness ____
    hearing loss ____   numbness ____   blurred vision ____
                                                    double vision

Other _____
None of the above ____

Amnestic disturbances: Yes ____   No ____

Disturbances of motor impairment:
apraxia ____   fatigability ____   muscle aches ____   shakiness ____
aphoria ____   hyperactivity ____   negativism ____   stupor ____

catatonia ____   jitteriness ____   paralysis ____   trembling ____
echopraxia ____   loss of control of: posturing ____   tremors ____
fainting ____   sphincters ____   retardation ____
                   voluntary
                   muscles ____

Other _____
None of the above ____

Somatic changes or physical complaints:

chest pain or   hot and cold flashes ____   sexual drive decreased ____
discomfort ____   hypersomnia ____   sweating ____
choking or smothering insomnia ____   trembling or shaking ____
sensations ____   menstrual difficulties ____   vertigo or unsteady
dyspnea ____   pain ____   feelings ____
dizziness, fatigue ____ palpitations ____   vomiting ____
faintness ____   paresthesias ____   weight gain ____
factitious complaints ____   weight loss ____

Other _____
None of the above ____

Autonomic hyperactivity:

Circulatory system:
   flushing ____   palpitations ____   pallor ____   pulse rate increase ____

Gastrointestinal system:
   diarrhea ____   discomfort ____   dry mouth ____   nausea ____   vomiting ____

Respiratory system:
   hyperventilation ____   increased rate ____

Miscellaneous:
   cold clammy hands ____   dizziness ____   paresthesias ____   sweating ____

Other _____
None of the above ____

Behavioral difficulties:

arrests ____   initiation of fights ____running away from   thefts ____
breaking rules ____   persistent lying ____   home ____   vandalism ____
delinquency ____   repeated drunkenness   sexual promiscuity ____
                       or substance abuse ____

Other _____
None of the above ____

REFERENCES

Appelbaum, P. (1984). The expansion of liability for patients' violent acts. *Hospital and Community Psychiatry, 35,* 13–14.

Bibring, E. (1954). Psychoanalysis and the dynamic psychotherapies. *Journal of the American Psychoanalytic Association, 2,* 745–770.

Birk, L., & Birk, A. (1984). Managing emergencies in the practice of psychotherapy. In *Emergency psychiatry, concepts, methods, and practices.* E. Bassuk & A. Birk (Eds.). New York: Plenum Press.

Caplan, G. (1964). *Principles of preventive psychiatry.* New York: Basic Books.

Chrzanowski, G. (1977). The occurrence of emergencies and crisis in psychoanalytic therapy. *Contemporary Psychoanalysis, 13,* 85–93.

Erikson, E. (1959). Identity and the life cycle. *Psychol Issues Monographs 1.*

Fensterheim, H., & Baer, J. (1975). *Don't say yes when you want to say no.* New York: Dell Publishing Company.

Klerman, G. (1986). *Suicide and depression among adolescents and young adults.* Washington, DC: American Psychiatric Press.

Kliman, A.H. (1978). *Crisis. Psychological first aid for recovery and growth.* New York: Holt, Rinehart and Winston.

Normand, W., & Bluestone, H. (1986). The use of pharmacotherapy in psychoanalytic treatment. *Contemporary Psychoanalysis, 22,* 218–234.

Perry, S., Cooper, A., & Michels, R. (1987). The psychodynamic formulation: Its purpose, structure, and clinical application. *American Journal of Psychiatry, 144,* 543–550.

Robbins, E. (1985). Suicide. In *Comprehensive Textbook of Psychiatry, Ed.* IV. H. Kaplan & B. Sadock (Eds.). Baltimore: Williams and Wilkins.

Robbins, E., & Stern, M. (1976). Assessment of psychiatric emergencies. In *Psychaitric emergencies.* R. Glick, A. Meyerson, E. Robbins & J. Talbott (Eds.) New York: Grune & Stratton.

Rothman, M. (1976). Evaluation and management of alcohol-related psychiatric emergencies. In *Psychiatric emergencies.* R. Glick, A. Meyerson, E. Robbins, J. Talbott (eds.). New York: Grune & Stratton.

Shneidman, E. (1985). *The definition of suicide.* New York: Wiley.

Stern, M., & Robbins, E. Unpublished data.

Wechsler, J., & Wechsler, N. (1972). *In a darkness.* New York: Norton.

Wolpe, J. (1978). *The practice of behavior therapy* (2nd ed.). New York: Pergamon Press.

Zeig, J. (1980). *Teaching seminars with Milton H. Erickson, M.D.* New York: Brunner/Mazel.

69

THE IMPACT OF GEOGRAPHY ON TECHNIQUE AND APPROACH— URBAN VS. RURAL, AS WELL AS REGIONAL DIFFERENCES

Minna Marder Genn, Ed.M.

I practice in two separate geographic areas. Approximately one-half of my practice is across the street from Lincoln Center in New York City in the upwardly mobile Upper West Side. The other half of my practice is in a middle to upper–middle class suburb in northern New Jersey. Some of the towns around me in New Jersey are distinctly middle class; certainly there is a sprinkling of blue-collar families. There are some similarities and some differences in patient-loads in the two areas.

The age range of the adults is similar in both areas. I see a few teen-agers in each office and most of the other patients range in age between 20 and 40. Seventy-three percent of my New York patients and 67 percent of my New Jersey patients are in that age group. In other words, there are a few more patients in my New Jersey practice who are past 40 than in my New York group. In both areas the percentage of females far outnumbers the percentage of males. In New York, the percentage of females is 87 percent; in New Jersey, it is 79 percent. The similarities end with these two features.

To begin with, there are differences in the marital status and in the level of education in the two groups. These factors, in turn, result in a profound difference in the type of therapy called for and in the length of treatment. Seventy-four percent of the New York patients are single; in New Jersey, the percentage is 45. There is a difference in educational level, but not as drastic as the difference in marital status. In New York, 52 percent had four years of college or more; in New Jersey, the percentage is 38. Although the distance between my two offices is no more than 20 miles, there is significantly more sophistication and more worldliness in the New York patient group than in the New Jersey patient group. Part of this difference may be due to economics, but not necessarily. Coming into New York City to have dinner, go to the theater, and park the car can add up to an expensive evening. However, the cost of movies in New Jersey does not differ appreciably from the cost of movies in New York. Yet there is much more movie-going, theater-going and museum trips in new York than in New Jersey. The pleasures in New Jersey are often tied in with family activities. Vacations tend to be spent near home.

New Jersey patients will frequently spend their vacations at the New Jersey shore. In contrast, New York patients are likely to travel abroad.

I have a general impression that some of the New Jersey patients tend to view psychotherapy as a "quick fix" which will deal with the problem of the moment, whereas more of the New York patients are likely to see the problem as coming from their emotional history. The New York patients seem to have some insight; they usually understand that they have to explore what their hidden motives might be. The therapy for them is psychoanalytic in style. They understand that therapy leads to more than just becoming aware of their feelings and expressing them. There is less complaining about the other people in their lives. They appreciate the fact that they have to look inside themselves. They are asked to try to remember their dreams. It is suggested to them that they keep a notepad at their bedside table and write down one or two key words of the dream so that they will not forget the dream.

In contrast, many New Jersey patients think that a cure should be obtainable through the therapist telling them what is wrong and then telling them what to do about the problem. Often the period of therapy is shorter for the New Jersey patients than the New York patients. A term of three to six months is not unusual for New Jersey patients. Most New York patients will stay in therapy for at least two years and often more. Among the clients from New Jersey, there is less understanding of the unconscious reasons which serve as a serious block to following so-called "rational advice."

I think of two very recent examples of the "quick fix school" of thinking. One is a married woman who is 46 years old and has agoraphobia. The other is a 40-year-old married woman who has let herself be tyrannized by a domineering husband. Each of these women left treatment gratefully after a short number of weekly sessions, the former after 16 sessions and the latter after 14 sessions.

The 46-year-old patient was brought up in a family with an alcoholic father and a mother who sought comfort and security in a close relationship with my patient. Needless to say, a symbiotic union was formed. The patient's first husband was an alcoholic, and when he had an affair with her sister, she broke up the marriage. Up to this point, she had been very much tied to her mother. For example, she could not even go out and buy curtains without her mother beside her. When she left her husband, she became somewhat autonomous: she worked, she earned some money, and she raised two children. One of them, the girl, is married. The boy, age 21, is addicted to crack. My patient married again and this time she married a man who took control of her and would not let her do anything. He did the marketing because he did not like the way she did it. He did all the family laundry as well. In fact, she is quite competent to perform these household chores. She re-formed a symbiotic union, this time with her husband. It was then that she developed the agoraphobia. She could not drive any distance. She became lightheaded. She felt as if she would faint. Even taking the dog for a walk upset her. She had trouble going to work at a nearby mental health center. Then her husband developed a brain tumor, which ultimately proved to be benign. While he was ill, while the surgery took place and while he recovered, she resumed her former competence. When he was totally well, she became agoraphobic again. In other words, she resumed the symbiotic position and became agoraphobic when there was someone to lean on. With the help she was given in understanding this position and in playing out a more assertive role with her husband, she shortly became symptom-free. Some work was also done on her fear of her phobia. To explore the unlikely possibility that the fainting was organic in origin, she was sent to a physician for a check-up. There proved to be no sign of neurological impairment. Needless to say, her symptoms may recur and she will then return to therapy. However, as of this writing, her therapy has ended.

The other patient came in because of troubles with her father and with her husband. She experienced each of these men as very domineering; this seemed to be especially true of her father, a highly critical, opinionated person. Her husband's style was less severe than her father's, but he was still prone to function as if his word were the only word that counted. My patient, in turn, who did have some strengths, would vary between yielding and fighting. Sometimes there would be some passive aggressive acting out. My work with her was geared, as with the other patient, to help her to be more assertive when appropriate and to understand that when she acted out in a passive aggressive way, she was re-enacting her life with her father.

For the sake of contrast, two New York patients will be described. The first of these is 32 years old. She first came to see me at the end of 1982, and she remained in therapy for about 14 months. Six months later in the summer of 1984, she returned to therapy. What brought her into therapy originally was the break-up of a relationship with a man with whom she had been living. She had wanted the security of the relationship, but she was not satisfied with him and had constantly criticized him. The patient felt critical of her boyfriend chiefly because he was not as successful, both personally and professionally, as she would have liked. A college graduate, she works in a creative aspect of the advertising business where she is quite successful. With that break-up she experienced a loss of a sense of her worth. Successful at work as she was, she felt inferior because she came from a poor background and had not had certain privileges and advantages that she valued and even overvalued. Her own home environment had been in sharp contrast to that of her neighbors', for she lived in an upper-middle class community. While her own home environment was impoverished, her classmates wore beautiful clothes, took music lessons and dance lessons, went skiing, went away to supper camp, and went away on wonderful vacations. She had none of this. My patient envied these classmates of hers; she saw them as having a magic aura. The fact that the lives of some of these young women had not necessarily turned out particularly well did not alter my patient's perception of herself. She did not value her own achievements at all. The first period of her therapy ended when she met a new man who worked in a field related to her field. They soon became close, and the patient felt that her life was soon to be settled. She had a great deal in common with this man professionally. She was enchanted with his affluence and his success.

The patient came back into therapy six months later. The relationship was not going well. She wanted a stronger attachment to him and more commitment from him; and she was getting less of both. She would leave him, hurt and angry, go home and cry, and then come back again. Finally, he broke up the relationship.

The patient met a third man, also in a creative field. That, too, seemed to go very well at the start. However, he, too, did not make a firm commitment to her. She would then become very anxious and very hungry, accepting anything he suggested. There were moments when she felt secure with him but then she would be critical of the fact that he was eight to ten years older than she and she was critical of his height and his looks. However, for the most part, she was concerned about maintaining the connection. The more distant he was, the more anxious she became, the more she idealized him and the more she felt as if she were nothing. She was caught in the traditional "vicious circle." She devalued herself by presenting herself as rather empty, at the same time overvaluing him. For a while, it seemed impossible to get her to understand this process. As stated, she felt as if she would be nothing if they broke up. And break up they did, several months ago. Since then, there has been some progress. She is beginning to see how she devalued herself. She is making overt changes as a result of her dawning understanding that she has value and that she has a right to enjoy things on her own. For example, she is allowing herself certain pleasures, she is buying appropriate clothes, and she is thinking about redecorating her apartment.

The second patient is 35 years old. She is an executive secretary, earning a good salary. She was referred by her employer, a senior vice-president in a large firm. She had incurred debts adding up to $15,000. She understands very well that she has some basic problems that have to be worked out. She had had some therapy previously and her problems remained untouched. At my suggestion, she went to Debtors Anonymous for a few sessions. Her employer has taken away all of her credit cards and a plan to pay off of her debts has been worked out. She is following through very well on that plan. She has been in therapy for nine months and she is doing very well in therapy. Her family history is an unhappy one. Her mother left home to be on her own when she was still a young teen-ager. This mother has played out a very selfish, demanding role with her husband, a quiet, self-effacing man, and with her children, three daughters and a son. She has seemed to see all of them as owing her service; and she has in turn been unable to give any love or affirmation. As a teen-ager, my patient would do anything to win her mother's approval: clean up the yard, clean the house, take care of her mother's special breed of dogs, and so on. It is only in the recent few months that she has understood that she will get nothing from her mother. However, up to now she bought herself things to make herself feel good and to make up for what she has not received from her mother. She has bought furniture, clothes, books, courses, and so on. She was an incessant shopper. She would spend her mornings at work thinking about what she would buy at lunchtime or after work.

In relationships with others, she was compliant, lest she lose love. She would not actually be mistreated; but she would sell herself short. She always assumed others were better than she, that they had more education than she, or that they came from better families. The concentration on this envy probably has been covering feelings of anger, of which she is not yet aware. In the meantime, she is "giving up" on her mother and has become more assertive in her dealings with others. She is beginning to value herself, something she had absolutely not done at all. She has not valued her competence, her organizing ability, her good taste, or her beautiful apartment. And, like the other New york patient, she has wanted a husband who came from a "good" family and had a "good" education. In the recent past, she went out with a man who ostensibly had these advantages. As she got to know him, she discovered that his range of interests was much narrower than hers, that he lacked manners, that he was untidy and that he was selfish. She is beginning to understand that a mature, healthy, integrated individual does not necessarily spring from a so-called "good" privileged family. As of this writing, I have been seeing this patient for about ten months, and her therapy is certainly far from completed.

It is evident then that I am doing two kinds of therapy. Some of my work is short-term therapy; and it is more likely to take place in the suburbs, rather than in New york City, although there is a mixture of both kinds of therapy, short and long, in both places. The short-term therapy is diagnostically understood by me according to psychoanalytic developmental principles. However, the therapy would not be described as psychoanalytic as it has a counseling quality and because occasionally it is in a characterological analytic style. (That is, if the patient characteristically acts out in a passive aggressive way, this might be pointed out to her or him.) The other therapy I do is, needless to say, longer term. The emphasis is on uncovering the emotional history and the unconscious origins of the neurotic patterns. Such therapy can last anywhere from two to four years.

C H A P T E R
70

SHORT-TERM VERSUS LONG-TERM TREATMENT

Martin S. Pollens, M.S.W.

THE MENTAL HEALTH PROFESSION FACES A REVOLUTION

The mental health profession is now in the midst of a revolution that was totally unforeseen several decades ago. Just listen to these indicators. The case loads of private practitioners who had always had full practices are reduced by an average 20 to 30 percent. Practitioners who generally had waiting lists and were even in a position to refer to their supervisors and colleagues report that their primary sources have almost dried up. The psychoanalytic institutes currently are struggling to fill their incoming classes. And the graduate schools of social work report that applications have dropped significantly. Adding salt to these open wounds, insurance carriers have been moving in the direction of setting lower per-session limits on reimbursement; in some cases, lifetime benefit levels as low as $7,500 have been instituted. And "peer review" has been established to determine whether "appropriate treatment" is being provided for a patient and reimbursement should be continued. Practitioners on all levels and their patients have all been feeling the effects of these rapidly-changing trends.

This chapter will endeavor to: (1) Examine the symptoms of this revolution. (2) Review the alternative treatments that have been suggested to cope with the new trends.

THE SYMPTOMS OF THE REVOLUTION: PRESENTING PROBLEMS

The following presenting symptoms have been reported by therapists on the "front lines":

1. More people are *refusing treatment,* indicating that they can solve their difficulties on their own. They prefer to:

a. Purchase "how-to" books that are very concrete, leading to immediate results.

b. Visit their local chiropractor for an immediate adjustment.

c. Visit their local acupuncturist.

2. Those patients entering treatment generally come in with specific goals and a time-frame in which they wish to accomplish these aims, very much like the structures set up in a good business. Fewer individuals are willing to enter a long-term, ongoing process like psychoanalysis, requiring four to five sessions per week and a large expenditure of funds over a decade or more. More to the point, fewer individuals are willing to accept the rigid parameters of the doctor–patient relationship required in psychoanalysis. And many patients have rejected the authoritarian nature and delivery of interpretations from their former analysts. The patients who are now leaving their physicians who are arrogant, emotionally withholding, and arbitrary in their treatment style are similarly terminating psychoanalytic treatment that is provided in the same style or looking elsewhere from the start.

TREATMENT SUGGESTIONS
FOR A REVOLUTIONARY ERA

The following questions frequently occur in the minds of both inexperienced and experienced practitioners.

What Proportion Of My Practice Should Be Comprised Of Long-Term Patients?

Far fewer patients are coming in the door in 1987 looking for long-term psychoanalysis. Furthermore, the large majority of those patients who directly seek out analysis are receiving third party reimbursement for this treatment. In my experience, and the experience of my colleagues, when, for one reason or another, the insurance support is denied to the patient, the patient will not on his or her own continue paying for this long-term treatment. At best, the patient will remain in treatment on a once per week frequency. If you have set aside 2 to 3 hours per week for this patient, it can, along with other patients in this category, represent a significant proportion of your practice week. In my opinion, modern practitioners cannot realistically devote more than 25 to 50 percent of their practice to the long-term analytic patient.

Government and private industry insurance contracts are now limiting their benefits to what is believed to be cost-effective: short-term crisis-oriented psychotherapy. At best, most insurance contracts provide only for once per week contact. Even if practitioners had predominantly analytic institute candidates in their practice, these students are subject to the same financial pressures as the general population. And there are fewer analytic institute candidates available as the economy becomes more restrictive. As the fountains of insurance reimbursement dry up, patients will enter treatment mainly on a short-term basis. When the insurance benefits are exhausted, they leave treatment. Often it is difficult for them to handle the deductible and the out-of-pocket costs.

Aside from the radical shift in insurance reimbursement schemes, you must be meeting patients in your practice who approach treatment in a much different manner than even a decade ago. As mentioned earlier in this chapter, patients are much clearer about their short-term goals (e.g., finding a new job, leaving a relationship, solving a parent–child difficulty), the financial limits of their endeavor, as well as the kind of therapeutic relationship they are looking for. And, if they do not sense that movement is taking place fairly early in the contacts, they will seek out a different practitioner. Modern clients are very sophisticated and knowledgeable; they know what to look for in a good therapeutic contact. And they are also aware that treatment can take place on a once per week basis and at times on an alternate week basis. As Robertiello pointed out, 2- to 4-times-per-week treatment is often prescribed for the therapist's needs, not the patient's best interests.

In summary, if fewer people are using horses for basic transportation, and they are shifting to other means of getting around, it is risky to devote the greater percentage of your daily work to shoeing horses. It just makes greater economic and rational sense to learn auto repair.

Which Patients Are The Best Prospects For Long-Term Treatment?

Psychotherapists almost always appreciate the patient who can walk in, describing various symptoms and dysfunctions in life, and then acknowledge awareness that there is a "deeper problem" that must be excavated. This patient is prepared, almost from the outset, for a long-term process that will require weekly sessions and several years of "working through." These patients will generally present themselves with disturbances more in the neurotic range. These patients are not looking for a "quick fix," just for the symtoms to go away. They recognize that the symptoms are just the "tip of the icebert." The person who is the best prospect for long-term treatment, then, is generally high-functioning, articulate, and often has a network of family, friends, and colleagues who, themselves, are in treatment. He or she recognizes that this support network has grown, has changed from their psychotherapy experiences. Such a candidate comes into treatment with a good preparation, a positive emotional orientation and expectation from the very beginning, settles into treatment with a minimal amount of resistance, and is prepared for the investment of time, energy, and money.

The long-term patient is relatively easy to recognize and to appreciate, but is becoming very scarce in the world of 1987.

What Proportion Of Your Practice Should Be Comprised Of Short-Term Patients?

Since the greater proportion of people will be approaching you and directly requesting short-term, goal-oriented psychotherapy, it is axiomatic that you reserve adequate time for these patients. And the more patients you treat, either on a long-term or short-term basis, the more people you have sharing their experiences with you within their networks. If these patients develop a positive transference to you and are satisfied with what they are achieving in their lives, they will undoubtedly refer their networks to you. As you see more patients on a short-term basis and they accomplish their goals, there is a greater likelihood of a larger volume of referrals. If your practice is limited to 10 to 15 patients whom you see on a 2- to 3-times-per-week frequency, you are not permitting the practice sufficient generativity. It can become an insulated, restricted environment that does not allow for optimal growth.

Which Patients Are The Best Prospects For Short-Term Psychotherapy?

The best prospects for short-term therapy are the people who come in directly requesting this form of treatment. Patients who are very well suited for this approach are often those who are looking for a specific reason for their problems. They do not appear to be looking for insight. Frequently, they approach their individual problems like they were business psopositions. Most often, these patients have a goal in mind that they want to achieve in a given time-frame, for example, getting married, getting a raise, becoming pregnant, alleviating migraine headaches, handling a child with less anger. Patients might even tell you directly that they do not want to delve into the past, that they want to work in the here and now. They may request help in just getting rid of headaches and stomachaches.

These patients are very amenable to various kinds of short-term methods which include, but are not limited to, biofeedback, hypnosis, crisis intervention, short-term brief dynamic psychotherapy, and so on. Long-term analytic patients can also be part of the group seeking short-term therapy, either as a supplement to their analytic work or as a completely separate experience. There may be symptoms and problems that the analytic work has not been effective in reaching. These long-term analytic patients come in genuinely looking for "something extra" to reach them on a very deep emotional level. In my hypnosis work with long-term analytic patients, the primary analyst has often told me that the patient's contacts with me made the analytic work easier and more rewarding.

Does It Often Happen That A Short-Term Patient Becomes A Long-Term Patient?

Yes, a short-term patient can often develop into a long-term patient. How does this process occur? For example, in my short-term hypnosis practice, I have recently had the experience of a woman seeking help primarily with the panic preceding and following herpes attacks. As we proceeded in the hypnosis work, the patient began to recognize, quite spontaneously, that during the symptom-free periods she would begin thinking about the symptoms, that she could not let go of them. She then asked to re-focus the therapy to explore why she could not "let go" of the herpes. She realized that holding on to the symptoms was psychologically significant. This "holding on" was preventing her from "getting on" with her life. I have had numerous experiences in which patients in short-term work began to realize the deeper emotional conflicts that were integrally related to their symptoms. And then, without my forcing or pushing them, they began working on an insight level. It all begins as a result of my "beginning where the patient is at," dealing with what he or she wants help with. And you never know where the path will take the patient.

What Are The Special Problems That Arise In Short-Term Treatment?

Short-term therapy requires the therapist to be very versatile and flexible and imaginative. For example, in my hypnosis work, I custom-tailor the imagery work and indirect suggestions to the individual requirements and response patterns of the patient. And I am constantly "fine tuning" the inductions with the feedback that the patient is presenting. Often, what works so well in the initial sessions must be modified as the patient's condition changes. Short-term work, then, requires that the therapist be very active and directive in the sessions. The demands are very different from the traditional analytic situation in which the analyst can be more passive as he waits for the free association and transference material to emerge.

In short-term therapy, by its very nature, patients are always in the process of terminating. The short-term therapist almost never has a "break" from dealing with his separation anxiety. The analyst has plenty of time to prepare for the patient's termination. In short-term work, the "interruption" can come at any time. Nicholas Cummings has suggested that if the therapist sees "termination" as an "interruption," the practitioner's anxiety diminishes rapidly. Cummings, the dean of short-term therapy, talks about having treated three generations of many families in his area.

What Are The Different Kinds Of Short-Term Psychotherapy Approaches?

There are a wide variety of short-term approaches that have been adopted by psychotherapists practicing across the country. The few that I will describe are the most representative of the strategies that have been evolving over the past decade. There are many more that could be listed, but space is limited.

Brief intermittent therapy throughout the life cycle   This is an approach that has been pioneered by Dr. Nicholas Cummings, a psychologist. In developing the brief targeted therapy approach, Dr. Cummings declares to his fellow professionals: "You have to give up the concept of cure." And he writes that "that concept has held back psychotherapy more than any other concept. . . . And so psychologists keep patients in treatment until they are sure that every recess of the unconscious has been analyzed as to its conflicts, because both patient and therapist get only one chance. If three years from now the patient has another problem, the psychologist hasn't done his job correctly." How then does Cummings relate to patients in his short-term strategy? Here is how he explains it to his colleagues:

> . . .so at Biodyne we employ what we call "brief intermittent psychotherapy throughout the life cycle." This means that when a patient comes

in with a problem, the psychologist takes the problem seriously but not necessarily at face value, and he or she treats that problem. When the problem is resolved, the psychologist interrupts treatment. (Cummings, 1983)

And Cummings indicates that at Biodyne there ar at least 50 different kinds of targeted therapies. To justify the requirement of such a vast number of different therapies, he asis, "Would you go to a physician that treated everybody who came in the door with penicillin, whether one person had a broken leg from skiing or another had pneumonia? Of course you wouldn't."

Cummings gives the following parameters to his therapists:

1. *Literally hit the ground running.* What Cummings means here is that something effective and therapeutic must occur in the first session. He makes it very clear that spending the entire session taking a history is as antiquated as the horse and buggy. The patient must feel that he or she has been touched in the first session or the contacts will probably not continue; the patient will not return for the second session.

2. *Perform an operational diagnosis.* This kind of diagnosis is as different as day and night from the conventional DSM-style diagnosis. As Cummings puts it, "The operational diagnosis asks one thing, "Why is the patient here today instead of last week or last month, last year, or next year?" The operational diagnosis is directly tied in with a treatment plan.

3. *Create a therapeutic contract.* It is very important for the therapist to hear the contract that the patient gives in the first session. As Cummings and others point out, resistance is often wrongly labeled. More than 80 percent of what therapists label as "resistance," Cummings explains, "is nothing more than a therapist's failure to recognize the patient's goals in treatment."

4. *Do something novel in the first session.* According to Cummings this "will cut through the expectations of the 'trained' patient and will create instead an expectation that problems are to be immediately addressed."

5. *Give homework in the first session and every session thereafter.*

A major problem in doing brief therapy, Cummings further cautions, is "that the therapist is always having separation anxiety. There's tremendous turnover of patients because you're terminating constantly, and as a therapist you're always depressed because of separation anxiety. I'm saying to you, under this model we don't terminate. Rather, therapy is interrupted."

In summary, Cummings writes:

> . . .you can free yourself from the concepts of the ideal therapist, where each of us has to be all things to all people. You can free yourself from the concept of cure, and you can free yourself from the troublesomeness of termination.

Ericksonian hypnosis   This is a close "cousin" of Cummings brief intermittent therapy throughout the life cycle. Not a magic show, but something you do for yourself.

As Grossbart (1986) lucidly explains:

> Regrettably, hypnosis still retains a magic-show aura that keeps many from appreciating its possibilities. No, hypnosis does not mean a Svengali putting dupes under his power, making them cluck like chickens and per-

form ridiculous stunts they'd never do while "awake." In fact, it's not something that somebody does *to you* at all, but something you do *for yourself*, perhaps with the help of another person.

The phenomenon of hypnosis is a naturally occurring talent, capacity, and skill that some practitioners suggest exists in nearly 90 percent of the population. The hypnotherapist, as the Spiegels (1978) point out, merely arranges for a comfortable ambiance in which an individual can discover and utilize his hypnotic capacity. The simplest way to describe hypnosis is by terming it as one variety of an altered state of consciousness. This does not mean that the individual goes into a real sleep, losing consciousness of what is going on around him. Rather, in the altered state of consciousness achieved through hypnosis, there is a focus, an alertness that is not generally experienced in the conscious non-altered state.

As Erickson and Rossi explain:

> The induction and maintenance of a trance serves to provide a special psychological state in which the patient can reassociate and reorganize his inner psychological complexities and utilize his own capacities in a manner concordant with his own experiential life. Hypnosis does not change a person, nor does it alter his past experiential life. It serves to permit him to learn more about himself and to express himself more adequately. . . . It is this experience of reassociating and reorganizing his own experiential life that eventuates in a cure.

More than a decade ago, there were heated debates at professional conferences between the behaviorists and the psychoanalysts, each group claiming that they were practicing something distinct, separate, and unique from one another. The analysts claimed that they were treating "cause" rather than "symptom," in contrast to the behaviorists who were very superficial in just going after the "symptom." Anybody could tell that the approach of "symptom relief" was only skin deep! The behaviorists, on the other hand, pointed out that they felt that "doing archeology for archeology's sake" only perpetuated the patient's problem: analytic psychotherapy required too much of an investment of time and money. The results of behavior modification were quicker and the cause of the problem was essentially irrelevant.

Hypnosis, a modality utilized generally within a psychotherapy format, is, by itself, neither "behaviorist" nor "reconstructive" per se. Hypnosis, as explained earlier, is a naturally occurring phenomenon that can be utilized in various ways to assist persons suffering from various kinds of difficulties. The manner in which hypnosis is utilized, under what conditions it is introduced, the emphasis and focus of the hypnotic treatment, are all dependent on the practitioner involved, his or her training, inclinations, and personal interests. As in conventional psychotherapy, some professionals practicing hypnotherapy adhere to a directive approach while other professionals prefer to utilize an indirect permissive format. Some combine approaches. There are also a growing number of physicians, surgeons and dentists who use hypnosis primarily in the management of pain and anxiety related to medical conditions and procedures. And there are behaviorists, closer to the pure model, who employ hypnosis as a means of desensitizing their patients to various kinds of phobic tendencies such as fear of heights, elevators, and closed-in places. The various applications of hypnosis to pain management, psychotherapy, and behavior modification are all legitimate and valid provided that the practitioner is operating within the scope of his or her professional training and competence.

Biofeedback This is still another close "cousin" in the brief psychotherapy family of strategies. Biofeedback borrows from information theory concepts. This strategy utilizes simple and more complex instrumentation in the service of teaching individuals how to communicate relaxation to their bodies. The instruments in this approach rely on the body's galvanic skin response (GSR) When the individual's organism is experiencing a high level of anxiety, the GSR level is correspondingly higher, and the instruments often attached to the individual's fingers transmit a high frequency noise. As the individual learns to relax, his organism, through imagery and other techniques common in hypnosis, the noise level goes down appreciably. This provides immediate and direct feedback to the patient that his tension level has decreased. And it represents a positive reinforcement.

Biofeedback represents a practical application, as does hypnosis, of the concepts of psychoneuroimmunology, that is, helping the brain to communicate healthy positive attitudes to the organism. The "suggestions," either in biofeedback or hypnosis, modulate the limbic-hypothalmic and endocrine systems of the body; the immune system is strengthened and reinforced as a direct consequence. Biofeedback has been very effective in helping individuals to cope with phobias and the sequelae of traumatic experiences in the past.

What Is So Unique And Special About Short-Term Techniques?

I am now calling short-term psychotherapy techniques *reapprochment strategies.* In a child's normal development, "separation" and "individuation" are achieved by a continuing series of both forward and return movements. The child leaves the parent but then periodically returns to "touch base" and then goes back out into the world. Short-term therapy is structured especially, it seems to me, for the separation/individuation needs of patients, as they emerge, throughout an entire lifetime. Patients enter treatment to deal with specified issues and "transitions" in their lives and, then, leave or "interrupt" treatment to go out and "practice." And in the process they discover more of their innate skills and talents. Then, at later stages, when they are having a child, on the verge of getting a promotion, changing careers, or confronting the empty nest, they can re-enter treatment to again find their bearings to absorb the support and nurture of the treatment "holding environment."

To call a particular set of strategies *short-term therapy* seems like a misnomer to me. Since these short-term techniques can be and are utilized over an entire lifetime, it is arbitrary to divide therapies into so-called "long-term" and "short-term" approaches. I believe Cummings makes the salient point that the short-term approach is always available and the patient and therapist always have more than once chance to grow and develop. Clearly, the concepts of techniques of the many short-term approaches are utilized both over the short term and over the long term.

C H A P T E R
71

THE APPLICATION OF THEORY TO PRACTICE

Phyllis Caroff, D.S.W.

The widely felt sense of crisis in contemporary psychoanalysis in part reflects public disenchantment with its unfulfilled promise. A range of therapeutic alternatives offer possibilities of help that are shorter term, less expensive, and more acceptable to the sensibilities of a wide variety of patients. Within the psychoanalytic ranks serious questions are being raised about the effectiveness of the alternatives as therapy, as well as about the adequacy of the theories. Concomitantly, rigorous efforts are under way to systematize and revise more recent contributions to psychoanalytic psychology to develop an epistemologically sound metapsychology, as well as to revise and develop further theories about clinical procedures.

At the same time, within the past decade, in the wider world of the psychotherapies there appears to have been a diminution of intense ideological struggles and a movement toward rapprochement among clinicians of all persuasions and disciplines. Perhaps this is a function of the growing awareness of the necessity to evaluate consistently whether what we know and value is working; that is, whether it fits what the patient needs and can use or whether something else is needed.

Currently, there is a group of psychologists who, while maintaining their own theoretical identifies, are exploring potential sources of enrichment and convergence among other systems of thought. Others are seeking a rapprochement of various systems and an integration of therapeutic intervention (Norcross, 1986). The proliferation of therapies and a period of intense self-examination in which the failures and limitations of pet theories are being reappraised have fostered the special credence and attention given to rapprochement.

The argument is made that despite a noticeable increase in the quantity and quality of research on psychotherapy, it has not been possible to show that one therapeutic approach is clearly superior to another. An additional factor in the rise of this eclecticism is related to the fact that success in therapy can best be predicted by the attributes of the patient, the therapist, and their particular relationship. These are still considered more crucial for outcome than is technique. Also, the move toward eclecticism is perceived as an adaptive response to external contingencies. Attacks from outside the mental health professions are forcing us to come togehter. The courts, insurance companies, and national health insurance planners are sources to be attended to. Third-party payers and the general public are demanding answers about the durability, quality, and efficiency of psychosocial treatments (Parloff, 1979). In another forum I have suggested that models of treatment discussed in the literature are rarely replicas of the actual work of practitioners who claim to be connected with a given approach, and that no one approach provides the theoretical grounding applicable to the full range of clinical practice (Caroff, 1982). As clinicians we are pressed to do what's needed. Nevertheless, to be a professional requires that treatment decisions be made within some framework that seeks to describe and explain our professional purposes and the use of knowledge and values.

Whatever the choice of practice model, most of us are in agreement that assessment and diagnostic processes are intrinsic to all clinical work and are the basis for determination of goals and techniques. In my view, notwithstanding the complexity involved, a treatment perspective that incorporates a biopsychosocial assessment will provide for the clinician undertaking the process with the client a reasonably good idea of what is needed, what the client wants, and what it seems possible to do. On the basis of this assessment, the experienced clinician may then determine what model is most applicable. While it is my projection that the advanced clinician will become increasingly pluralistic, or the general move in theory development will be toward integration, my current concern is that we retain a principle-based practice central to our learning of skill — notwithstanding our exposure to other models and techniques as relevant to needs of particular populations. Although principles do not specify the particular technique and thus do not provide uniformity and control, they do allow for innovation, individualizing the particular treatment situation. Highly prescriptive models such as some behavioral therapies do not offer guidance for decisions in uncertain or ambiguous situations; nor do they account for the unanticipated events that may arise in a case (Lewis, 1982). However, behavioral models have lent themselves readily to outcome research because of their explicitness. Models that rest upon practice wisdom and conviction, upon which many of us rely, embody porcesses that are not explicit and do not readily lend themselves to objective evaluation. With both professional and societal pressure to find better ways to measure effectiveness, attention to clinical research will offer clearer criteria for choosing among alternative methods. Achieving this goal, however, seems a way down the pike.

It seems to me that the appeal of one approach over another not only has much to do with the way we were socialized to our respective professions but also depends on one's view of the nature of man, one's value stance about what constitutes help, one's comfort or lack of it with uncertainty, as well as one's view of the importance of empirical validation in light of the state of the knowledge. But I think we must attend the implications of our chosen model and be aware of the potentialities of others lest we risk imposing on patients that with which we are familiar rather than responding to what our patients need.

In light of all of the above, what follows is the explication of my position that psychosocial therapy with a supporting theory of psychoanalytic ego psychology, including its recent additions, continues to provide the most comprehensively relevant framework for my own practice as a clinical social worker in private practice, treating a range and variety of patients who are seen once or twice a week, within a time span from one session to more than 5 years.

ABOUT PSYCHOSOCIAL THERAPY

Diagnosis, assessment, goal setting, mutual agreement about problems to be addressed, the planning of treatment, pusposeful treatment in relation to assessment and goals, as well as the evaluation of its effectiveness, are the processes adhered to by most psychotherapists. The conceptual content that informs these processes and the techniques utilized provide the basis for our theoretical differences. Psychosocial therapy stresses the necessity for an integrated focus on humans as psychological and sociological beings and on the intrapsychic, interpersonal, and intrasystemic processes and experiences that constitute the basis for understanding and helping (Turner, 1974). In the past, this integrated focus underscored one of the distinguishing features of clinical social work as compared with other kinds of clinical intervention. Howsever, this differentiation is dissipating as psychology and psychiatry are becoming more concerned with the social context within which problems occur and are altered.

To this integrated focus on the psychological and the social components, there is the necessity to add the biological component, including the role of biological vulnerability in the development of patients' symptoms, as in schizophrenia and the bipolar affective disorders, as well as the understanding of genetic endowment and cognitive intactness. Organic impairment affecting the ability to receive, process, and act on information significantly impacts on functioning. Dysfunction in any one of these systems disturbs equilibrium and creates or aggravates tensions in individuals and those close to them. When there is biological dysfunction, it is inevitable that psychosocial effects will also be experienced. The knowledge derived from this biopsychosocial focus provides an understanding of individual development, interpersonal influence, influence of significant others, and significant environments and systems and provides the diagnostic underpinning for skilled treatment in engaging effectively in a therapeutic relationship for planned change.

As a dynamically oriented system of thought, psychosocial therapy operates on the assumption that a person's past is important. Controversy has ranged from almost total dependence on understanding the past to almost total negation of its importance. For me, the practice principle is that historical material is elicited for the purpose of removing distortions in experiencing so that patients may deal more effectively with their realities.

Another major assumption relates to nonconscious phenomena. Within the spectrum of current clinical work, the relevance of the unconscious and preconscious for diagnosis and treatment is differentially accepted. Cognitive therapies, for example, hold that the problems patients bring to therapists are problems of consciousness, and the theory requires the practitioner to disregard the concept of an "unconscious" as a significant force in psychic life. Within psychosocial therapy, the significance of the unconscious in practice has been a focus of ongoing reassessment. In this process, however, there has been no lessening of the necessity to understand the potential influence of unconscious and preconscious content on behavior. What has happened is the recognition that enhanced functioning and growth can and often do take place without direct use of out-of-awareness and unconscious material.

Psychosocial practice has relied heavily on psychoanalytic theory as a major source for understanding individuals and their relationships to society. In my view, it has been a source of the strength of this practice at the same time that it has been a strong focus of criticism. The fault lies primarily with a lack of understanding about differentiating the theory of personality from the theory of therapy, and as a consequence, with the inappropriate application of the theory of therapy to what has been known as clinical casework. Even today many social workers who identify with this school of thought utilize only limited segments of the theory. They know little of the contributions made by other theoreticians who followed Freud who are identified as having built upon psychoanalytic thought and expanded the boundaries of theory.

Like psychoanalysis in the 1920s and 1930s, we were overinvested in instinctual drives and libido theory and had minimal understanding of ego processes, functions, and development. With ego psychology coming into its own, our practice began to reflect a reworked understanding of structural theory, ego, id, and superego and a new understanding of ego integration and functioning. What was better understood was that ego functioning was influenced and affected by a continuum of external and internal stimuli. And we really needed to know more about the impact of social and cultural forces. With the contributions of Heinz Hartmann, the development of the conflict-free sphere of the ego and related concepts and their implications for healthier functioning, it was the notion that ego functions can become independent of the drives that was of special interest. With Erik Erickson's concept of cogwheeling and mutuality, and the extension of psychosexual development to the entire life cycle, new understanding was brought to the interactions between the individual and society and the ways each society meets the phases of the life cycle through its institutions, thus influencing how the individual solves and masters the tasks of each phase. Since therapy followed theory, external reality was brought center stage and "adaptation" became an emerging focus. With these contributions, the additions by Jacobson and Mahler, and those of Horney and Sullivan as psychodynamic interactionalists, a theory of object and interpersonal relationships evolved. Thus, with greater understanding of ego psychology and its application, a central place was being given to the ego and the reality side of experience. However, response to external reality need and disregard for internal reality in too many instances undermined patients' potential for achievement and growth. For the failure to hear need expressed on many levels precludes understanding patients — their external and internal situations, as well as what goes on between patient ahd therapist.

So, those of us who use psychoanalytic ego psychology as our supporting personality theory do place more emphasis on adaptation to external reality than those of us who don't. Under the rubric of ego psychology, knowledge about role performance, object relations, concepts of the development of the self, and interpersonal transactional relationships has offered a wide-angle lens through which to understand our patients' functioning better. Communication patterns among members of a family, their individual and collective perceptions of assigned and prescribed roles, and the ability of family members to be open to new learning have enriched our diagnostic acumen.

Finally, knowledge about ego processes and functions has enabled the development of a complementary relationship between psychoanalytic psychology and developmental learning theory to the enhancement of both. For example, the work of Piaget has enriched understanding of the role of the intellect in ego development. The emphasis on the development of task achievement and motor skills has added to understanding the role of ego mastery and the ability to control one's environment. And ego mastery spurs motivation toward greater maturity (Wasserman, 1974).

OPERATIONALIZING PSYCHOANALYTIC EGO PSYCHOLOGY IN PSYCHOSOCIAL THERAPY

To recapitulate what I sought to illustrate in the previous section, the dynamically changing nature of psychosocial therapy is based in considerable measure on the evolving state of psychoanalytic ego psychology, its supporting personality theory. In clinical work, the focus is on understanding the human being within the context of the social environment. In the assessment of individuals, their personality, and their needs, emphasis on the ego and its adaptive capacities has proved most operational and useful. Thus, we seek to understand those aspects of the external world that impact on the individual, and treatment is geared differentially according to our understanding of individuals and their assessed needs. While the therapist is responsible for the diagnosis, what is available for work is the conflict-free portion of the patient's ego. It is essential, therefore, that diagnosis and assessment include intrapsychic and situational strengths and resources, as well as dysfunctional limitations and pathology.

In the treatment process, several of the central concepts and techniques from psychoanalytic therapy are more or less relevant to ego-oriented casework treatment, and a few are not relevant at all. Wood (1971) elaborates on eight of these, including free association, the therapist as blank screen, the recovery of the repressed, dream interpretation, the development of insight, working through, transference–countertransference, and resistance. For example, the therapist as blank screen as technique is inappropriate, though dynamic passivity tended to be used in our earlier search for a suitable method. In its place, relationship and its differential use according to the patient's needs and situation is core to the process of helping. Nor is free association an appropriate technique. However, active listening is, and is most important in helping the patient develop an observing ego. As regards the interpretation of dreams, this is yet another inappropriate technique for clinical casework. The therapist listens, however, to the dream content, underscores its pleasure or worry for the patient, elicits the meaning of the dream to the patient, and may tie it to events in the therapeutic interaction, but avoids interpretation of its unconscious content. Social work clinicians have great respect for the ego defense of repression. Thus, recovery of the repressed is not a treatment goal. On the contrary, where ego boundaries are precarious or diffused, as with borderline or psychotic patients, the expression of unrepressed content is discouraged and repression encouraged. Interpretation as a technique has been highly overemphasized in the development of clinical treatment. Though interpretation is used on occasion in modified form when appropriate to the individualized needs of the patient, for the majority of patients, change, modification, and growth come about through and as a result of the therapeutic relationship as a corrective experience. Working through is an important and highly applicable concept. Awareness of the time factor in learning and interpreting new behaviors and of the back and forth movement in treatment as essential to test out and relinquish old behavior patterns enables the necessary therapeutic stance to communicate to the patient that "change comes hard." While resistance as a concept has been associated traditionally with repression, in our clinical context it may reflect the ego's need for protection, an indication of its being overburdened. Understanding patients' need to ward off our help is essential to effective practice. For example, a lack of congruence in expectations of the process, perhaps based on class or culture, requires careful attention as a precaution against an inaccurate assessment of resistance. Appreciation of the positive adaptive aspects of patients' need to resist often frees them to engage in treatment.

Transference–countertransference continues to be passionately argued in some professional groups. For clinical casework it is central to the treatment process. Patients frequently transfer to therapists irrational elements from past relationships. However, encouragement of the transference neurosis and extensive regression are part of the analytic model. In clinical casework, reliving of past traumatic events and regression are not encouraged. While meeting some dependency needs is a necessary part of forming a therapeutic relationship, work with the transference is toward corrective handling, thereby furthering growth. Also, the concept has undergone development over time. For example, some components of the relationship previously viewed as transference reactions can be more adequately explained in cultural, life experience, and value terms. Transference, if ignored, can create problems in the treatment. It is not held, however, that all transference reactions that take place need to be identified for the patient or examined in the treatment. What is important is that "when the phenomenon is present its occurrence and strength be recognized, controlled if necessary, utilized when appropriate and worked out if required" (Turner, 1974, p. 91). The ability to understand unconscious transference phenomena and how to work with them to keep the relationship focused on reality requires that we be aware of our own responses out of past or present experiences that potentially free or interfere with the creation of a therapeutic climate conducive to patients' progress. Countertransference analysis, or in other terms, expanding self-awareness and self-discipline, appears to me to be a necessary, ongoing process for us to assure a differential use of self that operates to maximize patients' potential for ego maintenance or growth.

Psychosocial treatment requires the knowledge and understanding of persons and situations in their external and internal dimensions as the basis for decisions about which of the available procedures are to be used to achieve the goals mutually arrived at with the patient. Like all other components of practice, diagnosis and assessment will be related to the nature of the case. Thus, considerations about content and detail will vary with the type of problem, the nature of the request, the time available, the services available, and the therapist's competence. In my view, the law of parsimony must obtain. That is, the amount of information required should be regulated by the conclusions needed to respond effectively to the situation. Thus, the patient who requests help with finding institutional care for an aged aunt need not be expected to share a detailed history, nor is a lengthy detailed diagnosis required of the therapist. At the same time, however, ignoring other possible difficulties related to the request, the effect on other parts of the patient's life, or other questions the patient might want to ask is to do a disservice to what we know. In those instances where the primary treatment focus is on the alleviation of external stress, there needs to be reasonable evidence in the assessment of the potential not only for the restoration of the patient's ego functioning but also for growth. For we know what problems have differential impact and that our patients vary in their ability to cope and may disguise what it is they want in a variety of ways. Thus, while current research suggests that the patient, the therapist, and their relationship are the most significant vairables in predicting outcome, technique and the knowledge informing it must continue to be central to our concerns.

Although there are limits to the data collected in the diagnostic and assessment processes, if we are dealing with behavioral change, it is patients' ego functioning, defensive structures, ability to cope with stress and anxiety, tolerance for frustration, judgment, reality testing, object relations, autonomous ego functions, and superego functioning that provide the guidelines for differential treatment. In ego psychology parlance, in all patient situations it is the conflict-free areas that are identified, assessed, and engaged within the relationship, with the therapist becoming the alter ego/superego until the patient's ego is strengthened and consolidated for the patient's own improved self-directed functioning.

Practice wisdom has provided the ego-oriented psychotherapist with a number of treatment rules of thumb evolving from ego assessment. We know that the weaker the patient's defenses are the more actively the therapist will work to help support defenses, will encourage repression of irrational chaotic content, and will refrain from probing and uncovering techniques. This broad general approach has goals of ego conservation or ego restitution, aims at restoring defenses, deals with the conscious rather than the preconscious or unconscious, and dynamically focuses on the present rather than the past. Conflicts in relationship are addressed to current derivative figures rather than to those of a primary genetic nature. Techniques of mobilization, manipulation, and suggestion are frequently used in the repertoire. This approach has been most effective with patients whose egos are at risk of being overwhelmed. In those conditions where the ego can defend against the intensity of the drives only through use of psychotic mechanisms, psychotropic medications are indicated.

For patients whose behaviors reflect problems of a more characterological nature, including the personality disorders — acting-out or impulse-ridden behavior, lack of anxiety, or primitive superego development — considerable activity is required in terms of the environment, setting limits, teaching impulse control, and pointing out cause and effect, as well as the consequences of behavior. The objective is to make destructive, acting-out behaviors ego alien. It is these patients who most sorely challenge our self-awareness and self-management. For at one and the same time we are obliged to retain a therapeutic climate of acceptance of the person and readiness to meet need and to confront the repetitive, destructive behaviors. The ability to allow for and at times generate optimal anxiety within the patient necessary for ego growth, and risk being misperceived as being punitive and withholding, is frequently experienced by us as a considerable threat. Is it the possible rageful response from the patient that creates much of our own anxiety?

Treatment of more neurotic patients will reflect and be affected by their stronger ego development. Verbalization of feelings is encouraged; cause and effect connections, clarifications, and, at times, interpretations are prevalent techniques. With the diminution of superego guilt, previously unacceptable thought, feelings, and behaviors may be examined. What usually becomes available during the work is suppressed, preconscious material. Later in the treatment, depending, in a measure, on the strength of the patient–therapist relationships and patient readiness, content that was unconscious in the initial phases may enter consciousness and be amenable to working through.

Within the past few years, my practice has reflected increasingly the influence of object relations thought. In addition to the assessment of patients' ego strength and structure, as well as their interpersonal environment in the present and the past to discern sources of stress and satisfaction, understanding patients object relations is important in determining the most appropriate level of treatment. Among the questions to be answered are whether there are sufficient environmental supports and to what extent the therapist may have to supply them; and to what extent the patient can accept the therapist as a separate, real person or whether, based on object need and ego boundaries, the wish to be incorporated or fear of engulfment colors the relationship.

Weiner (1986) presents a useful formulation for comparing and contrasting techniques and components in three types of psychotherapy—repressive, ego supportive, and evocative—based, in part, on different views of dealing with unconscious processes. Thus, repressive therapies embody observations and psychological interventions that seek to reinforce repression; ego supportive therapies essentially foster selective exploration of ego defenses; evocative therapies address the exploration of repressed mental content. Treatment techniques cut across diagnostic lines, and vary in relation to patients' ego strength and structure, type of life crisis, level of motivation, and potential for self-awareness. This classification of treatment methods with its biopsychosocial framework and emphasis on ego functioning also demonstrates an approach to integrating selective concepts and techniques from behavioral and cognitive systems of thought within an essentially psychodynamic framework and, as previously discussed, is one example of the inevitable move toward theoretical integration.

In systematizing practice content and process and explicating treatment techniques with their respective emphases within each of the treatment modes, Weiner's work has contributed to increased clarity about my own clinical practice. In particular, I note the considerable number of patients with whom my work is essentially ego supportive, in contrast to the number in analytically oriented psychotherapy. Also I have become increasingly convinced that ego supportive work has been undervalued and inadequately understood by both patients and therapists as a treatment mode to effect cognitive, affective, and behavioral change. Consequently, what follows is a discussion of selected components and techniques in the ego supportive mode that I have found particularly relevant in relation to my own work.

Most of the people with whom I work in this mode enter treatment formulating their problems in terms of their wish for symptom relief or their difficulties in interpersonal relationships, about which they are uncomfortable. They cope adequately on a day-to-day basis and are psychologically minded in the sense that they can make connections between their behavior and recalled thoughts and feelings or those they anticipate. Also, they evidence at least some ability and interest in self-understanding. An important factor is that a large majority of these patients are able to contract for one therapy session a week. For those able to come twice a week, the process of change is often accelerated.

The focus of the therapy is on problems in the present that are created or exacerbated by the nature of patients' relationships in the various areas of their functioning. The proloms may be in work or school, in social or intimate relationships. In addition to low self-esteem, they may complain of nervousness, fatigue, indigestion, and insomnia. Also, many suffer with symptoms of anxiety or depression that are ego dystonic.

The agreement for work together is to develop self-understanding, essentially at an interpersonal level. As the therapy progresses and there is sufficient trust in the relationship, the therapist becomes part of the patient's interpersonal world through observing, commenting on, and sometimes participating in the interaction. The reaction of therapist to patient and the patient's response to this are important elements in the dynamics of change. However, effective use of the therapeutic mechanism of feedback (Wiener, 1986), which entails sharing with patients the impact of their behavior on their therapist, particularly for patients who have little awareness of their impact on others, requires an assessment of patient readiness. Readiness can oftentimes be measured by patients' ability to identify feelings that previously have not been owned up to or about which they have been unaware. The capacity for the development of self-examination is critical. For, in addition to a positive relationship, unless patients come into treatment with the ability to be self-observing or can develop it in the therapy, feedback will not be experienced as acceptance, an essential for change in this mode. It may be experienced as disapproval, as a command to stop given behavior, or as approval of it, rather than as a stimulus for reflection, which is its purpose. In part, it is through this mechanism that patterned behaviors that are sources of interpersonal difficulty are confronted. For example, dysfunctional ego defenses of blaming others, denying responsibility for action, or rationalizing behaviors as these occur in day-to-day interpersonal relationships are addressed with the objective of encouraging patients' awareness of and taking responsibility for feelings and behavior that are self-defeating. Reflection is intended to encourage patients to think in terms of cause and effect in relationships, to develop the ability to contemplate feelings and thoughts before acting and, in time, to communicate their feelings to their therapist about their reactions, positive and negative, to their therapists' responses.

It has been my experience that the patient's response to the therapist's communication, assuming that the therapist's input is in the service of the patient's growth, is an excellent indicator of the extent to which the therapist is experienced as a real person committed to guiding the patient toward greater mastery and satisfaction, and the extent to which the therapist is experienced transferentially. Understanding the patient's object needs as these are reflected at any given time in the process of treatment helps us as therapists to determine how much we make our presence felt as people. Unquestionably, the interactive nature of this mode in psychotherapy offers transference gratification. Managed optimally, erotic transference and transference anger are limited. While they may arise, the experience is sufficiently diluted so that they do not interfere with the main thrust of focusing on interpersonal relationships in the present. Optimal management involves the balance between the therapist's sufficient exposure as a real person to keep the transference in bounds and enough of a personal barrier so that social friendship is precluded and sufficient anxiety maintained for motivation to work in the therapy. When anger or admiration interferes with the inquiry process, it is usually called to patients' attention in terms that illuminate understanding of how these color relationships. However, therapists need to be alert to the potential for destructive acting out that requires decreasing patients' emotional pressure during sessions or increasing pressure on patients to face what's going on in the therapeutic relationship. Effective decisions about how and when to gratify the transference rest on the therapist's accurate empathy as well as alertness to the potential to satisfy our own needs. For, there are those times with patients when failure to satisfy object needs may lead to the repetition of the deprivations with unempathic or uncaring parents and block patients' ability to experience their therapist as on the side of their health.

In addition to feedback, identification with the positive, constructive attributes of one's therapist is a powerful element in the change dynamics, particularly for those patients who were unable to make constructive identifications at crucial points in their emotional development. Some patients are helped to discard old values and replace them with new ones based on their identification with their therapists — a process analogous to that of superego formation. Particularly through the technique of reframing, which views a thought, feeling, or situation from a perspective that reduces self-criticism and encourages constructive action, patients are enabled to avoid prohibitions of the superego or ego ideal that inhibit adequate functioning.

As with other terms originating from traditional psychoanalysis, the reconceptualization of the concept of insight has been salutary. I think the promise of achieving insight — that is, the awareness of the unconscious meaning of thoughts, feelings, or behavior with its implications for change — in once weekly psychotherapy has done a disservice to many patients. With the broadening of the meaning of the term, in the ego supportive mode patients can develop insight through examining their interactions with their therapist, thereby understanding patterns of behavior previously out of awareness. Thus, in the reconceptualization, insight exists at many levels and serves a number of functions. As Weiner (1986) indicates, its most important function is "attribution of meaning" — that is, the explanation of symptoms, feelings, and behaviors hitherto unexplained. What is essentially therapeutic is that it enables patients to place their thoughts, feelings, and behaviors into a frame of reference that may then be discussed from an internally consistent, logical context. In my practice I use exploration of the past focused to situations in which patients have experienced difficulties similar to their problemful interactions in the present, including therapeutic sessions. At times, these connections and clarifications provide understanding (knowledge for action) that produces change. Awareness of similar patterns at earlier stages of development has given me the opportunity to attribute the difficulties to faulty learning, which notion is used by some patients successfully to reduce self-criticism, facilitating change. With other patients, understanding and conviction about the sources of difficulty are not sufficient. I agree with Weiner that with such patients therapists may have to urge and actively support desired change because an act of will is required.

In terms of length of therapy, I have found ego supportive work particularly useful in dealing with transitional life stage crises where treatment has been successfully completed in less than 6 months. A few of my patients have been in treatment over 5 years. I believe that we are ethically obligated to help patients achieve their objectives as quickly as possible. Most patients do not choose to make therapy a way of life. For those few whose needs for a connection may keep them in therapy forever, I believe our role is to facilitate their finding this in the larger community.

SUMMARY AND CONCLUSION

To come full circle, I think we must confront the demands from within and outside the helping professions for greater accountability. It has been my projection that mental health treatment will inevitably become increasingly short term, episodic, and pragmatic. Many of us who are committed to ego-oriented work are encouraged by the efforts to develop brief psychotherapy models. For the present, I think that reimbursement for service will press us to be more precise about symptoms and problems in social functioning toward which psychotherapeutic interventions are directed. Goals to be achieved will be specified in behavioral terms. The level of treatment, process, and techniques utilized to achieve the goals will be explicated. Progress and the evidence to support it, as well as the projection of a time frame to achieve subgoals will be required. While for many these expectations may be experienced as alien, they have the potential to sharpen our practice. Also, we must confront the reality that considerable effort is being expended to develop protocols for specific symptom diagnoses.

In carrying out my assignment to consider the application of theory to practice I have chosen to discuss psychosocial therapy and ego psychology theory because of its relevance for my own work. But more fundamentally, I have tried to make the case for individualizing treatment through a principle-based practice. While efficiency and cost-effectiveness are necessary and desirable, they may not become superordinate in the face of the psychological needs of our patients. Expediency, whatever its source, must be rejected as a primary determinant by the helping professions.

REFERENCES

Caroff, P. (1982). Treatment formulations and clinical social work. In P. Caroff, (Ed.),*Treatment formulations and clinical social work.* Silver Spring, MD: National Association of Social Workers.

Lewis, H. (1982). *Tools for thought: The intellectual base of social work.* New York: Haworth Press.

Norcross, J.C. (1986). Eclectic psychotherapy: An introduction and overview. In J.C. Norcross (Ed.), *Handbook of eclectic psychotherapy.* New York: Brunner/Mazel.

Parloff, M.B. Can psychotherapy research guide the policymaker: A little knowledge may be a dangerous thing. *American Psychologist, 34.*

Turner, F.J. (1974). Psychosocial therapy. In F.J. Turner (Ed.), *Social work treatment: Interlocking theoretical approaches.* New York: Free Press.

Wasserman, S.L. (1974). Ego psychology. In F.J. Turner (Ed.), *Social work treatment: Interlocking theoretical approaches.* New York: Free Press.

Weiner, M.F. (1986). *Practical psychotherapy.* New York: Brunner/Mazel.

Wood, K.M. (1971). The contribution of psychoanalysis and ego psychology to social casework. In H.F. Strean, *Social casework: Theories in action.* Metuchen, NJ: The Scarecrow Press.

C H A P T E R
72

ETHNIC AND CULTURAL ISSUES IN PRIVATE PRACTICE

Gerald Schoenewolf, Ph.D.

Perhaps nowhere more than in America do ethnic and cultural issues come up in therapy. We are and always have been a melting pot, drawing people of varying ethnic and cultural backgrounds into our society; the result is that our society is far from homogeneous. Not only are the patients we see from differing origins with differing belief systems and values, but we ourselves are also the products of differing backgrounds, belief systems, and values. Obviously, when our background, belief system, or values clash with those of our patients, there will be problems.

I have coined the term "cultural counterresistance" to define the kind of counterresistance that is of an ethnic or cultural origin. For example, if a liberal-minded therapist is resistant to hearing a conservative patient's opinions about social issues, hence falls silent, changes the subject, or in other ways expresses a judgment about those views, such a therapist is acting out a counterresistance that is not an aspect of the countertransference per se but an expression of inculcated values rooted in the cultural milieu in which the therapist was brought up. The therapist not only has to help the patient over-come his or her biases, belief systems, and values insofar as they serve as resistances, but also must overcome his or her own biases, belief systems, and values that manifest themselves as counterresistances.

The problem is that counterresistances — like resistances — are largely un-conscious. This holds particularly true for cultural counterresistances because they are ego syntonic. We do not normally think of our biases, belief systems, and values as things that might get in the way of our being competent thera-pists; quite the contrary, we tend to cherish them and think of them as bene-ficial. And, if we encounter a patient who has the same biases, belief systems, or values as we do, there is the danger of collusion. That is, we will also tend to be blind to the way in which our patient's cultural resistances impede his or her progress.

To return to the example of the liberal-minded therapist working with a conservative patient, in such a case the liberal therapist will not think of himself or herself as being in any way biased; yet because the therapist has been brought up in liberal cultural surroundings (or has been brought up in such a way as to gravitate toward a liberal orientation), he or she will develop what Elsworth F. Baker (1967) calls a "liberal character." Baker, a disciple of

Wilhelm Reich, posited both liberal and conservative character types. He saw liberals as guilt ridden and out of touch with their feelings, and believed they defend against unconscious feelings of rage through excessive intellectualism and through altruistic activities on behalf of those they view as underdogs (a symbolic rebellion against their fathers). Consciously they appear to have noble aims, but unconsciously their psychodynamics indicate a need for vindication and self-aggrandizement. Conservatives, on the other hand, are described by Baker as excessively emotional and antiintellectual. They tend to side with the top dog, with those in power (an identification with the father), and to be contemptuous toward underdogs, blind to the inequalities of the world. They also have their share of unconscious guilt, and they compensate for it through religiosity and moral self-righteousness and a blind faith in traditional values. It is not hard to imagine what might happen if a liberal therapist works with a conservative patient, or vice versa.

A colleague reported a case that illustrates this point. This colleague was a middle-aged, politically conservative psychoanalyst, and his background was one that put a great deal of emphasis on personal achievement. In the cultural atmosphere in which he grew up, little value was given to matters of the person as a member of a group in the communistic sense. In fact, communists and others in the liberal camp were viewed as "bleeding hearts" who did not see the world realistically.

Into his office came a patient, a younger man, who had been brought up in an atmosphere that laid heavy stress on communism as the highest priority in life. His parents had both been officers and active members of the party; they taught the patient to believe that achieving a communist society was possible in America and represented the only opportunity for dealing with the many social and cultural inequities that plague the country. Although the patient was not actually affiliated with the party, as an adult he still held a communistic view of the world, eschewing the "culture of narcissism." His relationships were also colored by the socialistic need to help others who were disadvantaged rather than to pursue his own "selfish" goals.

Whenever the patient spoke about his relationship to the community-at-large and the need to espouse social reforms, the therapist tended to deal with such statements by analyzing them as self-effacing defenses against the patient's narcissism and grandiosity. "If you're *not* a communist when you're 20, you don't have a heart," he once told the patient. "And if you're still a communist when you're 30, you don't have a head."

Although his interpretations about the patient may have been valid, the therapist nevertheless used them to shut the patient up. Because of his counter-resistance to anything that smacked of communism or liberalism, he could not listen empathically to the patient until the patient had established enough trust for him to be able to venture these interpretations in a loving, rather than a subtly hostile, manner. Hence a stalemate developed and therapeutic progress was stymied for months.

Ethnic or cultural issues can arise in numerous contexts: when a white therapist works with a black patient or vice versa, when a male therapist works with a female patient or vice versa, when an affluent therapist works with a patient from an impoverished background or vice versa, when a therapist of one religion works with a patient of another religion, when a therapist of one nationality works with a patient of another nationality, or when a therapist of one ideology works with a patient of another ideology.

One of the more prevalent and potentially harmful forms of cultural counterresistance comes about when therapists identify their selves — particularly their ideal selves — with a cause, a religion, or a mass movement. Those who identify with such a cause, movement, or religion — whether or not they are actually "card-carrying members" — will often become self-righteous (they are right and those outside the cause are wrong), in which case they will feel justified in transferring, resisting, and acting out aggressive feelings to such outsiders without feeling any guilt. In these cases, the cause, religion, or movement becomes a projection of the therapist's ideal image, while those parts of his or her self that are disowned are projected onto outsiders; the therapist and the movement are good and outsiders are bad. In the therapy dyad, when a therapist receives a patient who appears to be an outsider, the therapist may unconsciously resist certain material from this patient that is considered bad or wrong, thereby derailing the therapeutic process.

In recent times feminism has become such a cause. Those who identify themselves with feminism, women and men, often come to feel their way is the only way. They are right and those who do not accept the gospel of feminism are wrong. Therapists who identify with feminism will resist male patients who they determine are sexists, female patients who are dupes, and any ideas contrary to feminist doctrine. In fact, feminist therapists perceive any threat to their belief system as an attack on their selves, which have become identified with the movement, and they will react with a narcissistic rage to all such threats. Because feminism is in vogue now and has become such an influential force, a case in point seems appropriate.

A young woman patient came to me after she had left another therapist, a female therapist who advertised herself in the local newspaper as a "feminist therapist." My patient went to this woman because she felt she would understand her plight; she complained to the feminist therapist that her husband continually battered her, and got a sympathetic hearing. "You've come to the right person," the therapist said empathically. "I've helped lots of women like yourself. Don't worry, I'll tell you exactly what to do."

The therapist proceeded to help the patient move out, first placing her in a women's shelter, then helping her find her own apartment. She also assisted her in pressing charges against her husband for assault and battery and in taking other legal actions. After about 6 months the therapist suggested that the patient was doing all right and did not need therapy anymore, and the patient agreed. The patient thanked the therapist profusely for the help, they hugged, and she left feeling quite grateful and strong. A few months later she met another man quite similar to the one she had just separated from, and moved in with him. Before long he had begun to batter her just as the previous man had done. Obviously, the therapist had not helped the patient to resolve the underlying psychic conflicts that led to her difficulties.

The patient was a very angry and provocative woman who was unconsciously castrating toward the men with whom she became involved. Her provocative and castrating behavior invariably induced a rage reaction from the men (who were prone to violence anyway). She was drawn to violent men like her father, while her mother, who had also been a battered woman, had modeled the role of the helpless martyr. Throughout her childhood she had been trained to have masochistic relationships with men and knew of no other kind. The feminist therapist had not helped her at all to resolve this masochism.

The therapist had a resistance to seeing the patient's characterological problems. As a feminist, she harbored the view that men were oppressors and women were victims. Even when a woman, say, murdered a man, this therapist would find reasons why the woman had been driven to it by oppression; while if a man committed any act of violence or the like it was always becuase he was simply "bad." There was no capacity on her part to understand that the man, too, might have been driven to it. The therapist had never resolved her narcissistic rage connected to the events of her childhood, a rage thät now had become transferred onto men in general; and the cultural atmosphere of the times, in which feminism was predominant, reinforced this rage at men. The therapist acted out her rage by using situations such as the one provided by this patient as a vehicle to go on a witch-hunt for "male chauvinist pigs." She had a need to see herself and her patient as right and innocent, hence a resistance to considering the patient's contribution to her dilemma or looking at her masochistic character structure. It was only after this patient came to me that we began to analyze these things.

After ideology-based cultural counterresistances, the next most prevalent in our society are probably those involving racial differences. Ralph Greenson (1967) writes of a case in which he worked with a black male patient who continually brought in dreams that indicated a great deal of mistrust and suspiciousness concerning the therapist. Greenson admits he was resistant to interpreting these dreams in terms of the racial issue; instead, he repeatedly interpreted them as transference reactions derivative of early feelings toward the patient's parents. The patient was resistant to bringing up the racial issue, perhaps out of politeness, or perhaps out of a need to show how progressive and "unblack" he was; and, at the same time, Greenson also had an unconscious reluctance to bring up the matter, as he had a need to think of himself as a liberal and a humanitarian and hence oblivious to what color a person's skin is. The result was that the analysis stayed on a fairly superficial level for a time, and many obvious clues, such as those in the dreams, were misinterpreted or ignored.

Gender-based cultural counterresistances are also widespread. We are often raised with one value system if we are male, and a different value system if we are female. A male therapist might hae difficulty relating to a female's attempts to break free from a culturally induced value system that stresses a traditional motherhood role for women; while a female therapist, on the other hand, might not be able to empathize with a male patient's culturally rooted need to be assertive in his relations with women.

At its minimal level, a cultural counterresistance can result in a therapist's being selectively inattentive to certain material brought in by a patient. A patient may then be kept from progressing as far or as fast as he or she otherwise might. However, on a deeper level, a therapist's biases, belief systems, or values can actually lead a patient astray and cause damage. I refer to cases where therapists have an unconscious (and sometimes conscious) agenda for their patients. Frieda Fromm-Reichmann (1950) makes note of "insecure" therapists who attempt to mold patients in their own image, making of them a narcissistic extension, or trying to convert them to their belief system. Richard C. Robertiello (1985) goes much further, cautioning potential patients to be careful in choosing an analyst: "Beware of gurus who 'know the world' and will subtly impose it on you. Watch out for the 'Invasion of the Body Snatchers.' The Surgeon-General says that analysis can be injurious to your "Self" (p. 83). In essence, we are talking about brainwashing.

This, of course, is the form of therapy most often associated with Russian psychiatry and with novels such as George Orwell's *1984*. However, unconscious forms of brainwashing (or, at times, not so unconscious) may be happening in our own therapeutic community more than we think. What takes place behind a therapist's office door is a secret between the therapist and the patient. Those case histories that are reported in journals and books represent only a selected few, and even those are presented in such a way as to illustrate a point. How do we brainwash our patients? Let us say, for example, that a black male therapist has been raised in a cultural environment that stressed black pride and togetherness. Suppose a black man enters therapy with this therapist, one whose goal is to become assimilated in the "white world." The therapist may have an unconscious agenda for the patient: to convert him to the cause of black togetherness. Hence, in subtle ways, the therapist will discourage all movements by the patient toward assimilation with whites, and will encourage a kind of black separatism. He may even suggest that the desire to assimilate with whites represents a form of betrayal. Let us suppose, further, that during the course of therapy the patient is regressed to a stage of infantile dependence on the therapist: In this state the therapist can literally hypnotize the patient into adopting whatever philosophy or political stance he wants. As long as he is still attached to the therapist, the patient may even fool himself into thinking he is happy; but once the connection is severed and the transference wears off, he will find that he is going against the grain of his own inclinations and, in addition, will feel totally confused as to his real identity. That is, he will be worse off than when he started therapy.

Similarly, a classical analyst might value the controlling of emotions, since in classical analysis it is taught that when one has been thoroughly analyzed one no longer is beset by emotionality; the ego, not the id, is in charge. However, what often happens to classical analysts is that they become dull, mechanical people who have, in reality, developed highly effective intellectual defenses against their feelings. The result is that they can no longer be spontaneous, which is held by most therapists to be one of the keys to emotional and mental health. Now, in working with their patients, classical analysts will unconsciously (and sometimes consciously) guide them to a similar state of dullness. Over the years, when individuals are cut off from their feelings and from spontaneity, these emotions often get displaced into the soma; that is, diseases such as ulcers, heart conditions, cancer, and the like occur. So the end result of this kind of brainwashing can often be a ciminishing of one's vitality and sometimes downright fatal.

Murray (1956) once analyzed a tape-recording of a session by the noted psychotherapist Carl Rogers. In this analysis, Murray focused on the subtle signals Rogers was giving the client, such as asking an encouraging question when he approved of what the client was saying., and remaining silent when he disapproved. Murray counted 68 client statements about independence that were met by subtle approval, while none was met by disapproval. On the other hand, 16 client statements about sex were met with disapproval, while only 2 were approved. By the end of the therapy, Murray reported, the client was concerned with independence and unconcerned about sex.

Given that these cultural countertransferences exist and that they are generally unconscious, how can we resolve them and prevent them from occurring? First of all, we need to raise the consciousness of the therapeutic community as to their existence. Unfortunately, at the present time many therapists and anlysts go through their entire training and supervision without once having anybody call attention to their biases, belief systems, or values insofar as they affect the way they do therapy. Obviously, it is much easier for a supervisor to comment on some problem of erroneous technique or even a characterological countertransference problem than to point out to a therapist trainee that he or she is, say, prejudiced. To compound this dilemma, it is also generally the case that trainees pick supervisors whose biases, belief systems, and values are similar to their own. Thus a Catholic trainee will most likely pick a Catholic supervisor; a Marxist trainee, a Marxist supervisor; a conservative trainee, a consevative supervisor; and so on. This in turn leads to a vicious circle that perpetuates, rather than resolves, such problems. And the same thing happens with respect to the choice of training analyst and the choice of institute: Trainees pick those analysts and institutes whose cultural resistances match their own either partially or entirely. Lastly, these trainees then become therapists and supervisors, and will most likely draw patients who have similar biases or attempt to influence those who do not, and they will also form bias-based collusions with their supervisees. Thus, a therapeutic bias may be passed on from therapeutic generation to generation. If we are to deal with issues of ethnicity and cultural differences, we must start in our own backyard.

Raising our consciousness about this problem might bring about a change in our training institutes, where a heightened sensitivity to therapists' cultural biases might be in order. More attention should be paid to this matter by both the analyst and the supervisor of the trainee, and a class or two on the subject might also be helpful.

Second, we need to provide therapists with techniques for coming to grips with and possibly resolving (or at least bringing under their awareness and control) their cultural and ethnic biases. How can therapists know if they are acting out cultural counterresistances? One important clue might be a lack of empathy for a patient, or a feeling of disapproval toward the same. Another clue might be the need of a therapist to express opinions frequently to a patient on a particular subject. Feeling bored with a particular patient or having the impulse to change the subject or redirect the patient's attention to other, presumably more important matters may also be a sign of countertransference. If a therapist finds himself or herself experiencing these feelings, a little introspection might be in order. And possibly a trip back into therapy.

This raises the question: Can introspection, or indeed can therapy, change, resolve, or get rid of a cultural or ethnic or sexual bias? How much is such a bias rooted in one's character? Is it an aspect of one's narcissistic defense? Of one's ego ideal? I have sometimes felt that there is a universal need by human beings to be right. Perhaps this could be seen as an offshoot of Adler's "will to power" motif; however, in my view it is not simply power that people crave, but the feeling that they are okay and have the right philosophy, the right religion, the right attitude, the right spouse, the right country. When we argue, we need to be in the right. Many if not most patients who come to us spend a good deal of their time talking about the injustices that are done to them; they view themselves as right, as good, and those who victimize them as wrong, as bad. There is not so much a need for power as a need to be right, to be good, to be vindicated.

Therapists also have this need: We need to go to the right institutes, to practice the right school of therapy, and to have the right or "correct" viewpoint. And there is also the need to join with others who have the same viewpoint, and to attempt to persuade those who do not to "get with it." Eric Hoffer (1963), the dockworker-sociologist, commented succinctly on this need to join with like-minded others: "The less justified a man is in claiming excellence for his own self, the more ready he is to claim all excellence for his nation, his religion, his race, or his holy cause;; (p. 14).

This need to be right is, I believe, deeply ingrained in our psyches, and for that reason very difficult to get at in therapy or supervision. To be sure, it may be part of our inferiority/superiority complexes, but at the same time it has become crucial to our identity and welf-worth, and therefore very hard to look at. Often, then, all our training, analysis, and supervision is merely a mockery; we seek out the program that will confirm our biases and give them a false validity, rather than the program that will challenge us.

The world is full of various viewpoints, prejudices, philosophies, belief systems, ideologies, and religions. These do indeed become issues in the therapy dyad. So, if we in the profession have not overcome our own ethnic and cultural "blindspots" — at least to the extent that we are aware of them — then they can affect the outcome of the therapy to one degree or another.

REFERENCES

Baker, E.F. (1967). *Man in the trap.* New York: Macmillan.

Fromm-Reichman, F. (1950). *Principles of intensive psychotherapy.* Chicago: Phoenix Books (University of Chicago Press).

Greenson, R.R. (1967). *The technique and practice of psychoanalysis* (Vol. 1). New York: International Universities Press.

Hoffer, E. (1963). *The true believer.* New York: Time Incorporated.

Murray, E.J. (1956). "A content-analysis method for studying psychotherapy." *Psychological Monographs,* 70, Whole No. 420.

Robertiello, R.C. (1985). *A psychoanalyst's quest.* New York: St. Martin's/Marek.

C H A P T E R
73

SPIRITUALITY VERSUS POWER: THE ART OF THERAPY AND THE BUSINESS OF PRIVATE PRACTICE

Gerald Schoenewolf, Ph.D.

This is me. I am talking to you. I am a therapist; you are a therapist. We are communicating. Will I be able to communicate to you what I consciously intend to communicate? Will you be able to hear what I consciously intend you to hear? That depends upon many variables: on my mastery of the language; on my mood the day I write this; on my training as a therapist; on my experience as a private practitioner; on my talents, intelligence, perception, and self-knowledge; on intangibles stemming from my unconscious; on your mastery of the language; and on your mood, training, experience, talents, intelligence, perception, self-knowledge, and unconscious intangibles. In more psychoanalytic terms, this communication between us depends upon how successfully I overcome my resistance to communicate clearly and precisely what it is I want to communicate, and on your overcoming your resistance to receiving this communication clearly and precisely as I have intended.

I would like to think there is a science of communication that would ensure that, were I to follow certain principles, I would be successful in this endeavor. However, there are too many intangibles — some conscious and some unconscious — for me to call it a science. It is an art. As with any form of art, there is a degree of subjectivity involved — to claim otherwise would be a folly.

Have I captured your attention so far? If so, I have succeeded in one of my conscious aims. Do you agree or disagree with what I've said so far? If you agree, please keep reading; if you disagree, please leave these pages immediately! (I am joking, of course, and thereby exposing a bit of my own humanity — perhaps even a bit of my own neurosis — in order to break down your resistance.)

Therapy, like written communication, is an art. My success as a therapist also depends upon many variables, both conscious and unconscious. And, in order to overcome both my own and my patients' resistances, I must use many techniques, some scientific, some not. Sometimes I may even use a joke aimed at breaking down a patient's resistance, charming and relaxing the patient so that he or she can hear me better. To be sure, not every patient will appreciate my sense of humor, and sometimes a joke may backfire; this is where the art comes in. In taking the risk to use a joke, in deviating from standard technique, I am becoming an artist. I am attempting to speak from my unconscious to the patient's unconscious. If it works, it may be seen as a brilliant tactic. If it fails, it may be seen as an unfortunate one. It is a calculated risk, based on everything I know and feel at the moment.

There are those in the field who might disagree with me about therapy being an art, those who wish to make it a science. For example, Gertrude and Rubin Blanck (1974) have attempted to make of psychoanalysis a science, with laws and principles that therapists are to follow if they wish to be successful. They define the specific techniques of psychoanalysis as free association, use of the couch, abstinence from any physical or emotional contact with the patient, use of the transference and transference neurosis, frequency of sessions (three or more times a week), use of interpretation and auxiliary tecniques, use of maximum anxiety, use of regression, and use of dream interpretation. They assert that in psychoanalysis infantile gratifications are never in order, and caution gainst the current fads that masquerade as therapy.

However, Freud himself never went so far as to suggest that the technique of psychoanalysis was a science. In one of his papers, he states that while "this technique has proved to be the only method suited to my individuality; I do not venture to deny that a physician quite differently constituted might feel impelled to adopt a different attitude to his patients and to the task before him (Freud, 1912, p. 323).

In another paper, Freud supports lay analysis, suggesting that therapy is not and never will be an aspect of medical science, and in fact might be better served by nonmedical analysts. He did not wish for therapists to be either doctors or priests, but rather lay curers of souls. In essence, what he was suggesting wat that therapists had to be true to themselves: artists. Neither science nor morality, according to him, had any place in psychoanalysis. "Such work as this is spiritual guidance," he says, "in the best sense of the word" (Freud, 1927, p. 211).

I would venture to say that most therapists today would agree with Freud about adapting one's technique to one's constitution; and most would also agree that therapy is an art. There is hardly a conference nowadays in which the word "art" is not used in connection with therapy, be it psychoanalytic therapy or another mode. I do not feel psychoanalysis must be defined the way the Blancks define it, nor that we should disparage out of hand other modes of therapy. What I do is an art: the art of reaching another human being's soul (unconscious), and bringing it out; the art of helping another human being resolve pent-up aggression or aggression that has gone awry; the art of teaching another human being how to love and trust again. Such, I am convinced, is the art of therapy. Like any artist, I must always be open to new discoveries, to spontaneity, to creativity, in the attempt to do whatever I need to do in order to bring about these aims.

In this respect therapy is a spiritual quest, not in the religious but in the humanistic sense. I am interested in achieving oneness, first with myself, then with another person. Martin Buber (1970) , the humanist philosopher, said it best: "In the beginning is the relation" (p. 69). We understand ourselves through our contact with others. When a patient and I achieve oneness, achieve agreement, achieve emotional connectedness and the associated spirit of cooperation, then we begin to truly relate. It is in this relationship that patients begin to understand themselves, their transferences, their resistances; and the ways they defeat themselves, defeat others, and impede their own deepest aims. When all this happens, both of us are gratified spiritually, fulfilled, contented. We feel good about *us* in the most human way. We feel loved, respected, perhaps even cherished. We are spiritually rejuvenated.

Therapy is a spiritual quest in that it is a form of platonic friendship. In this friendship, love can blossom apart from its erotic connections. When I reach patients spiritually (when they share their honest, most vulnerable feelings with me), I also reach myself; and when they reach me they also reach themselves. When we are able to love each other without acting out our erotic feelings, we are able to love one another in the most primary manner. In order to love in an erotic way—and to sustain it—one must first learn to love in a platonic way. But that is saying a lot, because in order to love in a platonic way, one must overcome, as Heinrich Racker (1951) notes, the anxiety and fear of one's disowned self and the hostile means one uses to defend against this anxiety and fear. One must stop splitting, mutililating, denying, annihilating, closing up, and projecting oneself onto the world and then quarreling with it in order to alleviate internal discord, or withdrawing from the world to maintain a semblance of inner peace. There is a long road to travel before patients can attain primary love, and still another long road before they can achieve secondary (erotic) love. The most rich and rewarding relationships, of course, are those that involve both primary and secondary love. This, as the poets have told us, is what makes life worth living.

To travel this road, undertake this spiritual quest, one must be an artist. Each therapeutic relationship is a little different, and each requires us to create anew a method for reching the patient. When I am seated face-to-face with my patient (or, if the patient is lying on the couch, seated behind him or her), I am no longer thinking of psychoanalytic technique. I am just traveling the patient's road with him or her, and doing and saying whatever I think I need to do or say at any particular time to help the patient along. If I am to help the patient reach his or her own most sensitive places, I must be in touch with my own. If I want the patient to share his or her aggressiveness, I may have to share some of my own. We are a team, and together we undertake the spiritual quest and make art, the art of relating in a true way.

This is what impelled me to be a therapist, this spiritual quest. This is what makes me get up in the morning looking forward to another day of work. This is what fuels me as a human being. This is what gratifies me in the deepest, most human sense.

And yet, and yet...there is another aspect to therapy, the business aspect, especially for those of us in private practice. We need to make money—enough money to feel comfortable and to take care of loved ones. Some of us want to be more than comfortable; some of us want to be rich and to have the power that lots of money can bring. The questions then arise: What happens when art meets commerce? What happens when spirituality comes into conflict with power? Each therapist who is in private practice has to answer these questions in his or her own way.

Being in private practice is a way of making a living. It can also be a way of making a pretty good living if you work it right. But there is always the difficulty in balancing the art of therapy with the business of therapy, making sure one does not overwhelm the other. If I concentrate too much of my attention on being an artist and forget about the business side of it, I may not collect enough money in fees to pay the rent. On the other hand, if I pay too much attention to the business aspect, perhaps out of a need to be very secure or very powerful, then I may end up without a "soul."

Then there is also the matter of how this art/business polarity affects my patients. "You don't really care about me," one told me last week. "You're just in it for the money."

"But I *said* I care about you."

"I know, but I don't believe you."

She was a young woman in her late 20s typical of many of my patients — distrustful of authority figures, emotionally frozen, unable to take in positive feedback, unwilling to take down the armor. "You're just saying that because you're a therapist and you're trying to get me to open up. But you don't really care. How can somebody charge $70 an hour to listen to another person, and then say he cares? You're just doing your job, that's all."

I attempted to reason with her. "How many doctors have you had dealings with in your life?"

"Why?"

"Are they all the same?"

"No."

"Are they all equally competent?"

"No."

"Do they all have equally wonderful professional manners?"

"Of course not."

"And do they all care equally about you? Or do some care more than others?"

"Some care more than others."

"Yet they all charge money."

"I see what you're saying."

"And where do I fall in this spectrum of doctors? Am I one of the caring ones, or one of the ones who don't care?"

"You seem to be one of the caring ones."

"Then can you accept that I really care about you, even though I charge a fee?"

"In principle. I mean, I think you're a caring doctor. But I think you do it because you get paid to do it."

"I see." I thought for a moment and decided on a different approach. "How do you think I feel about you?"

"Honestly?" She smirked with embarrassment. "To tell you the truth, I think I could be anybody to you. As long as I pay you the $70 each week, you care about me. But I still remember that session when I forgot my money, and we spent the whole session analyzing my resistance. You didn't seem very caring that day."

I continued to work with this patient, and eventually over a period of time I was able to steer her toward analyzing her defense against taking in positive feelings from me. In her case, it could be traced back to a relationship with her mother. Her mother had used her "love" to manipulate her. That was the transference resistance aspect of her hesitancy to accept my caring as real.

However, for my part of it, was there any reality in her perception of me as somebody who was only in it for the money?

To be sure, were she not in therapy with me, I doubt if I would have cared about her, for she was not somebody I would have sought out for friendship. (Some of my patients *are* people I would seek out for friendship, and those are usually the ones I work best with.) So, the fact that this patient paid me $70 an hour certainly contributed to my caring about her. This points up one of the ways the business end of therapy can intrude on the art end of it.

I have known therapists who have said they care more about patients who pay high fees than those who pay low fees. Other therapists have reported that they want to earn enough money so that they can turn down difficult patients in favor of those easy to work with. (The difficult patients frequently pay the lowest fees and are, at the same time, the most needful of therapy.) Some therapists, in an effort to make as much money as possible, will pack their patients one on top of another, doing 12 to 15 sessions a day, giving themselves few or no breaks. I knew one therapist who would eat during sessions in order to save time. Other therapists will give patients extra time in order to compensate for feelings of guilt about earning money through "helping" people.

Of course, the whole area of money is laden with symbolic meaning. One therapist may have a narcissistic need to prove to himself and to his patient that he is a valuable person (he charges the highest fee possible); another may have a narcissistic need to prove she is a generous, giving person (charging low fees); another may have an oral need to be fed by the patient; while yet another may have an anal need to horde; and so forth. When the business end of therapy gets out of hand and in some way adversely affects the therapeutic relationship, it is usually because of a neurotic attitude about money and power.

It is healthy to want money and the power it brings if the desire is used to free yourself; that is, if it is used to actualize your potential as a human being, not to yourself or to put up walls between yourself and others, but to have more time to love and be loved, and to create possibilities for self-expansion in human terms. In other words, it is not necessarily unhealthy or neurotic for a therapist to want to make a lot of money; it depends on the therapist's underlying motivation. And it may be equally unhealthy for a therapist to remain relatively poor, refusing to raise fees out of some principle rooted in narcissism. And, in either situation it may be harmful to patients.

I used to be afraid of raising patients' fees. Sometimes I told msyelf it was because they had been with me since the early days and I was obliged to be loyal to them. Sometimes I did not believe they could afford it. Sometimes I was afraid they would leave therapy if I raised their fee. After a time I realized I was not raising their fees in order to spare myself a confrontation, and I was actually doing a disservice to them by keeping the fees low.

For example, a patient who had been with me for many years used to complain continually about not having enough money to pay for her rent, her art supplies, her school loans, and other miscellaneous expenses. At the same time, she could not tolerate a permanent job, so she always did temporary work through agencies and her earnings were sporadic. She had originally come to me through a low-cost therapy clinic, and I had kept her fee as low as possible years aftert she had followed me into private practice. I thought

I was doing her a favor, but I was not. Her therapy crept slowly along. Although she did not complain directly about not making progress, every now and then she would whine (she did a lot of whining) about not being able to get in touch with her rage, which she suspected was considerable. Eventually I figured out how to help her get in touch with her rage; I raised her fee. By then I had grown enough as a therapist to be able to tolerate her rage. It was when she went through several weeks of lambasting me for raising the fee that she had her most meaningful breakthrough.

Aside from the Faustian aspect of the conflict between spirituality and power as it applies to private practice, there is also the practical aspect. There is the day-to-day maintenance of one's practice: networking for referrals, making key conferences and perhaps presenting papers at them in order to keep one's name in the light, advertising in respectable ways, maintaining suitable office space, paying bills, raising fees, and the like. Sometimes, as for example in summer months, one's practice may suddenly dip and one can at those moments begin to panic; then art goes out the window. What if all my patients suddenly take off? The anxiety of knowing that one's patient load is transitory can at times be large. And it can interfere with the way we do therapy—cause us to react in insecure ways to patients who, for example, come in saying they're not getting anything out of therapy and are considering quitting.

When therapists speak of being "burned out,' it is often due, I believe, to this conflict between spirituality and power, between art and business (between the id and the superego?). Therapists can no longer enjoy their work when they are no longer meaningfully connected to it on a spiritual level. At that point, patients sometimes become "work objects" and the therapy dyad loses its potential for emotional realness. And, also at that point, therapists are more likely to practice a form of "wild analysis," a term that Freud (1910) used to describe doctors who practice a brand of psychoanalysis that makes a mockery of sound therapeutic procedure. They start pressing instead of coming from their center.

Because of the human factor of psychotherapy, this particular means of livelihood is a bit different from any other form of business. Patients are somewhat justified in feeling that if we really cared about them we wouldn't charge fees; after all, is that not the way Mother Theresa does it? Many of us ask ourselves this same question throughout our training, perhaps throughout our career. Ours is the only business in which one is required to have a personal relationship with the client; in all others a personal relationship is to be avoided. We are surrogate parents to the misparented; but unlike real parents, we charge fees, sometimes exorbitant fees. We are curers of souls; yet we demand a "ransom" for our services. There is a built-in conflict of interests here, one that each of us has to solve, for himself or herself.

This gets us back to the balancing act I alluded to before. A successful private practice is a balancing act between art and business. It is a compromise between our need for inner gratification and outer security—that is, between spirituality and power. Sometimes it also entails a struggle between the healthy and unhealthy forces inside us, in which case it becomes a matter of counter-transference or counterresistance. At any rate, it is an art and a business unlike any other, and one that calls for a special kind of versatility.

Have I gotten my message across? Have I communicated to you what I have intended to communicate? I do not know; nor can you know—unless we meet and discuss it. This is definitely not a scientific treatise. Perhaps the Blancks can write scientific treatises, and perhaps they can practice the science of therapy. It may be that their particular constitutions require such an approach. My constitution requires a subjective approach. It requires the recognition that I am human, equipped with an unconscious over which I do not now and never will have complete control. If I have succeeded in getting my message across, then I will consider it both a matter of expertise and luck. I will consider it a work of art.

REFERENCES

Blanck, G. & Blanck, R. (1974). *Ego psychology: Theory and practice.* New York: Columbia University Press.

Buber, M. (1970). *I and thou.* New York: Charles Scribner's Sons.

Freud, S. (1910). Observations on wild psychoanalysis. *Collected papers* (Vol. 2). New York: Basic Books, 1959, pp. 297–304.

Freud, S. (1912). Recommendations for physicians on the psychoanalytic method of treatment. *Collected papers* (Vol. 2). New York: Basic Books, 1970, pp. 323–333.

Freud, S. (1927). Postscript to a dicsussion on lay analysis. *Collected papers.* (Vol. 5). New York: Basic Books, 1970, pp. 205–214.

Racker, H. (1951). *Transference and countertransference.* New York: International Universities Press.

74

TRENDS IN TECHNIQUE

Diana Cort, C.S.W.

For the past 17 years I have been an administrator of a large psychiatric outpatient clinic. During that time I have also maintained a private practice for psychotherapy. During the past 10 years, as part of my administrative duties, I have reviewed and read files of approximately 10,000 patients. I have seen many changes in the population and the needs and wants of the population that presents itself for psychotherapeutic intervention.

The acceptance of the need for psychological help has changed considerably. At one time patients saw treatment as a luxury, feeling they had untapped potential for richer, fuller lives. They wanted growth in terms of their senses and their emotions. In the past 5 to 10 years, as the costs of mental health care have soared, people seeking the services of a mental health professional have been much more interested in changing an aspect of their personal functioning and interpersonal relationships. Usually something is interfering with their social relationships; marriage, job performance, or relationships within the family structure. Most patients come for psychological help for specific issues. Many of them are conversant with the kind of treatment they want and seek a therapist with the hope that they will be given what they are specifically asking for. The following are the major areas of current concern.

ALCOHOL ABUSE

It would be difficult to be in the field of mental health and not be aware of the increasing incidence of alcohol and drug abuse as a major health problem. We have been besieged by statistics as to the ways in which alcohol abuse costs the nation billions of dollars every year. These statistics have had a huge impact on the individual practitioner.

Many alcoholics are referred by their employers, who are becoming educated about the disease of alcoholism. Many alcoholics are mandated for treatment by the court after they have been arrested for driving while intoxicated. Less frequently alcoholics refer themselves for treatment.

The practitioner must be conversant with the ramifications of alcoholism and must be able to differentiate between a patient who needs treatment for alcoholism and a patient who needs psychiatric hospitalization. The therapist should be able to assess the need for detoxification, and be familiar with detoxification centers. Upon patients' release from these centers, they will be referred to Alcoholics Anonymous. Patients may at this time refer themselves back to their private practitioner.

The number of patients in a private practice who are husbands, wives, or children of alcoholics has increased tremendously. Private practitioners are referring their patients to AA as well as making referrals to Alanon and groups for adult children of alcoholics. Referrals to these groups are made in order to provide support for the patients.

Any discussion of alcohol abuse must include the problem of adolescent alcohol and drug abuse. Nearly one-third of all high school students have experienced at least one serious negative consequence resulting from alcohol or drug misuse. Therapists are being asked to recognize the problem and then understand the personal, familial, and societal dynamics of the abuser.

EATING DISORDERS

Patients who have eating disorders have become an increasing concern in psychotherapy. These patients are usually women whose diagnosis of bulimia or anorexia nervosa has been made by a medical doctor. However, in the past 5 years there has been an increase of self-referrals. Many women with these life-threatening illnesses are unaware of the gravity of their illness. Close consultation with a psychiatrist is often necessary, and hospitalization, particularly in the treatment of anorexia nervosa, is not unusual.

These patients have been extremely difficult to treat, but group therapy with other patients who also have eating disorders has been successful. Cognitive treatment, with behavior modification techniques, has also been successful. Family therapy is another intervention that has been successful and is essential, particularly in the treatment of adolescents.

WOMEN'S ISSUES

Women today are faced with new challenges in nearly every area of their lives. Their self-concept has undergone profound changes, and they are confronted with new problems, concerns, and anxieties.

Women's issues have therefore come to the foreground in the practice of psychotherapy. With the success of women's consciousness raising groups in the 1960s and 1970s, the idea that people with similar difficulties can obtain comfort and support from each other proved to be effective. Women's groups, most often led by women, have been organized around the categories and issues that follow: women who love too much, the biological clock, older women who have children, midlife crisis, menopausal women, young widows, sexually abused women, battered woman, and victims of incest.

Female patients are requesting female therapists to be the leaders of these groups feeling that women resonate in a particular way with each other. Women are questioning male therapists as to their feelings about the feminist movement and may not be satisfied by a male therapist's saying he is a feminist. (Many women believe that the philosophy of feminism comes from the female experience, and they are not sure that men can learn that experience. Some women feel that to be a feminist one must be engaged in a political struggle, and do not see men as engaged in that struggle.)

AGING

As many more people are living to old age, therapy with elderly people has become a new specialty. As a culture we have become more versatile with the problems of aging. The extension of life of good quality has become a major focus. Older people come for treatment to find ways of coping with inner changes and outer circumstances. Frequently the onset of aging triggers long-standing problems with which individuals now have less ability to cope. The consequences of aging and the reality of death are issues with which the elderly are coping continually.

The elderly person often seeks an older therapist. The needs and rights of the elderly to maintain control over their lives have been championed by the elderly population and may, in many ways, best be understood by the older therapist.

Many older people seek treatment after the death of a spouse. The best adjustment for the loss comes in a good social support structure, and the formation of support groups is an excellent way to help people through this life crisis.

THERAPY FOR CHILDREN

There has been an increase in the number of parents presenting their adolescent children for treatment. Social turmoil and the lessening of the family as a support network have led to many disturbed family structures. Parents are bewildered as to how to cope with their feelings of ineffectiveness. The fact that the incidence of suicide in teenagers has nearly tripled over the past 10 years has created tremendous anxiety for parents.

Many more parents are now asking to be involved in the treatment of their adolescent children, and family therapy has become the treatment of choice for many adolescents. The orthodox family systems approach has had many modifications in the past 5 to 10 years. Families are seen in treatment as a unit, but individual family members are also seen individually on an as-needed basis.

One in eight children suffers from a mental health problem severe enough to require treatment, and parents and teachers are better educated now than they were previously to diagnose the need for psychological intervention. Many more children are now being referred for treatment by their schools.

One of the most important new trends is referrals for the evaluation of a learning disability. Learning disabilities now include many developmental difficulties, such as auditory processing impairment. Parents are now more aware of the possibility that their child may have learning difficulties and are following through on school referrals. Parents are being helped to understand that neurological impairment has a psychological impact on the development of their child. Parents are looking for practitioners who are able to both tutor and understand the psychological aspects of the neurological impairment.

SHORT-TERM PSYCHOTHERAPY

Many people feel the need for some intervention when a crisis occurs in their lives. These are usually well-functioning individuals who suddenly find themselves unable to cope. Events that might lead up to this crisis include a tragic accident involving a loved one, diagnosis of a life-threatening illness, or a spouse's announcing he or she intends to leave the marriage.

These patients are usually not interested in long-term psychotherapy. They can best be helped by short-term interventions based on psychodynamic understanding, cognitive behavioral techniques, and parameters that assess the time in which former functioning can be restored. Occasionally these individuals may become long-term patients, but more often, once the crisis is over, they are able to return to their former functioning. Short-term interventions have been successful with children and adolescents. Short-term therapy is a modality that deserves more attention. People are now less interested in the commitment of long-term treatment than they once were.

SUPPORT GROUPS

The popularity of support groups for people wo share specific problems has increased. Many patients start therapy asking to be seen individually, and then realize that a group could be of greater help to them. Groups have been formed around the following problems: surviving the break-up (for the recently divorced); help for step parents; coping with elderly parents; drugs in our culture (for parents of adolescent children); and suffering from life-threatening illnesses (cancer patients being a segment of the population that will need ongoing support, not always provided by medical doctors or hospitals).

STRESS MANAGEMENT

Many patients come for treatment because they are experiencing stress and have various symptoms of general anxiety, headaches, insomnia, and tension. Frequently, these patients are referred by their family doctor after a physical examination has been negative. Their doctor usually refers them for behavior therapy.

There are many stress-reducing modalities that have become popular for patients suffering from anxiety. There is biofeedback, to teach patients the self-regulation of physiological functioning. Biofeedback technology can provide information about normally unnoticed physiologic reactions. Many people respond to their psychological state through their cardiovascular, musculoskeletal, and gastrointestinal systems. Cardiovascular and muscular systems will most readily lend themselves to biofeedback intervention.

The use of behavior modification for weight loss, quitting smoking, and phobias has become increasingly popular for helping people change these behaviors.

PSYCHIATRIC REFERRALS

Many more therapists are being confronted these days with patients who not only feel they could benefit from a referral to a psychiatrist for pharmacological treatment but also have accurately diagnosed their condition themselves.

Current treatment for depression includes antidepressants. There has been much evidence relating psychological stress to sudden unexplained experiences of acute anxiety. A clinical assessment needs to be made by the therapist before a patient is referred to a psychiatrist. The psychiatrist is dependent upon the therapist's assessment, which usually includes a current mental status, psychosocial history, presenting problems, and medical and drug treatment history. After the referral has been made and the patient has been started on a course of medication, the therapist will be responsible for monitoring negative drug reactions because the therapist will see the patient more frequently than the psychiatrist will. The therapist needs to be aware of the side effects of various drugs and should consider owning a *Physician's Desk Reference.* Therapists are increasingly less opposed to drug therapy. Although many therapists feel their treatment should be enough, more and more are accepting the benefits of pharmacological therapy and this helps them to make a more professional referral.

FAMILY THERAPY

As we have become aware of the importance of keeping the nuclear family functional and as increases in personal stress have led to increases in family stress, family thereapy has become a popular alternative treatment method. Frequently a dysfunctional family member will be taken for treatment first. However, upon exploration, this "identified patient" will be diagnosed as a symptom of the family's distress.

Although there are at least four methodologies of family therapy—the cognition model, the communications model, the family behavior model, and the general systems model—they all have the same goal of making families functional by maintaining the integrity of the family. In treating families, the therapist needs to be able to make both a diagnostic assessment and a dynamic formulation in order that a modality can be utilized that will be most helpful to the family. The therapist should be conversant with an integrative and flexible approach to family therapy.

The concurrent use of family and individual therapy is often indicated in treating a family. This is particularly so in the treatment of very disturbed families. Family therapy has been successfully used in the treatment of incest and child abuse and with families of alcoholics.

The goals for family therapy involve the strengthening of the problem-solving and adaptive functioning of the family rather than the creation of a problem-free situation. Family therapy tries to mobilize the already existing mechanisms that have allowed the family to be successful. Treatment is often short-term and is often contracted to be for a certain number of sessions. Often at the end of the contracted time a family member other than the identified patient will stay on as an individual patient.

HYPNOSIS

Hypnosis remains a popular modality of psychotherapeutic intervention. When so much of our lives may appear to be out of our control, hypnosis offers us the feeling that we can be in charge of our lives and that our minds can work for us rather than against us. People are drawn to hypnosis because it is a technique that promises to change behavior simply and painlessly. All it asks is the motivation to change.

Individuals can decide whether they will feel happy or sad. Those who are habitually depressed, disorganized, or evasive can change these personality habits. All patients need to do is to face the problem and take some action. The feeling that they can do something with their mind to change behavior is extremely persuasive, and patients look to hypnosis for change and exploration of their problems.

Hypnosis has been used successfully in helping people to give up smoking and control their eating. It has also been used successfully in helping people to deal with fear of success; procrastination habits; self-pity habits; alcohol abuse; and various physical difficulties, especially those associated with pain (e.g., headache, arthritis, hypertension). Also, relaxation techniques, an aspect of hypnosis, have been used effectively, sometimes resulting in the boon of reduced medication.

Most hypnosis is short-term treatment and is seen as an ego-strengthening modality. The new Ericksonian method of hypnosis has become extremely popular as it assumes that people with the motivation to learn a new way of "thinking" can succeed in changing. This way of thinking is seen as a skill that can be learned with the proper guidance, if the patient is properly motivated.

VIETNAM VETERANS

In the years since the end of the Vietnam War, the psychological and social problems of the Vietnam veterans have permeated American life. Many veterans came home from the war in despair, feeling detached from their families and their world. Primarily they were very angry. Vietnam veterans had a high incidence of alcoholism, drug abuse, depression, and anxiety. They suffered from decreased interest in life, low self-esteem, and feelings of estrangement. They had few social sanctions and little reentry support to help them reorganize their lives. These veterans had had a devastating assault to their psychic strucures and have continued to face a number of therapeutic problems that have not been easy to resolve.

The use of the diagnosis post-traumatic stress disorder from the third edition of the *Diagnostic and Statistical Manual of Mental Disorders* has made it easier for the mental health professional to define the Vietnam veteran's problem and thus find ways to help him. The treatment modality that has been found to be the most effective is group therapy. The leader need not be a veteran, but must be knowledgeable concerning the ramifications of treating patients with post-traumatic stress disorders. Tretment that focuses on the relief of guilt and rage in order that the positive and productive parts of the veteran's character can function has been found to be most successful.

C H A P T E R
75

SELF-ASSESSMENT, BUSINESS ACUMEN, AND PERSONALITY

Minna Marder Genn, Ed.M.

A therapist beginning a private practice needs to assess his strengths and weaknesses, relative competence, business acumen, etc. For the therapist in private practice is obviously a one-person operation and everything he is, as a person, is going to have a bearing on the practice.

Starting a private practice, needless to say, calls for something more than opening an office and sending out announcement cards. Sitting and waiting for patients to come will obviously not work.

The obvious major question is: How does one go about getting patients? The therapist has presumably been in an internship or has worked in an institutional setting. In this case, the therapist will start with a small core of patients taken from that setting. Perhaps there are some colleagues who are finishing an internship and who are not going to remain in the same area. They could possibly be solicited for referrals. Obviously, a certain degree of marketing will have to be done.

The therapist must choose the methods that will work best according to his or her personality. If the therapist is outgoing and feels comfortable speaking in front of groups, he will seek opportunities to speak before clubs or church or synagogue groups. He might offer to give classes in adult education. If there is some special topic about which the therapist feels particularly knowledgeable, he might advertise and offer a parent workshop or a group workshop dealing particularly with that topic. Some topics might include: single working parents; elderly parents living with their adult children; rebellious adolescents; substance abuse.

The shy person or the person not adept at public speaking might write a column for a local newspaper or offer to serve on a "hot line" for crisis intervention.

It is a common practice to send out announcement cards when one opens an office. How much business is generated from that is questionable. On the other hand, a letter that describes one's background and one's special areas of expertise sent to professional people in the locale is a more focused kind of announcement. Calling on some of the professional people in the area could help also.

The therapist should have a business-like attitude about his fees. If he knows he does not handle bookkeeping details well, he may have to delegate the handling of them to an assistant. Assuming that the training meets certain expected standards and that one has the appropriate credentials, the fee one charges would be influenced by a number of factors. Much depends on how one assesses oneself and one's competence.

There are three factors which should be considered in setting your fees. Of course, one of these is what the prevailing rate tends to be. It seems that the fee in the cities, especially those where there are big teaching centers, tends to be higher than in the suburbs. A second important factor has to do with the extensiveness of one's training. Someone with a master's degree and possibly just a year or two of supervised experience will probably not be able to command the highest fees. The M.D. with a two- or three-year residency and the Ph.D. with several years of post-doctoral supervised experience will command higher fees. The years one has been in practice is a factor in determining fees. A person who has been in practice 20 years or more is likely to be expecting a top fee. The highest fees, deservedly so, are charged by those with many, many years of experience who also teach and supervise others.

The therapist should try to set the fee at the end of the first session. The patient deserves the structure and comfort derived from knowing what his obligations are. Of course, if the patient does not know whether he has insurance which will cover his therapy, or what percentage the insurance will pay, the decision regarding the fee will have to be delayed.

The therapist might want to have a flexible fee schedule if he wants to build a practice. He might have a top fee in mind that he would charge to people with a great income or people who have insurance policies that pay 80 percent of the fee. Many insurance companies pay less. Firms or unions who have their own in-house insurance arrangements will sometimes have quite arbitrary restrictions on what percentage they will pay or which practitioners they will cover. The flexibility in the fees would then be downward, for example, for students who might be on their own, for individuals with low incomes, or for families who have many medical expenses or who have several people in therapy. Once the fee is settled, if it is low, there should be no reservation, needless to say, in the therapist's commitment to the patient.

Like others, this writer bills once a month. If the balances are accumulating, the reason for this should be explored at the end of the session, not at the beginning, for one would not wish the topic of money to get in the way of the main business of the session. If there is no financial reason for the delay in payment, this writer is likely to press rather firmly. If there is a financial reason for the delay in payment, this writer will suggest that the patient pay for each session plus an additional set amount on the balance. This system has worked quite well.

If the patient has been in therapy for some time and the therapist's typical fee has gone up from the time the patient entered therapy, the therapist might wish to raise that patient's fee, assuming that the individual can afford the increase. It is not totally necessary for the lower fee to be locked in place. The possibility of an increase can be broached. Some patients will see the increase as reasonable. Others might be unhappy and even angry. At all costs, the patient's feelings must be respected, even if the reaction is unreasonable. For, of course, what is important is that the therapy should continue. Dealing with the unreasonableness must wait for an appropriate time, and that would be when this kind of unreasonableness is being dealt with in the therapy regarding other issues.

This writer feels that she deserves whatever the maximum fee would be for her length of experience because of her own assessment of herself as a therapist. The writer experiences a continuous concern for each patient. The writer spends time outside of the therapy hour assessing the progress, reviewing her notes, and generally not taking the patient for granted. One should make it a point to remember names and events. One should be honest and admit if one does not remember something. One should be on time and give the patient every minute of his assigned session. The therapist ought to be able to assess within himself whether he is doing a good job. After all, he is the more experienced, more sophisticated judge than his patients. The therapist must "bake his own cake"; the compliment from the patient is just the frosting.

If a patient wishes to change the time of the therapy session or sessions, this writer will make some effort to accommodate the patient. On the other hand, if the therapist would find a change convenient and the patient does not find it so, the therapist should respect the patient's need. A "contract" of a kind has been made with the patient regarding the time of his or her appointment and it should be respected.

This writer asks patients to call early in the morning if an appointment needs to be cancelled because of illness or some other difficulty about coming in. If the reason for not calling early is sheer carelessness, like not waking up on time or forgetting to call, this writer is likely to charge for the time. Sometimes the carelessness is part of a destructive pattern or characterological problem that is being worked on in the therapy. There could be a patient who might see the charge as punitive and the issue is something that is not timely in the current phase of the therapy; then the therapist might not charge for the session, but would remind the patient to cooperate. If a cancellation occurs late in the day because of a bad storm or a car breakdown, this writer will not charge for the session.

This writer wants to give her patients the feeling that she can be reached between sessions, especially if a beginning patient is in a crisis situation. The writer will tell such patients that they can have five minutes "on the house," if she is free and can talk. She will also tell patients that if the talk is longer and takes up a recognizable fraction of a session, the patient will be charged for an appropriate fraction of the session. This writer has hardly ever experienced an abuse of this arrangement. After the first few weeks, the calls generally cease. Some borderline patients will continue to call; this writer feels that some of these patients need this kind of continuous connection and therefore will accept the calls.

Many therapists do not take calls during a session. If the therapist prefers to function this way, several spaces should be left during the day to pick up messages. If the therapist picks up his messages at the end of the day, it may by then be impossible to reach the patient. This writer finds it easier to answer the telephone and respond with one phrase or sentence. If the patient needs more time than the 15 or 30 seconds that this kind of response takes, arrangements are made to talk another time. Needless to say, a patient might resent the interruption of the session. This writer has had two or three patients who resented the interruption; she has then not taken calls during that session.

Needless to say, the patient sustaining the interruption knows that he or she can telephone and get a quick response.

This writer feels it is very important to assess what is happening if the therapy bogs down. It there resistance? Is there a negative transference? Or is it that the therapist is missing something? Has the diagnosis been wrong? Or is he using the wrong approach? After thinking through all of these possibilities and still not arriving at an answer, the therapist will want to check on himself. Perhaps he will take his notes to a colleague he trusts and respects in order to obtain an objective view. Sometimes it might be good to suggest to the patient to see the colleague for a second opinion.

Some therapists are prone to have a particular occupational disease and that disease is narcissism. It is not too hard to feel grandiose when patients attribute God-like powers to the therapist. It is important to have assessed oneself and to know one's strengths and weaknesses. What are the therapist's strengths and how can these be used maximally? Is there any risk in using them? If the therapist is warm, friendly and outgoing, he could do a more interpersonal kind of psychotherapy. He could allow himself to be real. But then he must guard against a transference which is not seen objectively by the therapist. The truly friendly therapist possibly will have to guard against giving too much, interfering too much and perhaps making the patient too dependent on him. If the therapist tends to be cold or emotionally distant, he will want to practice in a more orthodox psychoanalytic way. Either way, one should not need adulation or compliments from the patients.

If the therapist adheres strictly to the orthodox psychoanalytic model, he will remain totally impersonal. He will present a "tabula rasa," a clean slate on which the patient can write anything he wants. That is, he transfers any feelings he has onto the therapist. The idea has been that if the therapist had any definition in his personality style, the patient would be blocked about transferring his unconscious attitudes and feelings onto the therapist. In more recent years, many therapists have come to feel that the patient will create whatever transference he needs, regardless of what the therapist presents. Those therapists who practice a less orthodox kind of psychotherapy find that there is some advantage in being more real, even in revealing some of one's own past problems that have been worked through. The patient might then feel that he has a model he could incorporate. Of course, the therapist in offering his real self must guard against creating a symbiosis or too great a dependency. This writer in over 30 years of practice has been fairly real with patients and has not found this method to hinder the therapy.

Accordingly, there are certain types of events in the lives of patients at which the therapist could be present. If there is some major occasion which is a milestone in the life of the patient, the therapist might want to acknowledge that with his presence. This writer is perfectly comfortable going to a gallery opening for a patient who is an artist, or to a play in which a patient is appearing, or to a wedding ceremony. This writer, in such a situation, would not want to identify her true relationship to the patient unless the patient wished it. This writer stopped briefly at a patient's sweet sixteen party and suggested that she be identified as the patient's great-aunt. The writer sends gifts, or flowers, or notes regarding such special occasions. A patient who has to be hospitalized for surgery or for some organic illness might appreciate a visit from the therapist. The writer might give teen-age patients birthday gifts.

Presumably some therapists can handle socializing with patients on a one-to-one basis. This writer would find it difficlt to do this, except with a borderline patient. With the latter, this writer can remain mostly in the role of the therapist. With other patients, this writer would find it a little strained and would have difficulty knowing which "hat' she is wearing, the hat of the friend or the hat of the professional.

Sometimes a patient will want to end the therapy and in the therapist's view the patient is not really finished with therapy. First, one must make sure that there are still issues to be worked on and that successful work can be done. The therapist would be ill-advised to hold onto a patient when the patient has gone as far as he or she can go. Sometimes there is a tendency to regard certain patients' ongoing therapy as a kind of annuity for the therapist. Needless to say, the therapist will try to explore the reason for stopping therapy. Sometimes the reasons are valid; sometimes they are not. One hears on occasion of therapists who become angry in such situations or who utter dire warnings. The therapist should be gracious, if the patient seems adamant. Sometimes the patient wants to terminate on the telephone and refuses to come in, even for a "wrap-up" session. Such a patient might fear he will be trapped into remaining in therapy when he really does not want to. In the writer's opinion, it works best to be gracious and to avoid coercion. The patient will then perceive the therapist as reasonable, as noncontrolling and is thus more likely to return to therapy.

In sum, if one works hard, if one respects the patient, if one truly works toward a therapeutic goal, the patient will make progress and, for the therapist, being in private practice will be gratifying and challenging.

76

DOING STRESS MANAGEMENT AS A PRIVATE PRACTITIONER

Esther Siegel, Ed.D., R.N., Ed.M.

I n the past decade, stress and its management have become voguish themes — one might say too voguish. The problem with fashionable concepts and their related buzz words is paradoxical. Repeated emphasis points to and reflects concern while simultaneously diminishing importance by overusage.

As a word, "stress" has assumed lexical significance. It depicts concept, experience, and response. Unfortunately, the tendency is to view it exclusively in terms of its negative effects, thus negating positive aspects that Selye (1977) termed "the spice of life." The reality is that stress is both ubiquitous and manageable. First it is necessary to understand it as a concept; second, to recognize it as process; and third, to learn and then apply specific strategies and methods to prevent, reduce, or alleviate its effects, whichever is applicable.

All three steps are essentially cognitive ones. The first two mentioned — understanding and recognition — require an ability to objectively examine the stimulus and then subjectively become conscious of its impact. The third step naturally follows in the form of a tailormade prescription for stress management — one that takes into account personal style and reaction.

This chapter will provide the reader with background material on stress as concept and stress as process. What stress is and what it is not will be discussed. A brief review of related literature will be offered. The use of stress management strategies and techniques will be presented within the context of a private practice both for individual clients and for groups. The difference between stress management and crisis intervention will be discussed. Description of the kinds of stress management programs that can be effectively established in the work setting will be presented. The focus will be on the general kind of program; this will be followed by a presentation of a specifically designed program conceived and implemented by the author for a department of nursing in a large urban medical center. Case material will be offered for explication of material.

THE STRESS RESPONSE: WHAT IT IS, WHAT IT IS NOT

Since stress is a word that is frequently overused and misunderstood, let us begin by defining it. Hans Selye, whose name has become synonymous with stress-related research, defined it in both simple and abstract terms. Simply stated, stress can be seen as the rate of wear and tear upon the body and as a nonspecific response of the body to any demand made upon it (Selye, 1974, 1976).

A basic paradigm for the physiological effects of stress upon the body is as follows:

1. An event occurs or is anticipated—it can be almost anything. Since the experience of stress is a highly subjective one, the variation of triggering events is as varied as the individuals involved.

2. Negative evaluations are formed about one's ability to cope with the event. The perceived threat may be real or imagined. Self-esteem is threatened, with concomitant pressure felt to alleviate the threat.

3. Negative self-talk produces emotions that can be painful, such as anxiety, frustration, aggression, fear, and anger.

4. The brain receives the signal that sets off a series of physiological changes to summon the body's resources to meet the danger. This is termed the general adaptation syndrom, or GAS. As outlined by Selye, this is the body's response to handling stressors by seeking out and calling into action the most appropriate channel of defense.

5. Adrenalin and other hormones are released, which results in increased heart rate and blood pressure. Stored sugar enters the blood stream, with increased blood flow to the limbs. Muscles tense in readiness for action.

The above represents a basic outline of the adaptation response. What has been termed an adrenalin jolt is an extremely effective and protective mechanism for the handling of actual danger. It goes awry, however, when activated in response to day-to-day stressors.

It should be noted that not all physiological responses are this extreme, nor do they inevitably lead to pathology. The potential for pathogenesis exists, however, and is more likely in response to chronic stress. The terms "acute," "intermediate," and "chronic" characterize the time course of a stress response. Acute stress reactions are marked in minutes, hours, or days. Signs and symptoms are related to the activated nervous and endocrine systems, although other organ systems may be involved. Intermediate stress may extend over days and weeks. Signs and symptoms may become varied and include those related to organ systems, and there is sufficient definition of response to be designated a syndrome. Chronic stress extends into months and years, causing marked strain on the body systems sufficient to indicate frank pathology (Jacobson, 1983).

Now let us examine what stress is *not*. According to Selye, it is not merely nervous tension. While emotional stimuli rank high in activating a stress response, it should be noted conversely that lower animal forms and even plants without nervous systems reflect the effects of stress (Selye, 1974).

Stress is not always a nonspecific result of or cause of damage. This becomes apparent when one looks at the wide array of activities that can serve as stressors without necessarily causing or resulting from damage. One has merely to be present at any celebratory event that marks a rite of passage to note the increased stress and tension levels and the adaptive capacities that are invoked responsively.

Finally stress is not something to be avoided. While this last statement may seem to be self-evident, it is an important one upon which to reflect. Since a total absence of stress is equivalent to death, it follows that goal setting regarding stress levels should aim at reduction and titration rather than elimination. The determination of what constitutes acceptable and manageable, while at the same time productive, stress levels is important and can be arrived upon by individual exploration, reflection, and decision.

In the basic language of stress, the fight or flight mechanisms coupled with adaptive and defensive reactions can be applied to all areas of response. Since neither fighting nor fleeing provides practical solutions for most stressful situations, it is necessary to sort out which events require yet another approach — one of adaptation rather than defense. One may argue that any gradation or alterante response on the flight/fight continuum represents a form of adaptation that becomes, in effect, the sine qua non in a complex social structure. Obviously an employee who is reprimanded by a manager has learned alternatives to either walking off in a huff or engaging in a battle royal on the spot. What will most likely occur is the employee will exercise some control against the wish to engage in battle or free from it.

While self-control is not to be eschewed — quite the contrary, it is necessary and desirable — it should be recognized that symptoms of chronic stress are frequently associated with stimulus (stressor), response (defense), and control (internal response). The writer advocates not a lessening of self-control, but rather a reduction in kind and number of issues that are perceived as stressors. Selye (1974) descried an alternative mechanism that he termed "syntoxic." Implied by this is a passive tolerance toward stimuli: a tolerance that permits a kind of peaceful coexistence with specific stressors. This will be talked about further in relationship to the brief review of the literature that follows.

MIND BODY RESPONSE: SELECTED LITERATURE

The literature on stress management is already vast and rapidly becoming more so. Since it is readily accepted that no one is immune to the effects of unmanaged stress, every professional and vocationsl specialty provides offerings concerning stress reduction and management. The corporate/industrial sector and its related services have become involed with offering stress management to employees at all levels of the corporate hierarchy. Included are on-site workshops, 1- and 2-day off-site training seminars with suggestion for follow-up and reinforcement of learned techniques on a regular basis (LaGreca, 1985; Jenner, 1986).

The workshop format (Wolfe, 1984) is geared toward elaboration of cognition with a focus on increased awareness of participants in what experiencing stress means, encouraging exploration of conditions under which stress is experienced and providing focus for existing coping mechanisms. Workshops, by virtue of group membership, offer advantages inherent in the process of sharing experiences. Participants are able to learn from one another to develop increased repretoires of coping skills.

The special interest group in which management of stress is placed within the context of the stressors specific to the group is well documented. Nelson (1985) described a group designed specifically for professional women. A senior citizen group using a stress management model has been described as an effective format for working with a well elderly population (Siegel, 1983).

The helping professions are readily recognized as susceptible to the negative effects of stress. Groups designed specifically to help nurses deal with stress are documented. Donovan (1981) reported in her research the positive effects of a stress management group designed for use with cancer nurses. Randolph (1986) also described research of the benefits for nurses from a 2-day stress and burnout prevention workshop format. The study concluded that a significant reduction of stress-related symptoms resulted for those who participated as compared to a control group who did not.

In the above-mentioned literature, the ingredients for inclusion in stress management groups/workshops are essentially the same and only the style and emphasis have variation: the maintenance of good health through good nutrition, exercise, adequate rest; goal setting; and time management all are integrally related to feeling well and staying well. These points and their importance will be reviewed again later in connection to actual counseling. For the purpose of the literature review, I call the reader's attention to relaxation and visualization techniques as an excellent and effective strategy for coping with stress. As additional and important dimensions in the approach to stress management, relaxation, visualization, and imagery fall in the domain of what Epstein (1980) referred to as the "so-called minor hemisphere," or right-brain, function. As techniques they are integrally related to hypnosis but, as pointed out by Zahourek (1978), they can be used with less formal knowledge than specified by hypnosis proper, which implies "formal induction of an altered state with specific suggestions accompanying the induction" (p. 225). The use of relaxation and imagery falls under the rubric of hypnotic techniques and can be used within a variety of contexts so long as the methods are appropriately adapted to the frame; that is, the goals are clear and the visualization techniques are tailored to those goals.

Relaxation and its benefits have been decribed in full by Luthe (1970) and by Benson (1976), who termed it the "relaxation response." Benson stated that relaxation activates an innate mechanism available to all, that can serve as an antidote to the flight/fight response activated by the sympathic nervous system, and as a method for using "one innate mechanism to counteract the effects of another" (p. 178).

The use of guided imagery and visualization has been documented in the psychiatric literature as an effective means for learning, experiencing, and increasing affectie response for self-exploration and as a means to expand imagination (Koshab, 1974).

Simonton et al. (1978), oncology specialists, demonstrated a relationship between the ways in which individuals cope with stress and the incidence of illness. In response to these findings Simonton et al. developed a treatment program that included learning a positive attitude toward life (cognition) in combination with relaxation and visualization techniques (imagination).

LeShan (1974) went a step further in prescribing meditation on a regular basis as an enabling mechanism for the individual to summon inner resources to counter stress. Meditation when practiced regularly produces a physiological state of deep relaxation coupled with an increase of alertness. Tension indicators are reduced and the metabolic rate and heartbeat slow down. This physiological state appears to be the opposite of the state brought about by stress.

SOME NOTES ON DOING
STRESS MANAGEMENT

First, you must believe it yourself! By this I mean, you must believe that stress can be controlled and that at least some of the control resides within the individual. Second, you need to practice what you preach. Your own beliefs and their implementation are a sine qua non for being effective with clients. The reasons for this are: (1) stress management is short term, (2) it is primarily in the cognitive domain as an educational process, and (3) the counselor takes an active and directive approach. Your own enthusiasm based on a genuine belief in the efficacy of the prescribed methods will go a long way toward encouraging the client.

By example, when I first began to conduct stress management groups in a medical center, I enrolled in a stress management weekend workshop. Prior to the workshop I had been advocating regular exercise as an important component in managing stress. I, however, only sporadically followed my own prescription. During the course of the workshop, one of the leaders came to a morning meeting still dressed in jogging attire. Her comments about regular jogging—how good it made her feel—were congruent with how well she looked. This incident occurred 7 years ago. I have been a consistent jogger since then. When I talk about the benefits of regular exercise, I can without hesitation and from firsthand experience heartily recommend it as a meaningful antidote for stress.

INDIVIDUAL STRESS
MANAGEMENT COUNSELING

It has frequently happened a client will call and say, "I've been feeling very stressed lately, but I don't want psychotherapy, just a way to handle stress," or words to that effect. My response is a form of clarification that the first meeting will provide an opportunity for assessment of what the problems and issues are and whether the stress management model is the treatment of choice. A client's clear expression of not wanting psychotherapy can have a variety of meanings: I will not speculate here on what those might be. Suffice it to say, it definitely implies the client's wish for brief intervention.

A beginning formulation attempts to determine whether crisis intervention followed by stress management strategies is indicated or whether either method would be best used singly. During the first session it is important to discover what happened at this particular juncture to prompt a call for help. Since a crisis is defined as an imbalance between a perceived difficulty or the significance of a threatening situation and the coping resources available to an individual, it is not difficult to decide whether the specific incident presented is, in fact, a transitory imbalance in the individual's habitual problem-solving repretoire or whether the presenting material is more indicative of the circularity encountered with unamnaged stress malaise (Claiborn, 1983).

The components of stress management intervention are as follows: It should be noted that the steps outlined are merely a guide rather than an inviolate format. The individualized aspect means just that! Some may require more of one component than another. What is being offered are the basic ingredients, the proportions of which will depend upon and vary with individual needs.

Step 1: Assessment And Determination Of Life-Style[1]

What are the stressors? What coping mechanisms are being employed in the present, and were employed in the past? How effective were they in the past, and are they in the present? Is there a difference now? To do this effectively, the counselor takes a stress inventory with the client. It is helpful to formulate a written questionnaire that is called an inventory of daily living. It linguistically establishes a concept for the client that implies a process — something that is ongoing, symbolizing voids that can be replenished. Taking a complete and detailed inventory is an important step in that it points both you and the client in the direction of an individualized plan. It also provides the client with an awareness of what needs to be rearranged, altered, added, subtracted.

By the end of the first session, the client should be feeling encouraged by the possibility of relief. A homework assignment betweeen sessions is an effective technique and should be varied with each phase of intervention. After the first session, you ask the client to keep some version of a diary in which stressful events and responses are recorded to be reviewed and discussed during the next meeting.

Step 2: Examination Of Life-Style

Begin with review of homework from previous session. Discussion should be directed toward a cognitive recognition of pattern and form and style of reacting to potentially stressful events. Discuss with client that segment of the inventory that pertains to the structure of a typical day. For example, if you learned that the client tends to turn off the alarm, oversleeps, is rushed leaving home every morning, skips breakfast, gulps a cup of coffee en route, and feels generally harassed before actually starting a day's work, then your intervention needs to begin at this level. The discovery of how to establish the locus of control within oneself becomes the foremost task in teaching techniques for managing stress. Consequently, you take seriously the client's dilemma created by the dissonance of both wishing to sleep late and wishing not to start off the day feeling "jangled." The issue of choice is introduced here. You describe an altered scenario, making what you surmise to be ego-syntonic adjustments in the daily plan.

The same approach is used with the discussion of an exercise regimen. The goal is to tease out from the client the most suitable, appropriate, and doable program on the basis of time constraints, personality, and so on.

This session's homework should be a reflection of the material covered, again asking that notation be made regarding the alteration in behavior and response to it.

Step 3: Teaching Relaxation And Visualization Techniques

It has been my experience that most people have at some time been exposed to a form of relaxation technique. Responses to the benefits of relaxation are varied. While there is seldom disagreement regarding relaxation as antidote for tension, many claim being unable to integrate the technique on a regular basis. It is helpful to offer a simple exercise as prelude to a visualization exercise. I use the following relaxation instructions.

Get into a comfortable position and take a deep breath; relax. Then count: (1) Roll your eyes up. Keep your eyeballs up and close your eyelids. (2) Inhale and hold your breath. (3) Let your breath out slowly. Roll your eyeballs down keeping your eyelids closed. Imagine yourself floating down.

Now take three deep breaths and exhale slowly. Continue to imagine yourself floating in a comfortable position, feeling light and buoyant. Now start to relax all of your body. Relax the muscles of your head and neck, then your arms, chest, abdomen, and legs. Take a deep breath, and as you let it out feel your whole body relax. Remain relaxed for 30 seconds. Be conscious only of your breathing: Inhale, then exhale fully. At the count of 3, open your eyes.

It is helpful to use this relaxation exercise at the beginning of each of the remaining sessions for purposes of relieving tension and providing practice.

If you are guiding the client into a visualization exercise directly after relaxation, the eyes remain closed to maintain the relaxed state.

Guided imagery or visualization exercises are numerous—the choice of where to lead someone in imagination will depend upon the clues made available from the data gleaned thus far.

For the purpose of providing an example, I include at this point one particular visualization exercise. Others will be provided in the discussion of a group format.

Exercise 1: Fantasy Trip to a Meadow. The leader directs the group as follows:

1. In this relaxed state with eyes closed transport yourself to a meadow; it may be remembered from childhood or from imagination. Find a tree in the meadow. Go to the tree and lean against it.

2. As you lean against the tree, imagine the sun shining on the leaves and warming you.

3. Imagine your feet firmly planted on the ground. Imagine yourself being able to sway with the wind as a tree is able to sway without falling because your feet are firmly planted.

4. Remain so for a few minutes. Take in all the smells around you; feel the sun; feel the coolness of the earth.

5. Remember the feelings; remember the tree in the meadow; you can return to it at other times.

6. Inhale fully; exhale slowly. Return to the room and open your eyes.

Discussion: The imagery of the meadow and a tree are sufficiently neutral, pleasant, and accessible to most people. The suggestions are both concrete and symbolic, representing a "return to nature" as restorative. The tree as identificatory object represents both strength and flexibility.

Following the exercise, process the material with the client. Encourage discussion of the experience with emphasis upon the sensory components. If the individual states feeling uneasy with this kind of assignment, give reassurance regarding increased ease with practice. Again reiterate the benefits to be gained from relaxation and imagery.

Step 4: Examination, Discussion, and Reworking Of Cognitive Distortions

Cognitive distortions or negative self-talk represents a real source of "distress." The material I use for this segment is based on the work of Aaron Beck, as interpreted by David Burns in *Feeling Good: The New Mood Therapy* (1980). I refer clients to this book as well as other appropriate bibliographic sources that may be helpful for self-review and reinforcement of the counseling.

The emphasis in examining cognitive distortions rests upon helping the individual become aware of the extent to which negative thinking affects one's outlook and view of the world and how this kind of negativism increases stress levels. The list of distortions identified by Burns (pp. 4041) are helpful to discuss with the client.

Homework assignment for the following session should include reviewing how often during the course of the week the individual used one or more of the cognitive distortions and how the negative spiral toward increased stress became activated.

Step 5: Managing Time

Time management and self-management are integrally related. It is difficult to manage time effectively and feel in control of it unless you are quite sure of how it is actually being spent. The first step in time management is to keep a record of how you spend it. Oftentimes clients will object to doing this for one of several reasons—e.g., "It's time-consuming" or "It's too compulsive." This is fallacious thinking with regard to learning how to manage time in a more effective way. A record of time use helps to identify time problems. Time problems can be internally generated or externally stimulated from within the environment.

Self-generated time problems are the more difficult to identify and resolve. Some of the categories outlined by Smith (1983) relate to the following issues: (1) poor self-discipline, (2) anxiety, (3) difficulty saying no, (4) procrastination, (5) disorganization, (6) griping, and (7) inattention.

An assessment of time problems with the client is an important aspect of stress management. Oftentimes the mere recognition of one's own complicity in generating time pressure becomes the important first step toward being in control of altering the situation. Thoughtful introspection and practice are required to gain control of time.

Step 6. Setting Goals: Short-Term And Long-Term

Formulating goals, both short term and long term, represents a key to one's direction in life. The determination of which goals are sufficiently realistic to be realizable while at the same time not overly limiting is significant. Selye (1974) described long-term goals as those synonymous with a philosophy of life—a sense of purpose that will give meaning and direction to one's life.

Although offered as the last step, the analysis and discussion of setting goals is paradoxically the most important aspect of stress management in that how we organize our lives essentially flows from how we define our goals. Its placement at the end is a reflection of its importance vis-à-vis the client's ability to better hear and reflect upon this aspect when feeling more in control of self as a result of intervention. This step in a sense serves as resolution prior to termination.

CLINICAL EXAMPLES

Before proceeding to a description and discussion of stress management in groups, I offer two examples of case material chosen to illustrate a differentiation between stress management and crisis intervention.

Case 1: Marian J.

Marian was a 28-year-old woman referred for stress management counseling. She had recently been promoted to a supervisory position, one for which she was appropriately qualified with credentials and experience. She therefore had readily accepted the position. But during 2 months in that role, she had become increasingly distressed with what she viewed as her inability "to do the job." She described feeling overwhelmed and terribly stressed. "Being the boss is not much fun," was her comment.

In taking an inventory during the first session, it became apparent to me she was in the throes of a crisis; that is, a temporary state of disorganization in which her customary methods of problem solving were not adequate for the demand. The other parts of her life were in order, although she expressed concern lest there be spillover based on how badly she was feeling on the job.

During the first session, I determined the treatment of choice to be crisis intervention for probably no more than four to six sessions at the end of which we could evaluate the progress and decide if more time would be necessary.

We met four times. The work in each of the sessions focused upon the significance of the promotion in terms of her private "cognitive map"—the internal drawing of how one views self, past, present, and future. She effectively used each session by using the work situation as a kind of laboratory to try new behaviors. At the end of the four sessions, she said she felt sufficiently in control of the situation to conclude treatment.

Case 2: Joanne L.

Joanne was self-referred. She worked in the medical center where I led groups in stress management but felt she needed help on an individual basis. At 26, single, working as a critical care nurse in a prestigious medical center with an apartment nearby that she shared with her sister, Joanne described feeling "pretty good" about herself and her life—that is, until recently. It was difficult for her to assess when it all started to turn sour: the job, her social life, and so on. She said she felt tense, frustrated, over-worked, too much of the time, with others noting the change in her, especially her sister with whom she was very close. In fact, it was her sister who urged her to get help.

A stress inventory revealed a clear precipitant to the recent awareness of a generalized malaise. Her sister's engagement and soon-to-be marriage triggered for Joanne a real discomfort with only marginal recognition of how much she depended upon her sister as the initiator, organizer, and energizer of her life. The upcoming marriage created a shift in a precariously balanced system. In reality Joanne could acknowledge an overdue need to rearrange and overhaul parts of her life, e.g., planning future career goals, altering her current work life, which she had been ex-periencing as overly stressful but for which she had not attempted to find constructive methods for alleviation. In short, a change in the system forced upon her a need to take control of her life, which is essentially the essence of stress management counseling.

Discussion: In each of the above cases, the client came for stress manage-ment counseling. For Joanne, the latter example, it was both suitable and ef-fective. For the former client, crisis intervention represented the preferable model. Although each presented a situational change that triggered a stress response, the total picture represented variables and consequent treatment variation.

GROUP FORMAT FOR
STRESS MANAGEMENT COUNSELING

The group provides an excellent format for presenting stress management strategies and techniques. Since it is primarily a cognitive process, the group experience lends itself well to exploration, comparison, suggestion, encourage-ment, and support by participants to one another. The entire format described earlier can be replicated within the group with the added dimension created by the process inherent within groups.

In Step 3, Teaching Relaxation and Visualization, I presented a relaxation technique and one example of a visualization exercise. In this segment, I will present a series in addition to the earlier offering. Their use in groups has been effective and documented in two other sources by the author.[2]

Begin with the relaxation exercise as outlined in step 3 above. Then con-tinue with exercise 1, Fantasy Trip to Meadow.

Exercise 2: Fantasy Trip to Inner Guide.

1. With eyes closed imagine yourself traveling along a path. It could be

---

[2]These exercises have been adapted from Siegel (1988) and Siegel & Liefer (1983) with permission of the publishers.

real or imagined. Travel the path slowly and take time to notice everything along the way. Notice the colors, smells, and sounds. As you travel along the path, try to imagine coming to a place — a safe, comfortable, accepting place, real or imagined, a place where you feel thoroughly at home.

2. Upon arriving there, look around you. Make note of what you see, hear, smell. Is it a familiar place or one that you imagine you would like to visit? In this place try to find a guide — someone you either know or perhaps knew at another time in your life or someone you would like to have as your guide.

3. Now talk to your guide. Ask the guide a question of importance to yourself. If your guide is impatient or unresponsive to you, ask him or her to be more patient and responsive.

4. Remain so for several minutes.

5. Look around you once more: at the guide, at the place, so you can remember it. You will be returning there again.

6. Come back to the room and open your eyes.

Discussion: With this exercise it is important for each group participant to be encouraged to set the frame in which the imagining took place. Ample time should be allowed for elaboration and in-depth description. The leader must also be alert to individuals for whom imagery and visualization present a problem and assist them in finding a safe place. The process, however, must be accomplished in a way that does not diminish self-esteem. Inevitably there is at least one person in the group who will express having difficulty with imagination by saying "I'm just not good at this kind of thing." My response to this type of comment is both neutral and educative. Rather than provide a more typical reassuring response, I find the neutrality of further explanation about the use of imagination to be in fact reassuring.

Exercise 3: Best Decision. Before proceeding with the exercise, the leader assists each individual in establishing the scenes from memory of the previous journeys. Participants are encouraged to elaborate the details. Doing this is both practical and salutary. Details from preceding exercises provide necessary context for the succeeding one. It has been my experience that unless encouraged otherwise, individuals have a tendency to abridge rather than elaborate. The leader's encouragement is helpful on two levels: It validates importance of the experience and also indulges each participant with equal time and attention. This kind of active leadership also protects members from revealing too much about themselves.

1, With eyes close, return to the safe place.

2. From the vantage point of feeling safe, return to a particular good time in the past. Try to remember the happy quality of that episode: the people who shared it with you, everything that made it a happy time for you. Stay in that time. Focus on the different aspects of the memory, on as many details as you can remember.

3. Now try to remember a decision you made at that time, bearing in mind that this was the *best* decision possible at that time.

4. Stay with the memory for a few minutes.

Discussion: Following this exercise, each participant is asked to describe his or her experience. In processing the material, the leader needs to tease out real or symbolic aspects of the best decision. One's best decision as it emerges in this context can be both illuminating and reassuring to the individual. It can serve to validate choices made in a variety of areas: vocational, interpersonal, and so forth. Frequently participants express surprise at the kind of images that present themselves: "Almost out of nowhere," said one nurse as she realted the context and experience of deciding to transfer from an unrelated field of study to pursue a career in nursing.

A STRESS MANAGEMENT CONSULTATION PROJECT

In the introductory portion of this chapter, I mentioned the specifically designed stress management program for special interest groups. The advantage to this kind of program lies in its personalized approach, which provides participants with a feeling of being genuinely understood. Problem solving assumes additional meaning. There is an inherent heightening of support from this kind of group.

To do this kind of consultation, it is imperative for the consultant to be knowledgeable about the particular stressors encountered within the field or vocation. Your credibility as a leader is markedly increased if you are familiar with the language commonly used by the participants.

As a consultant to a large department of nursing in a major urban medical center, I provided material to the groups that covered the stress management steps described above. In addition, it also included discussion and specific problem solving as they related to ongoing events within the system. For example, since nurses are consistently involved with and concerned about matters of life and death and their concomitant ethical issues, much time was spent clarifying values and beliefs as a strategy for relieving the stress provoked by the clash of conflicting beliefs and actions.

SUMMARY

This chapter has described the use of a stress management model for the private practitioner in the treatment of clients on an individual basis, in groups and as part of a consultation project.

It is the author's belief that in order to be effective in providing stress management in a private practice, the practitioner must accept, at the least, the following three precepts: (1) that stress is in fact manageable, (2) that the principles and strategies of stress management must be used on oneself prior to one's attempting to teach them to others, and (3) that stress management is a valid treatment choice in and of itself.

REFERENCES

Benson, H. (1976). *Relaxation response.* New York: Avon.
Claiborn, W.L., & Specter, G.A. (1983). In L.H. Cohen (Ed.), *Crisis intervention.* New

York: Human Sciences Press.

Donovan, M.I. (1981, April). Study of the impact of relaxation with guided imagery on stress among cancer nurses. *Cancer Nursing,* pp. 121-126.

Epstein, G. (1980). *Waking dream therapy.* New York: Human Sciences Press.

Jacobson, S.F., & McGrath, H.M. (Eds.). (1983). *Nurses under stress.* New York: John Wiley

Jenner, J.R. (1986, May). On the way to stress resistance. *Training and Development Journal,* pp. 112-115.

Kosbab, F.F. (1974, Sept.). Imagery techniques in psychiatry. *Archives of General Psychiatry,* 283-290.

LaGreca, G. (1985). The stress you make. *Personnel Journal, 64*(9), 42-47.

LeShan, L. (1974). *How to meditate.* Boston: Little Brown Co.

Luthe, E. (1970). *Autogenic therapy research and theory.* New York: Grune and Stratton.

Nelson, D.L., & Quick, J. (1985). Stress of professional women. *Academy of Management Review, 10*(2), 206-218.

Randolph, G.L., Price, J.L., & Collins, J.K. (1986). The effects of burnout prevention training on burnout symptoms in nurses. *Journal of Continuing Education in Nursing, 17*(2), March/April.

Selye, H. (1956). *The stress of life.* New York: McGraw-Hill, 1976.

Selye, H. (1974). *Stress without distress.* New York: Signet.

Selye, H. (1977). A code for coping with stress. *Association of Operating Room Nurses, Inc. Journal, 25*(1), 35-42.

Siegel, E., (Liefer, A. (1983). A staying well group. In M. Rosenbaum (Ed.), *Handbook of short term therapy groups.* New York: McGraw Hill.

Siegel, E. (1988). Stress management groups for nurses. In R. Zahourek (Ed.), *Relaxation and imagery: Therapeutic strategies for nurses.* San Diego: Grune and Stratton.

Simonton, O.C., Matthews-Simonton, S., & Creighton, J. (1978). *Getting well again.* New York: St. Martin's Press.

Smith, C.M. (1983). Principles of time management. In S.F. Jacobson & H.M. McGrath (Eds.), *Nurses under stress.* New York: John Wiley.

Wolfe, R. (1984, July). Coping with stress: A workshop framework. *British Journal of Guidance and Counseling, 12*(2), 141-153.

Zahourek, R.P. (1978). Overview—The context of clinical hypnosis in nursing practice. In R.P. Zahourek (Ed.), *Clinical hypnosis and therapeutic suggestion in nursing.* Orlando, FL: Gurne & Stratton.

C H A P T E R
77

THE PSYCHIATRIC CONSULTATION

Leonard J. Deutsch, M.D., P.C.

While 70 percent of my working hours is spent in the private practice of psychiatry, 30 percent of my time goes to psychiatric consultations of many varieties. In this chapter I will explain each type of consultation and its purpose.

Every psychiatrist at one time or another is a consultant in one form or another. It is a question of the amount of time one spends in being a consultant. In analysis, the patient may sometimes try to convert the session into a consultation, and for analytic purposes this may be inappropriate. But certainly in the initial contact the analyst plays the consultant role to a certain degree.

The function of a consultation is to communicate your findings and opinions in a way easily comprehensible to non-mental health professionals, such as doctors and surgeons, jurors, judges, and lawyers, as well as to mental health professionals, such as other psychiatrists, psychologists, social workers, and nurses.

I have been a consultant for more than 20 years, since completing my residency in 1967. I conducted liaison psychiatry during my hospital training, working with nonpsychiatric doctors, and have continued ever since as part of my consultative work. It fills a need in me, bringing much satisfaction and pleasure. When I first started, I was naive, idealistic, and altruistic. Then I began to feel part detective, part savior, part psychiatrist.

Consultation gives me a chance to explore areas other than those explored in the chairs or on the couch in my office. It gives me a sense of independence. It is challenging and sometimes lifesaving for a patient in desperate need of help.

The psychiatric consultant, after taking the history and doing the usual Mental Status Examination, arrives at a diagnostic impression and creates a treatment plan, sometimes under less than ideal conditions and sometimes quite adverse ones.

THE LOCALES OF WORK

My work as a consultant psychiatrist occurs chiefly in two types of settings: outpatient facilities and inpatient facilities. The outpatient facilities include my office, clinics, child care agencies. Even at cocktail parties I may be asked by a worried man or woman holding a drink, "I dreamed last night I was attacked by a blind man. What do you think that means, Dr. Deutsch?" Or a harried mother will corner me and plead, "I think my 15-year-old son is taking drugs, though he denies it. What do you think I should do?"

The inpatient facilities are of three main types. First, there is the mental hospital to which the psychiatrist is called as consultant to another psychiatrist, often for medical/legal reasons. The latter may have a litigious patient at a private or public mental hospital and for his or her protection may need a second opinion about the mental state of the patient. The psychiatrist asks me to see and evaluate the condition of the patient. This is a highly neglected area because, though psychiatrists in the past were not sued as frequently as other specialists, today this occurs more often, as statistics testify.

The second type of inpatient facility is the general hospital where a non-psychiatric medical specialist, such as obstetrician or surgeon, calls for a consultation. This is known as "liaison" psychiatry, as psychiatrists help other medical specialties. A woman patient, for instance, may have undergone removal of a breast and sunk into a deep depression. Her surgeon or admitting physician may wish me to evaluate how depressed she is and whether she needs to seek psychiatric help immediately.

The third type of inpatient facility, a growing setting for consultations, is the nursing home, where the mental ability of an aged patient may be questioned. Even television shows have fcused on this locale as a popular theme. In a recent 2-hour feature, Kirk Douglas portrayed a patient in a nursing home where the owners were exploiting patients. Consultations are held for the protection of both patient and staff.

THE IMPORTANCE OF A POINTED REQUEST

One of the most important factors in consultation is the nature of the request. Sometimes it comes from the patient who walks into my office for the first time. The patient has heard about me from another patient, a family doctor, another psychiatrist, or even a friend. Sometimes the consultation comes at the request of another therapist or from an insurance carrier who is being sued and wants me to assess the psychiatric condition of the person.

A doctor in a general hospital or mental hospital can leave an order on a chart asking for a psychiatric consultation. It is possible to go to a hospital and review the chart, only to find there is no clear-cut question identifying the reason for the need of a consultation.

Unless the question is clarified, in each instance, it is possible to do a complete psychiatric evaluation, but it will not be meaningful because I will not have answered the question the person failed to ask. Without such clarity, I may not provide a full, accurate answer.

For instance, sometimes I am asked by a social worker, nurse, or other intermediary to answer a question posed by a judge or a physician who suggested transmitting the request to me. The point of the question frequently gets lost or distorted in the transmission because it was not written down as the originator of the question formulated it.

It is impossible to meet the need or answer whatever question led to the request for consultation unless the question is spelled out in a direct way that will benefit the person asking it. But if that direct way eludes the person transmitting the question, I am forced to do the best I can with what is available to me. The party asking for the consultation may be deprived of the desired information, the patient may suffer, and the consultation may be viewed as a failure. To avoid this happening, it is necessary in such cases to go to great pains to clarify the reason for the consultation.

WHO IS PRIVY TO THE INFORMATION?

Obviously when a private patient walks into my office, the patient is the one who receives the information requested. But in other cases, who else receives that information? This is an extremely important point.

The issue of confidentiality between patient and therapist, which arises out of the ethical traditions of the medical profession stemming from the Hippocratic oath, was catapulted into the national limelight on October 27, 1969. The Hippocratic oath reads in part: "Whatever in connection with professional practice I see or hear in the life of men which ought not to be spoken of abroad, I will not divulge, as reckoning all such should be kept secret."

On that October evening, Prosenjit Poddar, a graduate student at the University of California at Berkeley, walked into the home of Tatiana Tarasoff, a young woman who had rejected his love. He was carrying a pellet gun and a large kitchen knife. Ms. Tarasoff, who lived in the house with her mother and father, was standing alone in the kitchen.

She screamed as she saw the murderous weapons in Mr. Poddar's hands. He aimed the gun at her and fired. Wounded but alive, she tried to escape through the back door. He ran after her, stabbed her repeatedly with the hunting knife until she lay dead.

A year before, Mr. Poddar, born into the Jarijan ("untouchable") caste in Bengal, India, had met Ms. Tarasoff at folk dancing classes at the university's International House, where he lived. On New Year's Eve she had given him the traditional holiday kiss, which he had interpreted as a sign she loved him as ardently as he did her. When she told him she was not interested in an intimate relationship, he became very depressed, wept for hours in his room, and neglected studies, appearance, and health.

At the suggestion of a friend, Mr. Poddar sought help at the university's Cowell Memorial Hospital outpatient clinic. There he confided to his psychologist, Lawrence Moore, that he hated Ms. Tarasoff for spurning his love and planned to kill her.

Believing Mr. Poddar was disturbed enough to carry out his threat, Dr. Moore wrote the campus police on August 20, 1969, and suggested they take his patient into custody. He said he would arrange for Mr. Poddar's hospitalization at the Emergency Psychiatric Detention Facility of Herrick Hospital. When campus police picked up Mr. Poddar and questioned him, he denied any violent feelings toward Ms. Tarasoff. The police believed him, made him promise never to contact her, and let him go.

Mr. Poddar promptly gave up therapy, furious at Dr. Moore for trying to hsopitalize him and for telling the police of his threats to kill Ms. Tarasoff.

She went on a short vacation to Brazil and when she returned, Mr. Poddar visited her that fatal October evening to carry out his threat.

At the trial he pleaded not guilty by reason of insanity, or "diminished capacity" as the California courts call it. Dr. Moore and three psychiatrists testified Mr. Poddar was a paranoid schizophrenic who could not have "harbored malice aforethought" at the time of the killing. But he was convicted of second-degree murder. The Supreme Court of California reversed the trial court's verdict. The supreme court ruled the judge had failed to make clear to the jurors the application of "the evidence of diminished capacity to the underlying issues" and "the error was prejudicial to the defendant."

Ms. Tarasoff's bereaved and outraged parents, Mr. and Mrs. Vitaly Tarasoff, brought suit against several defendants: Dr. Moore; Dr. Harvey Powelson, head of the department of psychiatry at the outpatient clinic, who had ordered Dr. Moore to take no further steps to commit Mr. Poddar when the police refused to take further action; the campus police; and their employer, the Regents of the University of California.

They all were charged with "wrongful death" in failing to warn the Tarasoffs that their daughter's life had been in danger. The suit also charged the defendants had "negligently" failed to commit Mr. Poddar to an institution. (He never was committed, or given another trial, and eventually returned to India.)

When the Superior Court of Alameda County dismissed the Tarasoffs' suit, ruling that the defendants, as public employees, were legally immune under California law, the Tarasoffs appealed to the Supreme Court of California. It handed down on July 1, 1976, the decision[1] that was to shake the world of therapy.

The decision stated that while the defendants were immune from the charge of failing to act properly to commit Mr. Poddar, the therapist had not fulfilled his "obligation" to protect a possible victim when his patient presented "a serious danger of violence to another."

The court stated: "Protective privilege ends where public peril begins." It ruled that a therapist should use "reasonable care to protect the intended victim against such danger.... It may call for him to warn the intended victim, or others likely to apprise the victim of the danger, to notify the police, or to take whatever other steps are reasonably necessary under the circumstances." The University of California settled with the Tarasoffs out of court.

For the first time in American history, a court mandated that a therapist has an *obligation,* rather than merely the option, to warn a potential victim of a murder threat. The therapeutic professions — psychiatrists, psychoanalysts, and psychologists — were alarmed not only because the decision involved breaking the traditional confidentiality between patient and therapist but also because this could be mandated without the permission of the patient.

---

[1] Tarasoff v. Regents of the University of California, 118 Cal. Rptr. 129, 13 Cal. 3rd 177, 529 P. 2d 553 (1974), *modified on rehearing,* 131 Cal. Rptr. 14, 17 Cal. 3rd 425, 557 P. 2d 334 (1976).

The Tarasoff decision, though binding as a precedent only in California, led to similar cases in other states. Another failure to warn of "dangerousness" brought tragedy to Ewa Berwid, of Mineola, N.Y., wife of Adam Berwid, who had been an engineer in Poland. He had a history of violence, of beating his wife, and finally she had him arrested and filed for divorce. He wrote death threats to her from the Pilgrim Psychiatric Center, at Brentwood, where he had been committed. He persuaded a psychiatrist at the center, after he had been there almost a year, to give him a 1-day pass, took the hour's train ride to his former home, murdered his wife with a hunting knife he kept in the basement, plunging it into her body four times until she lay dead at his feet.

The treating psychiatrist and his immediate superior at the center were charged by the hospital, their employer, with negligence in allowing the day pass to be issued. These charges were temporarily dropped when Nassau County District Attorney Denis Dillon said he wanted to seek a criminal indictment, but this action never went through. Mr. Berwid stood trial and received a 35-year-to-life sentence on January 26, 1982. The case led to a new state law requiring that police and possible victims be notified when a patient with a history of violence is released from a mental hospital.

What do I do when a private patient walks into my office or I see a patient in a mental institution and have to determine if he or she is suicidal or homicidal? To permit a violent patient to leave without first informing a family member or the authorities could be considered malpractice. It is necessary to inform someone of the danger.

In the case of child abuse, it is mandatory in New York City to report the abuse to the Special Services for Children, a city agency under the New York City Human Resources Administration. At times they ask me to investigate allegations of child abuse after I have reported them as consultant for child care agencies. When the obligation to report them first became law in 1977, my initial reaction was one of apprehension. I feared the law would destroy the therapeutic work already in progress with parents who abused their children. I also feared it would harm not only the parents but the children who were benefiting by the changes in their parents as a result of therapy. But these apprehensions, fortunately, were unfounded. My experience has been that in all cases it has been possible to continue the work with these distressed people.

One of the mechanisms inadvertently helpful in this regard is the fact that the agency to which the reporting of child abuse is done is so overloaded that frequently its response is not to intervene significantly but to allow the practitioner to continue treating the parents. Though the reporting must be done within 24 hours of learning of the abuse, this has turned out to be more of a paper tiger threat than a real threat.

My work as consultant to social workers reporting abuse of children by parents entails having them tell their clients they will be reported for this abuse. Both the social workers and the clients usually become distressed, but the agency in charge tells the social workers they may continue the treatment and both social workers and parents then feel relieved. In other words, this lack of bureaucratic functioning has proved beneficial to the parents, rather than penalizing them.

CONSULTANT TO THE COURT

The court initiates the request for my involvement in a case. I have been an impartial examiner in child custody cases and for the United States Department of Labor. But more often, I have been asked by an attorney representing either the claimant or the defendant (insurance carrier) to evaluate an individual. This may be limited to the writing of a report, but it may also include the act of testifying in court. The latter has become controversial today in the field of psychiatry, some psychiatrists defending its use, others protesting it.

Court work may also include an evaluation relating to commitment proceedings. The psychiatrist may either recommend a disturbed person's commitment to a state hospital or, after a consultation with the patient, recommend that the patient be set free or perhaps go to a clinic for help.

As consultant to the court my report sometimes suffices as my testimony. However, either party has the right to subpoena me for cross-examination. There are various courts before which I testify. Most of my cases concern workers compensation, but I also am consultant in cases involving social security benefits and civil and criminal suits, as well as suits revolving around child custody. In the latter, I am often asked to interview one or both parents and make recommendations to the judge. I may advise after interviewing both parents, that a mother would make the better parent, or that the father would, but it is the judge who decides, as in a commitment proceeding or any case in a court.

I have learned that my recommendations cannot be "wishy-washy." I have to be definite. Judges want an "either-or" answer, not one that is loaded with *ifs, ands,* and *buts,* which leaves the judge in a dilemma.

There are many types of court cases. I was consultant on one where a woman sold a cooperative apartment and then died right after the closing transaction. The lawyer for the estate represented the deceased relatives who did not think she received enough money for the apartment and were contesting the sale. They claimed she was not competent at the time of closing and consequently the transaction was not valid.

I was asked to review the records and decide whether the deceased had been competent at the time of the transaction. Records showed she was taken to the hospital, where she was deemed brain damaged as a result of a stroke. Her lawyer insisted this meant the woman was incompetent before the closing. But in my review of her records and talks with neighbors and friends, I established she had been competent at the time of the closing. A person is judged competent until declared "not competent" by a court. The judge failed to rule the woman incompetent at the time of the transaction.

CONSULTANT FOR INSURANCE PROBLEMS

A fair share of my time as consultant outside my office is spent on cases that pertain to insurance. Usually the insurance carriers ask me to verify the legitimacy of a claim, as I did in the following case. Sometimes the carriers feel the claims are outrageous and sometimes, on the other hand, it is a matter of my interpreting and explaining to the carrier why a claim that may not appear so, is really a legitimate one.

It is common practice for a lawyer to phone, make an appointment with me to evaluate a man or woman who is suing an insurance company, and ask to bring along a court reporter to take notes, as in a deposition, to which lawyers are accustomed. A courteous lawyer will call in advance and ask, "Dr. Deutsch, is it all right with you if I am present with a court reporter while you interview the claimant?"

Court rulings have upheld the right of the claimant to have a psychiatric evaluation with the opposing lawyer present. But this has been decided on a case-by-case basis. Psychiatrists have to decide for themselves, when this issue arises, whether they want in their office the lawyer representing the claimant, along with a court stenographer. A psychiatrist not wishing to accept the lawyer can ask the insurance carrier requesting this evaluation to go to court and get a ruling that the opposing attorney not be present during the claimant's evaluation.

One day when I was scheduled to evaluate a claimant for an insurance company, the lawyer for the claimant showed up without notice. He announced, "I won't interfere in any way with your interview, Dr. Deutsch." The man to be evaluated had not yet arrived at my office. He had been in an automobile accident and he claimed he had been harmed psychologically, had been disabled, and was unable to work. The lawyer arrived at 4:30 P.M. and we spent an hour arguing. I objected to the court stenographer being present without advance notice. The lawyer countered, "There are court rulings which show I may attend and bring my own stenographer."

I then said I would use my tape recorder, thinking, If the lawyer has his court stenographer, why should I not have equal opportunity to make a precise record of the consultation? He insisted that the recording not be entered as evidence in court. I refused to agree. He offered as consolation a copy of his transcript if I would forego the tape recorder.

I refused to give up the tape recorder. My office is my castle, the way a man's home is his castle. The issue boiled down to the question, Who wants this interview more—he or I? The moment I want the interview more than the claimant's attorney does, I put myself in the position of making compromises, and that I would not do.

He offered to call the judge to find out how he would rule. The hour was then 5:50, so I knew he was bluffing, for the judge would have long since left the court. But he dialed the court's number and there was no answer—to the lawyer's "surprise."

I then called the insurance carrier's attorney, who was still at work. He said he had no objection to the court stenographer being present, or the lawyer, if I had no objection. It was his opinion, he said, that the court would uphold the claimant's attorney in this matter.

By that time the claimant had arrived, and the lawyer and I agreed to go ahead with the interview, he with his stenographer and I with the tape recorder. He failed to keep his promise to send me the transcript. The case is still pending.

CONSULTANT TO CHILD CARE AGENCIES

Over the years I have been psychiatric consultant for several child care agencies, working at Carholic Charities, for instance, for 20 years. During that time I have found the most urgent requests are, as one might expect, the evaluation of suicide/homicide risks. More frequently, however, occur the consultations with social workers and staff of the agency to make recommendations regarding planning for child care. This usually involves deciding whether a child should be placed for adoption.

A big problem today, as it has been for some time, is the unwed mother on welfare who is involved with drugs or alcohol and is consequently unable to provide adequate care for her children—usually more than one child is involved. Most of these cases come to the attention of the authorities and are reviewed by the agency only because the parent is in conflict with the law. Neighbors' complaints (they usually call anonymously, for this is one area in which anonymous complaints are accepted) or observations by schoolteachers or nurses in a hospital emergency room are relayed to the police and the Special Services for Children of the New York City Human Resources Administration, who then investigate the complaint.

Children are often removed from the home and decisions must be made about their future. The question frequently asked is: "Is this mother capable of providing adequate care for her children?" In certain instances this leads to freeing a child for adoption, obviously an important decision that requires careful, extensive field work by the social work staff before the case is presented to the psychiatric consultant. The court's role is a difficult one, trying to walk a tightrope betwen preserving the constitutional rights of the mother and acting in the best interest of the child.

In more than one case I have found both parents were drug addicts, constantly in and out of jails, and the mother was a prostitute who neglected the child over long periods of time. Recommendations were made on the basis of the behavior of the parents, who, I knew, were not going to change in a 2-year period. A law in New York State holds that if a parent is not expected to be rehabilitated within 2 years, then, under certain conditions, the child can be freed for adoption. Again, I reiterate, it would be the judge who made the final decision. I could only make the recommendation that the child be placed for adoption.

Those are the easy cases. I had one difficult case that I followed 18 years for Catholic Charities. The child was placed in foster care a few days after birth. The mother was schizophrenic and mentally retarded; the father also was schizophrenic. He physically abused the mother, who at times had to flee to a shelter, to which I drove her on one occasion.

I had recommended adoption. The family with whom the child had been placed soon after birth provided the child with a "real" home environment that, in my opinion, was healthy. However, because of various technicalities the case dragged on in court through appeals and delays for over 18 years. It was finally decided to permit adoption. But by that time the "child" (now an adult) was quite paranoid about the agency, and me in particular, believing we were not trying to work for her adoption. Originally the court ruled that technical errors had been made in record keeping, which delayed the progress of the case, but she did not understand the significance of this. From her perspective, the agency was at fault and that was all that mattered.

On one occasion during this case I found myself testifying in court before what seemed a mass of lawyers. One represented the natural mother, by that time divorced. Another represented the natural father. A third represented Catholic Charities. A fourth represented the child; and a fifth, the New York City Human Resources Administration. There were so many lawyers that at times I did not know whom the lawyer questioning me represented.

The consultant's role in such cases is to a very large extent dependent upon the care and diligence of the social workers and staff who provide the consultant with the information needed. It is the consultant's function to exercise great care in making sure he or she has the information needed to do the evaluation properly.

The psychiatrist faces the dilemma that while the mother may be well-meaning and genuinely love her child, she may not be capable of caring for the child adequately, and outside intervention may be essential for the child's emotional, and sometimes physical, survival. The court's dilemma is to make the decisions; the psychiatrist's role, once again, is to provide clarification, advice, and direction.

CONSULTATIONS FOR PRIVATE PATIENTS

Many patients come to my office for consultations, intending to ask for either treatment or advice on whether they need treatment. The question "Do you think I need help?" is a common one.

Whether I accept the patient in therapy depends on the patient's choice and mine, also on my time availability and the state of the patient's finances. If money is a real problem, I may advise a clinic.

During some consultations, I am asked all kinds of questions that have to do with the mental health of the patient's relatives. A prevalent one pertains to the mental status of an aging parent as the son or daughter seeks my advice as to what to do.

But what is not asked about is the kind of help the son or daughter may need. An opportunity to help the son or daughter may be lost if this is not recognized. In asking about care for a family member, the persons who make the request should never be neglected. They may benefit from help suggesting therapy for themselves, therapy they have covertly sought, in addition to the recommendation they overtly sought.

MEDICAL RECORDS AND THE PSYCHIATRIC CONSULTATION

When you do a consultation there is the question of having before you the available medical records. Recently, a doctor was sued for releasing a patient from a mental hospital in which he had been confined for 30 years. The patient viciously attacked a member of his family, nearly killing him.

The victim and other family members sued the psychiatrist because he had not told them how dangerous the patient was. They won the case as the court ruled they were entitled to the medical history of the patient in order to protect themselves adequately. The doctor, in releasing the patient, did not review the medical records. It may be that after 30 years a review of the records seemed like an overwhelming task and probably unnecessary at that.

To cover oneself legally, as well as to provide better care for the patient, the psychiatrist should always review the medical records available. Psychiatrists are the first to recognize one person cannot do everything and has to operate under the conditions that exist, rather than the conditions one would like to have. As psychiatrists, we would like to possess all the information about a patient. But we work with *all the information available.*

The courts may view this as negligent in certain instances where there is evidence that there has been no attempt to obtain past medical records. At least one should make a diligent attempt to locate all possible information.

How far back do you have to go in examining medical records? This will depend primarily on the question being asked of the consultant. In cases where violence, including suicide, is the subject of the question, then the answer may depend on a prior history of violence, including suicide attempts. This may take the consultant to the point where history is not forthcoming from the patient and otherwise unavailable.

The consultant who sees the patient for only a relatively brief time may be asked to make recommendations for future therapists to focus on certain areas in the course of the patient's future therapy sessions — for example, those areas the consultant feels he or she was not able to adequately explore.

I find myself frequently in the situation where it is not possible to obtain all the records. Yet in only a small percentage of the cases do I find myself deferring a recommendation or a diagnosis pending receipt of more information, such as an opportunity to interview a family member. When this happens, it occurs most frequently in a nursing home or inpatient setting, and there the opportunity to have more time is greater. It is more structured and less open than the usual outpatient setting. After the first meeting, I will then return to complete the consultation at a later time. In the interim, an attempt to obtain records will have been made.

However, as a rule, the desired information is not made available, even after the consultation has been prolonged. One must weigh the disadvantage incurred or the cost in delaying. Most often, I find efforts to obtain records from other institutions or a private MD are fruitless.

One must also keep in mind that the delay can be more costly than it is worth in terms of additional information providing meaningful help. Promptness in the delivery of service is frequently invaluable even if it has to be provided with information limited to what is obtained at the moment of the consultation.

CONCLUSION

Thus there are many different kinds of psychiatric consultations, and as a psychiatrist one may specialize in a single type, several types, or most of the types, depending on the amount of time the psychiatrist wishes to give to consultations.

As I said at the start of the chapter, I find my consultation work very gratifying. The combination of private practice and consultations seems mutually complementary and satisfying to me as one flows into the other, providing new insights that help both the patient and myself.

The need for these kinds of consultations or communications between psychiatrists and others (specialists of all types) is growing. With the increased number of patients in nursing homes, for example, the need is most apparent. The new psychiatrists entering the field should see in this an opportunity for them to provide a valuable service to the community, as well as to advance their own careers.

REFERENCES

Confidentiality and third parties. (1975). A report of the American Psychiatric Task Force on Confidentiality as it relates to third parties. Washington, DC: American Psychiatric Association.

Levine, M. (1972). *Psychiatry and ethics.* New York: George Braziller.

Prevost, J.A. (1980, December). The Berwid case. *The Bulletin,* Area II District Branches, American Psychiatric Association, *23*(4), 1-3.

Robitscher, J. (1980). The law begins its reliance on psychiatry. In J. Robitscher (Ed.), *The powers of psychiatry* (pp. 19-28). New York: Houghton Mifflin.

Roth, L.H., & Meisel, A. (1977, May). Dangerousness, confidentiality, and the duty to warn. *American Journal of Psychiatry,* 134-135.

Stone, A.A. (1977, March). Recent mental health litigation: A critical perspective. *American Journal of Psychiatry,* pp. 133-134.

ORGANIZATIONAL CONSULTING FOR CLINICIANS

David Monroe Miller, M.B.A.

INTRODUCTION:
WHAT ORGANIZATIONAL CONSULTANTS DO

This chapter is addressed to helping professionals with little or no background in management and organizational theory who are interested in exploring opportunities to consult with organizations on an occasional basis. Three major themes are developed. One is the broad range of consulting opportunities that exist, provided the clinician is willing and able to go beyond his or her existing capabilities and become involved in fundamental issues of human behavior in organizations. The second is the desirability of functioning as a genuine consultant, not just as a supplier of standard services. The third is the need to adopt a businesslike approach to the marketing, pricing, and performance of consulting services.

Needs Of Organizations

Although we are primarily thinking of the business firm when we use the term "organization," most of what is said applies equally to the nonprofit sector. It is the opportunity, and flexibility for action, rather than the need, that is greater in the business world. In both cases, the fundamental human-resource needs are to select, train, motivate, supervise, and reward people to enhance productivity, job satisfaction, fulfillment of individual needs, good interpersonal relationships, and efficient organizational functioning.

Other critical organizational needs include adapting to changes in the environment, having good decision-making processes, and striking the proper balance between innovation and stability. Consultants in these areas come from all of the social sciences as well as the business and management area. For these higher-level survival and growth needs, the primary specialized contribution of the helping professional is in breaking down barriers to effective, open communication and examining the extent to which "cultural" factors in the organization promote or inhibit growth.

To emphasize the range of needs that organizations have for professional assistance, we use the term "consulting" in its inexact but broadest sense of any professional services rendered on a contractual rather than employee basis.

The term *pure consulting* refers to a project or a relationship in which the primary output is policy guidance and recommendations. *Design and development* may include needs analysis, formulation of objectives, training guidelines, content outlines, and detailed other creative and analytical work specifying how an organization is to go about solving some problem or creating some new procedure. The third general category of consulting work is the one- to three-day *topical workshop* on psychologically related topics such as stress management or negotiating techniques. Workshops might be offered on a generic basis: for example, to any organization with little or no modifications — or with considerable custom-tailoring, perhaps originating as a recommendation to fulfill a need uncovered in other types of consulting work with that organization.

A fourth category, which may be of greatest initial interest to the practitioner, is *direct provision of clinically related services,* such as assessments or outplacement counseling (but not actual therapy). An important theme of the present chapter is that services of this nature frequently require the clinician to utilize "pure consulting" skills to establish the rationale and approach of the clinically related services.

Any of these four types of consulting might also include *research* for such purposes as providing a database for consulting recommendations, assessing needs analysis for program design, or validating one's own workshop or any other organizational program. In general, however, validation research is not nearly as common in business as it is in the public sector.

Skills Required

Consulting projects in any of the above areas usually require a variety of skills, which are listed roughly in a combined order of frequency and importance.

1. A basic *knowledge of the fundamental theories* of behavior and motivation in work organizations — some of which are summarized in this chapter — or at least the ability to apply general psychological theory to concrete situations. Without this element, there is no genuine expertise.

2. *"Active listening" and inquiry* skills, and the ability to modify them appropriately for a variety of populations and in a variety of situations. Nonclinical interviewing of organizational personnel and problem-oriented discussions with the client are two uses of these skills that occur in almost any type of project.

3. *Project management skills,* such as the ability to estimate time and costs, plan for and adapt to contingencies, and deliver on time.

4. Good *expository writing skills* for the letters, proposals, memos, interim reports, or other documents that are generated in the court of any project.

5. *Oral presentation skills,* or even the more difficult *platform skills* of the workshop presenter, which have a way (like expository writing) of appearing in almost any kind of project.

6. *Basic computer literacy,* which could be considered a plus rather than a necessity, but is becoming more important every year.

The fundamental paradox facing readers of this chapter is that consulting may be defined as the application of expertise, but many of the consulting opportunities discussed here require the readers to ignore, go beyond, or sometimes even reverse their previous training and expertise. A second and related problem is that the underlying skills of all consulting work are also not necessarily correlated with the training and career choice of the therapist — some of the most successful of all organizational consultants and theorists have a background in therapy or personality theory (see later).

In fact, consulting is not for everyone, and solo consulting on a variety of project types and for the purpose of making a living is for practically no one. Assuming that consulting is purely a "plus" rather than an economic or professional necessity, those readers who lack some of the skills required may be able to make contributions (1) as a member of a university-based or other type of team; (2) working mainly with smaller organizations; (3) in a large organization, working up from one specialty to the broader consulting aspects; or (4) without any limitation at all, given the accumulation of experience over time.

CONSULTING SERVICES: CLINICALLY RELATED SPECIALTIES

Aptitude And Ability Testing

The same developments that have made testing less popular in industry over the past two decades — notably, potential prejudice against minorities, a decline in popularity of the "specific aptitude" construct, and a general distrust of pencil–paper instruments — have actually increased the need for consultants when tests are used. The Civil Rights legislation of the mid-1960s did not outlaw tests for minority groups. What it did, under later Supreme Court and Equal Employment Opportunity Commission guidelines, was to require demonstration of criterion-related and content validity, both of them based on the actual job and company rather than on national validation samples.

Thus, a need exists for psychometric expertise in evaluating (or selecting, and possibly even designing) tests with good content and construct validity, and in conducting validation studies. In addition to credentials in these areas, the consultant must also have a solid, up-to-date knowledge of EEOC and other guidelines.

Executive Assessment

The principle underlying executive assessment is that for higher-level managerial or sales personnel, less value is placed on technical skill and more on motivational patterns and good interpersonal skills. The predictive rather than simply descriptive aspects of assessment are based on the assumption that personality characteristics of this nature are stable throughout the life cycle. Assessment, therefore, might be used as part of a hiring decision, to evaluate the present ranks of middle managers for future potential, or (less commonly) as input to counseling and even training.

In the clinician's office, a typical battery generally requires a single two- or three-hour appointment, with breaks. (Here and throughout this chapter it must be kept in mind that this population is basically nonpathological, well defended, hardworking, and highly intelligent.) The nucleus is an interview, one projective instrument (Rorschach or TAT), a WAIS, and a standardized pencil–paper inventory specifically designed for a type of position (sales, management, etc.) or for particular trait(s) deemed necessary. This nucleus might be altered or expanded with a second, high-stress interview by another interviewer; a second projective instrument; a high-speed, high-power, culture-fair, or other intelligence test; and other pencil–paper inventories.

Even in this relatively cut-and-dried application of familiar work, the clinician has the opportunity to function as a "pure" consultant working in the area of human resource policy—and, in fact, may be obligated to do so. Is the battery selected on the basis of general principles, or should some research be done first on success and failure in the particular client organization? Under what circumstances should assessment take place—before hire, before promotion, and so on—and how are results to be interpreted? What place does the assessment battery have in the overall decision? Who, if anyone, will conduct longitudinal validation research? The clinician who was not the consultant in these areas should satisfy himself or herself as to the propriety of the decisions made in regard to these questions and the potential ethical problems noted immediately in the following.

The clinical-battery approach to executive assessment is still practiced on a spot basis, but has undergone a considerable decline in popularity. Although racial bias is less of an issue than with the entry-level population, sexual bias may be present in individual instruments or in the underlying trait or motivational theory. Moreover, even though the argument for interpersonal qualities might solve content-validity objections, most sophisticated organizations prefer additional job-related tests and exercises. A third problem with the clinical battery model is vulnerability of the individual (and the client organization) to the psychological interpretations of a single clinician with limited understanding of the business environment. Probably the most serious problem from a legal/ethical point of view is that the assessed individual frequently gets no feedback, and has no appeal, or even informational database for an appeal.

For all of these reasons, many large organizations prefer to utilize the *assessment center* technique (Finkle, 1976). Briefly, an assessment center is any combination of activities that involves a multitrait, multimethod, and multijudge approach (Miller, 1977). The traits are usually nonclinical, common-sense syntheses such as "initiative," "flexibility," and others following from the general analysis of executive success in a particular setting. The methods are in two categories: expanded clinical batteries, as described above, and business-type exercises such as an "in basket," a leaderless group discussion, or a business simulation game. The observers ("assessors") are interested not only in technical decision-making ability, but also in how the individual approaches the task, manages anxiety, reacts to frustration, and relates to others in the group. The assessors are usually senior executives in the organization, trained by consulting psychologists. At some point—not necessarily during the assessment center itself—feedback and career counseling are usually provided to the assessees.

Consulting opportunities for the clinician include selection of the clinical portions of the battery; implementation thereof, including interpretation; training of company assessors in observation and reporting techniques; validation studies; and training in providing feedback.

Coaching And Counseling

In the past decade, "coaching and counseling skills" has become a "hot" topic in organizations, spawning many books and articles and a variety of organizational programs. Though the two concepts are frequently confounded, we suggest that they are actually alternative modes. *Coaching* should refer to behavioral analysis, assisting in overcoming personal skill deficits or environmental obstacles, working out detailed objectives and subobjectives, and providing the "moral support" that comes from attention, optimism, and feedback as to progress. When *counseling* is gratuitously added to a coaching situation, excessive emotional considerations may needlessly come into play and, more important, it may constitute a misdiagnosis of the problem.

This implies that coaching, rather than counseling, is the initial remedy of choice to any performance problem, corresponding to the idea that ability, rather than motivation, should be the initial focus (Gilbert, 1978; Mager & Pipe, 1970). Coaching may also be the preferred remedy to a morale problem insofar as good performance itself is highly motivating. Therapists with a background in behavioral analysis, not necessarily "behavior therapists," can make a contribution in the coaching area. The target population is not the employee and the focus is not on substantive skills. Rather, the consulting opportunity is in design and development of training programs for supervisors to make them better coaches. In addition, any time a supervisory population is a candidate for a training program in personnel-related procedures, members of the personnel department are also candidates—as trainees themselves or as potential workshop leaders.

Counseling can be defined for narrow organizational purposes as communication that involves effective, empathetic, action-oriented discussion in a supportive attmosphere (Miller, 1976). In itself, this is nontherapeutic in nature since it lacks the elements of analysis of feelings, confrontation, or other resistance and working-through phenomena. But even this milder form of counseling is at the opposite pole from most organizational communications, which involve the neutral exchange of information or unidirectional transmission of assignments. It also, clearly, has nothing to do with coaching except that both modes require considerable patience and represent constructive alternatives to transfer or termination. Counseling rather than coaching is indicated (1) when a problem is general dissatisfaction rather than a specific inability to perform effectively; (2) when feelings need to be expressed; or (3) when the employee is apparently requesting it.

From the general and mild definition of counseling given above, it follows that it is neither necessary nor desirable to teach confrontation techniques, self-revelation, or process commentary. Limited but valuable goals can be achieved if the consultant is willing to accept the fact that even a little bit of attitudinal change and communication authenticity can go a long way. That little bit consists of (1) positive regard, with or without labeling it as such, or even deliberately mislabeling it as "benefit of the doubt," and (2) a genuine desire to help. In a somewhat more advanced direction, it is also possible to give brief training in (3) labeling one's own emotions during the interview without necessarily soliciting the same from the employee. To this must be added only (4) an appreciation of the value of listening as opposed to talking.

Using the above principles, derived primarily from Garrett (1945) and Maier (1958), the present author has trained hundreds of supervisors in coaching and counseling skills. To make this approach work, four elements are critical: (1) didactic explanation of the helping role of the supervisor, which can be justified on the basis that it is ultimately the easiest as well as the most constructive alternative; (2) role play, with or without videotape (the consultant should demonstrate, not just critique); (3) a module on coaching (as opposed to counseling) principles as summarized earlier; (4) a clear indication, either didactic, by example, or both, that no emotional confrontations or other therapeutic skills are required. As long as it is made clear that the supervisor is not being asked to be a "shrink," or to give up the right to make the final decision, the principles of mutuality and supportiveness usually receive genuine acceptance.

With respect to coaching, the same general suggestion applies as to counseling: aim for limited, but valuable and thoroughly presented objectives. In addition, suggestions 1 and 2 above also apply to coaching training, and suggestions 3 and 4 can be rephrased and summarized as a suggestion to clearly differentiate coaching from counseling.

Coaching and (less frequently) counseling might be considered as basic skills that can be employed by anyone in the organization at supervisory level or above. In practice, however, they are better taught and more receptively learned when they are presented in the context of some specific application, such as performance appraisal, effective supervision, career development, or assisting special-problem subpopulations. There is much more to these areas than just coaching or counseling skills, and they are discussed later under "Human Resource Policy."

In summary, the coaching and counseling areas offer an excellent potential opportunity for therapists to utilize some aspects of their existing expertise within a broader organizational context. Three major themes have been emphasized: (1) the need for a clear distinction between coaching and counseling and their best applications; (2) a "narrow and deep" approach to training, bringing many training modalities to bear on limited goals rather than attempting to make experts out of beginners; and (3) a distinction between a generalized skill approach and an applications-oriented approach.

Individual And Organizational Stress

There are several different approaches to the topic of stress as it affects individuals in organizations. The indicated remedies may partly overlap, but the goals and rationales are quite different. The following labels and analyses are the author's own (Miller, 1983), but the basic issues are familiar to all investigators.

From a *medical* model or orientation, the primary interest is in prevention of heart disease, hypertension, gastritis, and other serious illnesses to which the work environment may contribute. Among the many "organizational stressors" that have been identified in the research literature are physical environmental factors such as temperature and noise, supervisor-employee relationships, and all of the tensions inherent in climbing up the promotional ladder. One possible consulting approach is to identify the "stressors" in a given organizational setting and attempt to change them (Kahn, 1974). Another approach is group training in symptom-reduction techniques such as the relaxation response or biofeedback training. This might be combined with a stepped-up program (internally or externally based) of medical and psychological diagnosis (Warshaw, 1979).

From an *organizational* perpsective, the original and still dominant conception of stress is based on the concept that the individual's role requirements in an organization cause internal conflict, ambiguity and overload (Kahn et al., 1964). These can be linked to the medical model under the assumption that problems of this nature provoke the alarm, resistance, and exhaustion responses discovered by Selye (1976). A more general version of the Kahn model is the idea that stress is caused by a poor "fit" between the individual and the work environment (French, 1974; French & Caplan, 1973). Under this conception, stress might be caused not only by overload but also by under-utilization or any chronic dissatisfactions with the job.

In social agencies or educational institutions, the term "burnout" rather than stress is frequently used (Paine, 1982). The usual stress of the workplace is compounded by the additional difficulty of working with populations and situations which produce more frustrations than successes (Maslach, 1982). Another type of burnout occurs in certain jobs such as that of air traffic controller or anesthesiologist in which the individual must continually function at a level of alertness so high as to incorporate the physiological stress response as a constant rather than an occasional variable.

Consulting approaches to job-related problems might include (1) analysis of the role requirements of those jobs where stress symptoms seem to be greatest; (2) examination of management policies, human-resource policies, and "cultural" factors that might give rise to unattainable goals or conflicting demands; and (3) group workshops or other interventions aimed at reducing unnecessary role conflict and ambiguity.

Clinical approaches to stress start with the premise that any stimulus can provoke the "alarm reaction" that initiates the stress response (Selye, 1976). Since individuals also differ in their behavioral, cognitive, and emotional versions of Selye's "resistance" and "exhaustion" responses, it could be argued that the primary locus of stress is individual rather than organizational (Miller, 1983). From this it follows that the symptoms of stress are more likely to be attributable not to the job but to the adaptive or maladaptive capabilities of the individual (Haan, 1977), to idiosyncratic cognitive/amotional responses to stressful stimuli (Coyne & Lazarus, 1980; Hamilton & Warburton, 1979), or to the individual's tendency to magnify the original problem by unnecessarily blaming himself or herself for failing to solve it (Ellis, 1978). The idea that organizational (or other) stressors may affect people differently is supported by the fact that stress-induced symptoms are characteristic primarily of the chronically aggressive, angry, multiphasic "type A" personality (Friedman & Rosenman, 1974; Glass, 1977; Ivancevich et al., 1985).

Stress management workshops from the clinical perspective thus might include discussion and possibly self-diagnosis of type A symptoms, an understanding of the vicious stress circle where inability to cope magnifies the original problem and causes secondary symptoms, and teaching individuals to strike a proper balance between excessive self-blame and unproductive externalization of the causes of stress.

Though different remedial actions may apply, there is no necessary fundamental contradiction between the medical, organizational, and clinically oriented approaches to stress. Aspects of all three may well be combined in the same workshop or consulting project. The clinical professional is clearly at least as well places as the organizational expert or physician to make contributions in this area, and probably better since the clinician's background and training include some aspects of those other disciplines.

Outplacement

Unemployment counseling is the process of helping individuals (1) deal with their (and their families') emotional crises; (2) deal with financial matters, possible relocation and other concrete consequences of the new situation; (3) find and evaluate job opportunities, including the possibility of career change; and (4) actually conduct the job search, including but not limited to how and where to look, how to prepare résumés and conduct oneself in an interview, and how realistically to evaluate one's salary potential. *Outplacement* is simply the name given to this kind of counseling from the corporation's perspective. It is becomig routine for large organizations to utilize external outplacement counselors, simply as a benefit they are willing to provide in addition to severance pay.

Of all the topics covered in this chapter, outplacement counseling is the closest type of work to what therapists do in private practice — provided they normally deal with an intelligent, aggressive, well-functioning, primarily male population. Management of the defenses is a critical area because those same defenses that must be maintained may actually be major obstacles to the effective mobilization and decision making on which the welfare of the person and the person's family depends.

But because they are decpetively similar, some important differences between outplacement and therapy present potential pitfalls. In particular, the following cautions are recommended.

1. Multiply by a large factor whatever reservations you normally have against excessive interpretation, and in general resist temptations to go therapeutically beyond what is explicit or implicit in the contract with the client organization.

2. Make fine discriminations and maintain extreme flexibility with regard to the appropriateness of directive versus nondirective responses, depending on the context. For example, directive and specific recommendations as to self-presentation are essential in outplacement work.

3. In the absence of considerable business experience or specific training,

and assuming that this aspect is covered elsewhere in the process, avoid all substantive, job-oriented issues. The counselor who does not have a genuine undestanding of, say, the difference between managerial accounting and independent auditing or how sales promotion differs from advertising will lose all credibility when trying to "dip in" to job-related areas.

Against these important cautions, there are many positive factors that make outplacement counseling a good possibility, even for therapists with no business experience. One is the common practice of working as part of team in a specialized outplacement organization that will provide training and supervision. Second, the psychological aspects of the lost-employment problem are highly repetitive and generalizable, allowing for development of a rapid learning curve. Finally, this high generalizability and consensus as to what the key issues are have produced a large and growing literature in which even the popular authors offer helpful advice to clients and counselors alike (e.g., Morin & Yorks, 1982; Brammer, 1984).

In the basic outplacement model as summarized above, the employee is external to the organization and for that reason, even though the firm is paying the bill, the consultant can unambiguously consider the individual (rather than corporate management) to be the client. But there are also consulting aspects to outplacement counseling. A consultant rather than a counselor would redefine the problem from "How do we help individuals?" to "Why is outplacement necessary in the first place, and what can be done about it?"

When a merger, deconglomeration, or cost-cutting drive requires a large-scale reduction in force, there is little that can be done from a consulting point of view. But the majority of executive terminations or semiforced early retirements involve fundamental organizational phenomena such as selection, placement, performance appraisal, career counseling, midcareer training, and many others (some of which are discussed in the next section). Experience as an outplacement counselor can be a valuable background to consultation in these areas.

Summarizing this section, the four clinically related areas of organizational consulting are entry-level or other high-volume testing, executive assessments, training in counseling and coaching skills, and outplacement counseling. The first three, if done thoroughly, may require some of the consulting skills discussed in the introduction, and at the very least a willingness to become involved in the organizational context. The last can be aspired to by any therapist with a strong background in crisis intervention with normal populations. But even outplacement offers the opportunity to begin thinking as a consultant rather than as a practitioner.

BROADER-BASED ORGANIZATIONAL INTERVENTIONS

Organization Development

Organization development (OD) is a label for a number of related techniques and principles designed to increase organizational effectiveness through improvement of communications, working relationships, formal and informal power structures, change processes, and other internal factors that might impede the performance, adaptability, and quality of life in an organization. There are numerous approaches to OD work, usually having in common a broad set of goals, premises, and techniques that include the following.

1. Emphasis on diagnosis of disruptive or unproductive relationship patterns. Diagnostic techniques may include formal employee-attitude surveys, group sessions, individual interviews, and observation.
2. Analysis of conflict patterns, and an attempt to substitute productive for unproductive conflict resolution mechanisms.
3. "Team-building" approaches, both within and across organizational sublunits (Dyer, 1977).
4. Greater openness in communications — if not always significant and durable after the fact, then at least at a very high level during the diagnostic/consulting process itself.
5. Participant-centered research and interventions (Nadler, 1977).
6. Analysis of underlying cultural patterns.

OD has its roots in part in the classic Hawthorne work group studies of the 1930s (Roethlisberger & Dickson, 1939); the field theory and group dynamics of Kurt Lewin (Lewin, 1951; Cartwright & Zander, 1953); the many "humanistic" approaches to management such as Argyris (1964, 1971) and MacGregor (1960); the survey research methodology developed at the University of Michigan (Bowers & Franklin, 1972); and the sensitivity training and other group techniques developed at the National Training Laboratories and other institutions.

It is no accident that these references are old. While many of the techniques of "classical" OD are still applicable, the overall rationale has shifted in the past decade from a humanistic-psychology rationale and an almost exclusively group-dynamics approach to a more strategically oriented conception of the requirements of organizational effectiveness (Kotter, 1978). The contemporary OD practitioner defines relationships as much more than the surface communication and interaction patterns. The focus, rather, is on making the organizations more receptive to change and able to adapt to it, strategically as well as technically (Beckhard & Harris, 1977). A full-scale OD effort may involve job redesign, structural changes in reporting relationships, and partial redefinition of the organization's or unit's strategic mission as well as the classic group-oriented techniques (Marrow, 1973).

"Neurotic" Organizational Patterns

One clinically related application of OD, to which considerable attention has been given only in the past decade, is "organizational neurosis." The rationale for this metaphor is a broad conceptualization of neurosis as cognitive, emotional, or behavioral patterns that interfere with flexibility and reality-based decision making. Hence, the growing literature on barriers to organizational adaptability and learning (Duncan & Weiss, 1979; Hedberg, 1981) is addressed to this issue even without using the term "neurosis." The classic work on organizational learning (Argyris & Schoen, 1978) is more directly based on a neurosis model, although again the term is not used.

More explicitly addressed to clinical issues, Kets de Vries and D. Miller (1984) have suggested that the "fantasies, beliefs, and aspirations" of the key individual organizational decision makers are translated into cultural and communications patterns that may be destructive to optimal strategy formulation. Five destructive patterns are outlined: paranoid, compulsive, dramatic (apparently a synthesis of "manic" and "hysteric"), depressive, and schizoid. These styles are correlated with organizational processes with regard to structure, culture, decision making, and supervisor–subordinate relationships analyzed in a "transference" framework. The governing model, however, is only indirectly Freudian, based most strongly on Bion's analysis of shared group fantasies, itself derived from the psychoanalytic theories of Melanie Klein (De Board, 1978).

Merry and Brown (1986) analyze similar phenomena but from a Gestaltist rather than psychoanalytic perspective. The important diagnostic and descriptive categories are the Perlsian rather than Freudian versions of the defense mechanisms. The consequences of the dysfunctional patterns are similar to those described by Kets de Vries and Miller, but the causes are rooted more firmly in organizational rather than individual pathology. Nevis (1987) relates organizational functioning to more classically cognitive rather than strictly Perlsian Gestalt principles. (Irrespective of its theoretical basis, the Nevis book cited in the bibliography provides excellent advice on the consulting process.)

In all cases, the general remedy of choice is a number of OD-type interventions in which realistic communication is a major goal. Because of the sensitive nature of the issues raised and the need to include the very top managers in the program, consulting in this area requires considerable experience and prestige, as well as a strong background in organization theory.

Organizational Culture

Analysis of "neurotic" patterns is just a special case of a more general area of interest—organizational culture. This term refers to a "complex set of values, beliefs, assumptions, and symbols" (Barney, 1985) that might be highly explicit or, alternatively, not at all apparent to the organizational participants. Among the more important dimensions of culture (or its near-synonym "climate") are formality versus informality, emphasis on merit versus seniority and how "merit" itself is perceived, quality versus quantity orientation, attitudes toward risk taking, and individual versus group emphasis.

A bureaucratic culture tends to emphasize compliance with rules, aversion to risk and innovation, production of written documentation, and closely monitored hierarchical control. Other broad cultural types include the professional, entrepreneurial, and "missionary." Different cultural elements might tend to affect effectiveness of leadership style (Litwin & Stringer, 1968), strategic decision making (Nystrom & Starbuck, 1984), type of managerial personnel most likely to climb the ladder successfully (Miner, 1978), and many other elements of an organization's functioning.

The purpose of consultation in this area is not to come up with the proper label but to analyze those ways in which the culture is functional or dysfunctional to the organization. One possible dysfunctional element is the mixing of disparate cultural elements. Another is a misplaced culture in a particular external business environment. A third is a mismatch between the type of personnel hired and the underlying cultural values.

All of these elements are coming to the fore as the American economy becomes more and more based on innovative, hi-tech firms growing into industrial giants. With increasing growth and market penetration, the entrepreneurial values and missionary spirit tend to be replaced by the need for control of procedures and assets, formal personnel policies, emphasis on decorum and reliability rather than sheer brilliance, and accommodation to the needs of the marketplace rather than the best possible technical product. But the same creative personnel are still responsible for design and production.

Similar cultural conflicts are frequently observed in the nonprofit sector, as hospitals and educational institutions come under increasing pressure to emphasize financial rather than technical success criteria. There is no necessary conflict between the two, and if there is, it is not necessarily dysfunctional. But to some of the individuals caught in these situations, it may appear as if the organization is changing for the worse every day, and to others that the forces of progress are being kept back by the reactionary old guard, and so on.

It is not just in periods of rapid growth and change that cultural issues become prominent. Sometimes a new chief executive, or even department head, can cause cultural change and disorientation. Even in the most placid of times, there are usually chronic cultural conflicts among functional specialties such as sales, accounting, production, and others (Lawrence & Lorsch, 1967).

The goals of the consultant are not to change the culture, or even to resolve the conflicts, but to assist the participants in becoming aware of the underlying cultural patterns, to help the organization avoid incongruence between human resource policies and cultural realities, and, in some cases, to assist individuals in dealing with cultural issues.

It should not be concluded that culture, or more generally the "informal" aspect of an organization (Barnard, 1938; Kanter, 1977), is only a negative force. On the contrary, when cultural attitudes are institutionalized in clearcut, consistent policies for dealing with employees and customers, morale and performance are likely to improve (Peters & Watermann, 1983; MacMillan, 1983). Even without clearcut indications at the policy level, the myths, sagas, folklore, and unstated beliefs of an organization as shared and perceived by all participants are likely to exert positive force toward goal attainment and conflict reduction — provided, however, that they are applicable to realities of the present and are not just relics of the past (Deal & Kennedy, 1982; Nystromn & Starbuck, 1984).

For the nonspecialist, the most important implication of organizational culture is its potential pervasiveness throughout all aspects of organizational life. When consulting in human resource policy, it is always necessary to have an understanding of the underlying culture. At the individual level, executive assessment and outplacement counseling both involve implicit or explicit judgmnets as to how an individual will perform *in a particular type of environment.* In OD, work culture is more than just important background; it is a critical area ot analyze directly.

PSYCHOLOGICAL APPROACHES
TO HUMAN RESOURCE POLICY
AND WORK MOTIVATION

Theoretical Foundations In Clinical Psychology

Selection, training, maintenance of job satisfaction, work redesign, performance appraisal, career pathing, compensation guidelines, special-population problems, and similar areas are generally considered the province of the industrial rather than clinical psychologist. But much of the theory underlying many advanced personnel practices has come from psychologists with a background in clinical and counseling psychology, or personality theory. Maslow's *need hierarchy* (Maslow, 1943, 1962; Alderfer, 1972) is perhaps the best-known example of motivational theory aplied to industry. Herzberg's (1959, 1966) *two-factor* theory of motivation and job satisfaction actually began as a theory of mental health. Both theories have in common the idea that the motivational aspect of job performance does not come from pay alone. Rather, it is necessary to give employees the opportunity to satisfy higher-level needs such as belongingness and self-esteem (Maslow) or accepting of genuine responsibility and challenge (Herzberg). These theories have their widest application in work redesign ("job enrichment") programs.

McClelland's *need theory* of achievement, affiliation, and power motivation is widely used in motivational research, executive assessment centers, and management training (Boyatzis, 1982; Miller, 1985). His most recent and organizationally relevant theory of power motivation (McClelland, 1975) is strongly based in the developmental psychology of Freud and Erikson. Another noteworthy feature of McClelland's theory is that it requires a fantasy-based conception of motivation, which is measured by the TAT. Two of McClelland's associates and students, Richard Boyatzis (1982; McBer Corporation) and George Litwin (1968; Forum Corporation) are among the most successful practicing consultants in the 1980s.

With the notable exception of Harry Levinson (1964, 1970, 1973, 1974) and the recent interest in organizational neurosis discussed above, the direct influence of *psychoanalysis* in organization theory has been weak relative to its overall influence in intellectual history. Indirectly, however, it is built into applications of McClelland's work and (especially in Great Britain) the Tavistock approach to interpersonal relations. De Board (1978) emphasizes the latter but also provides a comprehensive introduction to psychoanalytic approaches in organizations.

Cognitive Approaches To Work Motivation

In the past decade, the forefront of psychologically based research has begun to shift from a need-satisfaction model to a combination of cognitive consistency and competence motivation. The underlying notion of "intrinsic motivation" (Deci, 1975, 1980) is that effort both comes from and enhances the sense of ability and self-worth. When the motivational basis is shifted to purely monetary or other extrinsic compensation, the individual loses the intrincis aspect of the motivation and performance may decrease. Intrinsic motivation is partly based on attribution theory, of which Julian Rotter's (1966) "locus of control" is the best-known concept. As later developed by Bernard Weiner (Weiner & Sierad, 1975), persons with a strong internal locus of control will tend to attribute their successes to their own efforts and ability. Persons with an external locus will tend to attribute their successes to luck or the easiness of the task. Another important basis for intrinsic motivation is DeCharms' (1968) theory of personal causation, itself based in part on White's (1959) "competence motivation."

Probably the most effective theory and practice in cognitive-based work-motivational theory is the goal-setting approach of Edwin Locke (1968). Goal setting is compatible with behaviorist notions such as successive approximation and positive reinforcement (Feeney, 1973), but is more fundamentally based on the newer ideas of intrinsic motivation and locus of control. The basic propositions, confirmed in a number of studies, is that performance will increase when goals are (1) higher, (2) specific, (3) accepted by the individual, and (4) the individual is given appropriate feedback as to progress.

Although these latter theories are very much cognitively oriented, they are all based on an underlying notion of the importance of self-esteem (Korman, 1975). While theorists and researchers in the organization field might tend to make self-esteem a more fragile, more easily manipulated, and more ephemeral variable than most clinicians would, a large area of common ground exists between the clinical and cognitive orientations.

A psychologist familiar with some or all of these theories will find that they can be brought to bear on a number of organizationally relevant issues, such as job redesign, effective supervision, productivity improvement (insofar as motivation appears to be the problem), compensation policy, and excessive unwanted turnover. For example, in order to attract the most able and ambitious management candidates, it may be necessary to offer high starting salaries, but in order to maintain their motivation, it is necessary to offer the kind of challenging assignments that enable them to demonstrate competence through their own efforts. What does this say about the wisdom of traditional job-rotation programs where trainees have little opportunity to do anything constructive on their own?

It is not suggested here that a psychological theory can easily be translated into organizational practice, or that the results are always justified by unambiguous validation research. The primary point made in this section is that within the total field of psychological applications to organizational functioning, the clinical and counseling disciplines have provided much of the underlying theoretical, and even philosophical, foundations — second, if at all, only to the cognitive area. Thus, the main concepts with regard to work motivation and human resource policy are familiar in one guise or another to all therapists: need satisfaction, responsibility and challenge, self-esteem, and individual differences in motivation and personality.

A second major point is that the cognitive, personality, and motivational constructs discussed in this section are only grossly, and even inaccurately, captured by naive notions of "patting on the back," "being nice to people," or even "industrial human relations." The theories discussed suggest that praise and good fellowship are meaningless, even counterproductive, if not accompanied by genuine structuring of the work conditions and effort–performance relationships to encourage internal attributions, satisfaction of achievement needs, intrinsic motivation, and other sophisticated rationales for better performance and satisfaction. [An excellent though research-oriented overview of the theories discussed in this section, and many others, appears in Miner (1980).]

Organizational Applications Of Coaching And Counseling Techniques

For any other readership, the author would not present performance appraisal and topics in this section as "applications of counseling and coaching techniques." They are, rather, important organizational procedures with a number of ramifications. Counseling and coaching techniques are only means to achieving some of the objectives of human resource policy. However, skill training in coaching and counseling represents the most likely avenue for the clinician to begin getting involved in the broader areas.

Performance Appraisal   The most common coaching and counseling context is in connection with the periodic (usually annual) performance-appraisal interview. It may appear ludicrous to expect a supervisor, with or without training, to adopt a person-oriented rather than problem-oriented mode of communication once a year—and then under circumstances that are usually characterized by a high degree of anxiety and defensiveness on the part of both parties (Meyer et al., 1965). While it is highly unlikely that a consultant will be able to persuade a large corporation to change such a widely practiced and long-institutionalized procedure, it might be possible to make certain specific recommendations about the process. In addition to the coaching and counseling aspects, clinicians can help train supervisors in avoiding common rater errors such as halo effects or idiosyncratic criterion definitions.

The performance-appraisal systems should ideally be tied in with human resource policies and programs with regard to promotion, career pathing, career counseling, "early identification" or "fast tracking" systems, and other aspects of human resource policy or procedure, some of which are discussed in this chapter.

Career Development   A second application of counseling, and to some extent coaching, is in career-development programs. The purposes of a career-development interview vary widely, but usually include (1) specific information as to promotional opportunities in the future; (2) summarization of the company's view of the employee at this time, including future prospects; (3) review of company policies with regard to relocation, retirement, educational benefits, and other personnel policies, especially those that may affect the individual in the near future; and (4) recommendations as to specific formal training and job positions that are necessary in the career path toward some desired goal.

Unlike many of the other topics discussed in this section (for example, assessment centers and outplacement), there is very little in the way of consensual theory or practice with regard to career-development programs. Among the important unresolved questions and issues are the following.

1. "Representation'—organization- or individual-oriented?

2. Counseling technique—primarily information, or genuine exploration of feelings?

3. Role of supervisors (as opposed to personnel specialists) in the process.

4. How and with what degree of finality are negative prospects to be communicated?

5. Timing and goals of the career development interview(s).

Thus, the consultant should not approach a career-development program as a routine application of counseling techniques. A "pure consulting" perspective is essential.

Needs of Special Subpopulations   A third application of coaching and counseling techniques is in assisting special-problem subpopulations such as female executives, racial minorities, formerly hard-core unemployed, or new employees. For example, as director of executive training in a large corporation, the author identified a number of special problems in recent junior- and senior-college graduates hired as part of an executive training program. Simply being on trainee status, drawing a full salary without a "real" job, was in some cases guilt provoking or otherwise emotionally disturbing, even though the situation had been predicted and explained intellectually many times. Turnover was sharply reduced with (among other methods) a counseling program that consisted mainly of (1) an increase in individual attention, (2) an opportunity to ventilate safely, (3) reassurance that these concerns (and others not mentioned here) were normal, and (4) investigation, and in some cases outright mediation, of difficult, policy-oriented trainee–supervisor conflicts.

For any of the special populations, *mentoring* is frequently seen as a helpful practice (Zey, 1984; Kramm, 1985). Should this be totally informal, or officially sponsored by the organization? Do mentors need training or does that destroy the essential nature of what they are and do? How are they to be allocated? Are all people equally adept at seeking out and making the best use of mentors? Is it important to have age, ethnicity, or sex match between mentor and mentee? A counseling psychologist is in as good a position as any other behavioral-science specialist to answer questions of this kind.

For females, programs are frequently given in assertiveness training (Zucker, 1983), coping with "tokenism" (Kanter, 1977), dealing with sexual harassment, and other special-interest topics. Once again, the psychological consultant might approach such areas in any or all of three different ways: (1) delivering workshops in these areas directly to the target population; (2) training personnal executives in how to conduct such workshops or otherwise be of counseling- or coaching-type assistance; or (3) examining the fundamental organizational and psychological factors and attempting to get at the root of the problems.

Employee Assistance   Probably the greatest use of counseling techniques in organizations is in connection with Employee Assistance Programs (Shain & Groenevelt, 1980; Masi, 1982). This broad term usually includes alcoholism, substance abuse, family or other casework-type advice and assistance, and, in some cases, diagnosis and referral for personality or behavior disturbances. The unit of analysis is the individual case rather than the broader organizational phenomenon, and, therefore, this topic is covered elsewhere. There are, however, a number of areas in which the underlying model is not pathology or deviance, but normality. Among them are retirement, relocation, problems of the working single parent, and psychological problems pertaining to midlife crisis. All of these may be realted, to some extent, to organizational personnel policies in such areas as compensation, training, career development, and promotion policies.

Summary: Human Resource Policy

Very few therapists can come into an organization and claim to have the specific expertise needed to design or revise a performance-appraisal system, a career-development program, or the structure of jobs in the organization. But very few personnel executives, much less the operating executives, have a background in the underlying psychological principles.

Rather than try to sell expertise where it is lacking—that is, specific experience with organizational functions such as job redesign or performance appraisal—clinicians are advised to emphasize what they presumably do have: an understanding of behavior and motivation from a number of theoretical perspectives and/or specific expertise in coaching, counseling, and other aspects of behavior change. After some experience is gained, however, it becomes feasible actually to begin designing or recommending specific systems and procedures.

ESTABLISHING AND MAINTAINING A CONSULTING RELATIONSHIP

Marketing Of Services

Overview   The term "marketing" may sound alien to helping professionals, but it is essential to understand the meaning of the term as used by management professionals. In this context, marketing refers to (1) understanding the needs of potential clients, (2) evaluating and developing one's capabilities to meet those needs, and (3) using a variety of methods to bring the customer in contact with the supplier. Marketing is a difficult job even for the experienced professional, but the task might actually be easier for the practicing therapist who is in no great hurry and is simply looking for broader opportunities, career enrichment, and supplementary rather than basic income. For these purposes, most of the necessary marketing work involves the use of affiliations, informal networking, and other third-party techniques based on word of mouth rather than direct solicitation of potential clients. We also consider the "work sample" approach (workshops, articles, etc.) and last, primarily to dismiss it, direct-response techniques.

Third-Party and World-of-Mouth Approaches   A *university affiliation,* even on an adjunct basis, can be quite helpful. Let the key people in the departments of psychology, management, and related areas know that you are prepared to do consulting work. Teaching itself, irrespective of the subject, is a helpful credential and good experience for consulting work, implying that you are able to make presentations to groups, prepare materials, and work toward achievement of concrete objectives on a three- or four-month planning horizon. Hospital or agency affiliations are less attractive to potential business clients, but still helpful for making contact with people who are doing consulting work.

Networking and cross-referring is a potentially valuable, low-cost activity. Occasionally, a person with an "in" to an organization is asked to do something outside his or her area of expertise, but within yours. Networking, especially in conjunction with the professional societies discussed below, is also an excellent way to become informed about the pricing of services and other practical aspects of consulting that are covered only on an overview basis in this chapter.

The best third-party technique, but not easy to attain in practice, is to examine the possibilities of working on an affiliated basis with an *existing consulting firm.* The large, well-known firms will probably not be interested, but every major city has a number of smallish firms specializing either in personnel-relevant work or in more concrete specialties such as outplacement or testing. Diligent perusal of the classified telephone directory will yield some eligible names, but the best approach is through networking and professional meetings.

Various *professional societies and interest groups* represent an excellent source of networking opportunities and, in some cases, provide valuable introductory or advanced knowledge of the topics discussed in the previous sections. The major academic societies are the Division of Industrial and Organizational Psychology of the American Psychological Association, and the Academy of Management. Among the relevant divisions in the latter are Organization Behavior and Development, Management Training and Education, Management Consulting, and Personnel and Human Resources. Through its membership rather than formal programs, the Association for Humanistic Psychology can be a helpful affiliation for networking and informational purposes, especially to consultants interested in OD.

The primary semiprofessional society for psychologically oriented consultants is the American Society for Training and Development. Its publication, the *Training and Development Journal,* is an excellent nonacademic guide to the type of programs currently of interest to large organizations. The local chapters are an important source of networking, and also sponsor workshops for members. In New York City, the Management Development Forum and the OD Nedtwork are typical interest groups consisting partly of consultants and partly of human resource managers. These societies, their counterparts in other cities, and others that may exist are best tracked down through word of mouth.

Work Samples *National workshops* represent a potential avenue to consulting. Workshop organizations always have a need for faculty, either presenting their existing programs or developing your own. Considering the total time involved in preparation and travel, the remuneration of $300–500 per day is not high — but it is a helpful credential and a possible source of future clients, provided you can legitimately deal with contractual provisions to the contrary (e.g., by waiting a certain number of years). However, do not even consider this option unless you are prepared to conduct workshops in cities other than your own, and you already have "platform skills" of a very high order.

Most consultants at one time or another find themselves giving a *gratis speaking engagement* or miniworkshop. Two principles should be observed. First, do not do it just for marketing reasons alone. Preparing and conducting a presentation should also help clarify your approach and sharpen your skills. Second, pick your spots carefully.

Publications can be extremely helpful, but the usual academic priorities are reversed. Very few clients are interested in the refereed journals, even those of a business orientation. A readable but technically sound book is best, but any publication at all serves the purposes of helping you define your approach, giving something more substantial than a business card to hand out, and establishing you as an expert. For these reasons, gratis or nominal-honorarium articles can be attractive, even more so than the corresponding gratis workshops (since there is a lasting product to show for it). The same principles apply that were given earlier in that connection.

Direct-Response Techniques   *Direct individual solicitation* of a potential client is not at all unprofessional for consulting purposes, but it is economically unrewarding except when you have a specific and somewhat unique approach or program to offer, as well as a rationale for contacting a particular organization and an appropriate named individual within it. Larger mailings of a form letter are not recommended, not because they are unprofessional, but because for the typical reader they will not represent a productive input/output ratio. The final direct-response mode, advertising, simply does not work and may involve considerable risk in the expenditure of funds. Even the small expenditure involved in a display ad (or even the basic listing fee) in the classified telephone directory under "Consultants" is usually not worthwhile.

To summarize our remarks on marketing, the major principles are (1) do not wait until you are equipped with what you hope will later be all of your consulting skills, (2) work initially through third parties using informal techniques, and (3) do not invest large amounts of time or money in the marketing activities described if they are not activities that are at least minimally rewarding or would be undertaken anyway. A second, consulting-oriented business card and some occasional lunch treats for "brain picking" and networking are the only marketing expenses necessary.

The final principle can be stated negatively: never adopt the many principles and methods given here in the assumption that consulting can turn into a reliable or major source of income. Economically, consultants resemble actors. *Everybody would like to make large fees doing interesting work on an occasional basis.* For that very reason, it is just not in the cards for everyone to do so. Thus, therapists who are unsuccessful in obtaining consulting business should not succumb to the myth that they would do so if only they worked harder at it. The author advises keeping financial, time-related, and ego commitments low as befits a secondary, part-time occupation. But it is also fallacious to assume that success comes from the luck of being in the right place at the right time. In consulting, as in therapy, practice development results from a gradual accumulation of contacts, prestige, and experience.

Pricing

Pricing of consulting work can be an extremely complex subject and cannot be treated here in great detail. There are three common types of billing — total project, daily, and hourly. The hourly model is appropriate only when the primary input is an actual session (as in outplacement counseling or clinical assessments). The suggested pricing method is to add at least one-third to one's existing session-fee rate to cover the additional costs of doing business as a consultant (which, in practice, reduce primarily to the time and effort spent in the marketing activities described above).

Except for the above circumstances, most organizational consulting is billed according to a *nominal daily rate.* The "day" in consulting work is the usual unit of analysis, but except when the project consists solely of discrete days spent on-site, there is no such thing as a "day." Despite the fictitiousness of the daily rate and the near-impossibility of an accurate project estimate, the consultant invariably is asked to state a daily rate and to gived an estimate of the total project costs. The consultant is urged to answer the first question with a range, depending on type and circumstances of work as described below, and the second question only after considerable thought and analysis.

A *fixed project fee* (usually paid in "progress payment" installments) is the method favored by most consultants and clients alike, but is quite risky for the inexperienced consultant. Even when some other method of billing is ultimately agreed on, the client will invariably ask for a "ballpark estimate" of total costs. It is advisable to defer answering this question until you have had time to think through the following considerations.

1. Estimate the amount of time to be spent on different types of activities, and consider pricing them differentially. For example, workshop presentations usually are priced at higher than the normal daily rate whereas preliminary interviewing and other activities undertaken primarily for your own learning and familiarization might be priced much lower.

2. In addition to the type of work, the circumstances and conditions have to be considered. A project that can be done at your own convenience can, and should, be priced lower than work done in a client's facility, which inevitably requires travel time and unproductive waiting around. Projects done (at the client's request) on a "crash" basis should be priced at a premium. Finally, it is perfectly legitimate to charge a higher base rate for a short-term project. and a lower one, perhaps considerably lower, for longer-term work.

3. The final and most important rule of thumb is, when in doubt, err on the high side. The most common mistake made by inexperienced consultants is to set their initial fees too low and then compound this by underestimating the total time required to complete a project. A related mistake is to absorb costs unnecessarily. No matter what method of pricing is used, certain expenses, such as non-local travel, high-volume duplicating, and toll calls, among others, are always reimbursable or done at the client's facilities.

Selected Aspects Of The Client–Consultant Relationship

Mutual Definition of Problems and Solutions   Most consultants begin by providing relatively well-defined services and then gradually work up to a pure consulting arrangement with their clients. However, the recommendation here is that the consultant should always begin thinking as a pure consultant—not as a supplier. From this perspective, the golden rule is: Clients know what is bothering them, but do not necessarily know what the problem is, much less what the solution is. Certainly no therapist would accept the conclusions of a patient with regard to diagnosis and indicated therapy. indicated therapy.

This is by no means the same as an inflexible "I'm the doctor" attitude. In many cases, the client's intuitive, experience-based diagnosis of an underlying problem or remedy may well be correct but still has to be verified by the therapist's own first-hand knowledge and thoughtful analysis.

Written Proposals and Other Documentation   A well-thought-out *proposal* is a vehicle for planning, pricing, and even "selling" the project. It may also serve as the only contractual documentation needed and additionally can be the design document for a complex project. It should contain, at a minimum, a statement of what you plan to do, how and when you plan to do it, what informational input and other support are needed from the client, the price and price basis (hourly, daily, total project), any contractual type of provisions you deem necessary (e.g., timing of payments, limitations on your availability), and statement of qualifications for the particular proposed project.

Most consultants are willing to write a proposal at no charge, compensating for the time spent by factoring it into the price. Others insist on charging half-rates or even full rates. It is appropriate to suggest this to the client when (1) a considerable amount of time is spent in preliminary meetings and familiarization, (2) the proposal is large and complex, and (3) it is not just a pricing vehicle but contains design or consulting recommendations.

For projects of large scope where the problems and solutions are unclear at the outset, a *design document* should be produced at the conclusion of the research and familiarization phase. This states, in greater detail and with greater information than was available in the proposal stage, the specific objectives, methods, and scheduling milestones. An important purpose of the design document is to secure the client's formal review and approval or other input.

Most projects end with a written *report* embodying conclusions and recommendations. This may substitute for or simply recapitulate an earlier (or subsequent) oral presentation. The time and effort spent on a written report may be a major expense item, so it is advisable to specify the form and content in the pricing stage.

Other Business-Related Aspects   Beginning consultants frequently ask if they need to have a separate office, mailing address, business name, or incorporated status for the purpose of appearing more substantial to clients. The answer is almost always "no." In this field, practitioners who work out of their own homes or home/offices is the rule, not the exception. The only item in this regard that is recommended is a second business card, and possibly a letterhead. Office facilities are irrelevant since there is almost never a need for a client to come to your office.

Physical production of typed materials—for example, proposals, workshop materials, interim or final reports, and other documents that a therapist normally does not produce—can be a problem if it catches the consultant by surprise. In the proposal (or equivalent) stage, it is essential to estimate the quantitative requirements, the form that materials must be in (preliminary, camera-ready, etc.), and the question of who will do them. Do not assume that a secretary who does bills or brief clinical reports has the ability, much less the time, to do this kind of work.

Another potentially thorny issue involves scheduling conflicts. The vast majority of business meetings are scheduled at mutual convenience. The consultant who has one morning and one afternoon free on different days will almost never have a problem. Make your hours of availability known at the beginning of a project and they will be respected. *Never reschedule a patient* or any other valuable professional activity for a routine business meeting that has a 50 percent probability of being changed at the last minute.

Results Orientation   Some clients are overly suspicious of academic or therapeutic credentials and others are overly impressed. But at either end of the spectrum and on the vast middle ground in between, clients always prefer consultants who show that they understand their problems and concerns. A consultant who proceeds on the basis of purely theoretical knowledge and has a lack of appreciation for what business people are trying to do will, quite rightly, have no credibility in spite of great technical skills.

The primary difference between a manager and a clinician has nothing to do with a "profit" versus a "helping" orientation. It is, rather, that professional managers are oriented toward the efficient, effective, and observable solution of concrete problems. In this regard, a short-term, contractually oriented therapist is more attitudinally in tune with a business executive than with another therapist of the traditional long-term, open-ended persuasion. Therapists of the latter type must constantly guard against the fallacy of thinking that input is equivalent to output. From your perspective you might think you are conducting a workshop in coaching skills (input), but from the client's perspective—the correct one—you are helping supervisors remedy performance problems (output). The results orientation, not revenue or profit, is what clients really mean by a bottom-like perspective.

Consulting Process and Style   Nevis (1987) distinguishes between the Sherlock Holmes and the Lieutenant Columbo approaches to consulting. Holmes formulates clear hypotheses and uses clues and rigorous deductive logic to arrive at the truth. But as Nevis and many other process-oriented authors point out, unambiguous clues are not always available in organizations, frequently there is no one clear solution, and the deductive logic of the consultant does not always match the internal logic of the participants (Nadler, 1977). Columbo proceeds by intuition. Frequently he learns more from a wrong guess than from a right one. Where Holmes errs on the side of arrogance, Columbo would rather err on the side of humility.

The present author, whose experience is primarily in testing, training, personnel policies, and organizational theory applicable to business firms, is unabashedly Holmesian. We advocate a clear definition of the problem and expected methods and results as early as the proposal stage, and a deductive approach whereby established theory and accumulated experience, modified by the individual circumstances, are used as a guide to action. Other authors whose experience is primarily in less structured settings and oriented to OD applications might be more Columbian.

In clinical practice, there is a similar distinction between the rigorous, problem-oriented approach of the psychiatrist or behaviorist and the holistic, relationship-oriented approach of the psychotherapist. Clearly, the best approach can only be determined by a conjunction of individual style, client preference, and type of problem at hand. Ideally, both approaches should be used. For example, we have noted the importance of understanding the underlying culture, even in the most cut-and-dried consulting projects. But we have also noted the importance of an overall results orientation even in the most process-oriented type of work. Ultimately, there is no necessary contradiction except when the individual preferences of the consultant limit flexibility.

SUMMARY

The difficulties involved in learning about organizations and marketing one's own services are indeed formidable, but not insurmountable. The task is impossible only if incorrect ideas and assumptions prevent the attempt from ever being made. Lack of paper credentials, or even of experience, is not as much of a drawback as the reader might expect. The business world is quite different from the university, hospital, or government environment in this regard. Business executives — at least the successful ones — are conditioned to look at tasks and problems as the units of analysis. The individual who can help them solve the problem, reliably and on time, is the one they want. The differences between the Ph.D., Ed.D., Psy.D., D.S.W. or other doctorates are of no consequence to them, and the doctorate level itself is by no means a prerequisite.

The second and related false assumption is that therapists must limit themselves to narrowly defined clinical specialties. We have discussed in some training can be helpful to organizations, based on the premise that an understanding of human behavior and motivation is actually the core organizational discipline. The second core organizational discipline is simply the ability to get things accomplished, on time and as promised. Therapists who view themselves as having those two kinds of expertise can find many opportunities to solve interesting problems, and so enhance their own knowledge as well as income and prestige. Others might prefer to stick closer to home and investigate opportunities in outplacement and similar areas.

With regard to all types of consulting services, the clinician has been encouraged to think like a consultant from the beginning. What are the purposes of the program or technique? Are the methods suggested actually the best for the purpose? Above all, what is the underlying organizational problem or pattern that is really the issue?

Organizational consulting offers the opportunity to learn more not only about organizational phenomena, but also about fundamental individual phenomena such as job choice, midlife crisis, job-induced stress, and personality characteristics that are amenable to certain types of jobs or organizations (Maccoby, 1976; Miner, 1878). Given the importance of work in the lives of almost all private clients, and the almost total lack of expansion anywhere in the therapeutic literature on Freud's afterthought *und arbeiten,* the experience gained can only be beneficial to the private practice.

REFERENCES

Alderfer, C. (1972). *Existence, relatedness, and growth: Human needs in organizational settings.* New York: Free Press.

Argyris, C. (1964).*Integrating the individual and the organization.* New York: John Wiley and Sons.

Argyris, C. (1971). *Management and organizational development.* New York: McGraw-Hill.

Argyris, C., & Schoen, H. (1978). *Organizational learning: A theory of action perspective.* Reading, MA: Addison-Wesley.

Barnard, C. (1953). *The functions of the executive.* Cambridge, MA: Harvard University Press.

Barney, J. (1986). Organizational culture: Can it be a source of sustained competitive advantage? *Academy of Management Review, 11,* 656–665.

Beckhard, R., & Harris, R. (1977). *Organizational transitions: Managing complex change.* Reading, MA: Addison-Wesley.

Bowers, D., & Franklin, J. (1972). Survey-guided development: Using human resources measurement in organizational change. *Journal of Contemporary Business,* 43–55.

Boyatzis, R. (1982). *The competent manager.* New York: John Wiley and Sons.

Brammer, L. (1984). *Outplacement and inplacement counseling.* Englewood Cliffs, NJ: Prentice-Hall.

Cartwright, D., & Zander, A. (Eds.) (1953). *Group dynamics* (3rd ed.). New York: Harper & Row.

Coyne, J., & Lazarus, R. (1980)?. Cognitive style, stress perception, and coping. In I. Kutash, L. Schlesinger, et al. (Eds.), *Handbook on stress and anxiety.* San Francisco: Josey-Bass.

De Board, R. (1978). *The psychoanalysis of organizations.* London: Tavistock Publications.

Deal, T., (Kennedy, A. (1982). *Corporate cultures.* Reading, MA: Addison-Wesley.

DeCharms, R. (1968). *Personal causation: The internal affective determinants of behavior.* New York: Academic Press.

Deci, E. (1975). *Intrinsic motivation.* New York: Plenum.

Deci, E. (1980). *The psychology of self-determination.* Lexington, MA: Lexington Books.

Duncan, R., & Weiss, A. (1979). Organizational learning: Implications for organizational design. In B. Staw & L. Cummings (Eds.), *Research in organizational behavior.* Greenwich, CT: JAI Press. Vol. 1, pp. 75–123.

Dyer, W. (1977). *Team building: Issues and alternatives.* Reading, MA: Addison-Wesley.

Ellis, E. (1978). What people can do for themselves to cope with stress. In C. Cooper & R. Payne (Eds.), *Stress at work.* New York: John Wiley and Sons.

Feeney, E. (1973). At Emery Air Freight: Positive reinforcement boosts performance. In K. Wexley & G. Yukl (Eds.), *Organizational behavior and industrial psychology.* New York: Oxford University Press, pp. 560–568. (Originally in *Organizational Dynamics,* Winter, 1973.)

Finkle, R. (1976). Managerial assessment centers. In M. Dunnette (Ed.), *Handbook of industrial and organizational psychology.* Chicago: Rand-McNally, pp. 861–888.

French, J. (1974). Person-role fit. In A. McLean (Ed.), *Occupational stress.* Springfield, IL: Charles C. Thomas.

French, W., & Bell, C. (1973). *Organization development.* Englewood Cliffs, NJ: Prentice-Hall.

French, J. & Caplan, R. (1973). Organizational stress and individual strain. In A. Marrow (Ed.), *The failure of success.* New York: AMACOM.

Friedman, M., & Rosenman, R. (1974). *Type A behavior and your heart.* Greenwich, CT: Fawcett Publications.

Gilbert, T. (1978). *Human competence.* New York: McGraw-Hill.

Glass, D. (1977). *Behavior patterns, stress, and coronary heart disease.* Hillsdale, NJ: Earlbausm Associates.

Haan, N. (1977). *Coping and defending: Processes of self-environment organization.* New York: Academic Press.

Hamilton, V., & Warburton, D. (Eds.) (1979). *Human stress and cognition: An information processing approach.* London: John Wiley and Sons.

Hedberg, B. (1981). How organizations learn and unlearn. In P. Nystrom & W. Starbuck (Eds.), *Handbook of organizational design.* New York: Oxford University Press, pp. 3–27.

Herzberg, F., Mausner, B., & Snyderman, B. &1958). *The motivation to work.* New York: John Wiley and Sons.

Herzberg, F. (1966). *Work and the nature of man.* Cleveland, OH: World Press.

Ivancevich, J., Matteson, M., & Preston, C. (1985). Occupational stress, type A behavior, and physical well being. *Academy of Management Journal, 25*(2), 373–391.

Kahn, R., Wolfe, D., Quinn, R., Snoek, J., & Rosenthal, R. (1964). *Organizational stress: Studies in role conflict.* New York: John Wiley and Sons.

Kahn, R. (1974). Conflict, ambiguity and overload: Three elements in job stress. In A. McLean (Ed.), *Occupational stress.* Springfield, IL: Charles C. Thomas.

Kanter, R. (1977). *Men and women of the corporation.* New York: Basic Books.

Kets de Vries, M., & Miller, D. (1984). *The neurotic organization.* San Francisco: Josey-Bass.

Korman, A. (1975). Hypothesis of work behavior revisited and an extension. *Academy of Management Review, 1.*

Kotter, J. (1978). *Organizational dynamics: Diagnosis and intervention.* Reading, MA: Addison-Wesley.

Kramm, K. (1985). *Mentoring at work.* Glenview, IL: Scott, Foresman.

Lawrence, P., & Lorsch, J. (1967). *Organization and environment.* Boston: Harvard Business School.

Lazarus, R. (1966). *Psychological stress and the coping process.* New York: McGraw-Hill.

Levinson, H. (1964). *Emotional health in the world of work.* New York: Harper & Row.

Levinson, H. (1970). *Executive stress.* New York: Harper & Row.

Levinson, H. (1973). *The great jackass fallacy.* Cambridge, MA: Harvard University Graduate School of Business Administration.

Levinson, H. (1974). A psychoanalytic framework for occupational stress. In A. McLean (Ed.), *Occupational stress.* Springfield, IL: Charles C. Thomas.

Lewin, K. (1951). *Field theory in social science.* New York: Harper & Row.

Litwin, G., & Stringer, R. (1968). *Motivation and organizational climate.* Boston: Harvard University.

Locke, E. (1968). Toward a theory of task motivation and incentives. *Organization Behavior and Human Performance, 3,* 157–189.

Maccoby, M. (1976). *The gamesman.* New York: Simon & Schuster.

Maccoby, M. (1983). *The leader.* New York: Simon & Schuster.

McClelland, D. (1975). *Power: The inner experience.* New York: Irvington Press.

McGregor, D. (1960). *The human side of enterprise.* New York: McGraw-Hill.

McLean, A. (Ed.) (1974). *Occupational stress.* Springfield, IL: Charles C. Thomas.

MacMillan, I. Corporate ideology and strategic delegation. Journal of Business Strategy, 1983, 71–76.

Mager, R., & Pipe, P. (1970). *Solving performance problems, or: You really oughta wanta.* Belmont, CA: Fearon Publishers.

Maier, N. (1976/1958). *The appraisal interview: Three basic approaches.* Palo Alto, CA: University Associates.

Marrow, A. (Ed.) (1973). *The failure of success.* New York: AMACOM.

Maslach, C. (1872). Understanding burnout: Definitional issues in understanding a complex phenomenon. In W. Paine (Ed.), *Job stress and burnout.* Beverly Hills, CA: Sage Publications.

Maslow, A. (1943). A theory of human motivation. *Psychological Review, 50,* 370–396.

Maslow, A. (1962). *Toward a psychology of being.* Princeton, NJ: Van Nostrand.

Merry, U., & Brown, G. (1980). *The neurotic behavior of organizations.* Cleveland, OH: Gestalt Institute of Cleveland Press.

Meyer, H., Kay, E., & French, J. (1965). Split roles in performance appraisal. *Harvard Business Review,* Jan.-Feb.

*Miller, D.M. (1976). Counseling in industry: An integrated approach. *National Retail Merchants Association Personnel News.* Fall.

*Miller, D.M. (1977). Managerial assessment techniques. In E. Lynch (Ed.), *Measuring executive and employee performance.* New York: National Retail Merchants Association.

*Miller, D.M. (1983). Process and personality in work-related stress. Baruch College, CUNY (unpublished).

*Miller, D.M. (1985). McClelland's theory of power motivation. Baruch College, CUNY (unpublished).

Miner, J. (1978). Twenty years of research on role motivation theory of managerial effectiveness. *Personnel Psychology, 31,* 739–760.

Miner, J. (1980). *Theories of organizational behavior.* Hinsdale, ILL: Dryden Press.

Nadler, D. (1977). *Feedback and organization development: Using data-based methods.* Reading, MA: Addison-Wesley.

Nevis, E. (1987). *Consulting in organizations: A Gestalt approach.* Cleveland, OH: Gestalt Institute of Cleveland Press.

Nystrom, P., & Starbuck, W. (1984). Managing beliefs in or ganizations. *Journal of Applied Behavioral Science, 20*(3), 277–287.

Paine, W. (Ed.) (1982). *Job stress and burnout.* Beverly Hills, CA: Sage Publications.

Peters, J., & Waterman, R. (1983). *In search of excellence.* New York: Harper & Row.

Roethlisberger, F., & Dickson, W. (1939). *Management and the worker.* Cambridge, MA: Harvard University Press.

Rotter, J. (1966). Generalized expectancies for internal versus external control of reinforcement. *Psychological Monographs, 80.*

Selye, H. (1976). *The stress of life* (rev. ed.). New York: McGraw-Hill.

Shain, M., & Groeneveld, J. (1980). *Employee Assistance Programs.* Lexington, MA: Lexingtron Books.

Terborg, J. (1976). The motivational components of goal setting. *Journal of Applied Psychology, 61,* 613–621.

Warshaw, L. (1979). *Managing stress.* Reading, MA: Addison-Wesley.

Weiner, B., & Sierad, J. (1975). Misattribution for failure and enhancement of achievement strivings. *Journal of Personality and Social Psychology, 31,* 415–421.

White, R. (1959). Motivation reconsidered: The concept of competence. *Psychological Review, 66,* 297–333.

Zey, M. (1984). *The mentor connection.* Homewood, IL: Richard D. Irwin.

Zuker, E. (1983). *Mastering assertiveness skills.* New York: AMACOM.

See also:
Academy of Management Journal
Annual Review of Psychology
Human Relations
Journal of Applied Psychology
Personnel Journal
Personnel Psychology
Training and Development Journal

---

*Abstracts, reprints, and/or bibliographies available from author.

C H A P T E R
79

HOW TO DEVELOP AN
EMPLOYEE ASSISTANCE PROGRAM

Jayne Eliach, R.N., M.S.

It is now well accepted that if personal problems are not attended to they can eventually affect an employee's job performance. Although historically employee assistance programs (EAPs) developed as an outgrowth of the alcoholism programs of the 1940s, they have now expanded to address the broader problems of today's worker. This includes helping employees with marital problems, substance abuse problems in their families, child care problems, and legal problems.

EAPs are different from traditional mental health clinics in that there is specific attention given to how problems may impact on job performance. Specifically addressing issues related to workers, job performance criteria, and the connection to personal problems has not historically been the focus of the professional training of most mental health clinicians, nor has it been a treatment focus. However, the most significant difference in approach involves the ability of a supervisor to refer an employee to the EAP. These referrals are based on deteriorating job performance that does not respond to normal corrective measures. The assumption is that if a well-functioning employee suddenly has a deterioration in job performance that does not respond to normal corrective measures, that employee may have personal problems that require attention. EAPs work because often workers are unable to see how their personal problems may be affecting their work performance. This denial of the severity of a problem may be the reason employees do not seek assistance on their own. Employers can use job leverage to assist employees in seeking help for problems they may be unable to see on their own. This approach is both humanistic and economic for the employer.

Today's EAPs also attempt to educate supervisors and workers to spot potential problems early and seek assistance before there is evidence of job performance problems. The new EAP encourages self-referrals in addition to supervisory referrals. The concept of self-referral emphasizes the new preventative component to the EAP model.

In order to develop an EAP program successfully, mental health professionals need to become educated about negotiating systems in the world of work. It is critical that the practitioners are also well trained in the area of substance abuse. This is important for two basic reasons: (1) the prevalence of substance abuse in the workplace has dramatically increased, and (2) employers are especially intersted in addressing this issue since there is good data to suggest that substance abusers increase costs within an organization.

BASIC INGREDIENTS OF AN EAP PROGRAM

There are several basic ingredients that must be present in order to establish a well-functioning and successful EAP program. The program's credibility and utilization by both employees and supervisors will depend on the presence of these elements:

1. Program support
2. Policy statement
3. Policy ensuring confidentiality
4. Appropriate staffing
5. Resource and referral network
6. Education and training component
7. Program publicity
8. Program evaluation

Obtaining a philosophical and financial commitment on the part of the organization is the kind of support necessary to implement successful EAP. At the beginning stages of program development, educating key officials in the organization about reasons to implement a program is a critical first step. This educational process should include information about how personal problems may affect an employee's job performance and the potential cost savings to the organization.

Having the support of top-level management as well as other key personnel in the organization is crucial to the success of an EAP. Administratively the responsibility for the EAP should be as high up in the organizational structure as possible. This will indicate that the program has the endorsement of top-level management and will ultimately give the EAP more influence and credibility. Early publicity about the EAP should be accompanied by a letter or statement of support from the presdient of the organization. When the organization has a union, the letter should be jointly signed by the union president and the president of the organization.

Having a well-written policy statement describing how the organization views personal problems and clearly stating how the EAP operates is a core component to program development. Every EAP policy statement should begin with an overall philosophical statement about the purpose of the EAP. Following this, all policy statements should acknowledge that substance abuse, family problems, emotional disorders, and other personal problems can have a serious negative effect on a person's job performance and that treatment rather than discipline is the organization's position regarding these problems. The policy statement should also assure employees that participation in the program will in no way jeopardize their professional status or opportunities for promotion. A description of the program — its scope, activities, and functioning — should also be included. Also, a brief statement should address self-referrals versus job jeopardy referrals and any differences in the program policy. It should be clearly stated that there is no cost to an employee for services at the EAP, but that if a referral is made, the employee may have to absorb any of the cost not covered by the employee's insurance. The language of the policy statement should be simple and clear and consistent with the style of the employees who work in the organization. Also, it is helpful to specify who is eligible for the service. For example, some programs are available to family members and retirees. The policy statement should be distributed to all employes.

Confidentiality is probably the most significant ingredient of an EAP program. If confidentiality is not provided, there will be no program because employees will not use the service. Several areas need to be addressed regarding confidentiality: disclosure of information, record keeping, and office location. Written rules specifying how, to whom, and under what circumstances disclosures of client information will be made are very important in being able to maintain a confidential program. Utilization of written consent forms prior to disclosures of client information is generally the best method for ensuring confidentiality. EAP records should always be kept separate from an employee's personnel file. Clearly stated policies should regulate how records will be maintained, for what length of time, and who will have access to them. In order to ensure confidentiality it is common practice to code EAP records with numbers rather than to use the employee's name. Records shoud always be kept locked, and only personnel working in the EAP program should have access to them. Decisions should be made about whether records may be used for purposes of research, evaluation, and reports. All EAP programs that receive federal moneys either directly or indirectly are required to adhere to the federal regulations protecting the confidentiality of alcohol abuse and drug abuse records. In the choice of location for the EAP office, every effort should be made to find a place that is convenient for employees and is most likely to maximize the confidentiality of the visit. For example, most self-referrals would be hesitant to use the EAP if it were located in the personnel department.

Staffing patterns in EAP programs vary. However, most programs are staffed by mental health clinicians who are trained in social work, nursing, or psychology at the master's level and have expertise in substance abuse. Many programs also employ alcoholism counselors, but the scope of their practice is much more limited. However, if the staffing pattern will permit or if the percentage of clients with a diagnosis of alcoholism is high, an individual with this background may complement the staff, especially if the person is a recovering alcoholic. Although clinical work is the foundation of many of the services offered, it is just as important to have staff who possess administrative, management, and training skills. These skills are necessary to coordinate the program, provide training, develop the program, and be adept in business and systems analysis.

The assessment and referral component of the EAP involves the counselor's ability to make an accurate assessment of the employee's problem and then an appropriate referral when necessary. Often the counselor's assessment of the problem may be different from the employees. For example, an employee may seek out services for a marital problem and request marital counseling. However, the counselor obtaining a history may assess that the employee has a substance abuse problem and that may be the real cause of the current marital problem. It is the responsibility of the counselor to assess the client's problem on the basis of clinical expertise and make an appropriate recommendation. When a referral is made the counselor should be sensitive to the needs of the client socially, culturally, and financially. Referrals should be made so that the employee can receive services at times that will not interfere with the employee's work schedule. Resources should be chosen that are either convenient to the employee's workplace or home. In order to match clients successfully with referrals, the program should establish an elaborate network of resources.

Training and educating supervisors on how to identify troubled employees is the foundation of a successful EAP program. Employees using denial about the severity of their problems are not likely to seek out services at the EAP on their own. In these cases the ability of the supervisor to recognize a job performance problem and make a supervisory referral to the EAP may be the only way employees using denial are likely to get help.

The EAP should develop and provide various lunchtime or after work programs that will train and educate employees about various issues that promote health. Health promotion and prevention are concepts that naturally fit into the concept of an EAP program. Helping employees to prevent problems from developing is the most progressive type of intervention an EAP can make.

If the EAP program is well publicized, it will increase utilization of the program. Various methods can be used:

1. Brochures describing the program can be mailed to employees or distributed with paychecks.

2. Posters advertising the program can be posted in key areas around the organization.

3. Supervisors, health service personnel, and personnel representatives can all be coached to inform people about the existence of the program.

4. Brief presentations about the program can be made at new employee orientations and at all EAP-sponsored seminars and workshops.

All opportunities should be used to keep employees informed about the availability of the EAP and the broad scope of the program's activities. All employees should be knowledgeable about how to use the service, what services are offered, and what the scope of the program's activities are.

Methods for evaluating the EAP should be considered in the earliest stages of program development. The program should be evaluated by a design reflecting the goals and expectations of greatest concern to the organization. Program evaluation may focus on cost reduction, utilization rate, or satisfaction levels of employees, management, or the union. Since one evaluation tool cannot measure all these variables, those in charge of the EAP will have to choose which area they are most interested in measuring.

The most common kinds of data collected for routine statistical reports include:

1. Number of employees who use the program. This figure should separate employees, dependents, and retirees.

2. Number of self-referrals and the number of supervisory referrals.

3. Demographic data including client age, sex, ethnicity, educational level, income.

4. Problem identification, including categories such as substance abuse, marital relationship, job-related, medical, and environmental problems.

5. Data reflecting whether employees feel the problems are affecting their job.

6. Data reflecting whether employees feel the problems are affecting their personal life.

7. Information about absenteeism, lateness, sick days, disability days, and visits to the personnel or medical departments should be collected by the client on self-referrals and from supervisors on employees who are supervisory referrals.

8. Data reflecting the numbers of referrals made and whether the employees accepted the referrals.

Any type of data may be collected and examined to evaluate program effectiveness. However, the most important issue is that the type of data collected should be consistent with the primary goal fo the sponsor organization.

SUPERVISORY TRAINING

A strong supervisor is the linchpin in a truly successful EAP. Developing a program that ensures appropriate supervisory intervention will establish the foundation for an effective EAP. Since supervisors are in close contact with employees, they are in an ideal position to evaluate and monitor job performance changes at the earliest stage possible. For a variety of reasons supervisors are often reluctant to address problems linked to job performance problems and then to use the EAP as a resource:

1. Supervisors may deny a problem exists.

2. Supervisors may feel helpless in dealing with employees.

3. Supervisors may feel responsible for employees' job performance problems.

4. Supervisors may feel sorry for employees.

5. Supervisors may feel angry at employees for the job performance problems.

6. Supervisors may be fearful about confronting employees.

7. Supervisors may try to handle the employees' problems on their own because they believe it is their job.

Despite supervisors' difficulties, their job is to identify troubled employees through job performance, to motivate employees through intervention and confrontation to address the problems, and to urge employees to seek help through the organization's EAP. Supervisors have one of the most powerful methods of motivating employees to seek help; that is, the leverage of possible job loss. However, the supervisor must recognize that the decision to use the EAP is a voluntary one. The supervisor should make it clear that corrective disciplinary measures will be instituted if job performance does not improve. However, the supervisor should not threaten discipline just because the employee does not use the EAP. An employee may choose to get assistance elsewhere, and the employee's job performance may improve. The supervisor can strongly recommend that employees use the program but cannot force them to use it.

In supervisory training sessions, supervisors must be taught to recognize that job deterioration may be a result of an employee's personal problems. However, in training sessions supervisors should be discouraged from attempting to diagnose their employees' problems. Diagnosing and treating personal problems are not the role of a supervisor. The training sessions should emphasize that the role of the supervisor is to monitor job performance.

When consulting with supervisors, the EAP counselor should emphasize the following supervisory responsibilities:

1. Monitoring job performance, attendance, tardiness, behavioral and attitude changes
2. Specifically and clearly documenting any deterioration in job performance
3. Informally discussing the need for improvement with the employee
4. Giving the employee a specific length of time to demonstrate improvement
5. Reevaluating the employee's job performance
6. Referring to the organization's EAP if there is no improvement
7. Evaluating job performance after referral is made
8. Implementing further disciplinary measures if there is no improvement in job performance

Supervisory training should be provided to supervisors at all levels of management. In some organizations it may be difficult to get the highest level administrators to attend trainings. However, every effort should be made to work with management from the top down so that when problems arise at any level, supervisors, managers, and administrators understand how to intervene. Anyone who is responsible for the job performance of at least one employee should be invited to attend training sessions.

Organizations will have different policies regarding attendance at trainings. Some organizations will require the attendance of all supervisors, whereas others may just strongly encourage supervisors at attend. Every effort should be made to maximize attendance. This is most easily accomplished if sessions are scheduled during times that are convenient for supervisory personnel. In an organization that has shift workers, sessions should be sensitively scheduled so that supervisors working all three shifts can participate in a training session.

Supervisory training sessions may be scheduled in a variety of ways. Generally, initial sessions run from 1 to 4 hours and may be followed by periodic refresher sessions designed to meet the particular needs of the group. For example, one group may want more time to discuss how to deal with employees who appear intoxicated on the job, whereas another group may want more practice in role-playing in order to be able to refer an employee to the EAP effectively.

Although the format for a particular group of supervisors and the individual style of the trainer will vary, the key issues to address in the training are:

1. Overview of the EAP concept
2. Definition of the "toubled" employee
3. Reasons for having an EAP in the organization
4. Overview of the EAP program in the organization
5. Review of EAP policy statement
6. Explanation of how employees can utilize the program: self-referral and supervisory referral
7. Role of the supervisor in encouraging referrals
8. How to identify a troubled employee
9. Importance of confidentiality
10. Availability of EAP as a resource for supervisors for their own problems and as a consultation service for helping supervisors handle difficult situations involving their employees

Training sessions vary in size, but small groups of 10 to 20 are probably best. A combination of lecture, discussion, small group exercises, role-playing, and audiovisual aids will probably produce the most effective training. The quality of the trainer is important to the success of the training session. The sessions are usually conducted by an EAP staff member who has excellent public speaking skills, is charismatic, and has some experience in training.

RESOURCES AND REFERRALS

An important component in developing an EAP is establishing a comprehensive network of quality resources. This system should include therapists, community agencies, substance abuse treatment programs, mental health centers, legal services, and so forth. Having located individuals for use as referral resources, the EAP must ensure clients receive quality services. Methods to evaluate services include interviews with individual practitioners, site visits, and follow-up with employees.

Devising a system to evaluate an individual therapist's competency to do psychotherapy and capacity to be responsive to the needs of the EAP is not an easy task. As an initial step, a detailed questionnaire can be sent to all therapists who are interested in referrals from the program. Include questions regarding office location, fees, reimbursement status, clinical orientation, knowledge of chemical dependency, and treatment modalities utilized. Once the questionnaire is completed and returned, an EAP staff member reviews it. If the therapist appears to be an appropriate resource, an interview is set up. During the interview the therapist can be asked detailed questions about his or her practice, areas of interest, theoretical orientation, and so forth. In addition, the therapist can present a case in treatment. The therapist could also be asked to respond to hypothetical clinical situations posed by the EAP staff member. The interview should also be used to help the therapist understand how the EAP program operates, how referrals are made, and what information therapists may be required to report to the EAP. Rules governing disclosure of confidential information must be discussed since the therapist's responsibility to a patient and the EAP's obligation to the sponsor organization may cause potential conflicts.

After the interview, the EAP staff member's impressions of the applicant are then presented to the staff and a decision is made as to whether the therapist should be added to the resource directory. Therapists may be removed from the directory at any time if the EAP staff finds the therapist uncooperative, inappropriate in treatment planning, or the like.

Making a site visit to a treatment program or community agency is an excellent way to begin to evaluate the quality and responsiveness of the facility to the needs of the individual EAP. A simple form to record basic information about the facility as well as impressions may be helpful. Include information regarding the name of the facility, location, telephone number, services offered, fees, and kinds of personnel involved n providing services. In addition, establish a liaison person at the facility who can act as a link between the facility and the EAP. This person can facilitate and expedite the referral process, assist in smoothing out problems that develop, and coordinate the flow of information that may need to be communicated back to the EAP. Following the visit, the EAP staff member can communicate all findings to the rest of the staff and attach the information collected to any other literature obtained and place this information in the resource file.

All resource files should also include the full array of self-help support groups. The EAP staff also needs to be knowledgeable about 12-step self-help programs, such as Alcoholics Anonymous, Cocaine Anonymous, Overeaters Anonymous, and Alanon. All these groups have some meetings that are open to the public; EAP staff members should visit as many of these groups as possible to gain a better understanding of the working and philosophy of these programs.

HEALTH PROMOTION, WELLNESS, AND PREVENTATIVE PROGRAMS

A comprehensive preventative approach to illness became popular in the late 1970s. This model replaced the old disease model that monopolized health care. At the workplace health promotion can be fostered when an organization supports behavior that maximizes the health of employees and their families.

There are two basic reasons why the workplace has been identified as an ideal setting for health promotion programs: (1) people are often willing to participate in health programs when they are free and convenient to attend; and (2) employers have an economic incentive to provide such programs since they should see a reduction in health care costs, absenteeism, disability, and improved employee productivity as a result of successful programs.

The most typical health promotion programs include those on nutrition and weight control, smoking cessation, alcohol and drug abuse education, stress management, fitness and exercise, and high blood pressure control. These programs range from inexpensive programs where employees are given information about various health matters to more expensive programs that involve screening, treatment, and follow-up.

Health promotion programs will also help to publicize the EAP to employees who might otherwise not use the program. For example, a top-level manager may enthusiastically attend a stress management program sponsored by the EAP and as a result be more receptive to contacting the EAP after the sudden death of his spouse. Positive, nonthreatening, nonstigmatized contact with the program staff will increase the likelihood that employees will seek out other EAP services if a crisis or problem develops at a later date.

Doing a needs assessment will help to determine what kind of health promotion program should be established within an organization. This may be accomplished in several ways:

1. Speak with top-level management and determine their major concerns regarding the health of employees.

2. Speak with the benefits personnel to determine the kinds of health problems employees are already experiencing.

3. Survey the general employee population to determine their needs and interests regarding various health promotion programs.

4. Examine the kinds of problems employees are seeking services for at the EAP, and determine whether health promotion programs could alleviate any of these problems.

5. Determine what are the kind of problems the employees who work in your organization might be experiencing by looking at statistics revealing age, sex, ethnicity, and so forth.

The EAP can sponsor health promotion programs alone or jointly with another department within the organization. Personnel and medical departments are often interested in cosponsoring programs. Employers can support the belief that well-educated, informed individuals can more effectively deal with the health care problems when they provide health promotion programs at the work site.

SUPPORT GROUPS

As a partial means of helping employees achieve and maintain wellness, EAPs can develop both self-help and therapist-led support groups. These groups may range from drop-in groups to time-limited structured groups to on-going groups that require group members to tackle more long-term problems. Although the EAP may use a staff person to lead a group or may merely serve as a catalyst in the development of a self-help group, another interesting model appropriate for EAPs begins with an EAP staff person establishing and leading a time-limited group and then helping the group function on its own. The staff person then functions as a consultant to the group by attending group meetings on a monthly basis to discuss group problems and membership issues.

These groups can be developed to help employees with problems as diverse as single parenting, caring for an aging relative, spouse abuse, and substance abuse among family members. By offering people a free core of support in a convenient location that does not conflict with their job or other personal responsibilities, such groups often provide assistance to those employees who are least likely to seek out services elsewhere.

CONCLUSION

The success of EAPs is based on the premise that these programs are beneficial to both employers and employees. In developing EAP programs it is critical to address the specific needs of the organization while still developing a program consistent with EAP philosophy. It is not unusual for EAP practitioners to feel pulled between their responsibilities to the organization and their responsibilities to the employee. Developing the skills necessary to achieve a sound professional balance to the sponsor organization and the employees served is the art in developing a successful program. This balance is not easily achieved since historically mental health clinicians have needed to consider only their responsibility to their patients.

The establishment of a successful EAP program will involve careful planning, the genuine support of the organization, and a real commitment on the part of the EAP staff to make the program work. Most EAPs gain credibility with management, employees, and unions over time. Providing quality, confidential, and professional services to all those involved with the program will be one of the best beginning steps to achieving a successful program.

REFERENCES

Abelson, P.G. (&1982). Employee assistance programs from the inside, from the outside. *Practice Digest,* pp. 5–8.

Blair, B.R. (1985). *Hospital employee assistance programs.* American Hospital Publishing Inc.

New York State Division of Alcoholism and Alcohol Abuse. *Employee assistance program...an overview.*

Masi, D.A. (1984). *Designing employee assistance programs.* New York: American Management Associations.

Santa-Barbara, J. (1984, September). Employee assistance programs: An alternative resource for mental health service delivery. *Canada's Mental Health,* pp. 35–36.

Scanlon, W.E. (1986). *Alcoholism and drug abuse in the workplace.* New York: Praeger Publishers.

Standards for employee alcoholism and/or assistance programs. *EAP Digest,* pp. 42–43.

C H A P T E R
80

HOSPICE:
CLINICAL CONSIDERATIONS

Elisabeth G. Everett, L.I.C.S.W., M.S.W.

To heal a person does not always mean to cure the disease.
—Logo, Hospice of the Good Shepherd, Waban, Mass.

In 1967, physician Cicely Saunders established St. Christopher's Hospice in Sydenham, England. The purpose of this institution was to offer hospitality to people who were dying, "much as the medieval hospice replenished, refreshed, and cared for pilgrims and travelers on their journeys" (Casperson, 1985, p. 15). St. Christopher's became the paradigm, the model, for the contemporary hospice.

One hospice existed in the United States in 1974; by 1980, 269 hospices were in operation in this country; and in 1987, there were over 1500 hospices at various stages of development. Hospice programs exist in each of the 50 states and serve more than 120,000 people a year (National Hospice Organization, 1987).

As defined by the National Hospice Organization (NHO), a hospice is a medically directed, interdisciplinary program of supportive services and pain and symptom control for terminally ill people and their families. One eligibility standard for hospice is that the patient have a prognosis of 6 months or less. The term "hospice" refers primarily to a philosophy of care rather than to a particular institutional model; the majority of hospice services are delivered in the home, with inpatient care available as needed.

Within the last decade, hospice has achieved recognition as a respected care alternative for people who are living with dying. In 1986, care by certified hospices became a permanent benefit under Medicare, and an optional benefit under Medicaid. Private insurance companies have also begun to provide hospice coverage, thus making it possible for hospice services to be more widely used.

THE INTERDISCIPLINARY TEAM

The core of the hospice concept is the interdisciplinary team. The nucleus of this interdisciplinary team is the hospice staff, which might include an administrative director, a medical director, a nursing department, a coordinator of volunteers, a social worker, a psychologist, a psychiatrist, a pharmacist, a pastoral coordinator, a home-health-aide department, and a bereavement coordinator. A cadre of volunteers, carefully selected and educated, enhances the efforts of the staff and greatly expands the possibilities for consistent and creative intervention. A dynamic system in itself, the hospice staff interacts with patient and family, the patient's physician, and sometimes with inpatient staff and other cooperating agencies to form a larger dynamic system.

An objective of the hospice team is to view the patient and family within the totality of their life context. Dym (1987), elaborating on George Engel's thought that physical illness must be viewed in the context of the "biopsychosocial field," observes that this is a broader context than usually encountered by physicians or psychotherapists. Dym and Berman (1986) state elsewhere that "the organic reality (the change in a family member's health) provokes reaction and change within the family, *and* the family's functioning markedly influences and shapes the nature and course of the illness. The biopsychosocial field presents a constantly changing, developing, interacting picture" (p. 11). The implication here is that the complexity of this field requires an equally complex response from the professional community. When various disciplines work in partnership, differences in language and working assumptions become both a challenge and a potential source of enrichment. Thus Dym and Berman stress the need for flexibility and a willingness to reexamine old beliefs and assumptions: "Patience, persistence, and mutual respect will be necessary for joint practitioners to coin their own new language to describe illness and health" (p. 18). While Dym and Berman propose a model involving collaboration between family doctors and family therapists to create a primary care team, their comments are equally appropriate for the hospice team.

Implicit in the sharing of language, assumption, and expertise is the need to educate; thus, educational exchange becomes the responsibility of each team member. Such exchange can illuminate and enrich the perspective of all care givers to the benefit of patient and family. This commitment to education on the part of the team has particular relevance for volunteers, who usually have more frequent contact with families than do the professionals on the staff. With consistent guidance and education, volunteers can develop their talents, becoming better and better able to observe, evaluate, and serve as compassionate and knowledgeable peers for patients, families, and the rest of the team.

The concept of release — of letting go — is obviously a pertinent theme in hospice. The family prepares to release the patient; the patient prepares to let go of life. It is a theme that applies to the hospice team as well. To be an effective team member often means being a catalyst for change — participating in a meaningful intervention and then releasing it into the biopsychosocial field. Here, the ability to let go of rigid role definitions and share therapeutic interaction across disciplines is essential.

What one care giver initiates with a patient may be continued by the patient with another care giver, who may not be the "appropriate professional." In issues that do not require specific medical expertise, boundaries of disciplines must be flexible. At a vulnerable stage it becomes impossible for patient and family to perceive and respect discipline boundaries. When a thought or feeling emerges, it is important that it be heard and responded to—in an appropriate manner—by any member of the care team. There may not be time to wait until the "appropriate" team member is available. That the team be viewed as a group of caring and competent individuals who share expertise and information is therefore of the utmost importance. The explicit and implicit message to families must be that disciplines are not guarded or territorial, and that communication is open and encouraged. The vitality generated by such a "complex response" on the part of the interdisciplinary team fosters growth, or coevolution, of all the dynamic systems involved.

THE UNIT OF CARE

Historically, the modern hospice has identified patient and family as the unit of care. In what has been referred to as the unified biopsychosocial-spiritual field "several levels of organization, including the cellular, organ system, individual, community, and cultural, all mutually influence one another in the presentation of and in the exacerbation and resolution of symptoms" (Dym & Berman, 1986, p. 10). If we accept this belief, then any definition of "unit of care" should assume the influence of each level or organization on the others, and on the larger context. Thus regarded, the unit of care with which any hospice must concern itself would encompass the members of and systems involved in the interdisciplinary care team as well as the patient and family. And it is true that support for and nurturing of the entire care team is basic to the well-functioning hospice. However, for the purpose of this discussion, the "unit of care" will be defined as the social unit living in the same home as the patient, plus friends and relatives involved in the care of the patient but not living in that home. That entire unit of care will be referred to as family.

Most hospice families consist of members of the nuclear family of the patient. Most patients are adults over 50 years of age; according to an NHO survey conducted in 1984, less than 10 percent of U.S. hospices have served children as patients. As more and more AIDS patients seek hospice services, the definition of family broadens to include lovers and friends.

Members of the unit of care may elect various services offered by hospice, including the psychological therapies.[1] Not all patients and family members

---

[1]In this discussion the term "psychological therapies" includes psychotherapy, family therapy, pastoral counseling, spiritual counseling, and bereavement counseling. There are clear as well as subtle distinctions between these disciplines. However, for the sake of simplicity and because many hospices do not offer all of these services, "psychological therapy(ies)," or "therapy(ies)" may refer to any or all of the above. The term "therapist" will refer to professionals in the above disciplines.

[2]For the sake of clarity and simplicity, the patient will be referred to as "he," the therapist as "she."

[3]In clinical examples names of patients have been changed, and situations slightly altered to maintain confidentiality.

choose to participate in these therapies; however, these services should remain constantly available to the family.

PRELIMINARY CONSIDERATIONS

Therapy In The Home

The majority of hospice services are home based, and this fact can evoke mixed reactions in the therapist. There is comfort in the continuity of familiar office space. Diagnosis and pattern may be more evident when the interviewing environment is consistent. On the other hand, working within the home of the patient, the therapist fully experiences her[2] client's context; she may be literally flooded with information. In this connection, consultation with team members before the first visit can provide a degree of predictability; in fact, there is no substitute for factual information about the disease process and about the family system as observed by colleagues.

Guest And Professional

In the home the therapist is at once guest and professional and as such must be sensitive to each role. As guest, she must understand spoken and unspoken family traditions. Knowledge of the culture of the family as well as any cues the family may provide are markers for behavior in the initial interview. The family will at the same time be looking for cues from the therapist, as they would from any professional. They may be confused as to procedure and look to the therapist for direction. If none is forthcoming, they will probably refer to some past situation that they feel is similar and act on information from that situation (Chasin, 1987). Sensitivity to their need for guidance can avoid confusion and possible embarrassment for the family.

> Theodora was a 6-year-old girl, the second and youngest child of a young Greek family that had moved to the United States 5 years earlier.[3] Three years after their arrival, Theodora was diagnosed as having a brain tumor; treatment did not cure the disease. The child was admitted to hospice with a prognosis of 3 to 6 months. When the therapist arrived at the family's home both parents were present. The father had left his construction business to "meet our new friend." A special dessert had been prepared; it was obvious that no serious discussion would take place before the parents both entertained and came to know and trust this new member of the team. After dessert and conversation, the parents were visibly uncomfortable, unsure of how to continue the visit. The therapist graciously thanked the couple for their hospitality; she then asked their permission to meet Theodora and show her some special puppets. She asked the parents to join her in the child's room, and added that she would like another opportunity to talk with them at the end of her visit. With direction, the parents relaxed. They eagerly introduced her to Theodora and to their 9-year-old son, who had been caring for his sister in her room during the initial part of the visit.

Here family and therapist provided some structure for one another, each reacting with sensitivity to create a comfortable interaction.

Family Culture

Culture has been defined as the shared beliefs, arts, and behaviors of a group of people. Most often these are ethnic groups that have in common linguistic, national, religious and racial characteristics. But other groups within the larger American culture—for example, the gay community—also share characteristic beliefs and behaviors.

The cultural heritage of patient and family forms a pattern tightly woven into the biopsychosocial and spiritual tapestry. For patients to be well cared for, their frame of reference must be understood. Ethnic and cultural groups exhibit marked differences on a number of issues pertinent to thorough hospice care:

1. How they experience pain
2. What they label as a symptom
3. How they communicate about their pain or symptoms
4. What they believe to be the cause of their illness
5. What attitudes they assume toward helpers
6. What treatment they desire or expect (McGoldrick et al., 1982)

In any given instance, the meaning of pain, illness, and death—to cite but a few examples—must be grasped within the cultural context by the team. The therapist's awareness of relevant cultural issues has critical implications for effective psychotherapy with patient and family.

Naming

Asking family members what each would like to be called is not only a sign of respect but also a matter of potential therapeutic import. A choice in this regard can be particularly critical to the patient who is struggling to maintain identity amid many role changes.

> A 59-year-old physician in the final stages of lung cancer preferred to be called Dr. Whitaker by the hospice staff, as he had been when he worked as a member of an interdisciplinary team at his hospital. His family was surprised by his sudden formality; the hospice staff perceived this request as a strategy to maintain self-esteem.

Space

At Home   Creating an environment for therapy within a home is a challenge. Sourkes (1982) found that "space—the physical setting—established concrete boundaries for the therapeutic process. As the therapy hour is a time apart, so the setting affords a private space apart from daily life" (p. 9).

Time apart from daily life is not easy to establish in the home of a family living with illness. However, privacy is essential when an individual or subgroup of the family talks with a therapist. Assuring that private space will be available and that unnecessary interruptions will not occur requires planning and cooperation on the part of the family and the team. When family sessions that include the patient are scheduled, it is important to ask the patient where he would like the meeting to take place. His room may be too small to accommodate the family comfortably, and he may not wish to discuss important issues with those he loves in a space where he is most often sick and uncomfortable (Jaffe et al., 1976). For these reasons the patient may prefer to have meetings somewhere other than in his private space. If he is not mobile, preplanning to have assistance available for his transfer may save the patient frustration and embarrassment.

It is equally imperative that conversations not meant to include the patient or a family member take place outside of that person's presence. It is often assumed that a person who is sleeping or a child who is playing in the next room will not hear what is being discussed close by. However, a high level of stress is often accompanied by heightened awareness of the dynamic environment. Thus, what is said in open space must be acceptable for all to hear.

As the patient's condition deteriorates, his discomfort may make access to him more difficult. At times the patient may need psychological as well as physical distance from family and care giver. If the patient is not able to speak, it is important to watch for subtle cues about closeness and distance.

> Pat, a 53-year-old woman, was dying at home. She was in much discomfort and was not alert enough to speak. By accepting or physically withdrawing from touch she communicated how much distance she wanted from family and care givers. On one occasion her husband and four adult children were standing near her bed. The pastoral coordinator joined the family at their request, and asked them to recall their most cherished memories of Pat. As her family began to talk and remember, Pat became more relaxed. Her clenched fist opened slightly. When this happened her husband took her hand in his and Pat seemed to smile.

At the Office   If the opportunity is available, family members may choose to meet in the therapist's office; sessions outside the home can provide a safe environment, apart from the intensity of their daily life. In such an environment they may feel free to express a broader range of emotion, with a corresponding clarity of thought and ability to solve problems.

Time

Unhurried Time   By conveying a sense of leisure to the patient and family, the therapist makes it clear that she cares about them. One of the most precious human qualities that can be shared is a feeling of unhurried time. So as to better communicate her availability the therapist may choose to prepare herself before meeting with a family by using relaxation techniques, meditation, or prayer. This preparation can be particularly relevant when the stress of seeing a number of families in 1 day collides with the pressures of highway driving in between visits.

Patients and family members may need assistance in adjusting their inner rhythm for the therapeutic encounter;

> Mr. Haynes, a 79-year-old hospice patient, asked for help in planning a family meeting. Though he lacked physical strength he participated

avidly in the planning, saying that he wanted to assume his patriarchal role one more time. His purpose for this meeting involving his wife, his four children, eight grandchildren, and five great-grandchildren was to tell them all how they had enriched his life and to give them his blessing for future generations. The patient requested that the therapist be present at the meeting "because I can't handle their tears." He was bedbound; his bed was in the living room of his home. With everyone present for the meeting, the atmosphere in the room was charged with the energy of young children and nervousness about what might happen. Mr. Haynes looked especially frail surrounded by all the energy and seemed perplexed about how to proceed. Sitting with the family, the therapist suggested as a good way to begin an exercise to help them all feel peaceful. With the patient's permission she introduced a simply relaxation exercise involving deep breathing. When the younger children laughed in embarrassment, she asked their parents to help them participate. With every breath the atmosphere became calmer, and Mr. Haynes seemed to gain strength. Soon Mr. Haynes cleared his throat, as was his custom, and the meeting began.

With the assistance of the therapist, the family and Mr. Haynes had found a common place.

Time of Referral   Several variables will significantly limit or enhance the possibilities for doing psychotherapy within the hospice structure. The most important of these is the point at which a patient is referred and accepted into a hospice program. Patients admitted with a 6-month prognosis will have the chance to get to know the hospice team members, and as the disease permits, to establish a routine that meets their needs and those of their family. When either patient or family chooses to participate in therapy at this point, there is time to establish a solid therapeutic alliance. However, often patients are not referred or do not choose hospice until the disease process is quite advanced; and with a prognosis of a month or less, therapeutic strategies will of necessity be directed toward crisis intervention.

Frequency, Duration, Scheduled Time

> The time commitment in psychotherapy has three facets: frequency, duration, and appointed time of sessions. In traditional psychotherapy, this structure is critical to the containment of the process. Thus there is both theoretical and practical adherence to the "fifty-minute hour." With illness and approaching death as the reality at hand, the scheduling of sessions may vary considerably. Whereas the traditional structure is optimal for the patient during certain phases, there are times when more fluidity is necessary. Effective availability is based upon this recognition, and implies the therapist's consistent and abiding presence. (Sourkes, 1982, p. 4)

Once the unit of care for psychotherapy has been determined, therapeutic goals are established. If the patient is involved in therapy, the frequency and duration of meetings will depend on (1) the goals established, (2) the patient's physical ability to participate, and (3) the patient's perception regarding his tolerance for emotional intensity. Sourkes (1982) states that patient-initiated regulation of the frequency of sessions can be a part of the therapeutic contract because, as she puts it:

> The patient who is facing the enormity of loss may at times need to control his or her emotional thermostat, and shut off confrontation and intensity. In exercising this option, the patient must be secure in the knowledge that contact with the therapist may be reinitiated without fear of reprisal. (p. 5)

It is important that the therapist carefully assess the meaning of a request for less frequent meetings. If the request is deemed appropriate to the therapeutic process, the patient must be secure in his belief that the therapist will be available again whenever he is ready.

During each session, keen sensitivity to the patient should determine the intervention strategy. At times, lengthy discussion may be in order; at other times, a calm presence. "The therapist's goal for a session may be as simple as providing reassurance of continued presence, or it may be to facilitate the patient's working through of an issue (Sourkes, 1982, p. 7).

Often sessions with family members can more readily be structured in terms of frequency, duration, and appointed time. The consistent structure of meetings can be an important intervention.

> Margot, the mother of a 37-year-old hospice patient with AIDS, welcomed her son Ralph back into her home to live out the last few months of his life. Two of Ralph's brothers took leaves from their professions to help with his care. After an initial session in which all family members participated, only Margot chose to continue with psychotherapy. She asked to have her sessions at the therapist's office every Monday morning from 10:00 to 11:00, as a way of marking the end of what were usually chaotic weekends at home with her grown children. She said, "I'm used to living quietly with my husband. It's wonderful that all our kids are here, but between the pain of living with Ralph's illness and the fact there is not a private, quiet place for me in my home, I'm going crazy."

In this case, a set time, a place away from home, and the therapist's presence combined to create the sanctuary that Margot needed. Here, as elsewhere, familiarity with the biopsychosocial and spiritual field of patient and family and a commitment to flexibility as an intervention strategy proved to be necessary tools for effective therapy in the unpredictable environment of patient and family.

Life Trajectory   The patient's life trajectory has provided him with significance and substance; to view him with dignity then, is to view him within the context of his life history. However, he may be so focused on the present, or his present situation may be so compelling or disquieting, that the therapist can easily lose sight of this broader frame of reference.

> Art, a 65-year-old man with metastatic disease, became enraged during an interview with his therapist. "You act like I was born with cancer; like it was always my life. This hell is new to me. I had a wonderful life of my own and with my family. You didn't know me then; you don't know me."

While the emotional stress of the moment may lead the patient to seek psychological support, a skilled therapist will evoke and interweave with present issues themes from the patient's life story.

Within the life trajectory, the moment of the patient's life-threatening diagnosis takes on great significance for him and his family as a marker and a point of reference. At the time of diagnosis, the family's experience of the flow of time is rudely altered. Their stability becomes turbulence; their sense of security diminished. Fear becomes a conscious presence in their lives. It is important that the therapist be aware of psychological and dynamic shifts that may have occurred at this time.

> Jim, a 68-year-old man, said that when he was diagnosed as having pancreatic cancer his two sons flew long distances to be with him. He complained that one son, who had always been in close contact, hadn't been back since that time. Jim's wife had died of cancer 1 year earlier, and he was feeling abandoned.

The therapist explained to Jim that family members who are "in sync" at a point of crisis often become reinvolved in their own lives as the illness enters a chronic and more routine phase. With Jim's permission she called the absent son. As a result of this call Jim learned that his son was so grief stricken over his mother's death that he could not bear to anticipate the loss of his father; he was actively choosing to be absent. Further intervention was planned on the basis of this dynamic change in family structure at the time of diagnosis.

Confidentiality

Policies regarding confidentiality of information about the patient and family are defined within each hospice. Admission forms usually include an information release, in which the patient gives the hospice team permission to share information for the enhancement of his care. However, confidentiality remains a complex issue within the hospice setting because so many people are involved in the care of each patient. Additionally, many team members may live within the patient's community and know family friends and acquaintances with whom information should not be shared. Finally, the therapist's responsibility vis-à-vis confidentiality is complicated by the fact that she may be seeing several members of the same family separately.

> In a family confronting life-threatening illness, the boundaries of confidentiality may be more permeable than is traditionally dictated. The therapist bears heightened responsibility for handling privileged communication within an emotionally intense system. Skill is required to convey the facts and implications of the therapeutic material, without exposing its essence. (Sourkes, 1982, p. 11)

While this observation refers to the management of privileged communication within the interdisciplinary team, it applies equally to the sharing of information within the family system. For a number of reasons, then, confidentiality should be a matter of ongoing concern and highest priority for providers of hospice care.

ISSUES IN PSYCHOTHERAPY

Stress Caused By Illness

> The diagnosis of a life-threatening illness leads many individuals to enter psychotherapy. Their focus is the emotional stress engendered by the illness, rather than more general intrapsychic and interpersonal concerns. (Sourkes, 1982, p. 3)

During the terminal phase of illness, emotional disruption is common for patient and family. Several recurrent themes that contribute to stress appear or reappear at the time of acceptance into hospice. Thus, the very fact of application for and acceptance into a hospice program has serious implications.

A prerequisite of admission into most hospices is the recognition by patient and family that the patient has 6 months or less to live. The patient acknowledges that he is losing everything in this life; the family is losing the patient and their life with him; all are experiencing their worst fear since the moment of diagnosis. At this time physical and emotional comfort become the goals of treatment.

Another implication of acceptance into hospice is a change in the medical management of the patient that can necessitate major emotional adjustments on the part of the family. In the majority of hospices the patient's oncologist continues to monitor his care; however, care is provided by the hospice staff. While meeting and getting to know and trust this new system of care givers, the patient and family are often grieving the loss of a clinic and hospital staff that have provided treatment and support for months or years. Because of the structure of most hospital systems, staff cannot continue to provide care on an outpatient basis. A psychotherapist may be among the staff members no longer available to the patient or family. This loss and the need for readjustment may remind the patient and family of the patient's impending death and may influence their initial reaction to hospice.

A further factor contributing to stress at the time of acceptance into hospice is the clear definition of family members as care givers, who share responsibility for the patient's physical and emotional well-being. During the chronic stage of a life-threatening illness medical staff usually encourage family members to maintain their individual and collective identities — apart from the illness. The goal during this chronic phase is continued individuation as opposed to a unit tightly organized around an illness. A critical shift occurs when the family elects hospice and the illness explicitly enters the terminal stage. At this time family members make a commitment to care for the patient. As this responsibility consumes more and more time, they may have to organize their lives around the care of the patient. They may have ambivalent feelings about providing care, as well as questioning their ability to provide adequate care. The patient may struggle with his increasing dependency on his family.

There are other issues that are common to hospice patients and their families. A change in the physical condition of the patient can affect the equilibrium of the family system.

> Allen, a 35-year-old patient with AIDS, was given methadone for his high level of pain. The drug was an effective pain medication; for Allen

it was also a stimulant. After being bedbound and passive he became energized. The exhausted family had difficulty shifting gears to accommodate Allen's energy. Allen grew angry at their seeming unresponsiveness; the family felt guilty and confused.

In this instance a desired change put more stress on an already tired system. The deterioration of a patient's condition can cause even more distress. The family may be frightened by the look or sound of a new symptom; they may feel inadequate in dealing with it. The patient's fears may escalate with his family's lack of confidence.

Family styles and patterns of communication persist and often grow more pronounced during the last months of a patient's life. If communication is already difficult, impending separation through death may make more direct communication increasingly risky. Expressions of love may be desired but feel awkward. Fear of the dying process, of separation, of what might be in store for family members as survivors and for the patient beyond this life may preoccupy individuals in the family. Guilt over past remarks or actions and the guilt that often accompanies helplessness may be present but unexpressed.

Anger is a source of stress. There are good reasons to be angry when one is faced with impending loss; however, its direct expression may be blocked to protect a family member from distress. In addition, anger often contributes to an inappropriate reaction to fear or grief. Unacknowledged or unmanaged, anger can escalate into harmful noncompliance with the medical regimen, or into psychological and physical abuse.

Living with the reality of limited time, the patient may wish to attend to tasks still undone. These tasks may be of an interpersonal nature — for example, a reconciliation with a family member or friend. Or they may be more concrete. Many patients want to share their thoughts about legal documents or funeral arrangements and services.

> Summer, a 9-year-old girl dying of leukemia, said to her mother, "This is so sad, Mommy. All I want to do is cry. I wanted to grow up with you. Thank you for loving me. I love you."

It is rare to have such a clear statement of farewell. Summer provided her mother with an opportunity for transition into bereavement with this statement of love and of leave-taking. Goodbyes matter. For the patient, saying goodbye can heighten his sense of completion of life tasks, as can hearing from others what he has meant to them. For family members, saying goodbye can be a precious experience from which to begin to reorganize their lives without the patient.

Exhaustion is a frequent experience during the terminal phase of illness: for the patient, because dying is difficult, often frightening, and uncomfortable; and for family members, because care giving can seem to drag on endlessly, often interrupting sleep and the general business of life. Because caring for a dying patient is so time-consuming, worry over finances and the limits of physical endurance often adds to the care giver's exhaustion. A quest for a sense of balance becomes paramount for each individual involved.

Grief

In patient and family alike, a terminal illness and its attendant changes can evoke sadness, anger, and a sense of longing for the past. These feelings are all components of the grief that accompanies losses occurring from the moment of diagnosis. Common among such losses are (1) usual patterns of family interaction, (2) feelings of general security, (3) a sense of predictability in life, and (4) a reduction of family income. In addition, the patient undergoes changes in his physical capabilities, his sense of independence, and his life structure. By the time it becomes clear that the illness will not respond to treatment, he and his family have experienced multiple losses. Their grief may either surge at a time of crisis or be intensely felt during a calm interval, when they have time to process events and the accompanying emotions.

Anticipatory Grief

C. K. Aldrich defines anticipatory grief as "grief expressed in advance when the loss is perceived as inevitable" (Sourkes, 1982, p. 67). Sourkes continues: "In contrast to its almost palpable presence at diagnosis, anticipatory grief now charts a subterranean course as the undergirding and pervasive theme of the living-dying experience (p. 67).

The patient grieves his impending loss of life and separation from those he loves. For the family, the grief of separation begins when they imagine what life will be like without the patient. While this can be emotionally wrenching, it is adaptive, and initiates the process that will continue in bereavement.

During the terminal phase of the illness, patient and family may react differently to the thought of separation.

> The family often articulates what appears to be a paradox; whereas they were prepared to let go of the patient earlier in the illness, they now feel less and less able even to imagine the loss. In contrast, the patient often describes a growing accommodation — albeit painful — to the idea of impending death. This is an anguished crossroads, for it indicates the recognition that the patient and family are moving in different directions. (Sourkes, 1982, p. 69)

The challenge is to maintain a shared family context, while permitting individuals to let go at their own pace.

Bereavement

Social rituals mark the beginning of bereavement. Within the familiar structure of ritual, the family first experiences life without the patient. Cultural and religious rituals validate grief and therefore can be of comfort to the family; they often become a marker in the family's continuing development.

During bereavement the family begins its reorganization to accommodate life without the patient. A wide variety of responses to grief can be expected. Major determinants of the grief responses are the nature of the bereaved person's relationship to the deceased, personality variables, and ethnicity and culture (Osterweis et al., 1094). In part, reorganization of the family involves mourning of the roles lost in relation to the person who has died, and creating or recreating roles — new ways of interacting and/or perceiving oneself.

Maternity

One wept whose only child was dead,
New-born, ten years ago.
"Weep not; he is in bliss," they said
She answered, "Even so,

Ten years ago was born in pain
A child, not now forlorn.
But oh, ten years ago, in vain,
A Mother, a mother was born."

Alice Meynell,1847–1923
(Arnold & Gemma, 1983, p. 58)

Bereavement involves all areas of life and leaves no part of it untouched. During the first years after the loss, sleep may be interrupted by thoughts or dreams about the person lost or about death. In these first years mornings tend to be the most difficult part of the day as the realization of loss breaks into consciousness upon awakening. During this period the process of mourning may include emotional swings, from numbness and an inability to focus with clarity to heightened awareness with aching feelings of isolation. In addition to the intensity of emotion, there is current belief that traumatic events, like the loss of a family member, may have an impact on the body's immune system. Therapy after the loss can help the survivors to articulate their overwhelming feelings of separation and loss, and thereby achieve some sense of mastery as they reconstruct their lives.

CONCLUSION

At a time of vulnerability psychotherapy within hospice can be an enriching experience. The general goal of therapeutic intervention is to help the patient and family achieve successive levels of stability after periods of emotional disruption. Modalities for intervention include individual therapy, family therapy, and group therapy.

REFERENCES

Arnold, J., & Gemma, P. (1983). *A child dies: A portrait of family grief.* Rockville, MD and London: Aspen Publication

Casperson, D.M. (1985, March/April). Family perceptions of hospice care. *The American Journal of Hospice Care,* p. 15.

Chasin, R. (1987, April). Lecture, Family Institute of Cambridge, MA.

Dym, B. (1987, March). The cybernetics of physical illness. *Family Process, 26,* 35.

Dym, B., & Berman S. (1986). The primary health care team: Family physician and family therapist in joint practice. *Family Systems Medicine, 4,* 1:11.

Jaffe, L., Jaffe, A., & Love, R. (1976). *Living with dying.* Videotape, Alfred University School of Health Related Professions.

McGoldrick, M., Pearce, J., & Giordano, J. (Eds.) (1982). *Ethnicity and family therapy.* New York and London: The Guilford Press.

National Hospice Organization. (1987). *Fact sheet.* Arlington, VA.

Osterweis, M., Solomon, F., & Green, M. (Eds.) (1984). *Bereavement: Reactions, consequences and care.* Washington, DC: National Academy Press.

Sourkes, B. (1982). *The deepening shade.* Pittsburgh: University of Pittsburgh Press.

C H A P T E R
81

WORKING WITH THE GAY MALE COMMUNITY: A Historical Perspective

William Wedin, Ph.D.

Twenty years ago we thought we knew a great deal about "practicing homosexuals."* We thought we knew, for example, what made them "that way" (Mitchell, 1981a). In general, we believed them to be the pathological product of a distant father and an invasive mother. Only the specific mechanism was a matter of debate. Were the Freudians right in maintaining that the family pattern "unnaturally" strengthened the young child's "natural" homosexual tendencies, due to an overstimulation of the negative Oedipus complex? Or should we rather follow the British school in seeing the family structure as creating an even earlier developmental arrest, namely, in the initial separation/individuation process vis-a-vis the mother? Whatever the answer, we were sure that the parents were to blame.

Twenty years ago we also felt extremely confident as to what our treatment goal should be. No matter what the patient wanted, no matter how non-conflictual his homosexuality seemed to him, our goal in treatment was always to "cure" him of his sexual preference and set him on the one "true" path to genital happiness. The means were beyond moral scrutiny (Mitchell, 1981b). Giving orders and advice, manipulating the positive transference, taking over reality testing for the patient, reporting confidential information to parents, wives, and institute training committees—all were considered acceptable parameters to stop the patient's "acting out." Even outright deception was sanctioned: for example, where the patient shows such "poor reality testing" as to believe that he was already *in* a loving, committed relationship with a man, and had no desire to "change." Here the therapist was expected to pretend to support the relationship until the patient gained the ego strength to see it for the sado-masochistic sham it "really" was. So far as professional ethics were concerned, the "practicing homosexual" was a man about to leap from a bridge.

The connection, of course, was not just projection. If some of us secretly wanted these patients to "take a flying leap" at times and rationalized our treatment strategies accordingly, it was born out of impotent anger over our inability to "cure" them of an "illness" which we seriously thought might kill

---

Note: For the sake of historical accuracy, terms such as "homosexual" are only used for the period in which they were current.

them. James Dean crashing his motocycle, Hart Crane plunging off the Brooklyn Bridge, come to mind. But then, twenty years ago, were the alternatives so much better? If there were any "happy homosexuals" back then, they certainly never came to see *us*. The only homosexuals we knew anything about were the lonely, the frightened, the broken: those who could no longer cope; those who dumbly accepted society's judgment that theirs was a "pathological choice," but still could not change that "choice"—not for all the power and wealth, not for all the rugged good looks in the world. To us it seemed so wanton and perverse: to choose a life of booze and backroom sex, phony marriages and live-in "friends," when with just a little "will" and enough analysis, we thought that *any* guy could become a real Rock Hudson with the girls! No wonder we sometimes wanted to murder them.

Today the world is a very different place. Today there are gay cable and radio shows, gay dance and film festivals, gay magazines and newspapers. There are gay clinics, gay clothing stores, gay health spas, gay high schools, gay hotlines, gay restaurants, gay resorts, gay study programs at universities. There are clubs for gay bikers, gay boxers, gay hikers, gay runners, gay wrestlers. There are gay baseball, football, rowing, soccer, and track teams, who compete together in a gay Olympics. There are organizations for gay Protestants, gay Catholics, Gay Jews, gay Hispanics, gay Italians, gay veterans. There are support groups for gay fathers, gay teens, older gays, parents of gays, wives of gays, the gay blind, the gay deaf, the gay obese, the gay wheelchair-bound. There are professional organizations and publications for gay accountants, gay anthropologists, gay attorneys, gay bankers, gay brokers, gay businessmen, gay civil servants, gay communications specialists, gay dentists, gay firemen, gay historians, gay librarians, gay musicians, gay nurses, gay physicians, gay policemen, gay priests, gay psychiatrists, gay psychologists, gay social workers, gay sociologists, gay teachers. There are foundations for the funding of gay-related artistic, educational, legal, and political affairs. There are gay antidefamation and antiviolence leagues. In short, within the last twenty years, a social revolution has occurred.

The revolution can be traced to a hot June night in 1969. On that night a band of New York City policemen, allegedly angered over a delay in payment of their weekly "protection" fee, staged a raid on a peaceful, transvestite bar, known as the Stonewall Bar (Teal, 1971). According to the unwritten code of the demi-monde at the time, the police were in the right and the owner in the wrong, as the supposed protection had been provided but not paid for. It was therefore the owner's responsibility to pay up and apologize so that the patrons who had been arrested could get back to the bar, instead of spending the night crying their eyes out in jail. Only this time, for the first time since gay bars began in New York City in the early 18th century, the code was ignored. As word of the raid spread through the Village like fire across a prairie, thousands of "practicing homosexuals" took to the streets, converging on the precinct house, where the patrons were being held. A riot broke out. Alarmed and out of control, the police charged the crowd with battle gear. There were arrests and bloody beatings. That same night the networks carried the amazing news to every "practicing homosexual" in the country. Out of the ashes of the old demi-monde a sense of open community had suddenly arisen. Gay liberation was born.

In hindsight we can see how gay liberation had been in the works since at least the beginning of World War II, when heretofore largely isolated homosexuals were brought together in large numbers from every corner of the country. With the close of the war many of these ex-servicemen chose to find new homes in the great seaport cities, like New York and San Francisco, where a thriving demi-monde was to be found, rather than return to the small towns where they had been brought up. Then came the civil-rights and antiwar movements of the 1950's and 1960's, in which many younger homosexuals found common cause on both a social and psychological level. Thus, by the end of the 1960's, the stage had been set for a routine "fag bust" to become an instant focal point for a radical redefinition of experience on a mass scale. Literally, at the same moment in 1000 different minds, what had always been seen as a legitimate act of enforcement of a mutually beneficial "gentlemen's agreement" became a horrible piece of police brutality against an oppressed *people*.

So where were we? Where were all the helping professionals the night that gay liberation was created by a bunch of dizzy drag queens? Where were all the papers, pamphlets, handouts, revolutionary texts, which we should have been writing for decades to bring about that particular night? If there is one thing that must be understood about the gay community before professionals should even think of working with and in that community, it is that community's individual and collective memory of the fact that when it counted the most, *we were not there*. We were not there in a real sense. We were not there in a transferential sense. Like so many of their own fathers, on both a real and transferential level, we kept our distance and let conventional attitudes determine what our thoughts and actions toward these our "children" should be — never seeing, until they finally showed us, how profoundly we had failed them.

The source of such empathic failure was, is, and ever shall be our professional hubris: in particular, our collective delusional belief system that we beings-bound-to-time can yet create a science of human behavior which exists outside of time for all time, at the same time that it is we ourselves, we beings-bound-to-time, who constitute both the subject and object of that timely science at any time. What narcissistic nonsense! And yet how we all do partake of that nonsense still — even as that queer genius, Alan Turing, did partake of a cyanide-painted apple, when his "suicide" was demanded by the British Secret Service (Hodges, 1983). It remains the downfall of every clinician to this day.

Consider the case of the very father of cultural relativism, Harry Stack Sullivan. When the issue of Sullivan's homosexuality is discussed in psychology and psychiatry courses even today, too often it is presented as a juicy piece of gossip, of the giant-with-feet-of-clay variety. On the rare occasion when the question is examined in print, it is usually to show that Sullivan was not a "practicing homosexual," after all, but just a confirmed "Irish bachelor," who just happened to have a handsome, live-in "friend," named Jimmie, whom he picked up on a Washington street corner one day (when Jimmie was 15 and Sullivan 35), and proceeded to live with for the last 20 years of his life (Chatelaine, 1981; Perry, 1982). Sullivan, in fact, was so smitten with Jimmie that he eventually left Jimmie his entire estate, at the same time he commemorated their relationship in a coat-of-arms which Sullivan insisted be inscribed on the cover of every book he published: namely his self-designed, yin-yang emblem of two horseheads, whirling round and round, in an eternal "69"— like Turing's apple, a marvelous metaphorical pun. Yet his biographers still contend that Harry never had a "yen" for Jimmie in all those twenty years?

What the gay community finds so damning about the Sullivan case is that it dramatizes once again how little, even now, we are able to empathize with *them*. For Sullivan's detractors, his homosexuality is an easy weapon at hand. For his self-appointed defenders, it is an accusation to be denied, however clear the truth, unless and until convincing glossy photos can be produced. But who among us ever thinks about the needs of gay people here? If all of the available evidence points to the conclusion that Sullivan was a homosexual man in a homosexual marriage within the social and psychological constraints of the 1930's and 1940's (Allen, 1989; Chapman, 1976), what right does the professional community have to keep that knowledge a matter of secret gossip, while publicly demanding a standard of proof more appropriately reserved for murder trials? Is it not rather our solemn duty to the living to publicize that knowledge as widely as possible that gay people may point to him with pride and shout: *"Ecce homo!"* ("Behold the man!")

How we answer those questions depends on how we privately view gay people. Publicly, we know, we are supposed to treat them as "normal." But how do we really see them in our professional heart of hearts? Do we privately continue to see them as sick *people*? Or have we managed to internalize the vision of Stonewall to the point where we actually do see them as *a people* made sick by their oppression? Clearly, if we take the former view, we may well feel justified in "protecting" Sullivan's memory, even at the cost of truth. (Let his "sickness" be buried with him that only the purity of his insights may remain, etc.) Whereas if we take the latter view—privately as well as publicly—then there is no escaping the judgment that our collective behavior in the Sullivan case is *morally wrong*. To deprive a people of their heroes is to deprive them of their self-respect.

Neutrality is not a moral option here. Either we approve of the way gay people and their heroes are treated in this society or we do not. There is no way out. If we are not part of the answer, we are part of the problem. Silence gives consent. Indeed, in terms of the Sullivan case, silence *is* the problem. Silence is the very thing which prevents the process of positive identity formation from occurring. Thus, we cannot take the analytic position of somehow being "above" the fray and still maintain ourselves as moral beings. As the deaths of so many tens of thousands of gay people in the Holocaust bear witness (Heger, 1980), Freudian "neutrality" has its moral consequences too. Profession makes no difference. Whether we are therapists or farmers, bankers or bricklayers, we still belong to the same moral universe, from which there is no existential exit. As beings-bound-to-time in a society which actively discriminates against gay people and their potential heroes, we are, all of us, just as much responsible for our *passive* choices as our active ones.

The same may be said with respect to treatment. If we attempt to practice a "value-free" form of therapy with people whom our society consistently devalues, we ineluctably participate in that devaluation, if only passively.

Whether or not the patient is aware of this participation, he still experiences it on both a real and transferential level in terms of abandonment and betrayal by the therapist as therapist and the therapist as parent. The only question is how the patient will handle and process the experience. Specifically, will he be healthy enough to recognize the nature and source of that experience and move forward to do something about it? Or will he take in the therapist's betrayal and abandonment as simply his just deserts? Clearly, it is a very tall order to expect the vast majority of patients to be able to comprehend and articulate how a "value-free" stance can actually be toxic to them when neutrality seems so benign and therapists so sincere. If anything, we should rather expect a gradual increase in symptomatology in keeping with the patient's individual character structure, followed by what the therapist would see as a "premature" termination — unless, of course, the patient is so masochistic that he would have the experience repeated forever in the form of an interminable analysis.

It is therefore incumbent on each of us to ask ourselves beforehand in as open and undefended a manner as we can: "Is this for me? Do I really want to work with such a scorned population if much of the work in treatment is actively combating that scorn? Do I really have the personality for it? If it means giving up my safe neutrality, if it means exposing *myself* to scorn, will I have what it takes to be there for them? Or when it counts the most, will I fail them too?" Sexual orientation has nothing to do with it. Just as one can be gay and white and still work effectively for black civil rights, the reverse is also true: one can be straight and black and still work effectively both with and for gays. To be a "good enough" therapist all that is required is a capacity for sustained empathy, combined with a certain caring iconoclasm. But first there must be the commitment.

At the same time, the sexual orientation of the therapist does have a bearing on the kind of "boundedness" he is bound to bring to the work. For straight therapists, the boundedness is in believing they can fully imagine the gay experience when they cannot even comprehend gay *oppression* — from never being able to hold hands in public for fear of physical violence to never having one's lover invited to one's parents' home for the holidays. The totality utterly escapes them. Gay therapists, by contrast, must deal with the boundedness of living within that universe of scorn so completely that they may begin to experience its "laws" as immutable when such things are simple reified fictions — like the self-fulfilling prophecy that gay relationships never work. In the days when gay therapists felt bound to rejoice in that Biblical sounding "law" — having "a different form of sexuality" was the secular version — it *was* largely true. Now that it is largely thought to be false, it largely is false. Thus, there is a boundedness that goes with sameness, just as there is a boundedness that goes with otherness. There is a boundedness to every being even now.

The concept of homosexuality is one such conceptual bound. To us the concept seems so basic that we take it completely for granted, to the point that we hardly conceive of it as being a concept at all. Like the concept of gravity, we assume that it somehow must have always been there, as a sort of Kantian idea, existing *a priori*, in every civilization and culture, down to the most primitive. To think of thinking of sexual behavior without it seems absurd.

Yet even our own proud civilization engaged in precisely that absurdity from the early Middle Ages until the mid-19th century, when the concept was introduced into Western thinking by an otherwise obscure Hungarian physician, K.M. Benkert (Steakley, 1975). Before that time, such nice distinctions would have been considered at best sophistical, at worst Satanical. So far as medieval Christian theology was concerned—which was essentially still *the* theology of the West in the 19th century—what mattered was the *fact* of sexual sin, not its specific nature. Sexual "congress" with man, beast, or child— "buggery" even between man and wife—it all came down to the same thing. Once a person fell into temptation and disorder, that person became, in the Elizabethan sense of the term, a "Sodomite," that is, a person who freely engaged in every manner of sin, according to opportunity (Bray, 1982). (Even today, the *Oxford English Dictionary* defines "sodomy" as any type of "unnatural sexual intercourse," including that "with animals.") How could it be otherwise? If only the Creator was able to create order, how could there possibly be any order to "sodomitical" acts, that, by definition, represented a turning away from God's natural order" towards Satanical disorder? To the medieval Christian mind, the idea that sodomy could be anything but totally chaotic and polymorphously perverse was anathema. To impose form on formless lust and name it "homosexuality" was to become a blasphemous Faust.

By the mid-19th century, however, things had become a bit "schizophrenic." While Darwin's discoveries were being excoriated as Satanical by Victorian moralists, the classificatory system of Linnaeus—which had led to those discoveries—was still being praised as showing the handiwork of God. To use a Freudian metaphor, science was now "in the saddle," however restless the horse. Indeed, in the hands of Goethe, Faust himsef had become the ultimate Romantic hero: the very embodiment of the scientific, observing ego—forever seeking knowledge for the good of mankind, forever striving to unbind the human spirit from time. So why not study sodomy too? Just imagine the possibilities for social control! If sodomy could be broken down into certain *stable* behavioral patterns, it might actually be possible for science to predict *in advance* which people were the most likely to repeat which sins, instead of treating these things as matters of random chance. For example, it might be found that certain Sodomites displayed such a consistent preference for sodomy with other human males that one might reasonably call them "homosexuals." By carefully studying the habits of these "homosexuals," science might then develop more effective ways to hunt them down where they lurked. In the not too distant future, it might even be possible to eradicate such "monsters" altogether. What a brave new world that would be!

For a time, the Faustian dream indeed seemed attainable. As Victorian psychiatry began to reveal the nature of the beast, existing sodomy laws were strengthened; Draconian penalties made more severe. The vice squad became a separate arm of the police. In 1896, the high-tech trial of Oscar Wilde for "crimes against nature" was instantly carried by transatlantic cable even to the tiny town of Smyrna, where Sullivan was already a child (Perry, 1982). The demand for treatment soared. Castrations and lobotomies proliferated. After a false start in the direction of nonprofit acceptance (Freud, 1951), Freudian analysts soon gained an even greater market share with promises of purely verbal "cures." The referral possibilities seemed endless.

That became the problem. By the Great Depression, the number of homosexuals seeking treatment for their "condition" was rapidly overwhelming the medical system. What was going on? Was it just that diagnosis was becoming more accurate? Was it a case of rampant recidivism? Or was the prevalence of homosexuality actually increasing? As Marx's Victorian view of homosexuality as the ultimate symbol of "bourgeois decadence" began to grip both capitalist and communist countries alike (Fernbach, 1981), "homosexual panic" emerged as a recurring nationalist phenomenon: first in the Soviet Union, with the mass extermination of homosexuals under Stalin; then in Nazi Germany, with the application of "the final solution" to homosexuals as well as Jews; and then in the United States, with the Nixon-McCarthy witch hunts against "commie queers." The irony was that, at least where homosexuality was concerned, both fascists and communists accepted the same Victorian Marxist view.

Then came Stonewall. Exactly 100 years after the term "homosexuality" was coined, Leviathan rose up from the deep and smashed to pieces the foundering Faustian dream. The moralists were aghast. Where had Marxist science, Freudian science, Victorian science gone wrong?

In 1851, before Freud was even born, another queer genius, Herman Melville, had already deeply contemplated the Victorian "ego" from the perspective of his own homoerotic experiences with men and arrived at a singularly prophetic, if chilling, conclusion in his allegorical masterpiece, *Moby Dick* (Martin, 1986): man is never more sadistic and insane than when he systematically seeks to destroy that which his bounded science condemns as "unnatural" — be it an "unnatural" creature (Moby Dick), an "unnatural" culture (Queequeg's) or an "unnatural" form of love (that between "sperm-squeezing" men). It is Freud's later image of that ego as a rational rider on a restless horse that is both prefigured and answered in Melville's horrific vision of a blood-drenched Ahab savagely hacking at his own animal nature in Faustian rage, even as he is dragged to his self-bounded doom.

So what is next? In a clairvoyant leap of mind that leaves the "lee shore" of morality far behind, Melville suddenly springs forward to Stonewall as he celebrates the indestructibility of male love in a wonderful parody of the Resurrection. Veritably, on the "third day," Ishmael rises from his watery grave, riding his cannibal lover's coffin. How quintessentially camp! How utterly gay!

What psychiatry has done to Sullivan, literary criticism has done to Melville. The bawdy jokes, the broad innuendos, the erotic descriptions of sailors and South Sea Island men, the passionate letters to Hawthorne — whatever might contradict the image of a conforming Victorian with wife and children has been surgically removed from view as both irrelevant and tasteless. ("Taste" is the ultimate form of Victorian censorship.) Only now, in the wake of Stonewall, are a few gay people finally beginning to ask: "Is this book meant for *us*? Is this book *about* us? Could as great a man as Melville actually be *one* of us?" These are not just intellectual questions. They are longing questions. They are the questions of a people yearning to create a future through a quest for a remembrance of things past. They are Rachel searching for her missing children. But what do Melville's self-anointed protectors care? The only queston they will entertain is: "Where are the glossy photos?" ("Standards of scholarship, you know!") It is a Catch 22. First they bury the evidence; then they demand to see it.

For his part, Ahab is portrayed as a Victorian tragic hero: indeed Melville's hero. He is not. For all of Ahab's energy and eloquence, his command of religious philosophy, his store of righteous wrath, he remains utterly lacking in the ability to love that which he also hates: hence any capacity for tragic conflict and ambivalence, such as Lear, Othello, Hamlet have. He is even devoid of the attenuated compassion of a Macbeth. Ahab is far too modern for that. In his view (which, of course, is the only "right" view) Moby Dick is nothing less than the living embodiment of all those countless, senseless evils that attack and torment mankind. How can pity, compassion, and acceptance be shown towards that? No. So harmful a thing must be pursued and destroyed without mercy or remorse, in cold blood, scientifically—the way one would remove a tumor or a Jew. That is the Faustian model.

Thus Ahab is himself the personification of human aggression directed toward the betterment of mankind. He is *that*—nothing less. If he is not Melville's hero, he is not some cardboard villain either. In his relentless quest to find and destroy that which he regards as evil, he is Faustian science at its best and worst. He is Faustian science in all its ambivalent complexity. He is Faustian science draining the tropical swamps to rid the world of malaria and yellow fever. He is Faustian science building death camps to rid the world of inferior races, classes, and lifestyles. He is Hubble and Hitler, Schweitzer and Stalin, all rolled into one. That is what makes Ahab so complex, so confusing, so compelling. How can we tell which causes, methods, outcomes are right? Starbuck counsels humility and harmony with nature, but then Starbuck's own sense of duty overwhelms his judgment, and he leads his men to certain slaughter, while nobly "following orders." Clearly, the Victorian ego is just not up to the task.

What the Victorian ego is up against is collectively expressed as Moby Dick. Moby Dick may be homoerotic love. Moby Dick may be a black hole sucking matter out of our own universe into God-knows-where. Whatever he may be at the moment, Moby Dick is whatever the Victorian ego cannot comprehend or control and so comes to loathe as an unassailable bound to its own grandiosity, its own delusional unboundedness from time. Yet Moby Dick remains unmoved. He neither attacks that ego nor avoids that ego. Be He quark or queer, Queequeg or quasar, Moby Dick just simply, incomprehensibly *is*. For the Victorian ego, Ahab's ego, the resulting narcissistic injury proves intolerable. When Moby Dick is finally confronted as The-Is-That-Is—yes, darling, The Simply Divine—the Victorian ego first implodes, then explodes, like a supermassive star that no longer can sustain the gravity of its own grandiose proportions, in a paroxysm of deneutralized aggression. Ahab, the cold-blooded scientist-hunter, madly hacks at the whale. The police charge a crowd of Village queers with battle gear. The illusion of reason is gone.

Not that there is any serious question whether Moby Dick will survive. Viewed from even the intimate distance of Barnard's star, man's capacity to do mischief to the Infinite is infinitesimal indeed. The only serious question is: will *we* survive with it? In the final non-Freudian analysis, will we be able to put our Faustian dreams behind us and live in harmony with all of nature, including our own? Or will we collectively self-destruct like the crew and captain of *The Pequod?* Clearly, in this nuclear age, it is the single most important question we can raise.

But *here*? In a chapter on *gays*? Exactly. It is exactly that note of puzzle-ment—that patronizing attitude of incomprehension—that makes the present chapter necessary. When we think of "working with the gay community" even today, twenty years after Stonewall, we still think in terms of "helping our little brown brothers." It never so much as occurs to us that *they* might help *us*. Such is our Victorian legacy, our Freudian manifest destiny. Though we may pay lip service to the notion that gay people should be shown acceptance and respect, we still do not accept or respect them *as* a people—with a culture, history, and perspective all their own. Much less are we prepared to acknowl-edge their rich achievements as contributions to our common well-being. Again, like so many of their parents, we ignore what they have to give us.

But then we also have a communication problem to overcome in that gay people, really, do not talk *straight*. At best, they sort of meander around, like Sullivan. With Melville, it is even worse. From the novel's queer beginning—"supplied by a late consumptive usher to a grammer school"—to the resur-rection of Ishmael at the end, Melville makes an obvious point of not going straight to the point as any straight-thinking novelist should. Oh, no, he is much too good for that! No, he has to go beyond the point, behind the point, above and below and beside the point. But the point itself keeps jumping around like a bombarded electron. In short(s) he is constantly *dishing*. Could it be some neurochemical imbalance in the gay brain? No, it would seem to be a matter of preference on Melville's part since he certainly can write like a Marx or a Freud when it takes his fancy. Ahab's speeches, for example, are a model of linear lucidity. So why this Mobius strip style of writing otherwise?

In her little jewel of an essay, "Notes on Camp," Susan Sontag (1983) states that camp: "incarnates a victory of style over content, of esthetics over morali-ty, of irony over tragedy." Elaborating on her theme, she continues:

> Camp taste is, above all, a mode of enjoyment, of appreciation—not judgment. Camp is generous. It wants to enjoy. It only seems like malice, cynicism. (Or, if it is cynicism, it is not a ruthless but a sweet cynicism.) Camp taste doesn't propose that it is in bad taste to be serious; it doesn't sneer at someone who succeeds in being seriously dramatic. What it does is to find success in certain passionate failures.

Adding:

> Camp taste is a kind of love, love for human nature. It relishes, rather than judges, the little triumphs and awkward intensities of "char-acter."...Camp taste identifies with what it is enjoying. People who share this sensitivity are not laughing at the thing they label as a "camp," they're enjoying it. Camp is a tender feeling.

What Sontag declines to mention because it could not be mentioned when she wrote her essay in 1964 (as is still the case today in the taste-setting *New York Times*) is that camp is and always has been a *gay* art form, artfully designed, like Queequeg's coffin, to rise above the surrounding doom and give gay people a private place to sun. As the originator and greatest practitioner of that form, Melville understood this only too well.

The therapist who would work with gay people must well understand it too. To see camp as too "silly," too "faggy"—even downright "sick"—is to see it from the outside, from the perspective of the unjudged, the unscorned. It is to see it from the standpoint of someone who never thinks twice about kissing in a restaurant or necking on a park bench because one has chosen the "right" gender. If camp is concerned with life's "little triumphs" and "passionate failures," it is because that is as much as most gay people have been able to hope for in *their* lives, at least until very recently. Camp is charity itself.

The alternative to camp is Harry Stack Sullivan, dead in a Paris hotel room at the age of 57, pills scattered around the corpse, his lover hidden away in their long shared closet, 3,000 miles away. The alternative is Melville himself, gradually ceasing to write after the commercial failure of *Moby Dick*, until the very last years of his life, just a year before Sullivan was born, when he began but did not complete *Billy Budd*: a gloomy and again, prophetic tale of an innocent young sailor, hanged for turning on a superior officer, praising the captain's justice as he dies. The alternative, in short, is the introjection of Western society's murderous rage toward The-Is-That-Should-Not-Be.

But why such rage in the first place? If homosexuality is simply a fact of life (and a harmless fact at that), why does Western society have such a pathological hatred toward it? In part, the answer seems to lie in our association of the homosexual with the feminine: namely, that gay men are supposed to "identify with women" and "respond as women." "Like women" they presumably want to "take in the penis" and "play the passive role" in bed. Outside of bed, it is said, they tend to want someone else to "take care of them," rather than "work for a living." In short, they are seen as lacking (phallic) "assertiveness" of the sort needed for success in business and war.

For a civilization as given to aggression as our own, especially since the Victorian era, this characterization of gay men as "less than men" and "womanly men" is damning indeed: the more so since gay men, by way of retaliation, at times make a point of "camping it up" in public. Victorian analysts, in turn, are quick to pounce upon such "feminine" behavior as evidence in support of their theories concerning mother fixation, hallucinated loss of the penis, and other such projective identifications. What they fail to "take in" themselves is that the association of the homosexual with the feminine is precisely that: an *association* — an association that is both time- and culture-specific. It is an association that does not exist in many cultures, and only came into our own culture towards the beginning of the 18th century, when cross-dressing (as "Mollys") first became a popular lark among the gay men of London and New York City (Burrough, 1976). Before that time, from ancient Greece to Renaissance imitations thereof, homosexuality was associated with "becoming a man" and/or "performing one's manly duties." In Dorian culture, a youth who refused to play the anal receptive role and "take it like a man" was considered a humiliation to his family — and a sissy (Vanggard, 1972). Thus while the association of the homosexual with the feminine may explain something about why our society sees homosexuality in such a negative light, we should be cautious in generalizing too far about such a recently acquired connection.

At the same time, we should also be careful not to confuse the magnitude of the oppression that homosexual behavior has elicited since the Victorian era with the importance of the trait as trait. That would be to give the Hitlers, the Stalins, the McCarthys of the modern world too much credit, too much rationality. Whatever we stand to gain from attempting to figure out why one trait is chosen as a basis for persecution as against some other, we must not let our interest in content distract us from function. So far as human survival goes, so far as even human progress goes, sexual orientation certainly ranks right down there with creed and color as irrelevant human traits. What gives them the significance they have is the use to which they are put, especially as sources of scapegoating.

The function of scapegoating, of course, is to relieve group tensions and frustrations by focusing all the "badness" that the group feels about itself and its current situation on one particular subgroup of individuals whom the rest of the group can safely hate because of the power imbalance between them. As this hatred begins to get expressed, the scapegoated subgroup is inclined, to a greater or lesser extent, to "identify with the aggressor" and "own" the projection, as we say. This, in turn, reassures the aggressor group that its hatred is justified. What happens next depends on the amount of "badness" that needs to be "dumped," not the intrinsic "goodness" of the aggressor group. In the Nixon-McCarthy era, for example, the amount of "badness" which had to be dumped onto "commie queers" for the "loss" of China and the development of the Russian A-bomb was relatively small, given the overall post-war boom. Thus, the American public was fairly well satisfied with the destruction of several hundred lives and a few electrocutions. Whereas the amount of "badness" which both the Russians and the Germans had to dump as a consequence of the Great Depression and the havoc of World War I required the extermination of literally millions of people, including tens of thousands of gays.

A facilitating factor in this process can be traced back to the technological and scientific advances of the early Victorian era, namely, the growth of a collective, grandiose ego, believed capable of overcoming all human problems and limitations, if given a free hand. The "fuel" for this ego, in turn, came from two sources. On the intellectual side, the sense of grandiosity was spurred by the development of scientific reductionism, which seemed to offer the possibility of turning all the heretofore baffling complexities of life into a series of simple polarities ("natural" vs. "unnatural," "progressive" vs. "decadent," "homo" vs. "hetero," "control" vs. "impulse," etc.) On the emotional side, the raw aggression required was provided by the breakup of the extended agrarian family into mutually deprived, individual units, massed together with other individual units of the same type, according to age and gender. Thus, when Ahab stands before his male-only crew, like Hitler before the Reichstag, and demands to know—"And what tune is it ye pull to, men?"—and they respond—"A dead whale or a stove boat!"—we see both the beginnings and clear direction of our own, increasingly borderline world.

For their part, gay people, particularly in the period prior to Stonewall, found it very difficult to resist identifying with the aggressor, except in marginal and/or parodistic ways, as evidenced by camp and "light" S&M. Since Stonewall, the assertion of "gay pride," combined with the formation of numerous gay organizations and institutions outside of the bar and bath scene of the old demi-monde has led to a noticeable decline in various forms of mental illness arising from self-hatred. However, the burden of continued societal oppression remains high. For example, it is estimated that even today the rate of completed suicides among gay men is 5 times that of their straight counterparts, while the rate of attempted suicide among gay youth is more than 20 times as high (Wedin, 1986).

How the AIDS crisis will affect both the gay community and society as a whole remains to be seen. on the one hand, there appears to be a greater incidence of anti-gay violence and denial of adequate medical care to gay patients. On the other hand, the heroism of gay people in the face of so much suffering and death has brought home to many families Sullivan's famous adage: "We are all more human than otherwise." In the past, we have not believed gay people quite were.

REFERENCES

Allen, M. (1989). *Harry Stack Sullivan: The Habit of Secrecy.* In press.
Allen, M. (1989). Personal communication.
Bray, A. (1982). *Homosexuality in Renaissance England.* London: Gay Men's Press.
Burrough, V. (1976). *Sexual variance in society and history.* New York: Wiley.
Chapman, A. (1976). *Harry Stack Sullivan: The man and his work.* New York: G.P. Putnam's Sons.
Chatelaine, K. (1981). *Harry Stack Sullivan: The formative years.* Washington, D.C.: University Press of America.
Fernbach, D. (1971). *The spiral path: A gay contribution to human survival.* Boston: Alyson Publications.
Freud, S. (1951). A letter to a grateful (American) mother. *International Journal of Psychoanalysis,* 32, 331.
Heger, H. (1980). *Men of the pink triangle.* Boston: Alyson Publications.
Hodges, A. (1983). *Alan Turing: An enigma.* New York: Simon & Schuster.
Martin, R. (1983). *Hero, captain, and stranger: Male friendship, social critique, and literary form in the sea novels of Herman Melville.* Chapel Hill, N.C.: University of North Carolina Press.
Mitchell, S. (1981a). Psychodynamics, homosexuality, and the question of pathology. *Psychiatry,* 41, 254–263.
Mitchell, S. (1981b). The psychoanalytic treatment of homosexuality: Some technical considerations. International Review of Psychoanalysis, 8, 63–74.
Perry, H. (1982). *Psychiatrist of America: The life of Harry Stack Sullivan.* Cambridge, MA: Harvard University Press.
Sontag, S. (1983). *A Susan Sontag reader.* New York: Vintage Books.
Steakley, J. (1975). *The homosexual emancipation movement in Germany.* New York: Arno Press.
Teal, D. (1971). *Gay Militants.* New York: Stein & Day.
Vanggard, T. *Phallos: A symbol and its history in the male world.* New York: International Universities Press.
Wedin, W. (1986, Aug. 25). High risk sex as an existential choice. *New York Native.* Reprints available from author.

C H A P T E R
82

THE ALCOHOLIC PATIENT IN DYNAMIC PSYCHOTHERAPY

Marion Gedney, Ph.D.

M ost of us dynamically oriented psychotherapists discourage the presence of alcoholics in our practices. We work in a circumscribed way. Our time is limited to rigidly scheduled sessions. We require that patients verbalize their feelings and tolerate strong affects — become anxious, sad, or angry, and at the same time be able to stand back, look at these feelings, reflect on them, and relate them to events both outside and inside the analysis, in the present and in the recent or remote past. All of this is accomplished with the analyst and in relation to the analyst in the transference. We expect patients to attend their scheduled sessions regularly, to keep only to these sessions, and to pay the bill, so as to maintain and protect their own therapy, while the therapist uses professional skill to facilitate the development and unfolding of a useful therapeutic experience.

Alcoholic patients do not do very well at any of these things. They cannot keep to schedules. They miss appointments and want to come at unscheduled times; they telephone at odd hours, break promises, and generally are difficult to work with. Sometimes they act out and get into serious trouble on the outside. But they do not seem overly anxious or appropriately concerned about the consequences of their accidents, violence, or other impulsive behavior. Moreover, although they may have insight into intrapsychic conflicts and make meaningful connections between past and present difficulties, nothing really seems to happen. Therapists gradually become aware that there is little progress. Perhaps the patients mention drinking or taking drugs, but mainly as secondary to other problems. Therapists begin to feel frustrated, or find themselves irritated with the difficulty in connecting with these patients. Perhaps the therapists find themselves becoming involved in hospital visits, or dealing with the results of patients' landing in jail for drunk driving. At the patients' homes, things seem always to be in a state of crisis because the spouse threatens to leave.

Very often the therapist, no less than the patient, is unaware of the importance of drinking in the patient's pathology. The therapist sees drinking as a means of dealing with anxiety or depression caused by other seemingly

Reprinted from *Issues in Ego Psychology,* 7, No. 1 & 2 (1984), with minor revisions, by permission of the publisher.

more important sources of disturbance in the patient's life. The purpose of this paper is to discuss the phenomenon of addiction in our practice, describe the alcoholic syndrome briefly, and offer some suggestions as to how to handle these patients.

Even though one may not believe in treating alcoholism by psychodynamic means, alcoholic patients keep turning up in our practices, or important people in patients' environments turn out to be alcoholics. The problem is much more widespread than most analytic therapists realize. Nicholas Cummings (1979) reported that in a random sample of psychotherapy patients seen in a large urban mental health center, 23 percent — almost one-fourth — were suffering from addictive problems or from emotional problems substantially exacerbated by alcohol or drug abuse. And of this 23 percent, only 3.5 percent were identified as problem alcohol or drug takers by their therapists.

It seems that an important problem is being overlooked. There is confusion about the nature of alcoholism and about the diagnosis. Everyone knows what alcohol is: Most of us drink it, we know the effects it has, and most of us can enjoy it. But some people do not seem to be able to handle it — about one in 10, according to most statistics. About one in 10 people become alcoholics, so that the 23 percent statistic in the mental health center population may not be so surprising.

In the psychoanalytic literature, papers on alcoholism are quite rare, and most were written relatively early in psychoanalytic history. Freud (1911), in his paper on the Schreber case, notes that alcohol removes inhibitions and undoes sublimations. In *Civilization and Its Discontents,* Freud (1930) discusses the various ways that unpleasure can be avoided and describes how pharmacological intoxication allows for the triumph of the pleasure principle in the face of adversity. Freud states,

> The crudest, but most effective among these methods of influence is the chemical one — intoxication. I do not think that anyone completely understands its mechanism, but it is a fact that there are foreign substances which when present in the blood or tissues, directly cause us pleasurable sensations; and they also so alter the conditions governing our sensibility that we become incapable of receiving unpleasurable impulses. (p. 78)

Not only does drink serve as a defense against unpleasurable affects and anxieties, but it also offers direct gratification of a libidinal drive.

Rado (1926), like other early psychoanalytic writers, stresses the libidinal significance of drug taking and describes the protracted state of well-being that is diffused throughout the organism. Rado finds that alcoholics in their early alcoholism or prealcoholic times respond to frustration with a painful tension combined with a high degree of intolerance of pain. In this state the future alcoholic is interested mainly in relief of the painful tension. Ingesting alcohol brings about a sharp rise in self-regard and an elevation of mood leading to elation, and a disappearance of the "tense depression." The elation is transitory, however. As the drug wears off, the individual comes down, is depressed, and returns to a state of tense depression, needing alcohol once again to return to a state of elation. A spiral is established in which increasing doses of the drug are needed to bring about what Rado calls the "pharmacogenic pleasure effect." Eventually, the drug can no longer bring about this pleasurable effect, and the patient, by now physically as well as psychologically dependent, is helpless to return to a predrug state. Rado notes that when addicts submit to withdrawal from a drug, they almost never are motivated by the wish to be well and free of the drug. What they really want is to return to a state in which small doses of the drug are once more able to gain for them the magical escape from unpleasure. Rado concludes that drug addiction is an artificial means of maintaining the ego's self-regard, evading the reality principle, and that the illness is a narcissistic disorder that gradually brings about the destruction of the natural ego organization.

Savitt (1963) emphasizes the role of oral dependence and impulsivity in the addict. He describes the individual's need to restore primary narcissism and the symbolic union with the breast — the early mother–infant relationship being the crucial factor in the addict's personality. Savitt acknowledges that many patients who are not addicts have had similar intrapsychic conflicts and early fixation points, but he does not offer an answer as to why some become addicts but others do not.

As Clifford Yorke (1970) points out in his excellent review on drug addiction, the literature tends to repeat itself. The emphases at different times have been on the role of oral libido and early oral fixations, sadism and the vicissitudes of aggression, impulsivity, regression to primary narcissistic states, or, more recently, withdrawal from object relatedness and regressions to narcissistic developmental levels. Anna Freud, in a comment to Yorke, observed that analysts have been baffled at all times by the addictions and have sought to explain them in terms of the prevailing interest of the period — for instance, in terms of the early mother–child relationship at the time when symbiosis was a leading psychoanalytical preoccupation. We now more often speak of ego defects, developmental deficits, and early narcissistic preoccupations. What seems clear is that many theoretical positions seem to describe aspects of the alcoholic patient, but no one seems to give a satisfying theoretical accounting that would provide a framework for both explaining and treating alcoholics.

Most workers have failed to find a consistent "alcoholic personality" or an identifiable "premorbid personality" of alcoholic patients. Vaillant (1981), Bean (1981), Blum (1981), Mack (1981), and others have argued convincingly the opposite position. They feel that ingesting alcohol over a long period is the cause rather than the effect of passive dependent traits and other deficiencies in ego and superego functioning.

Drinking damages the ego in many ways, one being the physical damage to brain cells, which causes confusion and memory loss. Alcoholic individuals are not, as the saying goes, playing with a full deck, and therefore have trouble putting together their experiences from day to day to evaluate events, remember what has happened, use their judgment, and act according to the reality principle. These patients' drug-induced regressive, infantile, omnipotent, and demanding object relations give the picture of a narcissistic or borderline personality. Accidents, lost jobs, troubles with the police, and failed marriages make for a sense of helplessness, hopelessness, guilt, and depression. With the chemical depression induced by the drug, one thinks of endogenous depression. All of these processes make alcoholic patients resemble each other and one sees the "alcoholic personality," the passive, dependent, inadequate personality, developing as alcoholism progresses.

The inability of these patients to control their impulse to drink baffles the professional as well as the layperson. As Mack (1981) points out, the ability to choose to act or not to act, to decide between alternatives, to direct and control one's life, is a highly valued function that is severely impaired in alcoholics. The inability to control whether one drinks is extremely frightening to alcoholics and is a major determinant in their low self-esteem. Drinking is accepted and welcomed in normal society, but at the same time there is the expectation that an individual can control and manage it. Uncontrolled drinking brings out fear and revulsion as well as strong disapproval in the rest of society. Sober people cannot understand why alcoholics continue to drink when it is obvious that the drinking is causing all manner of problems in their life. In this, the sober member of society, and perhaps the therapist, too, are reacting to their own fear of loss of control; and this fear on the public's part or on the therapist's part enhances the difficulty in dealing with the alcoholics' dilemma. It is even more alarming when alcoholics seem to show little concern for the consequences of their drinking, disregard the dangers involved, and maintain that they can be in control if they want to. Alcoholics use the defense mechanism of denial to escape from the recognition that they have lost control of their drinking and that they are powerless to abstain from this kind of instinctual gratification. Repeated loss of control, despair that they are powerless, fear of the loss of the pleasurable aspects of the alcoholic state should they stop, and shame at the results of their drinking all lead to an array of defenses, denials, magical thinking, and rationalizations that maintain the addiction while attempting to salvage some of the self-esteem that is lost when these patients realize what a mess they are in.

Alcoholism is set apart from neurotic disturbances in that ingestion of alcohol constitutes a direct gratification of a drive, not a compromise formation between a drive and the defense against it. Alcohol comes to serve as a love object for alcoholics. As they progress in the addiction, object cathexes are replaced by a narcissistic withdrawal and a concentration of libidinal energies on the artificial feeling of well-being and contentment derived from being intoxicated. Alcoholics' interests narrow until their main concern in life is maintaining an adequate supply of the drug, and in being able to continue to drink. Of course, this militates against forming any sort of workable transference relationship with the therapist.

These patients are left feeling hopeless and depressed at the realization that their drinking is out of control. At the same time alcohol continues, if only fleetingly, to give relief to anxiety and create a feeling of well-being — feelings that no longer can follow from relations with other human beings. These patients become afraid of how they would feel and what would happen to them if they did give up alcohol. They feel that there would be chaos and utter destruction. At the same time, amazingly, alcoholics continue to deny, rationalize, and minimize their drinking. And at this point, we professionals involved with alcoholic patients have to watch our step too, lest we deny the seriousness of the alcoholics' problem in the same way that they do themselves.

Most alcoholics come to therapy because they are depressed or anxious — they are having problems with their love life or their work, nothing seems to be going right in their lives, and they want help in getting a grip on things. Rarely do they come because of a drinking problem. They may say that they are drinking too much, but usually they see their drinking as a result of their other problems. They feel that alcohol allays their anxiety, gives them the occasion for social contact, and makes them feel better. They express varying degrees of uneasiness about their drinking. Often therapists go along with alcoholics' denial of the seriousness of their drinking. These patients are using alcohol as a defense against uncontrollable anxiety and a temporary escape from their conflicts. Therapists may feel that if they and their patients can attain some insight into current problems and what early experiences led the patients to react this way, the patients will no longer need to drink so much. Alcoholics are only too ready to go along with this. They don't want to give up drinking. Therapy can lull them into the feeling that something is being done about their problems and they need not worry too much about the destructive effects of their addiction. Often therapy goes on for two or three years with both patient and therapist expecting that in another six months or a year the patient will not need the alcohol so much. But it doesn't seem to happen. The patient may cut down, or even go for a period without drinking. Therapy moves slowly, if at all. Something is wrong with the treatment alliance. Although there seems to be insight into the need to drink, the patient may be getting into more trouble than he or she did at the beginning. Perhaps the patient gets hospitalized for physical problems. There may be automobile accidents or falls at home, perhaps even suicide attempts.

Some time ago a colleague from the Midwest told me of a patient who had made considerable progress in his five years of analysis but continued to drink heavily. He had insight into his drinking, which was understood as a means of coping with early deprivations and symbiotic needs. He resented his wife's demands on him for achievement, and her lack of support and warmth. The analyst refrained from pressuring the patient to relinquish the drinking; he felt the symptom would become unnecessary when the patient's anxieties diminished and he learned to cope better with his aggression. However, one night in December, the patient, angry at his wife, got drunk, went outdoors and fell into a pond. The wife found him, dragged him back home, and wrapped him in warm blankets, saving him from freezing to death. Although this man nearly died, he denied the seriousness of his drinking and continued to drink, all the time analyzing his need to drink. The therapist made the mistake of not giving top priority to the most dangerous symptom.

Things don't always go as they did in this patient's case. There may be only repeated quarrels at home or other interpersonal difficulties. A person may have trouble at work, or be a little erratic about keeping appointments, especially on Mondays. With all their difficulties, alcoholics do not necessarily lose their jobs. Very often they get to work on time and seem overconscientious on the job. But their work output declines, or rather contracts. Gradually they do less and less and take on fewer and fewer responsibilities. Often their supervisors unconsciously respond by assigning them less work, but they are unable to put their finger on what is happening to these employees. Finally, when patients start drinking on the job and become obviously intoxicated, it becomes impossible to miss, whereupon the individuals may lose their job, or be helped to get treatment.

For professionals, too, it is not always easy to make a diagnosis of alcoholism. If therapists have patients whom they suspect may be alcoholics, how should they proceed? How can one be sure of the diagnosis? Drinking is so much a part of the current social scene that the line between heavy social drinking and alcoholism is a fine one.

Some individuals can be heavy drinkers for long periods of time and not be true alcoholics in the sense that their drinking is out of control. When they say they can take it or leave it, it turns out to be true; they really can do so. If such people have to stop drinking, perhaps because of a physical illness, they are able to quit. This is not so for true alcoholics. Genuine alcoholics, even when threatened by serious illness that may be due to drinking, find themselves unable to quit for any length of time. Their powerlessness over their need to drink is severely demeaning to their self-esteem and sense of autonomy, so they resort to a strenuous use of denial to protect their feeling of self-worth and also continue to drink. Even though they may be able to quit for some time, sooner or later there will be a return to drinking. Memory lapses, or blackouts, are indicative of alcoholic drinking. The individuals report not remembering what happened the night before, either entirely or in patches. Perhaps the patients don't remember how they got from one place to another or how they got home. Often, promises are made but not kept because patients forget about making them.

Patients' denial of their inability to manage their drinking must be addressed by the therapists. Alcoholics' most serious impediment to recovery is their inability to admit that they are helpless in the face of their impulse to drink. It is important in diagnosis to notice whether patients repeatedly lose control of their drinking or whether there is marked denial. Do patients rationalize or externalize their drinking a great deal? Are untoward results minimized or even falsified or do patients avoid acknowledging their responsibility for them? It is important for therapists to comprehend the terror, confusion, and guilt that accompany alcoholic patients' perception of their loss of control and the humiliation connected with their inability to control the impulse to drink.

In discussion with patients it is wise for therapists to avoid questions such as: How much do you drink? or, Does your drinking interfere with your life? It is more useful to focus on alcoholics' own concerns about control, such as whether they have tried to limit their drinking in advance of an occasion where drinking will take place. That is, have they decided that this time they'll only have a certain number of drinks, or only one cocktail before dinner? Have they ever felt they should stop drinking for awhile? This avoids accusing patients and putting them on the defensive, and thus diminishes their need for denial.

One might try to make inroads on patients' denial by empathizing with their pain, but at the same time acknowledging and verbalizing the denial as such and as a defense. Therapists might then suggest that patients' problems may be caused in large part by drinking. Drinking can be identified as a disease in itself. This, in a sense, externalizes it, puts it outside the person's own self and thus may help the patient to be hopeful about coping with it; although it is a serious illness, it can be helped. If patients insist that drinking is not their main problem, one might suggest a procedure first formulated by Marty Mann (LeClair Bissell, personal communication). They should try to drink three measured drinks a day, no more and no less, for 90 days. It is important for patients neither to vary the amount of alcohol consumed nor to miss a day. If patients agree to give it a try, they usually find that it really is impossible to follow the instructions and they either must abstain completely or drink more than the agreed upon amount and get intoxicated beyond control. One might then be able to break through patients' denial and get them to acknowledge their helplessness over their drinking. Obviously, some volition remains, but it is more therapeutic to stress the lack of control than the remaining bits of control; an emphasis on the bits of control gives patients more cause to feel guilty and deepens their sense of failure. Here the concept of alcoholism as a disease rather than a moral failure or a weakness of the ego is very useful. Conceiving of alcoholism as a disease enables patients to preserve their self-esteem, to feel less guilty, and eventually to enter into an alliance with the therapist to deal with the drinking problem.

As was mentioned earlier, therapy for the active alcoholic cannot be based on the usual dynamic methods in which transference neurosis is encouraged. Treatment of transference in classical analytic practice involves mobilization of powerful wishes and affects that are not gratified. With alcoholics this leads to intolerable frustration and rage, which aggravate the drinking problem.

Therapists must note patients' difficulty in handling strong affects, and give ego support rather than interpretations at this point. Therapists can empathize with patients' difficulties, and also point out how drinking interferes with the ego's integrative and autonomous capacities, how it causes problems in relations with other people and lowers self-esteem. During this phase therapists can, as tactfully as possible, confront alcoholics with their denial, rationalization, and other defenses that prevent them from acknowledging their helplessness.

Alcoholics Anonymous can be of inestimable value to patients, and they should be encouraged to attend AA meetings. AA encourages replacing alcohol with the support of people, and it does this on a 24-hour basis, something impossible for therapy. In AA, people are available in a non-judgmental setting at the meetings, on a one-to-one basis in the practice of sponsorship, and in what AA calls "telephone therapy," in which members call each other during the day or night to lend support to each other. There are many helpful people involved rather than just one. This diminishes the risks of intense personal relationships and the danger of the strong transference affects that would emerge in classical dynamic therapy. If one person is not available for one reason or another, there are many others to take that person's place. Since all members of AA have been through the experience the patient is now going through, they can confront the patient with the denial, rationalization, magical thinking, and grandiosity without wounding the patient's self-esteem. AA provides objects, who are no longer drinking, for identification. The AA group as a whole can be internalized as a caring, nurturing, good object. In the end, AA enables alcoholics to abandon their narcissistic and maladaptive defensive positions for more object-related orientations. As alcoholics internalize the nonjudgmental, caring attitude of the group, they can overcome their own guilt feelings and low self-esteem, and in so doing abandon their need for alcohol.

When patients are newly sober, they remain for some time extremely vulnerable. It is difficult for them to deal with strong affects, and they have to relearn much adaptive behavior that they lost while they were drinking. It is wise for therapists to maintain an almost purely supportive role for the first year or so after alcoholics stop drinking. One should watch for what emerges in patients' ego structure. The personality may be quite intact in alcoholics after they stop drinking. Vaillant (1981) maintains that the apparently serious pathology often disappears when drinking is discontinued. Thus, it might become apparent that the ego weakness so prominent when a patient was drinking was a result of drinking rather than a cause of it. On the other hand, it also happens that people who have serious borderline, or even psychotic propensities can medicate themselves with drugs or alcohol and keep severe anxiety in the background. When these people become sober, the personality problems become visible and treatable. It is unreasonable to make a diagnosis in an active alcoholic because the drinking so strongly distorts the picture.

The therapist should avoid a competitive relationship with AA. Therapists complain that AA members advise new members to avoid psychotherapy. This is often true, and it is a real problem. But many members of AA who were in therapy during their drinking days remember years of therapy where nothing much was accomplished. They compare this with the dramatic improvement they see in 6 months or so of AA. It is logical for them to conclude that psychotherapy does not work. They are not aware that while they were drinking they were not giving psychotherapy a chance and could profit from it only minimally. Such patients often are happy to discover later, after they have been sober for a year or so, that they are able to use insights that they gained during their drinking days, even though they were unable to make use of them at the time.

In many cases alcoholics were diagnosed as depressed, anxious, or even psychotic, and were prescribed medication—Valium, Librium, or various antidepressants—that exacerbated their drinking problem by creating a secondary addiction to these drugs. The withdrawal, particularly from the minor tranquilizers, can be much more prolonged and painful than that from alcohol alone. If it did not happen to themselves, AA members often hear stories of its happening to other members, and they draw the conclusion that professionals are not to be trusted. When we recall Nicholas Cummings' contention that only 3.5 percent of the therapists of addicted patients are aware of the significance of the patients' drinking or drug taking we cannot blame the AA members too much. Maybe we have not been sufficiently aware of the implications of addictions in our practices.

REFERENCES

Bean, M.H. (1981). Denial and the psychological complications of alcoholism. In M.H. Bean and N.E. Zinberg (Eds.), *Dynamic approaches to the understanding and treatment of alcoholism,* 55–96. New York: Free Press, Macmillan Publishing Co.

Blum, E.M. (1981). Psychoanalytic views of alcoholism. *Quarterly Journal of Studies on Alcohol, 27,* 259–299.

Cummings, N.W. (1979). Turning bread into stone: A modern anti-miracle. *American Psychologist, 34,* 1119–1129.

Freud, S. (1911). *Psychoanalytic notes on an autobiographical account of a case of paranoia.* XII:9–82. London: Hogarth Press, 1964.

Freud, S. (1930). *Civilization and its discontents.* XXI:59–145. London: Hogarth Press, 1964.

Mack, J.E. (1981). Alcoholism, A.A. and the governance of the self. In M.H. Bean & N.E. Zinberg (Eds.), *Dynamic approaches to the understanding and treatment of alcoholism.* New York: Free Press, Macmillan Publishing Co.

Rado, S. (1933). Psychoanalysis of pharmacothymia. *Psychoanalytical Quarterly, 2,* 1–23.

Savitt, R.A. (1963). Psychoanalytic studies on addiction: Ego structure in narcotic addiction. *Psychoanalytical Quarterly, 32,* 43–57.

Vaillant, G.E. (1981). Dangers of psychotherapy in the treatment of alcoholism. In M.H. Bean & N.E. Zinberg (Eds.), *Dynamic approaches to the understanding and treatment of alcoholism.* New York: Free Press, Macmillan Publishing Co.

Yorke, C. (1970). A critical review of some psychoanalytic literature on drug addiction. *British Journal of Medicine and Psychology, 43,* 141–157.

C H A P T E R
83

FROM ADVERSARY TO ADVOCATE: COLLABORATION BETWEEN SCHOOL PERSONNEL AND THE PSYCHOTHERAPIST WHO WORKS WITH ADOLESCENTS

Thomas Edward Bratter, Ed.D.

EVOLUTION OF A ROLE

Shakespeare was correct when he wrote, almost 350 years ago, "In his time a man plays many roles."

I am a recovered adolescent academic failure who recently elected to create a residential therapeutic high school. I taught English at the Henry Abbott Vocational School in Danbury, Conn. For almost 10 years, I created and directed six community-based treatment programs in Westchester County that provided individual and group therapy for adolescents who engaged in self-destructive, drug-related behavior (Bratter & Hammerschlag, 1974; Bratter, 1973, 1972, 1971). In 1968, I served as a consultant to the White Plains public schools and helped write a reasonable and realistic drug policy. In 1969, I wrote the first proposal for an alternative school for the Scarsdale public school system which is still in existence. For 18 years, I (Bratter 1989A, 1981, 1980, 1973) maintained an independent practice in which I worked exclusively with alienated, angry, affluent adolescent substance abusers and their families. Periodically, I have been a part-time consultant to public schools. I have retired from my role of parent to school-aged adolescents as one of my children currently attends Columbia College, the other already graduated from there.

Four years ago, I discontinued independent practice to start The John Dewey Academy, which is a residential therapeutic high school (Bratter, 1987; Bratter, Bratter, & Radda, 1987). The academy offers a structured and supportive environment while providing intensive, individualized instruction (Bratter, Cameron, & Radda, 1989, Radda, 1988). Its objective is to place graduates in colleges of quality and, in so doing, to help erase permanently their bitter and painful records of mediocrity and failure.

I have been a casualty of the public school system (Bratter, 1977), a critic (Bratter, 1988, 1976), a consultant (Bratter, 1977; Collabolletta, Fossbender, & Bratter, 1983), and an advocate (Bratter, Fossbender, & Greenfield, 1985). I have been associated with schools as an adolescent consumer-failure, an employee, an outsider, and now as an insider who retains a proprietary vested interest (Bratter, 1989B).

Some of these roles have been contradictory. Similar in process is the evolution of a collaborative relationship with the school, which starts as an adversary, progresses to a double agent, and culminates as an advocate consultant. This chapter will detail these three phases and raise other issues pertinent to maintaining a harmonious relationship that benefits primarily the adolescent, and possibly the school or the psychotherapist.

THE SCHOOL: AN INVALUABLE CLINICAL RESOURCE

Second in importance only to family interactions, the total school expe-eience exerts a profound (positive or negative) effect on the adolescent's concept of self and future educational/vocational/social options. School performance becomes one of the most crucial diagnostic tools to assess the relative stability or the degree of pathology of the adolescent. Since the school plays such a central role in adolescent development, no effective treatment relationship can ignore what happens there academically and socially. The school is in a unique position to monitor the social network by providing invaluable information about individual attitudes and behavior.

Generally, adolescents spend most of their time particpating in school activities and forming social relationships with other students. Significantly, when adolescents are truant from class, often they go to the school and associate with classmates or former students. After hours, the school remains the center of social planning so adolescents congregate on or near the property. The school, moreover, has "custody" of adolescents for at least six hours a day, five days a week. Educators can furnish much clinical data based on individual performance in the classroom, social maturity (or immaturity), relationships with adult authority figures, and the like.

When the adolescent knows there will be ongoing communication between school personnel and the psychotherapist in independent practice, the opportunities for deliberate denial, distortion, and deceit are minimized. The sharing of information, furthermore, reduces the divisive "divide and conquer" manipulations so frequently associated with adolescents. Presenting a unified front can diminish the adolescent's need to test limits by acting out in a self-destructive manner, which places the student in a "no win/no exit" quagmire. When the psychotherapist knows there is a potential problem with a teacher, the issue can be examined and defused before the adolescent creates a crisis to which the school must react. Helping the individual to stabilize school performance is one of the priorities of psychotherapy with adolescents. Academic achievement, most assuredly, affects future educational and vocational opportunities, which determine the quality of life for the adult. Serving as a consultant-catalyst for the school to help the adolescent is a legitimate expenditure of therapeutic time and focus. Often the school can alert the psychotherapist to a potential problem as the adolescent may be unaware of the impact of his or her behavior.

THE PSYCHOTHERAPIST VERSUS THE SCHOOL: AN ADVERSARIAL RELATIONSHIP

It is important for both the psychotherapist and the school to recognize that the credentialed professional retains a primary allegiance to the adolescent, not to the educational institution. The converse is true for the educator who needs to consider the effect of the adolescent's behavior and subsequent decisions on policies designed for the management of the masses. The psychotherapist needs to understand the implicit and explicit constraints that affect decisions. Being able to appreciate the philosophical dilemma of the educator, in fact, may facilitate a positive resolution of the problem. Initially, there will be some inevitable tension because the psychotherapist seeks to redress an injustice, to stimulate change, or to request that an exception be made. The educator wants to maintain the status quo, seek security by citing a precedent, and be prepared to sacrifice one for the sake of the majority. It, thus, is incumbent on the psychotherapist to prove the validity of his or her request before the educator will accede. Simply stated, dynamically, the psychotherapist wants the answer to be "yes"; the educator, in contrast, is prepared to say "no!"

Complicating the situation is that most contact with the school by the psychotherapist occurs *ex post facto* when the institution already has reacted by punishing (disciplining) the offender. Frequently, a meeting has been convened when a number of school personnel — an administrator, a dean, the teacher — already have determined what they consider to be an appropriate outcome. The educational team members invariably will want to protect their colleague, who may feel insulted, hurt, angry, or unappreciated, or whose authority has been challenged. The school retains a vested interest in discouraging any further infraction for fear that anarchy will result.

The psychotherapist sincerely can mention that a goal of treatment is to help the adolescent exist harmoniously within the infrastructure to maximize further educational and professional options. Realistically, the adolescent must learn coping skills because the system, for the most part, will be resistant to change to accommodate idiosyncratic behavior. The psychotherapist needs to remember that it can be a profound learning experience for the adolescent to be "forced to endure" an incompetent teacher or one who is antagonistic because in the world of work not every supervisor or employer will be favorably inclined or sensitive to the individual. Rather than request or demand a transfer, perhaps more can be gained by helping the adolescent learn how to resolve a damaging or disastrous situation. The psychotherapist will need to assess carefully the probable gains and potential consequences. In any discussion with school personnel, the psychotherapist can communicate an appreciation and awareness of this realistic expectation — thus eliciting support from educators.

Rarely does any teacher encounter difficulty with only one student. While the school initially may appear defensive or deny, sometimes it will be conceded that the instructor inadvertently overreacted or is less than competent. The administration may wish to dismiss the educator. Obviously, when privy to this information the psychotherapist is in a position to negotiate a favorable settlement. *Quid pro quo* transactions can take place when the psychotherapist performs an invaluable service to the school that results in an advantageous outcome.

On the other hand, the student may clearly be at fault. Unless the student is prepared to show remorse — at the very least, to offer an apology — or to guarantee that "It will never happen again," the odds of achieving some sort of compromise are remote. The psychotherapist is advised not to offer to intervene because he or she can jeopardize future credibility. Before agreeing to contact the school, the therapist needs to achieve an understanding with the adolescent and to formulate a strategy for negotiating a solution.

The psychotherapist does retain significant leverage with the school, howeve,r The school views the therapist as having the expertise and power it lacks to control potentially disruptive and nonconforming students. The school would be most willing (and appreciative) to delegate the management of the student to the psychotherapist after receiving reassurances of the potential for and probability of a successful resolution. The psychotherapist needs to consider whether he or she wants to become so involved as to require continued contacts with school personnel, such as phoning, writing, and conferences.

EXTRAMURAL RELATIONSHIPS WITH THE SCHOOL

For any psychotherapist who works with adolescents, extramural contact with the school can be mutually beneficial. Obviously, any negotiation where one party functions as an advocate, personal contact certainly can influence the outcome positively. In a court of law, the attorney who personally knows the judge, in all probability, will be in a position to achieve a favorable disposition. Conversely, any attorney who needs to be an adversary candidly prefers not to know much about the personhood of the individual.

Any educator enjoys the opportunity, furthermore, to have a cordial and casual luncheon with any community resource. Educators like to discuss the pressure of their profession, and even their personal lives. Obviously, if the psychotherapist can clarify issues and provide helpful suggestions, the educator will remain grateful and favorably predisposed (I have declined administrator requests to treat school personnel because I wished to avoid any potential conflict of interest).

Before accepting any referral from the school, the psychotherapist needs not only to discuss the school's perception of the presenting problem(s) but also to articulate tentative treatment goals. Any potential for conflict and possible areas of collaboration can be discussed before meeting the adolescent. By making a referral to the psychotherapist, the school implicitly requests a favor — that is, to quell a potential problem. When placed in this position, before accepting the assignment, the psychotherapist can anticipate probable future concessions to facilitate resolution.

To enhance credibility and visibility, the psychotherapist can participate as a panel member at school functions or conduct workshops for teachers. In addition, the therapist can volunteer to serve on committees and, in so doing, interact with school personnel. All of these activities build a bond of mutuality that inspires cooperation and communication.

EXTENDING THE THERAPEUTIC ALLIANCE WITH ADOLESCENTS

Psychotherapy guarantees confidentiality. Having been sacrosanct, confidentiality needs to be redefined in view of the changing times and changing caseloads. There can be no justification for divulging the identity of any adolescent who acts responsibly and is productive.

In recent years, the stigma of seeing a psychotherapist has been minimized. In some communities, it is so common that it can be a status symbol to have "your own shrink." Adolescents often discuss their "shrink" and often quote, or misquote, the psychotherapist to suit their fancy. During its beginnings, psychotherapy was prescribed for individuals whose lives were stable, but who wanted to gain insight and understand themselves better. Now psychotherapy has been expanded to include people who engage in self-destructive, life-threatening acts or threaten the welfare and lives of others. The famous case of Tarasoff v. Regents of the University of California (1976) has modified the issue of confidentiality. There now exists a prima facie case for the "duty to warn." Recognizing the obligation of the psychotherapist to protect not only the individual being seen but also those who might be harmed, Bratter (1986) has written:

> Most professional organizations have explicit guidelines regarding confidentiality which state that this remains the purview of the individual in psycholotherapy. Yet when substance abusers engage in destructive and death endangering behavior, it remains countertherapeutic to enter into a conspiracy of silence because the individual so demands.

When the adolescent chooses to create a crisis by engaging in self-annihilative behavior, the psychotherapist needs to consider intervening, which, in extreme cases, might require informing others. While reviewing the impact of the Tarasoff decision, Kermani and Drob (1987) suggest that the individual needs to recognize there can be consequences to engaging in self-destructive behavior or threatening others. They believe the process of psychotherapy can be enhanced because:

> The trust that a patient has for his therapist not only involves a belief that the therapist will not breech his confidence, but also a faith that the therapist cares enough about him to take measures that will prevent the patient from causing serious harm to himself.... The therapist who reports a threat of murder, far from telling his patient that he cannot be trusted, is presenting a very different message, a message that he cares enough about his patient to set limits on his self-destructive behavior and demand that he act responsibly towrd the rights, and particularly the lives, of others.

Angry, alienated adolescents do not confess present or future self-destructive behavior because they feel discomfort or guilt. These adolescents disclose information because they recognize the potential for personal harm and want to be restrained. The psychotherapist who preserves confidentiality may encourage masochistic or saidstic acts by joining the conspiracy of silence. The psychotherapist who elects to work with self-destructive adolescents who have poor impulse control and are hedonistic to the point where they have little awareness about future consequences may need to expand the treatment team to sifnificant others who can help contain and control malignant behavior. It is not coincidental when friends and relatives contact the psychotherapist because often they know aobut the psychotherapist from the adolescent. There is no reason the psychotherapist needs to discourage these clandestine contacts, which can provide the necessary corroboration to gain perspective to help these adolescents stabilize and become more honest. The psychotherapist can listen and needs to say nothing other than to thank the caller for his or her interest. Any psychotherapist who adopts this pragmatic philosophical orientation can anticipate the inevitability of conferences with school personnel.

Before contacting the school, the psychotherapist can discuss candidly the rationale for doing so. The adolescent retains the prerogative to permit or prohibit collaboration if no emergency exists. It needs to be emphasized that there are only two legitimate reasons for the psychotherapist to contact the school. The first is the "duty to warn." The second is when the adolescent will benefit from collaboration. Mariner (1967) discusses the dual role of the psychotherapist, which has implications for those professionals who contact the school.

> If a therapist is guiding other agencies in their dealing with the patient, and in turn, is being guided by them. . .through the exchange of information and opinion, then he no longer has a therapeutic relationship with the patient in the usual sense. Indeed, it may be warranted for the psychotherapist to extend the treatment limits further

Awad (1983) assumes that it may be necessary to modify psychoanalytic techniques for antisocial adolescents and provides another justification for communicating with the school:

> Antisocial adolescents have the penchant to get into trouble and not talk about it. In addition, many parents, teachers. . .are troubled by the behavior of the adolescents and would like to discuss it with the therapist. Some therapists elect tohave no contacts with these people in order to protect the confidentiality and the transference. However, this attitude may provoke termination of therapy when these people get frustrated by the unavailability of the therapist. Instead, what seems to be more useful is to allow the important figures in the adolescent's life to have access to the therapist but on conditions that are clear to them and to the patient. Thus, it might be decided that the parents and/or significant adults could call the therapist if they are concerned. However, these calls are not confidential and every call will be discussed with the patient, even though sessions cannot be discussed with the parents. . . . Such contacts rarely affect the therapeutic relationship. In addition, they give the patient the message [that] every aspect of his life is a focus of therapy.

When the psychotherapist has some input, the professional can help the school devise a constructive strategy that may include reasonable consequences for continued disruptive and rebellious behavior. In so doing, the school can be converted into a catalyst for positive growth. The therapist retains more leverage and credibility than the parents to persuade the school to consider additional options. This kind of collaborative effort permits the psychotherapist to co-opt the school, which become a "sub rosa" adjunct to the treatment team. There can be a future serendipitous payoff. Acting-out, nonconforming, disrespectful, and disruptive adolescents permanently can antagonize individual teachers and administrators who, in turn, can affect adversely their colleagues' perceptions long after the annoying acts have ceased. Malicious gossip in the faculty room can result in unwarranted and prolonged reprisals. It is likely that the psychotherapist will be privy to this injustice and may be in a position to neutralize such acrimony by discreet discussions.

BEYOND THE DOUBLE AGENT ROLE: THE PSYCHOTHERAPIST AS ADVOCATE

Ironically, the psychotherapist initially serves as a liaison between two hostile parties — the adolescent and the school. Both remain suspicious because neither wants to change or acquiesce. As an incentive for the adolescent to change, the psychotherapist can pledge, "I'll negotiate on your behalf with the school and attempt to convince them to be less punitive and give you a final chance when you convince me you sincerely recognize the wrongness of your attitude and/or behavior." The preliminary communication with the school would be, "I promise to help persuade the adolescent not only to repent, but also to behave more reasonably from now on if a few concessions can be made."

The concept of protecting individuals from arbitrary and punitive administrative action is not new. The ombudsman, which originated in Sweden almost three centuries ago, provides the historical model for an impartial and independent person to investigate citizen complaints and subsequently to recommend solutions for resolving these conflicts and injustices. In 1809, as Rowat (1965) describes, the ombudsman was an officer of parliament who investigated the individual's allegations of unjust government treatment. If the ombudsman concluded that the complaint had merit, the official would propose corrective action. The ombudsman remained impotent, however, to implement any modification since the government legally was not forced to comply. More recently, perhaps as a reacton to the impotence of the ombudsman, binding arbitration has been introduced whereby both sides, when they reach an impasse, agree to abide by the resolution posed by acceptable third party. A judge often serves as the mediator who, in fact, legally is empowered to enforce compliance.

There is a realistic third model of conflict resolution that possesses the most significance for the psychotherapist in independent practice. Since in all likelihood the school would not view the psychotherapist as an ombudsman and surely will not relinquish its power, the concerned clinician can function as an advocate. The Joint Commission on the Mental Health of Children(1969) recognized the need for an advocate who can act on behalf of those who need services but are powerless to negotiate the bureaucratic labyrinth for themselves.

Advocacy is the unique relationship in which one party agrees not only to protect the interests of the other, but also to attempt to gain preferential consideration. At times, the advocate attempts to inluence a positive outcome to the detriment of another party (or parties). The dynamics of the advocacy relationship parallel those of the attorney and client, where the lawyer zealously guards and argues for the interests of the client. Bratter (1976–1977) describes an advocate as being "assertive and competitive. (S)he must be able to respond to a momentary defeat with a unique and more vigorous plan of action. . . . Periodically, the advocate must be prepared to challenge the system when (s)he believes there has been an injustice or discrimination. . . . The advocate, therefore, never remains neutral, but becomes a partisan who seeks preferential treatment."

LETTER WRITING: AN ESSENTIAL STRATEGY FOR THE ADVOCATE

Hallowitz (1974) lists some of the interventions that the psychotherapist-advocate can consider: telephone calls, correspondence, and direct meetings with personnel who command influence and power. The most potent weapon the psychotherapist possesses is writing letters and sending photocopies to appropriate significant others. When writing a letter, the psychotherapist can select the precise wording, knowing that it becomes a permanent record. School officials, like bureaucrats, can be influenced or intimidated by the written word because there is little opportunity to deny the contents. More often than not, bureaucrats will not respond in writing, which will weaken their case at a later time.

The psychotherapist can document progress persuasively by sending photocopies of letters of recommendation to appropriate school personnel. Any college recommendation at the very least ought to be sent to the school counselor. When sending the letter to college, it should be sent by certified mail/return receipt requested, so that the therapist knows the correspondence has been received. The psychotherapist presumably will write a more thoughtful and persuasive letter of recommendation than will the counselor, who not only will be overwhelmed by many requests to write similar letters, but also retains a primary allegiance to the school. Strategically, the therapist should write before the counselor does, as the counselor invariably will be influenced by the contents of the letter. Not infrequently, the counselor will confirm what the psychotherapist has written, which can have a most salutary impact on college admissions committees. If the psychotherapist enjoys a cordial relationship with a high-ranking administrator, it may be possible to enlist this support, which is prestigious and influential. Should the school administrator possess only second- or third-hand information about the student, it can be most effective for him or her to endorse and extol the virtues of the psychotherapist.

I had two objectives when I wrote the following letter. Primarily, I wanted to convince the college (not Sarah Lawrence, but one whose educational philosophy is compatible) to accept Lisa Brown (not her name), who is severely learning disabled. Second, I wanted to influence the letters of recommendations written by school personnel to validate my hypothesis. I recognized that this public school neither understood Lisa nor was informed about the unique educational philosophy and modus operandi of Sarah Lawrence College. I was fearful that this lack of comprehension would jeopardize my efforts to convince Sarah Lawrence College to admit this 18-year-old. This letter was sent to the director of admissions, Bob, whom I knew because I had recommended other students; the college president, with whom I coincidentally had lunched a month before; Lisa's high-school guidance counselor, who would write a letter; and each of her teachers, in an effort to "educate" them. I deliberately use the provocative word "love" in the first sentence to communicate to the reader that I am prepared to assume an aggressive advocate role for a special person. I also want to entice the reader to read this lengthy recommendation in its entirety.

> Let me start by stating that I love Lisa M. Brown. I have known this remarkable young woman for more than a year. I have come to trust, respect, and admire her. Lisa is a special person and we have a special relationship, which I am not sure exactly how to describe because it has the most idealized elements of so many dyads — i.e., father–daughter, older brother–younger sister, older friend–younger friend, mentor–student. My vested interest, Bob, in Lisa is different from any other adolescent with whom I ever had worked. In fact, I would like you to know that I give Lisa M. Brown the highest recommendation it is possible for me to write. Now all that remains is for me to convince you regarding the special circumstances that warrant her being given the opportunity to succeed at Sarah Lawrence College.
>
> Lisa has tremendous potential, Bob, because she has surmounted two tragedies that were beyond her control and probably even comprehension. The first problem was that suddenly, inexplicably, Lisa suffered from a rare illness that rearranged her brain waves, thus producing profound learnng disabilities. She was referred to Yale Psychiatric Institute for diagnosis but no definite cause or explanation has been found. At the time, Lisa was attending the Kent School, but was overwhelmed not so much by the work but by the time pressure. She studied to the point of exhaustion. Finally, school officials persuaded her family to withdraw her so she could attend public high school. Lisa has been in special classes for three years. Despite her profound learning disabilities, Lisa has remained highly motivated in her quest to complete the requirements for her diploma. Two years ago, Lisa's father died suddenly. Sadly, he was driving to school for a conference to discuss Lisa when he suffered a fatal heart attack. Lisa was dependent on her father who provided the nourishment and reinforcement that sustained her. Mr. Brown's death has created a void that never can be filled for Lisa. Her older brother, Len, is a superstar who is a gentleman, scholar, and athlete. Len currently attends Yale University on a full scholarship and continues to dazzle everyone. Given all of these factors, Bob, it is remarkable that Lisa still struggles to overcome her learning disabilities. The fact that Lisa is a sensitive, responsive, responsible, delightful, pleasant person is remarkable because it would be easy for anyone to become embittered by these tragedies and literally be consumed by so much self-pity; the individual would become depressed and quit. It is precisely because of this that I feel most comfortable writing that I find it possible to recommend Lisa for acceptance with absolute professional confidence.
>
> Lisa's learning disabilities are monumental. She took the untimed college board examination and spent almost seven and a half hours tortur-

ing herself. Her combined scores of less than 600 are so low as to invite an automatic rejection by any admissions committee that finds itself overwhelmed by applications of more academically qualified candidates. I did not cringe when Lisa tearfully reported her scores because I anticipated that they would not in any way reflect this young woman's intuition and special intelligence. What I did experience, however, was an intense and overwhelming anger regarding the injustice. I also experience an overwhelming sense of impotence because I knew there simply was nothing that I could do to rectify those scores that could produce such an insidious sense of failure and stupidity that encourages resignation to the point of terminating one's education. But not for Lisa. She continues to forge ahead, albeit painfully and slowly. Most assuredly, I urge you and the admissions committee to disregard the CEEB scores as legitimate indication of Lisa's ability to succeed. The college boards ignore the undisputable fact that Lisa subjected herself consciously to a senseless, brutally traumatic academic ordeal of tryng to decipher multiple choice questions knowing that there was but the remotest possibility of success. What kind of an individual willfully would engage in such behavior? A masochist would revel, of course, in such an inglorious way to punish himself or herself. Obviously, any sane observer would label this act as misguided and potentially awesomely self-destructive. The only rational alternative explanation is that there is dramatic prima facie evidence that the individual understands and values the need to become educated and is willing to pay the price to learn. I submit that Lisa M. Brown is such an individual who is incredibly motivated and wants to learn. Until this is understood, Lisa Brown remains enigmatic.

Lisa's situation can be best illustrated by recalling the Aesop fable about the race between the rabbit and the tortoise. Sarah Lawrence students are rabbits who possess quick, sharp wits. Lisa, of course, is the turtle. Lisa will win the "race" even though it will take her literally several times as long because she is disciplined and methodical. She knows herself academically and compensates for her learning disabilities by studying longer than anyone would dare to demand. Lisa often does not finish her studies until 2:00 a.m. Lisa will learn because she *wants* to learn. She is willing to pay the price of deferring gratification so that she can learn. Lisa will learn, Bob, because the so-called experts cannot assess or quantify the elements of motivation, of determination, and of courage.

Bob, I suggest that should Sarah Lawrence College take a different kind of risk, Lisa Brown will graduate. Lisa somehow will continue on to get a master's degree either in social work or education. Lisa will do so, Bob, because she possesses the consuming passion to learn and to achieve. Lisa has the maturity and the vision to see the light at the end of the tunnel and will continue to stumble forward. So what, Bob, if it takes her five or six years? I promise you she will be a most positive person in class and will inspire her fellow students to learn and make her professors feel good when they offer some encouragement. Lisa Brown will become living proof to so many parents of learning-disabled kids, showing it is possible to transcend deficiencies to succeed. Obviously, no one seriously will question why Lisa is taking longer than most. Hopefully, some will be motivated to give her a helping hand when they recognize that her will to learn is so fierce.

While it need not be stressed, I nevertheless wish to write that I recognize the fragility of this candidate's academic ego, which has been forced to endure many educational failures. Most assuredly, I do not wish to place this young woman in a "no win" educational situation. Yet when confronted with making a decision, I opt to place her in an environment where she will gain self-esteem and self-respect socially and hope that she will prevail academically. I am mindful of her learning disabilities and am fascinated why they have not discouraged Lisa, who remains optimistic and cheerful. I remain supremely confident that Lisa M. Brown will graduate from Sarah Lawrence College though she will take more than the prescribed four years. So what! Who really cares? This delightful young woman has paid her dues, and, therefore, has earned (and deserves) the chance to become a college graduate. I know there is a trade-off and together Lisa and I have decided that she is advised to attempt to succeed at Sarah Lawrence College rather than attending a specialized school for the learning disabled.

Lisa has read the candid and most realistic recommendations of her teachers. We have discussed this issue until we are all talked out. I guess what I am requesting, Bob, from Sarah Lawrence College, is that Lisa be given the chance to discover for herself whether she, indeed, can succeed. I know the temptation is great to write a compassionate letter saying, "Gee, Lisa, we like you but we think we know what is best for you!" Lisa no longer is a child. Lisa understands the potential for success and for failure. Lis wants to take the chance to see if she can continue to beat the odds and graduate from a competitively rigorous academic college rather than one that is not among the best. I certainly applaud her determination. I certainly hope I have convinced you and the admissions committee that, by virtue of her performance and determination, she has earned the right to prove to herself that she once again can and will succeed.

It has been a profound professional privilege for me to work with Lisa Brown. Rarely do professionals have the opportunity to be associated with decent individuals whom they love, trust, respect, and admire. Daily, Lisa struggles to surmount her incapacitating learning disabilities, but stubbornly refuses to submit. Lisa learns at her own rate and is a better, more sensitive person by virtue of her will to push herself and refusal to accept the limitations of her learning disability. Her diligence and discipline are remarkable. How can I help you understand the inordinate amount of courage and strength Lisa has developed to confront daily the painful reality that she simply does not learn as quickly as the other 99 percent who are college bound?

As both a psychologist and an educator, I have a dilemma to ascertain the most effective educational placement for Lisa. Clearly, she is academically incapacitated. Talking to Lisa, even the most sensitive and astute educator will not recognize she is learning disabled. Lisa has compensated for her learning disabilities by becoming an articulate, intuitive, positive person who gives absolutely no clue. I, therefore, favor Sarah Lawrence College where the students are "real" people rather than learning disabled. I sincerely believe that Sarah Lawrence College is the ideal environment because Lisa will be able to identify socially with the students and certainly has proved quite dramatically that she possesses an abundance of academic motivation to cope with the divisionals, etc. I like Sarah Lawrence College due to the small class structure where the emphasis is on interaction. I like Sarah Lawrence College because there are no formal tests that place an insurmountable burden on Lisa to the point where she simply cannot compete. Lisa will excel because she will seek out her professors and will do the required work. I believe that the human encouragement and admiration of her professors are more important to helping Lisa learn than a particular expertise in working with learning-disabled students. It is significant that Lisa is an adult and not an adolescent so she knows what she must do. Another crucial consideration is the fact that Sarah Lawrence College considers full-time attendance to include taking three courses rather than the more traditional five at other colleges. There is absolutely no reason why Lisa cannot elect to major in dance, drama, or photography and, thus, reduce a little more the academic load. Given all these unique assets, I honestly am excited about Sarah Lawrence College truly being the ideal learning environment for Lisa. Again, I repeat, for emphasis, that Lisa needs to interact with students, not with learning-disabled people. She made her decision several years ago and I applaud it. Undeniably, Lisa will be forced to devote many more hours than anyone else to learning. Lisa understands this and is prepared to make the necessary investment and sacrifice. In no way will the academic demands diminish the probability of her contributing positively to the quality of campus life. Lisa is a positive person who is responsible, respectful, and straight. Her determination will inspire others. I believe she will become a campus leader in the most idealistic sense of the concept.

The president of Sarah Lawrence College has mentioned that infrequently a student at risk will be admitted. Lisa is a risky student in a very special sense. I submit that since I have the unique advantage of knowing both the candidate and Sarah Lawrence College, my recommendation should be read and reread knowing that I write with the purest of motives in that I have the welfare of my young friend, Lisa, and that of Sarah Lawrence College as the motivating forces compelling me to write this admittedly aggressive letter of endorsement. I am not suggesting that the college ought to be humanistic to give Lisa the option to determine her educational future. I believe she has earned this right.

In conclusion, I hope it is clear that I believe that Lisa M. Brown ought to be admitted as a special student. I write with absolute conviction that if Lisa is permitted to progress at her own pace, I am prepared to stake my professional reputation that she will graduate from Sarah Lawrence College. So, for me, knowing both the candidate and the college, I see no risk whatsoever.

Thanking you and the admissions committee in advance for your faith in my judgment and anticipated cooperation...

When writing a letter of recommendation, the therapist can pursue one of two divergent strategies — to ignore or to confront the deficiency. In Lisa's case, I decided that her learning disability could not be concealed and thought it best to be direct and honest. By placing Lisa's problem in perspective, I thought I could aggressively function as an advocate since the reader understood I appreciated the magnitude of the incapacitating disability. Any recommendation, if it is to be credible, needs to discuss the applicant's strengths and weaknesses because dwelling on assets or liabilities implicitly conveys a message to any thoughtful reader.

Once the adolescent leaves the school with which the psychotherapist has worked, there is an opportunity for a continued therapeutic alliance.

AFTER MAKING THE REFERRAL

There is no geographical cure for either the adolescent or the family. Presumably, the student will continue to receive therapeutic support while attending a residential school. The treatment relationship established may be held in abeyance until the adolescent returns. The psychotherapist can continue communication by agreeing to see the student when he or she returns for weekend visits, vacations, and permanently (Bratter, 1981). To augment office visits, both parties can talk on the telephone weekly or correspond. When the adolescent returns home, the psychotherapist can conduct sessions to improve channels of communication among family members. In addition, the psychotherapist needs to help the adolescent terminate associations with those persons who still engage in self-destructive behavior, while concurrently assisting in the formation of more positive peer associations. It is not unusual for the returning adolescent to feel lonely and isolated since many have rejected him or her on the basis of previous acts or reputation.

The family, in contrast, is neglected and may stagnate in a myriad of unresolved feelings and dysfunctional communications. Often the family naively assumes that, with the removal of the son or daughter who is the identified patient, their problems magically will self-correct. There is a tendency for the family to minimize the intensity of pain, distrust, and anger created by the adolescent, who has defied limits, been deceitful, manipulated one member against another, or hidden behind the enabler. Shifting intrafamily alliances, furthermore, have damaged the constellation when one adopts a self-righteous (victim) posture while blaming others for exacerbating the adolescent's noxious or self-destructive performance. The family may have ceased to function as a cohesive unit. Communication patterns among family members, as Kolodny, Kolodny, and Bratter (1984) have written, can be characterized by acrimony, resentment, and mistrust.

The psychotherapist who has been a treatment agent for the adolescent might consider renegotiating a therapeutic contract with the family in an attempt to repair the damage and to restore stability for the eventual return from prep school. The family will appreciate the urgency of several sessions to ensure a harmonious reunion. The family may need not only to relate to, but also to resolve, a multitude of issues. Depending on the severity of pathology, the psychotherapist might be able to help the family:

1. Resolve feelings of separation trauma, hurt, impotence, guilt, and rage.
2. Recognize its complicity concerning the son's or daughter's malignant acting out.
3. Understand what caused the problem and what needs to be changed.
4. Correct dysfunctional communication patterns.
5. Strengthen the unit by eliminating contradictory and competitive contracts in order to facilitate the return of the prodigal son or daughter.

CONCLUSION:
THE BEGINNING, NOT THE END

The issue of confidentiality for adolescents needs not only to be revised, but also to define explicit therapeutic parameters. Sobel (1984) contends, "The limits of confidentiality need to be clearly defined. . . including what and how information if any will be released to their parents and other parties. . . . The issues of dangerousness and duty to warn are sensitive ones in any psychotherapeutic practice." The psychotherapist needs to consider innovative and humanistic ways to extend the treatment alliance and how to relate to school personnel in order to protect and promote the interests of the adolescent.

No longer does it appear to be in the adolescent's best interest for the psychotherapist to safeguard anonymity—and hence to avoid extramural contact with the school. To their credit, social workers recognized and reaped the benefits of collaboration with the school before their psychological and psychiatric colleagues did. Helping the adolescent learn to use his or her energy creatively, rather than being defiant and disruptive, obviously maximizes chances of future success.

This chapter, admittedly only preliminary, urges the psychotherapist and the school to explore ways that coordinative, but selective, collaboration can be applied constructively to help adolescents actualize their academic abilities. Benjamin Franklin was correct when he wrote more than 200 years ago, "United we stand, divided we fall." So it is with the adolescent in psychotherapy. Confidentiality needs to be redefined so that there can be collaboration with the schools to the benefit of the adolescent.

REFERENCES

Awad, G.A. (1983). The middle phase of psychotherapy with antisocial adolescents. *American Journal of Psychology, 37,* 193-194.

Bratter, T.E. (1989a). Group psychotherapy with alcoholically and drug addicted adolescents: Special clinical concerns and challenges. In F. Azima & L. Richmond (Eds.), *The Group Therapies for Adolescents.* New York: International Universities Press.

Bratter, T.E. (1989b). Uses and abuses of power: A view from the top. Residential Treatment for Children & Youth. 7:3. (In press)

Bratter, T.E., Cameron, A. & Radda, H.T. (1989). "Mentoring: Extending the psychotherapeutic and pedagogical relationship with adolescents. *Journal of Reality Therapy,* VIII:2, pp. 3-13.

Bratter, T.E. (1988). "The deplorable state of education in the 1980's: The need for radical educational reform." *Journal of Reality Therapy,* VIII:1, pp. 33-41.

Bratter, T.E. (1987). To be moral or not to be moral: The crucial educational imperative of the 21st century. In L. Bremberg (Ed.), *Proceedings of the Tenth World Conference of Therapeutic Communities.*

Bratter, T.E. (1985). Special clinical psychotherapeutic concerns for alcoholic and drug-addicted individuals. In T.E. Bratter & G.F. Forrest (Eds.), *Alcoholism and substance abuse: Strategies for clinical intervention,* 523-576. New York: Free Press.

Bratter, T.E. (1981a). Some pre-treatment group psychotherapy considerations with alcoholic and drug-addicted individuals. *Psychotherapy: Theory Research & Practice,* 18: 508-515.

Bratter, T.E. (1981b). After referring the addicted individual to a therapeutic community. In G. Loiselle (Ed.), *The therapeutic community in various cultures worldwide: Proceedings of the Sixth World Conference of Therapeutic Communities.* Manila, Philippines: Drug Abuse Research Foundation.

Bratter, T.E. (1986a). Negotiating the therapeutic alliance with unmotivated, self-destructive adolescent substance abusers in independent practice: Some pretreatment issues. In R. Faukinberry (Ed.), *Drugs: Problems in the 70's, solutions for the 80's.* Lafayette, LA: Endac Enterprises.

Bratter, T.E. (1986b). Educating the uneducable: The little "ole" red schoolhouse with bars in the concrete jungle. *Journal of Offender Counsel, Services and Rehabilitation, 4,* 95-108.

Bratter, T.E. (1979). The psychotherapist as a twelfth-step worker in the treatment of alcoholism. *Family and Community Health: Journal of Health Promotion and Maintenance, 2,* 31-58.

Bratter, T.E. (1977a). A letter to my children: Counsel on avoiding drug dependency in your teens. *Youth Magazine, 28,* 42-55.

Bratter, T.E. (1977b). From discipline to responsibility training: A humanistic orientation for the school. *Psychology in the Schools, 14,* 45-54.

Bratter, T.E. (1976-1977). The psychotherapist as advocate: Extending the therapeutic alliance with adolescents. *Journal of Contemporary Psychology, 9,* 119-126.

Bratter, T.E. (1976). The three "r's" of relevant educational reform: Responsibility, respect, reality. In A. Bassin, T.E. Bratter, & R.L. Rachin (Eds.), *The Reality Therapy Reader.* New York: Harper & Row.

Bratter, T.E. (1973b). Treating alienated, unmotivated, drug abusing adolescents. *American Journal of Psychology, 27,* 585-598.

Bratter, T.E. (1973b). Advocate, activist, agitator: New roles for drug abuse administrators. *Journal of Drug Issues, 4,* 144-154.

Bratter, T.E. (1972). Group therapy with affluent, alienated adolescent substance abusers. *Psychology: Theory, Research, and Practice, 9,* 308-313.

Bratter, T.E. (1983). Interaction groups. *Journal of Drug Issues, 1,* 17-32.

Bratter, T.E., Bratter, B.I., & Radda, H.T. (1986a). The John Dewey Academy: A residential therapeutic high school. *Journal of Substance Abuse Treatment, 3,* 53-58.

Bratter, T.E., Bratter, E.P., & Radda, H.T. (1986b). The evolution of the responsible role model. In A. Acampora & Nebelkov (Eds.), *Bridging Services: Proceedings of the Ninth World Conference of Therapeutic Communities.* San Francisco: Abacus.

Bratter, T.E., & Greenfield, L.J. (1985). Toward a theory of realistic, relevant, pragmatic education: Challenges and concerns for the 1980's and 1990's. In *Proceedings of the Eighth Conference of Therapeutic Communities.* Rome: Il Centro Press.

Bratter, T.E., & Hammerschlag, C.A. (1975). Advocate, activist, agitator: The drug program administrator as a revolutionary-reformer. In *Drug abuse control: Administration and policies.* Lexington, MA: D.C. Heath.

Collaboletta, E.A., Fossbender, A.J., & Bratter, T.E. (1983). The role of the teacher with substance-abusing adolescents in secondary schools. *Psychology in the Schools, 20,* 450-455.

Hallowitz, D. (1974). Advocacy in the context of treatment. *Social Casework, 55,* 416-420.

Joint Commission on the Mental Health of Children (1969). *Crisis in child mental health: Challenge for the 19870's.* New York: Harper & Row.

Kermani, E.J., & Drob, S.L. (1987). Tarasoff decision: A decade later dilemma still faces psychotherapists. *American Journal of Psychology, 41,* 282.

Kolodny, R.C., Kolodny, N., & Bratter, T.E. (1984). *How to survive your adolescent's adolescence.* Boston: Little Brown.

Mariner, A. (1967). The problem of therapeutic privacy. *Psychiatry, 60,* 66-72.

Radda, H.T. (1988). Extending the therapeutic alliance: Mentoring. *Journal of Reality Therapy,* VIII:1, pp. 45-51.

Rowat, D.C. (1965). *The ombudsman: Citizen's defender.* London: Allen and Unwin, p. 7.

Sobel, S.B. (1984). Independent practice in child and adolescent psychotherapy in small communities: Personnel, professional and ethical issues. *Psychology, Theology, Research & Practice, 21,* 112-118.

Tarasoff v. Regents of University of California. (1974). 13 Cal. 3d. 177, 529 P. 2d 533, 18 Cal. Rptr. 129.

Tarasoff v. Regents of University of California. (1976). 17 Cal. 3d. 425, 551 P. 2d 334, 131 Cal. Rptr. 14.

C H A P T E R
84

GROUP THERAPY FOR SINGLES AS AN ADJUNCT TO INDIVIDUAL THERAPY

Malka Sternberg, Ed.D., M.A., M.S.W., C.S.W.

A s the number of single people grows larger in proportion to the general population with each passing year, there is an increasing need for therapy to deal with their unique problems and concerns. It is our intention to investigate here the viability of group therapy as an adjunct to individual therapy in coping with the needs of singles. To make such a judgment, we must first look into the kinds of problems faced by contemporary singles, whom we will define as post-college-age single people who are widowed, divorced, separated, or never married.

One of the problems singles have today, of course, is that of meeting other singles and having a sense of belonging and intimacy. In a society that has been drained of many of its traditional, institutionalized means for single people to meet each other, it's conceivable that some people come into group therapy not only for psychological assistance but also, perhaps, or even primarily in some cases, for the purpose of finding compatible partners of the opposite sex. For these people, the proliferation of singles bars and discotheques has not filled that need — such places are too impersonal, their "meat market" aspect is humiliating, and the cast of characters changes constantly so that there is no way to connect with another person closely on an ongoing basis.

However, we are not concerned here with the effectiveness of group therapy as a socially sanctioned way for singles to search for a mate, but rather with its performance as a means of support and treatment of the psychological problems of single persons, acknowledging that these psychological problems may be related to that very inability to find people to build a relationship with.

PROBLEMS OF SINGLES

Loneliness

Generic to single people, it goes without saying, is loneliness. This doesn't mean that people who are married or living with lovers do not experience intense loneliness — but there is greater probability that singles will have this as an ongoing problem.

The lack of someone on a continual basis with whom to share the triumphs and disappointments of daily living, to exchange thoughts and feelings, and to give to and receive physical and emotional nurturing from — these and many other deprivations of loneliness are particularly germane to the lives of the isolated single. There is loneliness, and there is loneliness, it must be noted. There are single people who live with their children or parents or roommates who feel a tremendous lack of intimacy with another human being but who receive companionship to some degree from the people they share living space with. They would define themselves as seriously lonely, perhaps. But, then, there are those who live all alone. The depths of their loneliness, it can be assumed, are enormous. One West Side gentleman stated it poignantly when he commented, "It's so hard to accept that you'll never hear a key turn in the lock."

For single people, therefore, therapy of any kind must be extremely significant in helping assuage loneliness in that, whether group therapy or individual therapy, it provides a regular and dependable set or sets of ears in which to pour one's confidences, one's innermost feelings. The question we will be addressing here, however, has to do more with the ability of group therapy to help people cope with their loneliness than to alleviate it. We will attempt to analyze that issue later after reviewing more of the characteristic problems of the single.

Mourning

Lawrence Shulman (1985) points to other issues especially relevant to singles, like mourning, feelings of rejection, and lack of empathy from friends and family who do not perceive the nature of problems peculiar to or more prevalent among single persons.

The first of these, mourning, is certainly indigenous to single people. These people are single by default, so to speak, as the result of having lost a significant person to whom they had a strong attachment. The grief experienced by widows and widowers is very acute, and if they do not receive appropriate support of some type, it can be incapacitating. According to Lindeman and Caplan (1965), grief is a definite syndrome with combats and psychological symptomatology. The most striking characteristics are weeping, tendency to sighing, complaints about lack of strength, physical exhaustion, digestive disturbances, a sense of unreality, and detachment. The bereaved person is restless, has a short concentration span, and has low energy levels. Depression and insomnia are symptoms of grief.

The intense reactions of grief to the death of a spouse are exemplified in a group of widows the author studied for a doctoral dissertation, "The Long-Term Adaptation of Young and Middle Aged Widows to the Loss of a Spouse" (Sternberg, 1982). One of the women, a Holocaust survivor now living in Israel, in describing her grief stated, "My husband's death was a nightmare. It was a return to the isolation and to the feelings of aloneness in an alien world that I haven't experienced since I was in the concentration camps."

Lynn Caine, author of the best-seller *Widow,* eloquently details her emotions during the early phase of mourning in her follow-up book, *Lifelines*: "I had been transported to hell. My grief was a raw wound that would not heal. But grief was only part of it. I was desperately frightened and confused, panicky, angry, lost" (Caine, 1977, p. 11).

Widowers, too, feel much of the same emotional devastation, but also experience different sorts of distresses than do the women. For instance, widowers, unlike widows, who very often gain new status through taking jobs and participating in the community for the first time, feel a loss of status through the sudden necessity to take care of the children and the home in addition to continuing in their roles as providers.

Further, unlike widows, they are not conditioned to spending holidays and vacations with people of their same sex, nor are they often sufficiently liberated enough to travel with members of the opposite sex. Thus, they have fewer options for assuaging the extreme loneliness they experience in the wake of their wives' passing.

Rejection

Here we are dealing with a human emotion felt by all of us whatever our marital status, age, or living situation. But, in the case of singles, it can be speculated that it occurs more frequently and relentlessly. And being "dumped" as opposed to being widowed, be it through divorce, or "breaking up" a nonmarital relationship, has its own particular agony. A person who is rejected by another person not only must deal with the loss of the companion but also must confront the concomitant emotions of unworthiness and shame.

The experience of rejection, particularly if it is a repeated phenomenon, gives rise to other, more subtle problems for single people. They must confront the question of their own culpability in evoking rejection. They must try to face up to any subconscious compulsions to bring about these painful situations. Is there a hidden agenda, a destructive pattern, that is operating in their relationships? These are the kinds of dilemmas faced by single people in our society that urgently need attention.

Lack Of Empathy From Family And Friends

The feeling that family and friends do not really understand what a single person experiencing any of the aforementioned difficulties goes through and that consequently the single person cannot get sufficient support from them was articulated over and over by the women studied by the author in her Ed.D. dissertation on widows. Many of them spoke bitterly about not being able to talk to their family and their puzzlement at the insensitivity of close family members to the pain they were enduring. They spoke also of their great disappointment in their friends, their feelings of loss of support and being misunderstood, and their subsequent efforts to form new friendships with other single women.

Single Parenting

E. E. LeMasters (1974) in his article "Parents Without Partners" discusses the growing numbers of single parents and the disproportionate number of these families falling within the so-called poverty group. This deprivation is endured particularly among single women inasmuch as they are the bulk of parents without partners who have custody of the children.

In addition to the financial stress besetting single parents, there are many other kinds of woes attendant upon raising children alone. LeMasters' descriptions of the problems of single mothers is further confirmed by a study in a Canadian journal (Gulpan). Sixty-seven single-parent families were interviewed. These families were found to be economically disadvantaged and to go through a period of emotional disarray. LeMasters (1974) refers to the anguish felt by divorced fathers — for example, in the aftermath of divorce. Single fathers do not always suffer from the separation from their children; occasionally they are the parents who have gotten custody of the children. Greff (1985) has indicated that these fathers have particular difficulty in balancing the demands of work and child rearing and difficulty in adjusting to being single again and establishing a social life. They evince considerable anxiety in dealing with the legal system around issues of custody and support of the ex-wife.

Unmarried mothers have a whole range of problems that need not be delineated here, but not the least of them is that they are likely to be on public welfare and suffer a collateral lack of status. This stigma and the lack of regard for single parents are further confirmed by a study done of 82 elementary school children and their single parents (Epstein, 1984). The single parents indicated that they felt less listened to and less accepted by teachers and school administrators than were married parents of school children.

Not only do parents without partners already have an unusually heavy burden of stresses and responsibilities to cope with, but the writer has observed a new psychosocial phenomenon coming to light in the 1980s as the children of the liberated women of the 1960s grow up and leave the nest. These mothers, who may have spent a major portion of their child-rearing years as divorced, separated, or even never-married women, are finding now that it is particularly traumatic when the kids leave because they have depended upon their children emotionally and socially far more than they would have if they'd had mates to relate to. This lamentable situation adds yet another wrinkle to the host of singles' troubles requiring, in many cases, therapeutic intervention.

These, then, are some of the problems endemic to the contemporary singles population. Next we will attempt to see if group therapy has something to offer them in addition to what they can gain from individual psychotherapy.

GROUP THERAPY— HELPFUL TO SINGLES?

There are, broadly, two categories of group therapy available to the public today: therapist-administered and self-help models. It is our contention that either one is a valuable adjunct to private psychotherapy for singles. Because of the litany of problems single persons confront, it seems apparent to this writer that they have a greater need than others for a group structure within which to work through their problems.

To some extent, this conjecture was arrived at partly on the basis of Bennis Warren's (1983) theories about the general advisability of combining therapist-run groups with individual therapy. It is Warren's belief that since human beings are born into and function within groups inevitably throughout life, group therapy can only enhance private counseling in that it provides a controlled setting in which to further work through insights and deal with problems of interpersonal relationships that are worked on in individual treatment.

In support of his conclusion, Warren (1983) states:

> Another therapeutic advantage of combined group and individual psychotherapy lies in the potential for simultaneous, complementary therapeutic work at different levels of experience. Individual therapy provided the opportunity for an intensive dyadic relationship in which the patient could re-experience and work through developmental conflicts and failures of the early mother-child relationship. Group therapy provided the opportunity for consolidation and integration of the achievements of individual work in a safe, consistent environment where defenses were confronted in action and new object relationships tested and established. (p. 25)

It would seem that this would be no less true for single persons, and in all probability even more valid, inasmuch as it is supposed that singles have less access to settings in which to explore their capacity to achieve intimacy with others and generally to interrelate utilizing the insights they have gleaned from their private sessions.

For the therapist, also, much can be gained from observing the patient in a systems model encompassing group dynamics. Significant aspects of the patient's personality and functioning mechanisms are revealed that otherwise might not surface within the medical model of therapist vis-à-vis solitary patient.

SELF-HELP GROUPS

And what about the burgeoning trend toward self-help groups, which do not have a therapist supervising or even participating in the sessions? The groups for overeaters, Parents Without Partners, the AA-modeled groups for smokers and others, and all the other diverse peer-operated groups? These groups, also, have a definite value for single people as an adjunct to individual psychotherapy despite the fact that a therapist is not involved and can neither structure the treatment nor observe the patient. Kaplan describes these groups as members helping each other through providing information and constructive action, a resocialization process, and a temporary community, as well as through sharing common experience in giving each other mutual help and support. Singles have often been misunderstood and have been stigmatized — especially women who are alone. In this respect, the groups serve the purpose of raising self-esteem through the support and recognition provided by others in self-help and peer-support groups. The group members through sharing and suggesting help each other find new ways of dealing with living alone and provide a sustaining community. In this regard, it is interesting and important to highlight the distinct differences between traditional one-to-one psychotherapy and self-help support groups, and thereby hypothesize on the virtues of participation in such nonorthodox groups as a supplement to private therapy.

A comprehensive comparison of the two methods has been developed by Durkin (1968) citing 20 significant dissimilarities, among them the fact that a private therapist is not a role model and does not set personal examples, whereas in the group peers are role models and must set examples for each other; the fact that a personal therapist is often noncritical, nonjudgmental, and neutral and listens, whereas peers within the group are active, judgmental, supportive, and critical and talk as well as listen; and the fact that patients expect only to receive support in private analysis, whereas they must also give it within the self-help group situation.

HOMOGENEOUS OR HETEROGENEOUS GROUPS FOR SINGLES?

In the structuring of groups for single people, consideration has to be given to the question of whether they should be homogeneous or heterogeneous groups. There is disagreement in the field on this question, but the treatment of preference tends to be a homogeneous group (Yalom, 1975). Just as singles have, in all probability, a greater need than others for the kind of support offered in groups, so, accordingly, does it seem to work better for them if the groups are issue oriented toward their specific concerns, or at least limited to singles, which automatically narrows the focus to issues of mutual concern. These include, partly described already in these pages, (1) redefining their roles in a society that, even in a liberated age theoretically accepting singleness as a viable life-style, still discriminates against them in many overt and covert ways, (2) dealing with changes in status following divorce or death of spouse, (3) dealing with rejection in relationships, (4) similarly, coping with the transitory nature of relationships among today's singles, and (5) facing and overcoming one's own inability to sustain relationships, and one's own acts of rejection toward others. In a homogeneous group therapy situation, these issues can be concentrated upon, and a high degree of valuable support can be engendered beyond that emerging from a heterogeneous therapeutic structure (Yalom, 1975).

In the author's study on widows, this concensus that homogeneous groups are more helpful than heterogeneous ones was reinforced. One of the common themes in all the interviews of these widows was a feeling of difference from other single women — divorced or never married. While the interviewer was aware of great similarities between these widows and many of the divorced people she had talked to, in terms of their fears at being on their own, the sense of loss, the loneliness, all of the widows studied tended to emphasize their differences and their need to be with somebody who understood some of the differences.

OPINIONS OF GROUP THERAPISTS

Overall Positive Advantages

To help us judge the merits of the view that group therapy for singles as an adjunct to individual psychotherapy has distinct advantages, we did in-depth interviews with therapists who both see individual patients and conduct groups for single people.[1]

They were unanimous in their feeling that group therapy has definite value for single people as an adjunct treatment to one-on-one therapy. They expressed this belief with particular reference to the value of the group in alleviating the loneliness of single individuals, in providing a safe environment in which to air their true feelings, and in providing a space where unmarried people can get support and feedback that they don't obtain from the outside world.

As one therapist put it, "If I have them in individual therapy, they only get feedback from me. In the group, they have a lot of feedback from a lot of other people...that's extremely important! Other people may perceive situations differently from how I perceive situations. If you have 10 people who give you feedback, you can get 10 different viewpoints, which is all the more helpful."

She felt this kind of feedback was valuable to members of the group not only in terms of learning more about their behavior as perceived by others but also in very practical terms of providing suggestions on how to cope with particular situations. "A woman just lost her husband. Many alternatives on how to cope are presented by the group which she wouldn't have had if she'd seen only me."

Another therapist drew a similar conclusion. In discussing the usefulness of self-help groups, she stated, "You can learn other strategies. You can learn other coping mechanisms, learn other alternatives. You begin to see how other people feel about something, and you begin to say, 'Hey, that's another way of looking at something.'"

The particular worth of group feedback for singles, however, judging from the overall consensus of the therapists interviewed, seems to be its feasibility in providing a way for people to see themselves as others see them, and thereby to gain insight into the psychodynamics compelling their behavior. The value of this sort of mirror reflection of the self by members of the group is illustrated in a case cited by one of the therapists interviewed by the author.

She described a young woman, a nurse, who was unaware when she first came into the group that she projected an extreme amount of aggressiveness. She complained of problems with her coworkers, with patients and doctors, as well as a general inability to relate to people in her personal life. She got feedback from the group indicating that she was behaving in an unacceptably aggressive way, and after absorbing the feedback, and after the employment of some therapeutic techniques within the group such as role-playing, she gradually began to change her behavior. There was a tremendous improve-

---

[1]We interviewed group leaders who work with singles groups in the New York area, among them, Jeannette Haines, Lois Ackner, Bella Schaehfeld, and Elaine Rosen.

ment in her outside relationships, according to her therapist.

Another very favorable aspect of group therapy pointed out by the interviewed therapists was the kind of honest and open communication that exists. This is especially significant for singles, inasmuch as they lack a network of family support figures with whom they can intimately expose their deepest feelings and, at the same time, receive input, generally, on how their behavior affects others. All therapists with whom the author discussed this issue agreed that the degree and quality of this honesty and openness within the environment of group therapy is significantly greater than that achievable with people in the outside world.

In the group, people feel free to talk about their deepest feelings with respect to themselves, and people also feel free to express their honest reactions to others. With this kind of truthfulness, people can grow—not only in the sense of being able to confront themselves openly but also from the perspective of gradually seeing how they actually affect others.

People in groups also find a significant amount of supportiveness, which they don't often encounter among their family and friends. This is an outgrowth of the open quality of the group. People know they are accepted for the people they *truly* are, and this, of course, provides a genuine acceptance. But people in groups also receive a kind of nurturing, caring acceptance that they don't acquire in their ordinary lives.

Specifically, for instance, a therapist spoke of a divorced woman in her group whose family was very opposed to the divorce. The young woman had a lot of difficulty with the fact that her family would not accept her situation, but "in the group she's fully accepted and she finds a lot of understanding." Over and over, the therapists emphasized the importance of the kind of candor and veracity occurring in their groups. "In the outside world, people are more reluctant to be that open about their feelings, and in the group it's a much, much more accepting climate. The whole environment is much more conducive to openly discussing issues."

An additional favorable quality of group therapy for single individuals stressed by the group of interviewed therapists is the fulfillment of the need to know that one is not alone, that one is not unique or strange in the kinds of feelings and reactions one sustains in relationship to whatever crisis one is undergoing. For instance, one therapist outlined the case of a woman who had lost her husband 18 months before she entered the group. She was still in a state of mourning and grief and found that people in her regular life felt she was behaving inappropriately and should be fully functioning by this time. In the group, she encountered two other women who had lost their spouses. These women identified with her strongly and ressured her that her feelings were acceptable and normal, that they too still felt their losses keenly. This kind of group reinforcement is particularly important for single people, who are so often deprived of intimate communication with a concerned and supportive partner.

One of the therapists with whom the author consulted for this article suggested another positive element of group therapy in support of the basic premise that it is a worthwhile supplement to private therapy. She spoke of its therapeutic worth for people who've recently been traumatized by divorce or loss of spouse in that they get a sense of being *needed* by other group members at a point when they are at their most vulnerable. As the therapist put it, "You see that at a time of your life when you're questioning your value, you have something to contribute."

Group Therapists' Observations Regarding
Homogeneous Versus Heterogeneous Groups

There was mixed opinion from the interviewed therapists on the question of whether it is better for singles in group therapy to be in heterogeneous or homogeneous gatherings. One therapist ran a heterogeneous group in terms of the age, sex, professional status, and problems of the participants. However, there was the common denominator of their being single. She found that the group worked very well within that structure, and that there were many positive factors at work. For instance, she felt that the age differences made it more possible for group members to relate to each other transferentially — the older woman was regarded by younger people in the group as a mother figure, and so on. However, when asked if, ideally, she would prefer different groups for singles who've never been married and those who've been dirovced or widowed, she responded in the affirmative. She felt that there are significantly different issues for the never-married as contrasted with the widowed and divorced, and that this fact creates conflict within a mixed group.

Another therapist, who ran a group of male and female singles aged 25 to 45, felt it was good for patients to see other points of view generationally and also beneficial for the women in the group to learn that single men are lonely and scared in the same way they are. Still another concluded that it was very helpful to have homogeneous, specifically issue-oriented groups in the initial stages of crisis and trauma. This psychologist ran both a short-term crisis intervention group for divorced people and an ongoing group oriented more to providing long-range general therapy. She felt that the judgment as to whether to be in a short-term, homogeneous group or an extended heterogeneous one depended on "where you are and what you're looking to do. When what you're dealing with primarily is your widowhood, then maybe you need to be with other widows. If you're at a stage where you're dealing with being single, then you can be with singles."

Group Therapists' Observations Of Single Men
Vis-À-Vis Single Women In Groups

Some very interesting and diverse points of view about men and women in singles groups emerged in the interviews with group therapists. As mentioned, one therapist found it very useful for women in a heterogeneous singles group with men to learn that men experienced feelings of loneliness and fear similar to theirs. This theory was echoed by another group therapist who felt that one of the chief advantages to short-term crisis intervention therapy for divorced people was that they learn that there is no real difference between men and women relative to the way they react to the trauma of the split up. "Men go through the same fears, the same isolation. Last week, the group was talking about being alone when newly single — about walking down the street and all they notice are couples, or going into a restaurant with a sense of being only one person. A man said, 'Wherever I go I feel that people are looking at me,' and this woman said, 'Oh, I'm so glad to hear that, I thought it was only women who felt that way.'"

And yet, in contrast to that observation is that of the group leader who found notable differences between men and women with respect to the issues as singles that preoccupy them. She discovered from running her group that, generally speaking, the women are concerned with trying to find men with whom to have intimate relationships, and the men are experiencing difficulties in trying to become close to women. This suggests a rather ironic fact of contemporary life. There are far more available single men for the women — this stampede of women allows the men to indulge their avoidance of commitment. They are having too much fun being free and being involved with many different women. The men's concerns as expressed in this therapist's group have to do with problems they have with their ex-wives and their isolation from their children, not with seeking commitment with women. Unfortunately, if the therapist is correct in her perceptions, this indicates a possibly unresolvable sociological condition that individual psychotherapy and group therapy, together or separately, may not be able to relieve — that of women desperately seeking intimate relationships with men who are not disposed to wanting such relationships.

One of the therapists with whom the writer talked offered some wise guidelines for frustrated singles (mostly women, according to the previously mentioned therapist):

> What people should do is do what they like to do and do what they're interested in doing and make themselves available and open to new experiences so that the focus on the fact that they're single and the focus on meeting someone is only part of a whole pie. You're developing yourself as a person, you're enriching your life, you're enjoying your life. Having a mate is one part of your life that you would like to have fulfilled, but it's not all of you.

We can conclude that, to a great extent, group therapy is instrumental in making it possible for people to develop as she suggests, judging from the experiences and observations of those we interviewed about the validity of group therapy for singles as an adjunct to individual psychotherapy.

CASE HISTORIES OF SINGLES IN GROUP THERAPY

Two cases from the writer's own practice come to mind as good examples of the effectiveness of group therapy in helping singles cope with their unique problems as supplemental therapy to their individuual therapy.

Paula

> One case involves Paula, a pretty, quiet, young woman who had recently separated from her husband. She gave the impression of being a lost child who could easily be bullied and pushed around, submissive and eager to please, and this is exactly the role she played with the thera-

pist in private sessions. While it was apparent that rage and anger were the underlying dynamics, these emotions rarely surfaced in the individual therapy, and she continued to project the compliant, good child responding with gratitude to anyone who did not try to hurt her. In her relationship with her former spouse, it seemed that she had been victimized, and her decision to leave him was based on what she felt was the only response she could have to this aggressive man. She began in group shortly after her individual treatment had started. A very different picture of her emerged in the group. She was, as with the therapist, accepting, compliant, eager to please with the women in the group, but with the men her reactions were rather surprising. The unhesitating aggressiveness, the anger, the attacking quality were greatly at odds with the previously presented picture. In fact, she intimidated the men in the group. They were able to confront her about the hostility she displayed, and slowly, with some resistance, she became aware of the antagonism and controlling quality she displayed toward men. In the light of this awareness, she began to reexamine her relationship with her ex-spouse and subsequently began to take some responsibility for her own behavior. While there is no question that this would eventually have emerged in individual sessions, the process would, in all probability, have taken longer.

Harry

In the other case, a young man, Harry, became repeatedly involved in relationships with women with whom he had become intensely preoccupied. As soon as there was any hint of the relationship developing into a more long-term, stable one, he would reject the woman. His fear of these relationships was evident in private therapy, but in group therapy it became clear that he focused on the negative qualities of women in the group close to his age, to the exclusion of their good characteristics. He was empathic to the men in the group and to the older women, but his sense of balance and his ability to discern the various levels with which a particular young woman might function became distorted. As a result of this poor reality perception, the negative aspects of the women became, for him, their totality as people. As the group continually picked up his distortions about the young women in the group, he became aware of his fear of close relationships and his propensity to see individuals as all bad when there was a threat of permanency. What inevitably followed was his departure from the liaison. Ultimately, he began to realize, as he jokingly put it, that "others have a left side as well as a right side, and maybe now I'll be able to see them as balanced."

CONCLUSION

As a result of reviewing the literature, interviewing therapists who conduct therapy groups for singles as adjuncts to their private practice, and recalling the writer's one caseload with respect to this issue, it is reasonable to conclude that such group therapy is a useful supplement to individual psychotherapy.

All groups give an opportunity to work out various transferential relationships — mother, father, sister, brother, mate, partner — as various members of the group come to symbolize these figures. For singles, whose isolation is often a problem, the opportunity to work out these transferential relationships in a safe environment is crucial.

Group supportiveness is something they rarely find in the outside world, where they are often confronted by judgmental, unsympathetic attitudes. The accusation implicit in these reactions is, what is wrong with you that you are alone? If they are mourning the loss of a mate, they are made to feel that people are tired of hearing about it and they should stop. If they do not meet a partner, family and friends constantly infer that there is something wrong with them. The group, on the other hand, can understand both the psychological and social ramifications of being alone and can distinguish between individual pathology and societal insensitivity toward the single person.

The unique issues of the single person can be dealt with effectively and concretely in a singles therapy group, where all share such concerns as defining oneself in one's new role; loneliness; raising children as single parents; examining the intense conflict between ex-mates; practical matters such as legal considerations; sense of bewilderment and confusion; and generally finding one's place and status as part of a new and somewhat alienating community where the solid family network is available.

REFERENCES

Caine, L. (1977). *Lifelines.* New York: Dell Publishing Co.

Durkin, H. (1968). Relationship between individual and group psychoanalysis. *The group in depth* (pp. 131–143). New York: International University Press.

Epstein, L. (1984, March). Single parents and the schools. *Center for Social Organization of Schools,* Johns Hopkins University, Report No. 353.

Greff, G.L. (1985). Practice with single fathers. *Journal of Social Work Education, 7*(4), 231–243.

Gulpan, F. La Famille Monaparentale Matricentrique. *Revue Canadienne de Psych Education, 14*(1), 19–30.

LeMasters, E.E. (1974). Parents without partners. In A. Scolnick & J. Scolnick (Eds.), *Intimacy, family and society.* Boston: Little Brown and Co.

Lindeman, E., & Caplan, G. (1965). Symptomatology and management of acute grief. In H.J. Parad (Ed.), *Crisis intervention* (p. 7). New York: New York Family Services Association of America.

Shulman, L. (1985). *Skills in working with individuals and groups.* Itasca, IL: Peacock Press.

Sternberg, M. (1982). *The long-term adaptation of young and middle aged widows to the loss of a spouse.* Dissertation, Teachers College, Columbia University, New York.

Warren, B. (1983). Combined treatment for the borderline patient. *Group, 7*(3), 23.

Yalom, I.P. (1975). *The theory and practice of group psychotherapy.* New York: Basic Books, Inc.

C H A P T E R
85

THE PRIVATE PSYCHIATRIC PRACTITIONER, THE POLICE, AND THE COURTS

Sheldon Travin, M.D.

P sychiatrists and other mental-health clinicians increasingly are likely to interact professionally with outside agencies (Group for Advancement of Psychiatry, 1981), including the police and the courts. There are a multitude of ways in which not only clinicians in the public sector but private practitioners as well may become involved professionally with the police and the courts. The psychiatrist may cooperate with the police to arrange an involuntary admission for a dangerous psychotic patient. Psychiatric clinicians may also act as consultants to the police in screening candidates and evaluating or treating police officers. Psychiatric practitioners may be subpoenaed to give testimony in court about their private patients, or they may accept an assignment to evaluate a patient and testify as an expert witness.

This chapter reviews the various ways in which private practitioners become involved in, and can contribute to, the work of the police and the courts. Because differences between the institutional structure and goals of these professions can lead to misunderstandings, this chapter also discusses potential stumbling blocks to the practitioner working with the police and the courts, to enable the clinician to avoid such misunderstandings and work effectively with these agencies (Group for Advancement of Psychiatry, 1981). It also emphasizes that these interactions among the police, the courts, and psychotherapists are frequently mutually helpful to these professionals' common commitment to serving the interests of both the private patient and society in general.

Although psychiatric clinicians do not like to regard themselves as performing acts of social control, the reality is that many do so, for example, by their participation in the civil commitment of patients to hospitals. Commitment proceedings can readily be seen as an area in which psychiatric, police, and judicial activities overlap in a social control function whose common purpose is to benefit the individual patient and society. When we consider the change that has occurred in the kinds of patients now being seen by private psychiatric practitioners, the need for cooperation among the professions becomes clear. Psychiatric clinicians now treat in their private offices more disturbed patients, such as severe borderlines and chronic schizophrenics. Those patients may act out in dangerous ways, are frequently on psychotropic medications, and are sometimes simultaneously in treatment with other mental-health professionals in a variety of different settings, such as day hospitals or residential treatment facilities. Such patients are at good risk to decompensate, which increases the chances that the practitioner will become involved with outside agencies to bring about rehospitalization.

In treating these patients, the psychotherapist, although engaged in a private dyadic therapeutic relationship with the patient, must remain cognizant of shared societal obligations. All citizens have an obligation to abide by and uphold the rules of law and justice. Both the psychiatric clinician and the patient are part of society and thus are subject to a wide range of legal and judicial constraints. Today's trend toward the increased use of the courts to redress personal-injury disputes, resolve malpractice cases, and address a variety of civil-rights issues related to alleged psychiatric abuse makes the psychiatric professional's testimony increasingly needed by the courts. Private practitioners should consider a requirement to give testimony in court as a duty of citizenship and as a part of the routine of psychiatric practice. However, they must balance this duty to society with the obligation to preserve the confidentiality of their patients.

DOUBLE AGENTRY AND CONFIDENTIALITY

The major concerns that mental-health clinicians have in their professional interactions with the police and the courts are, in fact, related to issues of confidentiality and double agentry. The problems of double or multiple loyalties and complicating roles that confront clinicians employed in institutional settings, such as the military or prisons, also confront clinicians in private practice faced with the obligation of having to act at times as an agent of society (Hastings Center Report, 1978). In their private offices, therapists are relatively clear about their roles vis-à-vis their patients in that the therapist is the unambiguous agent of the patient who, in this relationship, is the master. With the introduction of a third party, the relationship becomes more complicated. For example, in a situation involving the civil commitment of a dangerous decompensated patient, the therapist is forced to act as society's agent, and to serve additional masters defined by society in general and the law in particular. For the clinician, the resulting complexities of divided agencies and allegiances are fraught with enormous ethical tensions and inescapable infringements on patient confidentiality (Gotheil, 1986).

Generally, clinicians are extremely wary about breaching patient confidentiality. They are, therefore, very cautious about disclosing information to outside agencies, including the police, and are circumspect in their involvement with the courts concerning their patients. Yet compelling circumstances do arise when even the private psychiatrist's participation is required by these agencies. The psychiatrist must then be unusually careful in protecting the patient's rights, a fact that most states have acknowledged in their laws.

Every state but South Carolina has passed into law a form of physician-patient or psychotherapist–patient privilege statute, more accurately called "testimonial privilege." This privilege bars the physician–psychotherapist from testifying in court about confidential information obtained from the patient unless the patient consents. However, there are so many exceptions to privilege that the clinician is often uncertain about what, if anything, can be disclosed. Among these exceptions are civil commitment proceedings, examinations and reports ordered by the court, criminal proceedings involving the patient, will contests, child-custody disputes, and patient-litigation exception when the patient raises his or her mental condition as an issue in the lawsuit. Therefore, it is important to understand that there is no absolute testimonial privilege and that, except for Illinois, the states have granted the privilege exclusively to the patient. This means that the patient may be able to compel the therapist to testify in court about the patient's mental condition.

PSYCHIATRIC PRACTITIONER AND THE POLICE

Some understanding of the historical development and current role of the police force is essential to the clinician who works with the police. The following sketch of the various roles and responsibilities the police face in their daily work suggests that private practitioners can offer assistance to the police primarily in the following areas: screening of prospective police officers, consultation on educational training, the psychiatric treatment of police officers, and working with them in the emergency hospitalization of a decompensated, dangerous patient. The ensuing discussion will explore the challenges each of these areas poses to the clinician.

In a comprehensive study, Bittner (1970) traces the establishment of the first modern police department in the United States to the London model in England. First used in New York City, this general plan of organization was soon adopted by many other American municipalities and established the preeminent pattern of police work. The modern police system in London was the last of the structures in the executive government of that city to have evolved, in part because of fears that creating a police force controlled by the executive branch could lead to a suppression of civil liberties. Eventually, it became obvious that inherited methods of police work were inadequate to manage crime control and peacekeeping. Even then, however, the exact location in the political system and the official mandate of the police were poorly defined (Bittner, 1967a). As a result, the degree of judicial control over police work is often overestimated. Bittner points out that the "judge is not the policeman's superior" and that the courts have only a limited degree of control over police procedure. In particular, in the broad area of disorderly conduct charges and other minor offenses, the police decision is not ordinarily challenged because the police are compelled by public pressure sometimes to act in ways that are outside strict legal interpretation. For example, the police sometimes neglect rules of legal restraint to proceed against certain types of illegal activity, as when they make harassment arrests to discourage further illicit activity. Moreover, police have to respond to a variety of situations that have nothing to do with legality or law enforcement, such as marital or family disputes. For these reasons, police behavior differs from community to community, and is influenced iin part by the viewpoint of the police administration and in part by local politics and community needs.

Police officers in the community are not merely engaged in fighting crime; they function in a wide range of activities that do not culminate in making arrests. Estimates as to the extent of police functioning in activities unrelated to crime control or law enforcement range as high as 90 percent; over half of all calls to an urban police department are made for help in some crisis situation involving personal or interpersonal problems. These calls are made because of the public's perception in most communities that the police department is the only service agency available on a 24-hour basis that is capable of handling such crises. And the police officers who confront this extraordinary range of social and mental-health-related problems are usually the lowest-ranking officers, who are empowered with enormous discretion in decision making but may be lacking in training, experience, and even personal qualities.

Screening Prospective Police Officers

The variety of tasks and extreme stresses related to police work necessitate considerable care in the selection of successful applicants for the job. Psychiatric clinicians can help in this selection process, according to Rhead et al. (1968), by conducting multiple interviews and performing psychological tests, including projective techniques, on each candidate. Mangelsdorf (1978) has utilized an assessment procedure consisting of a stress interview and an evaluation of the motivation, stability, prejudice, uncontrolled anger and aggressiveness, chemical abuse, sexual deviation, and judgment of prospective officers. Although the typical candidate is generally more suspicious, risk taking, and prone to act on impulses than the average person, Mangelsdorf argues that the success of a police officer in performing the job does not depend as much on his or her unconscious conflicts or ego defenses as on the extent to which his or her adaptive ego has remained undistorted in response to those conflicts. While it is clear that clinicians can offer valuable assistance to the police in their efforts to screen prospective officers, it is imperative that, whatever assistance the psychiatric consultant provides, the police should be the ones devising their own standards and ultimately deciding on the their choice of candidates.

Consultation With Police On Educational Training

An important contribution that clinicians can make to police departments in their community is to educate officers about basic mental disorders and to provide training in family-crisis intervention. Barocas (1973) has aptly characterized the police in the community as "the front-line 24-hour urban psychiatric G.P....an invaluable, though ill-prepared psychiatric manpower supply..."; because these officers are frequently called upon to intervene in the most difficult family crises, their need for appropriate training is obvious. Underscoring this need, a 1963 FBI report indicated that 22 percent of the police officers killed nationally were killed while intervening in family-crisis situations. Approximately 40 percent of injuries sustained by the police occurred in similar circumstances. Although not nearly as much as they ideally could, mental-health professionals have been working with police departments in providing training and in acting as consultants in various educational programs. These programs have focused on training in human relations, community relations and urban problems, community mental-health education, and family-crisis intervention. Friedman (1965) points out that in participating in these training programs, it is important for the mental-health consultant not to talk down to the police officer but to be sensitive to the officer's need to be recognized as a professional who also has had considerable contact and experience with mentally disturbed people. It is also helpful to appreciate that the police are essentially men and women who relate best to the consultant who can think quickly, who emphasizes action and experience, and who stresses what they have in common rather than how they differ.

Police and Emergency Psychiatric Hospitalization

The emergency hospitalization of dangerously disturbed patients exemplifies how mutual help on the part of the clinician and the police best meets the challenge of extremely difficult situations. Although the police have discretionary powers in emergency situations and generally take the more disturbed patients to psychiatric emergency rooms, there is a paucity of data about these police-initiated referrals. The major studies in this area have been made by Bittner (1967b) who concluded that police officers are generally reluctant to make emergency apprehensions of mentally ill people. Like most people, the police tend to employ denial in doing something about mental illness; they have frequent contact with a wide assortment of marginal characters who do not seem to require any intervention measures; they are often ambivalent about recognizing mental illness as a proper task for them; they dislike the ordeal of taking somebody to a hospital; and they are uncomfortable about taking someone who is not a criminal to a hospital to be locked up and are much more inclined to search for available alternatives in the community. However, Bittner (1967b) did find that the police were disposed to making emergency apprehensions on their own initiative in cases of clear suicide attempts; where there were serious signs of mental disorder with disorientation, agitation, and becoming a public nuisance; and when the complaints came from reliable people with some instrumental relationship with the patient, such as doctors, lawyers, and teachers. The police officer must have a detailed report from the complainant, and also needs to see the patient in an agitated, disordered state before taking action in order to feel protected from possible later legal and other repercussions.

Private practitioners may require the help of the police in hospitalizing their decompensated, dangerous patients who refuse medication or to accept treatment. In such situations, the police need the psychiatrist's help: the psychiatrist should be present to evaluate the patient and make the medical decision for involuntary hospitalization. This is often a crucial determination, especially if, at the time of the examination, the patient appears calm and relatively normal.

The present author has been for some years a psychiatric member of a rather unique crisis-intervention service program that provides psychiatric services on a 24-hour basis to county residents, and on many occasions has accompanied the police in making home visits. In general, this author has found the police to be extremely cooperative and appreciative of the fact that a psychiatrist is present to evaluate the patient, who is often already known to the police as a mental patient who periodically "acts up" and needs to be hospitalized. The police are grateful for being relieved of the anxiety of having to act on their own, especially in questionable cases.

The Private Practitioner and the Criminal Patient

A category of decisions that sometimes has to be faced by private practitioners regarding the police is whether or not to report to them their patients' revelations about either intended or committed criminal acts. It is not uncommon for patients to reveal to psychotherapists their unlawful behaviors and aggressive fantasies (Ochberg & Gunn, 1980), and it is not always easy to distinguish between the two. In all such cases, a careful review of the legal statutes in the jurisdiction is required, as well as careful consideration of the ethical obligations pertaining to breaching patient confidentiality in criminal matters.

In the landmark first Tarasoff decision of 1974, the California Supreme Court ruled that when the psychotherapist believes a patient to be dangerous to an identifiable victim the psychotherapist has a duty to warn the intended victim. Although this duty to warn was changed to the duty to use reasonable care to protect the intended victim in the second Tarasoff decision in 1976, the court was vague as to how this duty could be discharged. Depending on the circumstances, some reasonable steps that psychotherapists can take to carry out this duty include warning the victim, calling the police, and medicating or hospitalizing the patient. Although Tarasoff is a California case, the doctrine is increasingly being cited in other jurisdictions, and it is a factor that the clinician must deal with in practice.

The question of psychotherapists' obligations to report their patients' past criminal acts is the subject of a comprehensive article by Appelbaum and Meisel (1986). These authors consider this topic to fit primarily into the general category of "misprision of a felony," which obligates all citizens to report felonies they know about. However, they found that the federal courts' interpretation of misprision of a felony means active concealment of a crime and not just a failure to report it. State law concerning misprision of a felony varies considerably, but the trend in most states is not to impose liability for it as a common-law crime. Appelbaum and Meisel remind us of the fact that reporting a patient's revelation of a past crime is a breach of confidentiality, but note that if reporting were mandated by statute, it would serve as a defense against civil liability for disclosing this information. Interestingly, the passage in 27 states of "eavesdropping bills" that authorize the wiretapping and monitoring of conversations in the offices of doctors, lawyers, and clergy who are suspected of having clients suspected of a crime is clearly another assault on the privacy of the professional–patient relationship.

Psychiatric Collaboration With Police On Cases

Ochberg and Gunn (1900) describe some circumstances that call for the collaboration of mental-health clinicians with the police on criminal cases.

They argue that clinicians who have helped the police develop psychological profiles of mentally abnormal offenders have essentially worked in a highly questionable area on grounds of both validity and ethics. But if the police request help on a case involving a suicidally depressed or otherwise mentally abnormal individual, the clinician who enters the situation brings along a crucial psychiatric perspective. The question of what special contribution the clinician can make in a criminal hostage or political terrorism situation remains unanswered.

Psychiatric Treatment of Police Officers

Police work places unique demands on officers. They must exercise good judgment under the most stressful conditions; they frequently perceive negative feelings held toward them by much of the public, and the sense of isolation that they feel from the rest of the community (Symonds, 1972) can contribute to a need for psychiatric counseling. Private practitioners who treat police officers need to understand these unusual stresses inherent in their patients' work as well as their more common psychodynamics. Symonds has described the typical police officer as having a mixture of both conforming and aggressive behavioral characteristics combined with a reverence for authority (though recently he finds more questioning of authority). When faced with situations that compromise their self-esteem, such officers are especially vulnerable to depression, and even disorganization. While undergoing psychiatric evaluation, it is usual departmental procedure to have the officer's guns taken away, which is something much dreaded by the officer. Before examining or treating the police officer, the clinician must state in detail the extent of confidentiality and under what conditions it will be breached. The psychiatrist will probably be asked to write a report concerning the officer's mental condition and ability to return to duty. In such cases, Mangelsdorf (1978) argues, police officers should not be fired on psychiatric grounds for a variety of reasons, including the possibility of a recrimination that psychiatry was being used as a political tool. He notes that the police department can find enough technical reasons in the rules book to terminate the officer's employment without resorting to psychiatry.

PSYCHIATRIC PRACTITIONERS AND THE COURTS

There are two basic ways in which psychiatric practitioners can utilize their professional expertise in helping the courts. The first way is involvement as an amicus curiae or "friend of the court." This is a written argument, usually prepared by an attorney, that brings to the attention of the court certain points of law and other information the court should have in order to be fully informed about an issue under deliberation. The professional, usually representing the point of view of a special-interest group, may be able to give important psychiatric information to the attorney preparing the brief and thereby influence the court decision. This amicus curiae process is, therefore, actually a form of advocating a point of view in the judicial system. The second, and most common, way the practitioner becomes involved in the court system is by giving psychiatric testimony.

Except possibly for the relatively small group of specialists who are engaged in the practice of forensic psychiatry, most psychiatric clinicians experience varying degrees of uneasiness when giving testimony in a courtroom (Bromberg, 1979) since the courtroom represents unfamiliar territory and has a whole set of rules and procedures that are generally outside of the clinician's experience. Yet, because psychiatric testimony is increasingly being requested by the courts on a wide variety of issues such as competency, civil commitment, psychic impairment, and disability and compensation, the prospect of the psychiatric clinician's being called into court has increased (Resnick, 1986). Indeed, most mental-health-related testimony is provided by psychiatric clinicians who do not have any special forensic psychiatric training. The psychiatric clinician may be subpoenaed to appear in court and testify about the clinical findings of a patient as either a common witness or an expert witness. A common witness is merely expected to give testimony about facts and direct observations of the patient and symptoms, whereas the expert witness's testimony is broader and more flexible. It may involve giving an opinion with reasonable medical or psychological certainty or "probability" (or some variation of this formula in different jurisdictions) embracing the ultimate issue before the court.

The expert witness is also expected to give opinions on hypothetical questions based on all the relevant facts that have been or are likely to be introduced as evidence. The way the expert responds can help the trier of fact (judge or jury) to undrstand the basic premise of the expert's opinion. Although the treating clinician may be reluctant to give expert testimony about a patient, if properly subpoenaed and when legally unavoidable, he or she cannot decline testifying. The clinician who does testify as an expert witness should bill the side that subpoenaed the testimony for an expert-witness fee (Gutheil & Appelbaum, 1982). The court rules on whether the individual's particular background, training, or experience qualifies him or her to be accepted as an expert witness in the case. In the mental-health areas, the trend in recent years has been not to accept nonpsychiatric physicians but to allow psychologists, and even some social workers, to testify as expert witnesses (Gutheil & Appelbaum, 1982). It is, therefore, important for mental-health professionals who want to function effectively in the courtroom to become familiar with basic courtroom stratagems and procedures.

The Adversary System

An understanding of the adversary system, including some of the procedures and rules that control it, is fundamental to an appreciation of the American trial process. The system is not the cooperative effort in the pursuit of scientific truth that psychiatric clinicians are used to, but rather a fight between opposing sides conducted through intellectual arguments according to formal rules. The adversary system assumes that truth will emerge best in a courtroom when the two opposing sides, the prosecution and defense, each presents the strongest case for its respective side (Slovenko, 1973). It is particularly important to stress that, although he or she may have been retained by one of the sides, once sworn in as a witness, the psychiatric clinician must not see himself or herself as an adversary of either party, but only as the servant of the court giving testimony to the truth as he or she sees it, even if it may be damaging to the client (Halleck, 1980).

The Meaning Of Subpoenas

The word "subpoena" means "under penalty" and is the formal method used by the courts to obtain important information useful in the administration of justice. A general principle of law entitles the courts to have every person's evidence that can aid in the settling of a case. With the exception of the president of the United States, anyone believed to possess relevant factual information may be subpoenaed. There are two types of subpoenas: the *subpoena duces tecum,* which pertains to medical records, documents, or papers, and the *subpoena ad testificandum,* which requires the witness's appearance in court. Disregarding a subpoena is punishable as contempt of court. It is important to know that it is the clerk of the court, at the request of the attorney and the judge, who issues the subpoena. The attorney merely has to assert that he or she believes the individual has important information relevant to the case before the court. The subpoena, therefore, legally compels the individual to appear in court but does not compel the person to testify. Upon receiving a subpoena without an accompanying consent form signed by the patient, the clinician should consider his or her obligation to protect the confidentiality of the patient.

Consultation With The Attorney

If summoned to give testimony about a patient, the clinician should consult beforehand with the patient's attorney. The clinician who is subpoenaed by the opposing atttorney as either an ordinary or an expert witness, should discuss the issue of psychotherapist–patient privileged communication with the patient's attorney. If the subpoena is not quashed, the clinician should appear in court and either the clinician or the patient's attorney should raise this issue before the former testifies. Although opposing attorneys realize that reluctant expert witnesses may not present the evidence in a favorable way and thus may undermine the case, if they believe the clinician possesses significant information, they will probably subpoena such testimony (Gotheil & Appelbaum, 1982). If the patient's attorney requests the clinician's testimony and the clinician is willing to testify as an expert witness, then the clinician will need to consult with this attorney in order to prepare for the testimony. Although questions have been raised about whether the treating clinician should also be the forensic psychiatric evaluator, a role that requires the use of psychiatric expertise in helping to decide a legal issue, the courts often place a high value on this testimony because such a treating clinician is not viewed as a paid "professional" witness.

The treating clinician willing to testify as an expert witness will want the patient's attorney to clarify the specific legal issues (e.g., competency to divorce, competency to manage one's own estate, etc.) and the legal standard and criteria in the jurisdiction of the litigation. Unfortunately, not all attorneys fully comprehend the legal issues involved in these kinds of psychiatric cases and so may not be very helpful to the clinician. The attorney will most assuredly want to know the clinician's psychiatric findings and versions of the truth in order to decide whether to use the clinician's testimony in the case. Assuming that the clinician's views can be helpful to the attorney's case, the attorney and the clinician should go over the kinds of psychiatric and legal questions that the attorney will ask the clinician in the direct examination and the clinician's intended answers. They should also discuss points likely to be brought up by the opposing attorney in the cross-examination. The important thing is that there should be as few surprises as possible, as being unprepared for them may hurt the case (Sadoff, 1975).

Depositions

As part of the sequence of pretrial procedures, the psychiatric witness may be directed to make a deposition, statements under oath, either orally or in writing. Depositions are an aspect of the "discovery" process that permits each side to gain vital information held by the other before a civil action takes place in the legal dispute. This process is supposed to ensure that the outcome of the contest will be decided on the basis of all the available facts. In the oral deposition, it is mostly the attorney for the opposing side who conducts the examination, which is held outside the courtroom but in the presence of a court reporter. The examination is in form of questions and answers, with an opportunity for cross-examination resembling that which will occur in the courtroom. In a written deposition, the witness responds in writing to the list of questions submitted by the attorney.

It is important for the witness to remember that depositions are sworn statements about the psychiatric clinician's findings and opinions on the case. This information may impeach the credibility of witnesses whose testimony in court differs from that of the deposition. The deposition may also be used as evidence if the witness is unable to appear in court. Therefore, the witness is well advised to regard the deposition seriously. In the deposition, as in giving courtroom testimony, the witness should be concerned about revealing psychotherapist–patient privileged communications, and should provide thoughtful responses consistent with the psychiatric opinions without volunteering uncalled-for information.

The Written Report

The patient's attorney may ask the psychiatric clinician for a written report on the clinician's evaluation of the patient. This report may be of sufficient help to the court that the witness may not be required to testify in person. The witness who does appear will be required to clarify and defend the contents of the written report during the cross-examination in the courtroom. In preparing such a report, the clinician should be very careful about its precise wording. Although there is no universally accepted format, the basic qualities of any written report, as of any testimony on the witness stand, should be objectivity, completeness, and comprehensibility. The clinician should use plain language and a minimum of psychiatric jargon (Bromberg, 1979).

A systematic approach in preparing a written report is of value in ensuring that important areas will be covered. Forensic psychiatric specialists who evaluate patients at the request of the patients' attorneys usually incorporate into their reports the following specific topics: purpose of the examination, consent by the patient to the examination, time and place of the examination, conclusions, personal history, psychiatric history, surrounding circumstances or the patient's involvement with the legal issue or situation, results of mental-status examination and psychological testing, diagnosis, and a discussion of the conclusions. In this kind of forensic report, it is extremely important to document the patient's understanding of the purpose of the examination and his or her consent to it. Mention should be also made of how many times the patient was seen, where, and under what circumstances.

The question of where to place the conclusions, whether at the beginning (as some judges prefer) or at the end (the conventional psychiatric report), is a matter of personal style. What is important is that there be a report of the findings and a discussion of the reasoning and basis for the conclusions. Discussion of the topics listed need not necessarily be in paragraph form under specific headings, but can be integrated into the body of the report. The report should be extremely accurate in summarizing the pertinent data of the case. It should describe the psychiatric symptoms, problems, and impairments of the patient without going into a detailed discussion of psychodynamic factors. The report should allow the reader to gain a better understanding of the patient's psychiatric condition and the legal implications relevant to the case.

Testifying In The Courtroom

The courtroom presents unique challenges to the treating clinician summoned to give testimony about a patient, and to the psychiatric practitioner who agrees to evaluate a patient for forensic purposes and then to testify as an expert witness. In the first category, although psychiatric-fact witnesses are not ordinarily asked their professional opinions, in some jurisdictions, they may be required to state their opinions after being qualified as experts. A most difficult switch in roles is now expected of an expert witness. Whereas before the treating clinician sided with the patient, or, in the case of the forensic psychiatric evaluator, consulted with the patient's attorney to prepare the testimony, the expert on the witness stand is obligated to serve only the court in the interests of truth and justice. The witness is sworn to tell the whole truth in a neutral and unbiased manner. But, because the patient will also be present in the courtroom during the testimony, the treating clinician should understand that these truthful statements should be expressed as sensitively as possible in order to minimize potential trauma to the patient.

A common pitfall in serving as a forensic psychiatric expert in the courtroom is the countertransferential reaction of overadvocacy (Rada, 1981). This may take the form, in the expert, of arrogance, inflexibility, unwillingness to acknowledge the possibility of being in error, or histrionic pleading of the case. Such behaviors are not only inappropriate but frequently are counterproductive. The expert should understand that the unbiased findings and opinions about the case to be presented in court already represent an advocacy position on the patient's behalf, or the patient's attorney would not have called the expert to the witness stand. Ideally, expert witnesses should be able to distance themselves from the outcome of the trial, which is decided by the finders of fact (jury or judge). Experts who can maintain this dispassionate attitude should also be able to recognize that it is not themselves personally who are under deliberation, but only their opinions. This should help them to take the cross-examination by the opposing atttorney in stride rather than to react defensively and in a hostile manner.

To improve their credibility on the witness stand, and thus enhance the chances that their testimony will be properly accepted and contribute to the decision in the case, experts should pay attention to their attitude, demeanor, and style of dress and communication. An expert witness should dress conservatively; assume a confident, neither pompous nor overly humble stance; and speak respectfully to the participants in the trial, not at them, in clear statements free of psychiatric jargon. The expert should not volunteer gratuitous information, but during the cross-examination, if needed, should ask to be allowed to qualify a response rather than merely to give a yes or no answer. Above all, the expert should project honesty and reasonableness, and should be able to answer "I don't know" to questions beyond his or her knowledge. The expert should also be willing to acknowledge that he or she would modify an opinion if given new information, for example, in a hypothetical question.

After being sworn in, the expert will be engaged in at least the first two of the following proceedings. First, he or she will undergo direct examination by the attorney who called the expert to testify. Since this part of the testimony has been discussed beforehand with the attorney, it should present no great difficulty to the witness. At the outset, the expert is asked to describe his or her professional qualifications. The questions are then posed in a progressive manner designed to give the witness the opportunity to present his or her psychiatric findings, conclusions, and reasoning on the case. Second, the expert is required to submit to cross-examination by the opposing attorney. This phase is generally the most uncomfortable one for the inexperienced witness. The cross-examining attorney will attempt to undermine the credibility of the expert's testimony. As a legitimate tactic, the cross-examiner may even resort to an attack on the person of the witness; this is called an *ad hominem* attack. The attorney will try to discredit the expert's testimony by showing the expert to be less than candid and otherwise holding the witness up to ridicule. After this, the redirect examination allows the expert's attorney to clarify some points raised or repair damage to the case done in the cross-examination; finally, the re-cross-examination gives the adversary attorney the same opportunity to go over points raised in the redirect examination (Resnick, 1986).

CONCLUSION

The current state of private practice has increased the need for psychiatric clinicians to be able to work effectively with a variety of outside agencies. While working with these agencies poses challenges to the clinicians, and clinicians must take particular care to protect their clients' confidentiality in these cases, adequately prepared clinicians can work effectively with the police and the courts to the benefit of their patients, and of the larger community. To this end, this chapter has examined the potential pitfalls the clinician must avoid, and has pointed to the benefits that can result from the collaborative efforts of the police, the courts, and clinicians.

REFERENCES

Appelbaum, P.S., & Meisel, A. (1986). Therapists' obligations to report their patients' criminal acts. *Bulletin of the American Academy of Psychiatry and the Law, 14,* 221–230.

Barocas, H.. (1973). Urban policemen: Crisis mediators or crisis creators. *American Journal of Orthopsychiatry, 43,* 632–639.

Bittner, E. (1967a). The police on skid-row: A study of peacekeeping. *American Sociological Review, 32,* 699–715.

Bittner, E. (1967b). Police discretion in emergency apprehension of mentally ill persons. *Social Problems, 14,* 278–292.

Bittner, E. (1970). The functions of the police in modern society. DHEW Publication No. (ADM) 75-260.

Bromberg, W. (1979). *The uses of psychiatry in the law.* Westport, CT: Quorum Books.

Friedman, M.H. (1965). Community mental health education with police. *Mental Hygiene, 49,* 182–186.

Group for the Advancement of Psychiatry (1981). *Interfaces: A communications case book for mental health decision makers.* Mental Health Materials Center. San Francisco: Jossey-Bass.

Gutheil, T.G., & Appelbaum, P.S. (1982). *Clinical handbook of psychiatry and the law.* New York: McGraw-Hill.

Gutheil, T.G. (1986). Clinical issues in forensic psychiatry. In R. Michels (Ed.), *Psychiatry.* Philadelphia: Lippincott.

Halleck, S.L. (1980). *Law in the practice of psychiatry.* New York: Plenum.

Hastings Center Report (1978, Apr.). In the service of the state: The psychiatrist as double agent. *Hastings Center Report Special Supplement.*

Mangelsdorf, T.K. (1978). Psychiatric consultation to the police *Psychiatric Annals, 8,* 200–206.

Ochberg, F.M., & Gunn, J. (1980). The psychiatrist and the policeman. *Psychiatric Annals, 10,* 190–201.

Rada, R.T. (1981). The psychiatrist as expert witness. In C.K. Hofling (Ed.), *Law and ethics in the private practice of psychiatry.* New York: Brunner/Mazel.

Resnick, P.J. (1986). The psychiatrist in court. In R. Michels (Ed.), *Psychiatry* (rev. ed.). Philadelphia: Lippincott.

Rhead, C., Abrams, A., Trusman, H., & Margolis, P. (1968). The psychological assessment of police candidates. *American Journal of Psychiatry, 124,* 1575–1580.

Sadoff, R.L. (1975). *Forensic psychiatry. A practicel guide for lawyers and psychiatrists.* Springfield, IL: Charles C. Thomas.

Slovenko, R. (1973). *Psychiatry and law.* Boston: Little, Brown and Co.

Symonds, M. (1972). Policemen and policework: A psychodynamic understanding. *American Journal of Psychoanalysis, 32,* 163–169.

86

SHORT-TERM SPECIFIC THEME GROUPS AS AN ADJUNCT TO PRIVATE PRACTICE

Carol A. Chanco, A.C.S.W.

Clinicians in private practice can increase their exposure to a wider number of potential patients by organizing short-term specific theme groups. These groups are beneficial to the psychotherapist because they increase caseload numbers, introduce new clients to therapy in a low-key manner, and attract clients who may become potential individual therapy clients after or during the group.

Clients who are unfamiliar with therapy or who don't understand therapy may understand going to a group that has a theme that affects their lives. For example, clients who may not be ready to locate an intimacy problem may be ready to go to a group described as a "support group for singles." Once in the group, they may be ready to explore their difficulties in getting close to others.

These short-term theme groups also generate referrals in other ways. (1) The clinician begins to get identified with certain areas of specialization that attract future clients. (2) Groups tend to increase the clinician's exposure to a wide variety of contacts (e.g., patients refer friends). (3) Theme groups familiarize clients with therapy, and with the therapist. (4) Good theme groups identify therapy issues that clients may wish to explore in individual therapy at a later deate.

WHAT ARE SOME EXAMPLES OF SHORT-TERM THEME GROUPS?

There are many types of groups and many ways to structure these groups depending on the objectives of the clinician. Some suggested theme groups are the following:

- Singles support groups
- Groups for recently separated men and women

- Support groups for widows and widowers
- Infertility groups
- Endometriosis support groups
- Marriage enrichment groups
- Groups for incest survivors
- Groups to help women understand the importance of menopause
- Groups for victims of rape or for friends and family members of rape victims
- Phobia groups
- Alcoholics' groups:
  - The "recently sober alcoholic"
  - One-year anniversary (of being sober) groups
  - Adult children of alcoholics groups
  - Codependency groups
- Holocaust survivors group
- Gay, lesbian groups:
  - "Coming-out" groups
  - AIDS information, ARC information groups
  - Gay and lesbian support groups
- Illness-related support groups:
  - Support groups for cancer patients
  - Groups for mastectomy patients
  - Multiple sclerosis patients support groups
- Groups to prevent job burnout
- Stress relief groups
- Support groups for performers
- Support groups for women:
  - Women in business
  - Pregnant women
- Single parents support groups
- Supervisory groups
- Hypnosis groups
- Weight reduction groups
- Teachers support groups
- "Fear of success" groups
- "Supportive discipline" groups for parents
- Short-term sex therapy groups
- Support groups for "women who love too much"

Before organizing or selecting a group theme, the clinician needs to address the following questions:

- Am I qualified to lead this group? Have I had training and/or life experience that would help me lead this group?
- Is this theme group a "hot" or popular topic? Has there been a lot of recent media coverage on this topic? Is there enough interest in this topic to generate a group?
- Is this an area of specialization I'd like to develop?

• Can I get referrals for this group? How easy (or how difficult) will it be to get referrals?

• Do I already have patients who are interested in this group? Since it is easier to build a group from an interested "core group" of my own patients, is there a topic or theme my own patients have suggested?

• Do I know colleagues who will refer patients? Do I have colleagues who would like to refer patients and colead the group with me?

• Do I have access to an adult education center, or "audience" that I can give lectures to about this group topic and attract group members? For example, if I want to give a group for single parents, do I have access to the PTA or the group Parents Without Partners?

• Does the type of group I am organizing lend itself to future therapy referrals?

Once practitioners address the issue of what type of group to run, they need to consider how to get group members. There are various ways to build groups. Some ways are easier and less time-consuming than others. Obviously, the best way to build a group is to evaluate the needs of current clients to see if a "group theme" emerges. The next step is to contact colleagues in private practice as well as colleagues in social service organizations who may have clients to refer. Friends and colleagues who belong to voluntary organizations like AA or Al-Anon may also wish to make referrals for group.

Clients may also wish to refer friends to a group. In this case, clinicians need to evaluate the clinical appropriateness of such a referral particularly if a client refers a friend to the same group the client is in. Some clinicians keep an information sheet of upcoming groups in the waiting room for clients to read. The information sheet should explain the type of group, the type of questions and issues usually addressed in this type of group, and all basic information about the group.

Another way to get group members is to do lectures on a topic directly related to the group theme. For example, a clinician desiring to do a support group for women in business could set up a lecture titled "Preventing Stress: Rx for Women in Business" at local women's organizations. During the lecture the clinician could present the idea of a support group both directly and indirectly; directly by talking about the group and handing out flyers, and indirectly by giving examples during the lecture of how a support group might help lessen stress. The clinician might also want to pass around a sign-up sheet for women who want more information about either the support group or therapy.

SHOULD I ADVERTISE FOR GROUP?

Many clinicians in private practice ask in practice-building seminars whether it pays to advertise for groups. There are several advantages and some disadvantages to advertising for clients.

It is advantageous to advertise if the ad is well placed, well written, and located in a magazine or newspaper that caters to the type of population that would attend the group. The ad generally needs to run on an ongoing basis so that people begin to notice the ad over time. Clinicians who choose to advertise might want to do a cost-effectiveness study for themselves to see if the number of clients the ad attracts outweighs the cost.

The advantages of a "good" ad are the following: The ad circulates the clinician's name as a specialist in that area, it provides telephone contact with a variety of prospective clients who may call the clinician asking for information, it can provide group or individual referrals, and if the ad continues to run, it can generate an ongoing base of clients.

The disadvantages of advertising for a group include the following: (1) The clinician can spend hours of time on the phone with many people who are not very motivated for any group of therapy. (2) The clinician frequently encounters very seriously disturbed clients who may be more appropriate for clinics or even inpatient hospitalization or who require medication. (3) The referrals are not as "solid" referrals as those patients who are either referred by other colleagues or who have seen the clinician by attending a lecture.

Clinicians need to evaluate how their time can best be spent in acquiring either individual clients or group members. The methods of acquiring patients, arranged from the most effective to the least effective, are as follows:

1. Client referrals
2. Colleagues in private practice
3. Colleagues in social service organizations
4. Friends and colleagues in voluntary organizations
5. Lectures, teaching
6. Advertising

Obviously, referrals from clients are the easiest method of obtaining referrals; lectures and advertising are the methods hardest on the clinician. The clinician should work toward the easiest route.

Clinicians who choose to advertise should begin reading newspapers or magazines they are considering advertising in to see how many therapists place *ongoing* ads in them. Obviously, a therapist who places ads month after month is most likely getting referrals.

The wording and placement of the advertisement is extremely important. One clinician who built an extremely successful private practice ran an ad for singles support groups in a newspaper for singles. The ad copy read, "Make Friday Night the Most Important Night of Your Week." The ad then went on to give basic information about the group. A successful ad will most likely contain: a good eye-catching headline about the group, basic credentials of the clinician,a short basic outline of the type of issues the group will cover, the time and day the group runs (if known), and the clinician's phone number (preferaly an answering service, not a home or office phone if a large ad response is expected). Fee is generally not included in the ad.

After the clinician receives phone calls about the group, a good time-saving device is to schedule a full group information session for interested callers that lasts about 30 minutes. The purpose of the free group information session is to prescreen callers, to expose the callers to the clinician, and to provide additional information. It is this author's experience that most people who call for therapy through an advertisement will not commit themselves to paying a fee for a group interview unless some type of personal contact has been established with the clinician.

GROUP MECHANICS

One of the major considerations of the practitioner is group structure. Is this a support group? Is this a short-term psychotherapy group? Will this be a 10-session group? How many themes and issues does the practitioner hope to explore? What is the likelihood of getting people together for one, two, or 12 sessions?

Clinicians need to consider why they are doing the group. If the purpose of the group is mainly to increase exposure to a large number of people, then 10 one-night groups might be more advantageous than one group of 10 sessions. If, however, a practitioner wants to lead a group in which group members deal with issues in depth, and the practitioner enjoys more in-depth work, then 12 sessions are more appropriate than one session.

Practitioners also need to consider how many participants they want and how long they are willing to wait to get the proper group composition. The longer a group runs, the more important that the group be composed of members who are on similar functioning levels.

FEES

Group fees should be determined by several factors: What are local clinicians charging for group? How much money has to be made to cover office fees and my time? How many members will there be? Will the group have a coleader? Standard group fees in the New York area are $25 to $40 including a fee for the pregroup interview.

THE PREGROUP INTERVIEW

One of the most important clinical and business "tools" in short-term group composition is the prescreening interview. The main functions of the pregroup interview include: providing the client with information about the group, finding out the reasons the client is interested in group, screening the client to determine his or her appropriateness for group, making a clinical determination about what group the client need be placed in, and preparing the client for the first group session.

Of these functions, one of the most important is screening since the screening will help determine who belongs in which group. Schopler & Galinsky (1981) have found that group composition is the most important factor in group success. Practitioners therefore need to design a screening tool for themselves in which background material on each client is secured. Clinicians need to pay particular interest to vagueness on problems in a client's history. Direct questions should be asked: Do you have a history of depression? Have you had previous hospitalizations? Have you ever been on medication? What is your prior experience with group or individual therapy? General intake information should be gathered as well.

The only time when this information may not be necessary is when the clinician decides to do a "one-shot" lecture group that is highly structured. For example, if the clinician intends to advertise for a lecture on separation and run a brief group afterwards, he or she doesn't need to go through a pre-screening interview that is this thorough.

During the pregroup interview, clinicians need to consider factors conducive to good group composition and ask themselves which clients are on a similar functioning level socially, intellectually, and emotionally; which clients have issues in common; and which personalities and diagnoses will work best together.

If, during the course of the interview, the clinician determines that a client is appropriate for group, then the client needs to be prepared to enter group. The clinician needs to feed back to the client his or her explained reasons for entering the group and to be told how to work on these issues with other group memebers. With a short-term group, the client often needs help articulating issues for the first group, needs to be presented with general information about the type of people in the group, and needs reassurance about self-disclosure, confidentiality, trust, and confrontation levels. During the prescreenig interview, the clincian needs to "reach for the negatives," to find out what fears and hesitations the client has about entering group and to help the client work through those fears.

An important feature of the prescreening interview is the clinician's ability to make the client feel as comfortable, safe, and protected as is possible with the clinician. The client needs to know that the clinician will protect the client from genuine harm in the group (Galinsky & Schopler, 1977). This is conveyed nonverbally and verbally to the client. One way to handle the issue of "safety feelings" is to explain to the client in the beginning of the interview that both clinician and client have the same goals to provide the client with a sound group experience and to carefully explain what goes on in a group. Most clients coming from support groups are not looking for highly confrontational groups, although the client needs to know that sometimes one member will confront another with the clinician there to guide the interaction.

If the clinician determines that the client is not accepted for the current group or that the client is not appropriate for group, the issue needs to be handled with the client so that the client does not feel rejected. The client can honestly be told that this is not the best group for him or her and should be given a reason that is clinically appropriate. For example, the client can be told, "This group is not supportive enough" or "I recommend individual rather than group therapy" or "This is not the safest group for you."

If the waiting period for the group is longer than 1 week, the client should be contacted before the group starts. If there is a long waiting period, the client should be contacted by phone periodically and notified as to when the group will begin. Many clients are lost during the waiting period. Generally the clinician should start interviewing for group months ahead of the projected starting date.

THE GROUP CONTRACT

Once clinicians decide on the length of the group, they need to define for themselves what they hope to accomplish. A comment of a client recently referred to a short-term group reflects the failure of the group leader to define the group contract. He stated, "I keep asking the group leader, 'Why are we here? I thought we were here to discuss what it's like to think you might be gay. Everybody is discussing everything.' All he said to me was, 'We're here to discuss feelings.' I feel very scared in that group."

Clinicians need to have a fairly clear idea in a short-term group of what they hope to accomplish and to have an idea from the screening interview about what clients hope to accomplish. A working agreement that leaves most members clear about why they are in group should be made in the first session. A contract like, "We're here to discuss feelings" or "to talk about being single," is generally not effective. Practitioners who run a short-term group need to select a more active model of group treatment since the group needs to unfold in a few sessions.

CONSIDERATIONS FOR THE FIRST GROUP

If the first group meeting seems unusually tense, the clinician might consider some questions that would lower the level of anxiety, such as, "What was it like to walk through the door into group tonight?" or "What is your greatest wish or fear about what will happen in this group?" Clinicians need to be "tuned-in" to the level of anxiety that clients unexposed to therapy or group dynamics may feel. Clinicians may want to familiarize themselves with some of the literature on early group formation, particularly information on confrontation levels, group resistance, group intiation stages, and self-disclosure (Anderson, 1984).

RECONTRACTING

Sometime before the end of each short-term group (if the group is successful), members usually bring up the issue of extending the group. This is the time to present to the group the idea of a longer-term group either dealing with the same issues or moving toward psychotherapy issues. Again, this is generally determined by how the group is going. Since some members may wish to stay and others with to leave, the idea of introducing new members and a longer-term group should be raised.

SUMMARY

Although group information can be a lengthy and tedious process, short-term groups can be effective treatment strategies and exciting experiences for both client and practitioner. In addition, short-term groups, once formed, are a source of new referrals as clients become familiar with the clinician and the clinician's area of specialization and work.

REFERENCES

Anderson, J. (1984). *Counseling through group process.* New York: Springer Publishing Company, Inc.

Galinsky, M.J., & Schopler, J.H. (1977, March). Warning: Groups may be dangerous. *Social Work, 22,* 89–94.

Schopler, J.H., & Galinsky, J. (1981, September). When groups go wrong. *Social Work, 26,* 424–429.

Author Index

Subject Index

1033

About The Editor

In private practice for the past twenty years, Dr. Margenau has worked with a variety of populatons and settings including sports consultation, drug and alcohol abuse, hypnosis, and sex therapy. He is the Executive Director of the Center for Sports Psychology. His practice includes working with individuals, families, couples, and organizations.

Eric Margenau received his Ph.D. from New York University and did his post doctoral work at the Institute for Practicing Psychotherapists, Mt. Sinai Medical School and the Center for Ethical Hypnosis. He is currently practicing in New York City and Hackettstown, New Jersey. Dr. Margenau is a contributor to professional journals and writes a popular sports column called "Psyching It Out." He frequently appears on local and national network television and radio. His book publications include *The Handbook of Children of Alcoholics* (co-edited), *Sports Without Pressure*, and *Psyching It Out* (co-authored).

Dr. Margenau lives in New York City with his wife and two children.

Russell Bianca Production Editor
Editorial Consultation by Lorna Porter
Copyediting by Evelyn Tucker and Sally Van Duyne
Typesetting by S. Smith, Inc., New York
Printing and Binding by Hamilton Printing Company, Castleton, N.Y.
Index prepared by Barbara Farabaugh